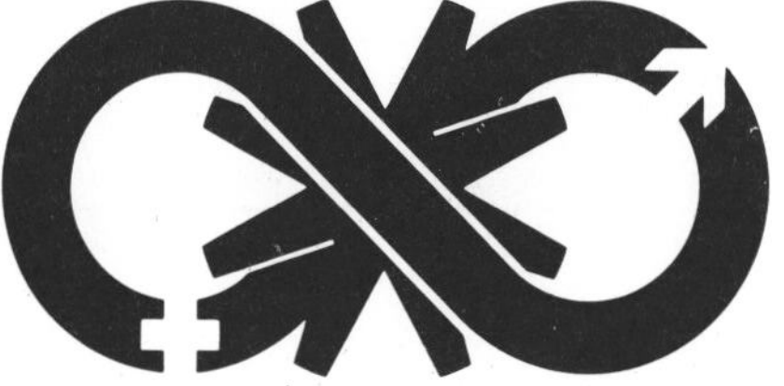

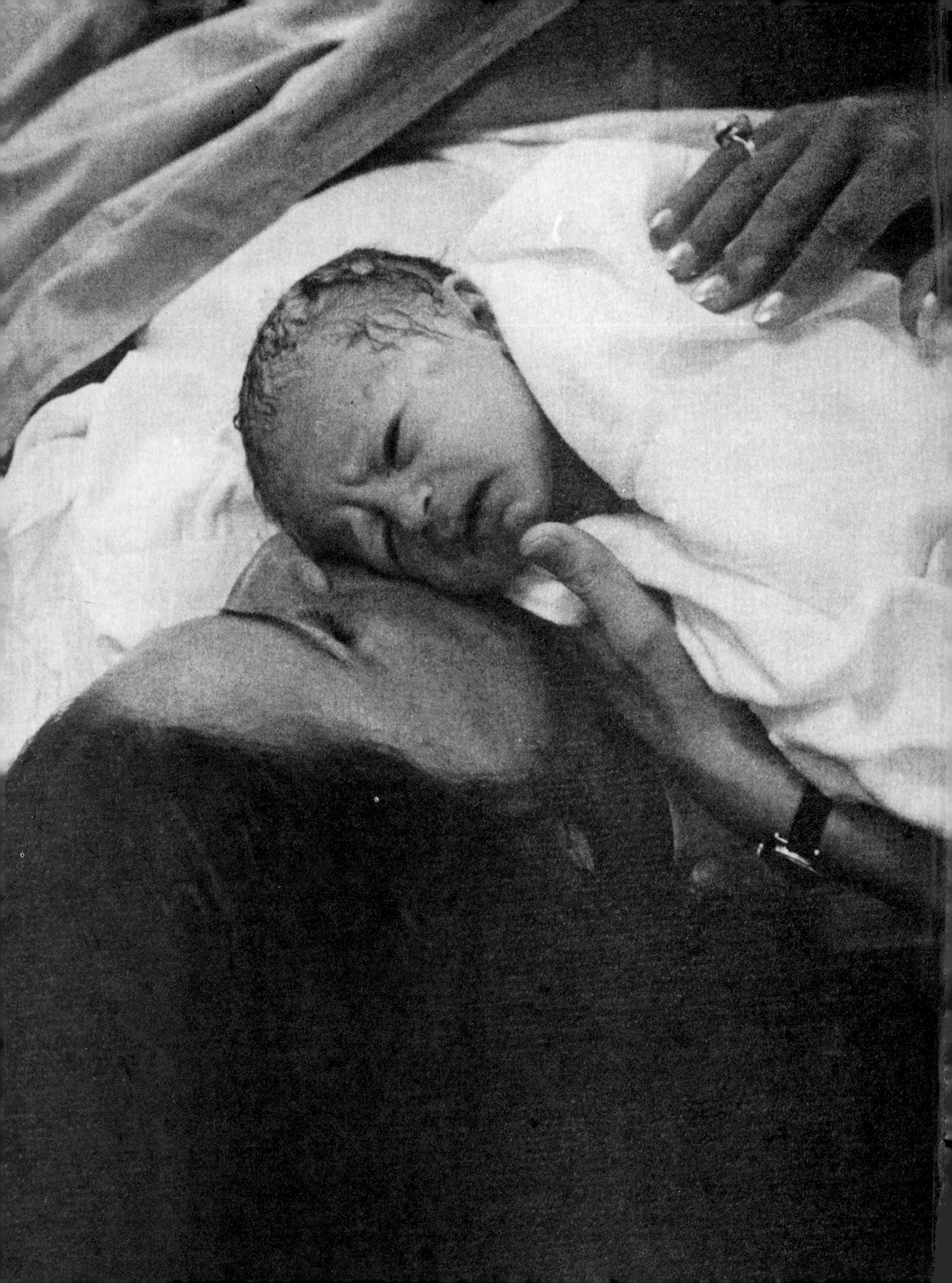

15th Edition

Maternity Nursing

Sharon J. Reeder, R.N., Ph.D., F.A.A.N.
Professor of Nursing, School of Nursing,
University of California, Los Angeles

Luigi Mastroianni, Jr., M.D., F.A.C.S., F.A.C.O.G.
William Goodell Professor and Chairman, Department of Obstetrics and Gynecology,
University of Pennsylvania School of Medicine, Philadelphia

Leonide L. Martin, R.N., M.S., Dr. P.H.
Family Nurse Practitioner, Professor, Department of Nursing,
Sonoma State University, Rohnert Park, California

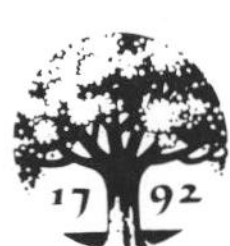

J. B. Lippincott Company Philadelphia
London Mexico City New York St. Louis São Paulo Sydney

Sponsoring Editor: Paul R. Hill
Manuscript Editor: Shirley Kuhn
Indexer: Julie Schwager
Designer and Art Director: Tracy Baldwin
Cover illustration: Sharyl Sand Carow
Production Assistant: Charlene Catlett Squibb
Compositor: John C. Meyer & Son
Printer/Binder: Murray Printing

15th Edition

6 5 4 3 2

Library of Congress Cataloging in Publication Data

Reeder, Sharon J.
Maternity nursing.

Includes bibliographies and index.
1. Obstetrical nursing. I. Mastroianni, Luigi. II. Martin, Leonide L. III. Title.
[DNLM: 1. Obstetrical nursing. WY 157 M424]
RG951.Z3 1983 618.2 82-21701
ISBN 0-397-54369-7

The authors and publisher have exerted every effort to ensure that drug selection and dosage set forth in this text are in accord with current recommendations and practice at the time of publication. However, in view of ongoing research, changes in government regulations, and the constant flow of information relating to drug therapy and drug reactions, the reader is urged to check the package insert for each drug for any change in indications and dosage and for added warnings and precautions. This is particularly important when the recommended agent is a new or infrequently employed drug.

The 15th edition of *Maternity Nursing* is dedicated to our past, present, and future students whose acquisition of knowledge makes this book worthwhile.

Contributors

Ida Stanley Bird, R.N., M.N.
Assistant Clinical Professor
Childbirth Educator
Medical Center UCLA
Los Angeles, California

Chapter 19: Parent Education

Roberta Gerds, R.N., M.N.
Visiting Assistant Professor
University of Hawaii
Manoa, Hawaii
Formerly Assistant Clinical Professor
School of Nursing
UCLA
Los Angeles, California

Chapters 20, 31, 32, and 33: Nutrition in Pregnancy; Assessment of the Newborn Infant; Care of the Newborn Infant; Infant Nutrition

Brett B. Gutsche, M.D.
Professor of Obstetrics and Gynecology
Professor of Anesthesia
University of Pennsylvania School of Medicine

Chapter 27: Analgesia and Anesthesia for Childbirth

Susan M. Ludington–Hoe, R.N., C.N.M., Ph.D.
Assistant Professor of Nursing
School of Nursing UCLA
Los Angeles, California

Infant Stimulation in Chapter 32: Care of the Newborn Infant

Jane McAteer, R.N., M.N.
Instructor of Nursing
Department of Nursing
Mount St. Mary's College
Los Angeles, California

Chapters 42, 43, and 44: The High-Risk Infant with Disorders of Gestational Age and Birth Weight; The High-Risk Infant: Developmental Disorders; The High-Risk Infant: Acquired Disorders

Margo McCaffery, R.N., M.S.
Consultant in the Nursing Care of People with Pain
Santa Monica, California

Chapter 24: The Nurse's Contribution to Pain Relief During Labor

Ann McDonnell, R.N.
Coordinator of Prenatal Genetic Diagnosis
Department of Obstetrics and Gynecology
University of Pennsylvania School of Medicine

Co-author, Chapter 16: Genetic Counseling and Diagnosis During Pregnancy

Michael T. Menutti, M.D.
Assistant Professor
Department of Obstetrics and Gynecology
University of Pennsylvania School of Medicine
Philadelphia, Pennsylvania

Chapters 16 and 41: Genetic Counseling and Diagnosis During Pregnancy; Electronic Fetal Monitoring and Fetal Intensive Care

Preface

The 15th edition of *Maternity Nursing* again reflects extensive revision. Several new chapters have been added, most of the chapters have been rewritten, and the remainder have been completely updated.

In the past five years, society has continued to change at a phenomenal pace and the institutions in our society continue to reorganize, particularly the family and the educational and health systems. As society changes, so must those who occupy roles in society. Thus, as clients change their orientations, values, and behavior, health providers must change in order to maintain a synchrony in their roles.

The family system continues to change and many new lifestyles are becoming more apparent. With these various lifestyles come a melange of attitudes and behaviors regarding reproduction, family planning, sexuality, birthing, and childrearing. These broaden the scope of maternal care. Moreover, the continuing innovation that is occurring in the health-care delivery system, especially in nursing, has an additional impact on the specialty. These current issues are examined in depth to enable students to gain a better insight into their importance so that this knowledge can be incorporated into their care of families during the reproductive process.

Unit I has been reorganized to provide a variety of fundamental concepts regarding the structure and function of the modern family and health systems, emerging multiple lifestyles, and various social factors relating to health. These concepts are explored in depth as a basis for discussion of the current thinking regarding sexuality, changing role relationships in the family, nursing and parenting, reproductive behavior, and use of maternity services. This information provides a broad conceptual base which the student must have in order to deliver high-quality nursing care to families.

A new chapter has been added to Unit II which deals with the human sexual response cycle. This chapter covers not only the physiology of the sexual response cycle but also the affectional and relational aspects that are so inextricably bound to the cycle. This provides a further elaboration of the concepts introduced in Unit I and provides the student with a sound knowledge base in this fascinating area. Sections on the development and physiology of the embryo and fetus have been revised to reflect current data and thinking. This unit supplies the basic anatomy and physiology upon which students can base their nursing care.

Unit III continues an in-depth examination of areas of sexuality and various facets of reproduction. Common concerns that individuals have regarding sexuality are addressed and the chapters dealing with contraception, pregnancy termination, infertility, and genetic counseling provide additional necessary information for the delivery of quality maternity care.

Units IV through VI deal with the normal reproductive cycle from conception through the postpartal period. All of these chapters have been revised and updated. A new chapter dealing with the immediate care of the newborn after delivery has been added. These chapters will enable the student to gain a knowledge of the total normal reproductive cycle and its management. Throughout these and the other chapters in the book, dimensions of effective nursing care for each phase of the reproductive cycle have been expanded, based on recent research and conceptual developments in nursing practice and related disciplines.

Units VII and VIII reflect current research and practice regarding the assessment and management of maternal and infant disorders. A full chapter has been devoted to electronic monitoring and its appropriate use. Fetal diagnosis and the management of the high-risk infant have been extensively updated to reflect current thinking and management.

Three chapters are now devoted to assessment and management of the infant with neonatal disorders. These chapters provide the student with an elaboration and an in-depth knowledge needed to care for these infants. The information in these chapters is essential as the fields of perinatal medicine and nursing burgeon.

Unit IX examines several special considerations in maternity nursing. The current issue of alternatives in childbirth is addressed and the topics of home deliveries, birth centers, lay midwives, and nurse midwives are discussed to enable the student to realize the place of these important events and the contribution of these providers in the total maternity spectrum. The section on the evolution of maternity nursing has been rewritten to reflect current trends. Health care is not carried out in a vacuum, nor did present-day maternity care spring from nothing. It was shaped and nurtured by a variety of economic and social factors. Thus, a good understanding of the history of the field will enable the student to appreciate current practice and predict future care patterns.

At our readers' request we have added a chapter on emergencies in maternity nursing. Nursing care during a precipitate or emergency delivery is examined in depth as is the maternity nurse's responsibility in large-scale disasters.

Maternity Nursing has been reformatted to provide greater readability. Many new photographs, drawings, illustrations, and figures have been added to reinforce points made in the text and to provide the student with quick reference information. Many of the tables in this edition have been identified as AT (Assessment Tool), NC (Nursing Care Plan), or PE (Patient Education) to further enhance the quick reference features of the text. Again, at our readers' request, we have included study questions and conference material at the end of the units in this edition. All of the suggested readings have been updated with references from current professional literature.

In this edition we introduce our logo. We have chosen the signs for woman, man, birth, and infinity. As woman and man combine their corporal and spiritual energy in the drama of birth, new beings are brought into existence which have, in turn, their own energy and existence. We know from principles of physics that once matter and energy exist they can never be destroyed, although their forms may change. Hence, once an individual's substance and energy are created, they exist infinitely. Indeed, the phenomenon of birth is the most awe-inspiring and dramatic episode of a lifetime and beyond.

Sharon J. Reeder, R.N., Ph.D., F.A.A.N.
Luigi Mastroianni, Jr., M.D., F.A.C.S., F.A.C.O.G.
Leonide L. Martin, R.N., M.S., Dr. P.H.

Acknowledgments

Once again, we wish to thank our contributors who have given a special dimension to the 15th edition of *Maternity Nursing* with their varied expertise. We wish to express our gratitude for the help and encouragement of our many colleagues and friends in the revision of this edition. In particular, we would like to thank Cheryl Hayes, R.N., M.N., Mary Dromi, R.N.P., M.N., and Mary Sullivan, R.N., M.N. for their scholarly and meticulous pursuit of the literature searches and revision of several of the care plans. We are also indebted to Linda Taeger for her expert typing and editorial services.

We would like to extend our thanks to the Maternity Center Association of New York for permission to publish the exercises taught by the Center in its prepared childbirth program. We would also like to express our appreciation to colleagues, publishers, and organizations for the use of illustrations, assessment tools, and other tools that are found in the text. We are especially appreciative of the many parents, nursing students, and staff members who granted their permission for photographs appearing in *Maternity Nursing*.

Finally, we take this opportunity to thank the J. B. Lippincott Company, particularly David T. Miller, Executive Editor, for his interest and cooperation. Most especially, we would like to thank Paul Hill, Editor, and Shirley Kuhn, Manuscript Editor, whose steadfast assistance helped make this edition possible.

Contents

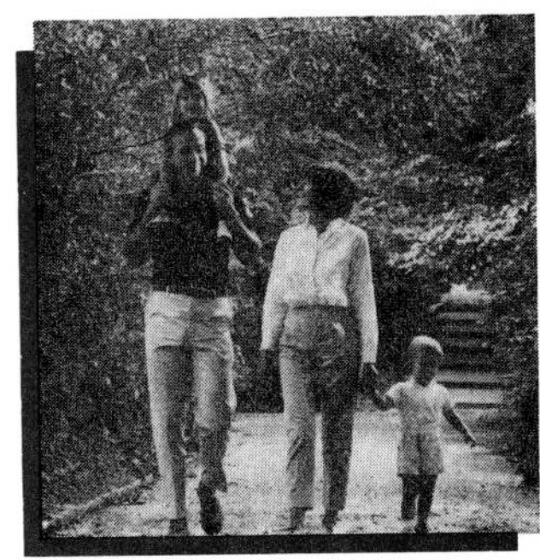

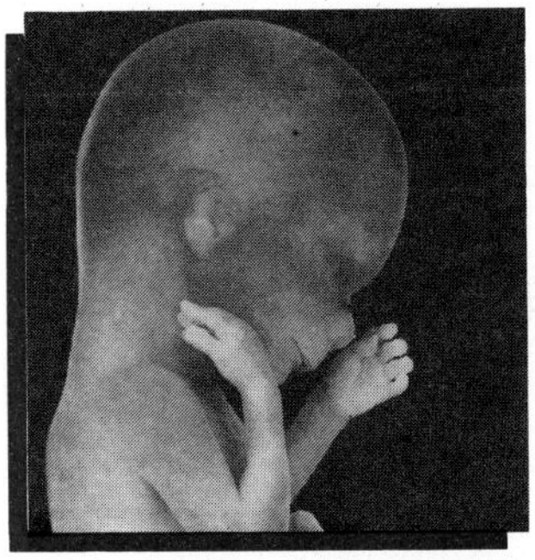

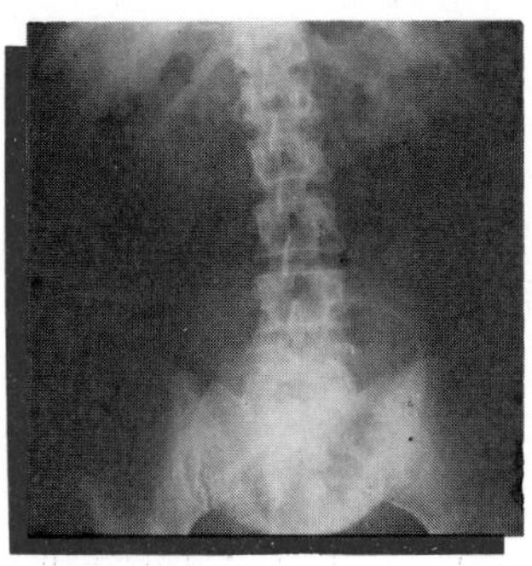

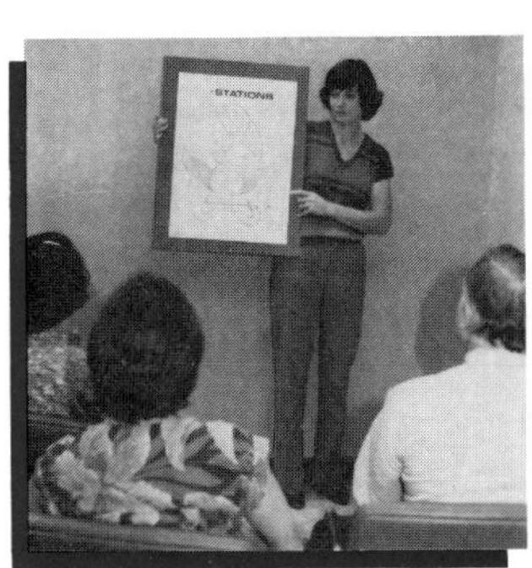

Unit IV Antepartal Assessment and Management 289

17 Biophysical Aspects of Normal Pregnancy 293

18 Psychosocial Aspects of Normal Pregnancy 309

19 Parent Education 323

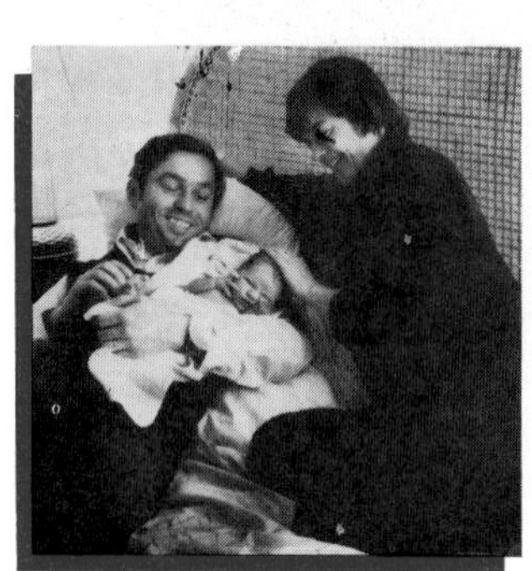

31 Assessment of the Newborn Infant 649

32 Care of the Newborn Infant 679

33 Infant Nutrition 701

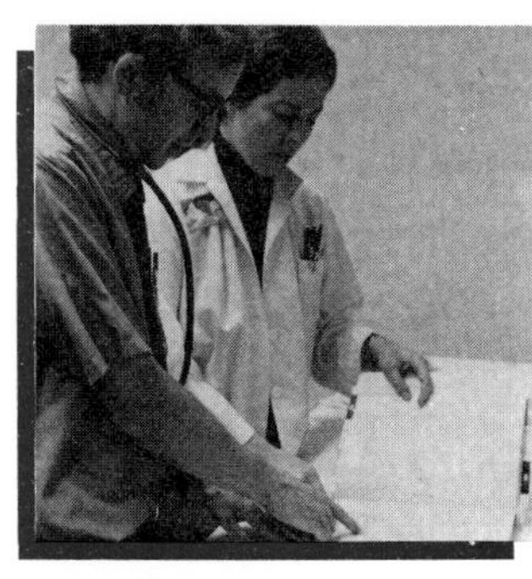

Unit VIII Assessment and Management of Perinatal Disorders 881

40 Fetal Diagnosis and Treatment 885

41 Electronic Fetal Monitoring and Fetal Intensive Care 905

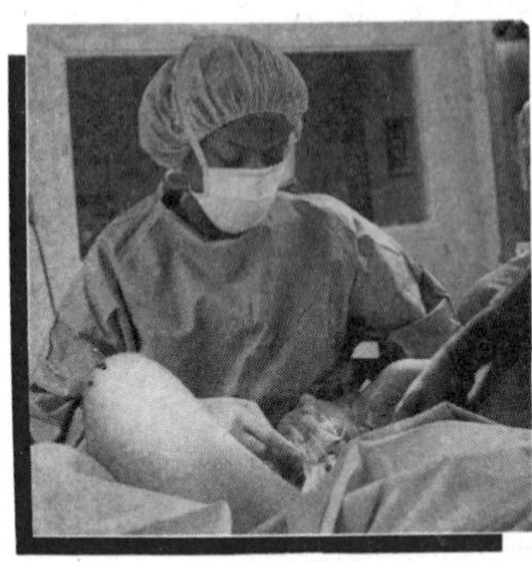

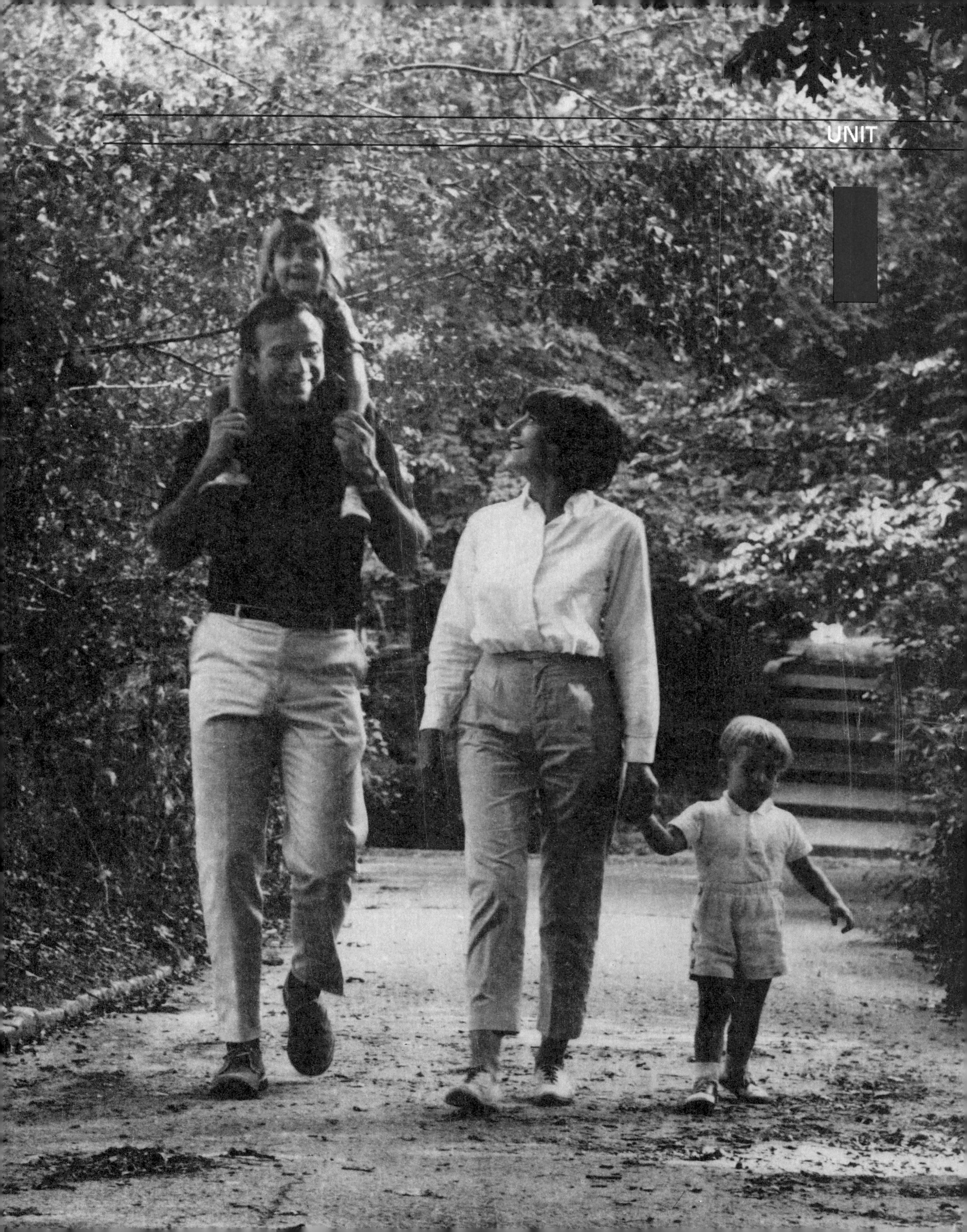
UNIT

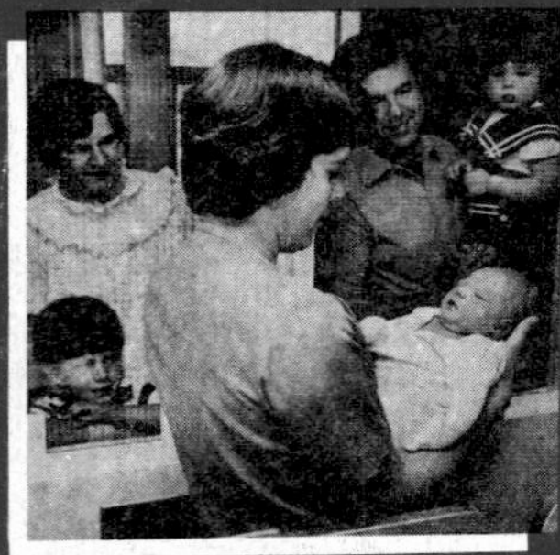

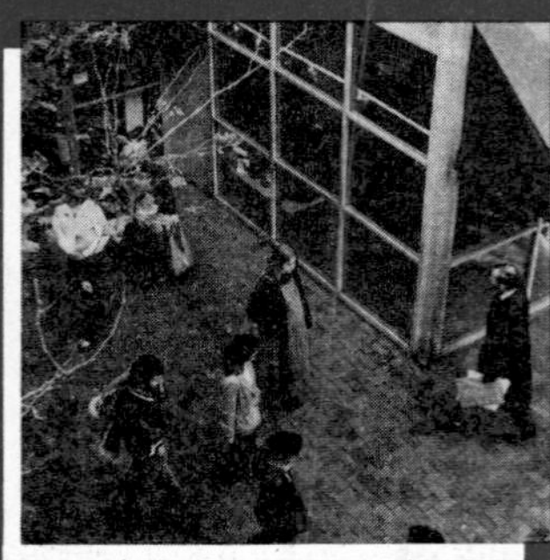

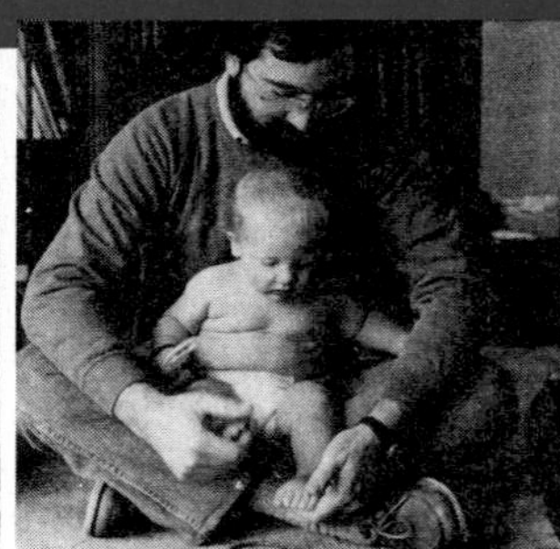

UNIT I

Family Health and Reproduction

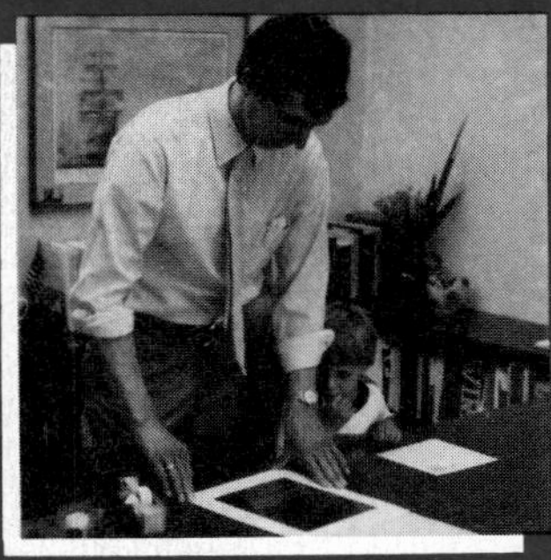

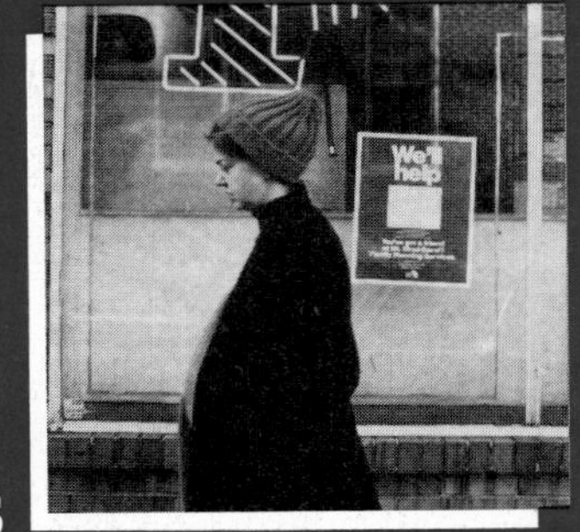

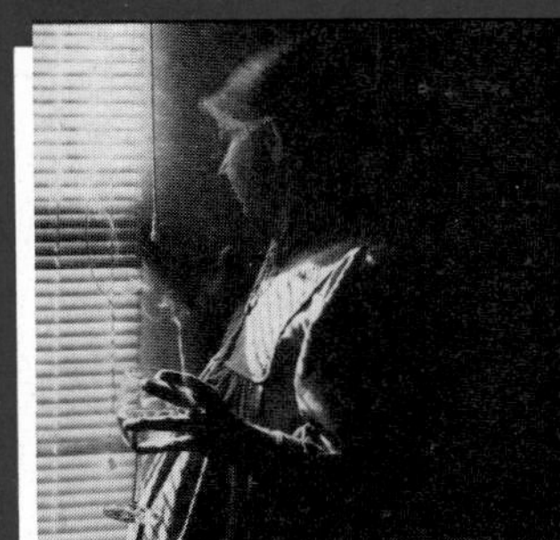

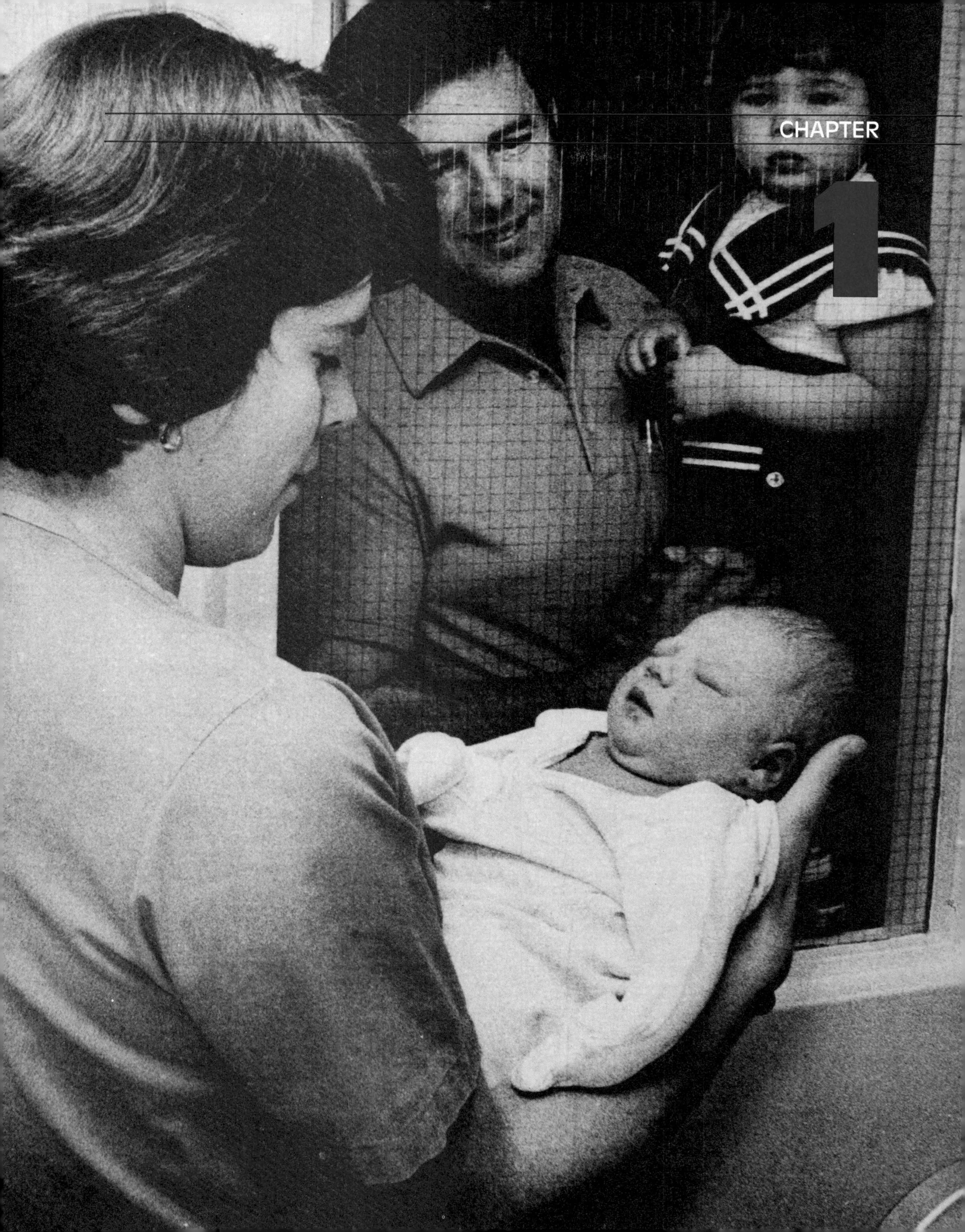

CHAPTER 1

CHAPTER 1

Philosophy of Family-Centered Care

Of all the phenomena that humans experience, birth is perhaps the most awe-inspiring, emotional, and dramatic episode of one's lifetime. It is, indeed, a family affair, and the reproductive health of the total family is the cornerstone upon which a healthy society rests. Thus, the study of obstetrics and the nursing care of women and their families during the various phases of childbearing includes not only the study of anatomical and physiological adaptations to human reproduction, but also the study of human growth and development and the many complex, interdependent relationships to the total society that are inextricably bound to this growth.

Knowledge of the anatomy and physiology of the reproductive organs and of the development of the unborn child from conception to birth is basic to the understanding required by everyone who participates in maternity care. The physiological mechanism by which conception takes place and the new human being develops is not only a fascinating story in itself, but also one that has far-reaching implications for the mother, the child, and the family. All that a person becomes depends on many factors—his or her heritage, the prenatal environment, the care at birth, and the care thereafter throughout infancy and childhood. Thus, it becomes apparent that the health, well-being, and safety of each mother, father, and infant must be protected, and simultaneously that the highest level of wellness possible for every childbearing family be achieved in the broadest sense of physical, emotional, and social well-being. Moreover, it is also important to understand the extent to which the structure and function of the family, as it relates to the larger society, influence the reproductive behavior and health of the childbearing family.

This chapter is planned to orient the student to maternity nursing. The philosophy and assumptions underlying care for the family during reproduction will be given and basic concepts of care will be examined. Basic and new evolving terminology will be defined. In the remainder of the unit, information and concepts relating to childbearing families and how they intermesh with society will be explored.

The Evolution of the Concept of Maternity Care

All definitions and modes of health care have a history. Maternity care is no exception. The student is referred to Chapter 46 for an in-depth presentation of the history of the field. For the moment, we will concern ourselves with a brief overview of some terms and the concepts of care that have become associated with them.

Obstetrics

Obstetrics is defined as that branch of medicine which deals with parturition, its antecedents, and its sequels. Thus, it is concerned principally with the phenomena and the management of pregnancy, labor, and the puerperium under both normal and abnormal circumstances.[1]

The etymology of "obstetrics" is mentioned here to serve as basic information. Briefly, the word *obstetrics* is derived from the Latin *obstetricia* or *obstetrix,* meaning *midwife.* The verb form *obsto (ob,* before, plus *sto,* stand) means to stand by. Thus, in ancient Rome a person who cared for women at childbirth was known as an *obstetrix,* or a person who *stood by* the woman in labor. In both the United States and Great Britain, this branch of medicine was called *midwifery* until the latter part of the 19th century. The term *obstetrics* really came into usage little more than a century ago, although reference to a variety of words of common derivation can be found occasionally in earlier writings.

The post-World War II era brought dramatic changes in the care of childbearing women and concomitant changes in terminology relating to them. In the then-current frame of reference, it seemed, and continues to seem, more appropriate to use the term *maternity* care because this term focuses on the *recipient* of care rather than on the *provider.* Moreover, it has come to imply a broader meaning of the care of the mother and her offspring; it emphasizes the importance of interpersonal relationships that are significant in the family and takes into consideration all the factors that are crucial in promoting the general health and well-being of the entire expanding family group.

The World Health Organization Expert Committee on Maternity Care has defined maternity care as follows:

> The object of maternity care is to ensure that every expectant and nursing mother maintains good health, learns the art of child care, has a normal delivery, and bears healthy children. Maternity care in the narrower sense consists in the care of the pregnant woman, her safe delivery, her postnatal examination, the care of her newly born infant, and the maintenance of lactation. In

the wider sense it begins much earlier in measures aimed to promote the health and well-being of the young people who are potential parents, and to help them develop the right approach to family life and to the place of the family in the community. It should also include guidance in parent-craft and in problems associated with infertility and family planning.[2]

Thus, from the rather narrow definition that focused primarily on the provider of care, we have come to expand our concept of obstetrics to include not only the childbearing woman herself, but all those in her social network who are significant to her.

Maternal–Child Health

Despite the fact that the use of the term *maternal and child health* seems to imply a relatively new concept of care, it was in usage more than 50 years ago. In 1912 the United States Children's Bureau was created by an act of Congress for the purpose of promoting maternal and child health "among all classes of people." It was said to be a community health nurse who first conceived the idea of a federal bureau of this kind and originally suggested the plan to President Theodore Roosevelt in 1905. The Children's Bureau continually stressed the importance of community health nursing in maternal and child welfare. Between the years 1921 and 1929, community health nursing consultants were employed by the Bureau, and their services were offered to the states for maternal and infant hygiene. In rural areas throughout the United States, community health nursing services were greatly extended, and 2978 centers for prenatal and child health work were established.

Until its reorganization into The National Institutes of Health, the Children's Bureau continued to make significant contributions to the promotion of maternal and child health in this country.

Trends in Maternal–Child Care

Trends in United States maternal and child health services were assessed in a report by the late Dr. Edward Schlesinger of the University of Pittsburgh, who had long been active in efforts to upgrade such programs. Writing in *Health and Society*, Dr. Schlesinger cited current and past developments to explain why those in the maternal–child health field have felt that they are in the throes of a profound "identity crisis."[3]

These developments are germane to maternity care because they exemplify a broad spectrum of thinking about delivery of health services in general. New systems of personal health services are being developed to serve entire populations regardless of age or categorical needs. Thus, expanding "special purpose" programs in early childhood and adolescence that tend to include their own independent health services have called into question the more traditional types of health services for mothers and children. The latter have tended to be separate and clearly identifiable programs in maternity and newborn care; in health-supervisory services for infants, preschoolers, and school-age children; and in rehabilitative services for handicapped children. The newer special purpose programs, because of their breadth, often lose specific aspects of care that are badly needed.

However, there have been certain reasons for the development of these newer programs, the most important of which is the unprecedented decline in the United States birth and fertility rates. Therefore, further expansion of maternal and child health services can no longer be justified *solely* by the argument of a continuing increase in the number of mothers and children to be served. Moreover, the United States infant mortality rate, although poorer in relation to the rates of other industrialized nations, has also reached record lows, thus making arguments for broadened services on this point no longer as compelling as they were. Hence, with a much smaller population to serve and a slightly better infant survival rate, what can be the rationale for continued expansion of maternal–child health services? It appears that the argument must be shifted to the need to provide adequate services in order to maintain and expand the gains of recent years, especially for those segments of the population that have not shared equally in these gains.

One other reason for the newer programs deserves mention because it is concerned with basic funding for maternal–child health services. In 1973, there was a drastic reorganization of the federal child development and child health services under the Health Services Administration. While necessary, this reorganization fragmented services and diminished the visibility of mothers' and children's health needs within the federal government. There is no longer a single, clear focus for the expression of concerns for those involved with the health of mothers and children. Before the reorganization, there was firm federal–local cooperation in the provision of special project grants for specific purposes in geographic areas of need, primarily inter-city neighborhoods. However, since the reorganization, the concept of revenue sharing has threatened to reverse this and other salubrious trends that had been growing since

1935 with Title V funding. Inherent in all of this is the hazard that the health needs of the inner-city and other special need populations will receive less emphasis. Moreover, in today's stringent economic climate with the recent reduction in all social programs, resources normally allocated for health and needs of mothers and infants can be expected to be diminished also.

Toward Better Maternal–Child Health

In view of these current outside forces and trends, we will summarize in the form of recommendations the major areas of concern in maternal–child health.

1. First, it is necessary to have integration of high-quality maternal–child health services within evolving comprehensive systems of prepaid group health-care plans. Moreover, services should include prevention, detection, and maintenance.
2. Second, adequate funding of preventive and ambulatory services, especially during the newborn period, must be included in all the mechanisms for financing maternal–child health services.
3. Third, the present services and special projects must be extended to meet the needs of specific high-risk and disadvantaged groups.
4. Fourth, there is a need to resolve the dilemma of providing health services in settings that do not focus primarily on health, that is, schools.
5. Fifth, there must be a focus on concern for maternal and child health within the federal government and for mechanisms for child advocacy both within and without the federal government. The recent fragmentation has left the federal government without a clear point of entry for those interested in maternal–child health services.
6. Finally, there is a need for continuing, critical evaluative research to explore innovations and alternative methods of delivery of care. For instance, it is necessary to have a much clearer idea about whether increased technology really results in higher quality of care.

Philosophy and Assumptions About Maternity Care

Philosophy

Health providers' responses to their clients' needs in both health maintenance and illness management must take into consideration current attitudinal, social, and cultural changes. Health care is not delivered in a vacuum; it takes place in a larger social context and is greatly influenced by current thinking and change manifested by the host society. Philosophies of care evolve from this thinking and change.

The authors of this text believe maternity care to be a philosophy of patient care rather than a special area of medical services or nursing. We believe that begetting children is a family affair; thus, the medical and nursing care of maternity patients is properly a family-centered activity. In most situations today the childbearing woman is a healthy individual in the normal physiological process of childbearing. However, like all individuals facing any other new experience in the family life cycle, the woman and her partner may begin the experience at various stages of preparation for pregnancy and childbirth, with various kinds of stress and different levels of contentment.

It is safe to say that in almost no other normal physiological process does one find such individual extremes of reactions within a normal context. For both the woman and her partner, these reactions may be based on events going back to childhood, as well as to those experienced as an adolescent and adult. Certainly, they are influenced by the immediate home environment from which the couple comes and to which they will soon return with their newborn. Moreover, the level of satisfaction with which the expectant parents leave the provider's presence, or the level of contentment with which the newly delivered mother and infant leave the hospital environment will be modified by the interpersonal relationships of those most significant to them in that environment.

Assumptions

Therefore, underlying the above philosophy are the following assumptions.

All individuals have the right to be born healthy, and to ensure this right, every pregnant woman and every fetus has the right to quality health care.

Individuals' sexuality is inextricably bound to reproduction but not subordinate to it; changing societal attitudes toward sexuality, role relationships, and childbearing, together with technological advances in fertility control, have combined to make parenthood increasingly a voluntary state.

Reproduction is not experienced alone; whatever the circumstances, it involves one or more individuals.

Reproduction is part of a normal psychophysiological process and can be physically and emotionally rewarding for the individuals involved.

The childbearing experience is a developmental opportunity; it can also be a situational crisis during which family members benefit from the solidarity of the family unit.

The profound physiological changes and adjustment that both the mother and her offspring experience during the childbearing process make them particularly vulnerable to changeable and noxious environments and situations that would ordinarily not prove hazardous.

Each individual's attitudes, values, and health behavior are influenced by the culture and society from which he or she comes; thus, each individual's reproductive outcomes and childbearing experience will be influenced by his or her cultural heritage.

Having stated our guiding philosophy and the assumptions underlying that philosophy, we will next examine our view of nursing's role in this philosophy of care.

Maternity Nursing/ Family-Centered Care

Definition

Maternity nursing can be defined as the delivery of professional quality health care while recognizing, focusing on, and adapting to the physical and psychosocial needs of the childbearing woman, the family, and the newly born offspring. The emphasis is on the provision of professional, quality care that fosters family unity while maintaining physical safety of the childbearing unit.

Implicit in this definition is the notion of a family-centered approach. This approach assumes that the family is the basic unit of society and, as such, is to be viewed as a total unit within which each member is a distinct individual entitled to consideration. It is further assumed that childbearing and the rearing and socialization of children are unique and important functions of the family. Therefore, the experience of childbearing is appropriate and beneficial to share as a unit.

It is important to note that, when we speak of the "family," we do not necessarily mean the traditional nuclear family composed of a married pair and their children. A family may be any constellation of interacting individuals who are considered to be "significant others" to the individuals involved. In Chapters 3 and 4 we will examine, in more detail, the various definitions and family forms that are emerging today.

Maternity nursing involves direct, personal ministrations to the childbearing woman and her infant, as well as the related activities of teaching, counseling, and supervising, during the various phases of the childbearing experience. A cornerstone of care is patient/consumer education with respect to health maintenance and reproductive health. It differs from the practice of nursing in other areas in that the clinical focus involves primarily the care of the childbearing unit—the mother, father, and infant (in contrast, for example, to the care of surgical patients or psychiatric patients). It is unique in that the nurse is called upon to attend, educate, and counsel all age groups, from the fetus through childhood, adolescence, and adulthood, since the childbearing unit may span all those stages in the life cycle.

How the maternity nurse meets the needs of mothers, fathers, and their infants cannot be spelled out in stereotyped activities any more than it can in any other situation in which individualized care is the underlying objective. She will intervene to relieve or reduce the client's problems caused by physiological, psychological, or social stress. In addition, she will consult with her clients and their families to make them aware of the principles of health maintenance so that they may incorporate these into their preventive health behavior patterns.

A significant aspect of maternity nursing on the professional level is that the nursing care involves purposeful, sustained interaction between the nurse and her clients. During this encounter, the nurse makes an assessment of the client's problems and resources, and then takes action to relieve the problem and support the strengths with appropriate nursing measures. If the condition requires additional services from the other members of the health team, referral or consultation is given.

Implementation

The successful implementation of family-centered nursing care includes recognition that the provision of high-caliber care requires a team effort by the woman and her family, the health-care providers, and the community. The composition of the team may vary from setting to setting and includes obstetricians, pediatricians, family physicians, certified nurse-midwives, nurse practitioners, and maternity clinical nurse specialists. While physicians are responsible for providing direction for medical management, other team members share appropriately in managing the health care of the family, and each team member must be individually accountable for the performance of his or her facet of care. The team concept includes the cooperative interrelationships of hospitals, providers, and the community in an organized care system so as to provide for the total spectrum of maternity/newborn care within a particular geographical region.[4]

Expanding Roles

The concept of expanded roles in maternity nursing is not new and, in fact, predates the expanded role concept now prevalent in nursing in general. Prior to the 19th century there was little interest by anyone in providing quality maternity care to mothers and families. Care was generally delivered by untrained women who had achieved a modicum of expertise by an apprenticeship/doer method. In the mid-1900s physicians became more interested in obstetrics. In Britain nurse-midwifery educational programs were implemented. In 1925 Mary Breckinridge, who had trained in England as a midwife, spearheaded the organization of the Frontier Nursing Service in Kentucky. Also in 1925 the Frontier Graduate School of Midwifery opened its doors and for many years was the premier school of midwifery in the United States. Today there are numerous educational programs throughout the United States that are undertaking the preparation of nurses for various expanded roles in the field.

A brief overview of the main categories of personnel in the expanded role will be useful to the student. At the time of this writing, several additional subspecialties are emerging. However, the following will provide a basis for later comparisons.

Nurse–Midwife

Certified nurse-midwives are registered nurses who have completed a specified program of study and clinical experience recognized by the American College of Nurse Midwives. They must also pass a certification test before beginning practice. They are qualified to take complete health histories and perform complete physical examinations for their patients. They can provide complete antepartal care, including teaching and counseling. They are qualified to give comprehensive care during the intrapartal period, including delivery of the infant. They are able to deliver care to the mother and infant in the postpartal period, including family-planning information and devices. Thus, they attend both the mother and infant throughout the maternity cycle as long as the mother's progress is considered normal and uncomplicated. The student is directed to Chapter 46 for a more detailed examination of the role and functions of this practitioner.

Obstetrical-Gynecological Nurse Practitioner

These individuals are registered nurses who have completed an additional formal educational program that meets criteria specified for state licensure and certification. Such programs may be at the master's degree level. The practitioners work in collaboration with physicians and may have varying degrees of supervision from their physician colleagues. They function in somewhat the same way that nurse-midwives do; however, they do not deliver infants.

Obstetrical-gynecological nurse practitioners provide immediate and continuing assessment of the newborn and its mother and aid the family in assuming the new parental role. Their focus of practice is on providing primary health care to normal pregnant and nonpregnant women with an emphasis on health maintenance. They can also diagnose and treat certain common abnormalities, such as uncomplicated cystitis or vaginitis, under the aegis of the collaborating physician's standing and contingency protocols.

Women's Health-Care Specialist

This level of practitioner may be a registered nurse or a licensed vocational nurse, or may have experience in another ancillary medical role. The length of training is variable, usually around three to six months, depending upon the entry level of professional education of the applicant. These programs do not have the in-depth preparation that the longer midwifery or master's degree programs do. Women's health-care specialists can screen for physical abnormalities in their patients; they then refer any person with suspected pathology to a physician. They can perform routine gynecologic examinations and provide family-planning counseling; they can also insert and remove intrauterine devices. Like the ob-gyn practitioner, they can, under physician's orders, treat simple gynecological problems. Their focus of care is primarily on women, as their name implies, but many of these practitioners expand their focus to include a more family-centered approach in their patient teaching and counseling.

Maternity Clinical Specialist

This specialist is a registered nurse who has completed a university-based, master's degree program of graduate courses designed to provide in-depth knowledge of the reproductive process and development of clinical expertise in the actual delivery of complex nursing care to the childbearing unit. Her functions include health education, counseling, dissemination of family-planning information, and assisting the family with their parenting role. These professionals may not have physical assessment (diagnostic) skills and hence would not do complete physical examinations or medically treat common disorders. Patient and family education, counseling, and delivery of complex, expert nursing care is the focus of practice. They are also resource persons for staff education and patient-care coordination.

New Directions/ Perinatal Nursing

As knowledge and technology continue to burgeon in the field of reproductive health, in the last decade an effort has been made to provide a conceptual umbrella to encompass maternal–fetal health care as a unit. Consequently, the term *perinatal care* has evolved. By definition, the word *perinatal* means the six-week period preceding or following birth. In actual usage, however, the connotation is much more encompassing. For instance, the term *perinatal* has been used to refer to the time from conception through the 28th day of life, the time from conception through the first year of life, and the time from the third trimester of pregnancy through the 28th day of life.[5] All of the definitions imply that both an obstetric and pediatric orientation is involved. Hence, perinatal care is a method of health-care delivery that would serve to decrease the segmentation and fragmentation of care for the mother and infant (Fig. 1-1).

Perinatal care has also become associated with the high-risk mother and infant in those hospitals designated as tertiary care, or Level III. These hospitals have the resources and expertise to manage any complication of pregnancy or of the newborn. The personnel in Level III institutions provide care for normal

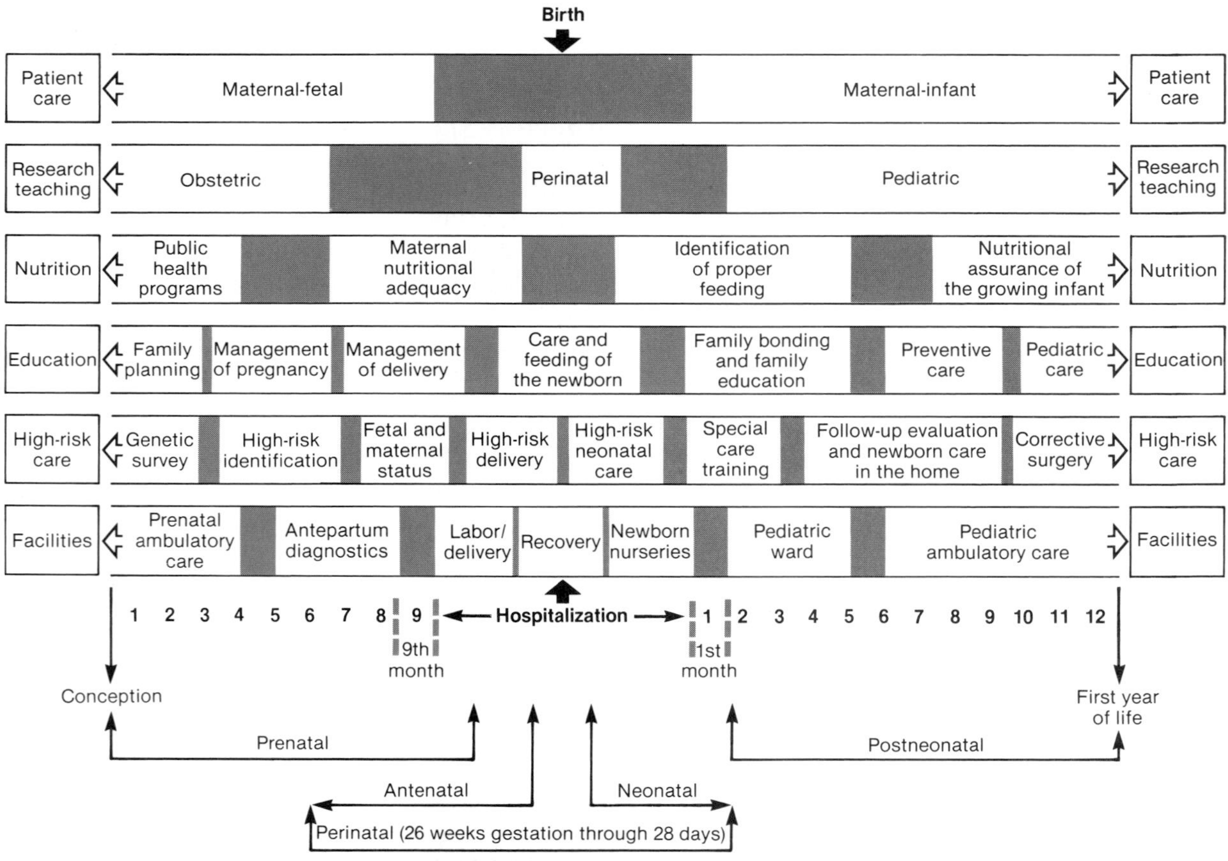

Figure 1-1.
Paradigm of comprehensive perinatal services for the expectant family. (Hospital Planning Associates: Planning and design for perinatal and pediatric facilities, Columbus, Ross Laboratories, 1977)

patients and for all types of maternal–fetal and neonatal illnesses and abnormalities. By contrast, Level I hospitals provide for management of uncomplicated maternal and neonatal patients, and in these institutions there should be a strong component of preventive services and early detection of existing or potential problems, which then may be referred to the Level III institutions. Level II hospitals provide the same services as the Level I hospitals; however, they can provide for uncomplicated obstetric problems and certain types of neonatal illnesses that do not require the wide array of expertise and technology that are found in the Level III hospitals.[6]

Perinatal nursing is therefore emerging as a new subspecialty of professional maternity nursing. It has evolved in response to a need that arose from past gaps, failures, and successes in the delivery of quality nursing care during the reproductive process. It encompasses many of the best features of the above roles, and the knowledge base is not significantly different from that of the midwife or master's-prepared maternity nurse/practitioner. It seems that this specialty will continue to flourish since professional nurses are capable of assuming new roles that are appropriate for new responsibilities and conceptions of nursing and for the health care of the childbearing unit in general.

The Nursing Process in Maternity Care

Implicit in the delivery of effective, professional nursing care is the ability to utilize a method that helps the nurse arrive at informed judgments about clients that have a sound data base. With the data base and these appropriate clinical judgments, nursing care can be planned and implemented so as to enable clients to maintain or return to a state of high-level wellness. This method has been conceptualized as *nursing process* by a variety of authors in an effort to describe a lucid, organized, scientifically based, problem-solving approach to professional nursing practice.[6–8]

Nursing process is the organizing conceptual framework used throughout this text to help the student learn to make nursing judgments appropriate to her nursing care. It supplies a mechanism that enables the nurse to arrive at a responsible valid judgment about clients from which to plan, implement, and evaluate nursing care that is responsive to the client's varied needs.

Components of the Process

The nursing process is composed of such phases as assessment, planning, implementation or intervention, and evaluation. Other authors have conceptualized the process as including observation, inference, validation, assessment, action, and evaluation.[9] Over the years, new terminology has evolved, and as nursing science develops, other terminology no doubt will be employed. Thus, we have in the literature such terms as *nursing diagnosis, clinical judgment, assessment, nursing prescriptions,* and so on. All of these terms refer in some way to the components of the nursing process and constitute the anatomy of nursing practice. Figure 1-2 presents a model for a contextual scheme of some current terms used in the conceptualization of the nursing process.

It is important to point out that, in the midst of the press and crush of everyday practice, where human lives may be at stake, calm fact-finding and judicial deliberation become increasingly difficult. Some of our most crucial nursing problems arise from conflicts between principle and expediency. Hence, we need to have a method so internalized as to be second nature so that we can arrive quickly at appropriate decisions and conclusions about our patients.

The components of the process also can help the student understand how nursing practice can be made operational. The various operations have been classified under headings derived from Bloch.[10] One is not to assume that these categories are mutually exclusive or stand alone. Rather, there are constant feedback loops in the process (see Fig. 1-2). Many authors might consider the data collection part of the nursing diagnosis stage. We present this interpretation as one means of conceptualizing more clearly the nursing process (See chart on Relationship of Scientific Method to Nursing Process).

The scientific method is used by other disciplines to provide a way of problem-solving for their members and as a basis from which to formulate research that will expand the theoretical base of the discipline. Since nursing also has the concern of expanding its theoretical knowledge to provide a sound basis for its practice, it is very important that the nursing process be scientifically grounded (See chart on Relationship of Scientific Method to Nursing Process).

In reviewing the process, it is seen that components 1 and 2 constitute a reconnoitering stage in which information is gathered and the diagnosis begun. Resources such as the chart, the family, the patient, members of the health team, and elements in the

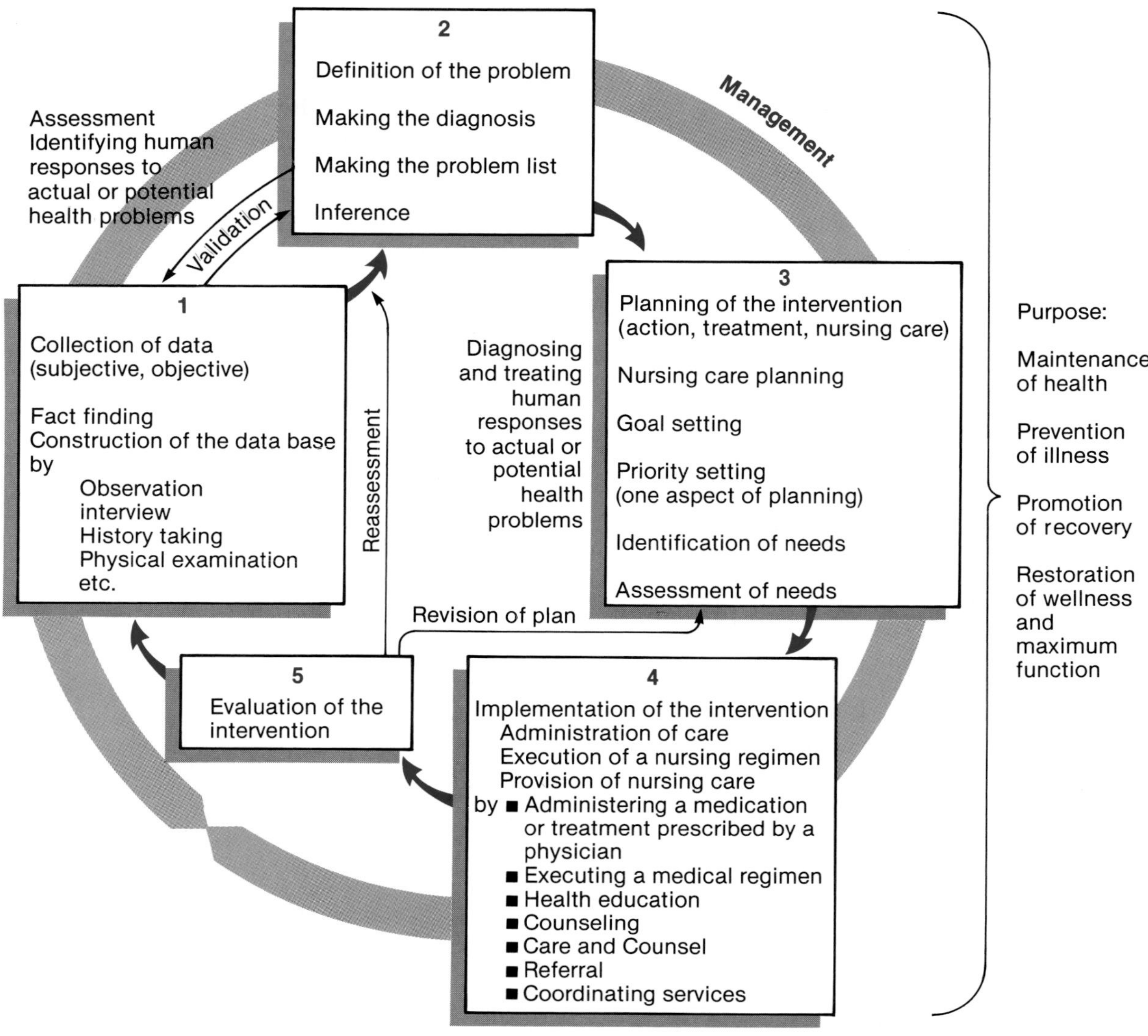

Figure 1-2.
Contextual scheme for some currently used terms in the conceptualization of nursing practice. (Block D: Some crucial terms in nursing: What do they really mean? Copyright © 1974, American Journal of Nursing Company. Reproduced with permission from Nursing Outlook, 22:4, Nov. 1974)

environment can be utilized. The nurse may also use the ability to "role take" to speed up the data collection.* This term refers to the ability to project oneself into the place of the patient in order to imaginatively construct the role of the patient, in order to provide appropriate cues for predicting and understanding the meaning of the patient's behavior, and thus, for determining appropriate behavior on the part of the nurse. The process by which the role of each particular patient is inferred stems from basic knowledge about the patient role in general, prior experience with the individual or others like her, or a specific bit of behavior that is being manifested. As the student gains more experience with various individuals involved in the patient role who are confronted with different kinds of health–illness conditions (including maternity patients), this role-taking ability will be facilitated.

*For a detailed definition and explanation of the concept of "role taking" and its application in maternity nursing, see the Reeder article in the Suggested Reading.

Relationship of Scientific Method to Nursing Process

	Components of the Nursing Process	Scientific Method
Assessment	1. Collect data (subjective, objective). a. Gather information on the physical, social, and psychological aspects of the health status of the individual and family. b. Construct the data base by observation, interview, history taking, physical examination, and role taking. c. Develop impressions.	1. Recognize general problem area. a. Survey pertinent information (literature, past experience, observation). b. Construct data base (organize, select). c. Develop "hunches."
	2. Define the problem. a. Make decisions regarding deficits or potential deficits in health status of the individual and family assigning resources. b. Make nursing diagnoses based on clinical judgment and inference, and review of related information, that is, theoretical formulations and research.	2. Define specific problem. a. Make decisions about relevance. b. Review related information (research already done, theoretical formulations).
Intervention	3. Plan the intervention. a. Make decisions regarding the actions believed to be appropriate to effect a solution of defined problems. b. Decisions include goal setting, priority setting, and nursing prescriptions.	3. Propose hypotheses.
	4. Implement the intervention. a. Execute a nursing regimen by administering a prescribed medication or treatment, executing a medical regimen, providing comfort measures and physical care, providing counseling, providing referral services, coordinating services for the patient, and providing health education.	4. Test hypotheses. a. Establish baseline data. b. State criteria for acceptance or rejection. c. Collect data.
Evaluation & reassessment	5. Evaluate the intervention. This in turn may lead to further reassessments. a. Determine the degree of effectiveness of the actions taken in solving the defined problems by observation, interview of patient status and conditions, physical examination, and reading of current records. b. Predict future nursing action and patient potential for change.	5. Analyze data and interpret results.
	6. Terminate or modify relationship.	6. Terminate or modify study. a. Make recommendations and predictions for future research.

Nursing Diagnosis

As we acquire our data, we become able to decide on the existence and extent of a problem. We can say in the most general terms that a problem does exist when there is a health goal to be obtained, but the client sees no well-defined, well-established means of attaining it. For instance, she may be too ill or too weak to help herself. Again, the goal may be so vaguely defined or unclear that the client cannot determine relevant means of achieving it. Thus, she may not understand or know how to accept conditions and instruction for achieving the goal of health.

A decision about the existence and extent of the problem initiates the diagnosis. There are many definitions of this term. For our purposes we shall regard a nursing diagnosis as a conclusion based on a systematic and scientific appraisal of an individual's health–illness condition, resulting from critical analysis of his or her behavior (alone and with others), the nature of the condition, and the numerous other factors (environmental, social, or psychological) that may affect the client's general state. This conclusion serves as a guide for our nursing care.

The statement of the diagnosis may be several words and more descriptive than etiological. As we find additional information about our patients, we may move from descriptive to more etiological statements. Moreover, there may be several diagnoses relating to a constellation of interrelated problems the patient has; for instance, if the nurse writes diagnoses regarding a labor patient, they might be as follows: "anxiety regarding process of labor," "elevated temperature," "inefficient but painful contractions."

Finally, one can have the same nursing diagnosis but have different pathological conditions that give rise to it. In the case of a newly delivered infant, for instance, the diagnosis might be "inadequate oxygenation," the cause of which for one infant might be a congenital heart defect, for another, immature lungs associated with prematurity. Thus, the total interrelationship of all the influencing factors is to be considered because it gives direction to our care plan.

Intervention

Components 3 and 4 are concerned with the planning and implementation of knowledgeable intervention in the form of nursing activities that encompass everything from the administration of comfort measures to counseling and health education. These activities are directed at moving the patient toward increased positive adaptation to the environment and high-level wellness.

Nursing prescriptions are given here. There are directions and suggestions that are incorporated into the nursing regimen or care plan. They constitute mutually agreed upon directives to the client that have bearing in furthering the well-being of the patient. They function much the same way as medical prescriptions but are often more elaborate and are formulated in consultation with the client and family.

Remember that the implementation phase is fluid because it is based upon a diagnosis or diagnoses which may be reassessed at any point in the process. Moreover, as we administer care, the patient's condition will be expected to change, which, upon evaluation, will necessitate possible new diagnoses and modification of care. Therefore, continuous feedback loops are built into the process.

In this phase, the nurse has the responsibility to disseminate her plan of care to her medical and nursing colleagues so that comprehensive care for the patient can be attained. This can be done by means of the Kardex, verbal reporting, charting, and nursing-assessment care plans. Most hospitals have instituted these care-plan forms, and they provide a thorough but brief summary of pertinent patient data together with space to write and record nursing prescriptions, interventions, evaluations, and patient response to care.

Evaluation and Reassessment

Component 5 includes both evaluation and prediction facets. A worthwhile evaluation includes an estimation of the results of our past nursing care activities to help predict the validity of our care for the future. Any statement of the effectiveness and reliability of our actions is best made with qualifications indicating the degree or amount of effectiveness and the reliability claimed:

1. What is the present state of the client?
2. Were all symptoms relieved?
3. What was the extent of the results?
4. On what evidence (observation of self, others, verbal response, cessation of symptoms)?
5. Who was involved (nurse, patient, others)?
6. In what contexts (what else was happening when the action was performed)?

When these points are established, we can begin to build categories of nursing action that are effective under certain circumstances for certain patients given certain conditions. As we ascertain the extent of our effectiveness we are then in a better position to predict the patient's potential for change toward stability or a wellness condition. Thus, we arrive at the nursing prognosis.*

The Social Context of Maternity Care

We mentioned earlier that maternity care is practiced in the context of the total society and, as such, is influenced by the values, attitudes, and practices of that society. Of late, society is adopting a new stance, particularly with regard to women. Since at least half of the maternity nurse's clientele will be women, attitudes and practices regarding them have great relevance for nursing practice. In concluding this chapter, we would like to leave the student with some information that, we hope, will be doubly thought-provoking for him or her.

Martin has pointed out in her book that the maelstrom of social change this country has experienced, particularly in the last 25 years, has greatly expanded the options open to women. At one time women had to make a choice between a family or a career; now women are increasingly combining the two, as men have always been privileged to do. Moreover, many types of occupations and professions formerly closed to women are becoming more accessible. Federal legislation now supports equal treatment of working women, and more mechanisms to challenge discrimination and unfair employment practices against women are being developed at the state level. Antidiscrimination laws have also had an impact on educational institutions. This is forcing a gradual change in the social biases toward a male privilege, perpetuated through values taught in primary and secondary schools, and culminating in the sex-linked admissions practices and career choices fostered by colleges and universities.[11]

Growing numbers of women and men no longer accept the traditional definitions of "feminine" and "masculine" identities and roles. They are seeking more individualized definitions of self that offer wider ranges of expression of their unique characteristics as *persons* rather than simply *woman* or *man*. Indeed, the common qualities shared by both women and men are felt to far outweigh their sex-related differences. Hence, social roles are developing that provide each sex with a much broader repertoire of behaviors. Women, in particular, expect more choices of lifestyle to be open to them. They may choose to marry or not, to have children or not, or to pursue any career or employment that is suited to their particular talent or interest. They expect to have a voice in the determination of their lives and well-being. And, increasingly, they are demanding a large decision-making role regarding economic and social policies that affect their lives and the larger society in which they live.

Women who choose to rear families spend significantly less of their lifetime in childbearing and childrearing. This fact, of course, has a direct impact on the structure and function of the family. Today's families are smaller and the last child is often born when the mother is in the mid- to late 20s or in the early 30s. The high degree of technology in the majority of American households has freed her from hours of household chores; thus, homemaking does not provide the fulltime occupation that it once did. With her lifespan lengthened and her health improved, the 35- to 40-year-old woman can be healthy and vigorous and can look ahead to at least another 25 years of productivity in a sphere outside the home.[11]

It has been said that roles are differentiated in pairs; that is, every role has its complementary role. Thus, as women's roles change and broaden, so too must men's. Slowly more egalitarian relationships are developing between the two sexes. Increasingly, men are assuming more responsibility in childrearing and running the household as their partners are forging ahead with careers. When both parties are pursuing a career, there is a growing tendency for household management, chores, and child-related activities to be shared equally. Thus, social power is very slowly being equalized and sex-linked exploitation is very gradually being diminished. However, there is still a long way to go before true equality can be achieved.

The authors hope that students will ponder these societal changes and the relevance that they have for nursing practice and for themselves as persons.

In the following chapters, we will examine some of the above ideas in more depth as we look at the various aspects of American families and the influence of a variety of social factors in the delivery of care.

*The student is encouraged to use the Suggested Reading for the articles on the nursing process and clinical judgment for a thorough and varied treatment of the subject.

References

1. Pritchard JA, McDonald P: Williams Obstetrics, 16th ed. New York, Appleton–Century–Crofts, 1980

2. World Health Organization Technical Report Series, No. 51. Geneva, Switzerland, World Health Organization, 1952

3. Schlesinger E: Health and Society 23:16–20, 1974

4. Committee on Perinatal Health, The National Foundation—March of Dimes. Toward Improving the Outcome of Pregnancy: Recommendations for the Regional Development of Maternal and Perinatal Health Services, 1976

5. Russell, C (ed.): Planning and design for perinatal and pediatric facilities. Columbus, Ross Laboratories, 1977

6. Orem DE: Nursing Concepts of Practice. New York, McGraw–Hill, 1971

7. Riehl J, Callista R: Conceptual Models for Nursing Practice. New York, Appleton–Century–Crofts, 1974

8. Little D, Carnevali D: Nusing Care Planning, 2nd ed. Philadelphia, JB Lippincott, 1976

9. Carrieri VK, Sitzman J: Components of the nursing process. Nurs Clin North Am 6: 115–121, 1971

10. Bloch D: Some crucial terms in nursing: What do they really mean? Nurs Outlook 22: 689–694, 1974

11. Martin L: Health Care of Women. Philadelphia, JB Lippincott, 1978

Suggested Reading

Aspinall MJ, Jambruno N, Phoenix BS et al. The why and how of nursing diagnosis. Mater Child Nurs J 2, 6:355–58, 1977

Barodish MS: Perinatal assessment. JOGN Nurs 10, 1:42–46, 1981

Curtin L, Petrick JA: Reproductive manipulation: Technical advances, options and ethical ramifications. Nurs Forum 16, 1:6–25, 1977

Durand M, Prince R: Nursing diagnosis: Process and decision. Nurs Forum 5, 4:50–64, 1966

Duxbury ML: Personnel and staffing needs for perinatal programs. Semin Perinatol 1, 3:267–277, 1977

Levine NA: Conceptual model for obstetric nursing. JOGN Nurs 5, 2:9–15, 1976

Mundinger MO, Johnson G: Developing a nursing diagnosis. Nurs Outlook 23: 94–98, 1975

Reeder S: Becoming a mother, nursing implications in a problem of role transition. ANA Regional Clinical Conferences, 204–210. New York, Appleton–Century–Crofts, 1968

Reiter FK: The clinical nursing approach. Nurs Forum 5, 4:39–44, 1966

Callista R: A diagnostic classification system for nursing. Nurs Outlook 23:90–93, 1975

Wilson RW, Schifrin B: Is any pregnancy low risk? Obstet Gynecol 55, 5:653–655, 1980

Editorial: Stop and think. . . what are we doing? Mater Child Nurs J 1, 3:146–151, 1976

CHAPTER

2

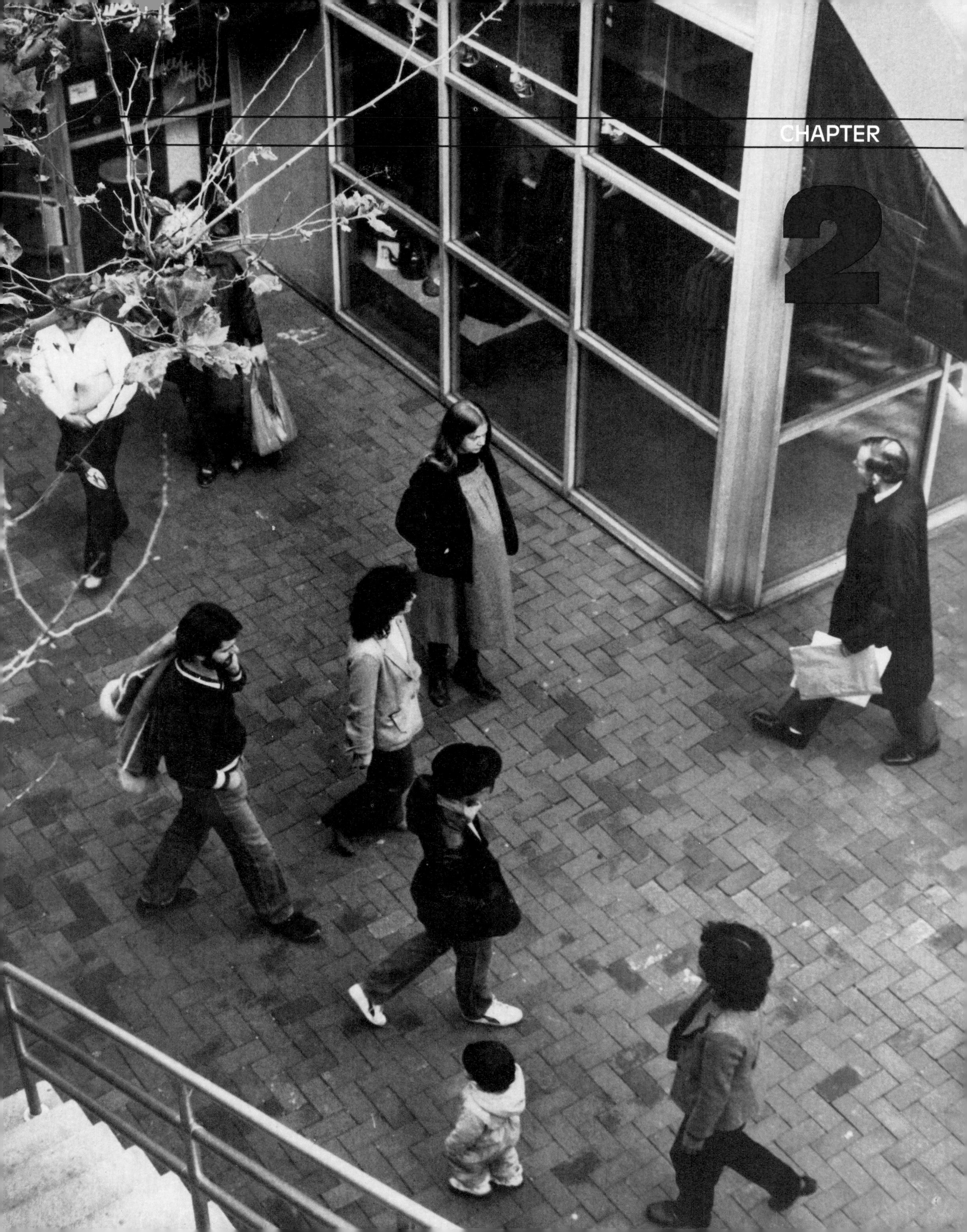

CHAPTER 2

Statistical Profiles

In the following paragraphs, we shall discuss several types of statistics that are relevant to the care of mothers and their infants and families. Statistical profiles are useful because they summarize a large amount of data about various populations and therefore supply health providers and policymakers with a valuable overview of needs and gaps in care.

Vital Statistics

Vital statistics reports give us quantitative data that have been systematically gathered and collated. Definitions relating to these data are presented here because they relate to statistical changes in the large body of people with whom we are concerned.

In this country these vital statistics reports are published officially by the United States Public Health Service, National Center for Health Statistics, Vital Statistics Division. The following terms have been defined by the National Center for Health Statistics. Mortality and morbidity terminology is classified according to the World Health Organization's Manual of International Classification of Diseases, Injuries and Causes of Death (ICD). The ICD is periodically revised; recently the ninth revision was published (1979–80). Some of the definitions below may change in subsequent revisions of the ICD.

Birthrate. The number of births per 1000 population. Also known as the crude birthrate.

Marriage rate. The number of marriages per 1000 total population.

Fertility rate. The number of births per 1000 women aged 15 through 44 years.

Neonatal. The period from birth through the 28th day of life.

Neonatal death rate. The number of neonatal deaths per 1000 live births.

Stillbirth or fetal death. A death in which the infant of 20 weeks or more gestational age dies *in utero* prior to birth.

Perinatal mortality. The current definition approved by WHO, includes all stillborn infants whose gestational age is 28 weeks or more, plus all neonatal deaths under seven days per 1000 births. The 1979 revision of the ICD, however, uses birth weight rather than gestational age as a criterion. It also recommends two different categories of reporting. For national data collection, the recommendation is that 500 g be used as the minimum weight of stillborn and live-born infants. For international comparisons, however, the weight should be 1000 g or more. When weight is unknown, either gestational age (28 weeks) or body length corresponding to 1000 g may be used. Obviously, these different criteria will make comparisons with previous data impossible and will also make national and international statistical comparisons difficult. There is current debate as to the efficacy of using the newly developed criteria.

Infant mortality rate. The number of deaths before the first birthday per 1000 live births.

Maternal mortality rate. The number of maternal deaths resulting from the reproductive process per 100,000 live births.

Race and color. Births in the United States are classified for vital statistics according to the race of the parents in the categories of white, black, American Indian, Chinese, Japanese, Aleut and Eskimo combined, Hawaiian and part-Hawaiian combined, and "other nonwhite." In most tables a less detailed classification of "white" and "nonwhite" is used.

The white category includes births to parents classified as white, Mexican, Puerto Rican, or "not stated." If one parent is Hawaiian and the other is not, the birth is classified as part-Hawaiian. If one parent is black, and the other is not Hawaiian, the birth is classified as black. In other cases of mixed parentage in which both parents are nonwhite, the child is assigned the father's race; if the father is white, the child is assigned the mother's race.

Natality

Overall the number of registered births in the United States has decreased in the last three decades from over 4 million live births in 1957 to 3.5 million in 1968 and 3.15 million in 1975. However, there was a small rise, about 1%, in the number of live births in 1976 as compared to the previous year. Moreover, provisional data from the National Center for Health Statistics indicate that in 1981 there was another 1% rise over 1980.[1] It is too early to predict whether this will continue to be a trend. However, these data are important for the planning of adequate maternal services in an era of diminishing resources.

Birthrates

The increase in the number of births is the result of the increase in the number of women in the childbearing ages (15–44). This number has risen rapidly due to the high birthrates of the 1940s and the 1950s—the so-called baby boom of the post-World War II era. Although the fertility rate reached a record low in 1976 for the fifth consecutive year, the decline was not enough to offset the 2% increase in the number of women of childbearing age. Provisional data for 1981 indicate a rate of 15.9 per 1000, which is an increase from the 1980 rate of 15.8 per 100.[1]

Thus, an important consideration that influences the number of children being born annually is the size and the age composition of the female population of childbearing age. Although the fertility rate is computed on the basis of births per 1000 women between ages 15 and 44, most of the childbearing is concentrated among women in their 20s. In 1973, for example, three out of five births were to women who were between 20 years and 29 years of age.

Another factor that influences the number of births is the number of marriages. In general, there has been a slight rise in the rate of marriages since 1968. However, more married couples are electing not to have children, and there are children being born more often now from social contract and other nonlegal unions. Thus, marriage is not as accurate a predictor as it was formerly.

Multiple Births

Over the years there has been a slight decline in the frequency of multiple births in the United States. The frequency of these births is another factor that bears on the natality rate. The rate was about 10 per 1000 deliveries.[2] Changes in age and the racial composition of the population, as well as the use of certain ovulation-producing drugs for infertility, contribute to fluctuations in the rate over time. There are differences, for instance, in the occurrence of twins, depending on the number of births the mother has had before delivery of the multiple birth. It should also be mentioned that there are differences between the rate of monozygotic, or identical twins, and dizygotic, or fraternal twins. The relative proportions of monozygotic and dizygotic twins are not the same for all races. The incidence of dizygotic twins is white 60%, black 70%, Japanese 40%. In the United States the twinning rate varies slightly from one region to another; the region with the highest rate of 10.5 is the Northeast; the lowest rate, 9.4, is in the West.

The Birth Certificate

In 1915 the federal government began to collect data on registered births and organized birth registration. At first only ten states and the District of Columbia were included in this method of reporting births, but it gradually expanded so that by 1933 the entire country was included. At the present time all 50 states and the District of Columbia demand that a birth certificate be filled out on every birth, and that it be submitted promptly to the local registrar. After the birth has been registered, the local registrar sends a notification to the parents of the child. Also, a complete report is forwarded from the local registrar to the state authorities, and then to the National Office of Vital Statistics in Washington.

Complete and accurate registration of births is a legal responsibility (Fig. 2-1). The birth certificate gives evidence of age, citizenship, and family relationships and as such is often required for military service and passports and to collect benefits on retirement and insurance. On the basis of birth certificates, information that is essential to agencies concerned with human reproduction is compiled by the National Office of Vital Statistics.

Population

The population of the United States more than doubled during the first half of this century and has continued to grow in tremendous proportions as was predicted. Between the time of the 1950 census and 1970, the population of the United States grew from 151 million to over 200 million. The predominant growth factor resulted from natural increases rather than international migration. This growth has required huge public and private expenditures for such basic facilities as shelter, schools, and highways. The high birthrates of the 1940s and the early 1950s first produced pressures for expansion of elementary education, then for the expansion of secondary education facilities, and, as we are aware now, for college facilities and jobs.

Three vital factors determine the rate at which population grows—births, deaths, and migration. The decline in the death rate that was so apparent in the first half of this century has fluctuated near the same relatively low level (9.7 deaths per 1000 population)

H105.142 Rev. 5-78

COMMONWEALTH OF PENNSYLVANIA
DEPARTMENT OF HEALTH
VITAL STATISTICS
CERTIFICATE OF LIVE BIRTH

TYPE OR PRINT IN PERMANENT INK

PRIMARY DIST. NO. ____________ STATE FILE NO.

A. ____
B. ____
C. ____
D. ____
E. ____
F. ____
G. ____
H. ____
I. ____

CHILD—NAME FIRST MIDDLE LAST 1. | SEX 2. | DATE OF BIRTH (Mo. Day Year) 3a. | HOUR 3b. ____ AM PM

HOSPITAL NAME (If not in Hospital, Give Street and Number) 4a. | City, Boro, or Twp. of Birth 4b. | COUNTY OF BIRTH 4c.

I CERTIFY THAT THE STATED INFORMATION CONCERNING THIS CHILD IS TRUE TO THE BEST OF MY KNOWLEDGE AND BELIEF 5a. (Signature) | DATE SIGNED (Mo, Day, Year) 5b. | CERTIFIER—NAME AND TITLE (Type or Print) 5c.

Name and Title of Attendant at Birth if other than Certifier (Type or Print) 5d. | CERTIFIER'S MAILING ADDRESS (Street or R.F.D. No., City or Town, State, Zip) 5e.

MOTHER—MAIDEN NAME FIRST MIDDLE LAST 6a. | AGE (At time of this Birth) 6b. | STATE OF BIRTH (If not in U.S.A., Name Country) 6c.

MAILING ADDRESS STREET AND NUMBER CITY AND STATE ZIP CODE 7.

WHERE DOES MOTHER ACTUALLY LIVE? STATE COUNTY CITY, BORO, TWP. (Specify) 8.

FATHER—NAME FIRST MIDDLE LAST 9a. | AGE (At time of this Birth) 9b. | STATE OF BIRTH (If not in U.S.A., Name Country) 9c.

INFORMANT 10a. | Relation to Child 10b. | REGISTRAR'S SIGNATURE AND DATE RECEIVED 11.

CONFIDENTIAL INFORMATION FOR MEDICAL AND HEALTH USE ONLY

Death Under One Year Of Age — Number of Death Certificate For This Child

RACE—MOTHER (e.g., White, Black, American Indian, etc. — Specify) 12. | RACE—FATHER (e.g., White, Black, American Indian, etc. — Specify) 13. | EDUCATION—MOTHER (Specify only highest grade completed) ELEMENTARY OR SECONDARY (0-12) | COLLEGE (1-4 or 5+) 14. | EDUCATION—FATHER (Specify only highest grade completed) ELEMENTARY OR SECONDARY (0-12) | COLLEGE (1-4 or 5+) 15. | IS MOTHER MARRIED TO FATHER? ☐ Yes ☐ No 16.

PREGNANCY HISTORY (Complete each section)

LIVE BIRTHS (Do not include this child): 17a. Now living Number ___ None ☐ | 17b. Now dead Number ___ None ☐

OTHER TERMINATIONS (Spontaneous and Induced): 17d. Before 16 wks. Number ___ None ☐ | 17e. After 16 wks. Number ___ None ☐

17c. Date of Last Live Birth (Mo. Year) | 17f. Date of Last Other Termination (Mo. Year)

Date Last Normal Menses Began (Mo. Day, Year) 18. | Month of Pregnancy Pre-Natal Care Began (1st, 2nd, etc.) (Specify) 19a. | Pre-Natal Visits — Total (If none, so state) 19b. | Length of Pregnancy in weeks. 20.

BIRTH WEIGHT 21. | THIS BIRTH—Single, Twin, Triplet, etc. (Specify) 22a. | If NOT Single Birth — Born First, Second, Third etc. (Specify) 22b. | APGAR SCORE 1 Min. 23a. 5 Min. 23b.

Multiple Births Enter State File Number for Mate(s)

Method of Delivery 24. | COMPLICATIONS OF PREGNANCY (Describe or write "none") 25.

CONCURRENT ILLNESSES OR CONDITIONS AFFECTING THE PREGNANCY (Describe or write "none") 26. | COMPLICATIONS OF LABOR AND/OR DELIVERY (Describe or write "none") 27.

Live Birth(s)

BIRTH INJURIES OF CHILD (Describe or write "none") 28. | CONGENITAL MALFORMATIONS OR ANOMALIES OF CHILD (Describe or write "none") 29.

Fetal Death(s)

Figure 2-1.
Certificate of live birth used by Pennsylvania Department of Health. Similar forms are used by other cities and states.

for the last decade. Control of immigration began in this country about a half century ago. However, recent modifications will undoubtedly exert an influence on this factor in our population growth.

One should not be deceived by the previous falling birthrate, which at first glance gives the impression that there is no need to have any concern about a population problem in the United States. The impression left by the tabulation of birthrates is that the number of live births has been relatively stable. However, it must be remembered that the birthrate is related to the number of births per 1000 population.

The former decline in the annual number of births was partly related to the age and sex structure of the population. The majority of Americans are young. More than half are under 28 years of age, but the proportion is shifting because of the fluctuating birthrates. The young adult group, composed of persons between ages 18 and 34, is now the fastest growing portion of the population, reflecting the high birthrates that followed World War II. This group, increased to 28.5% of the total as of 1980. The 40- to 50-year-old segment of the population is not expected to increase proportionately, but moderately large increases are anticipated in the older age groups, that is, persons 65 years and over.

According to population projections made by the Bureau of the Census, during the next ten years the number of women of childbearing age will probably rise in this country.

The uncertainty as to how much the population will grow rises from the unpredictable number of children who will be born to contemporary young couples. Though their fertility potential is huge, much will depend upon whether they choose to increase or decrease their family size.

Mortality

Maternal Mortality

Maternal mortality refers to deaths that result from childbearing; that is, the underlying cause of the woman's death is the result of complications of pregnancy, childbirth, or the puerperium.

In 1968 there were 950 maternal deaths registered in the United States. Over the past decade, there has been a decline so that now complications from pregnancy and childbirth account for about .03 of all the deaths per 1000. The maternal mortality rate in 1974 was about 15 per 100,000, in 1976 12.3 per 100,000, and in 1978 9.6 per 100,000. Provisional data for 1980 indicate a further decline to 7.6 per 100,000.

The reduction in maternal mortality rates has been rather consistent since 1951. The dramatic decline in these rates began about the mid-30s and continued until 1956. During the succeeding five years, the maternal mortality rate declined more slowly, reaching the all-time low in 1962. In 1963 the rate rose slightly to 35.8 per 100,000 live births but resumed its decline the following year and reached a record low in 1978.[1,3]

The risk of maternal death for all mothers is lowest at ages 20 to 24 (15 per 100,000 in 1970). It is slightly higher under age 20 and from age 25 on. Increasing age is associated with a steep rise in maternal mortality. At 40 to 44 years of age, the mortality rate is six times greater than at 20 to 24. At the oldest age in the reproductive age span, 45 years or older, the mortality is about 12 times greater than the low figure.

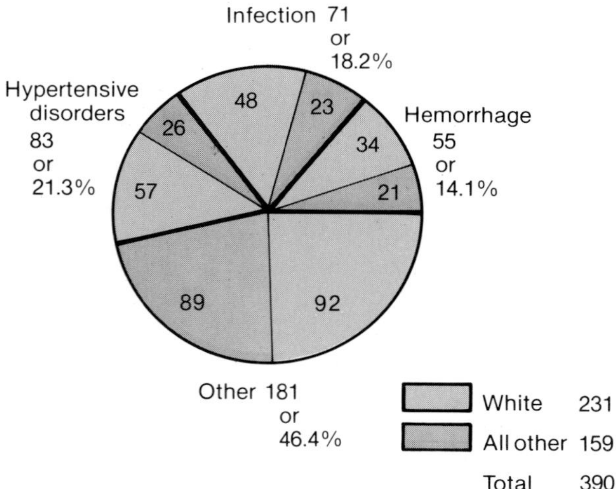

Figure 2-2.
Percentage distribution for causes of maternal mortality. (Data from Vital Statistics of the United States, 1976, Vol II—Mortality, Part A, Table 1-15, U.S. Department of Health, Education, and Welfare, Public Health Service, 1976)

Causes of Maternal Mortality

The reduction in maternal mortality from the hemorrhage disorders of pregnancy and childbirth was the largest single factor responsible for the reduction in the total maternal mortality rate (from 82.7 per 100,000 live births in 1949-1951 to 9.6 in 1978. The hypertensive disorders and sepsis (cases other than abortion) were next in importance as conditions affecting the mortality rate (Fig. 2-2). Subsequently, these three conditions will be discussed in detail, but it is important to stress the fact that deaths from these causes are for the most part preventable.[3]

It is also important to note that although hemorrhage is no longer the primary cause of maternal death as it once was, it still remains an important factor in the morbidity of mothers and in the underlying cause of death. For instance, according to the official classification, only the direct cause of death is considered, even though the predisposing cause may be an important factor. For example, in a case in which the mother has a massive hemorrhage and then (in her weakened condition) develops a puerperal infection that eventually causes her death, the death is classified as due to puerperal infection. Hemorrhage is often a predisposing factor, and in this manner its toll in maternal mortality cannot be underestimated.

Puerperal infection is a wound infection of the birth canal after childbirth, which sometimes extends to cause phlebitis or peritonitis. The nurse can play an important role in helping to prevent such infections by maintaining flawless technique in performing nursing procedures.

The *hypertensive disorders of pregnancy* are certain disturbances peculiar to gravid women, characterized mainly by hypertensive edema, albuminuria, and in some severe cases by convulsions and coma. Antepartal care is an important part of prevention or early detection of symptoms, and with suitable treatment the disturbance often can be allayed.

Reduction in Maternal Mortality

Many factors are responsible for achieving the overall reduction in maternal mortality in this country during the past 25 years.

Medical management has improved. The widespread use of blood and plasma transfusions and antibiotics, together with careful maintenance of fluid and electrolyte balance and sophisticated anesthesia management, has changed obstetric practice substantially. Legalized abortion has also helped reduce the number of maternal deaths associated with abortion.

Perhaps more important is the development of widespread *training and educational programs* in obstetrics and maternity care, which have provided more and better qualified specialists, professional nurses, and other personnel to deliver care in this area. Better hospital facilities and the increase in hospital deliveries have also helped reduce maternal mortality. The development of alternate hospital facilities to meet consumer demands for a more homelike setting for parturition may also prove to be a helpful factor.

The distinct change in attitudes of physicians, nurses, and parents has also contributed to this progressive saving of mothers. Childbirth is no longer an event to be awaited helplessly by the expectant mother with what fortitude she is able to muster; instead, it is the climax of a period of preparation—a true state of preparedness attained through the cooperation of the physician, the nurse, and the expectant parents. As indicated before, this preparation for childbirth, based on careful medical and nursing supervision throughout pregnancy, is called *antepartal,* or *prenatal care.*

Antepartal care has been an important achievement in maternity care during the present century. It will be of interest to the nurse to know that this salutary contribution to the mother's welfare was initiated by the nursing profession. It had its beginning in 1901 when the Instructive Nursing Association in Boston began to pay antepartal visits to some of the expectant mothers who were to deliver at the Boston Lying-In Hospital. This work gradually spread until, in 1906, all of these women prior to confinement were paid at least one visit by a nurse from the association. By 1912 this association was making about three antepartal visits to each patient. In 1907 another pioneer effort in prenatal work was instituted when George H. F. Schrader gave the Association for Improving the Condition of the Poor, New York City, funds to pay the salary of two nurses to do this work. In 1909 the Committee on Infant Social Service of the Women's Municipal League in Boston organized an experiment of antepartal work. Pregnant women were visited every ten days, more often if necessary. Blood pressure readings and urine tests were made at each visit. This important work was limited because of the effort to make it as nearly self-supporting as possible; therefore, only mothers under the care of physicians and hospitals were accepted. This began the movement for antepartal care that has been extremely important in promoting the health and well-being of many pregnant women.

Another important factor in the reduction of maternal mortality has been the development of maternal and child health programs in State Departments of Public Health, particularly the work of community health nurses. These nurses visit a large number of the mothers who otherwise would receive little or no medical care, bringing them much-needed aid in pregnancy, labor, and the puerperium. This service fills a great need not only in rural areas, but also in metropolitan centers.

Perinatal Mortality

The two groups of problems in infant mortality that are of chief concern in maternity are (1) those in which the fetus dies in the uterus prior to birth, and (2) those in which it dies within a short time after birth (neonatal death). The term *perinatal mortality* is used to designate the deaths in these two categories.

Fetal Death

In an effort to end confusion arising from the use of a variety of terms, such as *stillbirth, abortion, miscarriage,* and so on, the World Health Organization (WHO) recommended the adoption of the following definition of fetal death:

> Fetal death is a death prior to complete expulsion or extraction from its mother of a product of conception, irrespective of duration of pregnancy; the death is indicated by the fact that after such separation the fetus does not breathe or show any other evidence of life such as beating of the heart, pulsation of the umbilical cord, or definite movement of voluntary muscles.[4]

WHO further defined fetal death by indicating four subgroups, according to gestational age in weeks.

Infant Mortality

Two decades ago a total of 103,390 infant deaths before the first birthday was reported. By 1970 the infant mortality rate was 20.0 per 1000 live births in United States. As is shown in Figure 2-3, in the last decade the rate has dropped from 16.1 in 1975 to an estimated 11.8 in 1981.[1] The leading causes of infant

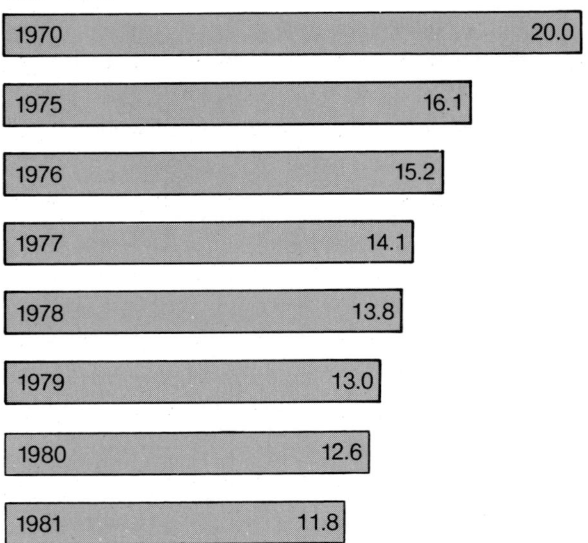

Figure 2-3.
Infant mortality rates per 1000 live births, 1970–1981. (National Center for Health Statistics, Annual Summary for the United States, 1979. Monthly Vital Statistics Reports 28:13, November 13, 1980 DHHS Publication No. (PHS) 81–1120)

mortality are listed in Figure 2-4. A falling fertility rate, better contraceptive practices, and increasing availability of safe abortion, together with a higher standard of living in the general population, have been suggested as factors in this decline in infant mortality.

However, it has been pointed out that this national figure does not accurately reflect trends in the large urban areas and the southern states where the rate has declined less.

Many factors are responsible for infant mortality. The vast number of infant deaths is the result of several main causes—respiratory distress syndrome, preterm birth, asphyxia and atelectasis, congenital malformations, and birth injuries.

During the first four weeks of life early gestational age and low birth weight are the chief causes of death. Birth injuries, another of the main causes of infant loss, accounted for almost 7000 infant deaths in 1970. Almost one third of these deaths were due to intracranial and spinal injury at birth. In the vast majority of these cases, death occurred within less than seven days of life. These conditions will be discussed in detail later. It suffices to say that one of the first and most important of them, immaturity, is largely a nursing management problem. Indeed, in all the wide range of nursing care there is no area that offers such a challenge to the nurse or such lifesaving possibilities as that of caring for the preterm infant.[5]

The welfare of some 4,000,000 babies born annually in the United States is very much the concern of maternity nurses and obstetricians and one of the main objectives of the entire field of maternity care. To reduce the enormous loss of newborn lives, to protect the infant not only at birth but also in the prenatal period and during the early days of life, and to lay a solid foundation for his health throughout life are the problems and the challenge of maternity care.

Reproductive Wastage

The vast number of infants lost by spontaneous abortion is a matter of grave importance. About 10% of all pregnancies terminate in spontaneous abortion because of such factors as faulty germ plasm, unsatisfactory environmental conditions, hormonal and many other unknown etiological causes.[3,5]

As our knowledge of determining and diagnosing these factors becomes greater, more definitive inroads are being made in this area.

Today the concerns for the United States stemming from the overall problem of maternal and fetal reproductive wastage reflect a symptom of far-reaching social change. The tremendous reduction in maternal and infant mortality rates presents concrete evidence of the noteworthy progress that has been achieved in maternity care in this country. Nevertheless, the current major concern is that a large segment of our population is not receiving maternity care.

The needs resulting from problems of maternal and child health in rural areas continue today, but what is alarming is that now there is a parallel situation in the larger cities.

Since World War II there have been major shifts in population: urban middle-class families have migrated to suburban areas, whereas large numbers of families from rural areas have moved to the large urban industrial areas. Despite the increase in employment and in income generally, the population still includes a large segment of disadvantaged, low-income families, as well as foreign immigrants, who recently have concentrated in the major cities. With the increased cost of health services in general and the cost of hospital care in particular, these low-income families are straining the local resources of the communities in which they reside. Also, the number of maternity patients in these areas has greatly

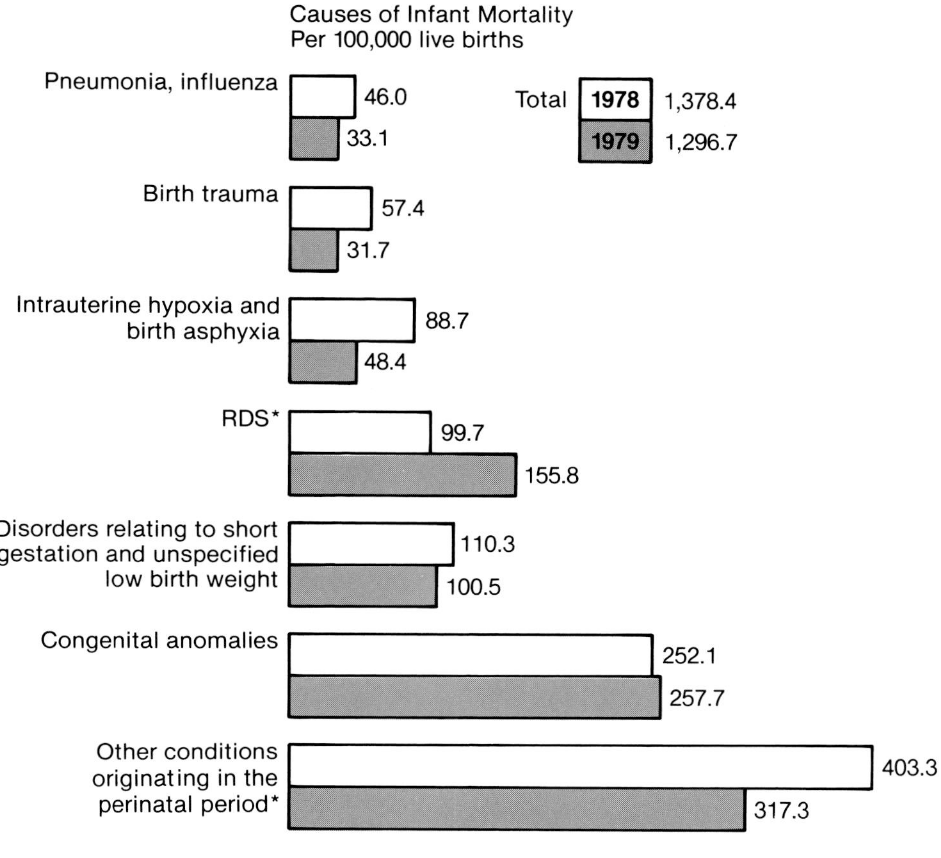

Figure 2-4.
Causes of infant mortality per 100,000 live births in 1978 and 1979. (National Center for Health Statistics, Annual Summary for the United States, 1979. Monthly Vital Statistics Reports 28:13, November 13, 1980 DHHS Publication No. (PHS) 81–1120)

increased as a result of migration, producing overcrowding of clinics and hospital maternity in-service divisions. To accommodate such large numbers of patients, many of the hospitals with large maternity services have had to resort to limiting the mother's hospital stay, some women being discharged 24 hours after delivery. The most serious problem by far is that many of these women are receiving poor or, often, no antepartal care, due in part to dissatisfaction with the kind of care provided. Inadequate care during pregnancy has been demonstrated to bear a direct relationship to the rate of immaturity.

Moreover, with spiraling inflation, it has been pointed out that middle-class couples are feeling the impact of not being able to afford adequate health care. They are not eligible for welfare coverage, yet not affluent enough to seek the kind of care that is appropriate.

It has been mentioned previously that social factors play a role in morbidity and mortality and, in fact, influence the reproduction efficiency of childbearing women.

Much of the difficulty in providing adequate care is due to a shortage of professional personnel in the maternity field. The rapid growth of the population has not been accompanied by a proportionate increase in physicians and nurses who are attracted to this area of specialization. Student nurses might well investigate the reason for this apathy and in good time provide some solution to this problem. These factors will be explored in greater detail in subsequent chapters.

References

1. National Center for Health Statistics: Annual Summary for the United States, 1979. DHHS Publication No. (PHS) 81–1120. Monthly Vital Statistics Reports 30:12, March 18, 1982

2. United States Department of Health, Education, and Welfare: Characteristics of births: United States 1973–1975. DHEW Publication No. (PHS) 78–1908. Sept 1980

3. Vital Statistics of the United States, 1976, Vol. 11, Mortality, Part A Table 1-15. United States Department of Health, Education, and Welfare, Public Health Service

4. National Summaries: Fetal deaths, U.S., 1954, National Office of Vital Statistics 44:11, Aug 1956

5. Op. Cit NCHS Annual Summary

6. Center for Disease Control: Abortion surveillance. Annual Summary, 1976

Suggested Reading

Hickey LA, et al: Maternity day care program offers economical, family-oriented care. Hospitals, JAHA 51, 23:85–89, 1977

Klein MC, Papageorgiou A: Can perinatal regionalization be reconciled with family-centered maternal care? J Fam Pract 5,6:969–974, 1977

Lawson J: Avoidable factors in maternal deaths. Nursing Mirror 139, 11:48, 1974

Osofsky H, Kendall N: Poverty as a criterion of risk. Clin Obstet Gynecol 16:103–119, 1973

Savage JE: Obstetrics through the retrospectroscope. South Med J 73, 11:1516–1520, 1980

Schneider L: Changing concepts of prenatal care. Postgrad Med 53:91–97, 1973

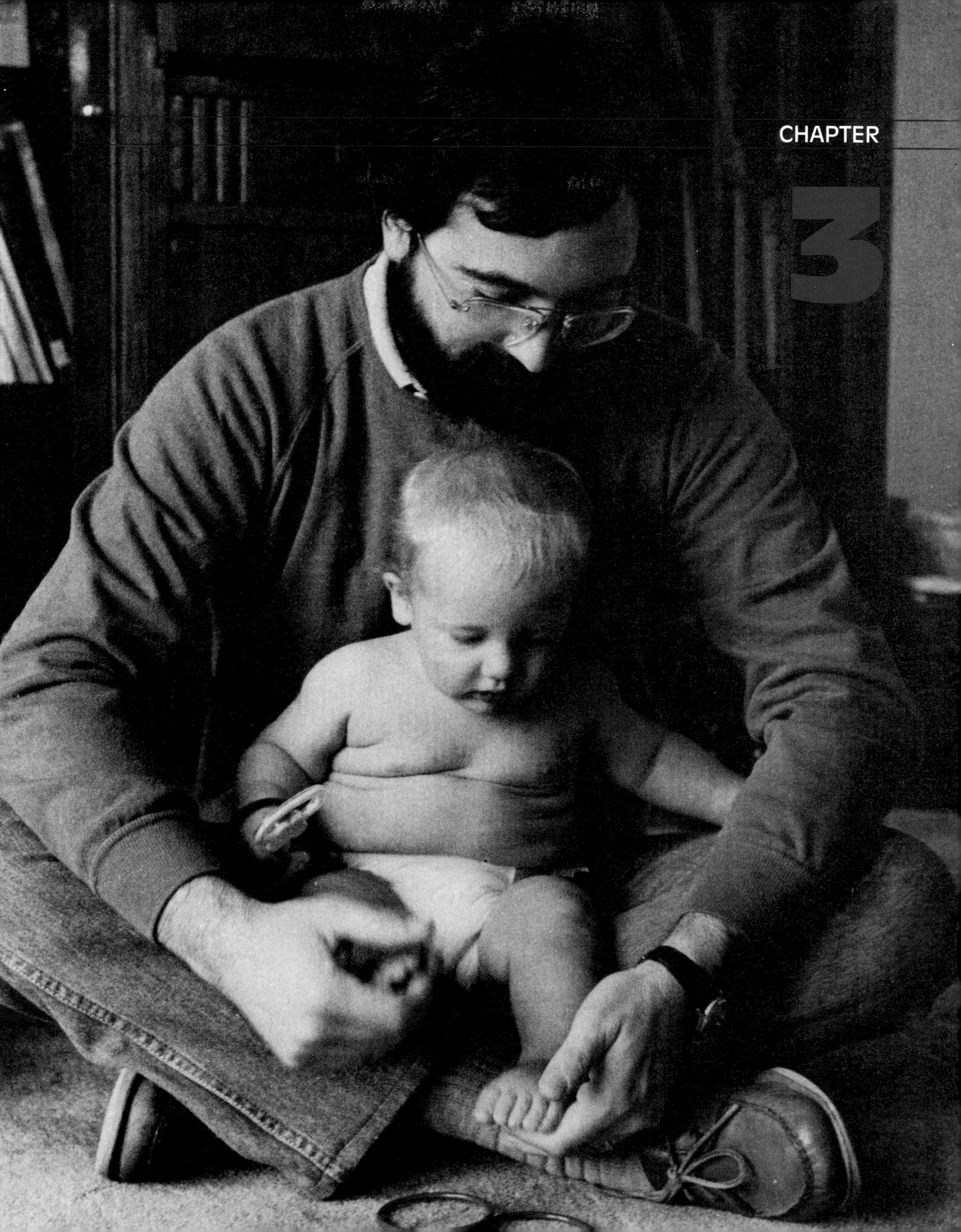

CHAPTER

3

CHAPTER 3

The Family in a Changing World

What is the Family?

Most people know intuitively what they mean by "the family." They have known families throughout their lifetime and intuitive definitions are sufficient for everyday conversation and action. However, when we begin to define what constitutes a family, or analyze this unit as a social institution, or attempt to deliver comprehensive care to it, it becomes apparent that what we have considered as *the* family is inappropriate for systematic treatment. The characteristics of the families of our own personal experience often do not fit "families" of other segments of society. Family life in different cultures exhibits even greater contrasts.

The family has been defined in a variety of ways. Torbett refers to it as "a group of two or more persons who are united by blood, marriage, or adoption residing in a common household wherein they create and maintain a common culture and interact with each other by way of familial roles."[1] Other authors have defined the family as a unit of interacting personalities or as a system of roles.[2,3] Common to all of these definitions is the fact that the members, whether they be a married dyad or a single parent and child, have anonymous role relationships, or belong to a union unsanctioned by law, relate to each other in some way; that is, they *interact* with specified patterns of behavior, and in so doing differentiate or structure roles for themselves.

The Relationship of Family Theory to Nursing Practice

Since nurses in their interaction with families will come into a situation in which there is a set of ongoing role relationships, it is important that they consider a number of factors when providing care for their clients. The structure and functioning of the family determines their use of health services. Hence, all members of the health team need to be aware of a variety of theories regarding human behavior and how families develop their various patterns of behavior. This awareness necessitates using knowledge from other specific disciplines where it is appropriate in order to deliver optimum health care.

Family-Centered Care

The concept of family-centered care and its logical extension, family nursing, has always been a part of nursing. Some areas of practice, notably that of community health, have traditionally claimed more interest, expertise, and responsibility for total family care than others. Delivering care in the client's home has allowed the nurse more insights into the family and its workings and the implications its structure and function have for the health of its members. Moreover, it has allowed the nurse to assess the problems and progress of the family members as a whole.

However, other nursing specialists, notably those in maternal-child health, have also demonstrated interest in family care, focusing initially on the mother–child dyad and later on parenting. In addition, midwifery has used a family-centered approach to home delivery services by utilizing family resources to prepare for care of the mother-infant couple in the home setting.[4] Parents' classes under the auspices of the Maternity Center Association and the Child Study Association in conjunction with the former Children's Bureau have also promoted the development of nursing care of the total family.[5] The philosophy behind this approach has been to meet expressed needs and concerns of parents through the nurse's group leadership role, not necessarily through a course of preplanned instruction. Thus, as nursing has evolved to keep pace with today's health needs, it has become apparent that concepts from other disciplines are badly needed in order to supply a total picture of the family unit for which high-quality care is to be provided.

Probably no force has been so potent or recent in supplying these valuable concepts as the theorists and researchers in the social and behavioral sciences. Efforts to theorize and to conduct research about the family as a social phenomenon have brought together many disciplines and encouraged cooperation and collaboration in the study of that complex social entity. These multidisciplinary contributions have stimulated many teachers and students of nursing to seek advanced preparation and to conduct research about families that have implications for their practice.

The comprehensive overview of family study by Christensen in his *Handbook of Marriage and the Family*,[6] as well as the identification and classification of conceptual frameworks relating to the family unit done by Hill and Hansen, and Nye and Berardo,[7,8] have been invaluable resources for helping to delineate content in clinical nursing courses and for providing conceptual frameworks for the development of assessment tools and the testing of nursing intervention techniques.

Perhaps most significant, nursing is now joining with other related disciplines whose basic interests and expertise in the family may someday ensure team approaches to research in clinical matters, multidisciplinary educational programs, and, most important, team effort in family care.[4] Society's demands, needs, and aspirations are causing rapid changes in all health fields, including nursing practice and educational programs. Tired of fragmentation in service, high costs, barriers to the entry into health services, and the inertia and unresponsiveness of the health care system in general, consumers are taking action in what amounts to a social movement.[4,9]

As a result, health professionals find themselves in the center of a revolution in the health care system. Only by multidisciplinary collaboration will they be able to rise to the occasion and provide adequate health services.

Roles, Role Theory, and Implications for Nursing Practice

As background for understanding the family, we must deal with another concept that permeates both lay and professional language today. That concept is role, and it is an integral part of the structure and function of the family.

As with the concept of family, we have an intuitive sense of what a "role" is, but when attempts are made to systematically study the construct, we find a broad latitude in definitions and understandings of it. Psychological and sociological approaches to role are closely interrelated because an individual's personality develops within a social system which, in our culture, is the family. Hence, roles may be viewed from a psychosocial viewpoint that enables us to focus on the individual and how he integrates his role relationships, and also from a sociological viewpoint which guides us in focusing on group or social relationships, primarily those within the family. We must also deal with culture, for the "self" can be viewed as either the unit of personality, an individual's "status" or position in a unit of society, or as a role enacted in the culture.[10]

Role and Status

Basic to any discussion of role are the definitions of role and status. *Status,* or position, generally refers to a person's location in a system of interaction. On the other hand, *role* applies to behavior that reflects the goals, values, and sentiments operating in a given situation. A further clarification of these definitions can be made by contrasting role as defined by two major theorists, Ralph Linton and George Herbert Mead. According to Linton, roles tend to be defined as constellations of rules or expectations for behavior associated with a given status or position.[11] In the Meadian, or interactionist tradition, however, roles are defined, created, stabilized, or modified as a consequence of interaction between the self and others.[12]

Role vs Interaction

From an interactionist frame of reference, role is more than a series of do's and don'ts for the behavior expected of a person occupying a given position. Rather, it is a constellation of behaviors that emerges from interaction between the self and others that constitutes a meaningful unit, and that is an expression of the values, goals, or sentiments that provide direction for that interaction. It is true that these constellations of behaviors become patterned over time and that the actors proceed as if there were prescriptions for performance.

However, there is much more latitude in the Meadian conception of role because it allows for innovative, individualistic designing of a person's role performance on the basis of assignment of some sentiment or goal to the behavior of relevant others.

This conception of role is particularly salient for nursing practice as it allows for a broader interpretation of the behavior of all actors than do more traditional concepts. Moreover, it does not limit either the interpretation of the behavior or the nurse's response to the behavior to a prescribed set of do's and don'ts. Hence, it permits creativity and innovation in interaction with clients.

Complementary Roles

Another basic concept in role theory is that of the *complementarity* of roles or the fact that all roles are learned in pairs. Thus, a role does not exist in isolation but is patterned to mesh with that of a role partner. For instance, the nurse's role meshes with the patient's role, the husband's with the wife's, the child's with the parent's, and so on. Some of these roles that are basic in society, such as husband, wife, child, and so on, have become more patterned in the various cultures than others, and thus, firmer expectations have come about. But we need only look at the innovative variation in recent family lifestyles to appreciate how traditional role prescriptions and expectations can, and often must, be modified.

Whether there be firm or loose expectations, this pairing or complementarity of roles provides for reciprocal arrangements in interaction and therefore allows social interaction to proceed in an orderly fashion, since there emerges a predictability in interaction. The actors "know" what they are to do. Without this complementarity, it would be difficult to maintain stable interaction networks such as exist in the family system. Indeed, the family's equilibrium depends on this role pairing.

Socialization of Roles and Role Models

Roles are learned through the process of socialization. In socialization, individuals learn the ways of social groups so that they can function within these groups. Socialization takes place through both intentional and incidental instruction, that is, by providing specific instruction regarding a certain facet of behavior and by providing examples of desired behavior, in other words, role modeling. All of the various socialization agencies—the family in the beginning and later the church and schools—teach the child certain role behaviors through intentional programs of learning and study.

However, operating conjointly may be incidental learning in which the child adopts the ways of others in his environment through play acting, peer group relations, and observations of adult and peer role models.

Thus, the significant others in the child's world teach him, both by defining the world for him and by serving as models for his attitudes and behavior. The child learns through a system of rewards and punishment and, if he behaves as the significant others desire, he receives positive attention and invitations to continue his participation and interaction. If, on the other hand, he behaves otherwise, he is refused attention, reprimanded, or physically punished.

It is important to remember that much of the role learning that takes place in the family is indirect. The child learns by observing and participating in the interpersonal relations patterns established by the family, the examples set by the other family members, and the role that he develops for himself within the family. Hence, he learns and adopts basic role skills from family members and concurrently adapts to the roles of the other family members.[10]

Emotional Basis of Role Learning

Another important aspect of role learning is that it is not merely a cognitive process. It is associated with multiple emotional or affective ties that the individual makes with others. These attachments begin with the mother and gradually include increasing numbers of persons with whom the child interacts and comes to identify with. As these attachments grow, the child develops a sense of "self," in that he can take a position from the outside and view his own thoughts, feelings, and actions. In this way, he gradually internalizes the behavior that is expected of him as he figuratively stands back and looks at himself and guides, judges, and reflects on his own behavior according to his perceptions of others' expectations for his behavior.

It has been noted that, while individuals learn role behavior in much the same way, there are differences in respective role performances. This differential role performance may be due to differences in the ways persons respond in interpersonal situations, their knowledge of the role in general, their motivation to perform specific roles, their attitude toward themselves, and finally, their response to the behavior of other persons in the interaction.[10]

Tension in Role Relations

Tension and discontinuities in role relations must also be considered when considering the concept of role. Many terms have been used to illustrate the idea of tension or interruptions in a smooth process of interaction. Terms such as role conflict, role strain, role change, and role transition have been used to convey the various aspects of tension that can occur in a role system.

We have made the point that role interaction is dynamic. As theories of the development of human nature change, so do socialization patterns. As these latter change, variant family life systems evolve, which in turn redefine reciprocal role relationships. Tensions and disruptions in smooth and rewarding role interaction may occur at any point.

Summary

The major determinants of the degree of adjustment an individual makes to a role can be summarized as follows: (1) the clarity with which a specific role and its complementarity is defined and demonstrated; (2) the clarity or definiteness of the transitional procedures in the acquisition of a new role; (3) how well the role is learned and enacted—this is partly dependent on 1 and 2 and the strength of the socialization process to the new role; (4) the consistency of the responses a role evokes; (5) a role's compatibility with the other roles in the individual's set of roles; (6) a role's congruity with the emotional needs of the individual; and (7) the degree of complementarity that exists between reciprocal roles.

When there is a high degree of adjustment, the enactment of an individual's set of roles can be rewarding in that they define for him his niche, his self-concept anchorage, a sense of belongingness and purpose. They give him social recognition and support which, in turn, allow him to buy or earn desired conditions or things in the world and to view himself as a worthwhile, contributing member of society.[10]

Family Roles and the Nurse

Concepts from role theory encompass a body of knowledge that is vital for the nurse who works with families or individual family members. The application of these concepts can greatly increase the nurse's understanding of the role strains and changes inherent in the phenomenon of family stress that can be precipitated by childbearing, chronic or acute illness in the family, or death of any of the family members.

For example, consider the change in the interaction patterns that must be accomplished when a new infant is incorporated into the household—restructuring of all of the members' roles is necessitated, and this is doubly complicated when there are other children present. Sibling rivalry is only one aspect of the impact of a new infant on the family.

Also, consider the situational crisis when parents bear a mentally retarded or otherwise defective child. Following the grief reaction and concomitant frustration, conflict, and high anxiety, the family equilibrium can be regained only when parents restructure their roles to either encompass or reject the afflicted member and learn to cope with the situation.

Finally, consider acute catastrophic illness in the father of a family with several children. When such an illness occurs, the man is thrust into the role of patient which is, in essence, a dependent role. This necessitates a reorganization of the role behaviors of the other family members. The wife must become more dominant, the children generally must assume more responsibility, and hence, their positions change vis-à-vis other family members. These few examples point out the necessity for the nurse to consider family role relations if she is to intervene in a holistic way.

The Role of Mother

Each society provides many cues and signals that tell individuals how it defines a role and identifies appropriate behavior for the role. These cues may be overt

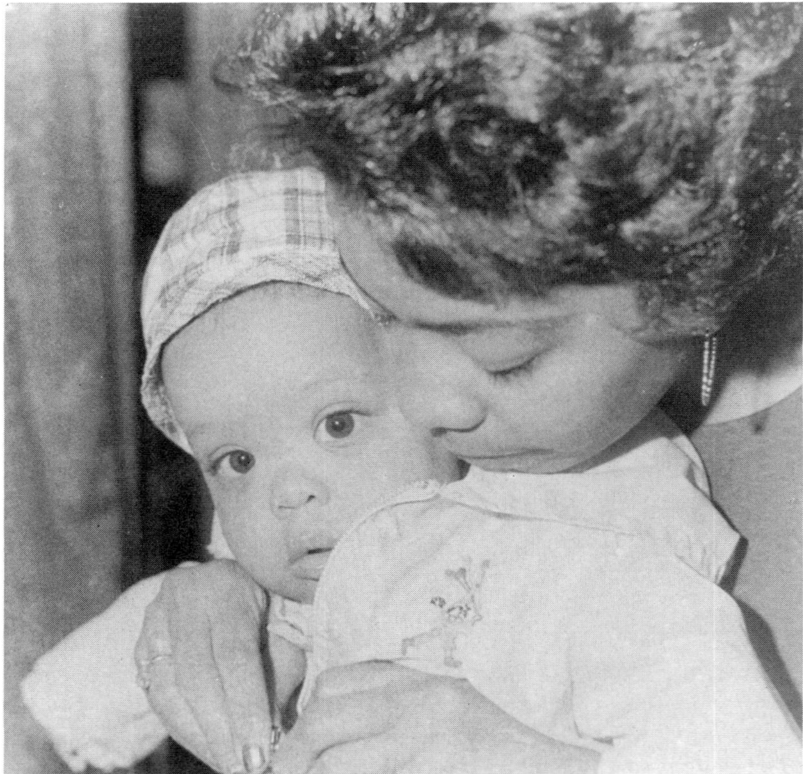

Figure 3-1.
In our culture, the ideal mother has been traditionally the nurturer.

or covert and may be perceived in a subliminal way. In our culture, the ideal mother has been traditionally the nurturer, the one who gives sustenance and unconditional love (Fig. 3-1).

A woman's concept of the mother role is based on the norms of the culture, the social class and ethnic group to which she belongs, and the type of socialization she has received from her immediate family.

Motherliness

It is important to remember that there is a difference between the role of mother and feelings of motherliness. In a sense, both are learned, but mothering, the enactment of the role of mother, involves skills and a certain understanding of the developmental process of the child. Thus, *motherliness* can be thought of as an emotional feeling that develops over time as the mother has increasing contact with her infant (see Chap. 29, Fig. 3-2). It is a feeling that the child is emotionally hers, and there is a need to identify the infant with the rewarding values and qualities that she considers part of herself and her life.

This development of motherliness begins with the maternal claiming process and is evident in the initial and early mother–newborn contact when the mother touches (at first timidly) and later enfolds her infant and exclaims, "Oh, he is finally here! How did I ever produce that?"[13]

Our hospital procedures often militate against this early claiming behavior, but fortunately we are now beginning to relax many of the restrictions that tend to disrupt the reality testing of this ownership process.

Anxieties and Conflicts in Motherhood

All mothers need reassurance that they are, indeed, mothers, and adequate if not excellent ones. The disappointment the mother feels when the infant sleeps at the breast instead of nursing is very familiar to everyone. Mothers excoriate themselves with criticism when they are awkward in handling their first born. They try desperately to "pull themselves together," to assume care of the infant only hours after delivery. Although seemingly small and unimportant, these initial anxieties are the basis of the future rela-

Figure 3-2.
Motherliness is an emotional feeling that develops over time as the mother has increasing contact with her infant.

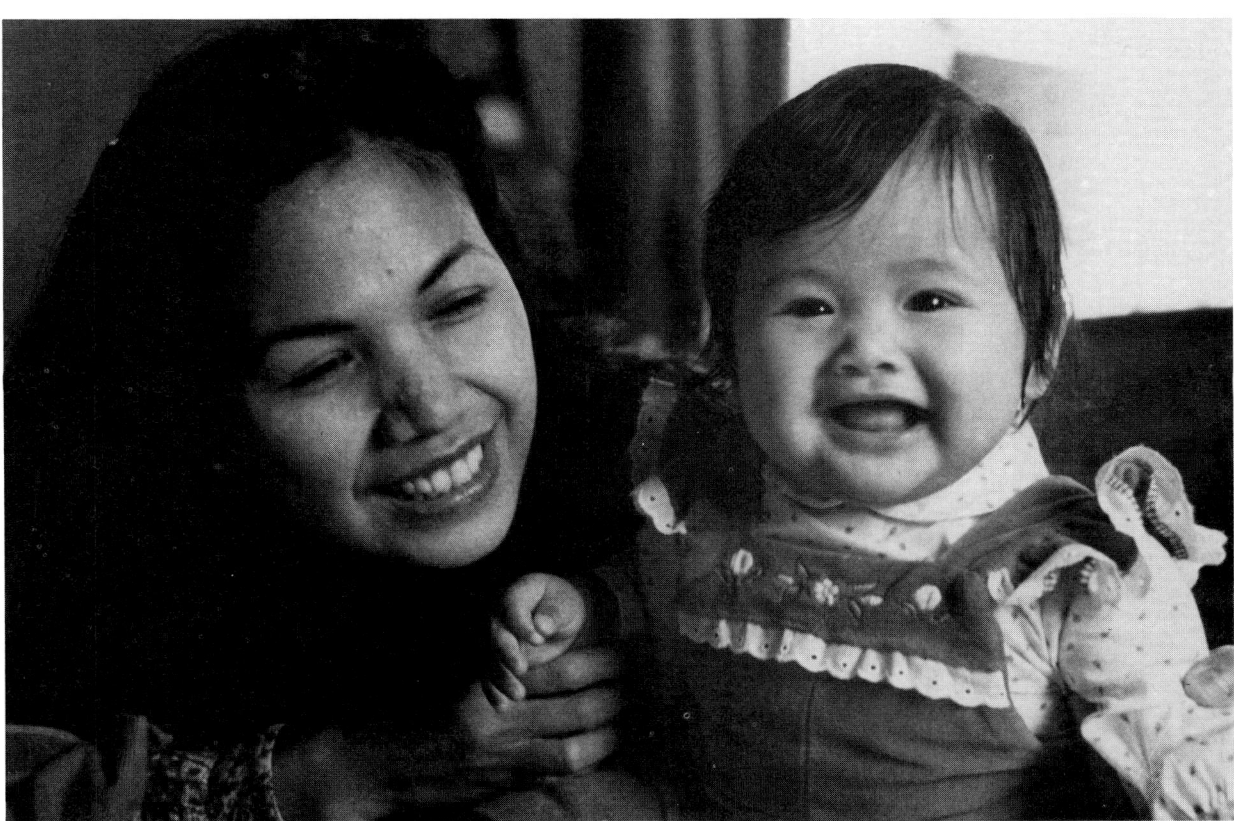

tionship between mother and child. Moreover, they are complicated by the many conflicts in modern society where the role of mother has come into increasing competition with other social roles a woman may enact. Paramount among these conflicts are fantasies of idealized motherhood versus feelings of inadequacy in actual role performance; the need for dependency versus the adult goal of independence and responsibility; love versus resentment for the baby owing to fatigue and increased responsibility for such a dependent being; feelings for the baby versus feelings for the husband; and self-actualization versus the demands of motherhood.[10]

If the mother has had problematic relations with her own mother during the early socialization years, these may affect her role enactment. She may project many of these negative feelings onto her own child or, conversely, bend over backwards to avoid socialization techniques her mother used, thereby limiting or missing important features that she might have kept and used. Also, if the normal and increasing dependency needs of pregnancy and the early postpartum are not met, she may not be able to easily care for and give love to her dependent child.

One final point deserves mention. For many, children of one age are more appealing than those of another. A mother may be able to respond to the needs of a dependent infant but not adapt readily to the four-year-old's search for and insistence on autonomy.

Thus, the role of mother and its enactment is shaped by many interacting factors and therefore will have a wide range of behavioral manifestations.

The Role of Father

It has been said that, if the 20th century is proclaimed the "Century of the Child," it certainly will not be remembered as the "Century of the Father."[14] Research on the dynamics of the father role or the development of fatherliness has received much less attention than that of motherhood. Recently, there has been some impetus in research, but it will be some time before there is solid empirical evidence regarding this topic.

Fatherliness

As with the mother role and motherliness, there is a difference between the father role or fatherhood and feelings of *fatherliness.* The role of father is learned as is the role of mother, but feeling tones are not initiated physiologically as with the mother. And this may be a very important difference. Moreover, the admission and enactment of fatherliness in our culture is still wrought with conflicts stirred up by discontinuities in cultural conditioning. This is gradually changing with the more modern attitudes toward relaxed sex role structuring. However, we still have a long way to go. By and large, the image of the virile male is still not compatible with the demonstration of tender feelings that have usually been attributed to the female domain.

Traditionally, the father in our society was supposed to be a leader, a hero, a disciplinarian, a mentor, an authority figure, and the family bulwark against the outside, reality-oriented world. Yet fatherliness must involve feelings of tenderness and gentleness, empathic capacity, the ability to respond emotionally, the valuing of a love object more than the self and, finally, the finding of a gratifying living experience in the experiences of others (Fig. 3-3). Obviously, these feelings are quite different from the simple pride of a man in his child as a symbol of his virility, or his feelings that the child represents a challenge to his own adequacy.[14]

It becomes apparent that, as long as women have an emotional investment in men, they will not be free to express their motherliness wholeheartedly until their relationships with their mates are integrated into men's fatherliness. It would seem that the coordination of the feelings of motherliness and fatherliness in those who choose to be parents is essential to the mature, creative psychosexual development of both parents and eventually their children's development.

Conflicts in Fatherhood

It may be that the same basic problems that confront a woman in delineating her role as mother also face the man in defining his role as a father. Interviews with young fathers indicate that they are immersed in many instrumental problems, such as rearranging work or study schedules, finding or preparing adequate housing, or taking on extra jobs to ease the finances. They also have basic questions and fears about their preparation for the parenting role, as well as changes in their wives during pregnancy and the postpartum periods. In some, the prospect of fatherhood also rekindles thoughts of the less happy aspects of their childhood and their relations with their parents. Their fears and concerns about their rest, quiet, and privacy, sexual relationships, and their wives' increasing demands for attention all become realities with the advent of childbirth.

We can speculate that these developments and problems may be due, at least partly, to our current lack of systematic obstetrical care of the father. It is true that we invite him to childbirth classes (and this has been a big step), and that we are allowing him

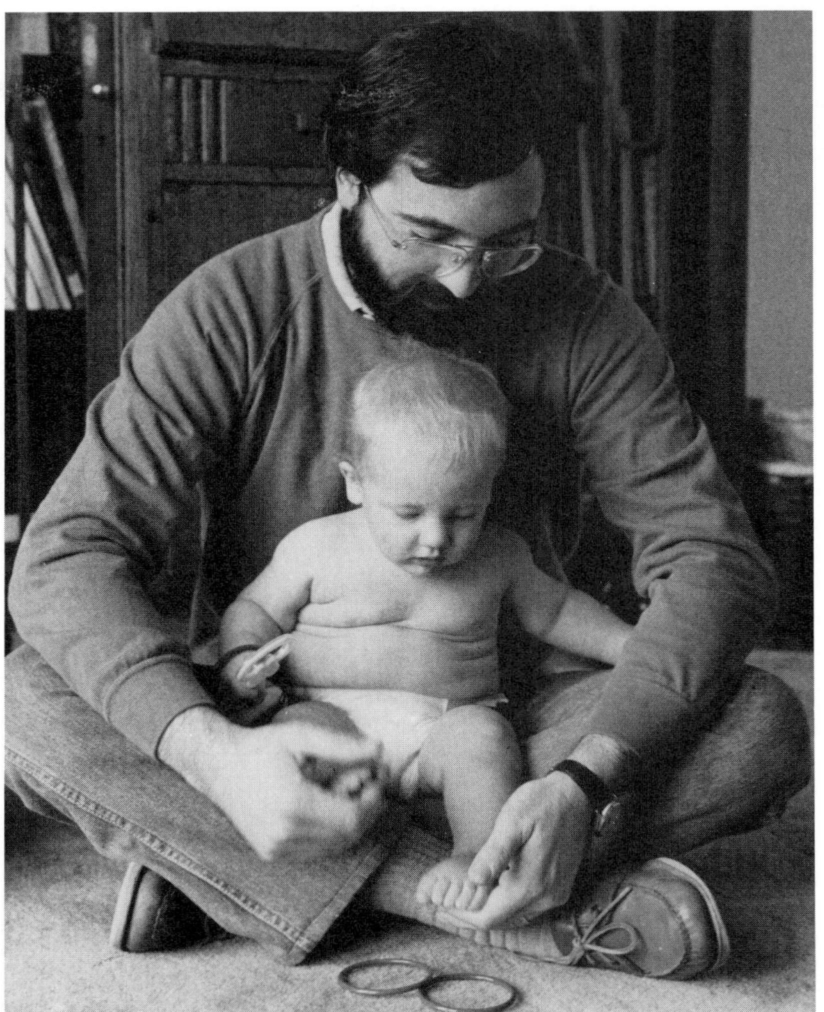

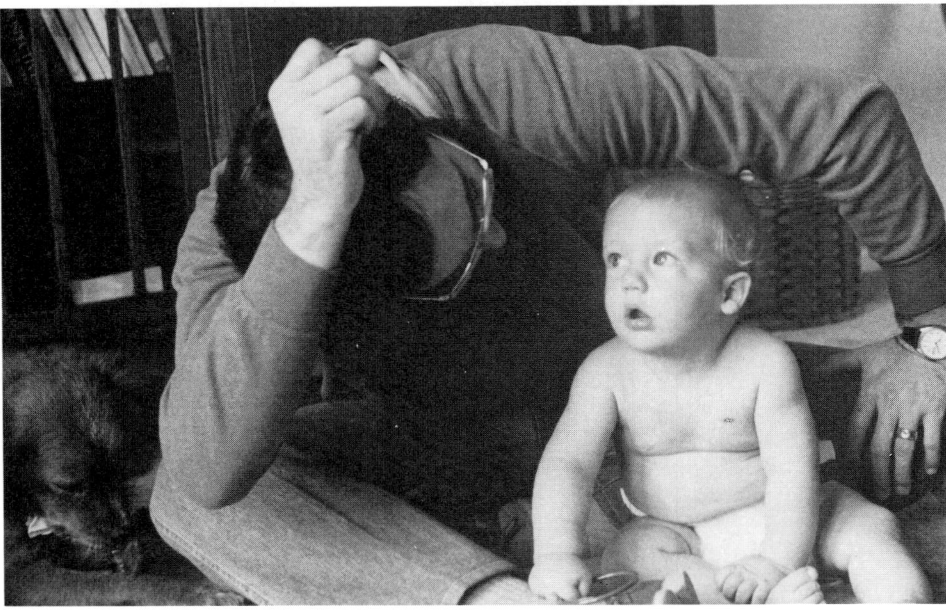

Figure 3-3.
Although the father has traditionally been viewed as an authority figure and breadwinner, fatherliness must also involve feelings of tenderness and gentleness and a gratifying personal involvement with his children.

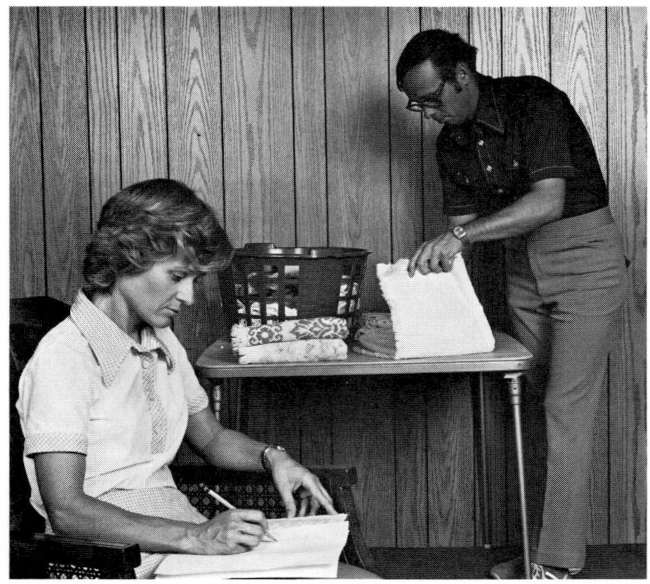

Figure 3-4.
Traditionally, women were homemakers and men were breadwinners. However, many fathers are now assuming more household duties, providing both parents with more time to parent. This sharing of duties may also provide the mother with a better opportunity for self-actualization by pursuing her own career-oriented goals.

greater participation in the actual birthing process. However, there is still no systematic attempt (or even acknowledgment of the necessity) to prepare him for his father role. All of these problems are the common components of severe role conflict and how they are resolved becomes the key to ultimate appropriate role transition.[10]

Creative Fatherhood

Josselyn has delineated several functions that a father can creatively undertake to enrich and maintain a healthy family life. First, a father can be a true companion, help-mate, and inspiration for the mother (Fig. 3-4). Second, he can be an awakener of emotional potential for his child as well as a beloved friend and teacher. Third, he can present a role model for masculine love, ethics, and morality. Fourth, he can be a stabilizing influence as the child proceeds through his maturational stages. Fifth, he can be a model and mentor for social and occupational behavior. Sixth, he can provide a model, as mentor and protector for children in general, and finally, he can be a counselor for and friend of the adolescent.[13] While each of these activities will be modified to meet the needs of a rapidly changing society, it is apparent that they provide more of a basis for sound family interaction than does the traditional role of father as sire, disciplinarian, and breadwinner.

The Role of Child

Of all the family roles, the child's role is perhaps the most dynamic because it is constantly evolving through techniques of socialization (Fig. 3-5). These techniques are essentially future oriented, since they focus on and emphasize what the child is to become rather than what he or she is. Helping the child learn appropriate social roles requires that the parents be emotionally healthy and stable enough to keep the anxiety level at a point that will allow the child's self-esteem to be in relative equilibrium with the environmental demands that are made. This does not mean that there will be no demand or no anxiety; without these, no learning takes place. However, they must not be excessive or incompatible with reality.

Socialization of the Child

There are many techniques of socialization, and the evidence indicates that no one technique is better than another. Rather, each set of parents must choose and modify what is best for them, and this will depend on the many factors that we have previously alluded to. Spiegel has attempted to delineate the various steps in the maintenance of role complementarity so that the family can balance the demands society's expectations place on it, the family's attitudes, and the child's needs, and eventually arrive at a progressively healthier family role equilibrium. He conceives of these steps along the torturous route of socialization as comprising two major groups of five steps, each linked by a sixth, or middle step (Fig. 3-6).[15]

Role Induction Procedures

The first group consists of *role induction procedures* by which compliance of the child is elicited. These are primarily manipulative and ensure that the child grad-

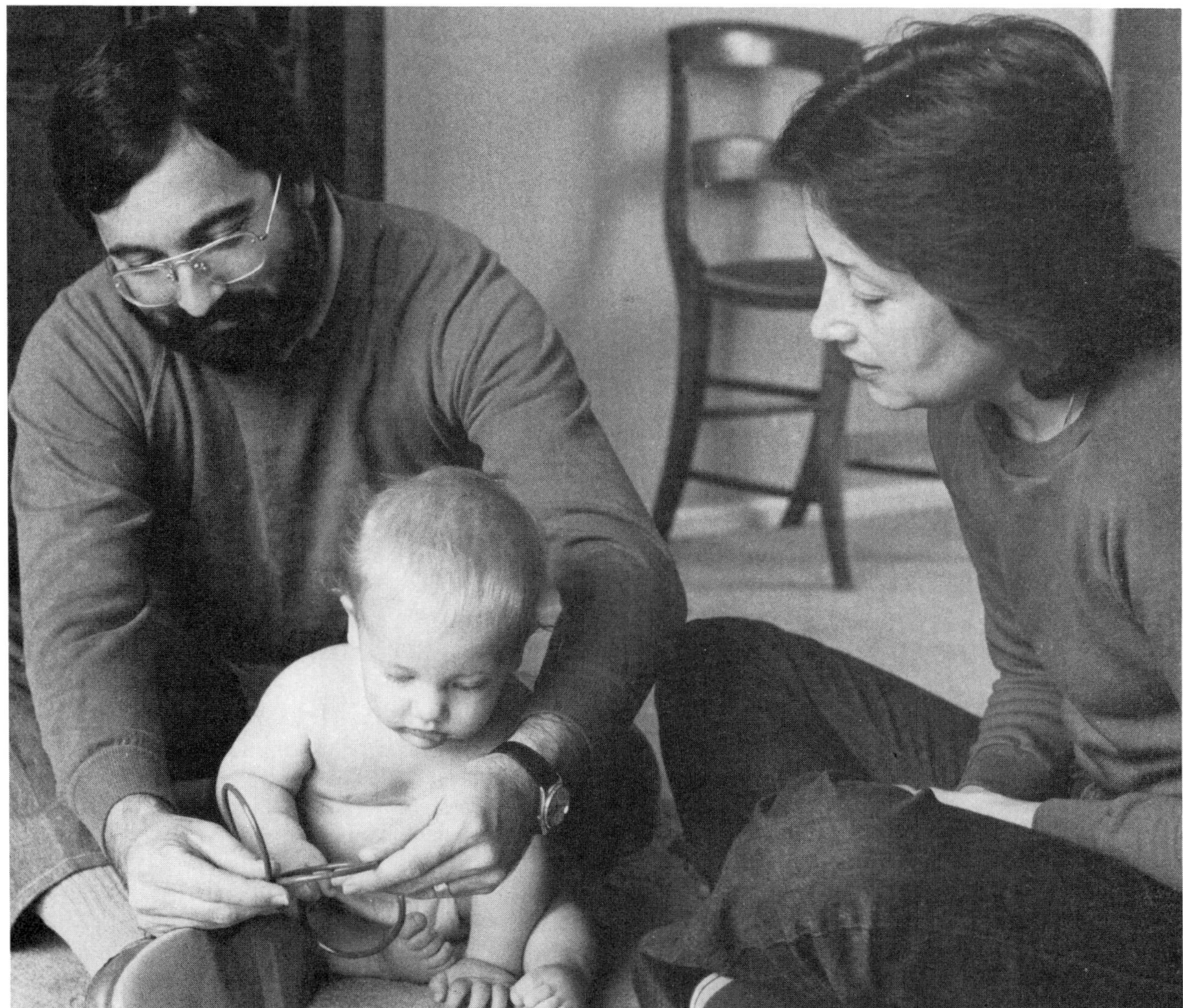

Figure 3-5.
Of all family roles, the role of the child is perhaps the most dynamic because it is constantly evolving.

ually realizes that he must learn and that his parents are the chief source of learning.

The first and second steps are *coercion* and *coaxing* in which punishment and rewards are used respectively to focus the child's attention on the fact that there are rules that must be observed and that the parents are the enactors of these rules.

The third step is *evaluation* in which a value judgment of good or bad is placed on the behavior and implies or directly gives praise or blame to ensure appropriate behavior.

The fourth step is *masking,* or withholding correct information or giving wrong information for the sake of settling a conflict. This can be pernicious and a crisis may occur if the child uncovers the truth; trust can be lost and reality is distorted.

Fifth, is the technique of *postponing* which can be useful because it puts off dealing with a conflict until a fresher look can be taken at the situation. Of course, if this maneuver is overused, it will intensify and prolong the difficulty.

The sixth step is the transitional step and has been called *role reversal* or *role taking;* that is, putting oneself in the role or position of the other and looking at the situation from the point of view of another. Some call this empathic ability. It is the first glimmer of adult thinking and requires a rather well-developed understanding of self and reality. The ability to perform this maneuver early and successfully depends on the degree of masking that goes on in the family. The less the extent of masking, the better the success of role taking.[15]

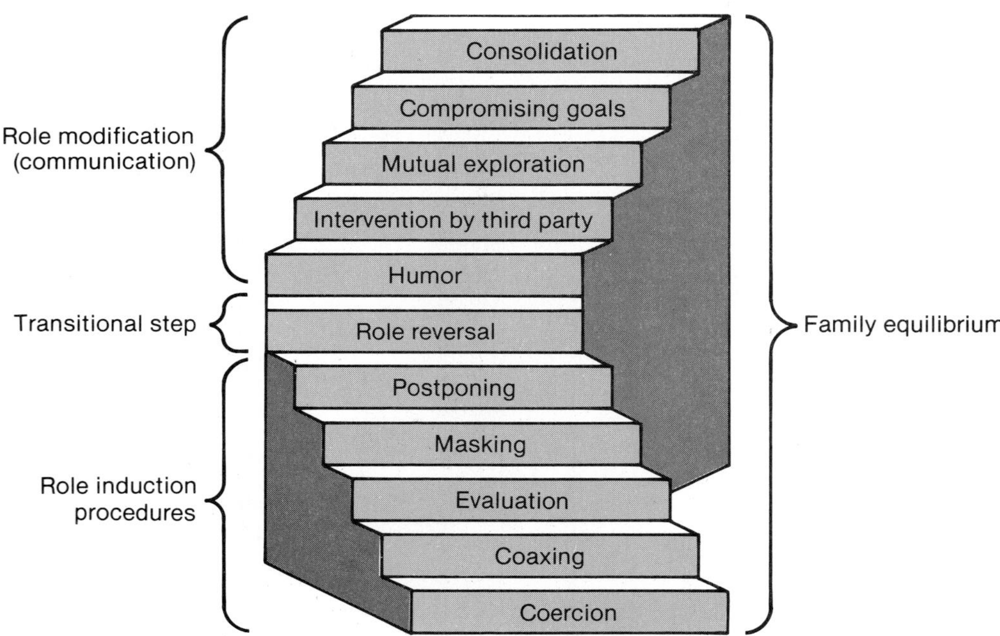

Figure 3-6.
Steps in resolving role conflict during childhood socialization.

Role Modification

The second group of procedures has been called *role modification* maneuvers. The basic characteristic here is *communication* and how individuals learn to complement each other in role change.

Role modification begins with the seventh step of *joking,* or *humor,* in which individuals develop the ability to laugh at themselves and each other (but affectionately). It is felt to be an outgrowth of role taking and the first of several tension-relieving mechanisms that families employ.

The eighth step employs the *intervention of a third party* (not necessarily a professional) who brings to the situation certain skills, a point of view, or knowledge that is not available to the parents or child within the family unit.

Mutual exploration is the ninth step, in which each person probes the capacity of the other to come to a solution regarding a conflict or problem. Here, trust and regard are expressed and invested in all members, including the children (to the extent of their capacity).

The tenth step, *compromising goals,* is an extension of mutual exploration. Here, goals are altered but to no single person's detriment.

Similarly, the last step, *consolidation,* is the refined, integrated effort of learning to compromise successfully. It is associated with adjustment, redistribution of rewards, and role clarification.

Needless to say, the evolution through these various steps does not necessarily proceed smoothly, nor at times are all accomplished, especially steps 8 through 10. However, the more frequently they can be used, the easier each subsequent role adaptation and transition will become.[15]

The Role of the Nurse

The understanding and application of role theory in nursing practice provides a conceptual base for understanding the populations that we serve and gives some anchorage to our therapeutic method. It increases our capacity to view the forces of personality, family interaction, social systems, the health condition, and nursing intervention as a unit. It provides a needed framework for studying motivations for childbearing, reproductive behavior, childrearing techniques, and cultural goals. In addition, it provides a basis for understanding ourselves and our colleagues who provide health care.

Nursing is an applied science. The broad implications of its scientific nature challenge its practitioners to document this aspect with intellectual experimentation, innovations in practice, and constant research. If we in maternity nursing define the family as the unit to be served, we must have a thorough knowledge of its dynamics, and that includes much more than the physiological and psychological stages the mother passes through during pregnancy, labor, delivery, and the postpartum. The use of role theory provides a vehicle to tie all of these disparate aspects of childbearing into related units amenable for study and practice.

Aspects of the Nurse's Role

There are multiple facets or aspects of the nurse's role (Fig. 3-7). First, the nurse is a practitioner—she assesses, prescribes, and implements nursing regimens for her patients and assists the physician in implementing his medical regimen for his patients. Another facet of her role is that of role model or mother surrogate. Maternity nurses and community health nurses have long been experimenting with providing role models for mothers who are inexperienced or exhibit maladaptive behavior in childrearing and child care. Again, in high-risk situations of child neglect or rejection, techniques of mothering the mother are implemented. Basically, the nurse meets the dependency needs of the mother, and in so doing, allows her to move on to mothering her own children. The nurse may also provide a role model for her peers and other professional colleagues as she initiates newcomers into the institutional or agency routines and practices and demonstrates an interest in delivering high-quality care.

Another facet of the nurse's role is that of teacher and, more recently, that of counselor. Nurses are becoming increasingly involved in parent education on all levels in order to socialize groups of parents expeditiously, thus avoiding the role strain and conflicts that can occur with the assumption of new roles. The counselor aspect has come into the fore with family-planning services and abortion and genetic counseling. Similarly, this aspect has become apparent in parental counseling with regard to health problems of the school child, management of sibling rivalry, and childhood and maternal nutrition.

Finally, in her "expanded role" the nurse may bring new physical diagnosis-clinician skills to her basic role. She finds in many instances that her work in an ambulatory care setting provides the bridge between the family in the community and the institution to which they must go from time to time for more severe conditions.

The potential for developing these multiple facets of the nursing role is unlimited and will only be fully realized when nursing recognizes its own unique and independent contribution to health.

When delivering care to individuals and families, nurses must observe and analyze the role behaviors of the persons involved, including their own. Cognizance must be taken of the various dimensions of the roles—the behaviors, values, expectations, and attitudes of the actors, as well as their underlying motivations and emotions. Role conflict and perceptions of inadequacy in role performance have the potential to undermine emotional and physical well-being. On the other hand, satisfactory role performance is a vital self-concept enhancing experience and can promote growth and emotional well-being.[10]

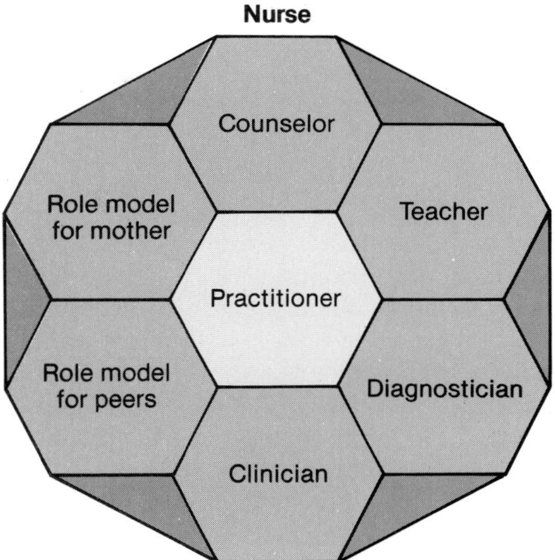

Figure 3-7.
Maternity nursing is a multi-faceted role.

Theoretical Approaches to the Study of the Family

In attempting to systematically study and delineate patterns of interaction in the family, scholars of the family, primarily sociologists, have developed several interpretive approaches to variations in family life, each one generating unique understanding about family organization while at the same time emphasizing a different aspect. These variations in emphasis result in slightly modified definitions of the family in each approach. For instance, some students of the family try to define the family in terms of a set of ends, others in terms of a kind of social structure organized to gain more general ends in societies, and still others in terms of structure and ends emerging in the unique history of each society.[16]

Conceptual Frameworks in Family Study

Five different conceptual frameworks have been designated that can be useful to nurses who deal with families. These have been summarized by Hill and Hansen as follows.[7]

The *interactional approach* views the family as a unit of interacting personalities. Each person has a position in the family in which he perceives the norms or role expectations held by the other individuals (or by the family as a whole) as the basis for his attitudes and behavior. The individual will define his role expectations primarily in light of their source and his own self-conception. The family is studied through analyzing the interactions of the role-playing members. The primary focus is on the internal structure of the family; this framework, however, neglects the family's relation to the community.

The *structural functional approach* views the family as a social system and one of the components of the complete social system, that is, society. It analyzes the functions that the family performs for society as a whole. The emphasis in this approach has been upon the statics of structure with a concomitant neglect of change and dynamics.

The *situational approach* is based on the assumption that all behavior is purposive in relation to the situation that triggered it. The situation itself or the individual's behavior in the situation is the focus for the study of families by means of the situational approach.

The *institutional approach* takes the perspective that the family must be considered a social unit in which individual and cultural values are the prime concern. The individual's values and learned needs are transmitted from one generation to the next within the family system.

The *developmental approach* focuses upon the study of the developmental phases of the family from the wedding to old age, and finally the dissolution of the family through death. The changing developmental tasks and role expectations of parents and children as they go through the family life cycle, as well as the developmental tasks of the family as a whole, are the basis for this approach.

As previously stated, any of these frameworks can be used depending upon the problem under study. It is important to remember that these frameworks are helpful tools and are not to be considered "right" or "wrong." In choosing a framework, an individual must consider the assumptions he makes about human behavior, how he views people in relation to the environment, and the problem that he is trying to solve.

The Interactional Approach

One of the most useful of the above frameworks for those who must deal with the family as a unit is the interactional framework. This conceptual scheme provides a system for viewing the personal relationships between the man and woman and parents and children, as well as the impact of various health conditions on the family unit. The family is conceived of as a unit of interacting personalities and, as such, is a living, changing, growing thing. This conceptualization does not view the family in a legalistic way or in family contract sense, but rather as it exists by virtue of the interaction of its members. Thus, a single parent with a child is a family unit, a household with several monogamous couples with children is a family unit, as is an unmarried couple with or without children.

Within the family, each member occupies a position or positions to which a number of roles are assigned or allocated. Through socialization and role differentiation (structuring a role) the individual perceives certain norms (rules) or role expectations that the other members of his family have set for his behavior in his role performance. The response of the others in the family reinforces or challenges this conception that he is developing. Thus, a person defines his role expectations in a given situation in terms of a reference group (others who are important to him) and also by means of his own self-concept.

Implicit in this formulation is the fact that human beings interpret or define one another's actions instead of merely reacting to them. For instance, a woman's response to her mate is not made merely on the basis of his actions; it also depends upon the meaning which both partners attach to such actions. Thus, the family members act and react by using symbols, and the key concept involved in the use of symbols is *communication.*

Interpersonal relations among family members based on communication is one of the major distinguishing aspects of the interactional approach. Foote and Cottrell have pointed out that the emphasis in this framework is on the development of competence in interpersonal relations and as such describes a *process* rather than a *state.*[17]

Family Interaction and Crisis

Several problems for investigation have grown out of these concerns and emphases on family unity, communication, and interpersonal competence. The one that is particularly important for health practitioners is that of the study of discontinuities in family life, particularly family crises or stress. This includes the impact of the reproductive process and parenthood on the family, stress created by acute or chronic illness of the various family members at any time during the life cycle, and the crisis brought about by death of a family member, particularly during the reproductive years.

Using this approach to the family, a practitioner can get inside the family group and analyze its coping as far as it involves interaction among members. Each family member, therefore, can be viewed as a developing member in a changing group. This approach can be particularly useful to the helping professions not only because it provides a practical way of inspecting the family, but also because it allows the professional to isolate and specify the potential sources of difficulty as family members relate to one another and to their society.[2]

Pregnancy as Crisis

Much of the "pregnancy as crisis" literature has developed from this orientation. LeMasters, Dyer, and Hobbs have been contributors in this vein. The extent to which parenthood is a crisis is likely to vary according to definitions (*i.e.*, crises as a crises, or simply a critical event or abrupt change. In addition, measurement techniques and other methodological aspects used in the studies also influence the extent and definition of crises (see Chap. 18).

There is little doubt that when a dyad of a man and woman becomes a triad of a mother, father, and child, a major reorganization of positions, roles, and interaction patterns takes place. The effect of the birth of a child and the preschool years of children on the adjustment of the parents seems fairly well established. General marital satisfaction of couples tends to decrease after the birth of their children through the preschool and school years, until the children are getting ready to leave the nest. Thus, the experiences of childbearing and childrearing appear to have a rather negative effect on marital satisfaction, particularly for the mother, who may even feel her basic self-worth is affected.[18]

All of this has grave implication for maternity health professionals with respect to our family-planning counseling, assistance during the reproductive process, and especially in delineating those successful aspects in the parents' coping behavior that can be useful in lessening this "critical" event.

In summary, there are several conceptual frameworks for the study of the family. Of particular use to practitioners is the interactional approach which strives to interpret family phenomena in terms of internal processes. These processes consist of role enactment (role playing) status or position relations, communication problems, decision making, stress reactions, and socialization processes. Little attempt is made to view the overall institutional or crosscultural relationship of family structure and function, and this has been one of the criticisms of this approach. However, this framework can be used to study the relationship of the family unit to the community, but it is more difficult because one must move from the microlevel of the small cluster of interacting persons to the larger macrolevel sweep of the community. However, where the interface of these units occurs is important for health practitioners.

Other critics feel that the interactional approach fails to recognize the biogenic and psychogenic influences on family behavior. This criticism seems destined to be short lived since these influences are recognized by the interactionist as factors that indeed set limits but are not determinants with respect to family interaction patterns. The focus is on the family in process, irrespective of the biological or personal makeup of its members, not on a static entity. What appears to be needed at this point for this framework to reach its greatest utility is better agreement and more precise definitions of its assumptions and concepts as well as extension of the framework through application and research. In this way, the interactional approach will function for the study of the family and eventually will mesh with other frameworks into what could be called a general family theory.[2]

References

1. Flook MH, Ford B, Torbett D: The single-parent family. In Clausen JP, et al., Materny Nursing Today. New York, McGraw–Hill, 1977

2. Schvaneveldt J: The interactional framework in the study of the family. In Reinhardt A, Quinn M (eds): Family Centered Community Nursing. St. Louis, CV Mosby, 1973

3. Turner RH: Family Interaction. New York, John Wiley & Sons, 1966

4. Ford L: The development of family nursing. In Hymovich RD, Barnard M (eds): Family Health Care. New York, McGraw–Hill, 1973

5. Corbin H: Development of parent classes in the United States. The Bulletin for Maternal and Child Health, A Symposium: Education for Parenthood. New York, American Association of Maternal & Infant Health Incorporated, 1960

6. Christensen HT: Handbook of Marriage and the Family. Chicago, Rand McNally, 1964

7. Hill R, Hansen D: Marriage and Family Living, 22:299–311, 1960

8. Nye I, Berardo F: Conceptual Frameworks for the Study of the Family. New York, Macmillan, 1966

9. Reeder LG: The patient-client as a consumer: some observations on the changing professional-client relationship. J Health Soc Behav 13:400–412, 1972

10. Robischon P, Scott D: Role theory and its application in family nursing. Nurs Outlook 17:52–57, 1969

11. Linton R: The Cultural Background of Personality, New York, Appleton–Century Co, 1945

12. Mead GH: Mind, Self and Society from the Standpoint of a Social Behaviorist. Chicago, University of Chicago Press, 1934

13. Josselyn I: Cultural forces, motherliness and fatherliness. Am J Orthopsychiatry 26:264–271, 1956

14. Hines JD: Father—the forgotten man. Nurs Forum 10:177–200, 1971

15. Spiegel JP: Resolution of role conflict within the family. Psychiatry 20:1–16, 1957

16. Farber B: Kinship and Family Organization. New York, John Wiley & Sons, 1966

17. Foote N, Cottrell LS: Identity and Interpersonal Competence. Chicago, University of Chicago Press, 1955

18. Eshleman JH: The Family: An Introduction. Boston, Allyn & Bacon, 1974

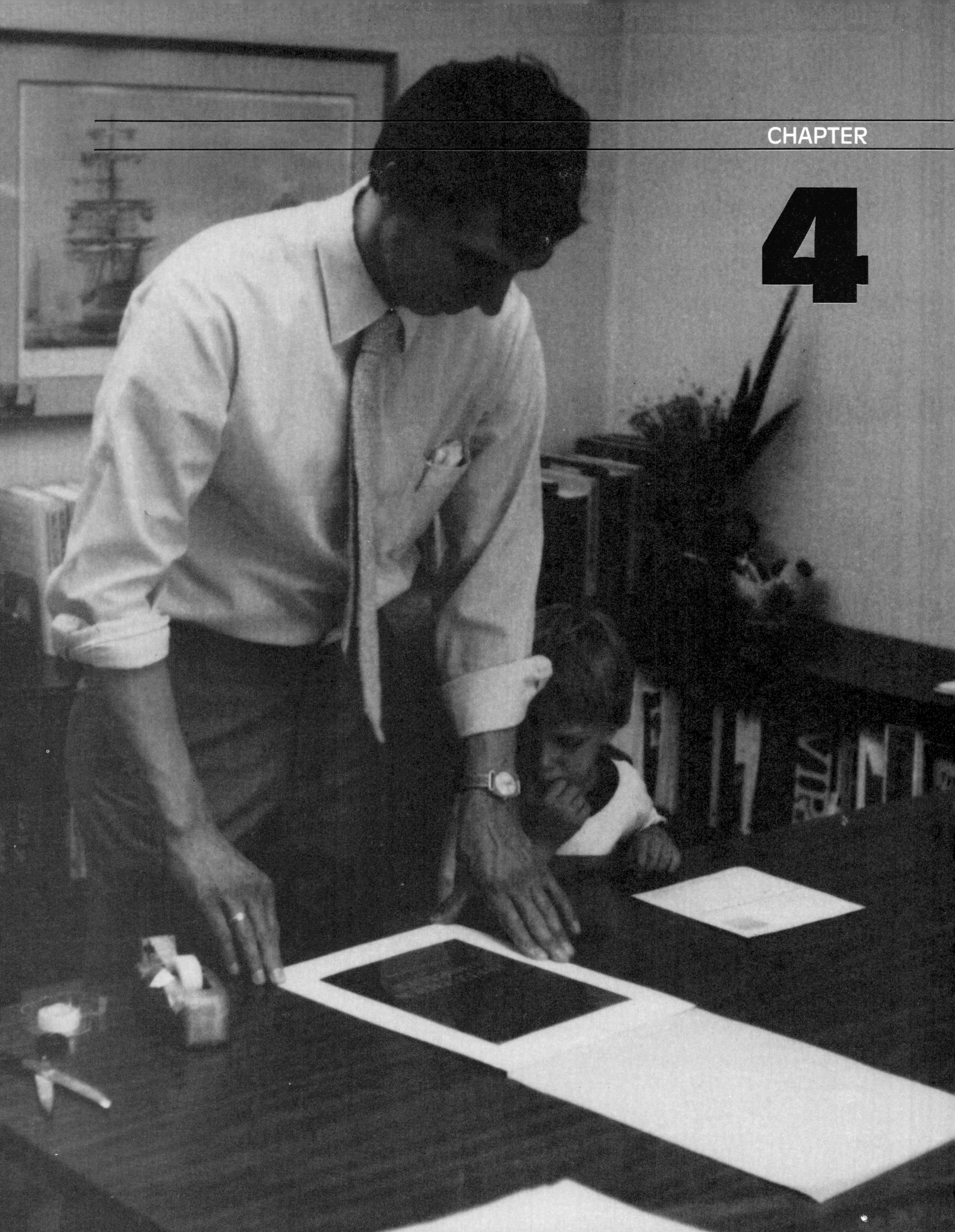

CHAPTER 4

CHAPTER 4

Evolving Family Forms

Family Forms of the Eighties

Ethnic historians and scholars of race relations and the family have emphasized the pluralistic character of American society. Over the years there has been a good deal of discussion as to whether this society was a melting pot cooking an amalgam of ethnic and cultural distillates called "American," or a salad bowl with a variety of shapes, hues, and various ethnic, religious, and racial identities. The argument continues, but the salad bowl concept appears to be winning.

It is interesting to note that the acceptance of pluralism and especially variability and differences has never been strong among those with an interest in the family, including health practitioners. This may be because the family, the bulwark of society, is a sensitive area surrounded by many judgmental and normative statements about what "ought to be." So often the family is still thought of as having some "ideal" form, which is preordained, often religiously sanctioned, and adhering to an ideal set of values. Thus, forms that vary from the traditional nuclear family of husband, wife, and children living together in their separate residence with the male as breadwinner and female as homemaker have been viewed as deviant. Research in the 1950s and 1960s on single-parent families, working mothers, or dual-work families was, for the most part, concerned with the deleterious effects of the absence of spouses or the effect of gainful employment on the children. The implication was, of course, that the woman should be in the home "where God intended her to be" and if a spouse was alone for any reason, he or she had the obligation to remarry (not just live with someone) as soon as possible.[1]

Several factors have been identified as responsible for the changes that we now are seeing in the structure and function of the modern family. A number of social indicators suggest that changes in the roles of both women and men have come about extremely rapidly beginning in the 1960s and are continuing into the 80s. The changes in women's roles particularly have been caused primarily by three interrelated factors—changes in the economy affecting labor–force participation; changes in the age structure of our society; and finally, changes in values.[2] Thus, there are more younger women who may delay marriage, and who, after commitment to a partner, work outside the home and choose to do so out of desire to realize themselves as individuals. Moreover, there is restructuring of values and roles within the home toward a more egalitarian or democratic orientation. Pickett has noted that the control base in families has shifted from patriarchal domination to egalitarianism and sometimes women centered. He points out that a new "ideal type" of democratic family has emerged which he calls "romantic monogamy" where partners are expected to be dutiful parents, dual wage earners, restrained but fascinating lovers, and finally, and most important, providers of unqualified emotional support. Since the goals of this relationship are incredibly demanding, a highly flexible divorce system has arisen as if in response. Partners may shift, but the *monogamous ideal* remains.[3]

Obviously, some have used divorce as a safety valve quite readily, but others have tried to modify the new ideal model from within or have attempted to build or select a model that better suits their needs. Thus, we see the phenomenon of a pluralism in family forms existing side by side, with members of each of these forms having different problems to solve and issues to face.

It is important to remember that not many persons remain in one type of family structure throughout their lifetime, although most have some experience in the more traditional nuclear family.[1] Thus, we see, along with the traditional family structures, emerging experimental structures that can have an effect on the socialization and health of their members and, hence, on their reproductive motivation and performance.

Traditional Family Structures

There are a variety of forms in traditional family structures. The most prominent among these are the following.

The nuclear family in which husband, wife, and children live in a common household. A single or a dual career may be pursued, and, in the case of the wife, her career may be continuous or interrupted as the children are born.

The nuclear dyad in which a husband and wife live alone. They may be childless or not have children living at home. Again, there may be a single or dual career or a "second career" where the wife enters the labor force after the children have left home.

The single-parent family in which there is one head as a consequence of death, divorce, abandonment, or separation. Here there are usually preschool or school-age children. There may or may not be a career; when financial aid is not forthcoming from the absent spouse, there is usually some form of occupation pursued by the parenting spouse.

The single adult living alone.

The three-generation family or extended family. These may be characterized by any variant of forms 1, 2, or 3.

The kin network in which nuclear households or unmarried members live in close geographical proximity and operate within a reciprocal system of exchange of goods and services.[1]

Each of these will have its problems and resources with respect to health needs and utilization of services. Generally, traditional households are looked upon more favorably by society because they are considered stable and provide a legitimating anchorage for the children born of these unions.

It has been said that nuclear families suffer from isolation and cannot cope with illness, repeated pregnancy, or reproductive wastage; hence, they must turn to professionals for sustenance and care. However, current research indicates that the nuclear family probably has less isolation and better coping ability than formerly was thought.[4] This is due to the fact that there appears to be great role adaptability and flexibility in time of stress as well as a greater utilization of kin and other social networks for advice and sustenance during childbearing as well as for other health conditions.

It is apparent that extended family forms can be helpful to counter isolation and to provide help during periods of stress. It must be remembered, however, that kin and friends can also deter family members from appropriately defining themselves in need of care as well as prohibiting or deterring them from prompt and continued utilization of health services.

Experimental Family Structures

1. The commune family. This form can be further divided into the following:
   a. A household of more than one monogamous couple with children, sharing common facilities, resources, and experiences; socialization of the child is a group activity. Each member is a responsibility of the other members, and there is mutual concern for the various aspects of the members' lives including health matters.
   b. A household of adults and children in which there is "group marriage"; that is, all the individuals are "married" to each other and all parent the children. A status system usually develops with the leaders believed to have charisma. These are very small in number and sometimes involve cultism.
2. The unmarried parent and child family, often a mother and child for whom marriage is not desired or possible. Children can be natural offspring of the parent or adopted.
3. Unmarried couple and child family. Again, these may be of two varieties.
   a. A social contract marriage in which there is an ideologic commitment to a relationship not sanctioned by law, which must be constantly worked at in order to maintain its vitality and meaningfulness. Common value systems are shared that strongly emphasize humanism and personal relationships. A great deal of time is spent by the members, including the children, in sharing mutual emotional experiences and ideas. The father plays a prominent role in the caretaking and socialization of the children and both parents have intimate, continued, and sustained contact with their children.
   b. The second type of unmarried couple and child family is that usually referred to as common-law marriage with the children either born to the partners or informally adopted. These unions are often found among the poorer strata of society who experience exceptional problems and constraints associated with legal marriage.[1]

It is with the experimental forms of family styles that today's nurse may have the least experience. Therefore, we will discuss some basic principles of care that have special relevance for these families. It is worth noting that as little as eight years ago these families were known as "alternate" lifestyle families. However, their ethic and philosophy have become so much a part of the mainstream of society that they no longer can be so classified. While we still use the term alternate or alternative from time to time in reference to them, it is more appropriate to consider their lifestyle as evolving rather than alternative.

Social Contract Families or the Unmarried Marrieds

As stated previously, social contract families are composed of two partners whose structure exists as a social rather than a legal contract. We in maternity nursing become acquainted with these patients when giving family planning counseling and services during pregnancy and childbirth. The literature and current research suggests that in many ways this group shares the philosophy of the "turned-off," middle-class countercultures. Living together in this form, however, has little similarity to the "shacking-up" of previous generations, or with the large number of common-law marriages found among some of the poor who experience constraints and problems associated with legal marriage, such as no finances to obtain a divorce or inability to manage the bureaucracy to facilitate legal severance. Rather, this form of marriage involves an ideologic commitment to a relationship instead of joint living by virtue of a legal status. Basic to this rejection of a legal marriage is the conviction that the bond of love and trust that binds the partners is more important and stronger than the legal bond authorized by church or state.[5]

In the family setting, parents spend long periods of time with one another and share emotional exchanges of closeness and rejection, desire and repulsion, and all of the certainties and uncertainties involved in living together and bearing and raising children. There is, for the most part, a great deal of frankness and openness about these statuses which include the children. There is little secretiveness about their approach to life, and both names may be displayed on the mailboxes, in financial arrangements, and the like. There are no hang-ups on their part regarding the legitimacy of the children.

Since the possible instability of the relationship can be critical to pregnancy outcomes and the children's development, researchers have explored these facets of alternate family forms. Motivations for this lifestyle are very important. Some partners do not accept the civil contract per se; others do not accept the relevance of the civil marriage contract to their relationship as it exists for them at the moment, wanting no civil constraints on their "splitting" if things change between them. Others seek to avoid the obvious unhappiness in their own family life and upbringing. In general, from the participants' point of view, living together in this family structure is seen as representing true maturity and an acceptance of the faith placed in one another.

The women's liberation movement and the raising of women's consciousness have played a strong philosophical role in determining reproductive behavior and childrearing activities. The choice of having a child appears even more determined than in the traditional nuclear family. Contraception services appear to be used and the option of termination of pregnancy is freely available and utilized without the apparent guilt associated with such termination in some of the traditional families. From this point of view, and because of the close interaction and caretaking when the children are born, this family style has been considered a very motivated form of parenting.[5]

The Single Parent

The Single Mother

The single or unmarried mother is far from a new phenomenon in our society. In decades past, the unwed mother bearing the so-called illegitimate child was synonymous with single parent. However, with today's high divorce rate, the term has added a new dimension. Glick and Norton, in a review of national statistics, report that the proportion of children living with one parent has more than doubled from 1960 to 1978. A little more than 5.5 million American families (19% of the 30 million families with children) were headed by a single adult.[6] In fact, the popular notion of the intact, conventional family of mother, father, and children is a minority family form in the United States today (Fig. 4-1). This form accounts for only 45% of Americans, whereas 55% are represented by single parents, couples without children, and reconstituted families (remarrieds with and without children).[7]

Bane estimates that almost 30% of children born around 1970 will experience parental divorce by the time they are 18, and an additional 15% to 20% will live in a single parent household because of death, birth to an unmarried mother, or long-term separation of the parents.[8]

The quality of the single parent experience will depend on the circumstances that result in this type of household. In the case of widows and widowers, for instance, where there is adequate insurance coverage and the remaining spouse has a high paying occupation, there may not be the economic stringencies and social stigma that are often associated with households where divorce has been the cause of single parenting. However, it is important to remember that the one common characteristic shared by almost all female-headed, single-parent families is poverty or at best very reduced economic circumstances. A 1976 report from the United States Department of Labor showed that only 28% of female-headed households had incomes in excess of $10,000. Forty percent of such households had incomes of less than $5000. In contrast, comparable families headed by a man showed 70% had incomes of above $10,000 and only 10% were in the less than $5000 range.[7] The inadequate incomes of most female-headed families arise from the loss of the male wage earner who traditionally has been paid higher wages overall and is paid at a higher rate for comparable work. The single

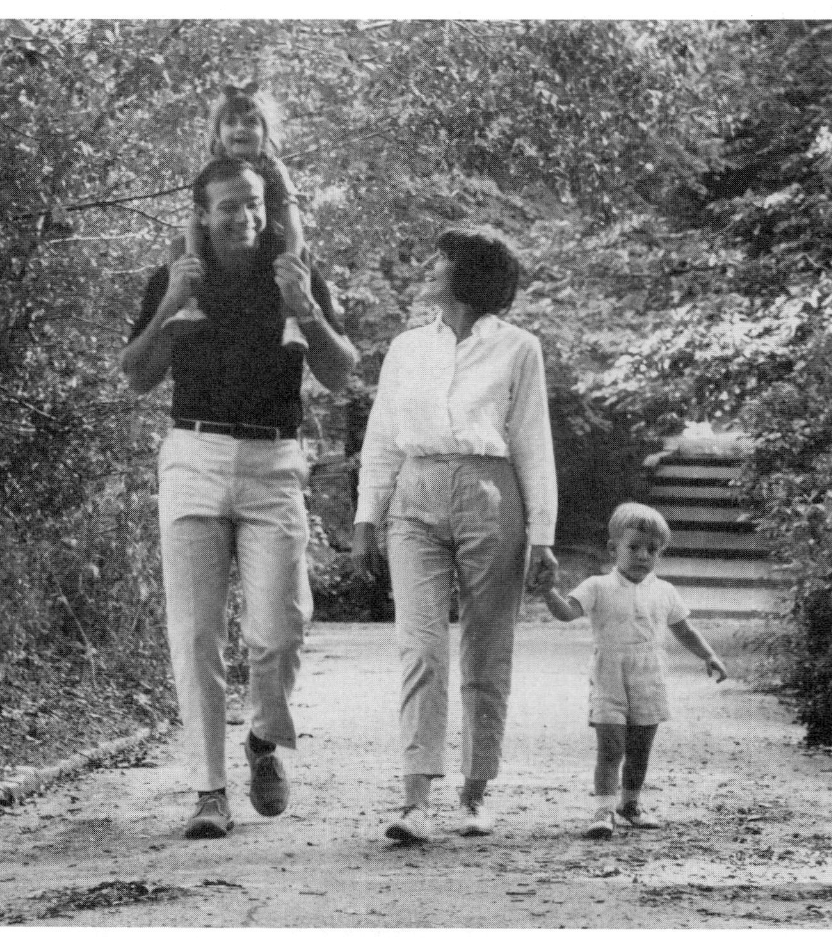

Figure 4-1.
The traditional nuclear family, consisting of a mother, a father, and their children now accounts for only 45% of the families in the United States today.

parent mother must also continue to care for her children who are often young and require high-cost child-care services when the mother works. Even with supplemental insurance or alimony and child support payments, the economic situation is often grim. And it is the mother who most often must be the ultimate financial support for her children. Even in today's so-called enlightened society, mothers are still awarded custody of the children in over 90% of all divorces.[7] Moreover, Ross and Sawhill state that child support and alimony supplements are less than commonly believed and, in any event, inadequate to keep the divorced mother and her children from a poverty subsistence level.[9]

Unfortunately, our society is still dominated by the assumption that families headed by a single parent, particularly when that parent is a woman and in stringent economic circumstances, are deviant and pathological. Such families continue to be characterized as broken and disorganized rather than being recognized as a viable alternative family form. Instead of being seen as a solution to circumstances and assessed in terms of their strengths, they are often viewed negatively, particularly by health professionals, with an emphasis on their alleged weaknesses. This uncritical acceptance of the above assumption has led to biased governmental, employment, and social policies that have been very detrimental to these families. Moreover, many separated and divorced women have incorporated these negative images into their self-concepts and this has become an obstacle to their readjustment to their new circumstances.[7]

Under such conditions, a variety of options need to be used because different supports are needed by these parents who are alone. Most importantly, the mother must enlarge her social support networks if she is to become economically independent and socially involved. The following paragraphs discuss several options and resources for the single parent that can be used to provide support and strategies.

Family Style Dwelling

Among the family styles that have been encountered among the single mother group are small group homes or boarding homes where a small number

(4–10) live together with their children, foster homes for mother and child, and apartment complexes where each family lives in its own unit.[5] The actual physical arrangements for the child differ among residences but, in general, there are separate sleeping quarters for the parent and child with common dining and living facilities. The opportunity for the children to eat and play together, share toys, and have a shared caretaker is considered one of the advantages for children in groups such as these.

Community Support Programs

Many communities have developed programs that facilitate a mother's return to school or work so that she can gain skills that will enable her to be independent. These programs are still in the early stages and are largely experimental but do indicate that society recognizes the complex needs of women who rear children alone. Child care facilities, caretaking arrangements, and infant caretakers in the home reflect the kinds of assistance the community has developed, which means that children of single parents can be exposed to multiple caretaking as early as six weeks of life.

Organizational Support

Societal recognition has also encouraged single parents to move toward developing organizations and social networks that provide them with tangible supportive contacts. The expansion of such organizations as Parents Without Partners, the Momma League, and the LaLeche League, into activity programs, information and training centers, and consciousness-raising efforts suggests that the middle-class parent has become more sensitive to his or her needs as a person as well as a parent.

The Single Male Parent

While voluntary single male parents are still much in the minority, they are becoming more numerous. Their living arrangements include group living as well as living alone with the child. Because the male's economic status is generally better than the female's, he has more options for child care and living quarters. Thus, caretakers in the home are found more frequently, although ample use is made of child care centers and children programs.[5]

In the case of divorce, it is still unusual for the majority of fathers to assume custody of the children. However, the beginnings of the breakdown in parental roles and postdivorce parental roles have begun to have some effect on custodial outcomes. Hence, a small but growing number of fathers are now requesting and getting both joint and sole custody of their children following divorce. In his study of fathers seeking custody and those who did not, Gersick has found that four interacting variables appear to be determinants of whether or not fathers consider assuming custody of their children. First, the father's own family relationships color his outlook toward his responsibility to his children. Many want to overcome, in their relationships with their children, the problems and the emotional detachment they experienced with their parents. Secondly, feelings toward the ex-wife affect the father's orientation. When he believes that the wife has betrayed him in some way, he is motivated to seek custody by a combination of a desire to punish his wife and a concern for the well-being of the children. The third variable is the fact that the wife gave pretrial consent, hence a court "battle" was not necessary and the father could assume custody with a minimum of conflict. The final factor has to do with the attorney's attitudes. If the attorney is reluctant to press for custody, the father tends to let the wife have the children.[7, 10]

As with the voluntary single male parent, divorced fathers generally have sufficient material wherewithal to provide at least an adequate lifestyle for their children. Interestingly, research shows that many of the difficulties that the men experience are the same as those of the single parent women. Economic circumstances become more stringent (but not as dire as for the women); arranging child care becomes a problem. Visits from the wife were anticipated with anxiety and, in general, for many of the men, the strain of the divorce coupled with the new demands of total responsibility for the children made readjustment to the single lifestyle difficult. However, none of the fathers studied regretted their decision to assume custody of their children.[10]

Thus, single parenting is not without its difficulties. For both men and women, it is important that they use the support systems discussed in the preceding paragraphs.

Communes

The creation of a communal alternate to the isolated nuclear family is not new in this country. Generations have sought a new start and protested the status quo. Causes of their dissent and the ways in which they chose to organize their new communal existence varied in the past as they do with today's communards. Some were based upon religious conviction, some on economic idealism, and some on rebellion against authority. Some attempted to establish a model of government based upon an absence of central authority; others sought a strict line of hierarchical authority with the rejection of those members who did not adhere to the authority prescribed. Some had relatively long histories, such as the Bruderhof, while others, such as "Brook Farm," an intellectual community in Massachusetts, dissolved rapidly.

Current Communal Lifestyle

Lifestyles displayed by the current commune movement are perhaps even more varied than those of the historical models. This makes attempts to define this alternate lifestyle difficult. Communes vary today in type of membership, organizational structure, and general purpose. Some are involved in agricultural subsistence seeking a closeness to the land characterized by the early close-knit communities reported to have existed in history, while others are composed of middle-class young professionals who do not wish to disengage from the urban scene and its various technological comforts. Size also varies from 12 or less to hundreds.

A significant number of present-day communes is based upon religious commitments of various persuasions. Eastern philosophy is often a guiding force in many of these religiously oriented communes. In others, the "Jesus movement" is central, with the members searching for a new way to live out the traditional Judeo–Christian convictions. Of late there have been some tragic happenings in some of these communal group living arrangements. It remains to be seen what effect these events will have on the total commune movement.

Communes are often formed around common interests, crafts, or some unifying goal. They start with people who like each other and share similar value systems, orientations, and convictions. This aspect is extremely important in these intentional communities, and some see their alternate family arrangement as the beginning of a social revolution that will bring about radical change in society.[5]

Family Structure Within the Commune

Some communes are reported to be group-marriage oriented, but they are in the minority. One such group lives in Taos, New Mexico, and another exists nationally with a sizable base in Los Angeles. Children are shared with the group and there is little concern about knowing or caring which individuals have been biologically responsible for the conception of the child. The rearing of the child is considered more important than who the parents are.

Other groups are oriented as extended families, with couples remaining essentially monogamous in their own private quarters, although partners may change from time to time. Still others live together under a community concept rather than a family unit, sharing resources that are more effectively achieved in multiple family cooperatives, such as expenses, household chores, and child care responsibilities. The women's consciousness movement has given particular impetus to these groups.

As we stated previously, the life span of the current communes varies. Such issues as organization of work and other aspects of living, interpersonal relationships, mutual values, economic feasibility, and ability to cope with outside community harassment have been suggested as important to the stability of communal arrangements.

Parent–Child Relationships

Living arrangements largely determine parent–child relationships. Great ingenuity is shown—tents, lean-tos, and cabins in the rural areas; apartment houses, motels, and sometimes single family dwellings in the city.

The number of children varies from commune to commune. In general, the adults are conscious of the population explosion, and few parents with more than three biological children are in evidence; however, there are some "families" who have eight to ten children. Birth, pregnancy, and children are esteemed and joyously regarded as an expression of a natural and ecologically appropriate experience.

Adult–child relations are often determined by proximity of living and sleeping quarters. Relations with biological parents may be infrequent, with children being physically separated from them and assigned to caretakers, as is the case in some instances. In addition, the child's relationship with other adults is related to the extent of the existence of a hierarchical structure. In a family, multiple dwelling arrangements can permit a child to move among households, as when he is in conflict with other members, lonely for playmates or when his family is "splitting" for a time.

Childrearing Practices

Investigators have found a wide range of childrearing practices among the communards. Some of the attitudes and value systems that are likely to affect the child's development and, hence, have relevance for health professionals are summarized here.[5, 11]

Breast-feeding appears routine and there is usually close tactile contact between mother and child in the first year. Strapped to the mother's back, the baby goes everywhere with her and is touched frequently.

There is often a clear break in the intense mother–infant relationship at around two-and-one-half years, when there is a push in the direction of independence and self-reliance. The mother begins to think of her own needs and returns gradually to activities.

Good health, together with a desire for wholesomeness, are revered. Natural foods are stressed and "junk" foods are restricted. Institutional medical and dental care may be limited to emergencies with self-help medical and pharmacological expertise encouraged. Few preventive measures are sought from organized medicine, except prenatal care. The emphasis is on prevention through healthful, natural living.

Nonviolence is generally espoused among the counterculture groups, although assertiveness among the children, especially the girls, is sanctioned. Children are often left to work out peer relationships and direct interrelations are fostered. Only the demands of safety take precedence. Children are disciplined, however, and a broad spectrum of this exists from verbal admonition to physical punishment.

Humanistic and interpersonal relationships and the direct expression of affectional needs are valued. Artificial repression of sexuality and intimacy are eschewed. Thus, exposure to nudity and observation of adult sexual activity may be permitted.

Children socialize each other, since, when the child gets into his own groups, he is dependent upon his peers' support. There is a great deal of age specific role peer modeling.

Early decision making is encouraged in the child. This is related to the philosophy that the child has individual rights and thus has a role in participatory democracy. This group decision making by parents is often modeled by children as an important mode for solving problems even though their decisions are by necessity immature.

The parents experience some difficulty with serving as role models for their children. They appear to be quite reluctant to "lay their trip" on the child. Yet, they admit to value and lifestyle preferences that are consonant with their attitudes, and, because of their verbal admonishings and role modeling, reinforce those behaviors of the child that are consonant with their attitudes. Another problem is that the parents may not be willing to serve as sex role models because of their general acceptance of an antisexist philosophy. Yet many of the males are out and out sexists. There is also ambivalence about having the girls identify with the not completely emancipated women.

Competency to handle daily life is stressed, while competition and achievement striving are played down; thus, individual potential and creativity are felt to be promoted. Sensory impressions, intuition, and the occult, as opposed to the rational, are data that are considered an enhancement of creativity. Children, because of their competency, are expected to distinguish between what is appropriate behavior within the "family" and the "outside world."

The materialistic values are seen as tied in with technological advances and nonhumanistic goals; thus, dependence on material possessions is minimized whenever possible. Shared objects, toys, and utensils are far in the majority. Some of the children see the adults "ripping off" the outside society and ignoring the social contracts involved in personal ownership (*i.e.*, stealing). There is such great variability in these groups that it is evident that follow-up is indicated to see what the impact is of these childrearing practices.

One of the other findings of the studies that have been done indicates that many of the practices within these lifestyles and relating to childrearing are also practiced in the present-day nuclear family. Much of what appears in the mass media (TV, newspapers) logically finds expression in many of these evolving lifestyle families.[5]

General Considerations in Working with Parents

There are several principles that health professionals will want to remember when delivering services to any couple, particularly those who may be involved in a variant lifestyle. A general rejection of so-called traditional values pervades our culture with more and more emphasis placed on the right of each individual to find values and a philosophy that is meaningful to him or her. Thus, couples involved in variant lifestyles may assume a more questioning attitude which may prove disconcerting to some health providers.

Evaluating Health Information

Health professionals often expect patients to accept their information as true because it is drawn from a scientific body of knowledge. However, thoughtful patients may not necessarily accept Western scientific knowledge. They may, indeed, regard modern science as attempting to bring forth more and more "laws" aimed at finding absolute truth in a relative world and, hence, having little to do with health and, more important, happiness.

On the other hand, information from other sources, including health information, is also subjected to scrutiny and evaluation before acceptance. Thus, many practices that could be potentially harmful are often rejected. If patients have any kind of relationship with a professional to whom they can turn for criteria against which to compare advice, they will usually make appropriate choices.

The tendency to evaluate medical information given by the health professional on an experiential rather than a scientific basis does not preclude an interest in what the health professional has to say. In our experience, particularly in the free clinics, we find that the nurse is respected as a person who has knowledge in her field and who shares some of the patient's concerns and feelings. Expectant parents will have many questions and, when the nurse responds to their inquiries, they may go on to relate information that they have gathered from other sources. It becomes important to discuss this information seriously and with respect because it is valuable to the parent. Health teaching documented with rational explanation and practical experiences is much more readily accepted. The advice and teaching must be practical also. To insist that a vegetarian eat meat, even if she may have anemia, is simply too impractical, especially if there are others in the family to consider.

Moreover, patients who follow evolving lifestyles are, for the most part, well educated and, because of this and their value system, expect a fuller and more complete explanation than many other patients. If a mother prefers a vegetarian diet and wants to know the food values of the foods she wishes to include in her diet, she will not be satisfied with only a suggested menu. Exchanges and equivalents must be discussed. It is not sufficient to tell a mother in an antepartal clinic to return in so many weeks for another blood test without telling her the reason for returning and the purpose of the procedure. If patients reject some of the advice, this, too, is to be treated with respect.[12]

Choosing Antepartal Services

The factors that affect the couple with an evolving family lifestyle also affect the traditional lifestyle couple. These include past experience with health personnel, geographic location, feelings about the pregnancy, the influence of significant others, and the parents' physical condition. Increasingly, there is a high priority placed on ambience and interpersonal relations during the pregnancy and at the time of delivery. Modern up-to-date equipment and technological expertise may be much less important than an environment that simulates the home. The rise of alternative birth centers which provide a homelike atmosphere and the rise in the number of home births attest to this value.

Selection of services is made on the basis of consultation with friends, referrals from professionals, and past experience with health providers. In general, couples are taking a more militant stand regarding participation in the planning and execution of their care and tend to seek out health professionals who allow them this right. It becomes important then to be sure that the patients be duly informed about the nature of their care, including their right to sign themselves out of the hospital. This information together with a genuine indication of regard for the couple is usually sufficient to lessen the apprehension about having a hospital delivery or seeking antenatal care from a "traditional" establishment provider.

Choosing the Place and Method of Delivery

Selecting a hospital for delivery or choosing between a hospital and home delivery involves many of the same factors as those considered in the selection of antepartal services. For most couples today, childbirth is regarded as a natural process; thus, prepared childbirth classes and the Le Boyer method of delivery are very popular. Today, parents come to their deliveries much more knowledgeable than previously. This is due, in part, to the large variety of books now available dealing with nutrition in pregnancy, the physiology of pregnancy, labor and delivery, and even "how to" books on home delivery. Parents therefore expect their requests to be considered. Hospitals that have the reputation for having a great deal of restrictions and "hassle" are avoided, regardless of the quality of technological expertise offered.

The need for control over one's own life may also be a strong motivating factor in the choice of a home delivery.[13] These types of deliveries still remain controversial due to a variety of factors. Safety of the mother and infant continues to be a grave concern for the health professionals, and there are data that indicate that this concern is well founded. However, birth carries a strong symbolic meaning and the home typifies this meaning. The traditional hospital setting is seen by many couples as a sterile place with little room for intimacy and family integration.[12] Many hospitals are now instituting birthing rooms or birth centers which simulate a homelike atmosphere that is free from many of the restrictions and rigidities imposed by the traditional delivery suite. It is hoped that this alternative will encompass both the symbolic atmosphere that is desired and adequate safety features for the mother and infant.

Ethnic, Social Class, and Cultural Variations

The recent emphasis on cultural pluralism and ethnic heritage in America seems to contradict the contention that ethnic groups tend to shed their distinctive family patterns as they become socially mobile. It can be seen, however, that the move toward the celebration of national origins represents an extolling of distinctive ethnic art, language, dress, and food patterns for the purpose of promoting a positive identity and ancestral pride in those who have had little of either.

If we examine the contemporary family roles of various ethnic groups, we see that the process of acculturation has been accelerated or delayed by several factors, including opportunity available in the new environment, the extent of discrimination, and the degree of cultural and physical similarity or difference between the acculturating group and the dominant society. There are many groups that comprise the "salad bowl" of America and, unfortunately, we cannot include all of them here. However, we will highlight some of the groups to give an indication of the current state of thought on contemporary family roles.

We would like to make clear at the outset that the variations among the different ethnic groups in family styles, health beliefs and practices, and utilization of health services, are a function of the socioeconomic status of the individuals far more than their particular ethnicity. Since minority groups in general are often poorer than their white counterparts and because more individuals within each group tend to be poorer than the same proportion of whites, there has been an inability to gain access to education and other resources that money can buy. Thus, behavior and beliefs which differ from the mainstream white middle-class dominant society have come about or been retained, and misconceptions have arisen attributing these behaviors to ethnicity.

Native American Families

Of all the ethnic groups that abound in this country, the American Indian has perhaps the most remarkable history—one that reflects severe exploitation, astounding endurance, and incredible capability for adaptation. The name "Indian" itself was a European appellation and was applied indiscriminately to the several thousand tribes that inhabited the North American continent at the time of its discovery by Columbus. From that time onward, the native American's history has been marred by disease, starvation, deliberate attempts at genocide, and blatantly inconsistent treatment by governmental agencies.[14]

Even today, there is no single accepted definition of American Indian or native American. Governmental agencies and the Census Bureau rely on the individual to define himself as Indian; some require proof of at least one quarter Indian blood. Hence, even enumerating the number of tribes and individuals is difficult. In 1976 it was estimated that this population was increasing so that now there may be around one million Indians in the country who are associated into over 300 tribes.

Approximately one half of the Indian population lives on reservations whose development was a result of a racist governmental policy of "exclusion." Reservation lands were much less acceptable than the lands originally inhabited by the various tribes. Life on the reservation, even today, is fraught with the twin plagues of poverty and substandard housing which, in turn, gives rise to myriad health problems.[15, 16]

An urban resettlement program was attempted in 1952 which was supposed to aid the assimilation of the Indian into the mainstream American culture. Participants were given job training and limited aid in finding jobs and housing. The program is generally regarded as a failure. Because of bureaucratic red tape and disinterest, financial and other aid was so meager that it did not begin to achieve the goals originally outlined. Those who did leave the reservation often found themselves separated from their families because the housing allowance was inadequate to accommodate an entire family. Moreover, the traditional social supports found on the reservation disappeared in the city. Thus, the urban Indian became a true "marginal" man. He was distrusted by his own people and unable to participate in traditional tribal life. Moreover, he was stigmatized and ignored by those with whom he was supposed to assimilate. It is estimated that about half of those who attempted the urban move have returned to the reservation.[17]

An attempt is being made through the use of Urban Indian Centers to meet some of the needs of these urban migrants. These centers supply health services, educational services, and job counseling. It is still too early to comment on the success of this innovation, but it does seem as though these programs are achieving at least a modicum of success.[17]

The cultural background of the native American

varies according to tribal affiliation. Thus, generalizations about the American Indian family must be made with caution. In the main, family life is influenced by tribal beliefs and there is a great deal of variation among the tribes with respect to holding to traditional values and customs. This variability occurs in both the reservation and urban Indian communities.

For the most part, the family remains the basic unit of native American society. The Indian idea of family is the extended family that includes grandparents, aunts, uncles, and even close friends. Children are valued and admired and all members participate in the childrearing. Each has certain things that must be taught to the child and the responsibility is taken seriously.

In many tribes, the lineage is matriarchal and the child automatically becomes a member of the mother's clan at birth (Fig. 4-2). Indian women have traditionally worked very hard, but they have also been very influential in tribal affairs. Indeed, they have been "the heart of the home" and several have also been leaders of their tribes.[16, 18]

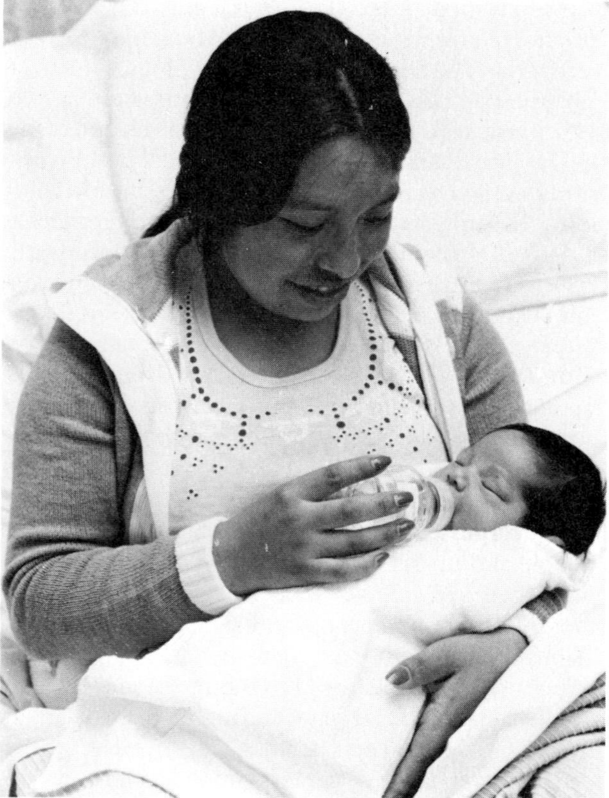

Figure 4-2.
In many tribes, the lineage is matriarchal and the child automatically becomes a member of the mother's clan at birth.

Health beliefs also vary according to tribal identity and religion is a powerful force in giving direction to childbearing, childbirth, and childrearing. Again it is difficult to make generalizations, but a few principles will be attempted here. For the most part, pregnancy is thought of as a natural process in the normal cycle of life and death. In general, a harmonious prenatal period is stressed with an attempt to help the mother be content, keep away from ill or evil persons and things, and think good thoughts. When facilities permit, prenatal care and hospital delivery is sought from obstetricians or other physicians. Tribal midwives are also used. The tribal medicine man is relied upon also to provide special foods and beverages that are believed to be helpful in increasing strength and preventing illness. He also supplies charms and amulets to aid in a healthy delivery.[19]

In spite of the fact that the majority of native American women deliver in hospitals, their maternal mortality rate is nearly 2% higher than the overall maternal mortality rate for the United States.[20] It is becoming glaringly apparent that health providers who work with these clients must make more of an effort to become familiar with the customs and needs of these patients if they are to provide adequate services. A recent positive development has been a rapprochement between traditional western medicine and the native healers. Programs have been developed that permit sharing of each's beliefs and techniques. Thus, the best of each tradition can be incorporated into the care of patients, which results in an upgrading in the quality of care delivered.

Black Families

One of the most significant factors affecting the family roles of the black population of the United States has been the concentration of a majority of these families at income levels that are grossly inadequate. This has largely been caused by discrimination, which is more severe for blacks than for other less visible groups. New opportunities have opened up for the black community in recent years; however, these have mainly benefitted upper-working-class and middle-class families. The poorest strata have not gained proportionally.

Another factor that has been woven into the fabric of what some have called mythology about the black community has been the lack of a strong patriarchal tradition among the black family. The mother is seen as the head of the household and provider, while the father is seen as mostly absent, a nonprovider, and a powerless parent. However, research has indicated that, among the middle-class and upper-working-class families, there is no significant difference from whites with respect to family role differentiation and the acceptance of a middle-class value system.

In a thoughtful review and evaluation of the empirical research findings regarding lower-class black families, TenHouten concluded that the bulk of the findings do not show these fathers and husbands to be powerless in either their conjugal or parental roles. Black wives do appear to be powerful in their parental roles, but there is no indication that this emasculates the black father.[21] Indeed, there is a healthy effect in that fathers tend to be more expressive in their marital and parental roles and are helpful and willing to share in childrearing and homemaking chores. Moreover, this freedom from patriarchy has enabled the black woman to be more pragmatic, resourceful, and flexible than her counterparts from other cultures in which the tradition of authoritarianism and patriarchy is strong.

Since they typically do not have authoritarian fathers, black children do not experience one of the psychological stresses of low-achievement motivations. The increased economic opportunities that will allow black fathers to become economic role models for their children, combined with an early emphasis on independence typical among black families, and confident setting of standards by black mothers should result in higher levels of achievement motivation among black children than those among children whose fathers play a more repressive role. There is already evidence that middle-class black children have higher levels of motivation and aspiration than do their white counterparts.[21]

Blacks in the lower socioeconomic strata, especially when confined to the ghetto or rural areas and deprived of educational and other acculturating opportunities, tend to hold a traditional value system that includes a strong sense of family (or familism), superstition, religiosity, and fatalism. This is in contrast to the "middle-class" value system generally held by highly industrialized urban societies. These values—rationalism, pragmatism, individualism, equalitarianism, secularism, and achievement—have also become known as the dominant American values.

Whether the individual's value system is traditional or middle-class urban, it becomes part of his belief system and is incorporated into the roles of husband, wife, parent, and child.[22] Thus, when dealing with these patients, health professionals often find their values competing with those of the patients. When the basic values are examined, it becomes clearer why certain health beliefs, differential use of health services, delay in seeking care and often nonadherence to prescribed regimens are established.

Mexican-American Families

Mexican–Americans have been the forgotten minority in the United States, possibly because the Southwest has been somewhat neglected by both academicians and writers with the exception of John Steinbeck. There are more than 5 million Mexican–Americans, who are mainly second-generation offspring of peasant immigrants from Mexico. They are concentrated in the border states of Texas, Arizona, New Mexico, and California, and comprise the second largest minority group in the United States.

Since World War II, the isolation of the Mexican–American has been declining; owing to the fact that many participated in the war and gradually new perspectives and opportunities have come about which have had an impact on family roles and traditional value and belief systems (Fig. 4-3). Neighborhood enclaves (barrios) still exist, of course, and in some small rural or isolated urban areas, even the middle-class Mexican–American tends to reside in them.

Familism appears to be the strongest surviving traditional value within the older Mexican-American community, along with patriarchalism and machismo, the cultural ideal of masculinity which equates maleness with sexual prowess.[22] These traditional values and certain folk beliefs persist, particularly because of the isolation of the barrios, and the persistence of these values and beliefs make the acceptance of modern health knowledge and practice difficult.

Mexican–Americans in the barrios who are educated and have had a positive experience with health services, have accepted the ideas of scientific medicine and health care, allow their children to be immunized, attend clinics and, in some cases, have accepted some kind of family planning. However, there are many others who have their own set of folk beliefs about illness and its treatment which they practice in conjunction with medical care or before seeking scientific health care. These beliefs about diseases and their cures are derived from experience and experimentation and are handed down from generation to generation. Two or more cures may be recognized for one disorder and disorders generally fall into two categories—those of emotional origin and those of magical origin. Folk healers (primarily curanderas [women] or curanderos [men]) are often used and some have an important and respected standing in the community. It is felt by the majority of the uneducated that physicians do not know how to treat folk disorders because they lack either faith, knowledge, or understanding of them.

Among those with little education, there is no distinction between the natural and supernatural and

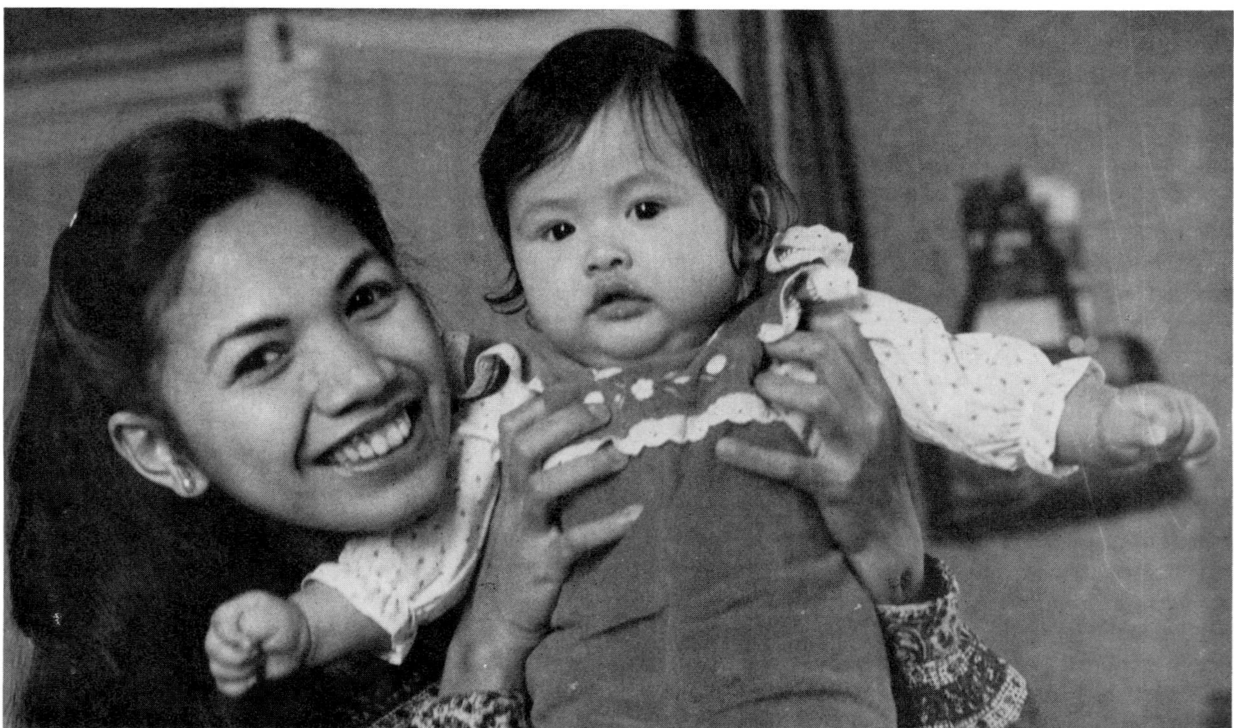

Figure 4-3.
Since World War II many Mexican-American families have become less isolated as new perspectives and opportunities have had an impact on family life.

many illnesses can be a result of evil forces, witches, spells cast by other persons, or punishment for some sin committed either knowingly or unknowingly. One common condition that health professionals should be aware of is the following: *mal aire* or bad air, especially night air. It can enter through any of the body cavities under certain circumstances and results in illness of both mother and child. *Mal ojo,* or the evil eye, is a culturally defined disease, primarily of children. It is caused when someone looks admiringly or covetously on the child or adult. Its symptoms are restlessness, crying, and headache, as well as other nonspecific symptoms. *Susto,* or fright, can be caused by a frightening experience that can result in excessive nervousness, loss of appetite, and loss of sleep. *Mollera calda,* or fallen fontanel, is a common disorder among infants. It is believed to be due to a fall or from taking the nipple out of the baby's mouth too suddenly, thus causing the fontanel to be sucked in. Symptoms include irritability, crying, diarrhea, sunken eyes, and vomiting. There are other afflictions as well as their home remedies that it is wise for the nurse to know if she will be dealing with these patients. The reader is referred to the books by Hymovich and Barnard, and Reinhardt and Quinn for excellent presentations of these conditions and specific nursing intervention.[23, 24]

Japanese-American Families

The modernization of the Japanese family in America has proceeded more slowly in some respects than in Japan because the isolation of the Japanese–American from the effects of technological development and rapid social change has been more pronounced here. However, in California, where the largest concentration of Japanese ancestry occurs, this segment of the population has the highest median levels of income and education of any minority group. Japanese–Americans also have very low rates of crime and delinquency, indicating at the same time the greater persistence of the traditional values of obedience and conformity to parental values and norms. The generational pattern of increasing acculturation is very clearly illustrated in the contemporary Japanese-American community since other factors such as urban-rural residence do not vary significantly.

A majority of the Issei or first-generation immigrants who were born in Japan arrived here some time between the end of the 19th century and 1924, when immigration from the Orient and Eastern Europe was sharply restricted by the Johnson Act. While the Issei came largely from rural agricultural areas and occupations, they were unusual in that they were relatively literate, compared with peasant immigrants from Europe, and they valued education even before their arrival in this country.

Second-generation Japanese–Americans, the Nisei, born largely before 1940, experienced an unusual push into modernity not only by the parents' preexisting emphasis on education, but by the West Coast evacuation of Japanese–Americans during World War II. Familistic values were weakened by the loss of confiscated family homes and businesses, which removed an important source of Issei control over their second-generation offspring. Thus, after the war, the Issei, who were forced to seek out independent, nonfamily occupational opportunities, were thereby more speedily acculturated into the modern values of individualism and equalitarianism in family relationships, although a cultural lag in this respect is still quite pronounced among many Japanese–Americans.

The third generation, the Sansei, born largely since World War II and now in high school, college, or in the adult occupational world, are the most totally acculturated of all. However, certain subcultural differences remain in family role conceptions, even within the third generation, which are traceable to the survival of traditional ethnic values in marital roles and in childrearing practices.

In the Orient, the patriarchal tradition has been much more crystalized than in the West. The deference and obedience of wife and children toward husband and father, and of the younger generations toward elders, was more intense and more formalized in ritual, ceremony, religion, and law in the Orient than in Western society.

The extended family form, the ancestral clan or house as the basic family unit, was far more salient in the Orient as reality and as cultural ideal, for all social strata. Arranged marriages and emphasis on lineage, important indicators of the value of familism, were common even among the poor in Japan. The values of obedience, deference, duty, and responsibility were constantly reinforced by pervasive mechanisms of control that elicited shame and guilt for the slightest deviation from established convention.[25]

Frequent sources of role conflict, in the Sansei generation especially, are found in the greater prevalence of strict disciplinary measures in childrearing, the greater emphasis on conformity and unconditional obedience, on humility and emotional reserve (particularly the suppression of anger), the continued extensive use of shame and guilt as mechanisms of control, the greater submissiveness of women, even within the higher strata, and the greater strength of extended family pride and intergenerational emotional dependence. These are the residual of traditional values of the parents.

Male dominance is stronger in Oriental homes, at all class levels, than in any other ethnic group in this country. While the emphasis within Japanese-American homes on achievement and competitiveness has promoted educational and occupational success, the continuing stress of familism and authoritarian values has retarded the flexibility, independence, and the self-reliance that are important attributes of individualistic achievement in highly industrialized society.

While recent studies of the Sansei generation have indicated a shift toward greater independence in this generation, both males and females remain, typically, less assertive, more deferent and conforming, and more emotionally reserved than their Anglo peers. The rigid conformity, status distinctions, and authority relations of traditional Japan that continue to affect family roles of Japanese–Americans in this country are likely to disappear with time, but more quickly in the occupational world than in the world of the family, where they appear less immediately dysfunctional.[22]

There are few folk beliefs and, in general, scientific medicine is accepted especially by the second- and third-generation Japanese–Americans. Preventive medicine is solicited and, because of the high educational levels as well as high achievement aspirations, health and medical regimens are usually followed. There may be some reliance on herbal medicine and an interest in acupuncture among the older generation.

Vietnamese Families

In April 1975 South Vietnam capitulated and almost 150,000 refugees from all walks of life sought new homes and a new way of life in the United States. All of the states generously received these people, but the highest concentration, around 27,000, is found in California.[17] This rather sudden influx of persons has caused some problems for both the refugees and the host society.

A great deal has been written about the Vietnam war, but there is very little recent material on the culture and mores of the people while they still remained in their homeland and endured the rigors of the war. The available data are experiential and anecdotal and derive from interviews with the families as they make their adjustment in their new country.[17, 26] Grasso and Stringfellow point out that the Vietnamese social concerns and problems including health needs are not significantly different from those of many Americans, especially those who live in reduced circumstances. Economic opportunities may be limited for the unskilled and for the educated former urban dweller. Economic opportunites may not be commensurate with the Vietnamese's considerable skill and expertise. Culture shock and a language barrier may also prove troublesome. Moreover, the economic and emotional exigencies that the single parents, who are waiting for news or the arrival of their loved ones, face impact on their lifestyle just as severely as on an American family.[17]

The development of community agencies to assist these families to become acculturated has been helpful to some extent. Social support systems including friend and family networks have also eased the transition to the American culture.[17, 26]

The Vietnamese family is not adverse to utilizing the existing American health care delivery system, including hospital care during parturition if the providers are sensitive to the family structure and try to utilize family members as resources for the care of the child in an extended family manner. The use of a telephone outreach program based in the maternity ward and a well-monitored referral system to public health agencies have been found to be beneficial in the delivery of health services.[26]

References

1. Sussman M: Family systems in the 1970's: Analysis, policies, and programs. Annals of the American Academy 396, 1970

2. Lewis GL: Changes in women's role participation. In Frieze I et al (eds): Women and Sex Roles, A Social Psychological Perspective. New York, W W Norton, 1978

3. Pickett RS: Monogamy on trial part II, the modern era. Alternate Lifestyles 1, 3:281–301, 1978

4. Reeder SJ: The Impact of Disabling Health Conditions on Family Interaction. Unpublished Ph.D. dissertation, UCLA 1974

5. Eiduson BJ et al.: Alternatives in childrearing in the 1970's. Am J Orthopsychiatry 43:720–731, 1973

6. Glick P, Norton AJ: Marrying, divorcing and living together in the U.S. today. Population Bulletin, 32, 5, Washington, D.C., Population Reference Bureau.

7. Hutter M: The Changing Family, Comparative Perspective. New York, John Wiley & Sons, 1981

8. Bane MJ: Here to Stay—American Families in the Twentieth Century. New York, Basic Books, 1979

9. Ross HL, Sawhill IV: Line of Transition: The Growth of Families Headed by Women. Washington, D.C., The Urban Institute, 1975

10. Gersick KE: Fathers by choice: Divorced men who receive custody of their children. In Levinger G, Moles OC (eds): Divorce and Separation: Context, Causes & Consequences, pp 307–323. New York, Basic Books, 1979

11. Johnston C, Deisher R: Contemporary communal childrearing. Pediatrics 52:326, 1973

12. Bancroft AV: Pregnancy and the counterculture. Nurs Clin North Am 8:67–76, 1973

13. Maralee J: Our Babies, Our Lives, Our Right to Decide. Chicago, Chicago Seed, 1972

14. Taylor TW: The States and Their Indian Citizens. Washington, D.C., U.S. Government Printing Office, 1972

15. Levitan S, Hetrick B: Big Brother's Indian Programs; With Reservations. New York, McGraw–Hill, 1971

16. Billard JB (ed): The World of the American Indian, pp 311–382. Washington, D.C., National Geographic Society, 1974

17. Clark AL: Culture Childbearing Health Professionals, pp 20–33. Philadelphia, FA Davis, 1978

18. Foreman, CT: Indian Women Chiefs. Muskogee, OK, Hoffman Printing, 1954

19. Vogel G: American Indian Medicine. New York, Ballantine Books, 1973

20. U.S. Department of Health, Education and Welfare. Report of a Regional Task Force: Health of the American Indian. Washington, D.C., U.S. Government Printing Office, 1973

21. TenHouten W: The black family: Myth and reality. Psychiatry 33:145–173, 1970

22. Yorburg B: The Changing Family. New York, Columbia University Press, 1973

23. Hymovich DP, Barnard M: Family Health Care. New York, McGraw–Hill, 1973

24. Reinhardt A, Quinn M: Family Centered Community Nursing. St Louis, CV Mosby, 1973

25. Benedict R: The Chrysanthemum and the Sword. Boston, Houghton–Mifflin, 1946

26. Grosso C et al: The Vietnamese American family . . . and grandma makes three. MCN 6:177–180, 1981

Suggested Reading

Balik B, Foley MK: Developing a community-based parent education support group. JOGN Nurs 10, 3:197–199, 1981

Blanton J: Communal child rearing, the Synanon experience. Altenative Lifestyles, 3, 1:87–116, 1980

Farris LS: Approaches to caring for the American Indian maternity patient. MCN 1, 2:82–87, 1976

Greenberg JB: Single-parenting and intimacy. Alternative Lifestyles 2, 3:308–330, 1979

Grosso C et al: The Vietnamese American family . . . and grandma makes three. MCN 6:177–180, 1981

Hanson FM: Single custodial fathers and the parent–child relationship. Nsg Research 30, 4:202–204, 1981

Rosenthal KM, Keshet HF: The impact of child care responsibilities on part-time or single fathers. Alternative Lifestyles 1, 4:465–491, 1981

CHAPTER 5

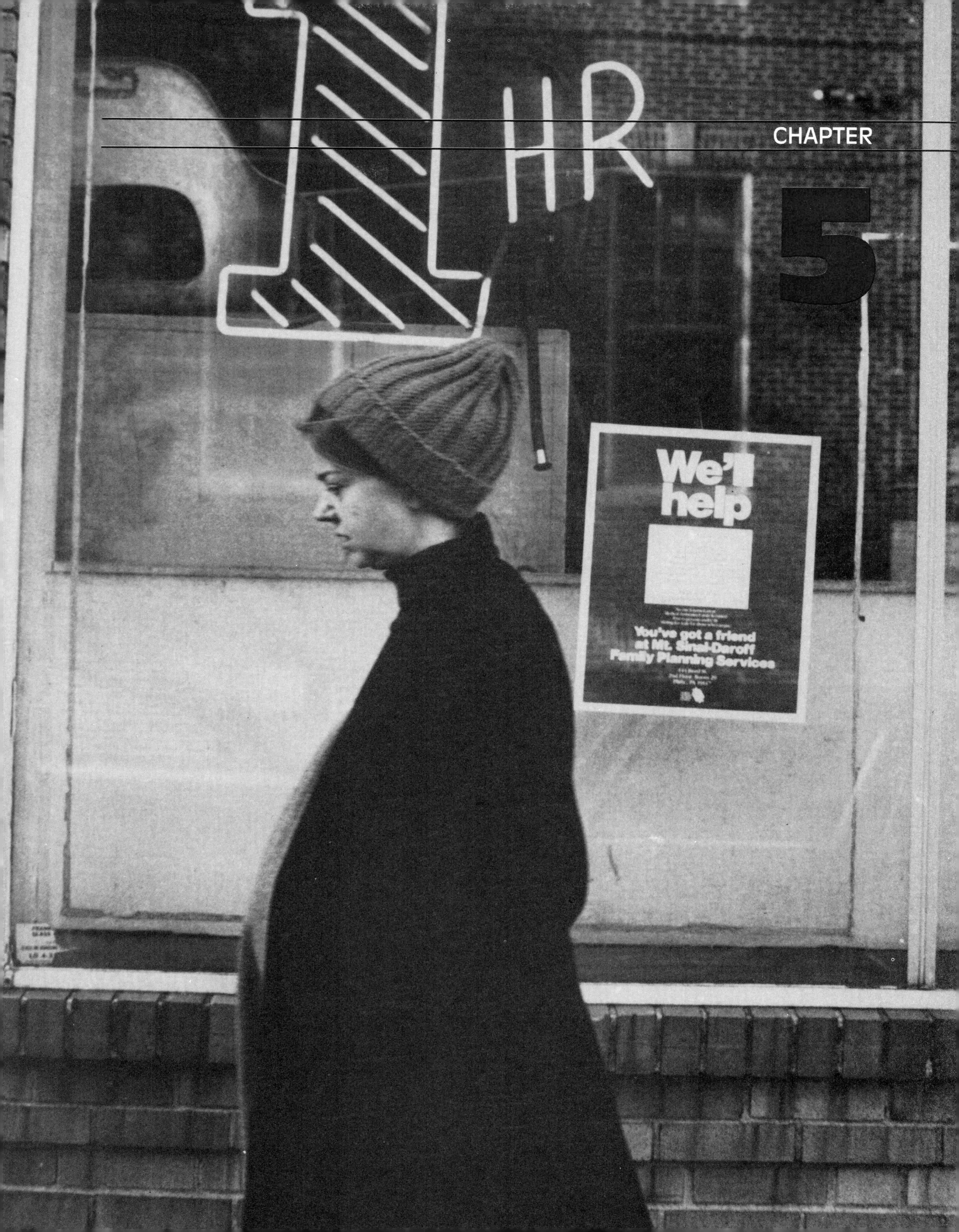

CHAPTER 5

Culture, Society, and Maternal Care

In most societies, conceptions of health and well-being reflect the orientations of the person's social class or group membership. Values, attitudes, perspectives, and the behavior that we engage in are formed and conditioned by the social groups in which we participate from earliest childhood. Consequently, there are differing orientations to health and health care reflecting memberships in differing ethnic, racial, religious, and social class groups. These varying health orientations become manifest both in the behavior of individuals and the institutions that are organized to deliver health services.

In recent years, there has been a heightened awareness of the importance of social and cultural factors in health status, specifically maternal care. Although Americans are accustomed to thinking of their health status as being the best and highest in the world, their health care is still far short of its potential. Large segments of the population either do not have access to adequate medical care or are deprived of quality care in the services that they do receive. There has been a great stimulus to improve the prenatal care system, in particular, in order to improve the delivery of maternal care services and thus reduce preterm, low birth weight, and infant deaths. Essentially, there has been an expansion and elaboration of the existing system of maternity services. Whether such an approach to maternity problems will have the desired effects depends on a variety of factors, not the least of which are those concerning the health values, beliefs, orientations, and, ultimately, behaviors of the target populations.

In this chapter the focus is upon those forces and features in society that influence the field of maternity services. First, it is important to examine the social and cultural meaning of pregnancy. What are the current social, cultural, and economic forces that influence motivations for childbearing? Second, we will discuss some of the critical issues in access and use of maternal services and finally present some aspects of the nurse's role in these matters.

The Social and Cultural Meaning of Childbearing

For nurses to function appropriately, to use their talents more creatively than in the past, they must have an understanding of the social and cultural meaning of pregnancy. As discussed in Chapter 1, pregnancy itself needs to be considered in terms of the social context in which it occurs, namely, the family and the larger society. Moreover, pregnancy and childbearing in general have different meanings in various societies and even within any given society.

In Western society the expectations and the prescriptions for behavior surrounding pregnancy are relatively ill defined, and in some situations they do not exist. Consequently, women are often uncertain when and how often they ought to visit the physician, whether they can continue employment, and what is expected of them by significant others. Part of the reasons for these loose definitions is related to the lifestyles of population subcultures and part of the answer lies in factors related to the social structure of society.

The Sick Role, Illness, and Pregnancy

How a society or groups within a society define pregnancy and cope with pregnancy tends to vary considerably. In some societies, pregnancy is regarded as a "normal" situation—a kind of status passage through which most women, at some time or other, will pass. In other societies, pregnancy may be regarded as an illness and is reacted to as other illnesses are. Moreover, there is considerable variation, even within societies, in the way health and illness are perceived by different social classes, ethnic groups, and age categories.

The Sick Role Concept

The sick role has been developed as a concept by sociologists to study the role behavior of persons who are considered to be sick or to have an illness. In brief, the sick role concept refers to the process by which every society ensures that an adequate level of health and normative conformity exists among the majority of its members most of the time. Society has various mechanisms for accomplishing this purpose. It accommodates individuals or groups who are ill by placing them in a special position or status. The term "social role" refers to both the regular way of acting, which is expected of persons occupying a given position, and the social position itself. Typically there are certain rights or privileges, as well as expectations, associated with given social positions. Parsons has presented an insightful and systematic analysis of the expectations associated with occupancy of the sick role.[1] There are two main rights in the sick role. (1) The sick person is allowed exemption from the performance of normal social role obligations, and (2) the sick person is allowed exemption from the responsibility for his own state. There are also two main obligations—(1) the sick person must be motivated to get well as soon as possible, and (2) the sick person should seek technically competent help and cooperate with medical experts.

The sick role is generally thought of as only a theoretical model for the purposes of understanding the processes contributing to and the various conditions to be fulfilled in the legitimation of illness conditions. In reality, the concept is not universally applicable to all who claim to be ill; it varies depending on the unique background of the person, the particular illness involved, and the social context within which legitimation is sought.

Behavioral scientists have made a number of criticisms concerning the sick role, including the fact that Parsons has left open the problem of the chronically ill, as well as some illness that is not considered serious enough to warrant more than a slight reduction in normal activities. Furthermore, much illness never reaches the stage of formal consultation with a qualified physician. Individuals who are ill may receive what they consider to be competent help from other than professional medical personnel. Finally, Parsons's formulation may not be relevant to all societies, and various studies have demonstrated that there are both intercultural and intracultural variations in the definitions of the conditions to which the sick role is thought to be applicable.

The Sick Role and Pregnancy

The state of pregnancy in its usual or normal situation, where there are no resultant obstetrical or delivery complications, must be considered in the discussion of the applicability of the sick role concept. If a woman is experiencing complications of pregnancy, certainly this would make her eligible for the sick role as discussed above. The question that arises is whether pregnancy is in fact a "normal" state.

One may conceivably take the position that illness, or sickness, is statistically normal in most members of the population at some point in their lives; similarly, pregnancy can likewise be considered statistically normal in that most of the population of possible conceivers at some time are in this state. Pregnancy can also be considered normal in the sense that it is a necessary biological function for the species. Indeed, it can even be considered a desirable state of affairs. In this latter sense, it is not similar to illness at all. McKinlay has noted that pregnancy differs from illness by "calling forth in both the woman and her significant others a set of responses which are in many ways different from those elicited with the onset of an illness."[2] Considering whether the sick role expectations noted previously apply to pregnancy, McKinlay suggests that for a variety of reasons the state of pregnancy is in some ways different from illness and cannot be analyzed in terms of any of the expectations associated with the sick role.[1]

There is a tendency in the more advanced societies to consider some point during pregnancy as illness and to treat it in a manner similar to that of illness. For example, women are discouraged from home deliveries and are hospitalized for delivery. Blood pressure, height, weight, and other vital signs are usually checked at several points during the pregnancy. Treating women as if they are ill may perhaps encourage the adoption of certain behaviors because the women perceive this type of treatment as being similar to that for an illness. In sum, the state of pregnancy and the expectations covering it differ from routine illness behavior and the situation is relatively unstructured. This relatively unstructured situation may produce a sense of role ambiguity in pregnant women. Women may take matters into their own hands and reduce the strain from ambiguity by structuring the situation in particular ways, including adopting the sick role.

For women who are at greater risk and who react excessively or unfavorably under the strain of pregnancy, the sick role becomes meaningful and relevant.

Thus, both in the "normal" circumstances of pregnancy and in pathological conditions, the sick role plays an important part in maternal care.

Childbearing Motivations

One of the most important factors in human reproduction that is determined and influenced by culture and society is the *motivation* for childbearing. In the past 15 years, numerous studies have appeared concerned with factors influencing the number of children desired by and born to married couples. Most of these studies have focused on the number of children desired rather than on the attitudes held by women regarding why they want children. A brief consideration of some of the social and psychological aspects motivating childbearing will be discussed.

No biological event has greater significance for society than reproduction and its outcome. Reproduction is important in family dynamics and population dynamics, which, in turn, have a heavy impact on individual and national welfare. Women begin their preparation for childbearing early in life. In a sense, they begin it at the time of their own conception.

As mentioned previously, society is primarily organized for families with children and the argument for having children can be very persuasive. Even in this newer era of voluntary childbearing, couples without children are still generally made to feel "out of place," especially if they have been married very long. Research has indicated that the value of having children remains generally accepted by the vast majority of Americans.[3]

Judith Blake, an internationally known demographer, has coined the term "coercive pronatalism" to encompass society's insistence that the marital pair bear children. She argues that even in modern western societies where effective contraception and enlightened attitudes toward women are becoming more prevalent, motherhood, far from being voluntary, is in fact a mandatory directive. Blake believes that two pronatalist coercions characterize American society. First, there is the prescribed primacy of parenthood in the definition of sex roles; thus, the parameters and content of adult sex roles are defined in terms of parenthood. Secondly, there is a prescribed fitting of personality traits with the demands of the sex roles as they are defined. Here it is mandated that Americans socialize their girls and boys to become the proper kinds of people that the cultural stereotype says good mothers and fathers should be.[4] In this context, it is understandable that all levels of society should be organized in favor of children. Rossi has also noted that the cultural pressure to become parents is great enough that a couple may plan to bear children in spite of a latent desire to the contrary. For the female, the pressure to become a mother may be the equivalent of the cultural insistence that the male assume a productive occupational role.[5]

The availability of acceptable means for preventing conception should theoretically permit childbearing today to be a consequence of motivated human action rather than mere biological happenstance. However, regardless of when pregnancies occur or if they are planned, the number of children a couple has and the time at which they have them are to a large extent a function of the couple's childbearing motivations which, in turn, are influenced by cultural imperatives.

Present Societal Trends Affecting Childbearing Motivation

Fertility Control

Elsewhere in this book we discuss techniques of contraception and family planning from a more technical perspective. Here we wish to highlight certain social implications of fertility control. A number of important trends have occurred in the United States and have resulted in lower fertility. As previously mentioned, the birthrate in 1974 reached an all-time low. Although it is on the rise, Americans are still restricting their families to about two children. This is particularly true of the middle class. Thus, in the opinion of many demographers, a revolution in the fertility regimen of American women that has profound implications for society, including maternity services, is taking place. At the core of the fertility changes is an apparent reassessment of the values associated with fertility control. Thus, the widespread use of the pill and the intrauterine devices (IUDs) has resulted not only in a more effective means of fertility control but has also made an apparent change in the rules under which fertility decisions are made.

First, it must be recognized that the extensive use of these more reliable contraceptives, not only vastly improved contraceptive protection, but also separated contraception from sexual activity. Now childbearing can be voluntary in a radically different sense than ever before. Under the previous fertility regimen, women could not confidently plan a lifetime of childlessness nor the prevention of unwanted pregnancy. Not surprisingly, under this regimen the role expectations of women were structured around motherhood. In fact, cultural values with respect to fertility can be thought of, in part, as rationalizations of the inevitable. For example, in the early 1960s about one half of all births were accidental and one fifth were reported by their mothers as unwanted.[6]

The widespread use of the pill has facilitated the adoption of other effective means of preventing unwanted births (the IUD, sterilization, and abortion) and has led to reductions in the number of children intended by women in the United States. Contraceptive sterilization had been a relatively infrequent occurrence in the population prior to the introduction of the pill. In recent years there has been a dramatic reversal of this pattern with majority approval and greater use of this procedure. By 1970 sterilization was the most prevalent contraceptive method among women older than 30.[6]

Competing Social Roles

All of the foregoing processes in contraceptive practice indicate a drastic realignment of values in fertility. These new fertility control values have given more support to the equal opportunity concept by making nonfamilial roles a realistic and viable option for women. Thus the potential for complete fertility control makes childbearing a matter of choice in a sense never before realized. Motherhood itself can now become a matter of rational evaluation. The costs as well as the virtues can now be weighed. This is, of course, not a new discovery. There has always been a large literature on the psychological and emotional costs of motherhood. They have, however, become more relevant and prominent particularly in the context of increased concern with equal opportunity for women.

Thus, as other social roles become more feasible, the opportunity costs of childbearing are increased. One of the consequences is to place motherhood more directly in competition with these alternative, socially desirable roles. As fertility becomes more a matter for decision, greater emphasis is placed on planning. Among the factors that must be taken into account in the decision are the direct social, psychological, and economic costs of children themselves, and also the loss of the wife's earnings and intrinsic satisfaction with her occupation (Fig. 5-1).

This is no small matter. Modern lifestyles are significantly dependent on the wife's earnings. In a majority of the families in which both the husband and wife have incomes, the wife's income represents over one fifth of the total family income.[7]

Impact on Maternity Services

The implications of all this are enormous, for fertility statistics influence almost every facet of our lives. Consider the following as examples: (1) elementary school enrollment has been dropping since 1970 and this is now being seen in high schools and colleges; (2) a slowdown in the birthrate affects the Social Security system of the country; (3) there will be changes in the consumption patterns that may influence smaller cars and even smaller houses; (4) last, but not least, there is an impact upon maternity services.

Two trends in particular are worth mentioning. First, not only are some hospitals closing their maternity units, but perhaps more important, hospitals are

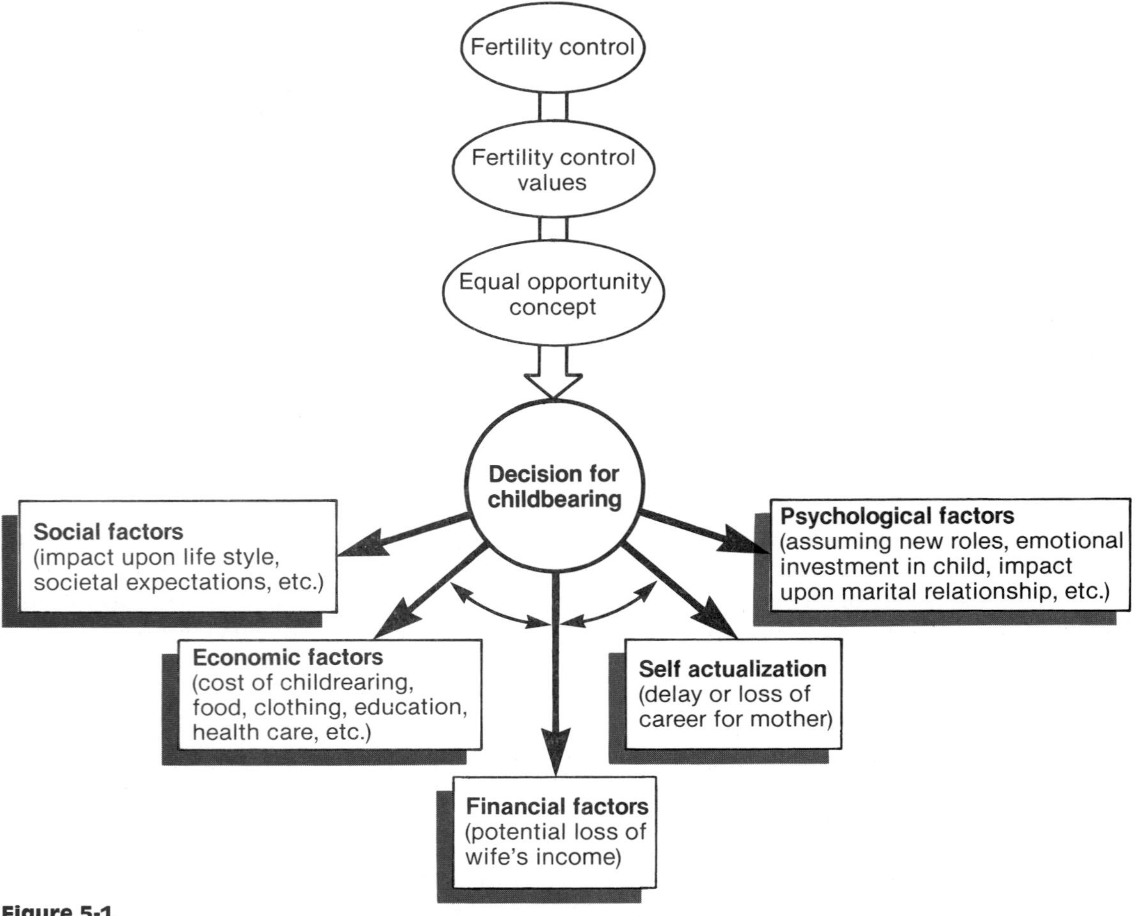

Figure 5-1.
Fertility control has made childbearing a matter of choice. This illustration shows some of the factors that may be included in the decision for childbearing.

merging their obstetrical units. This will hopefully improve the quality of obstetrical care for mothers and newborns, in addition to controlling costs and avoiding duplication of services. In addition, the experience of fertility control may make women more sensitive and aware of the need for better maternal care during pregnancy. Indeed, the increased availability of safe abortion after 1970 has been temporarily associated with a reduction in pregnancy-associated maternal mortality.[8, 9] There is also good reason to connect the trends in fertility control to the recent rapid decline in infant mortality.

It should be recognized that no one knows for certain that the current pattern of fertility control will continue indefinitely. Nevertheless, it is important to note that the "baby boom" children of the 50s are now forming their own families. Consequently, within the next few years, there will be an increase of approximately 20 percent in the number of women in the childbearing age groups of 15 to 44 years. Thus, the absolute number of births is rising even if the birthrate may not. This occurred in 1974 for the first time in four years, and will have relevance for continued, high-quality maternity services.

Sociocultural Factors Affecting Childbearing

Sociodemographic Factors and the Use of Maternity Health Services

Social Class

Social class is an important determinant of maternal reproductive behavior and maternal use of services. Since socioeconomic status or social class has such a pervasive influence upon health and health care, it is important to briefly describe the central features of this concept.

Social class, or socioeconomic status, is a complex concept referring to a theoretical formulation of relationships between subgroups in our society. It is a term frequently used by sociologists and epidemiologists in medical research in an effort to subdivide populations into a few descriptive categories that differ in a variety of social and economic characteristics, background, and behavior.

Typically, in determining socioeconomic status, the usual procedure is to select as indicators of social differences one or several characteristics, each of which are closely related to income, education, occupation, housing and place of residence, social values, and the general lifestyle of population subgroups. By far the most widely used indicator of socioeconomic status or social class is occupation. It is the best indicator of a person's income, education, standard of living, social values, and a variety of other attributes.

However, not all social differences stem from socioeconomic status. Dividing a population along one social dimension does not automatically provide categories that are socially meaningful in other respects. It can be demonstrated that such social variables as age, geographic region, height, parity, and ethnicity each contribute independently to the total picture of social variation in pregnancy outcome. The same may be said of other more complex social influences.

It is generally accepted that adequate medical care during pregnancy, particularly in the early stages of pregnancy, reduces the incidence of neonatal mortality, congenital malformations or other birth defects, maternal mortality, prematurity, and so on. The relationship between low socioeconomic status and failure to receive adequate antenatal care has been well documented. The data appear to be similar in the United States, Great Britain, and in various other Western nations. Not only do the lower-class women typically comprise the highest proportion of those who have not received antenatal care, they are also the women, as a group, who contribute to the highest proportion of underusers of antenatal care.[2]

According to data for the United States, the average white mother had 60% more visits for medical care than the average nonwhite mother. This is undoubtedly related more to the influence of socioeconomic status than to the ethnicity of the mother. According to these data, as family income increased, the number of visits for medical care also increased. On the average, women living in families below the poverty level made 9.3 visits for medical care; women from middle-income families averaged 13.7 visits. Most of the women in the lowest income group visited medical facilities (clinics, hospitals) for their care as contrasted to the women in the highest income group where the majority visited physicians for medical care.[10]

Thus, income appears to be a major factor in the number of visits for prenatal care. There is a large jump in number of visits when the income goes over the poverty line (*i.e.*, $5000 and over).

Medical Organization and Social Class

Before discussing how the characteristics of lower-income persons influence their behavior in connection with the issues of health, illness, and the use of medical services, it is appropriate to discuss briefly some aspects of health care organization and care for the lower-income groups. In the 1970s there was a national commitment for equality of medical care for all citizens which led to a variety of important legislative acts. The emphasis was on extending and improving the system of medical organization so that care could be offered more efficiently to the poor as well as to those more economically advantaged. For example, the federally subsidized maternal and infant care projects (MIC) were instituted to help reduce the incidence of mental retardation and other handicapping conditions caused by complications associated with childbearing and to help reduce infant and maternal mortality. These programs have been concentrated in the low-income areas of large and small cities and have emphasized early, comprehensive prenatal care for all patients in the geographic area served. The results, however, have been somewhat equivocal although they have been considered to have had some success. With the current era of economic austerity in governmental subsidies, it remains to be seen whether or not these kinds of programs will continue to be viable and whether or not there will continue to be a national commitment to quality health services for all strata of society.[10] There is also a serious question as to whether the inequities in the medical care system can be overcome unless changes are made reflecting greater understanding of lower socioeconomic lifestyles. It is well known that when medical facilities are set up in convenient proximity to lower-income housing, they do not automatically draw clientele.

There are two factors that contribute to inequities of medical care. The first of these relates to the way in which health organization facilities are structured; the second is concerned with the characteristic lifestyles of lower-income groups.

Medical Organization

What are the features of health-care organization that tend to blunt the effectiveness of medical care for lower-income patients? These negative features include the following: first, there is the massiveness of medical organization itself. As noted earlier, most of the lower-income women tend to visit medical facilities such as hospitals and clinics. These are often large and complex organizations, characterized by great specialization and a fair degree of impersonality. Lower-class patients are ill equipped by lack of education and experience to cope with complex bureaucratic organization.[10]

Professionalization

A second feature of medical organization that tends to decrease the quality of care for lower-income patients is professionalization. Its perspectives toward work and patients result in a gap between the patients and the professionals. Lower-income people are less skilled in obtaining information from professionals. They tend to be less aggressive in demanding explanations. On the other hand, higher-income patients have greater aggressive and interactional skills and can cope more effectively with the professional's failure to communicate.

Lower-income patients also suffer from other, more subtle disadvantages stemming from professional stances. These have been discussed by a number of investigators in the field of mental disorders. That is, middle-class patients are preferred by most providers and are viewed as more treatable. In other words, there may be a distinct bias expressed against the lower-income patient, based honestly on professional conceptions. Also, many regimens are impossible for low-income patients to carry out. The simple order that medication is to be taken "with each meal" may not recognize that many lower-income families eat irregularly and may not have three meals a day.

Middle-Class Bias

Another characteristic of medical organization that influences the quality of medical care is the middle-class bias of most professional health workers. The staff members, typically, do not understand the perspectives, attitudes, customs, and lifestyles of the lower-income patients. They often take for granted that the patients have the same attitudes about health as they do. Hence, they tend to issue orders that are not understood or cannot be easily followed by lower-income patients. Furthermore, there is a tendency to think of lower-income people in stereotyped terms—"they cannot keep appointments; they have little sense of time or responsibility, and so on." Lower-income patients may perceive these class biases, and this may affect the underutilization of medical services.

The many hours of waiting, the impersonal routines of institutional care in large hospitals or clinics, particularly in the municipal and county hospitals, the real or imagined perceptions of racial and class bias all tend to maximize dissatisfactions of lower-income patients and reduce the possibility of use of health facilities. Furthermore, the distances that patients must travel to the medical facilities and the cost of transportation are realistic matters. Customarily, poor people organize their lives so as not to go far for the necessities of living. This is one of the factors in the relative success of the MIC program that reached into the lower-income communities and brought the clinic facilities into the neighborhood. Similarly, the neighborhood health centers have been relatively successful for this reason.[10]

Lifestyles and Social Class

It is important to take into account the characteristic lifestyles of the poor. The lower-income person's experience of himself and his world is highly distinctive in our country. It is also distinctive for its problems and crisis-dominated character. As Miller has commented about these people, "their life is a crisis life constantly trying to make do with string where rope is needed."[11] In other words, health concerns are minor to those who feel they confront much more pressing troubles. Health problems are just one crisis among many that they must try to cope with, control, or just live with.[11]

Indeed, the value orientations of the medical system reflect the values of the middle- and upper-middle classes. These have been characterized as activistic, rational mastery, future-time orientation to life. A large body of empirical research data suggests that the values of the middle class tend to result in a specific outlook on life that is reflected in health beliefs and behavior. Conversely, the lower classes, whose position in the social structure does not support a belief in the rational mastery of the world, tend to have quite a different orientation of the world. There is a feeling of lack of control over events; occurrences are viewed as "luck" or fate rather than as planned by rational design. Planning, education, and involvement in organized activity are less important in this framework; they seek help from those in their social network rather than from "experts" or professionals.[11,12]

Another problem is that many lower-income households are often much more understaffed than those of higher incomes. Understaffing of households means that each individual's health receives relatively little attention as far as preventive measures are concerned, and when someone is sick it is more difficult to care for him or her at home. When the main family member is sick, he or she will be in a disadvantaged position in caring properly for himself or herself. There is a necessity for poor people to learn to live with illness rather than to use their limited financial and psychological resources to do something about illness.

Lower-income people also do not conform to the expectations of how "good" and "considerate" patients should behave in medical settings. Their behavior is often frustrating and annoying to medical and nursing personnel for a variety of reasons.

In short, the cultural values and health beliefs tend to shape the maternal behavior of pregnant women just as they influence other types of health practices. These values are not easily mutable; thus, in the absence of either powerful attempts to change behavior or the system itself, it is important to recognize the differences in assumptions, values, beliefs and behaviors, and attempts to adjust the structure of the maternal health service delivery system.

Ethnicity and Geographic Area

The evidence we have to date indicates that white mothers receive care earlier in pregnancy than nonwhite mothers. There is a consistent difference between white and nonwhite mothers in the receipt of medical care during each of the trimesters of pregnancy. There is evidence that women living in metropolitan areas receive care earlier than those outside metropolitan areas; this holds true for both white and nonwhite women. Furthermore, more nonwhite women in metropolitan areas are known to have received care than nonwhite women residing outside metropolitan areas. It is worth noting, though, that for any given income or educational group the differences between metropolitan and nonmetropolitan areas are insignificant with respect to the time when mothers first receive medical care.[13]

Age and Parity

Furthermore, there is a differential by age and parity; women in the younger age group tend to come later than women in the other age groups. This may be owing to the fact that the highest rates of illegitimacy are in the youngest age groups. Both the young mother and the unwed mother tend to be late-comers to prenatal care. Multiparas who have had little trouble with previous pregnancies also tend to come later and be more lax in keeping appointments.

Additional Factors in the Use of Maternity Services

The issues discussed here are also related to the changing relationships between the client–patient and the providers of maternity services, physicians and nurses. Walker has succinctly summarized the changes in maternity nursing caused by changing social factors and consumer demands.[13] She notes, as we have, the use of different terminology in the profession from "obstetrical nursing" to "maternity nursing" to "family-centered maternity care." Consumers complain that it is becoming more and more difficult to find a primary care physician who will give them the personal attention they want. Regardless of the social class level of the woman, it is very difficult for her to receive continuity of care from the personnel who provide maternity services. Regardless of its other merits, group practice sometimes disrupts the relationship between patient and physician; hospital structure requires nursing personnel to change with shift changes; patients have difficulty determining the status of the person in the medical office to whom they are speaking on the telephone. Patients feel that the obstetrician seems to relinquish his responsibility for the neonate during the post-partum period. Similarly, in this period, the pediatrician (from the mother's perspective) does not appear to be centrally involved with the needs of the mother. All of these features of the medical care system are reflected in the concept of "fragmented health care" and consumer dissatisfaction.

Consumer Satisfaction

Consumer satisfaction, that is, the satisfaction of pregnant women, refers to the attitudes toward the medical care system of those who have experienced a contact with the system. It is different from the medical and health beliefs of the patient in that it is concerned with the satisfaction of the patient with the quantity or quality of care actually received. There are several dimensions to this concept including (1) accessibility-convenience of services (convenience of care and emergency care); (2) availability (family physicians, hospitals, specialists, complete facilities); (3) continuity (regular family physician, same physician); (4) physician conduct (consideration of feelings, explanations, prudent risks, quality, regular checkup); (5) financial aspects (cost of services, insurance coverage, payment mechanisms). However, little is known about the relationship of these features of patient satisfaction to other social-psychological dimensions such as perceived health, values, psychological well-being, and general sentiments about life.

Communication

A crucial feature of this aspect of maternity care is the quality and quantity of patient-provider *communication*. Here we refer not only to the physician, but also to the nurse in communicating with the patient and her needs. One of the more important transactions that occurs in the provider-patient relationship is effective communication from the provider to the patient concerning the nature of the patient's condition and the actions to be taken. The degree to which the patient has understood the physician and can verbalize the physician's advice and instructions depends on the quality of the relationship.[14] Similarly, good medical care results in communication from the patient to the physician. In particular, the degree to which the patient's concerns, worries, and fears about her condition have been perceived by the physician are equally important.

Commentators on the physician-patient relationship frequently have discussed the social class and value differences between providers and patients as one barrier to communication and ultimately to utilization of medical services. Numerous studies have demonstrated that working-class patients tend to be diffident in questioning physicians, especially about their health or illness condition. These studies indicate that middle-class patients tend to obtain most of their information about illness by asking their physicians and nurses direct questions. In contrast, working-class patients receive their information from a passive process in which they are given information without asking; they also tended to receive less information.[15]

Despite their reluctance to request information, working-class maternity patients are not much different from upper-class patients in their desire for information.[12] Although upper-class patients may desire more technical details regarding their health condition, there is no general social class difference in patients' desires for as much information as possible presented in nontechnical language.

Part of the issue of better communication between provider and patient results from a reflection of a general social class difference in language use which was alluded to previously. Working-class patients sense that physicians do not expect them to ask questions; they tend to hold the physicians in awe, and there is social distance. But even middle-class patients hesitate to freely communicate with their physician about troublesome problems or symptoms. A virtual legend has been created by the media about the hard-working, busy physician. It has become generally accepted throughout our society that all physicians are extremely busy professionals. Thus, although there may be some apparent social class differences in the quantity and quality of communication with physicians, it is a matter of degree of communication.

The Role of the Nurse as Communicator

Given this situation, the maternity nurse has a crucial role to play. By and large the nurse is not perceived by the patient in the same manner as the physician. Patients perceive the nurse as filling a substantially different role, with accompanying differences in expectations. Thus, the nurse has an opportunity to fill a much-needed role in the delivery of health care by seizing the initiative and closing the communication gap in the patient-provider relationship. Such action would be congruent with patient expectations; moreover, several studies have indicated that the nurse can perform roles involving the receiving and giving of information to patients far more effectively than physicians.[13]

These problems of communication have been emphasized here because, among other things, the patient's perceived difficulties in communicating with medical providers has a direct influence upon the use of health services.

References

1. Parsons T: Definitions of health and illness in the light of American values and social structure. In Parsons T (ed): Social Structure and Personality, pp 257–291. Glencoe, IL, The Free Press, 1964

2. McKinlay JB: The new latecomers for antenatal care. British Journal of Preventive Social Medicine 24:52, 1970

3. Hutter M: The Changing Family: Comparative Perspectives. New York, John Wiley & Sons, 1981

4. Blake J: Coercive pronatalism and American population policy. In Davis E (ed): International Population and Urban Research Berkeley, pp 17–22. Berkeley, University of California Press, 1972

5. Rossi A: Transition to parenthood. Journal of Marriage and Family 30:33, 1968

6. Bumpass LL, Westoff CF: The "perfect contraceptive" population. Science 1969:1177, 1970

7. Lipman–Blumen J: Demographic trends and issues in women's health. In Olesen V (ed): Women and Their Health: Research Implications for a New Era. Washington, D.C., HEW, #HRA 77-3138, 1977

8. Pakter J et al: Impact of the liberalized abortion law in New York City on pregnancy associated death: A two-year experience. Bull NY Acad Med 49:804–818, 1972

9. Wright NH: Family planning and infant mortality rate death decline in the United States. Am J Epidemiol 101:182–187, 1975

10. Strauss AL: Medical organization, medical care in lower-income groups. Soc Sci Med 3:143–177, 1969

11. Hyman H: The value systems of different classes. In Bendix R, Lipset S (eds): Class, Status, and Power, pp 426–442. Gencoe, IL, The Free Press, 1953

12. Milio N: Values, social class and community health services. Nurs Res 16, 1, Winter 1967

13. Walker L: Providing more relevant maternity services. JOGN Nurs, Mar/April, 34–36, 1974

14. Waitzkin H, Stoeckle JD: The communication of information about illness. Adv Psychosom Med 8:180–215, 1972

15. Pratt L et al: Physicians' views on the level of medical information among patients. Am J Public Health 47:1277–1283, 1975

Suggested Reading

Abril IF: Mexican American folk beliefs: How they affect health care, MCN 2,3:168–173, 1977

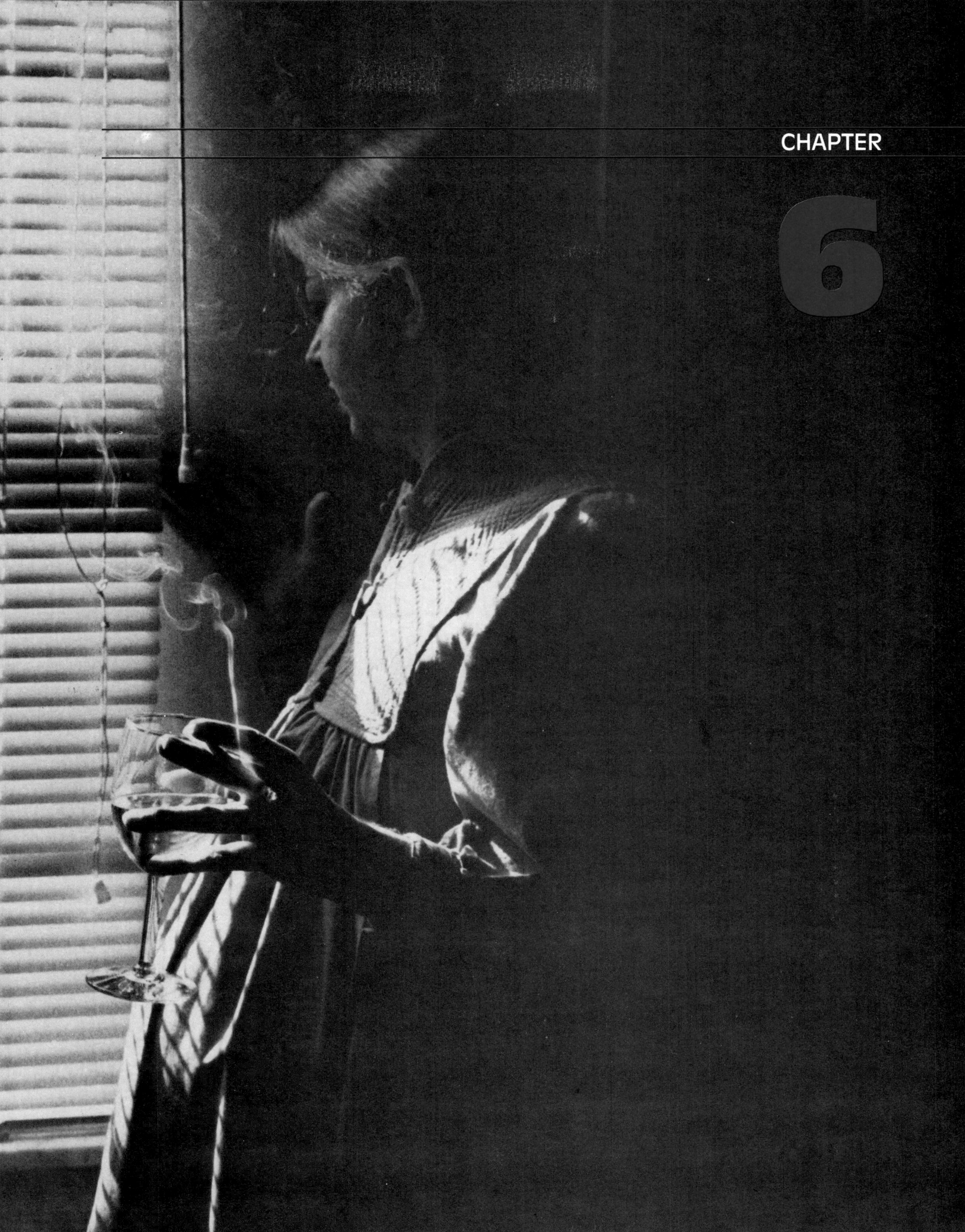

CHAPTER 6

CHAPTER 6

Social Risk Factors and Reproductive Outcomes

In this chapter the focus is upon selected risk factors that are associated with such reproductive outcomes as infant and maternal mortality, low birth weight, and other complications of pregnancy.

Sociodemographic Risk Factors

Maternal Age

The relationship between the age of the mother and infant mortality has been observed many times in the past and continues to hold true.[1] These findings indicate that there are higher mortality rates among infants of both the older primipara and multipara mother and among those of very young mothers. Moreover, there is a strong correlation between socioeconomic status and age of mother. Births to parents with more education or higher family income tend to occur to older mothers. The lower the socioeconomic status, the greater the tendency for the mother to be younger.[2]

Although women age 35 and over account for only about 5% of all births in the United States and statistics reveal that the number of births to women over 40 was 33,804 out of the total number of 3,136,965 live births, births to these women are viewed with interest and apprehension because they have come to be viewed as "high risk."[3,4] Heretofore attention has usually been focused on the maternal rather than the fetal results. More recently, because of the availability of sophisticated antenatal fetal assessment technology, the focus has gravitated to the fetal risk. Older women are considered "high risk" because they have more chance of neonatal mortality and morbidity, maternal mortality and morbidity, and spontaneous abortion.[5–7]

Thus, age and parity are two biological categories that have specific social significance since they contribute to a general picture of poor reproductive outcomes for both mother and infant. The role of the maternity nurse becomes particularly important here in terms of counseling women with respect to the problems they may encounter in such late pregnancies and the risks associated with some of the antenatal diagnostic techniques. Some popular articles give the impression that these diagnostic tests somehow cure fetal defects and can make pregnancy safer.[8,9] This is erroneous and the mother and father need to be apprised of the limitations associated with these tests. They are not a panacea for a safe pregnancy outcome. They are useful because they can determine if some fetal defects do exist and thus, the parents have the option of an abortion. They can also give a good indication of the age and well-being of the fetus, which helps if early delivery is indicated. Thus, these parents need meticulous antepartal care from all health providers as well as careful patient education, particularly from the nurse.

Teenage Pregnancy

Adolescent pregnancy is one of the problems associated with maternal age. Notable among the social and health costs of these pregnancies are the following: (1) about one half of school age mothers will have a subsequent unwanted pregnancy within two years of the birth of the first child; (2) evidence indicates that approximately 60% of those who had their first baby at school age become welfare recipients; (3) young mothers have a disproportionate number of babies of low birth weight, which is associated with mental retardation and other handicapping conditions; (4) problems associated with pregnancy are particularly acute in mothers age 15 and younger.[10]

We cannot consider this issue systematically without placing it within a broader social context. The teenage sexual revolution is related to a number of concurrent trends. For example, there is an increased number and proportion of births to women under age 20. One third of all births are to girls 17 or younger and about two fifths of these births are out of wedlock.[2] Thus, we shall consider out-of-wedlock births jointly with the problems of teenage or adolescent pregnancy.

Out-of-Wedlock Births. Out-of-wedlock birthrates have been increasing since 1940 among girls age 19 and younger. Among nonwhite individuals the birth rates for girls age 14 increased between 1940 and 1950 but have been rather stable since then. Similarly, there are variations for both white and nonwhites in the period 1940 to 1976; the rate for nonwhites seems to be declining recently, but the rate for whites appears to have risen steadily since 1940. The fact that the rate continues to increase is considered prima facie proof of increased sexual activity of revolutionary proportions.[11] In a definitive study of the problem, however, Cutright casts doubt on this conclusion.[12]

There are alternative explanations for rising out-of-wedlock births in addition to the simple one of a sexual revolution. In an examination of this issue, Cutright suggests that recent health status changes may explain a great deal of the recent increase in teenage out-of-wedlock births. He presents evidence of two health status changes—those that affect the ability of young girls to conceive (fecundity) and those that affect their capacity to avoid spontaneous abortion.

In addition, Cutright examined the interrelationships of customs, laws, and mean age of menarche. Data indicate that the mean age of menarche has decreased in the United States and western Europe. There is a general agreement that one major factor responsible for the decline is improved nutrition and health during preadolescent years.[12] Recent research suggests that improved nutrition increases the rate of physical growth, which in turn, decreases the age of menarche.[13]

Problems in Teenage Pregnancies. Childbearing at any age is a momentous event. For the teenager, however, it is often accompanied by a different set of problems from those experienced by older mothers. For very young mothers, at least those under age 15, risks that the baby will be stillborn, die soon after birth, or be born with a low birth weight, are much higher than those for women in their 20s.

The relationship of infant mortality to maternal age has been noted earlier. In a recently published study, matching infants' death certificates to infants' birth certificates, the National Center for Health Statistics reported that, at all ages, the infant mortality rate is considerably higher among nonwhites than among whites.[14] Moreover, neonatal mortality in infants of young mothers is much higher than that for infants of older mothers in both groups.

The increased risk of low birth weight may be the most important medical aspect of teenage pregnancy. Increased mortality risk is only one of the dangers facing infants of low birth weight. There are apparent linkages to epilepsy, cerebral palsy, mental retardation, and to higher risks of deafness and blindness.[2]

Various studies are not conclusive about the relationship of age of the mother to the intelligence of the child or physical and mental handicaps. Despite this inconclusiveness, these data document that the infant born to a teenage mother has a much higher risk of suffering severe handicaps than infants of older mothers.

For the mother, there are increased risks of complications of pregnancy, including toxemia, prolonged labor, and iron-deficiency anemia. Poor diets, inadequate prenatal care, and immaturity are probably all contributing factors. The primary concern appears to be with social rather than biological factors.[2]

The Role of the Perinatal Team. What is the role of the health professional in preventing early childbearing? Any action must start with the assumption that these are not inevitable consequences. Many women wanted to become mothers but the data indicate that a substantial proportion wish that their first child had come later.[15] What then might be the goals for dealing with adolescent pregnancy? Hayes and Crovitz have delineated two phases in goal setting for this population—(1) providing optimal services for adolescent unwed mothers and their families and (2) helping make real the option of "more mature" parenthood for adolescents in general.[16]

In the first phase of providing services, the researchers suggest that inexpensive pregnancy testing be made available by a nonjudgmental, well trained staff who can inform the adolescent of the options available to her—termination of the pregnancy, adoption, or keeping the infant. Details of the advantages and disadvantages of each option as well as how to go about each option also need to be discussed. Each visit is to be personalized so that realistic short-term goals are set, preferably by the same health personnel.

Temporary foster home care is another facet of services. For the youngster who wishes to keep her infant but cannot manage adequate baby sitting to allow her to continue school or get a job, this service is a life saver.

A third service would be a comprehensive team approach to antepartal care which includes the services of an array of personnel including a pediatrician who would be available for infant follow up and to give anticipatory guidance as needed. Group educational and counseling services are recommended so that the adolescent takes responsibility for self-care and feels free to interact with professionals. Self-esteem is enhanced and marketable skills are acquired. Thus, astute physical care as well as comprehensive counseling with referral to needed services lies within the purview of this perinatal team. It is also essential that the mother be encouraged to remain in either the public school system or in affiliated schools especially for pregnant adolescents.[16] Punitive efforts on the part of school systems to deprive the adolescent of schooling are anachronistic and have not worked in controlling the problem of unwed adolescent pregnancy.[17]

In the second phase, helping the younger generation realize "mature parenthood," the emphasis is on prophylaxis. Hayes and Crovitz suggest that there be early education in the area of life and health sciences. Ideally, there should be periodic parent–child discussions that begin as soon as the child expresses curiosity about sex and related matters and can comprehend accurate explanations. They recommend introduction of simple material as early as the third grade with the content becoming more complex and detailed as the child grows. The overriding object is to assure that by the time the child is a teenager, he or she has a clear understanding of how fertilization occurs and the events from fertilization through delivery and the postpartum periods, including both the biological and social consequences of pregnancy. In addition, the education should be handled by those knowledgeable and skilled in discussion groups. Parents need to be encouraged and given the chance to participate in these discussions.[16] See the chart below.

We cannot close this discussion without recognizing that knowledge, accessibility and contraceptive technology are not the only variables in adolescent pregnancy. More than one study has documented that a large proportion of young mothers say that they had not used contraception because they did not care whether or not they became pregnant.[2,18] Thus, some do not appear to be motivated to take advantage of the opportunities to control their fertility, no matter how accessible they are. Altering their motivation appears to be a major undertaking for society

Socioeconomic and Ethnic Indicators of Risk

Certain indicators of socioeconomic status such as family income, education of mother and father, and ethnicity can be risk factors in pregnancy. Low-income individuals are considerably more predisposed to lowered health status and obstetrical complications during pregnancy. Low birth weight is particularly prevalent in the lowest socioeconomic status groups, especially the black population. The role of ethnicity becomes readily apparent when one analyzes data which have accrued since 1935 on racial background. Throughout this period marked differences have occurred on the basis of racial background, with nonwhites faring much worse than whites. Indeed, the relative differential has actually risen during this period. The racially related differentials in mortality have also been noted beyond the first year of life. It should be stressed that virtually all of the racially related differentials in mortality are socioeconomically related.[19]

Undernutrition

One of the most important sequelae of low-socioeconomic status is undernutrition. Government studies have revealed that, compared to more affluent persons, the poor are twice as deficient in four essential diet ingredients. Most striking, poor persons had about four times as much clear-cut iron deficiency anemia and twice as many borderline cases as had the nonpoor. In three categories of essential diet ingredients—vitamin A, vitamin C, and riboflavin—the poor were found to have about twice as much of the clear-cut deficiency as the nonpoor. The survey also found a greater percentage of low height and weight measurements for children living below the poverty line than for those who were more affluent.[20]

Obviously, there is a complex interaction between undernutrition, poverty, and other environmental or genetic factors.

Health Care Goals for the Pregnant Adolescent

Optimal Health Services

1. Inexpensive pregnancy testing
2. Information regarding placement options
3. Information regarding operationalizing an option
4. Temporary foster home care for the infant
5. Comprehensive perinatal team approach providing for continuity of care, which includes obstetrician, pediatrician, perinatal nurses, and nutritionists skilled with adolescents
6. Educational and personal group experience which convey information and support for developmental and educational needs
7. Encourage parents to complete education
8. Supportive measures for enhancing self-esteem and developing marketable skills

Realization of Mature Parenthood

1. Emphasize anticipatory guidance before pregnancy occurs (prophylaxis)
   a. Early education in the life and health sciences
   b. Periodic parent–child discussion sessions regarding facts about sexuality
   c. Continue education during teen years to ensure accurate information regarding sexual facts and responsible sexuality
   d. Continual participation of parents

Effects on Fetal Brain Development. Studies have shown that deficiencies in the diet of a pregnant woman can have profound effects on a number of pregnancy outcomes (Fig. 6-1). For example, it has been shown that nutritional and genetic factors may interact during prenatal development with consequent irreversible results on the development of the baby's brain. This is one of the most important recent discoveries in the field of mental retardation. It is estimated that one tenth of the children born today are seriously affected as a consequence of malnutrition. Recent work at the former National Institute of Health suggests that there is a correlation between the level of the amino acids in the blood of a pregnant woman and the subsequent intelligence of her baby.

Low Birth Weight. Undernutrition has been identified as one of the causes of low-birth-weight infants born to poor urban mothers.[20] Extremely low birth weights have been reported among poorly fed groups in Asia and Africa. The relationship between low birth weight and malnourished populations may be more complex than a simple nutritional explanation. Rather than dietary deficiency in pregnancy, one specific factor, the small size of the baby, may reflect long-term maternal undernutrition dating back to the early childhood of the woman. Conceivably, malnutrition over many generations in underdeveloped societies may have favored the emergence of genetically different kinds of women with lower dietary requirements. This, however, is highly speculative and needs much carefully designed research to confirm such a possibility.

Hypertensive Disorders. The effect of socioenvironmental influences was most dramatically illustrated during World War II in Great Britain. During this period, the mortality from the pregnancy hypertensive disorders (toxemias) fell dramatically. The underlying reason for the drop in mortality resulting from this condition in England and Wales was that large numbers of women were evacuated from their homes in the cities into the country. The antenatal clinics were understaffed and improvisational. The major advantage brought about by this change of social environment was that the rationing system benefited expectant and nursing mothers and children. For the first time, women of the lower socioeconomic groups were fed as well as other population groups. Suffice to say that these disorders as a syndrome are most commonly seen in poor and badly nourished populations and that there is some evidence that the incidence has been modified by environmental changes, either situational or behavioral.[21]

The Role of the Nurse. What can be done to improve the nutritional and other risk factors associated with socioeconomic status and ethnic groups? Clearly, the role of the maternity nurse is relatively limited but not inactive. The nurse can be a force both

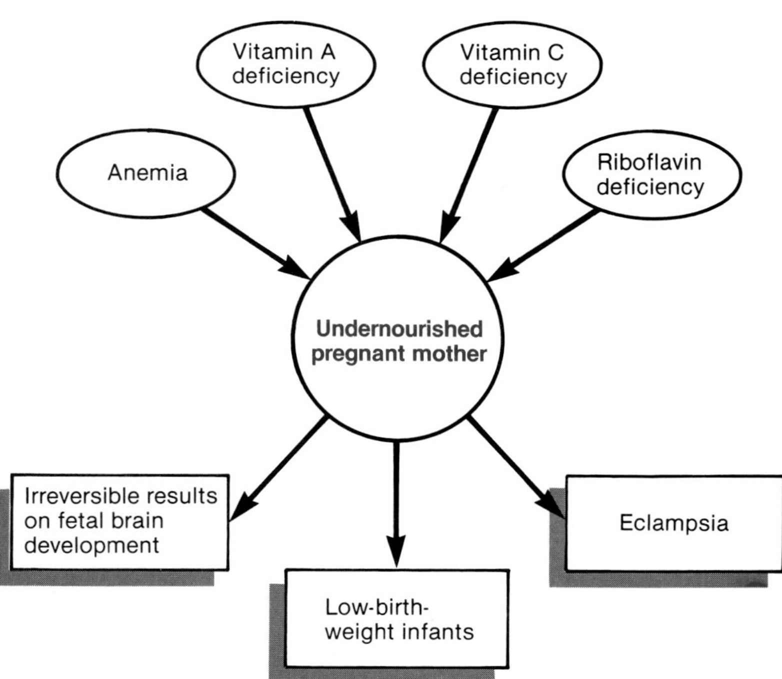

Figure 6-1.
Some of the effects of undernutrition on pregnancy outcomes.

in the community and in the clinic setting to help improve preventive services to those at highest risk because of situational factors. Better ways can be devised to use the nurse and other health personnel to provide health education to the individuals at risk. This assumes that the nurse herself is equipped with the knowledge concerning nutrition and other precursors of problems of pregnancy to provide the appropriate knowledge to the patient. Moreover, the nurse can be a positive force in the community to exert influence on other institutions such as the schools, health departments, government agencies, and voluntary agencies to provide preventive measures to the population at greatest risk.

Behavioral Risk Factors

Up to now, the discussion has been concerned primarily with factors that are not easily controlled by the nurse or other health personnel. A person's social position in society cannot be easily influenced by nursing intervention. As the following section will show, however, the risk factors of smoking and substance abuse are mutable, and hence, the nurse can have a greater degree of influence on the patient.

Smoking

In recent years literature has grown substantially, reflecting a heightened awareness of the important and substantial effects of smoking on pregnancy outcome. Earlier studies demonstrated that mothers who smoked cigarettes had smaller babies than nonsmoking mothers and subscribed this finding to the direct effect of smoking.

Unfortunately, cigarette smoking continues to be popular among women of childbearing age and many of these women are not being advised by their physicians to stop. It is estimated that one half of pregnant women smoke.[22] Much of the research to date has focused on the relationship of maternal smoking to fetal and infant outcomes. Diebel has pointed out, however, that smoking has direct effects on the maternal organism which in turn affects the fetus. The metabolism of several minerals including calcium, a variety of vitamins, hormones, glucose, fatty acids, and amino acids may all be interfered with by smoking.[23]

Recent evidence, based on prospective studies and other well-designed research, has substantiated the fact that fetal size, growth, and mortality are related to smoking of cigarettes by the mother. According to the United States Public Health Service, some 4600 stillbirths each year in the United States probably can be attributed to women's smoking habits. Research indicates that women who smoke have a 30% higher rate of stillbirths than those who do not. These women also have a 26% higher rate of perinatal mortality.[24]

A pòsitive association between maternal cigarette smoking and reduced infant birth weight emerges from every study of these two characteristics. The hypothesis that the relationship between smoking and weight reduction in the infant is one of cause and effect is supported by several types of evidence. This relationship has been consistently observed in a wide variety of populations differing by geographical location, race, and social and economic circumstances. Furthermore, there is an inverse relationship between mean birth weights and the number of cigarettes smoked during pregnancy, an evident dose–response effect.[24]

However, there have been a few studies that have not confirmed these findings. Since smoking is a preventable behavior, the focus of concern is to determine whether babies who would otherwise be alive and healthy might die, before or after birth, because their mothers smoked.[25]

Meyer and her colleagues found that mothers who are young, reasonably healthy, having their first or second child, and smoking less than a pack of cigarettes a day have an increased risk of perinatal loss of less than 10%. "At the other extreme, heavy smokers who are high parity, public patients, those who have had previous premature births, or whose hemoglobin is under 11 g have an increased risk of perinatal loss of over 70%. Other groups are intermediate—perinatal mortality increased with maternal smoking, with the magnitude of increase ranging from 4% to 97%." Thus, their data suggest that maternal smoking may interact with other factors in its influence on perinatal mortality.[26]

Meyer and her associates have further examined the contrary evidence from other studies and suggest that these selected studies study populations that were, in one way or another, not typical of the general population or did not impose appropriate statistical controls on the study population.[26]

Thus, in conclusion, the weight of evidence indicates that maternal smoking during pregnancy increases the infant's perinatal morbidity and mortality risk. This risk increases directly with the number of cigarettes smoked. The presence or absence of other risk factors alters the risk.

The Role of the Nurse

The implications for prevention are clear. Counseling the patient at the first visit, particularly in the case of mothers with other risk factors, can be done by the maternity nurse. Health education, although it needs to begin early in life, must be an essential part of prenatal care and smoking is one behavior that is preventable. Moreover, the nurse can provide an appropriate role model for the mother and father through her own behavior.

Drugs

There has been considerable interest in the potential genetic and teratogenic effects of a variety of foods and drugs for the mother and her offspring. Teenagers and young adults now comprise the majority of the population for whom this interest applies. Many of these patients will admit to use of drugs or else give some evidence of drug use. Detection of maternal addiction is based on history or physical evidence of administration, particularly puncture marks.

The true prevalence of drug-addicted mothers is unknown. But the indications are that, in large urban centers at least, the ratio of drug-addicted mothers to total deliveries has increased in the past 20 years. This is particularly true for those deliveries that take place in public hospitals.

Use of Services

Most drug-addicted patients are latecomers for prenatal care. Indeed, most patients delay until they feel that they are ready for delivery in order to avoid a long labor without drugs and in order to satisfy their need for a last "fix" before submitting to "authority." As a result, there is evidence that a substantial proportion of deliveries to this population occurs at home, in the ambulance, or on the stretcher.[27] This is especially true of the heroin addict. Also, addicts make considerable efforts to nourish their addiction during enforced periods of confinement in a hospital. Such patients will either hide the drug or obtain it from others in or outside the hospital. A portion of these patients supplement their supply with barbiturates or tranquilizers.

Another unfortunate complication is that very often the drug abusing mother is also an alcohol abuser as well as a smoker. The combination of these three risk factors can have dire results for perinatal outcomes in both mother and infant.[28]

Effect on Mother and Infant

As far as heroin addicts are concerned, there is some difficulty in evaluating the data on total length of labor, but available evidence indicates that labor is not prolonged. Greatest difficulties tend to occur after delivery when withdrawal in the infant and mother is a risk factor. Symptoms of withdrawal in the mother include nausea, tremors, sweats, abdominal pain, cramps, and yawning. (Chapter 44 discusses withdrawal symptoms in the infant.)

The attitude of the medical and nursing staff becomes a critical factor at this stage. The pregnancy outcomes of heroin-addicted mothers are typical of any nutritionally deprived groups of low-socioeconomic status receiving inadequate prenatal care, with one important exception, congenital addiction of the baby.[29]

There is some suggestion in the literature that narcotic use by the mother may lead to intrauterine growth retardation. The long-term effects on growth and development are now being observed and evaluated in at least one prospective study. As yet, the effects of narcotic addiction on the reproductive process are not clearly reflected in our standard measures of maternal and perinatal mortality rates. Available evidence indicates that the addicted individual, even after withdrawal, detoxification, or rehabilitation, remains at risk in that subsequent intake, even years later, may result in the immediate urge for more drugs.

Thus, a pregnant woman who is a user of narcotic drugs of unknown potency and amount is carrying a potentially addicted fetus, and while detoxification of the newborn infant seems to be initially successful, a detoxified baby is still a problem infant. Even with use of methadone in the management of the pregnant addict, it is possible to magnify the effects on the fetus.[29]

It is important to note that the problem of drug *usage,* as distinct from drug addiction, is of considerable magnitude. Although the former is seen more often in private and community hospitals, the addictive patient is a growing problem there also. It is increasingly apparent that our *drug-using* population is encompassing greater numbers of individuals from the middle- and upper-socioeconomic segments of our society. For these reasons, all maternal service personnel need to be familiar with both the maternal and neonatal aspects of drug use.[29]

Alcohol

Women cannot assume that it is safe to drink even small amounts of alcohol during pregnancy. Research in recent years is indicating that there is no "safe" level for alcohol consumption during this time. The Institute of Health has warned that an alcoholic intake of six drinks a day (3 oz of absolute alcohol) can lead to birth defects in the infant.[30]

Since ancient times, alcohol has been suspect as an agent of poor reproductive outcomes. In ancient Carthage, drinking was banned on the wedding night for fear of producing a defective child. In the 18th century a report to the English parliament called attention to the fact that the children of alcoholic mothers had a wizened, shriveled look. At the turn of the 19th century, Sullivan reported high perinatal mortality among the infants of 120 alcoholic women in the Liverpool jail. More recently, in 1968, Lemoine described a syndrome of prenatal and postnatal growth deficiency, mental retardation, developmental delay, cardiac defects, and a variety of skeletal–facial–limb pathology. Although he attributed these findings to the effects of maternal consumption of alcohol on the fetus *in utero,* his observations were neglected until Jones and associates coined the term "fetal alcohol syndrome" (FAS) in 1973. His description of the anomalies approximated that of Lemoine and subsequent studies document its existence.[31–33]

It is known that ethanol freely crosses the placental barrier, but it is not known whether or not it is the alcohol or the breakdown product (acetaldehyde) that causes the harm.[31]

This syndrome has become the third most commonly recognized cause of mental retardation in the United States, exceeded only by Down's syndrome and an incompletely enclosed spinal cord. It is estimated that the incidence is two to three per 1000 live births. As stated previously, it is characterized by mental retardation, low birth weight (2500 g or less), short stature, small head, and a variety of joint and heart defects, as well as fine motor dysfunctions (Fig. 6-2).[32]

It is important to note that a woman does not necessarily have to be an alcoholic to place her infant at risk for this condition. However, women who are chronic alcoholics run a much higher risk of having defective infants. Jones and Hansen found that women who drink 2 ounces to 4 ounces of hard liquor per day run a 10% risk of having an abnormal child. Women who drink 4 ounces or more per day have a 19% risk. If the average daily consumption is less than 2 ounces, the apparent risk is low but still present.[34]

Heavy alcohol consumption is most likely to affect fetal structure during the first trimester when organogenesis is taking place. Frequently abortion will take place. During the second trimester, when there is mostly an increase in cell size rather than cell volume, the infant's weight is most likely to be affected.

The Role of the Nurse

If the nurse suspects that her patient has a drinking problem or even drinks moderately but consistently, it is important that she explores her reasons for drinking and refers the mother for counseling if necessary. Often patients' lifestyles are such that "social drinking" is expected, and the mother may not realize the impact of her behavior on her fetus. The hazards of the syndrome can be clearly explained and various counseling and assistance avenues can be used.[35]

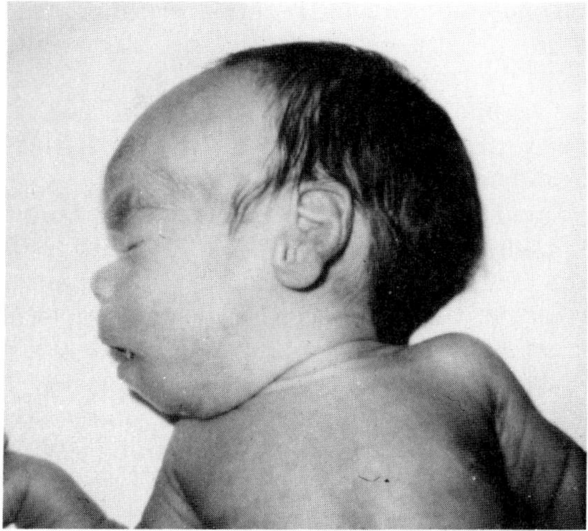

Figure 6-2.
Infants born with fetal alcohol syndrome exhibit an altered pattern of growth and development, low birth weight, short stature, small heads, and a variety of joint and heart defects, as well as mental retardation and fine motor dysfunctions.

Life Events and Life Crises as Risks

Life events and life crises in the sense used here refer to such events as divorce, illness, death of a significant other, such as a family member, and job loss, rather than to the occurrence of the actual pregnancy itself, although this too may be a factor in pregnancy outcome. Appropriate intervention by nursing staff can be especially effective in meeting the needs and reducing the risks associated with such life crises. The interest in the relationship between the psychological and social world of the individual and human disorders and disease have a long history. But even the findings of carefully designed and conducted investigations have not always yielded clear-cut and unambiguous results concerning this relationship. This is in sharp contrast to the dramatic results that have been obtained with animal experiments in which the various elements in the social environment have been correlated. Nevertheless, there is accumulating evidence of the intimate interaction between the social environment, physiological reactions, and pathological outcome in the individual. This is particularly true of the chronic diseases, such as heart disease and cancer.[36–38]

Data on the relationship between disorders of pregnancy and life changes and experiences that may be stressful are relatively scanty.

It should be clear that an outcome such as low birth weight is the result of multiple interactions between the human organism and the environment. As early as 1963, Gunter focused on the psychological and stressful environmental factors operative in the mother before conception and during pregnancy.[39] Almost ten years elapsed before another study appeared that was related to the Gunter study, although the importance of the variables had long been recognized and applied in research directed toward other problems.[40] The emphasis in Gunter's research was on critical life events that occurred before the onset of pregnancy, such as death within the immediate family of orientation or procreation; desertion by husband or by one or both parents of the subject; economic need; interpersonal problems, such as difficulties with husband (including divorce), difficulties with in-laws, family, or neighbors; and physical disability including illness, accident, and bodily harm incidents.

Gunter also had obtained data on events that occurred *during* the gestation period. She found that the "social and life situation of the mother are related to and may, in part, determine the outcome of pregnancy in terms of the birth weight of the infant."[39] A decade later, Nuckolls and her associates at North Carolina went beyond an attempt to assess only the effects of life experiences on pregnancy outcome. They included, in addition, the supportive or protective psychological or social elements of the patient, which was termed the adaptive potential for pregnancy (TAPPS). In short, Nuckolls and her group were attempting to assess the "balance" between the protective and the deleterious social and psychologic processes and the relationship of this balance to various health parameters of pregnancy and the puerperium.[40]

The results showed that considering the multiple life changes and the psychosocial assets separately, neither one alone was related to complications of pregnancy. When taken together, however, Nuckolls found that in the presence of mounting life changes, women with high psychosocial assets had only one third the complication rate of women whose psychosocial assets were low. In the absence of such life changes, particularly for the period before pregnancy, the level of psychosocial assets was irrelevant.

As these investigators point out, additional research is needed, but their data help to explain some of the discrepant results in literature. In short, the research and the approach cast serious doubt on the utility of specificity (as far as current clinical syndromes are concerned) in research concerned with psychosocial factors in disease etiology. Similar psychosocial factors may be related to different disease syndromes. At the present, this research approach is very promising and additional work needs to be done using this approach.

Attitudes and Emotions

Much has been written in recent years on the role of emotional and attitudinal factors and psychological stress during pregnancy, as these may be related to pregnancy outcomes. The evidence is inconclusive, but more important, much of it is based on poorly designed research and inadequate samples of the population at risk. Despite this poor state of affairs, there is a general consensus in medical science that psychological factors are in some way associated with various aspects of the maternity cycle. Indeed, some investigators have asserted that early psychological assessment of pregnant women holds promise of being predictive of the course and outcome of pregnancy. Most of the literature makes an attempt to measure the attitudes of the woman toward her pregnancy and to measure other psychosocial factors as these may influence the outcome.[41]

Surely there are attitudinal differences among women toward their individual pregnancies. There is also an intimate interaction between the psychological stress experienced by the person and psychological reactions, as Heinstien has noted.[41] Complications of pregnancy, labor, and delivery are obscured by this interaction. Thus, physiological changes and discomfort may trigger psychologically negative attitudes toward the pregnancy and, conversely, life stress may precipitate somatic problems.

There is no doubt that many, perhaps a majority, of women experience some psychological stress and anxiety during pregnancy. However, the literature in medical and nursing journals alike tends to assume that some of these conditions are psychosomatic or emotional in origin. In a paper critical of the cloudy thinking that has characterized such conditions as menstrual pain, nausea of pregnancy, and pain in labor, as caused or aggravated by psychogenic factors, Lennane and Lennane suggest sexual prejudice as the basis for such thinking. Such scientific evidence as exists clearly suggests organic causes for these conditions.[42]

The point here is that nurses must not unwittingly and uncritically accept long-established attitudes that are rooted in prejudice rather than in scientific evidence. Stereotypic thinking is not only poor in scientific terms, but, equally important, it tends to influence the course and quality of treatment of women patients.

The Role of the Nurse

Nursing staff has an important role to play in assisting the pregnant woman to use her psychosocial assets to the fullest in coping with the fears, anxieties, somatic complaints, and other problems associated with the pregnancy in the prenatal and intrapartal periods. Emotional and social support during and following the pregnancy cannot only be a comfort to the patient but may also assist in reducing problematic outcomes.

References

1. National Center for Health Statistics: Annual Summary for the United States, 1979 DHHS Publication No. (PHS) 81–1120 Monthly Vital Statistics Reports 28:13, Nov 13, 1980

2. Phipps–Yonas S: Teenage pregnancy and motherhood. Am J Orthopsychiatry 50,3:403–431, 1980

3. Hogan LR: Pregnant again—at 41. MCN 4:174–176, 1979

4. National Center for Health Statistics: Vital Statistics of the United States, 1973. Vol. 1, Natality (HRA) 77–1113. Washington, D.C., United States Government Printing Office 1977, 1–12

5. Jolly C et al: Research in the delivery of female health care: The recipient's reaction. Am J Obstet Gynecol 110,3:291–94, 1971

6. Bird CC, Mcelin TW: The premenopausal gravida: A study of 23 obstetrical patients age 45 and older. J Reprod Med 6:223–225, 1971

7. Biggs JS: Pregnancy at forty years and over. Med J. Aust 1:542–545, 1973

8. Siegal M: A first baby after 40—it's safer now. Parade: Sunday Supplement, pp 6–7. Detroit Free Press, Aug 1976

9. Calton L: Prenatal tests help cure defects and save babies. Parade: Sunday Supplement, pp 10–12. Detroit Free Press, April 1976

10. Card JJ, Wise LL: Teenage mothers and fathers: The impact of early childbearing on the parents' personal and professional lives. Fam Plann Perspect 10,4:199–205, 1978

11. Garmezy E: Communication on conception: A reply to Dr. Stearn. Social Work 14:101–102, 1969

12. Cutright P: Illegitimacy in the United States: 1920–1968. Final Report to the Commission on Population Growth and the American Future. Washington D.C., United States Government Printing Office, 1972

13. Tietze C: Teenage pregnancies: Looking ahead to 1984. Fam Plann Perspect 10,4:205–207, 1978

14. Infant mortality rates: Socioeconomic factors, United States. Series 24, No. 14, Vital Health Statistics. Washington, D.C., 1980

15. Presser H: Early motherhood: Ignorance or bliss. Fam Plann Perspect 6,1:8–14, 1974

16. Hayes L, Crovitz E: Adolescent pregnancy. South Med J 72,7:869–874, 1979

17. Chenoweth AD: The school-age pregnant girl (editorial). J Sch Health 41:347–348, 1976

18. Lindemann C: Birth Control and Unmarried Women. New York, Springer, 1974

19. Brooks CH: Social, economic and biologic correlates of infant mortality in city neighborhoods. J Health Soc Behav 21:2–12, 1980

20. Ten-State Nutrition Survey in the United States, 1968–1970. DHEW Publ. No. (HSM) 72–8129 through 72–8134, Washington D.C., 1972

21. Porapakkam SA: An epidemiologic study of eclampsia. Obstet Gynecol 4:26–36, 1979

22. Kretzehmar RM: Smoking and health: The role of the obstetrician gynecologist. Obstet Gynecol 55:403, 1980

23. Deibel P: Effects of cigarette smoking on maternal nutrition and the fetus. JOGN Nurs 9,6:333–336, 1980

24. United States Department of Health, Education and Welfare. A report of the Surgeon General. DHEW Publ No. (PHS) 79–50056, pp 1 ff. Washington, D.C., 1979

25. Lipman–Blumen et al; Maternal cigarette smoking and perinatal mortality. Am J Epidemiol 96:1–10, 1972

26. Meyer MB et al: The interrelationship of maternal smoking and increased perinatal mortality with other risk factors: Further analysis of the Ontario perinatal mortality study, 1960–61. Am J Epidemiol 100:443–452, 1974

27. Stone ML et al: Narcotic addiction in pregnancy. Am J Obstet Gynecol 109:716–723, 1971

28. Eriksson M et al: Abuse of alcohol, drugs and tobacco during pregnancy—consequences for the child. Paediatrician 8:228–242, 1979

29. Connaughton JF et al: Perinatal addiction: Outcome and management. Am J Obstet Gynecol 129:679–686, 1977

30. Alarm sounded on alcohol pregnancy. American College of Obstetrics & Gynecology Newsletter 21:3, 1977

31. Lindor E, McCarthy AM, McRae MG: Fetal alcohol syndrome: A review and case presentation. JOGN Nurs 9,4:222–228, 1980

32. Herrmann J et al: Tetraectrodactyles and other skeletal manifestations in the fetal alcohol syndrome. Eur J Pediatr 133:221–226, 1980

33. Clarren SK, Smith DW: The fetal alcohol syndrome. N Eng J Med 298:1063–1067, 1978

34. Jones KL et al: Pattern of malformation in offspring of chronic alcoholic mothers. Lancet 1:1267–1271, 1973

35. Luke B: Maternal alcoholism and fetal alcohol syndrome. Am J Nurs 12,12:1924–1926, 1977

36. Syme SL, Reeder LG (eds): Social stress and cardiovascular disease. The Milbank Memorial Fund Quarterly, April 1967

37. Gore S: The effect of social support in moderating the health consequences of unemployment. J Health Soc Behav 19:157–165, 1978

38. LaRocco JM, House JS, French JR Jr: Social support, occupational stress, and health. J Health Soc Behav 21:202–218, 1980

39. Gunter LM: Psychopathology and stress in the life experience of mothers of premature infants. Am J Obstet Gynecol 109:716–723, 1963

40. Nuckolls KB et al: Psychosocial assets, life crises and the prognosis of pregnancy. Am J Epidemiol 45:431–441, 1972

41. Heinstien MI: Expressed attitudes and feelings of pregnant women and their relations to physical complications of pregnancy. Merril–Palmer Quarterly 1:217–236, 1967

42. Lennane KJ, Lennane RJ: Alleged psychogenic disorders in women—A possible manifestation of sexual prejudice. N Engl J Med 6:288–292, 1973

Suggested Reading

Howley C: The older primipara, implications for nursing. JOGN Nurs 10,3:182–185, 1981

Lindor E, McCarthy AM, McRae MG: Fetal alcohol syndrome: A review and case presentation. JOGN Nurs 9,4:222–228, 1980

McCauley CS: Pregnancy After 35. New York, Elsevier–Dutton, 1976

Mercer R: Becoming a mother at sixteen. MCN 1,1:44–52, 1976

Peoples MD, Barrett A: A model for the delivery of health care to pregnant adolescents. JOGN Nurs 8,6:339–345, 1979

Silverstein B, Field S, Kozlowski LT et al: The availability of low-nicotine cigarettes as a cause of cigarette smoking among teenage females. J Health Soc Behav 21:383–388, 1980

UNIT II

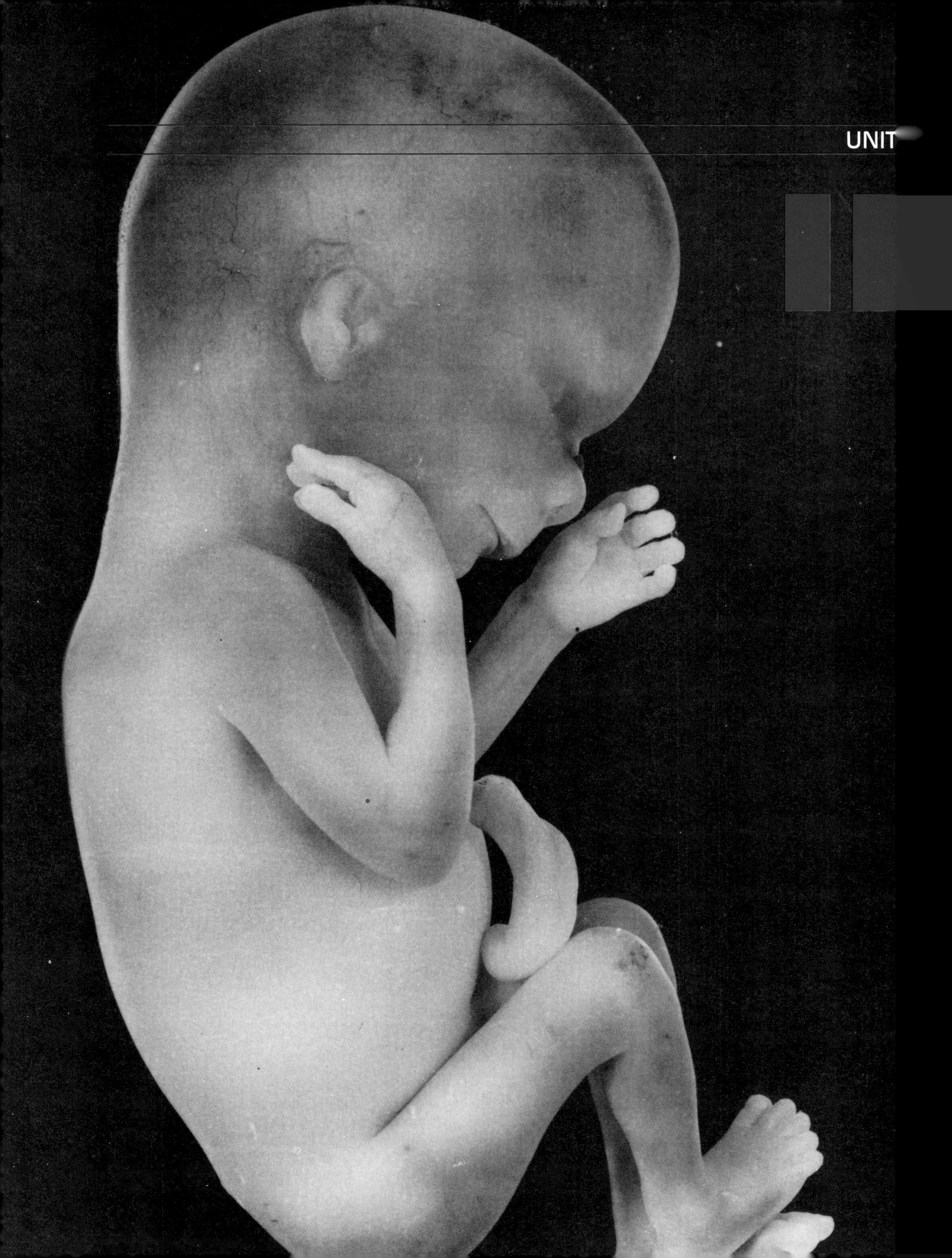

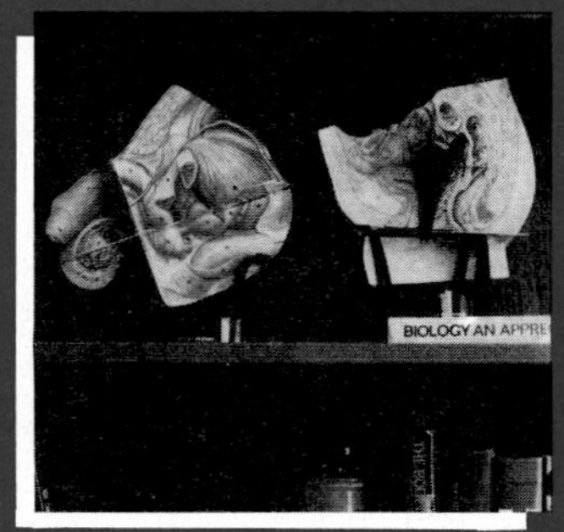

7
Sexual and Reproductive Anatomy

Pelvis

Female Organs of Reproduction

Mammary Glands

Male Organs of Reproduction

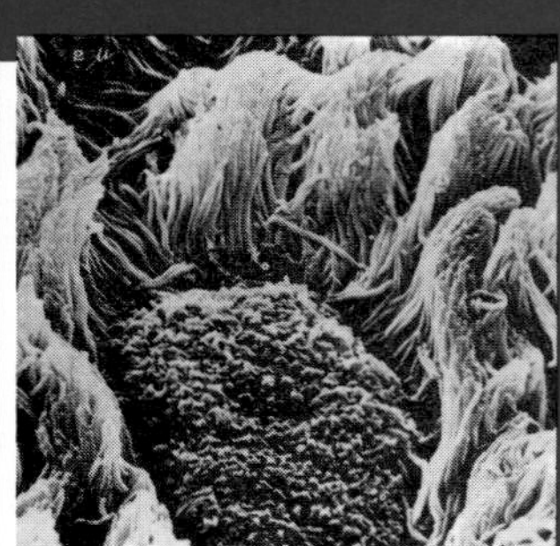

8
Sexual and Reproductive Physiology

Sexual Maturity

Menstrual Cycle

Bodily Manifestations of Ovarian Function

Menopause

Physiology of the Male Reproductive Tract

Female and Male Reproductive Capacity

Biophysical Aspects of Human Reproduction

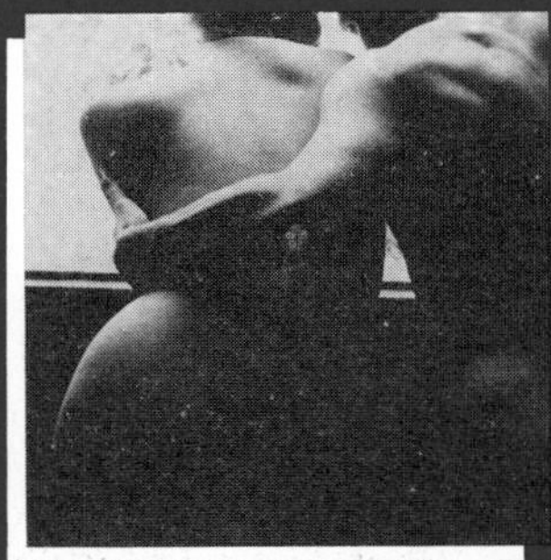

9 Human Sexual Response

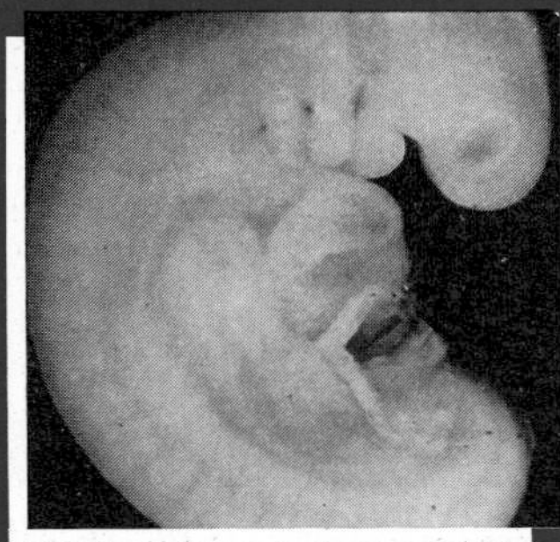

10 Conception and Ovum Development

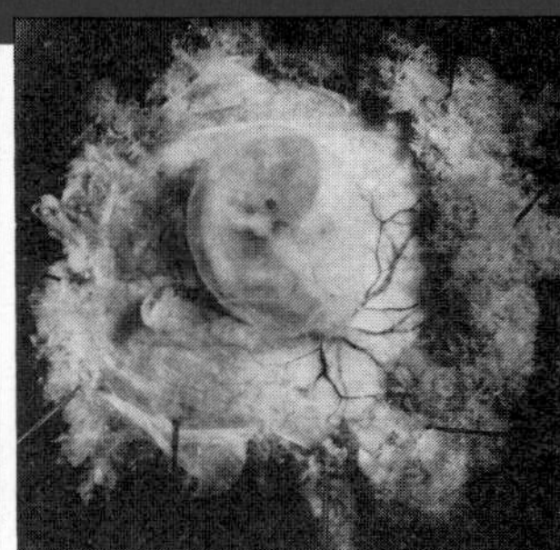

11 Development and Physiology of the Embryo and Fetus

CHAPTER 7

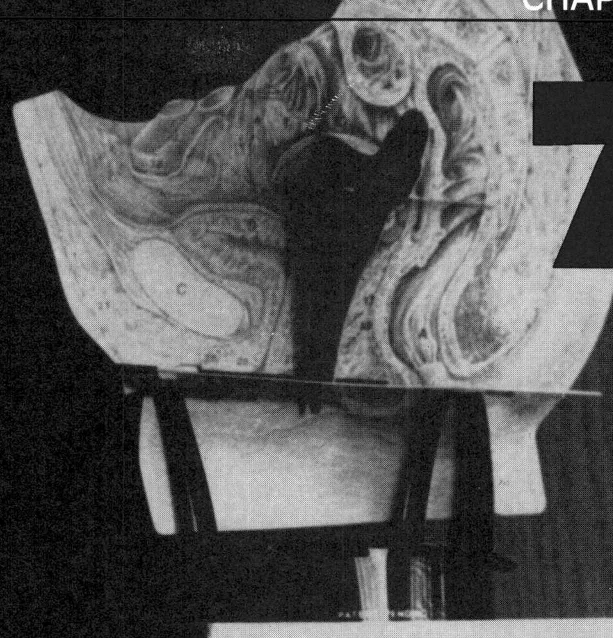

CHAPTER 7

Sexual and Reproductive Anatomy

- **Pelvis**
  - Bony Structure
  - Articulation and Surfaces
  - True and False Pelves
    - Pelvic Inlet
    - Pelvic Outlet
    - Pelvic Cavity
  - Pelvic Variations
  - Pelvic Measurements
    - Types of Pelvic Measurements
    - X-Ray Pelvimetry
- **Female Organs of Reproduction**
  - External Organs
  - Internal Organs
    - Ovaries
    - Fallopian Tubes
    - Uterus
    - Vagina
  - Related Pelvic Organs
    - Bladder
    - Anus
- **Mammary Glands**
  - Internal Structure
  - External Structure
- **Male Organs of Reproduction**
  - Penis
  - Testes
  - Transport of Spermatozoa

Pelvis

The pelvis, so named because of its resemblance to a basin, is a bony ring interposed between the trunk and the thighs. The vertebral column, or backbone, passes into the pelvis from above and transmits the weight of the upper part of the body to it. Then the pelvis in turn transmits weight to the lower limbs. From an obstetrical point of view, however, we must consider it as the cavity that contains the generative organs and, particularly, as the canal through which the fetus must pass during birth—the birth canal.

Bony Structure

The pelvis is made up of four united bones—the two hipbones (*os coxae* or innominate), situated laterally and in front, and the sacrum and the coccyx, situated behind (Fig. 7-1).

Anatomically, the hipbones are divided into three parts—the ilium, the ischium, and the pubis. These bones become firmly joined into one by the time the growth of the body is completed (*i.e.*, between the ages of 20 to 25) so that when the pelvis is examined, no trace of the original edges or divisions of these three bones can be discovered. Each of these bones may be briefly described as follows.

The *ilium,* the largest portion of the bones, forms the upper and back parts of the pelvis. Its upper flaring border forms the prominence of the hip, or crest of the ilium (hipbone).

The *ischium* is the lower part below the hip joint, and from it projects the tuberosity of the ischium, on which the body rests when in a sitting position.

The *pubis* is the front part of the hipbone; it extends from the hip joint to the joint in front between the two hipbones, the symphysis pubis, and then turns down toward the ischial tuberosity, thus forming, with the bone of the opposite side, the arch below the symphysis, the pubic or subpubic arch. This articulation of the two pubic bones encloses the pelvic cavity anteriorly.

The *sacrum* and the *coccyx* form the lowest portions of the spinal column. The sacrum is a triangular wedge-shaped bone that consists of five vertebrae fused together. It serves as the back part of the pelvis. The coccyx forms a tail end to the spine. In the child, the coccyx consists of four or five very small, separate vertebrae; in the adult these bones are fused into one. The coccyx is usually movable at the point of attachment to the sacrum, the sacrococcygeal joint, and may

Figure 7-1.
Front and lateral view of the pelvis showing major bones and articulations.

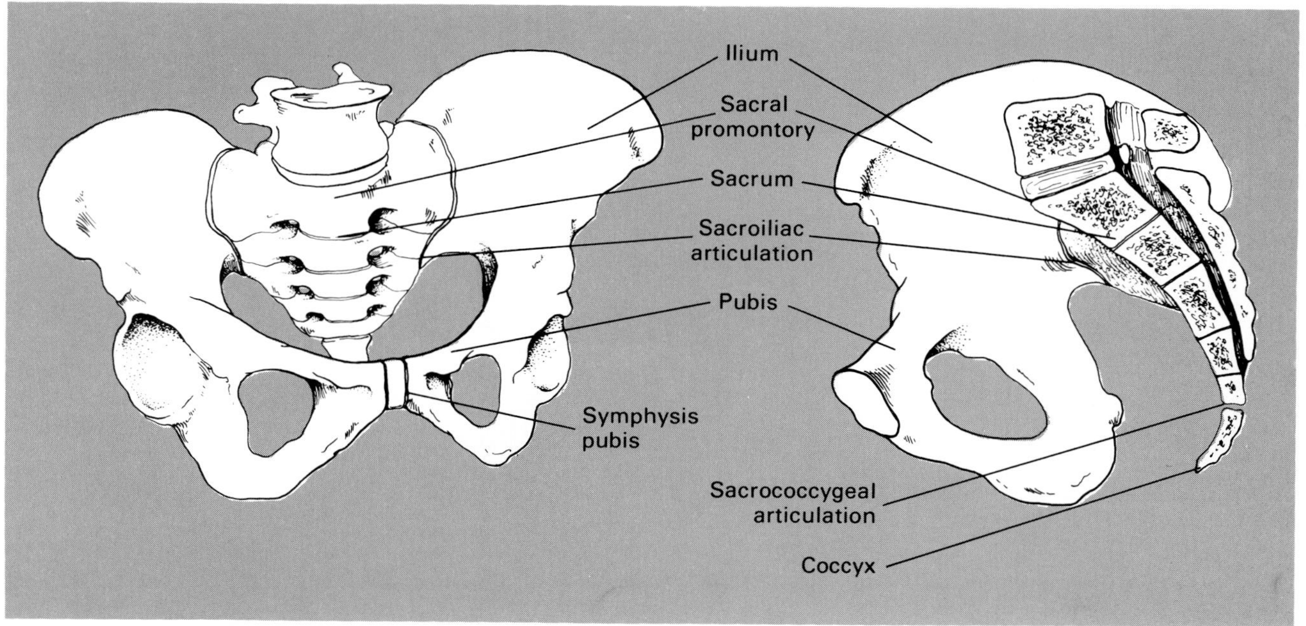

become pressed back during labor to allow more room for the passage of the fetal head.

The marked projection formed by the junction of the last lumbar vertebra with the sacrum is of special importance. This is the *sacral promontory,* one of the most important landmarks in obstetrical anatomy.

Articulation and Surfaces

There are four *articulations,* or joints of the pelvis, that have obstetrical importance. Two are behind, between the sacrum and the ilia on either side, and are termed the *sacroiliac articulations;* one is in front between the two pubic bones and is called the *symphysis pubis;* and the fourth is the *sacrococcygeal articulation,* located between the sacrum and the coccyx.

All of these articular surfaces are lined with fibrocartilage, which becomes thickened and softened during pregnancy; likewise, the ligaments that bind the pelvic joints together become softened, and as a result greater mobility of the pelvic bones develops. A certain definite, though very limited motion in the joints is desirable for a normal labor; however, there is no change in the actual size of the pelvis. From a practical standpoint, the increased mobility that these joints develop in pregnancy produces a slight "wobbliness" in the pelvis and throws greater strain on the surrounding muscles and ligaments. This accounts for much of the backache and legache in the latter months of pregnancy.

The pelvis is lined with muscular tissue that provides a smooth, somewhat cushioned surface which the fetus passes over during labor. These muscles also help to support the abdominal contents.

True and False Pelves

Regarded as a whole, the pelvis may be described as a two-story, bony basin that is divided into two parts by a natural line of division, the *inlet* or *brim.* The upper part is the false pelvis and the lower part is the true pelvis (Fig. 7-2A).

The *false pelvis,* or upper flaring part, is much less concerned with the problems of labor than is the true pelvis. It supports the uterus during late pregnancy and directs the fetus into the true pelvis at the proper time.

The *true pelvis,* or lower part, forms the bony canal through which the fetus must pass during parturition. For descriptive purposes it is divided into three parts—an inlet or brim, a cavity, and an outlet.

Pelvic Inlet

Continuous from the sacral promontory and extending along the ilium on each side in circular fashion is a ridge called the *linea terminalis,* or brim (Fig.7-2A). This bounds an area or plane, the *inlet,* so named because it is the entryway or inlet through which the fetal head must pass in order to enter the true pelvis.

The pelvic inlet, sometimes called the pelvic brim or superior strait, divides the false from the true

Figure 7-2.
(A) side view of true and false pelvis. *(B)* front view showing linea terminalis (pelvic brim).

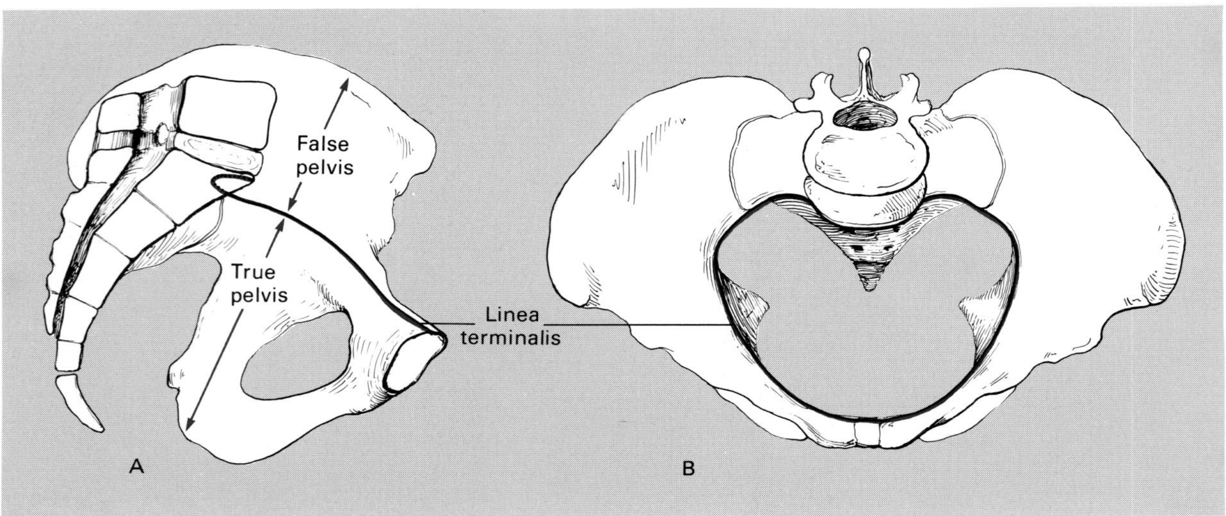

pelvis. It is heart shaped, and the promontory of the sacrum forms a slight projection into it from behind (Fig. 7-2B). Generally, it is widest from side to side, and narrowest from back to front (*i.e.,* from the sacral promontory to the symphysis). It should be noted that the fetal head enters the inlet of the average pelvis with its longest diameter (anteroposterior) in the transverse diameter of the pelvis (Fig. 7-3A). In other words, as shown in Figure 7-3B, the greatest diameter of the head accommodates itself to the greatest diameter of the inlet.

As the inlet is entirely surrounded by bone, it cannot be directly measured with the examining fingers in a living woman. However, the measurements of its anteroposterior diameter can be estimated on the basis of the diagonal conjugate diameter (see Fig. 7-7). The measurement of the diameters is very important, because variations from the normal (*e.g.,* smaller in size or flattened) may cause grave difficulty at the time of labor (see Chap. 25).

Pelvic Outlet

When viewed from below, the *pelvic outlet* is a space bounded in front by the symphysis pubis and the pubic arch, at the sides by the ischial tuberosities, and

Figure 7-3.
Views of pelvic inlet and outlet with fetal head in place. *(A)* Inlet of normal female pelvis showing transverse and anteroposterior diameters. *(B)* Largest diameter of the fetal head passing through the largest diameter of inlet; therefore, it enters transversely. *(C)* Pelvic outlet and sacrosciatic ligaments. *(D)* Largest diameter of the fetal head passing through the largest diameter of the outlet; therefore, it passes through anteroposteriorly.

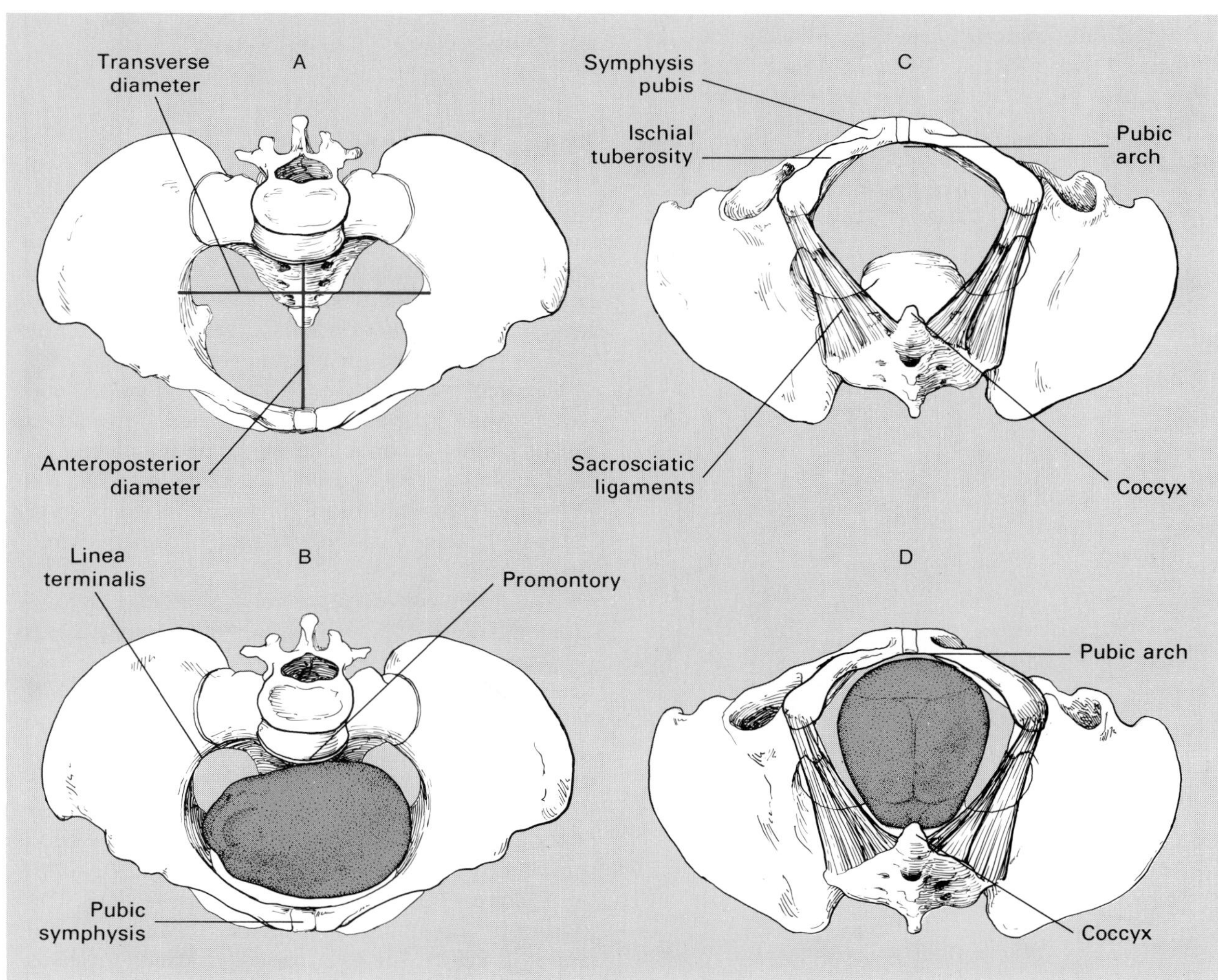

behind by the coccyx and the greater sacrosciatic ligaments (Fig. 7-3C). The front half of the outlet resembles a triangle, the base of which is the distance between the ischial tuberosities, and the other two sides of which are represented by the pubic arch. From an obstetrical point of view, this triangle is of great importance because the fetal head must use this space to exit from the pelvis and the mother's body (Fig. 7-3D). Nature has provided a wide pubic arch in females, whereas in males it is narrow (see Fig. 7-6). If the pubic arch in women was as narrow as it is in men, vaginal delivery would be extremely difficult because the fetal head, unable to traverse the narrow anterior triangle of the outlet, would be forced backward against the coccyx and the sacrum, where its progress would be impeded.

In the typical female pelvis, the greatest diameter of the inlet is the transverse (from side to side), whereas the greatest diameter of the outlet is the anteroposterior (from front to back, see Fig. 7-3A and 7-3C). As the fetal head emerges from the pelvis, it passes through the outlet in the anteroposterior position, again accommodating its greatest diameter to the greatest diameter of the passage. Since the fetal head enters the pelvis in the transverse position and emerges in the anteroposterior, it is obvious that it must rotate approximately 90° as it passes through the pelvis. This process of rotation is one of the most important phases of labor and will be discussed in more detail in a later chapter.

Figure 7-4.
Pelvic cavity showing plane of inlet and outlet. The direction the fetus takes through the pelvis is determined by the axis of the cavity.

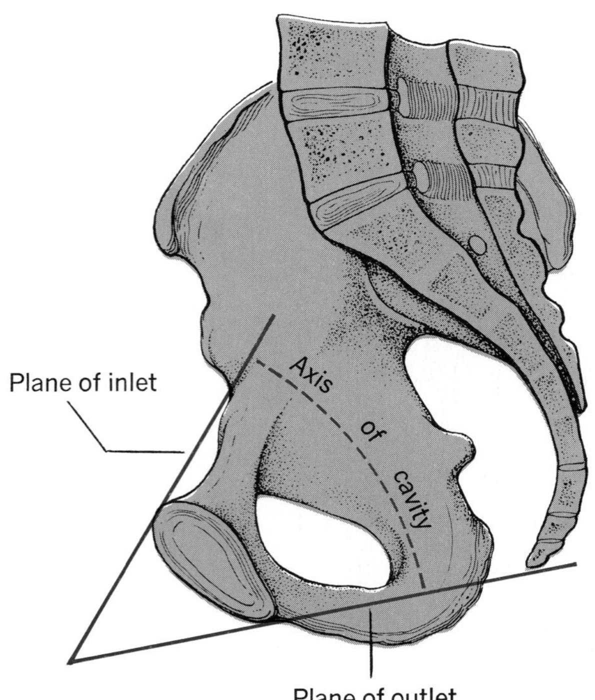

Pelvic Cavity

The *pelvic cavity* is the space between the inlet above, the outlet below, and the anterior, the posterior, and the lateral walls of the pelvis. The upper portion of the pelvic canal is practically cylindrical and the lower portion is curved. It is important to note the axis of the cavity when viewed from the side (Fig. 7-4). During delivery, the head must descend along the downward prolongation of the axis until it almost reaches the level of the ischial spines and then begins to curve forward. The axis of the cavity determines the direction that the fetus takes through the pelvis in the process of delivery. As might be expected, labor is made more complicated by this curvature in the pelvic canal because the fetus has to accommodate itself to the curved path as well as to the variations in the size of the cavity at different levels.

Pelvic Variations

The pelvis presents great individual variations—no two pelves are exactly alike. Even patients with normal measurements may present differences in contour and muscular development that influence the actual size of the pelvis. These differences are due in part to heredity, disease, injury, and development. Heredity may be responsible for passing on many racial and sexual differences. Diseases such as tuberculosis and rickets cause malformations. Accidents and injuries during childhood or at maturity result in deformities of the pelvis or other parts of the body that affect the pelvis. Adequate nutrition and well-formed posture habits and exercise have much influence on the development of the pelvis.

Also, the pelvis does not reach the final stages of maturity until the age of 20 to 25 when ossification is completed.

There are several types of pelves. Even pelves whose measurements are normal differ greatly in the shape of the inlet, in the proximity of the greatest transverse diameter of the inlet to the sacral promontory, in the size of the sacrosciatic notch, and in their general architecture. These characteristics have been used in establishing a classification of pelves that has been of great interest and value to obstetricians. The four main types according to this classification are shown in Figure 7-5. The manner in which the fetus passes through the birth canal and, consequently, the type of labor vary considerably in each pelvic type.

In addition, there are many pelvic types which result from abnormal narrowing of one or the other diameters. These contracted pelves are described in Chapter 25.

In comparing male and female pelves, several differences are observed (Fig. 7-6). The most conspicuous difference is in the pubic arch, which has a much wider angle in women. The symphysis is shorter in women, and the border of the arch probably is more everted. Although the female pelvis is more shallow, it is more capacious, much lighter in structure, and smoother. The male pelvis is deep, compact, conical, and rough in texture, particularly at the site of muscle attachments. Both males and females start life with

Figure 7-5.
Caldwell–Maloy classification of pelvic types. *(Top)* the typical shape of the inlet for each type is shown. A line has been drawn through the widest transverse diameter, dividing the inlet into an anterior and posterior segment. The longitudinal line illustrates the anteroposterior diameter of the inlet. *(Bottom)* the typical interspinous diameter of each type is depicted.

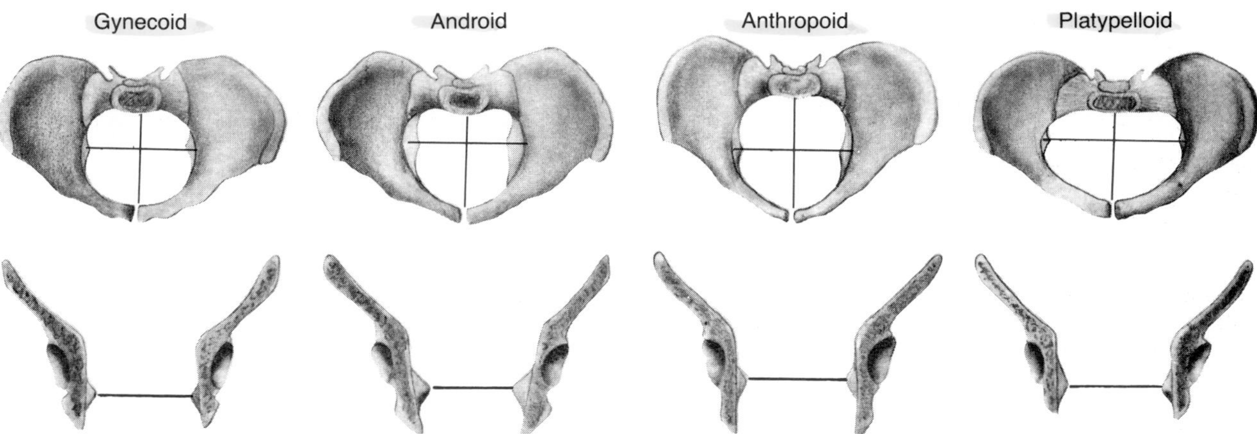

Figure 7-6.
Comparison of male and female pelvis. *(Left)* male pelvis, narrow and compact; pelvic arch is less than right angle. *(Right)* female pelvis, broad and capacious, pubic arch is greater than right angle.

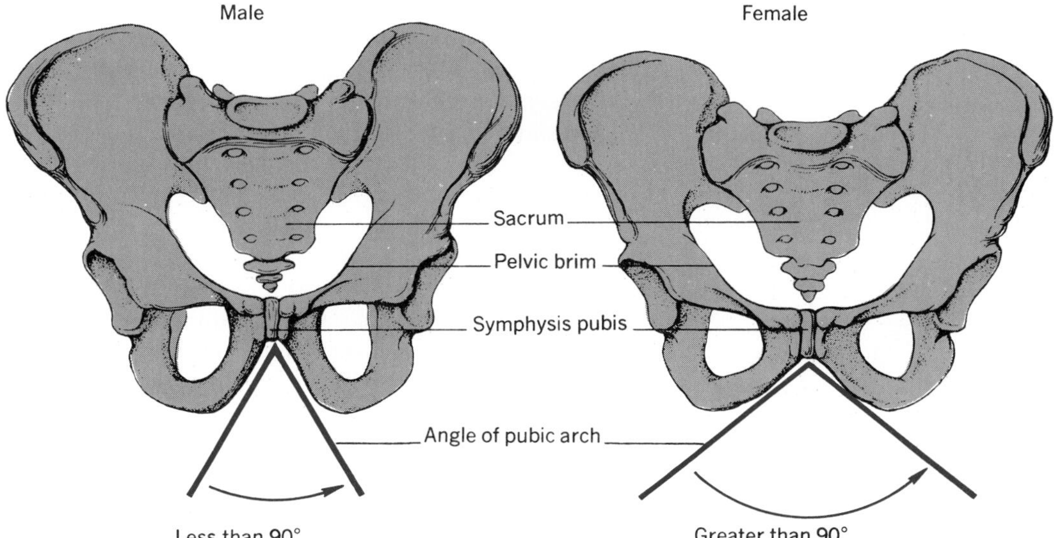

pelves that are identical in type; the major differences do not appear until puberty and are created by sex hormones. (For the definition and description of the sex hormones see Chap. 6.)

Pelvic Measurements

The entire childbirth process centers on the safe passage of the fully developed fetus through the pelvis. Slight irregularities in the structure of the pelvis may delay the progress of labor, and any marked deformity may render delivery through the natural passages impossible.

The pelvis of every pregnant woman should be measured accurately in the antepartal period to determine whether or not there is anything about the condition of the mother's pelvis that may complicate the delivery. This examination is a part of the antepartal evaluation.

Types of Pelvic Measurements

Internal pelvic measurements, made manually, are an important means of estimating the size of the pelvis. In the past, a number of external pelvic measurements were recorded. Except for measurement of the outlet, these are of dubious value in evaluating the true pelvis; thus, they are no longer used. In the majority of abnormal pelves, the most marked deformity affects the anteroposterior diameter of the inlet.

Diagonal Conjugate. Internal pelvic measurements are made to determine the actual diameters of the inlet. The chief internal measurement taken is the *diagonal conjugate,* or the distance between the sacral promontory and the lower margin of the symphysis pubis. The patient should be placed on her back on the examining table, with her knees drawn up and her feet supported by stirrups. Two fingers are inserted into the vagina and, before the diagonal conjugate is measured, the contour of the pelvis is evaluated by palpation. Included in this evaluation are the height of the symphysis pubis, the shape of the pubic arch, the motility of the coccyx, the inclination of the anterior wall of the sacrum and the side walls of the pelvis, and the prominence of the ischial spines.

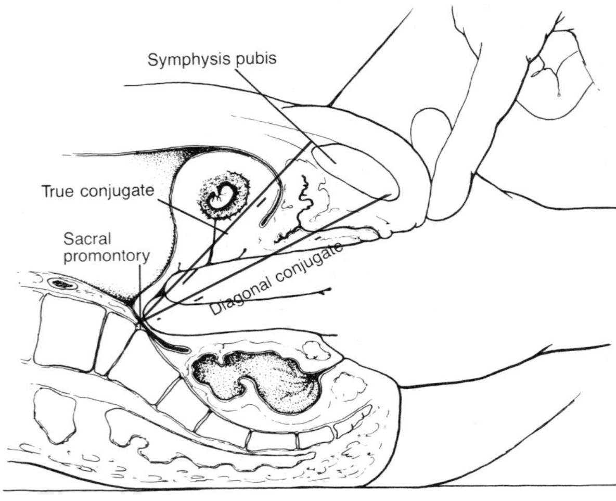

Figure 7-7.
Method of obtaining diagonal conjugate diameter.

To obtain the length of the diagonal conjugate, the two fingers passed into the vagina are pressed inward and upward as far as possible until the middle finger rests on the sacral promontory. The point on the back of the hand just under the symphysis is marked by putting the index finger of the other hand on the exact point (Fig. 7-7). Then the fingers are withdrawn and measured. The distance from the tip of the middle finger to the point marked represents the *diagonal conjugate measurement.* This distance may be measured with a rigid measuring scale attached to the wall or with a pelvimeter. If the measurement is greater than 11.5 cm, it is justifiable to assume that the pelvic inlet is of adequate size for childbirth.

True Conjugate. An extremely important internal diameter is the *true conjugate* or, in Latin, the conjugata vera, which is the distance between the posterior aspect of the symphysis pubis and the promontory of the sacrum. However, direct measurement of this diameter can only be made by means of an x-ray study; consequently, it has to be estimated from the diagonal conjugate measurement. It is believed that if 1.5 cm to 2 cm, according to the height and the inclination of the symphysis pubis, is deducted from the length of the diagonal conjugate, the true conjugate is obtained. For example, if the diagonal conjugate measures 12.5 cm and the symphysis pubis is considered to be "average," the conjugata vera may be estimated as about 11 cm. In this method, the problem consists of estimating the length of one side of a triangle, the conjugata vera; the other two sides, the diagonal conjugate and the height of the symphysis pubis, are known. If the symphysis pubis is high and has a marked inclination, the examiner takes this into consideration and may deduct 2 cm.

The length of the conjugata vera is of utmost importance, because it is about the smallest diameter of the inlet through which the fetal head must pass. Indeed, the main purpose in measuring the diagonal conjugate is to give an estimate of the size of the conjugata vera.

Obstetrical Conjugate. Students sometimes are confused when they are confronted with the term *obstetrical conjugate.* This term identifies a diameter that begins at the sacral promontory and terminates on the inner surface of the symphysis pubis, a few millimeters below its upper margin. The obstetrical conjugate is in reality the shortest diameter through which the fetal head must pass as it descends into the true pelvis. A distinction is rarely made between the conjugata vera and the obstetrical conjugate, except in x-ray pelvimetry.

Biischial Diameter. Next to the diagonal conjugate, the most important clinical dimension of the pelvis is the transverse diameter of the outlet, the diameter between the ischial tuberosities. This is sometimes called the biischial diameter or intertuberous diameter. This measurement is taken while the patient is in the lithotomy position, well down on the table and with the legs widely separated. The measurement is taken from the innermost and lowermost aspect of the ischial tuberosities, on a level with the lower border of the anus. The instruments usually used are the Williams's pelvimeter (Fig. 7-8) or the Thoms's pelvimeter. The intertuberous diameter may also be estimated by inserting the closed fist between the tuberosities. The known diameter of the hand can then be used as a reference. A diameter of more than 8.0 cm is considered adequate.

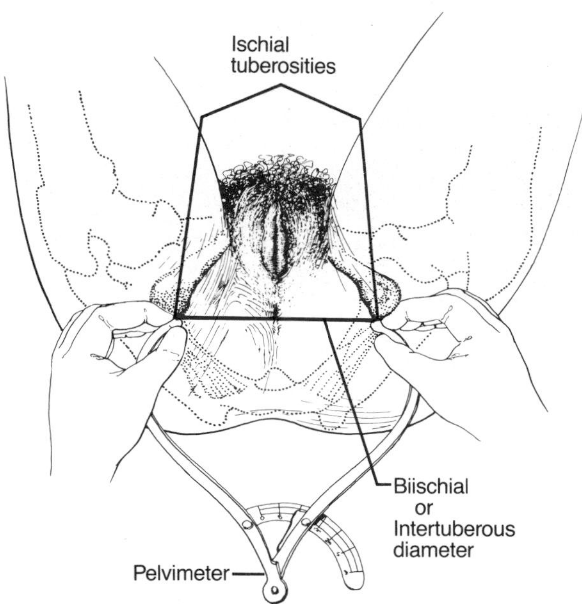

Figure 7-8.
Method of measuring biischial or intertuberous diameter of the outlet.

X-Ray Pelvimetry

X-ray pelvimetry is the most accurate means of determining pelvic size. The method subjects the maternal ovaries and fetal gonads to a certain amount of irradiation. Although the amount involved is minimal, exposure of pregnant women to irradiation should be avoided unless the procedure is absolutely necessary. X-ray pelvimetry is no longer used prior to labor, except in cases where there are sound reasons for suspecting pelvic contraction, such as small manual measurements or a history of previous injury or disease which could have affected the bony pelvis.

Pelvimetry may be indicated when there has been failure to progress during labor. It is also important to evaluate pelvic size in breech presentations when vaginal delivery is anticipated. The head is the largest part of the fetus, and the adequacy of the pelvis is not really tested until the body has already been delivered. It may also provide helpful information when there is a face or other abnormal presentations.

A variety of pelvimetry techniques has been developed. These provide views of the inlet and the interischial spinous diameter of the mid pelvis (Fig. 7-9), as

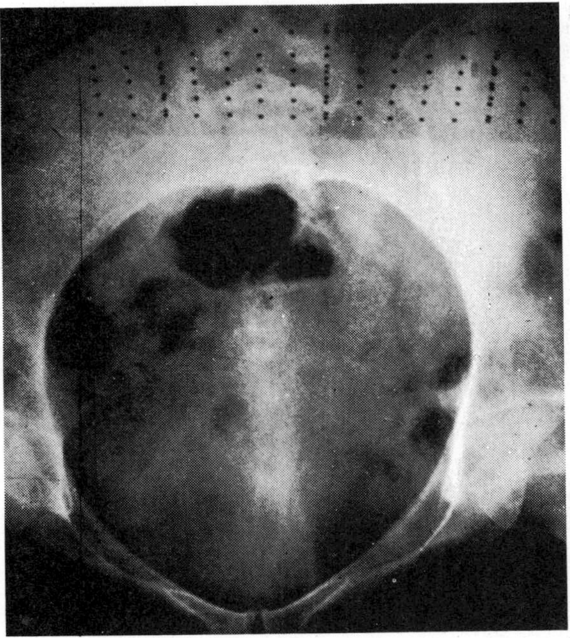

Figure 7-9.
Pelvic inlet roentgenogram. The scale represents corrected centimeters for various levels of the pelvic canal. The top line is used for measuring the diameters of the inlet. The other levels are established on the lateral roentgenogram. Pelvic morphology is readily established by viewing both lateral and inlet views. This is known as Thoms's technique.

well as the anteriorposterior dimensions of the pelvis including the obstetrical conjugate (Fig. 7-10). When x-ray films are made late in pregnancy or in labor, it is also possible to gain an impression of the size of the fetal head. When this is considered in relation to pelvic structure, helpful information may be obtained in forecasting whether or not the pelvis is large enough to allow the fetus to pass through.

Female Organs of Reproduction

The female organs of reproduction are divided into two groups—the external and the internal.

External Organs

The external female reproductive organs are called the *vulva,* from the Latin word meaning covering. This includes everything that is visible externally from the lower margin of the pubis to the perineum, namely, the *mons veneris,* the *labia majora* and *minora,* the *clitoris,* the *vestibule,* the *hymen,* the *urethral opening* and various glandular and vascular structures. (Fig. 7-11). The term vulva has often been used to refer simply to the labia majora and minora.

The *mons veneris* is a firm, cushionlike formation over the symphysis pubis that is covered with crinkly hair.

The *labia majora* are two prominent longitudinal folds of adipose tissue that are covered with skin and extend downward and backward from the mons veneris and disappear in forming the anterior border of the perineal body. These two thick folds of skin are covered with hair on their outer surfaces after the age of puberty but are smooth and moist on their inner surfaces. At the bottom they fade away into the perineum posteriorly, joining together to form a transverse fold, the posterior commissure, which is situated directly in front of the fourchette. This fatty tissue is supplied with an abundant plexus of veins that may rupture as the result of injury sustained during labor and give rise to an extravasation of blood, or hematoma.

The *labia minora* are two thin folds entirely covered with thin membrane that are situated between the labia majora. The outer surfaces join with the inner surfaces of the labia majora. The labia minora extend from the clitoris downward and backward on

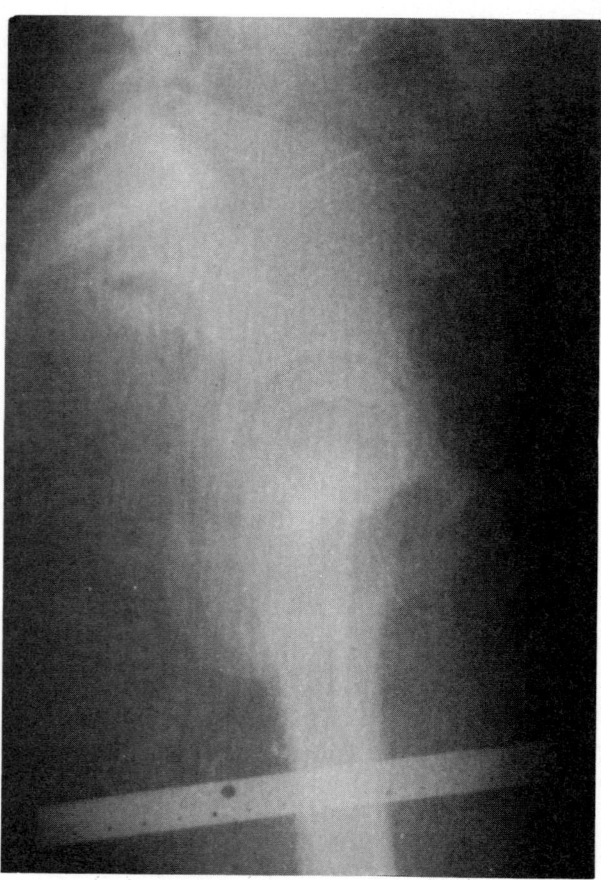

Figure 7-10.
Lateral roentgenogram. The scale represents corrected centimeters in the midplane of the body. The various diameters may be measured with calipers. The lateral morphologic aspects are readily visualized.

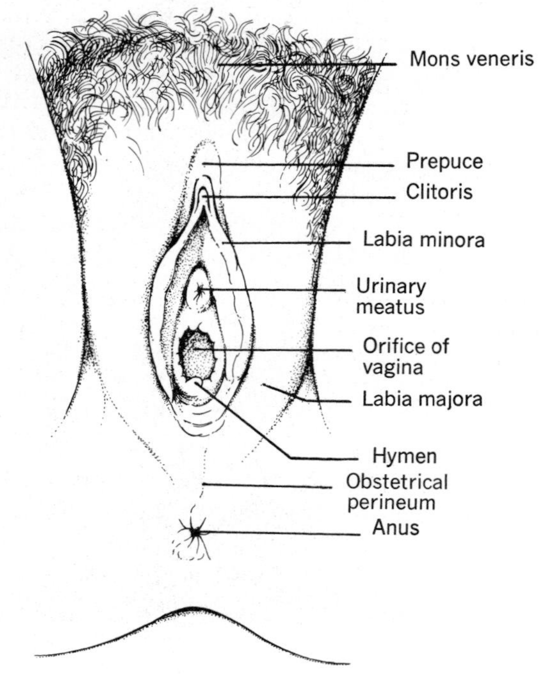

Figure 7-11.
External genitalia of female.

Female Organs of Reproduction

External	Internal
Vulva	Ovaries
Mons veneris	Fallopian tubes
Labia majora	Uterus
Labia Minora	Corpus (body)
Clitoris	Cervix (neck)
Vestibule	
Perineum	

either side of the orifice of the vagina. In the upper extremity, each labium minus separates into two branches which, when united with those of the opposite side, enclose the clitoris. The upper fold forms the prepuce and the lower fold forms the frenum of the clitoris. At the bottom, the labia minora pass almost imperceptibly into the labia majora or blend together as a thin fold of skin, the fourchette, which forms the anterior edge of the perineum or perineal body.

The *clitoris* is a small, highly sensitive projection that is composed of erectile tissue, nerves, and blood vessels and is covered with a thin epidermis. It is analogous to the penis in the male and is regarded as the chief area of voluptuous sensation. The clitoris is partially hidden between the anterior ends of the labia minora.

The *vestibule* is the almond-shaped area that is enclosed by the labia minora and extends from the clitoris to the fourchette. It is perforated by four openings—the urethra, the vaginal opening, the ducts of Bartholin's glands, and the ducts of Skene's glands. *Bartholin's glands* are two small glands situated beneath the vestibule on either side of the vaginal opening. *Skene's glands* open on the vestibule on either side of the urethra.

The *hymen* marks the division between the internal and the external organs. It is a thin sheath of mucous membrane situated at the orifice of the vagina. It may be entirely absent, or it may form a complete septum across the lower end of the vagina.

The hymen changes in shape and consistency throughout the life cycle. (Fig. 7-12). In the newborn child it projects beyond the surrounding parts. In adult virgins it is a membrane of varying thickness that presents an aperture that varies in size from a small opening to one that readily admits one or even two fingers. The opening is circular or crescent shaped. In rare instances, the hymen may be imperforate and cause retention of menstrual discharge if it occludes the vaginal orifice completely.

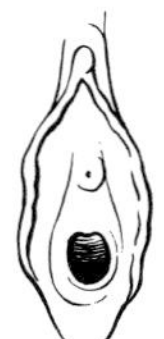
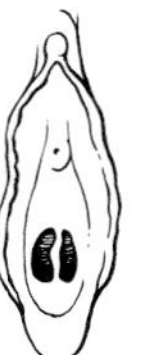
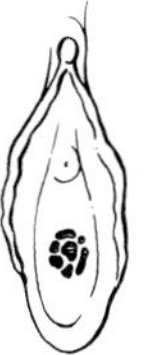
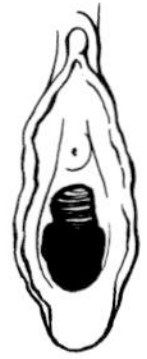

Figure 7-12.
Variations of the hymen. (From left to right) virginal, nondilated; septate, septum may or may not stretch; cribriform; parous, at least one full-term delivery.

The *perineum* consists of muscles and fascia of the urogenital diaphragm and lies across the pubic arch and the pelvic diaphragm, which consists of the coccygeus and the levator ani muscles. The levator ani consists of three portions that form a slinglike support for the pelvic structure, and between them pass the urethra, the vagina, and the rectum (Fig. 7-13). Between the anus and the vagina, the levator ani is reinforced by a central tendon of the perineum where three pairs of muscles converge—the bulbocavernous, the superficial transverse muscles of the perineum, and the external sphincter ani. These structures constitute the perineal body and form the main support of the perineal floor. They are often lacerated during delivery.

Internal Organs

The internal organs of reproduction are the vagina, the uterus, the fallopian or uterine tubes, and the ovaries (Figs. 7-14, 7-15, and 7-16).

Ovaries

The *ovaries* are two almond-shaped organs that are situated in the upper part of the pelvic cavity on either side of the uterus. Their chief functions are the development and the expulsion of ova and the provision of certain internal secretions, or hormones. These organs correspond to the testes in the male. They are embedded in the posterior fold of the broad ligament of the uterus and are supported by the suspensory, the ovarian, and the mesovarium ligaments (see Fig. 7-16).

Each ovary contains a large number of germ cells, or primordial ova, in its substance at birth. This huge storage of primordial follicles present at birth more than suffices the woman for life. It is believed that no more are formed and that this large initial store is gradually exhausted during the period of sexual maturity. Beginning at puberty, one of the follicles that contain the ova enlarges each month and gradually approaches the surface of the ovary and ruptures. The ovum and the fluid content of the follicle are liberated

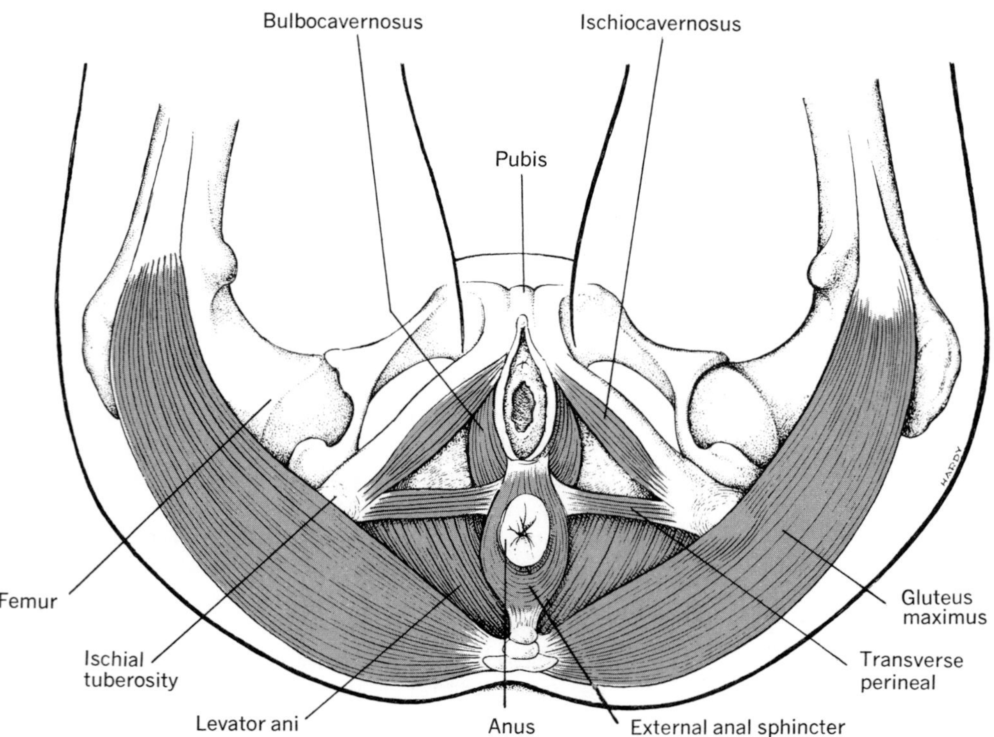

Figure 7-13.
Muscles of the pelvic floor (female perineum).

on the exterior of the ovary; then they are swept into the tube. The development and the maturation of the follicles containing the ova continue from puberty to menopause.

The arteries that supply the ovaries are four or five branches that arise from the anastomosis of the ovarian artery with the ovarian branch of the uterine artery (see Fig. 7-17). The veins that drain the ovary become tributaries to both the uterine and the ovarian plexus. Superiorly, the ovarian vein drains into the inferior vena cava on the right and into the renal vein on the left.

The nerves supplying the ovaries are derived from the craniosacral and the thoracolumbar sympathetic systems. The postganglionic and visceral afferent fibers form a plexus that surrounds the ovarian artery, which is formed by contributions from the renal and the aortic plexuses and corresponds to the spermatic plexus in the male.

Fallopian Tubes

The fallopian tubes are two trumpet-shaped, thin, flexible, muscular tubes that are about 12 cm long. They extend from the uterine cornua, along the upper margin of the broad ligaments to the ovaries. They have two openings, one into the uterine cavity and the other into the abdominal cavity.

The opening into the uterine cavity is minute and will admit only a fine bristle. The abdominal opening is larger and is surrounded by a large number of fine fringes or fimbriae. The fimbriated extremity lies near the ovary, but it is not necessarily in direct contact with it. It is generally believed that the cilia on the fimbriated end of the tube create a current in the layer of fluid that surrounds the various pelvic organs.

The tubes convey the discharged ovum by peristaltic action from the ovaries to the cavity of the uterus. By their tentaclelike processes the fimbriated ends of the tube draw the escaped ovum into the tube.

The tubes are lined with mucous membrane which contains ciliated epithelium. The muscular layer is made up of longitudinal and circular fibers which provide peristaltic action. The serous membrane covering the tubes is a continuation of the peritoneum, which lines the whole abdominal cavity.

The fallopian tubes receive their blood supply from the ovarian and the uterine arteries (Fig. 7-17). The veins of the tubes follow the course of these arteries and empty into the uterine and the ovarian trunks. The nerves that supply the uterus also innervate the tubes.

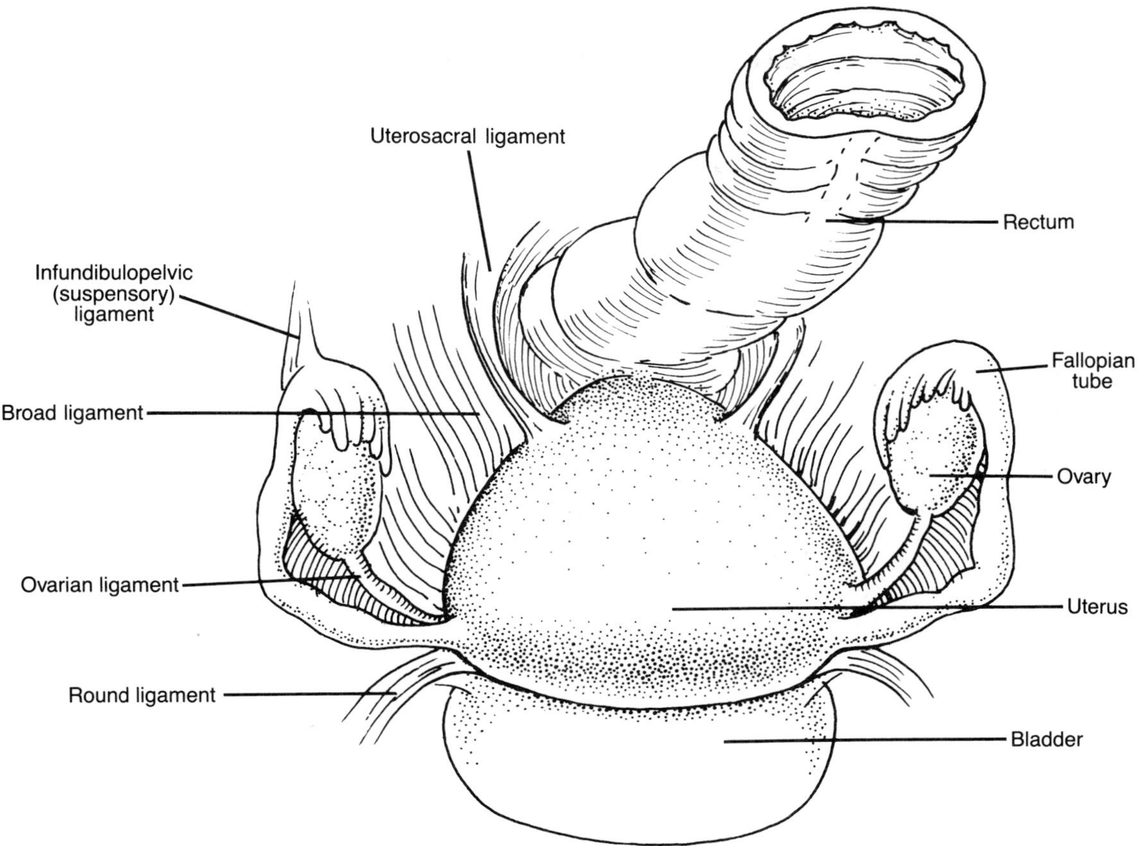

Figure 7-14.
Pelvic contents viewed from above.

Uterus

The uterus is a hollow, thick-walled, muscular organ (see Fig. 7-16). It serves two important functions—(1) it is the organ of menstruation, and (2) during pregnancy it receives the fertilized ovum and retains and nourishes it until it expels the fetus during labor.

The uterus varies in size and shape according to the age of the individual and whether or not she has borne children. The uterus of the adult nullipara weighs approximately 60 gm and measures 5.5 cm to 8 cm in length. It resembles a flattened pear in appearance and has two divisions—the upper triangular portion, the *corpus,* and the lower constricted cylindrical portion, the *cervix,* which projects into the vagina. The fallopian tubes extend from the *cornu* (the Latin word meaning *horn*) of the uterus at the upper outer margin on either side. The upper rounded portion of the uterus between the points of insertion of the tubes is the fundus (see Fig. 7-16).

The nonpregnant uterus is situated in the pelvic cavity between the bladder and the rectum. Almost the entire posterior wall and the upper portion of the anterior wall is covered by peritoneum. The lower portion of the anterior wall is united with the bladder wall by a layer of loose connective tissue. The lower posterior wall of the uterus and the upper portion of the vagina are separated from the rectum by the Douglas cul-de-sac, or pouch of Douglas.

Because of its muscular composition, the uterus is capable of enlarging to accommodate a growing fetus; at the termination of pregnancy it weighs about 1 kg or 2 lb. It is made up of involuntary muscle fibers that are arranged in all directions, making expansion possible in every direction to accommodate the products of conception. The arrangement of the uterus enables the fetus to expel at the end of a normal labor. Arranged between these muscular layers are many blood vessels, lymphatics, and nerves.

The cavity of the uterus is somewhat triangular in shape. It is widest at the fundus, between the small openings into the fallopian tubes and narrowest at the opening into the cervix. The anterior and posterior

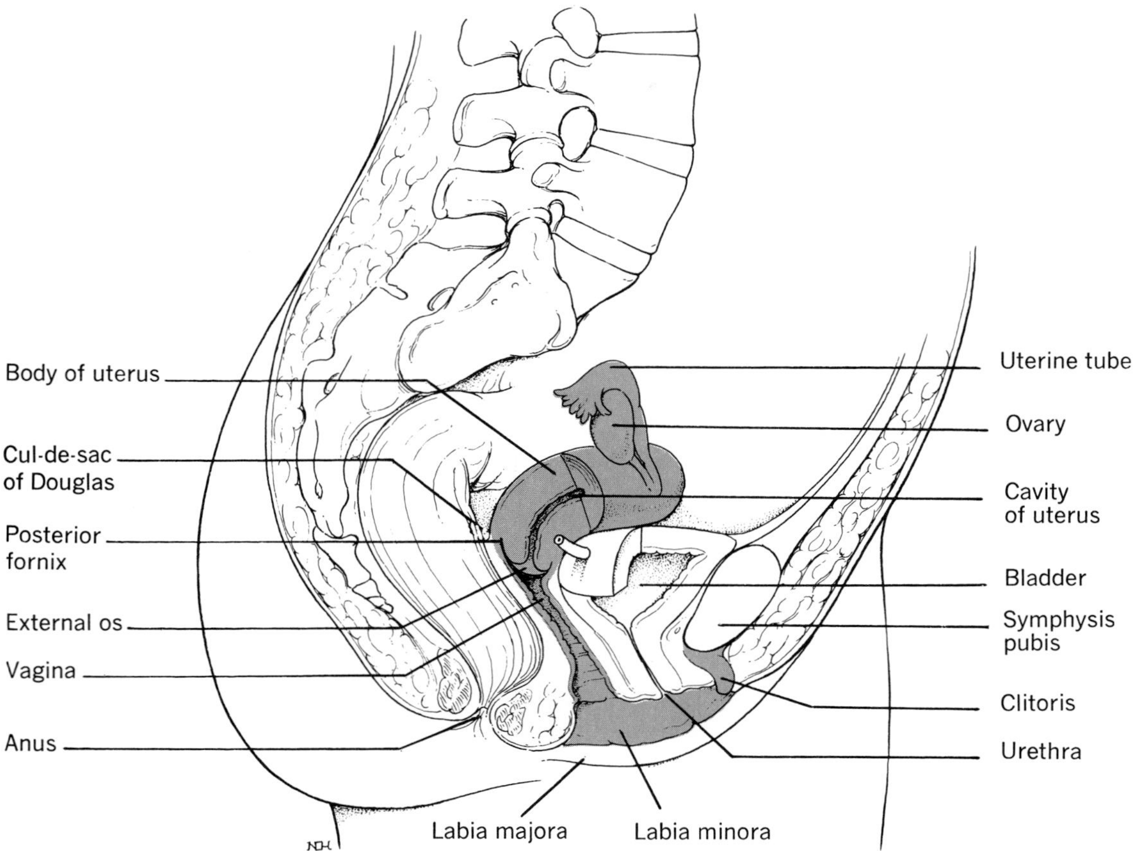

Figure 7-15.
Female reproductive organs as seen in sagittal section.

walls lie almost in contact, so that if a cross section of the uterus could be examined, the cavity between them would appear as a mere slit.

The uterus is lined with mucous membrane, the endometrium, and is divided into two parts—the cavity of the body of the uterus and the cavity of the cervix.

Cervix. The *cervix* is less movable than the body of the uterus. Its muscular wall is not as thick, and its lining is different in that it is much folded and contains crypts, that produce mucus and are the chief source of the mucous secretion during pregnancy. The cervix has an upper opening, the *internal os,* leading from the cavity of the uterine body into the cervical canal, and a lower opening, the *external os,* opening into the vagina. The cervical canal is small in the nonpregnant woman, barely admitting a probe, but at the time of labor it dilates to a size sufficient to permit the passage of the fetus.

Ligaments. The uterus is supported by ligaments extending from either side of the uterus and by the muscles of the pelvic floor. The ligaments that support the uterus in the pelvic cavity are the broad ligaments, the round ligaments, and the uterosacral ligaments (see Fig. 7-16).

The *broad ligaments* are two winglike structures that extend from the lateral margins of the uterus to the pelvic walls and divide the pelvic cavity into an anterior and a posterior compartment. Each consists of folds of peritoneum which envelop the fallopian tubes, the ovaries, and the round and ovarian ligaments. Its lower portion, the *cardinal ligament* is composed of dense connective tissue that is firmly joined to the supravaginal portion of the cervix. The median margin is connected with the lateral margin of the uterus and encloses the uterine vessels.

The *round ligaments* are two fibrous cords that are attached on either side of the fundus, just below the fallopian tubes. They extend forward through the inguinal canal and terminate in the upper portion of the labia majora. These ligaments aid in holding the fundus forward.

The *uterosacral ligaments* are two cordlike structures that extend from the posterior cervical portion

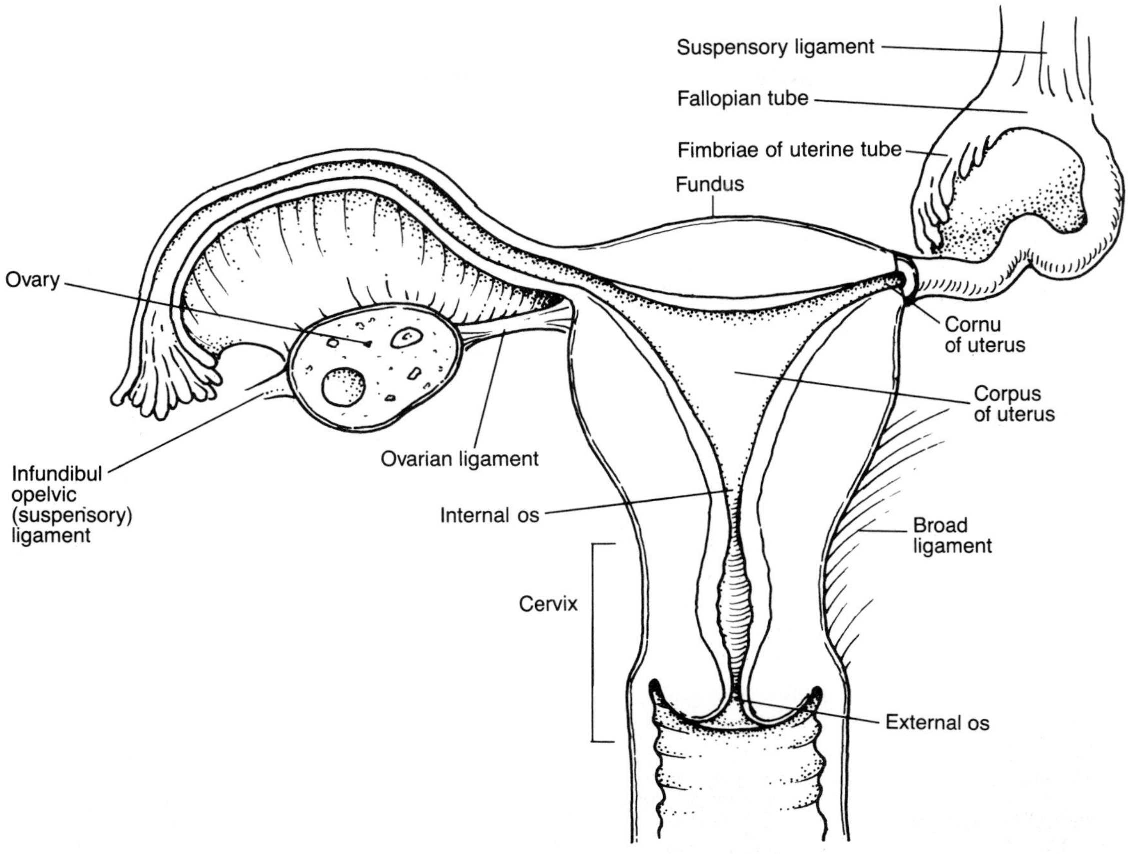

Figure 7-16.
Anterior view of the uterus and related structures.

of the uterus to the sacrum. They help to support the cervix. The uterovesical ligament is merely a fold of the peritoneum that passes over the fundus and extends over the bladder. The rectovaginal ligament is a fold of the peritoneum that passes over the posterior surface of the uterus and is reflected upon the rectum.

Uterine Blood Supply. The uterus receives its blood supply from the ovarian and the uterine arteries (see Fig. 7-17). The uterine artery, the principal source, is the main branch of the hypogastric artery, which enters the base of the broad ligament and makes its way to the side of the uterus. The ovarian artery is a branch of the aorta. It enters the broad ligament and as it reaches the ovary it breaks up into smaller branches that enter that organ, while its main stem makes its way to the upper margin of the uterus, where it anastomoses with the ovarian branch of the uterine artery.

The uterovaginal plexus returns the blood from the uterus and the vagina to the venous circulation. These veins form a plexus of thin-walled vessels that are embedded in the layers of the uterine muscle. Emerging from this plexus, the trunks join the uterine vein, which is a double vein. These veins follow on either side of the uterine artery and eventually form one trunk that empties into the hypogastric vein, which makes its way into the internal iliac.

Uterine Nerve Supply. The uterus possesses an abundant nerve supply which is principally derived from the sympathetic nervous system and partly from the cerebrospinal and parasympathetic system. Both the sympathetic and the parasympathetic nerve supplies contain motor and a few sensory fibers. The functions of the nerve supply of the two systems are in great part antagonistic. The sympathetic system causes muscular contraction and vasoconstriction, and the parasympathetic system inhibits contraction and leads to vasodilatation.

Position of Uterus. Since the uterus is a freely movable organ that is suspended in the pelvic cavity between the bladder and the rectum, the position of the uterus may be influenced by a full bladder or full rectum. The uterus could be pushed backward or

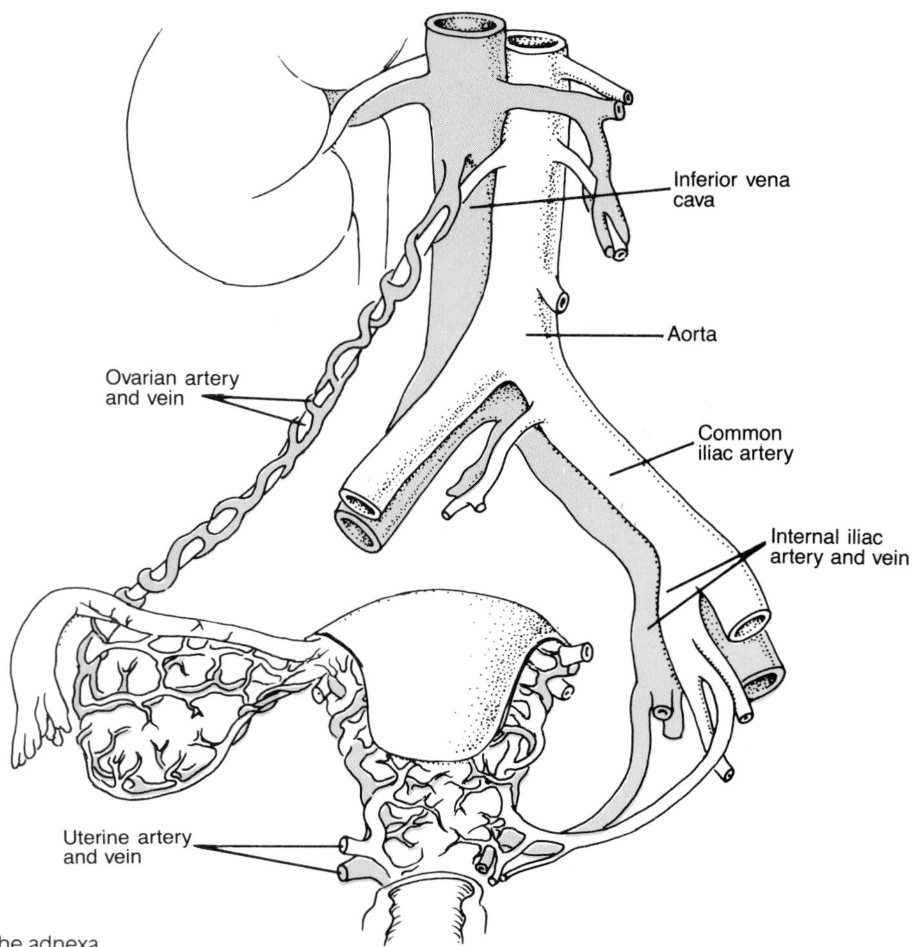

Figure 7-17.
Blood supply of the uterus and the adnexa.

forward. The uterus also changes its position when the patient stands, lies flat, or turns on her side. Also, there are variations in position, such as anteflexion, in which the fundus is tipped far forward; retroversion, in which the fundus is tipped far backward (Fig. 7-18); and prolapse, which occurs when the muscles of the pelvic floor and the uterine ligaments are attenuated.

Lymphatic Vessels. The lymphatic vessels drain into the lumbar lymph nodes.

Vagina

The *vagina* is a dilatable mucous membrane-lined passage between the bladder and the rectum. The vaginal opening occupies the lower portion of the vestibule. The vagina is from 8 cm to 12 cm long, and at the upper end is a blind vault, commonly called the *fornix,* into which the lower portion of the cervix projects.

The fornix is divided into four parts for descriptive purposes. The lateral fornices are the spaces between the vaginal wall on either side and the cervix; the anterior fornix is between the anterior vaginal wall and the cervix; and the posterior fornix is between the posterior vaginal wall and the cervix. The posterior fornix is considerably deeper than the anterior fornix because the vagina is attached higher up on the posterior than the anterior wall of the cervix. The fornices are important because the examiner is usually able to palpate the internal pelvic organs through their thin walls.

The vagina serves three important functions—(1) it represents the excretory duct of the uterus through which secretion and the menstrual flow escape, (2) it is the female organ of copulation, and (3) it forms part of the birth canal during labor. Its walls are arranged into thick folds, the columns of the vagina, and, in women who have not borne children, numerous

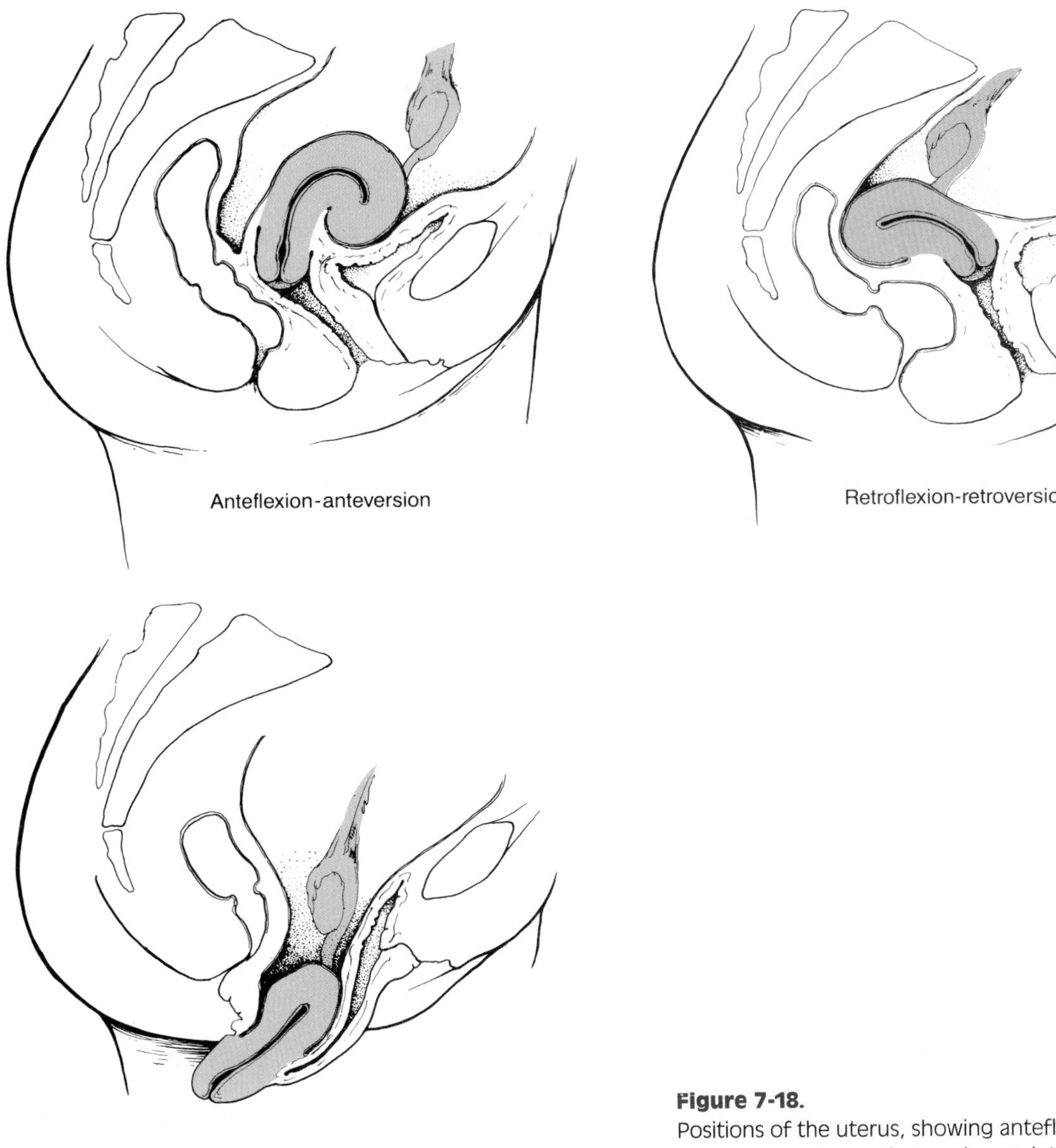

Figure 7-18.
Positions of the uterus, showing anteflexion-anteversion, retroflexion-retroversion, and complete prolapse.

ridges, or *rugae,* which extend outward and almost at right angles to the vaginal columns and give the surface a corrugated appearance. Normally, the anterior and the posterior walls of the vagina lie in contact, but they are capable of stretching to allow marked distention of the passage, as in the process of childbirth.

The vagina receives an abundant blood supply from branches of the uterine, the inferior vesical, the median hemorrhoidal, and the internal pudendal arteries. The passage is surrounded by a venous plexus; the vessels follow the course of the arteries and eventually empty into the hypogastric veins. The lymphatics empty into the inguinal, the hypogastric, and the iliac glands.

Related Pelvic Organs (See Fig 7-15)

Bladder

The *bladder* is a muscular sac that serves as a reservoir for urine. It is situated in front of the uterus and behind the symphysis pubis. When empty or moderately distended, it remains entirely in the pelvis, but if it becomes greatly distended, it rises into the abdomen. Urine is conducted into the bladder by the ureters, two tubes that extend down from the basin of the kidneys and over the brim of the pelvis beneath the uterine vessels to open into the bladder at about the level of the cervix. The bladder is emptied through the urethra, a short tube that terminates in the urethral meatus. Lying on either side of the urethra and almost parallel with it are two small glands, less than 2.5 cm long, known as Skene's glands. Their ducts empty into the urethra just above the meatus. Often in cases of gonorrhea, Skene's glands and ducts are involved.

Anus

The *anus* is the entrance to the rectal canal. The rectal canal is surrounded at the opening or anus by its sphincter muscle, which binds it to the coccyx behind and to the perineum in front. It is supported by the muscles passing into it; these are the muscles that help to support the pelvic floor. The rectum is considered here because of the proximity to the field of delivery.

Mammary Glands

The *breasts,* or mammary glands, are two highly specialized cutaneous glands located on either side of the anterior wall of the chest between the third and the seventh ribs (Fig. 7-19). They are abundantly supplied with nerves. The breasts contain tissue which responds to hormones. Thus, breast development at puberty and lactation during pregnancy occur as a result of endocrine influences.

The internal mammary and the intercostal arteries supply the breast glands, and the mammary veins follow these arteries. Also, there are many cutaneous veins that become dilated during lactation. The lymphatics are abundant, especially toward the axilla. These breast glands are present in the male, but exist only in the rudimentary state.

Internal Structure

The breasts of a woman who never has borne a child are conic or hemispheric in form, but they vary in size and shape at different ages and in different persons. In women who have nursed one or more babies, the breasts tend to become pendulous. At the termination of lactation, certain exercises aid in restoring the tone of the breast tissue.

The breasts are made up of glandular tissue and fat. Each organ is divided into 15 or 20 lobes, which are separated from each other by fibrous and fatty walls. Each lobe is subdivided into many lobules, which contain numerous acini cells. The *acini* are composed of a single layer of epithelium, beneath

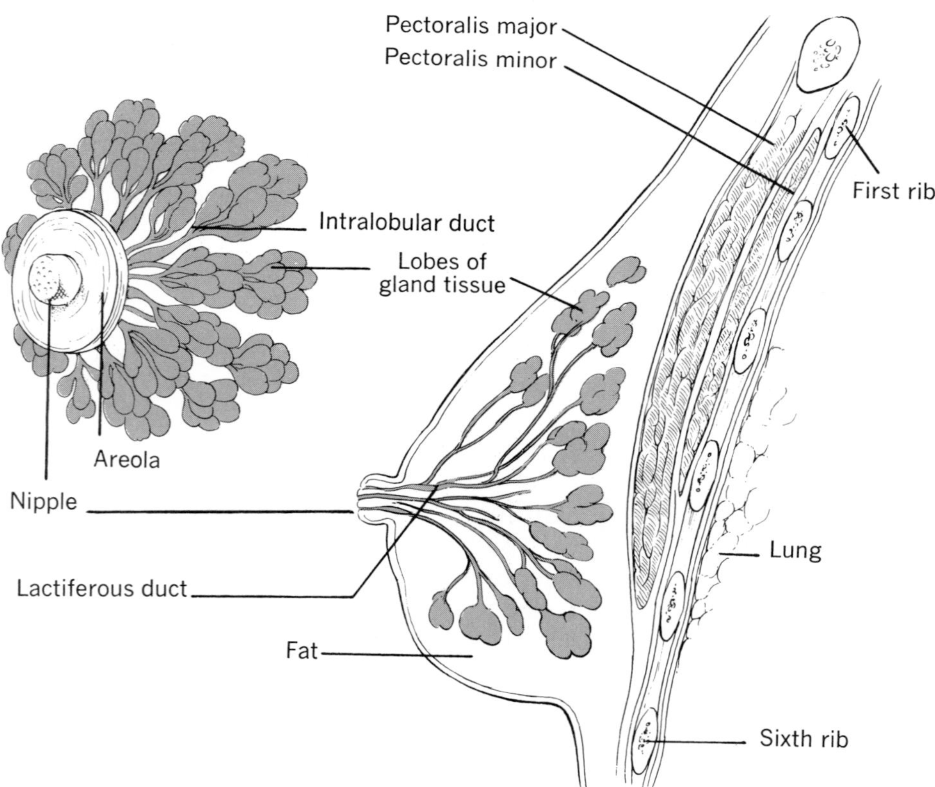

Figure 7-19.
Glandular tissue and ducts of the mammary gland.

which is a small amount of connective tissue richly supplied with capillaries. The products necessary for the milk are filtered from the blood by the process of osmosis, but the secretion of the milk really begins in the acini cells. As the ducts leading from the lobules to the lobes approach the nipple, they are dilated to form little reservoirs in which the milk is stored; they narrow again as they pass into the nipple. The size of the breast depends on the amount of fatty tissue present and in no way denotes the amount of lactation possible.

External Structure

The external surface of the breasts is divided into three portions. The first is the smooth and soft area of skin extending from the circumference of the gland to the areola.

The second is the *areola,* which surrounds the nipple and is of a delicate pinkish hue in blondes and a darker rose color in brunettes. The surface of the areola is roughened by small fine lumps of papillae, known as Montgomery's glands. These enlarged sebaceous glands, white in color and scattered over the areola, become more marked during pregnancy. Under the influence of gestation, the areola becomes darker, and, in many cases, this pigmentation constitutes a helpful sign of pregnancy.

The *nipple* is largely composed of sensitive, erectile tissue and forms a large conic papilla projecting from the center of the areola and its summit is at the openings of the milk ducts. There are 3 to 20 milk duct openings.

Breast care (see Chaps. 21 and 30) constitutes one of the important phases of the nursing care of the maternity patient throughout pregnancy and the puerperium.

Male Organs of Reproduction

The male reproductive system consists of the penis, the testes, and an excretory duct system with their accessory structures (Fig. 7-20).

Penis

The *penis,* the male organ of copulation, consists of the cavernous bodies (erectile parts) and a urethra through which the seminal fluid passes during ejaculation. The cavernous bodies contain blood spaces which are usually quite empty, and the organ is flaccid. When these spaces fill with blood, the organ becomes turgid. The flow of blood is controlled by the autonomic nervous system (vasodilator fibers) and varies with sexual arousal. The enlarged conic structure at the free end of the penis which contains the external orifice of the urethra is called the glans penis. Unless it has been removed by circumcision, the glans is covered by a fold of retractable skin, the foreskin, or prepuce.

Testes

Like the ovaries, the testes have a dual function—hormone production and the formation and release of gametes, in this case, spermatozoa. Unlike the ovaries, the testes are located outside the abdominal cavity in the scrotum (meaning bag). During early fetal life, the testes are abdominal. As the fetus develops the testes move downward and enter the scrotum through the inguinal canal shortly before birth. The testes are approximately 5 cm long and are contained in a fibrous protective covering, the tunica albuginea, which subdivides the testes into lobules (Fig. 7-21). Each lobule contains seminiferous tubules, coiled ducts in the walls of which spermatogenesis occurs. The testes also contain testosterone-producing cells, the interstitial cells of Leydig, as well as larger supporting cells, the Sertoli cells, which are important for sperm transport within the seminiferous tubules.

Spermatogenesis is a heat sensitive process. The 2° to 3° difference between scrotal and abdominal temperatures allows spermatogenesis to proceed normally in the cooler environment. Testosterone production is not affected by temperature. When there has been failure of the testes to descend, spermatogenesis is severely impaired, but testosterone production remains unaffected.

The *canal system* consists of the epididymis, which is made up of numerous seminiferous tubules, the vas deferens, which passes from the epididymis to the ejaculatory duct, the ejaculatory duct (formed by the union of the vas deferens and the duct of the seminal vesicle), and the urethra, which is surrounded by the prostate gland and traverses the penis (Figs. 7-20 and 7-21).

The accessory structures consist of the seminal vesicles (sacculated structures located behind the bladder and in front of the rectum), the prostate gland, which surrounds the base of the urethra and the ejaculatory duct, and the bulbourethral glands, or Cowper's glands, which lie at the base of the prostate and on either side of the membranous urethra. Cowper's glands produce a mucinous substance that lubricates the urethra and coats its surface.

Figure 7-20.
Organs of the male reproductive system.

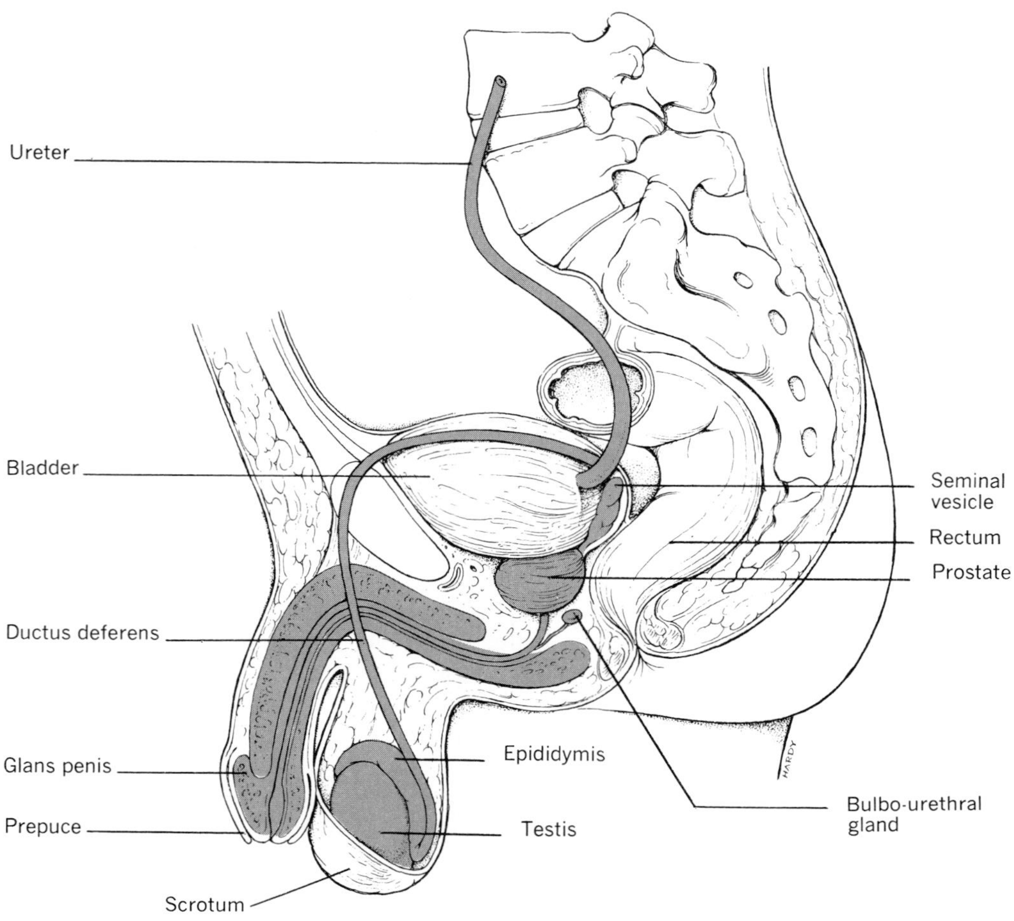

Figure 7-21.
Diagram of structural features of the testis and epididymis.

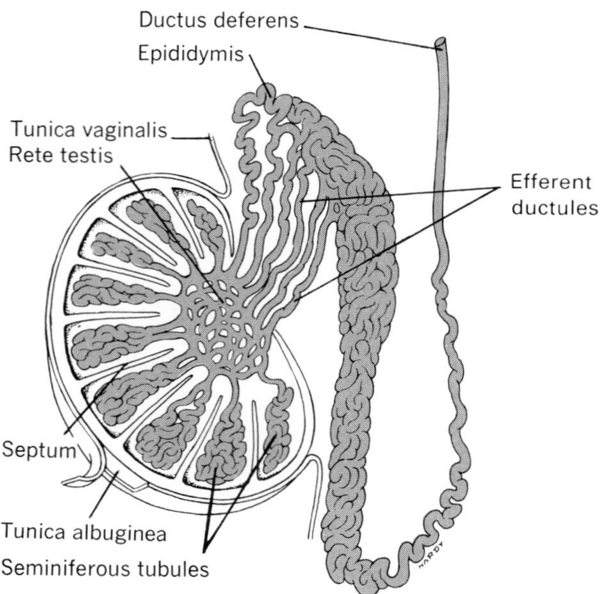

Transport of Spermatozoa

When spermatozoa are released into the seminiferous tubules, although endowed with tails, they are not yet capable of motility. They acquire motility as they pass along the epididymis, where they are stored. The ducts of the epididymis lead to the vas deferens, which provides the transporting passage along which spermatozoa traverse to the base of the penis. The ductus deferens or vas deferens has contractile power that allows it to propel the spermatozoa upward to the base of the penis. Seminal plasma, the fluid in which spermatozoa are transported during the ejaculatory process, is made up of secretions from accessory glands of the male reproductive tract. These include the seminal vesicles that empty into the ejaculatory duct, which in turn empties into the urethra, the prostate gland which surrounds the urethra, the ejaculatory ducts at the base of the penis, and the bulbourethral glands. During ejaculation, the seminal vesicles discharge their contents and propel spermatozoa that are already in the vas deferens along the urethra. The seminal plasma also receives a discharge from the prostate gland, which expels a thin alkaline secretion into the base of the urethra. The function of the secretions of the accessory glands is to facilitate transportation of spermatozoa along the urethra during the ejaculatory process and to provide a temporary milieu where the spermatozoa can survive. On intravaginal ejaculation, spermatozoa almost immediately begin to traverse the cervical mucus and within a matter of minutes some are on their way to the site of fertilization.

Suggested Reading

Chaffee EE, Lytle IM: Basic Physiology and Anatomy, 4th ed. Philadelphia, JB Lippincott, 1980

Goss CM (ed): Gray's Anatomy of the Human Body, 29th ed. Philadelphia, Lea & Febiger, 1973

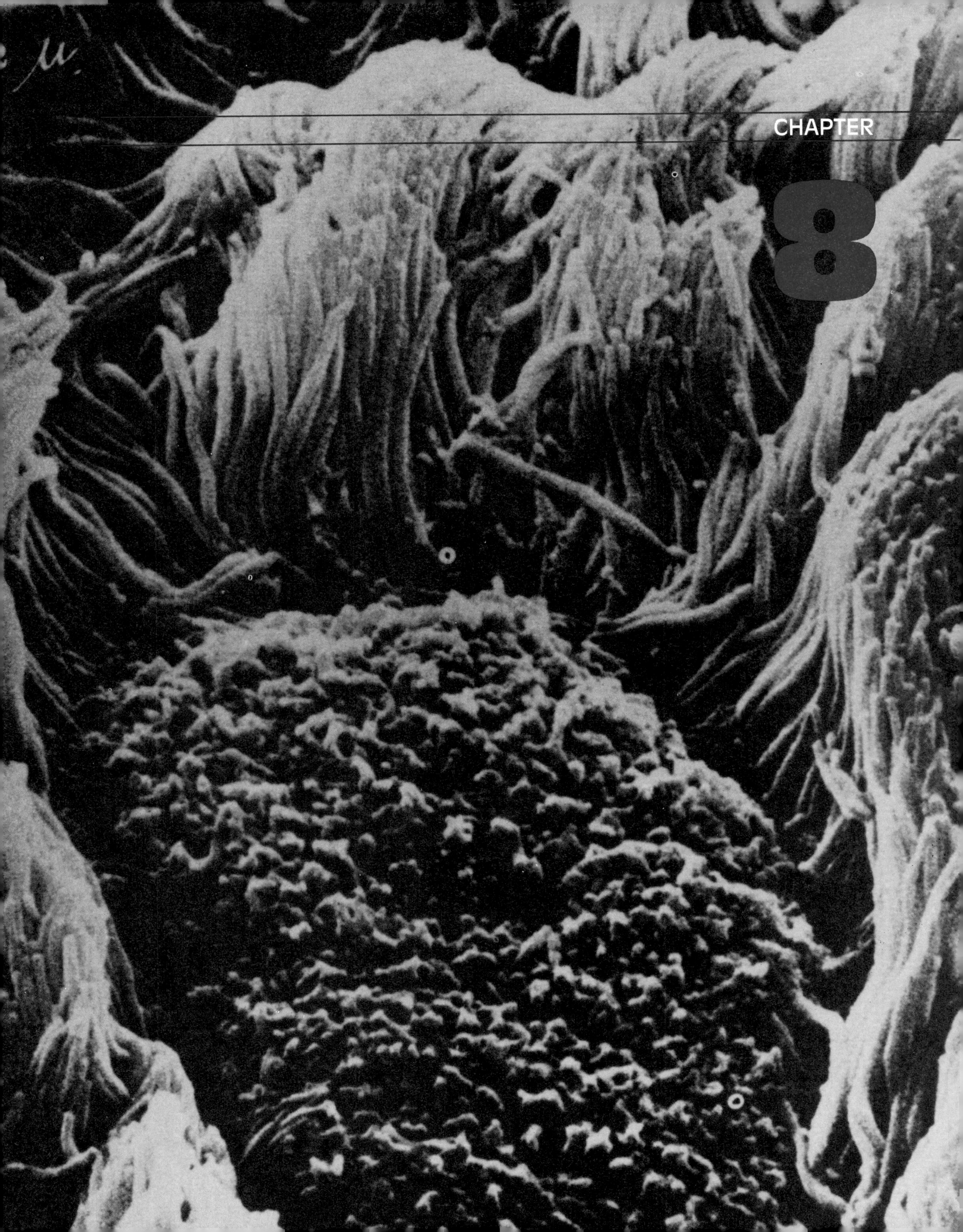

CHAPTER

8

CHAPTER 8

Sexual and Reproductive Physiology

A general review of reproductive physiology is included here to serve as background for the more practical aspects of maternity nursing. An understanding of physiology is essential, so that the nurse may recognize the special relation of physiology to problems in obstetrics.

Sexual Maturity

Female

Sexual maturity in the female begins at the time of puberty, with the onset of dramatic bodily changes. Early in the course of puberty, axillary and pubic hair appears. Shortly thereafter, there is a gradual change in the contour of the labia. The breasts also begin to mature at this time and there is a sudden increase in bodily growth.

These changes usually precede the onset of the first menstruation—the *menarche.* Establishment of the menstrual cycle is the most clearly identifiable sign of puberty and serves as an indication that the internal sex organs are approaching maturity. These physical changes are accompanied by emotional changes. The whole process of puberty spans about three years and is completed with the menarche.

The time sequence of changes that culminates in the attainment of reproductive potential varies considerably among individuals (Fig. 8-1). Bodily manifestations of puberty, such as the beginning of breast development, the appearance of pubic hair, and a spurt of growth, precede the actual onset of menstruation by a variable amount of time.

Throughout puberty there is an interplay of physiological and sociocultural forces, and often the nurse is called upon to explain the bodily and psychological changes in puberty to mothers who have daughters approaching their teens. There is often anxiety about the onset of pubertal changes that are thought to be occurring too early or too late. Therefore, it is important to recognize the wide variability from one young woman to the next.

Male

On the average, changes associated with puberty in the male occur somewhat later than in the female and span an interval of about four years. These include development of axillary, pubic, and body hair, and maturation and growth of the testes and penis over a two-to-three-year period, accompanied by a growth spurt and general muscular development.

Development of internal glands (prostate, bulbourethral, seminal vesicles) occurs synonymously with penile and testicular growth. These provide the seminal fluid in which spermatozoa are delivered during ejaculation. Ejaculation of fluid with penile erection may occur as soon as a year after the beginning of growth of the penis, even before it is of mature size. Generally, the ability to grow a full beard signifies the completion of male sexual maturity.

Menarche

Menarche usually occurs between the ages of 12 and 16, although heredity, race, state of nutrition, climate, and environment may influence early or late appearance. For example, maturity tends to occur earlier in warm climates and later in cold regions. The reproductive period spans about 35 years, from some point after the beginning of menstruation until its cessation during menopause, between ages 45 and 50.

Throughout childhood the *gonadotropins,* hormones produced by the pituitary gland to stimulate the ovaries, appear in very low concentrations. Estrogen, produced by the ovaries in the adult, remains undetectable. Puberty begins when there is a rise in the release of gonadotropins from the pituitary gland. These stimulate the ovary to secrete increasing amounts of *estrogen,* the hormone responsible for many of the bodily changes of puberty.

An orderly sequence of endocrinological events resulting in ovulation may not occur initially. The first few menstrual cycles following the menarche may not be associated with ovulation. However, once menstruation has occurred, it must be assumed that there is ovulation and, therefore, fertility and the potential for pregnancy.

Ovulation and Menstruation

Each month, with considerable regularity, a blisterlike structure about 1 cm in diameter develops on the surface of one of the ovaries. Within this bubble, almost lost in the fluid and cells around it, lies a tiny speck, scarcely visible to the naked eye (a thimble would hold 3 million of these specks). This speck is the human ovum—a truly amazing structure. It not only has the potential to develop into a human being, but it also embodies the mental as well as physical

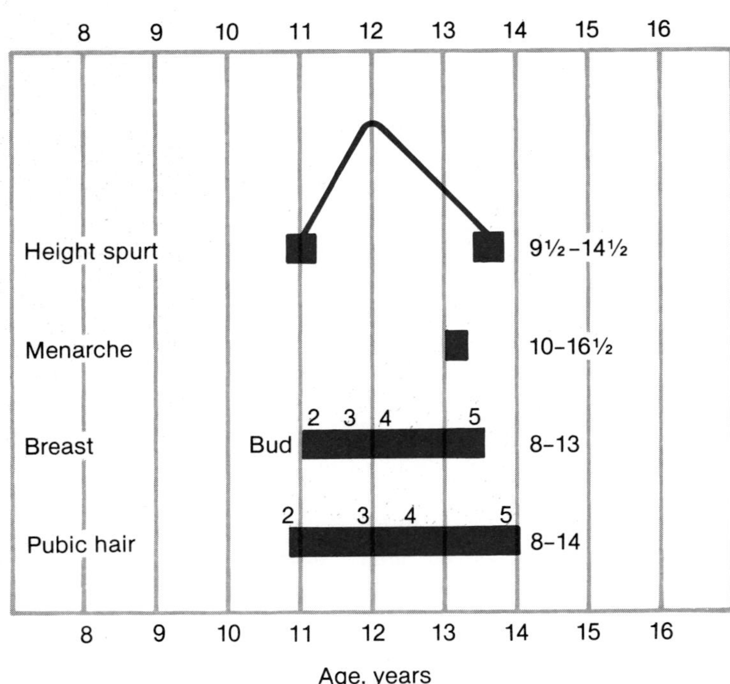

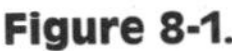

Figure 8-1.
Sequence of events at adolescence in girls. An average girl is represented; the range of ages within which some of the events may occur is noted. Breast development progresses from the development of the breast bud (2) through full development (5). There is progression from downy pubic hair (2) through complete development of hair over the mons (5). (After Tanner JM: Growth at Adolescence, 2nd ed. Oxford, England, Blackwell Science Publication, 1969. Pierson EC, D'Antonio WV: Female and Male: Dimensions of Human Sexuality. Philadelphia, JB Lippincott, 1974)

traits of the woman and her forebears (*e.g.,* her own brown eyes, her father's tall stature, her mother's genius at mathematics, or her grandfather's love of music). These and a million other potentials are contained in the ovum, which is so small that it is about one fourth the size of the period at the end of this sentence.

In the process of ovulation, one blister on one ovary ruptures at a given time each month and discharges an ovum. The precise day on which ovulation occurs is a matter of no small significance. For instance, because the ovum can only be fertilized (impregnated by the spermatozoon, or male germ cell) within hours after its escape from the ovary, the day after ovulation a woman is no longer fertile. However, a woman is potentially fertile for a number of days preceding the actual time of ovulation because spermatozoa survive in the female reproductive tract for hours, even days, awaiting the arrival of the ovum.

In a given cycle, the time of ovulation is unpredictable. Even the woman who consistently has regular menstrual periods could experience a delayed or early ovulation in any one cycle. This possibility of irregularity, combined with the potential for fertility any time prior to ovulation owing to the fact that spermatozoa retain their ability for fertilization, makes it difficult to identify accurately the fertile phase of a given cycle.

It should be remembered that the only really infertile interval is after ovulation has occurred. The time between ovulation and menstruation is relatively constant (14 ± 2 days); the time between menstruation and ovulation is variable enough that ovulation cannot be accurately predicted from one cycle to the next. It should be assumed that intercourse will result in conception unless some means of contraception is used, or if the patient is assured, by the use of the temperature chart described later, that she is past ovulation.

Graafian Follicle

In delving further into the process of ovulation, we find that at birth each ovary contains a huge number of undeveloped ova, probably more than 400,000. These are rather large, round cells with clear cytoplasm and a good-sized nucleus occupying the center. Each ovum is surrounded by a layer of a few small, flattened or spindle-shaped cells. The whole structure, ovum, and surrounding cells is a *follicle,* but in its underdeveloped state at birth it is a *primordial follicle.*

The formation of primordial follicles ceases at birth or shortly after, and the large number contained in the ovaries of the newborn represents a lifetime supply. The majority have disappeared before puberty, so that there are then perhaps 30,000 left. This disintegration of follicles continues throughout reproductive life until menopause when, usually, none are found.

Meanwhile, from birth to the menopause a few of these primordial follicles show signs of development.

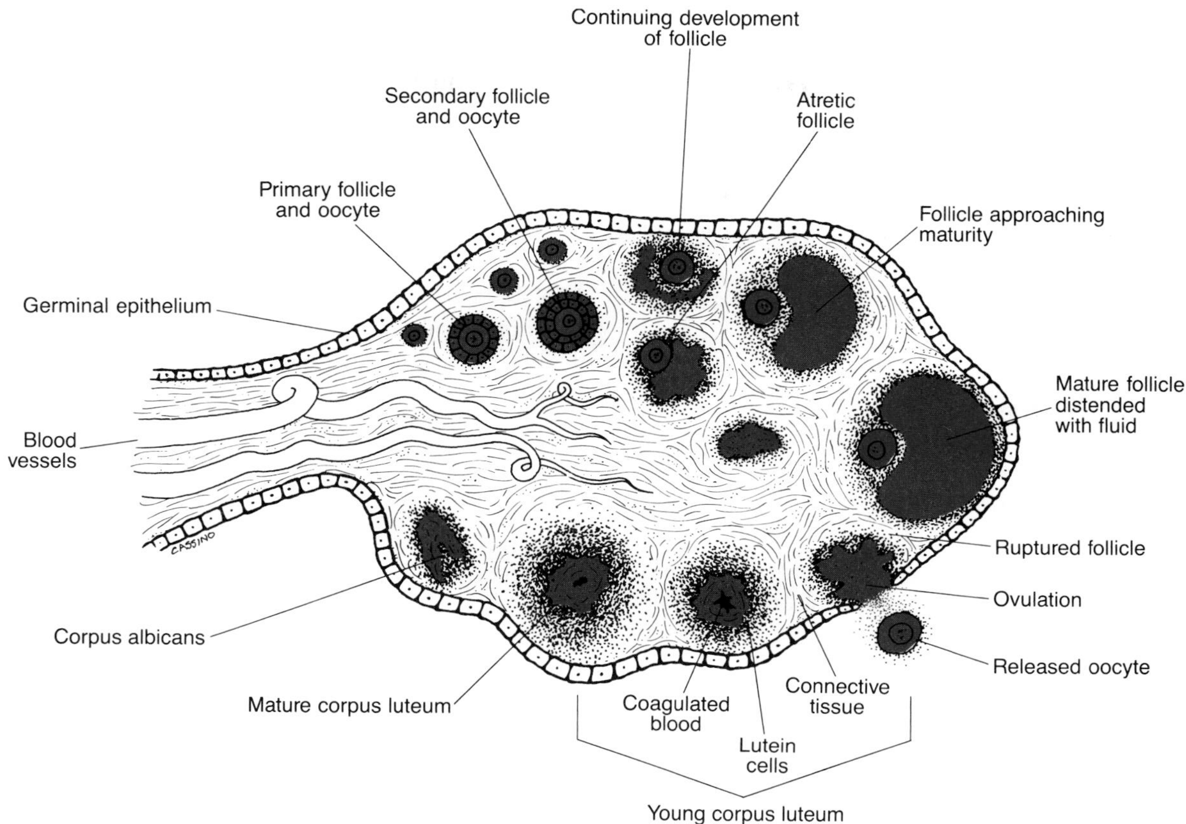

Figure 8-2.
Schematic design of an ovary, showing the sequence of events in the origin, growth, and rupture of an ovarian follicle. (Modified from Patten BM: Human Embryology, 3rd ed. New York, McGraw-Hill, 1968)

The surrounding granular layers of cells begin to multiply rapidly until they are several layers deep and, at the same time, become cuboid in shape. As this proliferation of cells continues, a very important fluid develops between them—the *follicular fluid.*

After puberty, the cells within the developing follicles produce estrogenic hormones, which in turn act on the reproductive organs and bring about cyclic bodily changes. During each menstrual cycle, several follicles develop further. One of these is finally selected by a process, not as yet completely understood, for complete maturation and ovulation.

Follicular fluid accumulates in such quantities that the multiplying follicle cells are pushed toward the margin; the ovum itself is almost surrounded by fluid and is suspended from the periphery of the follicle by only a small neck of cells. The structure is now known as the *graafian follicle,* named after Von Graaf, a Dutch physician who first described it in 1672.

As it increases enormously in size, the graafian follicle naturally pushes aside other follicles that form each month and a very noticeable, blisterlike projection appears on the surface of the ovary. At one point the follicular capsule becomes thin, and as the ovum reaches full maturity, it breaks free from the few cells attaching it to the periphery and floats in the follicular fluid. The thinned area of the capsule now ruptures, and the ovum is expelled from the ovary in the process of ovulation (Fig. 8-2).

Changes in the Corpus Luteum

After the discharge of the ovum, the ruptured follicle undergoes a change. It becomes filled with large cells containing a special yellow matter. The follicle then is known as the *corpus luteum,* or yellow body. If pregnancy does not occur, the corpus luteum reaches full development in about eight days, then retrogresses and is gradually replaced by fibrous tissue, the *corpus albicans.*

If pregnancy occurs, the corpus luteum enlarges somewhat and persists throughout the period of gestation, reaching its maximum size about the fourth or fifth month and retrogressing slowly thereafter. The corpus luteum secretes an extremely important substance, progesterone, which will be discussed later in this chapter.

In the absence of pregnancy, the corpus luteum remains active for about two weeks. The corpus luteum produces progesterone for the standard duration of the postovulatory phase of the menstrual cycle, 14 ± 2 days.

Menstrual Cycle

Menstruation in Relation to Pregnancy

Menstruation is the periodic discharge of blood, mucus, and epithelial cells from the uterus. It usually occurs at monthly intervals throughout the reproductive period, except during pregnancy and lactation, when it is usually suppressed. Accordingly, the span of years during which childbearing is possible, that is, from about ages 12 to 45, corresponds to the period during which ovulation and menstruation occur. In general, a woman who menstruates is able to conceive, whereas one who does not is probably infertile. Ovulation and menstruation are closely interlinked, and because no process of nature is purposeless, menstruation must play some vital and indispensable role in childbearing.

If day by day we were privileged to watch the *endometrium,* the lining membrane of the uterus, we would observe some remarkable alterations. Immediately following the termination of a menstrual period, this membrane is very thin, measuring a few millimeters in depth. Each day thereafter it becomes a trifle thicker and harbors an increasing content of blood. Its glands become more and more active and secrete a rich nutritive substance. About a week before the onset of the next expected period, this process reaches its height; the endometrium is now of the thickness of heavy, downy velvet and has become soft and succulent with blood and glandular secretions. At this time the ovum, if it has been fertilized, is embedded into this luxuriant lining.

All of these changes have only one purpose—to provide a suitable bed for the fertilized ovum to secure nourishment and to grow. If an ovum is not fertilized, these alterations serve no useful function. Accordingly, the swollen endometrium disintegrates, and the encased blood and glandular secretions escape into the uterine cavity. Passing through the cervix, they flow out through the vagina, carrying the tiny unfertilized ovum with them. In other words, menstruation represents the abrupt termination of a process designed to prepare lodging for a fertilized ovum. It forecasts the breakdown of a bed that is not needed because the "boarder" does not materialize. Thus, its purpose is to clear away the old bed so that a new and fresh one may be created the next month.

Hormonal Control of Menstruation

The menstrual cycle is regulated primarily through the highly coordinated function of the brain, the hypothalamus, the pituitary, the ovaries, and the uterus. If it was possible to inspect the ovaries from day to day during the menstrual cycle, it would be noted that the uterine alterations are directly related to certain changes that take place in the ovary. If it were possible to look further, it might be seen that the alterations that occur regularly in the ovarian cycle are directly related to certain phenomena that take place in the anterior pituitary gland and the hypothalamus, a portion of the brain that lies above the pituitary. Thus, the whole sequence represents the harmonious, integrated reactions of several processes within the human organism, all of which are necessary to maintain proper relationships in the menstrual cycle.

Phases of the Menstrual Cycle

Proliferative Phase

Again, immediately following menstruation the endometrium is very thin. During the subsequent week or so it proliferates markedly. The cells on the surface become taller, while the glands that dip into the endometrium become longer and wider. As the result of these changes, the thickness of the endometrium increases six- or eightfold.

Each month during this phase of the menstrual cycle (from approximately the fifth to the fourteenth days), a graafian follicle is approaching its greatest development and is manufacturing increasing amounts of follicular fluid. This fluid contains the estrogenic hormone *estrogen.* The word *hormone* comes from a Greek word that means *I bring about,* and in the case of estrogen, it brings about (among other things) the thickening of the endometrium described.

Each month after the cessation of menstruation, the cells in and around the developing graafian follicle produce estrogen which acts on the endometrium to cause it to grow or proliferate. For this reason, this phase of the menstrual cycle is commonly called the *proliferative phase,* although it is sometimes referred to as the *follicular,* or *estrogenic phase.*

Secretory Phase

Following the release of the ovum from the graafian follicle (ovulation), the cells that form the corpus luteum begin to secrete another important hormone, *progesterone,* in addition to estrogen. This supplements the action of estrogen on the endometrium in such a way that the glands become very tortuous or corkscrew in appearance and are greatly dilated. This change occurs because the glands are swollen with a secretion.

Meanwhile, the blood supply of the endometrium is increased, and it becomes vascular and succulent. Since these effects are directed at providing a bed for the fertilized ovum, it is easy to understand why the hormone that brings them about is called progesterone, meaning *for gestation.* It is also clear why this phase of the cycle, occupying the last 14 ± 2 days, is commonly called the *secretory phase* and why occasionally it is referred to as the *progestational, luteal,* or *premenstrual phase.*

Menstrual Phase

Unless the ovum is fertilized, the corpus luteum is short lived. Since corpus luteum cells secrete both progesterone and estrogen, cessation of corpus luteum activity means a withdrawal of both of these hormones. As a result, the endometrium degenerates. This is associated with rupture of countless small blood vessels in the endometrium with innumerable minute hemorrhages. Along with the blood, superficial fragments of the endometrium, together with mucin from the glands, are cast away, all of which constitutes the menstrual discharge (Fig. 8-3). Naturally, this phase of the cycle (from approximately the first to the fifth days) is called the *menstrual phase.*

Role of the Pituitary Gland

The pituitary gland is essential in the function of the reproductive system.* The anterior lobe of the pituitary, the "master clock," releases the gonadotropins, to stimulate the ovary, as well as other hormones. These hormones produce the ovarian alterations associated with ovulation. There are two principal gonadotropins. One is *follicle-stimulating hormone (FSH);* as its name implies, FSH stimulates the development of the follicle. The other is *luteinizing hormone (LH),* which is principally active during ovulation and the luteal phase of the cycle.

The release of the gonadotropic hormones by the pituitary is regulated by the *hypothalamus,* a specialized structure within the brain located just above the pituitary. The hypothalamus has a vascular connection to the pituitary gland, as well as nerve connections to the central nervous system. Indeed, its function can be modified by influences within the central nervous system. Thus, the function of the pituitary gland may be affected by the brain. The cyclic release of gonadotropin by the pituitary gland is controlled by a hormonal agent released by the hypothalamus. This is called gonadotropin-releasing hormone or LH/FSH-releasing hormone (GnRH or LH/FSH-RH), since it triggers the release of both FSH and LH from the pituitary gland.

*The posterior lobe of the pituitary gland produces oxytocin, a hormone that has an important role in obstetrics but one that differs altogether from the purpose of the present discussion.

Other Functions of Estrogen and Progesterone

In addition to their role in controlling menstruation, estrogen and progesterone serve other important functions. Estrogen is responsible for the development of the secondary sex characteristics, that is, all those distinctive sex manifestations that are not directly concerned with the process of reproduction. Thus, the growth of the breasts at puberty, the distribution of body fat, the size of the larynx and its resulting influence on the quality of the voice, as well as mating instincts, are all the results of estrogenic action. Thus, it may almost be said that a woman is a woman because of estrogen.

Aside from its action on the endometrium, progesterone also helps to relax the uterine muscle. Thus, it plays an important role in preserving the life of the embryo in early pregnancy, by preventing its expulsion from the uterus and by preparing the endometrium to receive and nourish it.

Sensitive laboratory methods now allow accurate measurement of day-to-day changes in circulating pituitary and ovarian hormones (Fig. 8-4). The interplay between the pituitary and the ovary, influenced in turn by the central nervous system through the hypothalamus, brings about orderly development of the follicle and ovulation.

At the end of a given cycle and at the beginning of the subsequent cycle (see Fig. 8-4), the pituitary gland releases increased amounts of FSH. With the help of small amounts of LH, FSH stimulates maturation of several ovarian follicles. Together LH and FSH produce modest amounts of the estrogen, estradiol. The levels of estradiol in the bloodstream begin to rise and estradiol in turn acts negatively on the central nervous system at hypothalamic-pituitary level by inhibiting the release of additional amounts of FSH. Consequently, the level of FSH in the circulating blood begins to fall. FSH also acts on the follicle to make it more sensitive to LH.

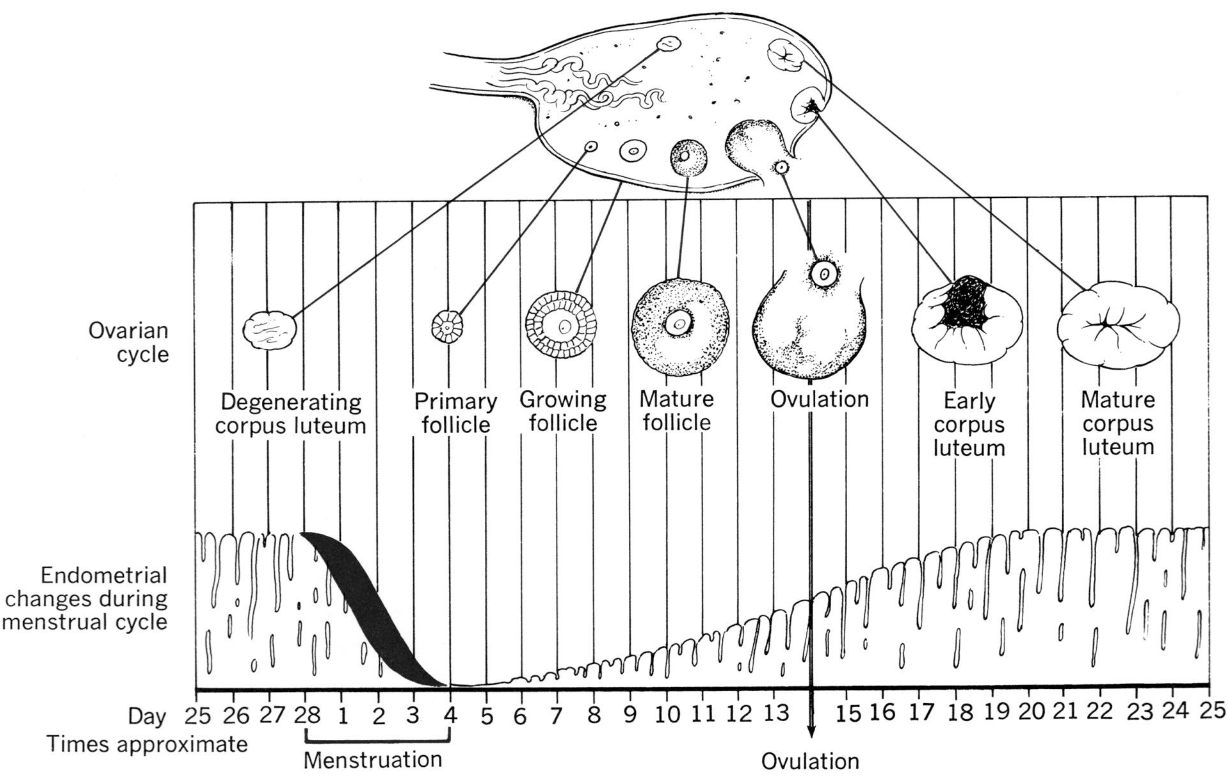

Figure 8-3.
Schematic representation of one ovarian cycle and the corresponding changes in thickness of the endometrium. It is thickest just before the onset of menstruation and thinnest just as it ceases.

About two days before ovulation, all but the one follicle that is destined to ovulate begin to regress in a process called atresia. That one follicle undergoes rapid growth, and estrogen production rises sharply. The increased amount of estrogen produced at this point then acts positively at the central nervous system-hypothalamic level, stimulating a rapid increase in GnRH levels. In turn, GnRH causes large amounts of LH, as well as additional FSH, to be released from the pituitary gland. This dramatic rise in LH stimulates the completion of maturation of the follicle and within 24 hours after the LH surge, ovulation takes place.

The increased levels of preovulatory estrogen prepare the genital tract for sperm migration. The secretions of the cervix, scanty and viscous early in the cycle, become thin and watery and more receptive to spermatozoa. The vaginal wall also reflects the effects of estrogen. A vaginal smear taken at this time reveals a large percentage of mature, or "cornified," cells. The endometrium displays maximal proliferation (see Fig. 8-3).

Following ovulation, the cyclic pattern continues. The ruptured follicle is transformed into a corpus luteum. The second function of LH is to maintain the corpus luteum. These endocrine events are associated with further modifications in the cervical mucus, vagina, and endometrium. The mucus becomes thick, "tacky," and viscous, and is no longer as receptive to spermatozoa. The vaginal smear reflects the influence of progesterone with a decreasing "maturation index." The endometrium takes on secretory changes preparatory to implantation.

Progesterone secretion by the corpus luteum reaches its maximum about five to seven days after ovulation (see Fig. 8-4). This is the time when the fertilized egg, now a *blastocyst,* is ready to implant. If pregnancy has occurred, another hormone, *human chorionic gonadotropin (hCG),* appears within two to three days of implantation. This hormone, which is produced by the conceptus, acts on the corpus luteum, maintaining its progesterone-providing function, and transforms it into a corpus luteum of pregnancy. If pregnancy has not intervened, the corpus luteum begins its demise at this time. Approximately 10 to 11 days after ovulation, progesterone levels decline precipitously, and on about the 14th

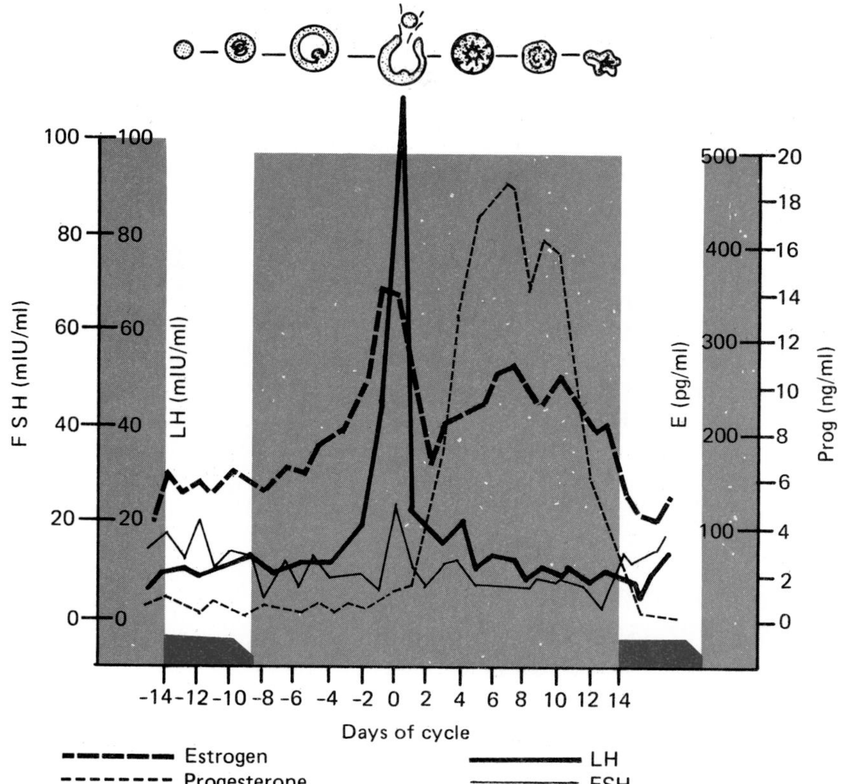

Figure 8-4.
Plasma hormones in the normal menstrual cycle.

postovulatory day, no longer receiving hormones, the endometrium begins to shed in the process of menstruation.

Bodily Manifestations of Ovarian Function

From what has been discussed concerning the underlying mechanism of menstruation, it is clear that the monthly flow of blood is only one phase of a marvelous cyclic process that not only makes childbearing possible, but also profoundly influences both body and mind. For this reason, the time of the onset of menstruation is a critical period in the life of a young woman.

The average age at which the onset of menstruation occurs is between 12 years of age and 14 years of age. It may be as early as the ninth year or as late as the eighteenth year and still be within normal limits. Although the interval of the menstrual cycle, counting from the beginning of one period to the onset of the next, averages 28 days, there are wide variations even in the same woman. Indeed, a woman rarely menstruates exactly every 28 or 30 days each month. This has been the subject of several studies on normal young women. These investigations show that the majority of women (almost 60%) experience variations of at least five days in the length of their menstrual cycles; differences in the same woman of even 10 days are not uncommon and may occur without explanation or apparent detriment to health.

The degree and intensity of the outward manifestations of the ovulatory cycle vary from one individual to the next. Some women consistently experience pelvic discomfort during ovulation, or "mittelschmerz," so named because it typically appears in the middle of a 28-day menstrual cycle. Slight staining or occasional bleeding may occur in association with ovulation. In the postovulatory interval there may be breast tenderness and fullness which typically reaches a peak just before menstruation. Premenstrual "tension" characterized by increased irritability may also occur after ovulation.

Cyclic changes in the quality of the cervical mucus may be observed and are often easily detected by the patient when she is made aware of this possibility. In some cases, a clear translucent mucus appears at the labia or may be wiped from the cervix to provide suggestive evidence of impending ovulation. In the postovulatory phase of the cycle, the mucus becomes sticky and less abundant. Daily observations of cervical mucus changes have been suggested as a useful parameter in using the "rhythm" method of contraception.

Normal menstruation should not be accompanied by pain; however, there may be some general malaise, together with a feeling of weight and discomfort in the pelvis. Painful menstruation is known as *dysmenorrhea.* If there is a great irregularity, extremely profuse flow, or marked pain, a pathologic condition may be present. Absence of menses is known as *amenorrhea.* The most common cause of amenorrhea is pregnancy, but sometimes it is brought about by emotional disturbances, such as fear, worry, or fatigue, which work through the central nervous system and hypothalamus, or by debilitating disease (*e.g.,* anemia, tuberculosis).

Variations in Basal Body Temperature

Beginning about the first year of life, slight daily variations in body temperature normally occur in all human beings. These temperature variations are relative to the time of the day and the nature of the circumstances surrounding the individual. For example, the body temperature is lowest in the morning before breakfast, after a good night's rest, and before activity. After a day of normal activity, the body temperature is usually highest toward afternoon and early evening. The fact that physiological variations in basal body temperature also occur in relation to the menstrual cycle is important here because it can be useful in estimating the time of ovulation. Such an index becomes extremely important in studies of fertility and sterility.

In the woman who is ovulating, there is normally a rhythmic variation in the basal body temperature curve during the course of the menstrual cycle (Fig. 8-5). The basal temperature is lower during the first part of the menstrual cycle, the proliferative phase. It rises in association with ovulation and remains relatively higher during the luteal phase of the cycle. The rise in the basal temperature occurs as a result of the influence of progesterone, produced by the corpus luteum following ovulation. Progesterone causes this thermogenic effect through its influence on the central nervous system. The basal temperature rises as much as 0.5 of a degree, and a relatively higher temperature is sustained until just before the onset of the menstrual period. This interval occupies the 14 ± 2 terminal days in the cycle.

If pregnancy occurs, the progesterone level is maintained, and under its influence the basal temperature remains high past the expected time of the period. In the absence of pregnancy, the basal temperature usually drops a day or so before the menstrual period.

The Use of the Basal Temperature Graph

The basal body temperature is one of the most practical means of diagnosing ovulation. It is the relative difference in basal body temperature during the course of the cycle which is the important diagnostic criterion for ovulation. It is only useful in the timing of ovulation retrospectively. Thus, when there is infertility, efforts to time intercourse to coincide with changes in the temperature chart have not proved worthwhile. In fact, such regulation of coital habits is not recommended. However, for the diagnosis of ovulation, the temperature chart has proved valuable. The temperature chart is also useful as an adjunct to the rhythm method of family planning (see Chap. 12).

Directions

1. The first day of menses is considered to be the first day of the menstrual cycle. The duration of menstrual flow is recorded, beginning on cycle day 1, (see Fig. 8-5). The date of onset of flow is recorded, and each subsequent date is recorded in the spaces provided. Following cessation of flow, the morning temperature is taken. Oral temperatures are as satisfactory as rectal recordings and are certainly more convenient. The temperature should be taken immediately after waking and before getting out of bed, talking, eating, drinking, or smoking. Ideally, it should be taken at about the same time every morning.
2. The thermometer is read to within 0.1 of a degree, and the reading is recorded on the chart.
3. Any known cause for temperature variation should be noted on the chart, for example, interrupted or shortened sleep, a cold, indigestion, or emotional disturbance. If intercourse has occurred, that fact should be recorded with a circle around the recording the following morning.
4. Some women can recognize ovulation by mittelschmerz; others have vaginal bleeding or clear preovulatory vaginal discharge. Such manifestations should also be recorded on the chart.

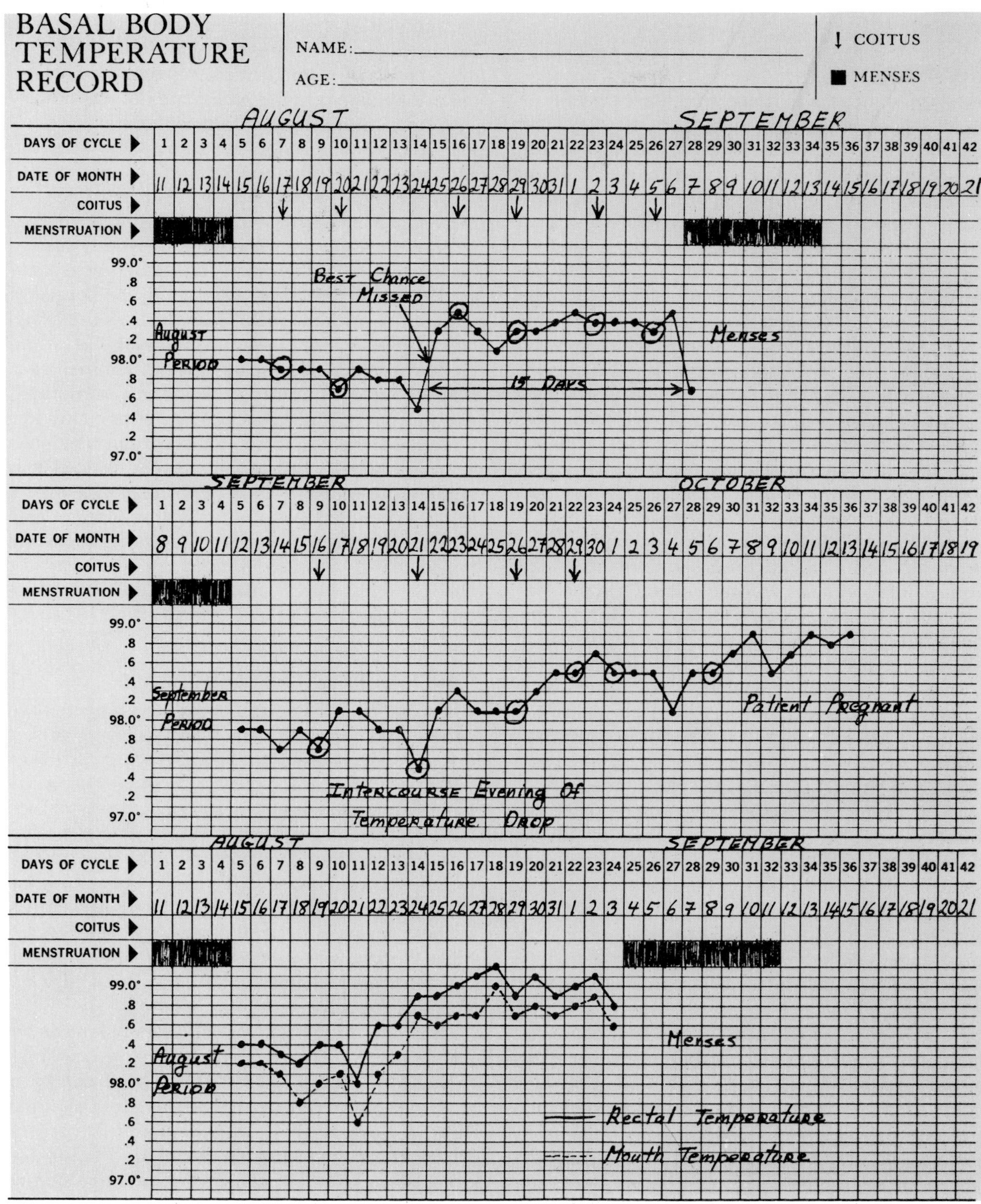

Figure 8-5.
Basal temperature chart. Directions for using this chart are given on page 120. (Published by Merrill-National Laboratories, Div. of Richardson-Merrill Inc., Cincinnati, Ohio 45215.)

Menopause

Menopause means the cessation of menstruation. In about 50% of women this usually occurs between the ages of 45 and 50. About 25% will reach menopause before the age of 45 and 25% after the age of 50. In commmon usage, menopause generally means cessation of *regular* menstruation. Since this is a normal process of aging and takes place gradually, the periods may become scanty or irregular, or intermittantly heavy before ceasing altogether. Cessation of ovarian activity, that is, estrogen production and ovulation cause menopause. Often the term menopause and climacteric are used synonymously, but the usage is not accurate. Climacteric encompasses the total syndrome of endocrine, somatic, and psychic changes occurring at the termination of the reproductive period in the female. It is derived from the Greek meaning *rung of the ladder,* or critical point in human life. The termination of estrogen production associated with the cessation of ovarian function cause the ovary, the uterus, and the breasts to decrease in size. The external genitals become flattened and the vaginal walls lose their folds, elasticity, and lubrication, becoming shiny and smooth. The decrease in estrogen levels may also produce intermittent "hot flashes" and some emotional instability, for example, irritability and sudden outbursts of tears much like the emotional lability associated with premenstrual tension. Increasing dryness of hair and skin are also associated with the menopausal years.

Each woman reacts somewhat differently to this withdrawal of estrogen. These reactions are unpredictable, vary from woman to woman, and depend, to some extent, on her previous emotional history, her present support systems within the family, and to a very real extent, on the fact that the menopausal reproductive-endocrine system may be quite labile during this interval, which may last as long as eight or nine years.

Hot flashes are not an old wives' tale; they are real and a result of vasomotor instability. This instability also results in sweating and brief sensations of being cold "all over." There may be redness and perspiration that are visible, or the sensations may be equally intense but with no visible signs. Their daily frequency may vary and there can be long intervals, sometimes weeks with no symptoms at all.

Menopause may result from other than the natural physiological alterations of the climacteric. The term *artificial menopause* describes the cessation of menstruation produced by some artificial means, such as an irradiation of the ovaries or surgical operation for the removal of the ovaries (oophorectomy) or the uterus (hysterectomy). As a result of either surgery, the woman will no longer menstruate, but beyond this the manifestations in the patient are not identical.

Certain misunderstandings based on incorrect interpretation of terminology are rather widespread and should be clarified. The fact that a woman has had a hysterectomy and ceases to menstruate does not mean that her healthy ovaries will not function. Hysterectomy involves only the removal of the uterus. On the other hand, if the ovaries are also removed surgically or are treated by irradiation, the source of estrogen is withdrawn abruptly and thus the symptoms caused by the sudden withdrawal of this hormone will occur. Because there is much misinformation among the public on this point, sometimes intensive preoperative and postoperative counseling is required. Abrupt interruption of ovarian function in a woman who is still having regular periods may create more withdrawal symptoms than in a woman who is in her menopausal years. The younger woman may need estrogen replacement to alleviate signs and symptoms of estrogen withdrawal. The need for estrogen replacement in the older woman after surgical removal of ovaries will vary from patient to patient.

Physiology of the Menopause

When one considers that menopause is experienced by all middle-aged women, it may seem surprising that the endocrine and metabolic changes associated with it are still not completely understood. This lack of information is due, in part, to difficulties associated with long-term, longitudinal studies spanning many years. In addition, the sensitive endocrine assays which would allow study of the endocrinological events associated with menopause have only recently become available. Because of this, estrogen replacement therapy with its possible short- or long-term effects has created much controversy in both lay and scientific literature.

It is now known that several years before menopause there is an increase in circulating levels of both FSH and LH. The actual levels of estrogen and progesterone produced by the ovaries are decreased. These are only slight changes, and in spite of them, ovulation and menstruation continue to occur. The decreasing production of estradiol and progesterone undoubtedly allows release of increased amounts of gonadotropins from the pituitary, resulting in higher circulating levels of FSH and LH.

In normal postmenopausal women, FSH and LH levels are consistently high. The ratio of FSH to LH is always greater than one. Both of the gonadotropins are released in a pulsating fashion, similar to that seen in younger women but much more pronounced, with bursts occurring every 10 minutes to 20 minutes. There is also periodic fluctuation in gonadotropin levels that occurs about every two hours. After removal of the ovaries in regularly menstruating women, gonadotropin levels begin to rise within two days. The rise in the FSH is more dramatic than that of LH.

Estrogen production by the postmenopausal ovary is minuscule. Surgical removal of the ovaries after menopause does not affect circulating estrogens in any significant way. However, the postmenopausal ovary does continue to produce androgens, and in increased amounts. The appearance of dark hair on the upper lip and chin is seen in some women. Since varying amounts of circulating estrogen are found in the postmenopausal women, it has been suggested that estrogen may be produced elsewhere in the body and also that other tissues are able to convert the circulating androgens to estrogen. Fat, the liver, and some areas of the hypothalamus are capable of this conversion. Such estrogen production varies from one postmenopausal woman to the next, and this variability may account for some of the variations in menopausal symptoms.

The mechanism responsible for *vasomotor symptoms* is not known. Obviously, neuroendocrinological factors are at work. It has been suggested that catecholamines that act as neurotransmitters in the brain—they transfer information from one neuron to another—may respond to fluctuating gonadotropin or ovarian hormone levels. Catecholamines are responsible for modulating behavior and motor activity as well as the function of the hypothalamus and pituitary. Disturbance in catecholamine activity produces vasodilatation in the brain that could bring about hot flashes. Many other environmental influences operate on the life of a postmenopausal woman and it is difficult to separate these from the physiological events associated with decreased ovarian function. Although it is clear that emotional and physical stress can be related to increased frequency of vasomotor symptoms and signs, this relationship does not always occur in a predictable fashion. Hot flashes are the result of vasomotor instability and are clearly related to the estrogen deficiency associated with the cessation of ovarian function.

Changes in the vaginal mucosa also vary among menopausal women. Even minimal changes may result in painful intercourse *(dyspareunia)*. Thinning of the vaginal lining and the decrease in lubrication can be corrected with estrogen administered orally or locally with vaginal suppositories or cream. Dyspareunia is a common symptom that should not be overlooked in the management of the postmenopausal woman.

Osteoporosis, demineralization of the bones, commonly occurs following menopause. Decreasing levels of estrogens are known to be associated with loss of bone calcium which is evidenced by high levels of circulating calcium in the plasma. This circulating calcium is excreted by the kidneys, leaving the body in a negative calcium balance. Osteoporosis is a serious medical condition in elderly women, as hip fractures in this age group are common. Healing is poor when there is osteoporosis, leading to long hospitalization and the morbidity associated with a nonambulatory status. Unfortunately, osteoporosis is seldom discovered in its beginning stages; often it goes undetected until a fracture occurs. Evidence of osteoporosis in the postmenopausal woman generally indicates a need for estrogen therapy.

Estrogen Replacement

A good case could be made for routine use of estrogen in all postmenopausal women were it not for some of its side-effects. The most serious of these is a greater incidence of endometrial carcinoma among estrogen-treated women than in the nontreated. Such factors must be carefully weighed and a risk–benefit ratio established for each individual patient.

One must consider the severity of the symptoms against the potential hazards of estrogen treatment and the quality of life. Signs and symptoms that interfere with working outside or inside the home or with a good sexual life are clear indications for treatment. Absolute contraindications to estrogen treatment include liver disease, cerebrovascular disease, venous thrombosis and embolism, and an estrogen-dependent malignancy of the breast or uterus. The use of estrogen in the menopausal years requires a carefully considered medical decision and, if instituted, careful monitoring during the course of treatment.

Physiology of the Male Reproductive Tract

The functional capacity of the male reproductive tract is governed principally by the testes. Like the ovary, the testis is dependent on an interplay between the brain, the hypothalamus and the pituitary gland. The testes have two functions—secretion of the male hormone, testosterone, and spermatogenesis, the production and release of spermatozoa. Both are initiated at about the time of puberty and, under normal circumstances, continue well into senescence. Testosterone production can occur independently of spermatogenesis, but spermatogenesis cannot occur independently of testosterone production.

Spermatogenesis

Spermatogenesis is initiated and maintained in the seminiferous tubules of the testes. The seminiferous tubules are long coiled structures containing a lumen into which spermatozoa are released from their epithelial wall where they are produced. (Fig. 8-6). During this process, meiosis occurs, and the number of chromosomes in each cell is reduced to half, which is the haploid number (see Fig. 9-2). A structurally mature spermatozoon is produced, complete with head, midpiece, and tail (see Fig. 10-5). The maturation of the human spermatozoon occupies an interval of 60 days.

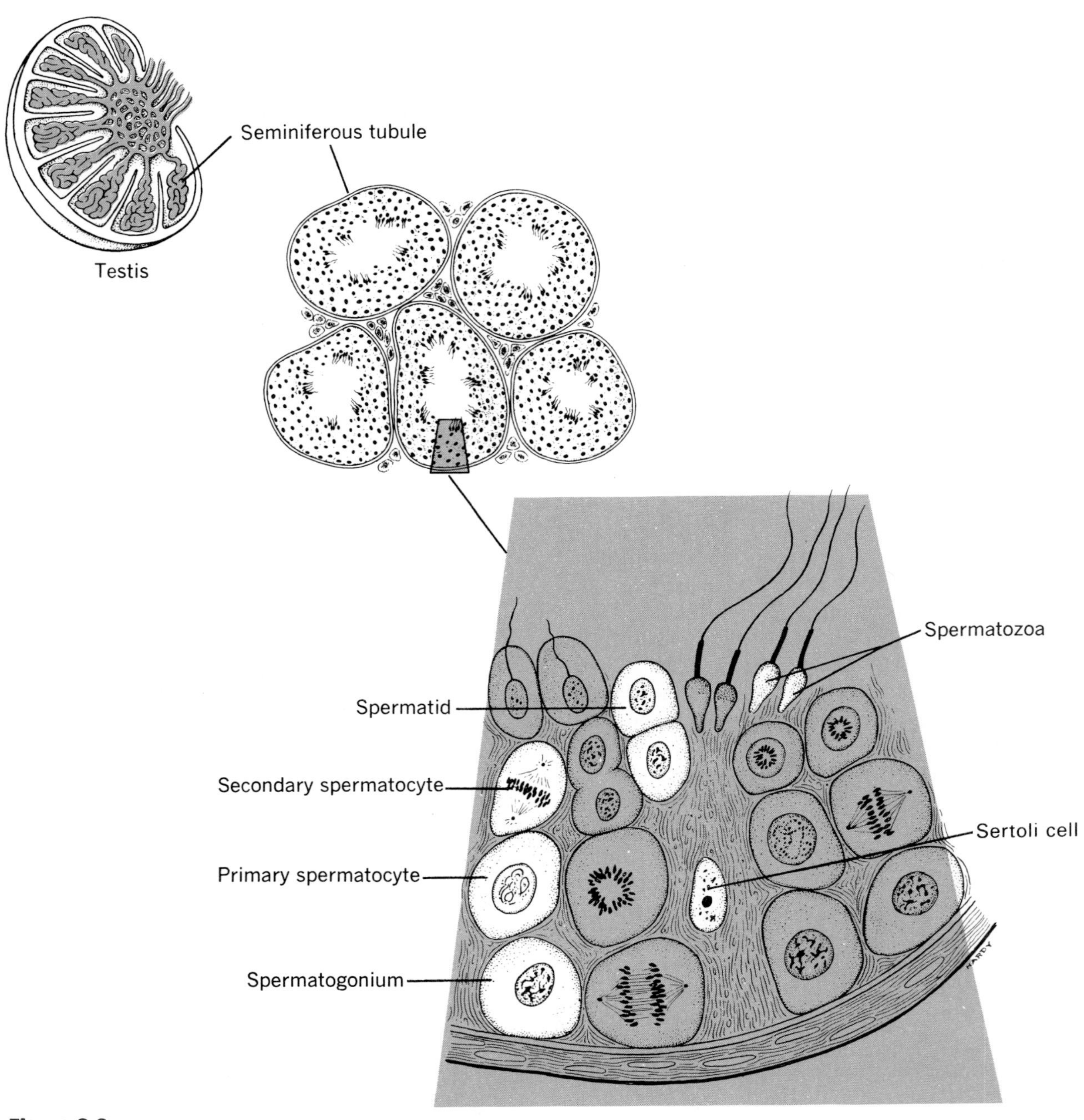

Figure 8-6.
Section of a seminiferous tubule, showing various stages of spermatogenesis.

Testicular Hormone Production

The adult testes produce a continuous supply of the male hormone, testosterone. Testosterone is synthesized and released by the interstitial cells, also referred to as Leydig cells. The interstitial cells are located in the interstitial connective tissue that surrounds and supports the seminiferous tubules (see Fig. 8-6). The interstitial cells are stimulated to produce testosterone by LH, which is released from the anterior pituitary gland. This is identical to the LH that is released in large amounts at midcycle to trigger the onset of ovulation in the female. In the male, LH is sometimes referred to by another name, interstitial cell stimulating hormone (ICHS). ICHS does not display the marked cyclic variation in concentration seen during the menstrual cycle, although as in the female, its release from the pituitary gland is controlled by releasing hormones from the brain and hypothalamus. There is a reciprocal relationship between LH release and testosterone production by the interstitial cells.

Testosterone establishes and maintains the secondary sex characteristics of the male, such as development and maturation of the external genitalia, prostate and seminal vesicles, growth of body and facial hair, and maturation of the larynx. It also contributes to body growth and general muscular development.

The principal role of testosterone in terms of reproduction is maintenance of spermatogenesis. Unless it is present in normal amounts, fertility is impaired.

Testicular Transport of Sperm

The wall of the seminiferous tubules is separated into two physiologically distinct compartments by specialized supporting cells, the Sertoli cells. These cells

Figure 8-7.
Diagram of the stages of sperm release. The conjoined cell bodies of the advanced spermatids are retained in the epithelium while the nucleus, neck region, and tail are gradually extruded into the lumen. The narrow stalk connecting the neck region with the cell body becomes increasingly attenuated and finally gives way. Individual spermatozoa are thus separated from the syncytial cell bodies. (Redrawn from Greep RO, Koblinsky MA (eds): Frontiers in Reproduction and Fertility Control. MIT Press, Cambridge, 1977)

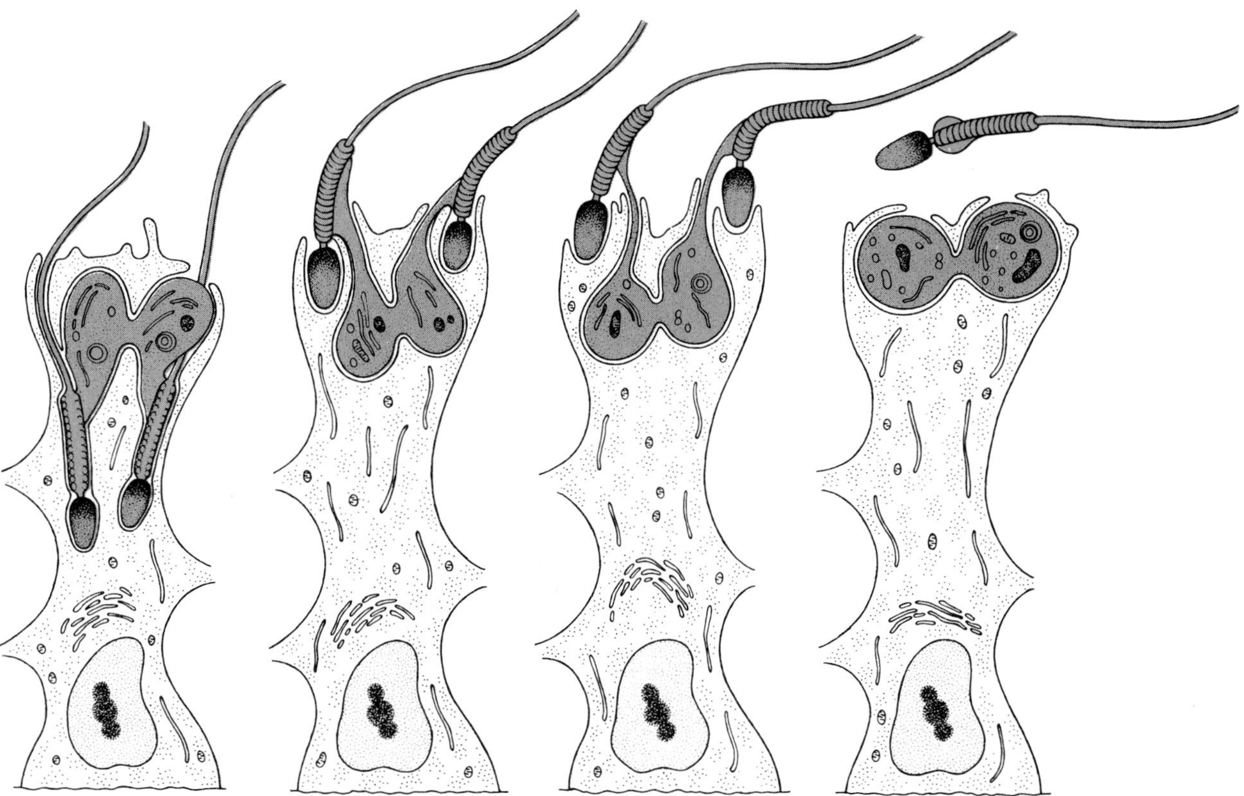

are large, easily identifiable structures that are joined to each other by firm cell to cell connections. They separate the epithelium into a basal and a luminal compartment. This arrangement produces an effective separation of the basal compartment from the circulation and provides a blood–testes permeability barrier. In this way the early developing sperm-forming elements are protected from harmful substances that may be circulating in the blood stream.

The Sertoli cell plays an active role in the release of spermatozoa into the lumen of the seminiferous tubules. The tight junctions between the Sertoli cells break down transiently to permit upward movement of spermatocytes into the compartment adjacent to the lumen. They are then drawn into the cytoplasm of the Sertoli cell, moved upward toward the surface of the cell, and finally extruded by contractions of the cytoplasm of the apex of the Sertoli cells (Fig. 8-7).

Duct System

Leading from the testes are the transporting and storage ducts of the male reproductive tract. The seminiferous tubules coalesce at the rete testis. These in turn enter the epididymis, a separate structure located adjacent to the testis (Fig. 8-8). The epididymis serves as a reservoir for spermatozoa where they are further conditioned. The epididymis is divided into a head portion (caput) and a tail (cauda). The cauda is connected to the vas deferens, which in turn leads to the ejaculatory ducts. The ejaculatory ducts empty into the urethra at the base of the penis. Spermatozoa are stored in the epididymis and vas deferens and are released during ejaculation and accompanied by seminal fluid.

During ejaculation the semen receives a contribution from the seminal vesicles and the prostate gland. The seminal vesicles are paired glands located dorsal to the neck of the bladder. They deliver their secretions to the urethra through the ejaculatory ducts, discharging a fructose-rich product. The prostate, located around the base of the urethra, transmits its contents into the urethra during ejaculation through a number of small ducts. It secretes a clear fluid with a slightly acid *p*H that is rich in acid phosphatase, citric acid, zinc, and a number of proteolytic enzymes.

The function of the accessory sex organs is maintained by testosterone. The role of seminal vesicular and prostatic secretions is to transport spermatozoa during ejaculation. They may also contribute briefly to the metabolism of spermatozoa. The ejaculate, or semen, consists of spermatozoa and seminal vesicular and prostatic secretions.

Two additional accessory glands, the bulbourethral, or Cowper's glands, empty into the bulbous urethra. They provide a lubricating fluid that main-

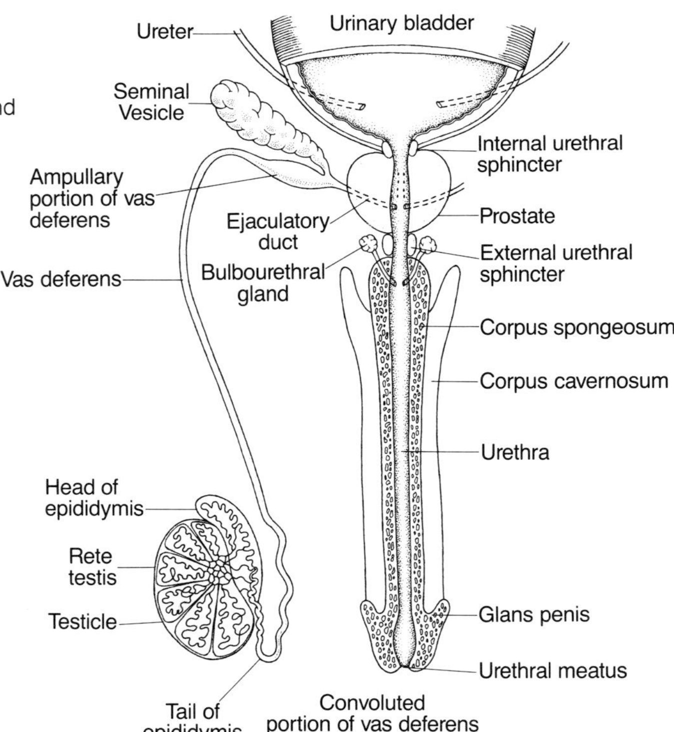

Figure 8-8.
Schematic representation of the male genital organs, illustrating the relation of the prostate and ejaculatory ducts to the internal and external sphincters, bladder, and urethra. (Redrawn from Amelar RD: Infertility in Men. Philadelphia, FA Davis, 1966)

tains moisture within the urethra. At the height of sexual excitement and full erection, their contents may be released, sometimes carrying with them a few spermatozoa.

The penis, which consists of two lateral bodies, the corpus cavernosum, and a central core of erectile tissue, the corpus spongiosum, becomes turged during erection. The glans of the penis, an extension of the corpus spongiosum, enlarges greatly during erection. When the erect penis is stimulated further, impulses from the autonomic nervous system trigger pulsatile release of semen along the urethra.

Female and Male Reproductive Capacity

Women have a limited reproductive life span, beginning soon after menarche, declining somewhat in the late reproductive years, and finally terminating at the menopause. No more than 500 ova may be released during the course of reproductive life. In the male, spermatogenesis is initiated at the time of puberty and sperm production continues well into senescence. The number of mature spermatozoa produced by the testes during this very long interval are in the billions, and the reproductive capacity of a given fertile male is nothing short of phenomenal.

Another important difference is that in the male the capacity to reproduce is necessarily associated with sexual excitement, erection of the penis, and ejaculation. As a requisite for procreation, the male must have an erection and the associated stimulation required to produce it. However, the capacity of the female to reproduce may be disassociated from sexual excitement and receptivity. Consider that conception can occur by mechanical placement of the ejaculate through artificial insemination. The capacity of the woman for sexual pleasure, however, is extremely important. There is no doubt that the physical aspects of a relationship play a critical role in the communication process that brings a couple closer together. The physiology and psychology of human sexual response is considered in detail in Chapter 9.

Suggested Reading

Greep RO, Koblinsky MA: Frontiers in Reproduction and Fertility Control. Cambridge, The MIT Press, 1977

Greep RO, Koblinsky MA, Jaffe FS: Reproduction and Human Welfare: A Challenge to Research. Cambridge, The MIT Press, 1977

Gwatkin RBL: Fertilization Mechanisms in Man and Mammals. New York, Plenum Press, 1977

Speroff L, Glass RH, Kase NG: Clinical Gynecologic Endocrinology and Infertility, 2nd ed. Baltimore, Williams & Wilkins, 1979

Yen SS, Jaffe RB: Reproductive Endocrinology: Physiology, Pathophysiology and Clinical Management. Philadelphia, WB Saunders, 1978

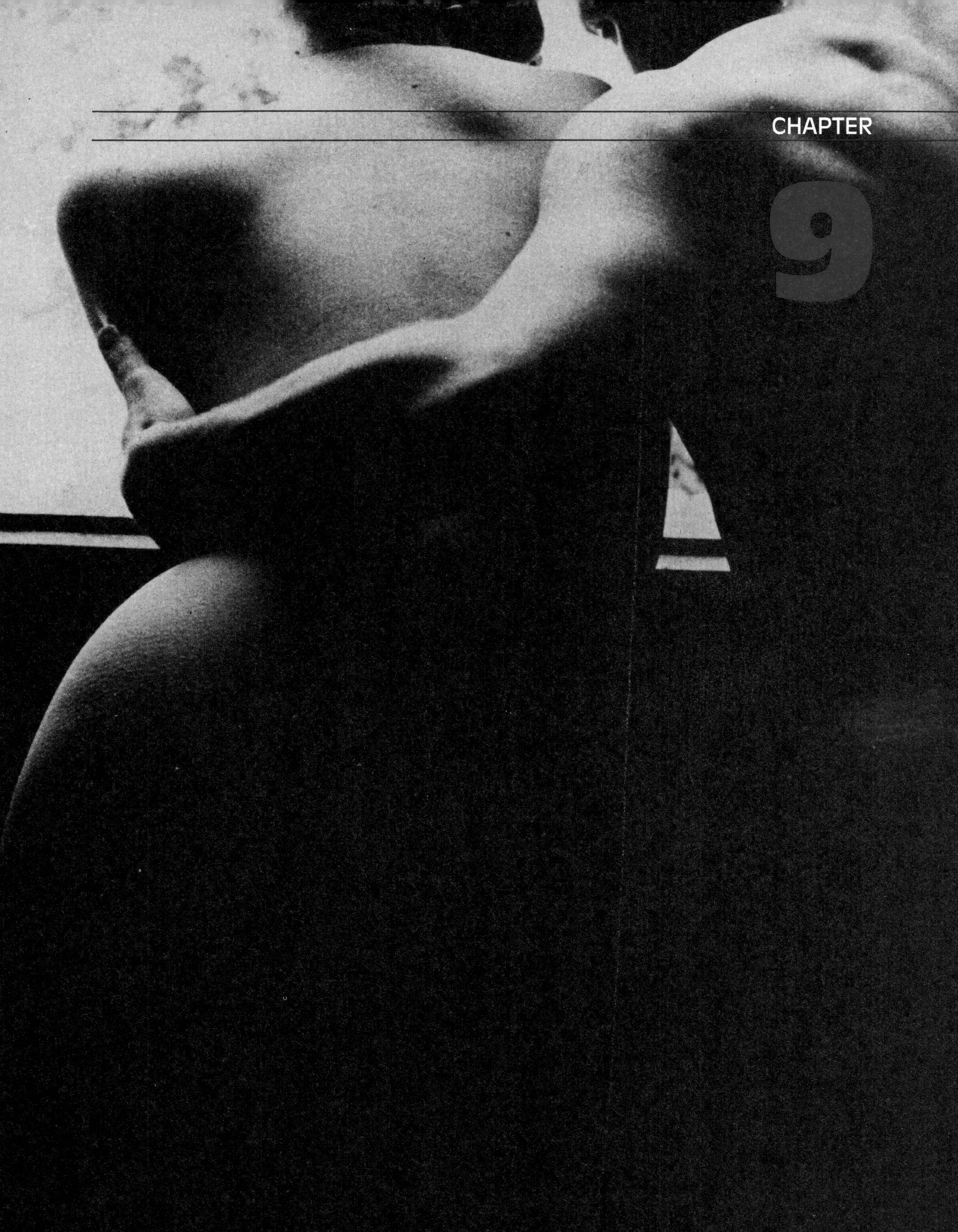

CHAPTER 9

CHAPTER 9

Human Sexual Response

Sexual response in men and women is a complex process with both psychological and physiological components. Sex can be considered one of the basic human drives, but is much more malleable in expression than food and sleep, for example. Although a nearly universal behavior among humans, sex can be postponed for long periods or, in some instances, never activated, without adverse effects. Although cultural expression leads to a wide variety of sex-related behaviors, the biological roots of sexual interaction lead to more underlying similarities than differences among peoples.

The apparent sexual differences between men and women have received much emphasis, and have been viewed as both a source of delight and pleasure and a cause of conflict and strain. However, since the advent of sex research, it has been found that male and female sexual responses are more alike than different. The woman's sex drive, in an era of greater social support and openness, is assumed to be as powerful as the man's, although an adequate measurement is lacking. The common stereotype that women need affection and intimacy to respond sexually, while men respond regardless of the relationship has been found to have numerous exceptions. Sexual responses of both men and women are direct and simple at times, and mysterious and complex at others.

The basic similarities of physiological sexual responses between both sexes has been stressed by such researchers as Kinsey and Masters and Johnson. Aside from the obvious anatomic differences, men and women are homogeneous in their physiological responses to sexual stimuli. There are direct parallels in male and female anatomic responses to effective sexual stimulation, and the same underlying physiological mechanisms are involved—vasocongestion and myotonia.[1] For example, vaginal lubrication in the woman is parallel to penile erection in the man, and both responses occur as a result of vasocongestion. Increases in muscle tension *(myotonia),* changes in heart rate, blood pressure, and respiration are common to both men and women during sexual excitement. The reflexive contractions of orgasm are virtually identical in both sexes, although there are variations in the results that these contractions produce. And, there is a considerable overlap in the subjective experience of orgasm.

The psychological and physiological components of human sexual response cannot really be separated because these are intricately interrelated and create numerous feedback loops that can enhance or inhibit sexual response. The changes in bodily function and the perceptions and emotions that precede or accompany these will both be included, although greater emphasis is placed upon physiological processes.

Components of Sexuality

A person's sexuality may be thought of as a complex of emotions, attitudes, preferences, and behaviors that are related to erotic expression. Among the many components of sexuality are a person's genetic (chromosomal) sex, gonadal sex, hormonal sex, morphological sex, gender identity, behavioral sex (sex role), and sexual partner preference. Usually there is congruence among these components, but this is not necessarily true. *Homosexuality* is an example of genetic, gonadal, and hormonal sex being incongruent with behavioral sex and sexual partner preference, at least by the dominant social definitions. *Transsexualism* (desiring to have the body, sexual organs, and sex role of the opposite sex) is an example of conflict between gender identity and genetic, gonadal, hormonal, and morphological sex.

In the more common case where there is congruence among the components of sexuality, it appears that the person's biological equipment provides a frame through which sociocultural definitions of sexuality can be expressed. There is considerable evidence that the expression of sexuality is largely learned, although the significance of relations among gonadal hormones, anatomic structures, and sexual behavior is only in the beginning stages of exploration.[2,3] Among humans, there are very few imperative, or unalterable, sexual behaviors, including ejaculation in the male and menstruation, pregnancy, and childbirth in the female. These are necessary to carry out reproductive functions. All other sexual behaviors are, in a sense, optional. They are subject to environmental influences and comprise a very large sociocultural expression of sexual behavior. The following are key components of sexual expression that are largely shaped by culture rather than biology.

Gender Identity

Gender identity is the personal and private sense of being male or female—the personal experience of one's sex role. The sense of being male or female begins by the time a child is three and a half years of age. This is also the age a child develops conceptual language, which is involved in establishing a gender-differentiated self-concept. Information about the development of gender identity was gained from studies of children born with ambiguous genitalia, where it was impossible to clearly distinguish the baby as male or female. Sometimes a child is initially assigned the wrong sex according to its chromosomal sex. If during the first 12 months to 18 months of life an error is discovered through chromosomal analysis, the child's identity may be changed to the opposite sex. With each subsequent month, however, changing gender identity becomes increasingly difficult.[4] Although the range of behavioral expression is extremely wide, this basic sense of maleness or femaleness persists throughout life (Fig. 9-1).

Sex Role

Sex role is the public expression of gender identity. A person's sense of what is appropriate behavior, attitudes, beliefs, and emotions for a female or male constitutes sex role identification. In most western

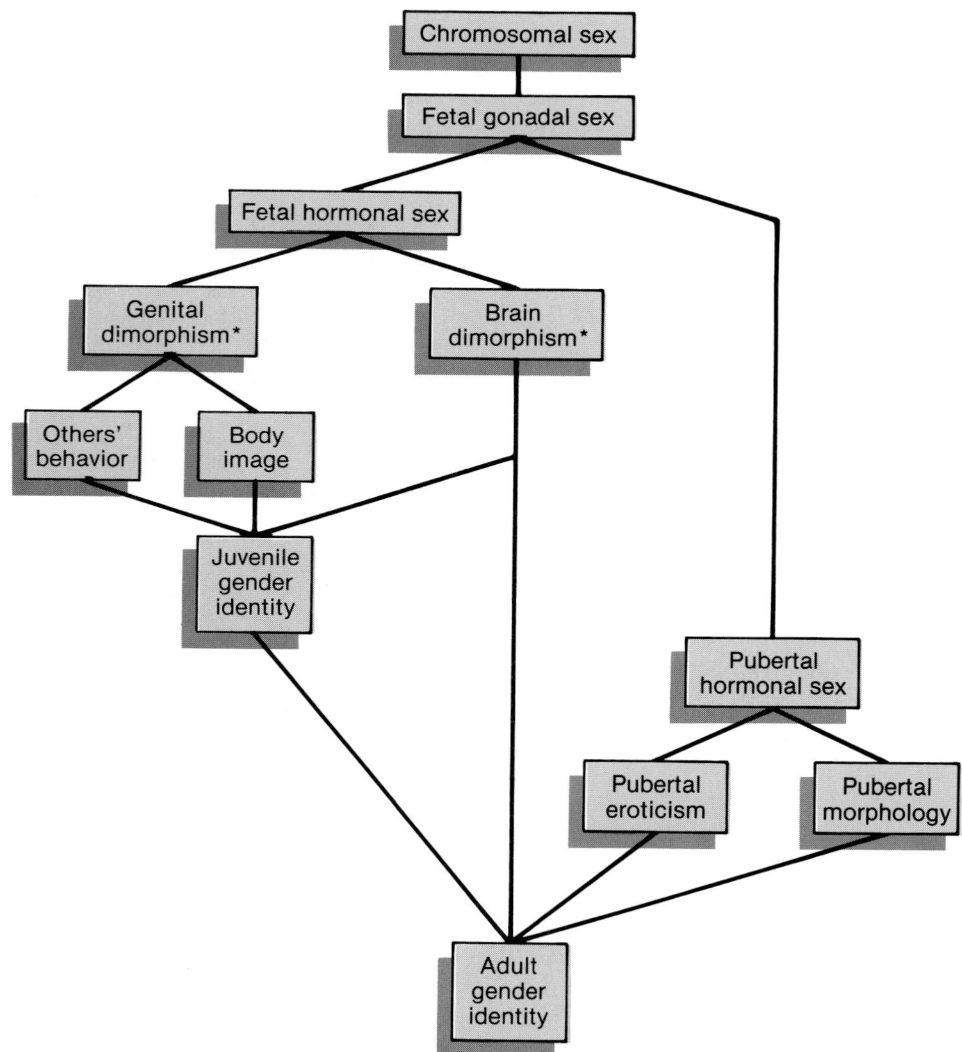

Figure 9-1.
The sequence and interaction of components involved in development of gender identity are diagrammed, showing the interaction of genetics and the environment. *Dimorphism is the manifestation in the same species of two forms, such as male and female; it refers to both bodily form and appearance and to sex differences in behavior and language. (After Money J, Ehrhardt AA: Man & Woman, Boy & Girl. Baltimore, The Johns Hopkins University Press, 1972)

societies, masculine (male sex role) behavior has been considered to be more aggressive, independent, and logical, while feminine (female sex role) behavior is seen as more submissive, dependent, and emotional. However, expressions of masculinity and femininity vary widely among cultures, and there are some societies in which what is considered male and female is exactly opposite of the western stereotype.

Although most cultures place the women in the role of caretaker to children, and men in the role of breadwinner, there is no necessity that roles be assigned in this manner. Sex roles and definitions of masculinity and femininity are based on arbitrary criteria, rather than anatomical and physiological differences. Femininity and masculinity are not absolute conditions, and they can have overlapping behaviors. All humans are a mixture of maleness and femaleness and have the same types of impulses, wishes, attitudes, and basic emotional and physiological equipment (except those imperative parts of sexual function and behavior, and the obvious anatomic differences). The different expressions of sex role observed in various cultures is a result of society's selective development of behavioral potentials. Sex roles are developed through family interactions, the effects of peers, social codes of dress and manners, all forms of media communication, and numerous social structures that encourage certain behaviors and inhibit others for males and females.

Sexual Partner Preference

Preference for a sexual partner may be heterosexual, homosexual, or bisexual, and this preference may change during one's lifetime. Despite considerable research, it is far from clear how preferences for a sexual partner develop, even among heterosexuals. Sexual partner preference also appears to be on a continuum, rather than an all-or-none situation, and it probably varies with the circumstances for some people. There is a difference between actual sexual experiences and sexual responsiveness in regard to partner preference. For example, a person may be exclusively heterosexual in actual experience, but feel somewhat sexually attracted to people of the same sex.

There is enormous variety in sexual partner preference and associated sex role behavior. A homosexual man may appear very masculine, carry out the role of a typical man, and have a strong gender identity as male, yet prefer a person of the same sex as an erotic partner. An effeminate-appearing male working at an occupation dominated by women may have a clear sense of male gender identity and opposite-sex erotic preference. A woman who appears and acts very masculine may have male gender identity and prefer women as sexual partners.

Many studies have examined social, psychological, and biological factors as possible causes of homosexualiy, but none are conclusive. It is well established that many people have sexual experiences with same-sexed individuals, usually during childhood and adolescence. Homosexual preferences often develop before any actual sexual experience, however. Most people who have same-sex encounters do not develop homosexual partner preferences. Recent biological research suggests that there may be a "sex center" in the fetal brain that is influenced by prenatal hormones, and affects later sex role behavior and choice of sexual partners. The mothers of some homosexuals were found to have atypical hormonal events during the critical period of sex center development during pregnancy, and it has been found that emotional stress during pregnancy causes reduced maternal androgen output which might have contributed to feminization of male infants.[4]

The biological linkage of sex role and sexual partner preference in humans is far from established. "Tomboy" girls and "sissy" boys do not necessarily, or even usually, become homosexuals. The development of sexual partner preference is probably shaped by such diverse and complex factors as the prenatal hormonal environment, early mother–infant interactions, imitation by the child of the most valued parent, family dynamics and interstructure that selectively fosters and inhibits behaviors, the privileges and drawbacks of social sex roles affecting value formation, and society's tolerance of variation in sexual expression.

Sexual Psychophysiology

Psychophysiology is a term that describes the interaction between psychological and physiological processes, between higher mental processes and the responses of muscles, glands, and organs. Two important fundamental psychophysiological principles are that a physiological response to a stimulus is influenced by past experiences and that current experiences and emotions are influenced by the body's responses. For example, a woman whose past experiences include frequent, intense orgasm may respond rapidly to sexual stimulation, while a woman who has learned not to expect to reach orgasm may have little response to the same type of stimuli. Also, awareness of the body's responses, such as vaginal congestion and lubrication in women and erection in men, can heighten pleasure and sexual feelings.

Human sexual response is determined by a delicate interaction between psychology and physiology. The nervous system has a central role in mediating sexual response by processing sexual signals of both cognitive and somatic origin. The causes of sexual arousal may be sought in the interplay between the brain and the sexual organs, to gain an understanding of the characteristics of sexual stimuli and the wide individual variation found.

Reflexogenic and Psychogenic Stimuli

Direct stimulation of erogenous areas, usually genitals and breasts, causes sexual arousal in a reflexive, or automatic, manner. When the penis or clitoris is stroked, the peripheral nerves send a signal to a relay center in the lower part of the spinal cord, which in turn sends a signal back to the penis for erection and to the clitoris and vagina for congestion and lubrication. The cerebral cortex and higher brain centers are not involved in this transmission of signals; it is a reflexogenic response that is mediated in the same way as the knee-jerk response. This is the mechanism through which some men with spinal cord injuries are able to have erections even though they have no sensation in the pelvic area.

Psychogenic stimuli are processed through the higher brain centers and can include sensory input such as sights, sounds, tastes, smells, and touches, as well as cognitive events such as thoughts, fantasies, memories, and images. Without direct stimulation of the genitals, it is possible to become sexually aroused through any one of these types of psychogenic stimuli. Watching an erotic movie, having the earlobe stroked, listening to a song with provocative lyrics, fantasizing a favorite sexual drama, or remembering a sexual encounter can all produce sexual arousal.

Most often, a combination of reflexogenic and psychogenic stimuli are used to produce sexual arousal, and they work in a synergistic way to enhance the level of excitement. Many men have found women more rapidly responsive sexually after an evening of candlelight, soft music, and romantic interaction. After seeing an erotic picture or movie, a man will often need considerably less (maybe no) direct stimulation to have an erection. On the other hand, feelings such as anger, guilt, or anxiety inhibit sexual response when direct stimulation is being used.

Neurologic Pathways

The neurologic pathways of reflexogenic stimuli are easier to trace than those of psychogenic stimuli, which involve complex mental processes and functions such as learning, emotions, and memory. The past experiences of an individual are very important in determining which types of psychogenic stimuli are perceived as arousing. Early childhood experiences of pleasurable genital touching occurring in an environment with certain smells, sights, or sounds may lead to later association of these sensations with sexual arousal. The process continues during adolescence and adulthood as sexual experience widens and different stimuli are associated with negative or positive sexual consequences. Being interrupted during sex by parents can lead to associations of anxiety or guilt with future sexual encounters. Circumstances in which a man has difficulty with erection can result in future erection problems under similar conditions. Situations in which intense sexual pleasure was felt tend to be sought again.

The central nervous system plays a key role in processing psychogenic stimuli and mediating the interplay between these and the activity of the peripheral nervous system. Central nervous system output travels through either the somatic or autonomic branch of the peripheral nervous system (Fig. 9-2). Generally speaking, the somatic nerves connect the central nervous system (CNS) with the striated muscles. The muscle tension (myotonia) during sexual arousal is caused by stimulation of the somatic nerves. The autonomic nervous system, however, is responsible for most of the physiologic changes during sexual arousal. In general, the autonomic nervous system controls the smooth muscles of the heart, internal organs, and glands whose functions are largely involuntary or not under conscious control. Thus, sexual response has a large involuntary component, with conscious inhibition generally more effective than conscious activation.

The sympathetic and parasympathetic branches of the autonomic nervous system, with their different anatomical pathways and chemical activators of the smooth muscles and glands, are the immediate mediators of sexual response. The parasympathetic branch is also called cholinergic because its nerve endings release acetylcholine to transmit their messages, and the sympathetic branch is called adrenergic because it releases adrenaline and nonadrenaline. These two branches serve different functions, with the sympathetic nervous system usually responding during times of stress, when there is a need for vigorous activity (thus the release of adrenaline), and the parasympathetic system dominating during periods of relaxation.

The sexual organs receive messages from both the sympathetic and parasympathetic systems, as do most other body organs. Penile erection and vaginal lubrication are caused by the effects of the parasympathetic system which produce vasodilatation. As arousal pro-

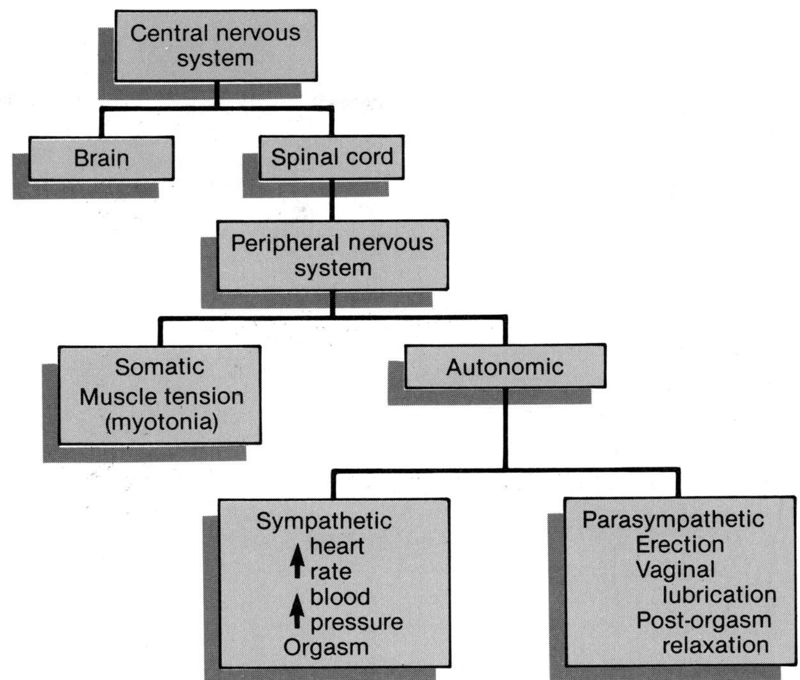

Figure 9-2.
Neurologic pathways of sexual response.

gresses, the sympathetic system plays a larger role, causing increases in heart rate and blood pressure. The sympathetic system may take over completely at orgasm, with ejaculation and vaginal spasms set off by a sudden discharge of adrenaline. The autonomic imbalance produced by this sudden release of adrenaline is quickly compensated for by a release of acetylcholine that comes from the parasympathetic system. This parasympathetic rebound phenomenon, with its vasodilatation, contributes to the subjective feelings of warmth and relaxation that many people feel after orgasm.

Psychological Mediators of Sexual Response

The psychogenic stimuli effects that affect sexual response work largely through the relatively simple process of conditioning by association, or conditioned response. However, sexual meanings can be attached to stimuli through more complex psychological processes. The mental state in which people are likely to initiate or respond to sexual advances is created by a complex interplay of many factors. Sometimes a person can identify why he or she is "in the mood" for sex or why he or she is not, but at other times the sources of a reaction to sexual stimuli are elusive. Sexual feelings can be spontaneous and uncomplicated at times, but in other instances there may be conflicts, uncertainty, resistance, or hesitation. Human emotions and thoughts are very complex, so it is not surprising that sexual responsiveness varies greatly among different people, and in the same person at different times.

Four major psychological mediators of responses to sexual stimulation have been identified as informational responses, emotional reactions, imaginative capacity, and attention. These factors interact with each other and exert a direct influence upon experiences in one area or another or create conflicts in responses to stimuli when there is disagreement among them. There is also a feedback loop between physiological response and the erotic stimulus; upon becoming aware of physical arousal, the stimulus causing arousal will be perceived as increasingly arousing (Fig. 9-3).

Informational Responses

The informational component that acts as a psychological mediator of sexual response consists of beliefs, knowledge, and labels concerning various aspects of sexuality. If a certain sexual practice is considered a perversion, such as oral-genital stimulation, then a person is unlikely to engage in this behavior and the idea of doing it would be repulsive, acting as a sexual "turn-off." If a sexual partner suggests or initiates oral-genital sex, this would effectively decrease sexual arousal and probably generate a number of negative feelings or expressions.

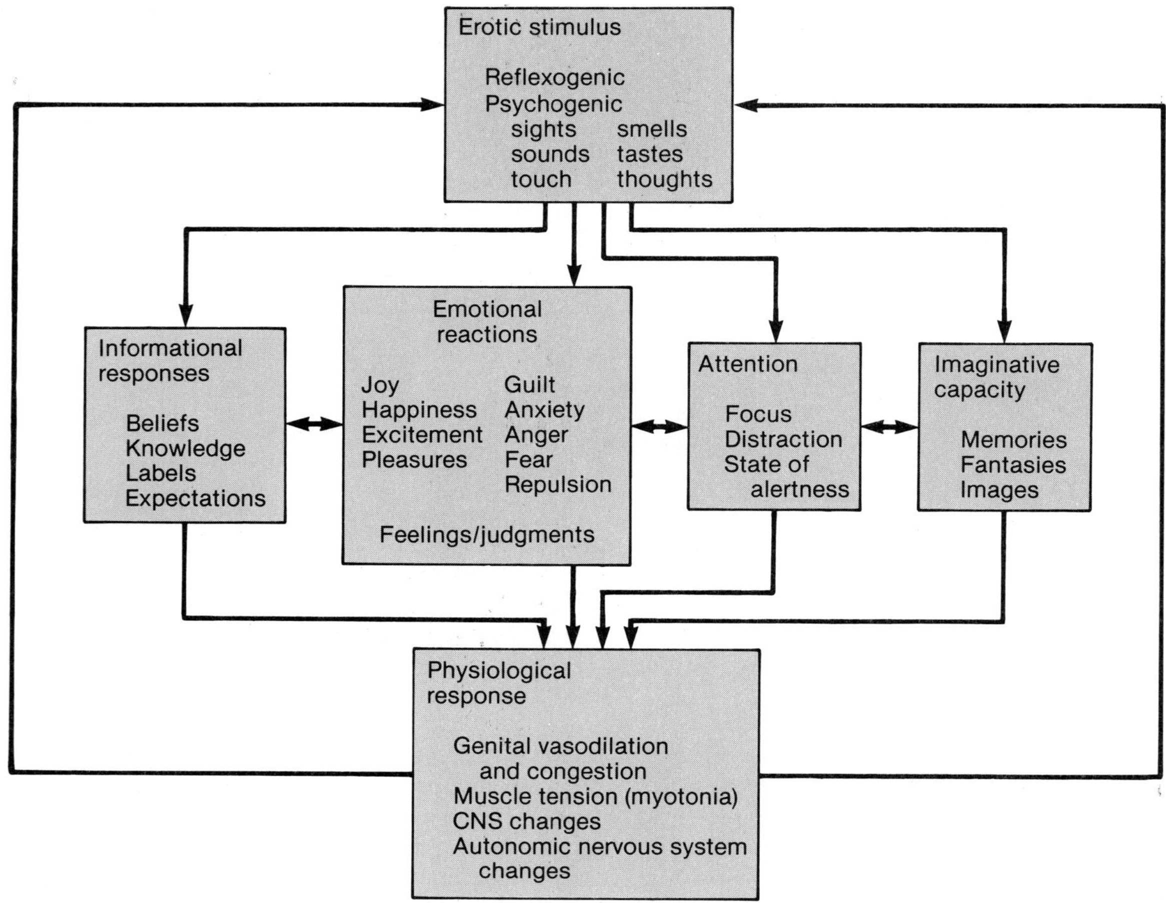

Figure 9-3.
Psychological mediators of sexual response and the processing of erotic stimuli. (After Rosen R, Rosen LR: Human Sexuality. New York, Alfred A Knopf, Inc., 1981)

A person without this belief, however, who sees oral-genital sex as healthy and desirable, and who has had pleasurable past experiences, would respond with increased arousal to the idea, suggestion, or initiation of this activity. The expectations that are built upon beliefs, experiences (experiential knowledge), and the labeling-categorizing process exert powerful influences upon sexual responsiveness. These can either effectively shut down the physiological response or greatly enhance it.

Emotional Reactions

The emotional components in psychological mediation consist of subjective feelings and perceptions about a sexual stimulus. These follow beliefs and expectations very closely; emotions are the affective expression of values and beliefs. Feelings about sexual stimuli can range from the very positive, such as joy, happiness, and excitement to the very negative, such as guilt, anxiety, repulsion, anger, and fear. A man exhibiting very "macho" behavior with the flavor of male superiority would probably evoke anger and repulsion in a feminist woman; therefore, he would be an ineffective visual and auditory sexual stimulus.

Many people report heightened arousal and increased intensity and rapidity of sexual response when there are deep, powerful feelings of love and commitment between partners. The boredom and diminished intensity of sexual experiences that are common among long-time married couples probably derive, at least in part, from a flattening of emotional response to each other. The sense of knowing someone too completely so there is no excitement of the unknown and unpredictable, and the little resentments that build up over years of unexpressed or unresolved conflicts so there is a smoldering anger just under the surface, constitute emotions that detract from sexual rsponse. The directness, honesty, and humility necessary to grow out of such traps require conscious cultivation by both partners.

As previously mentioned, guilt is one of the most effective inhibitors of sexual response. Many men and women with sexual problems find early inculcation of guilty feelings about themselves as sexual beings and sex-related activities at the base of their difficulties. Making judgments about oneself or one's partner, whether related to appearance or behaviors, sets up an acceptable or not acceptable dichotomy which may screen out many sexual stimuli. Judging something as "good" or "bad" is a way of expressing values and beliefs and lays the foundation for associated feelings.

Imaginative Capacity

The imaginative component in psychological mediation of sexual response includes the memories, images, and fantasies that are invoked by sexual stimuli. Almost everyone has sexual fantasies. Some people can create or enhance arousal by just thinking about them. Because some fantasies are bizarre, there is often guilt associated with them, producing a conflict in psychological input. Sexologists state that any fantasy which increases arousal is acceptable as long as it is not acted out in a way that will harm others, physically or emotionally.

Mental images have been found by sex researchers to be very important in determining sexual response. Arousal tends to be greatest with evocation of memories of the individual's own past sexual acts, when what was personally experienced produced significant pleasure in sexual encounters. Imagery is so powerful that people can quickly learn to arouse themselves sexually or turn off sexual response, just by using appropriate fantasies and images.

Attention

The importance of attention in mediating sexual response is so direct and obvious that it is often overlooked. If a person is not paying attention to a sexual stimulus, then it will have very little effect, if any. Sexual response will be limited, or may not occur at all, if a person is unattentive or distracted. This was well demonstrated in a laboratory experiment in which subjects listened to an erotic tape recording through one side of an earphone headset, while simple mental arithmetic problems were played through the other earphone. Using instruments to measure the subjects' penile erections, it was found that the distraction of the math problems definitely reduced the amount of erection produced in response to the erotic tape.[5]

The effects of distraction have been felt by most people at some time. They do not respond as readily to sexual stimuli when also aware of the noises of their children in a nearby room, when thoughts of housework or office work to be done arise, when hungry and smelling food cooking, or when dissatisfied with something about their appearance or the circumstances of sex. When no environmental distractions are present, the ability to focus on the sexual encounter becomes an important part of attention processes. For no apparent reason, a person may find his or her mind wandering to totally unrelated subjects. Although the body is physically going through the motions, the level of arousal may be quite low, delaying or inhibiting orgasm when a person is not focused upon the sexual experience. The state of alertness is also important; if a person is drowsy and drifting off into sleep, sexual responses will also be sluggish. This applies to the effects of certain drugs such as alcohol, which decreases mental alertness as well as depressing physiological responses.

The Sexual Response Cycle

The systems of sexual anatomy and physiology that are organized around the clitoris in women and the penis in men are exact homologues of each other. Each part in one sex has its counterpart in the other. These counterparts may be structurally the same in both women and men, or modified to perform the same function in a different way, or perform a different function. The sexual response cycle, with its two basic physiological mechanisms of vasocongestion and myotonia, progresses through identical phases with corresponding changes in genital and other body organs in both women and men. There are certain differences in timing and patterns characteristic of each of the sexes within this common physiological process.

Prenatal Sexual Differentiation

The physical similarities in sexual anatomy stem from the first few months of embryonic life. The XX (female) configuration or XY (male) configuration of the chromosomes after conception passes the sexual program to the primordial gonad. The primitive genital ducts of the embryo are identical until about six weeks gestation. At that time, under chromosomal influence, the gonads of the embryo become ovaries with the XX pattern or testes with the XY pattern. In the male embryo, androgenic hormones secreted by the

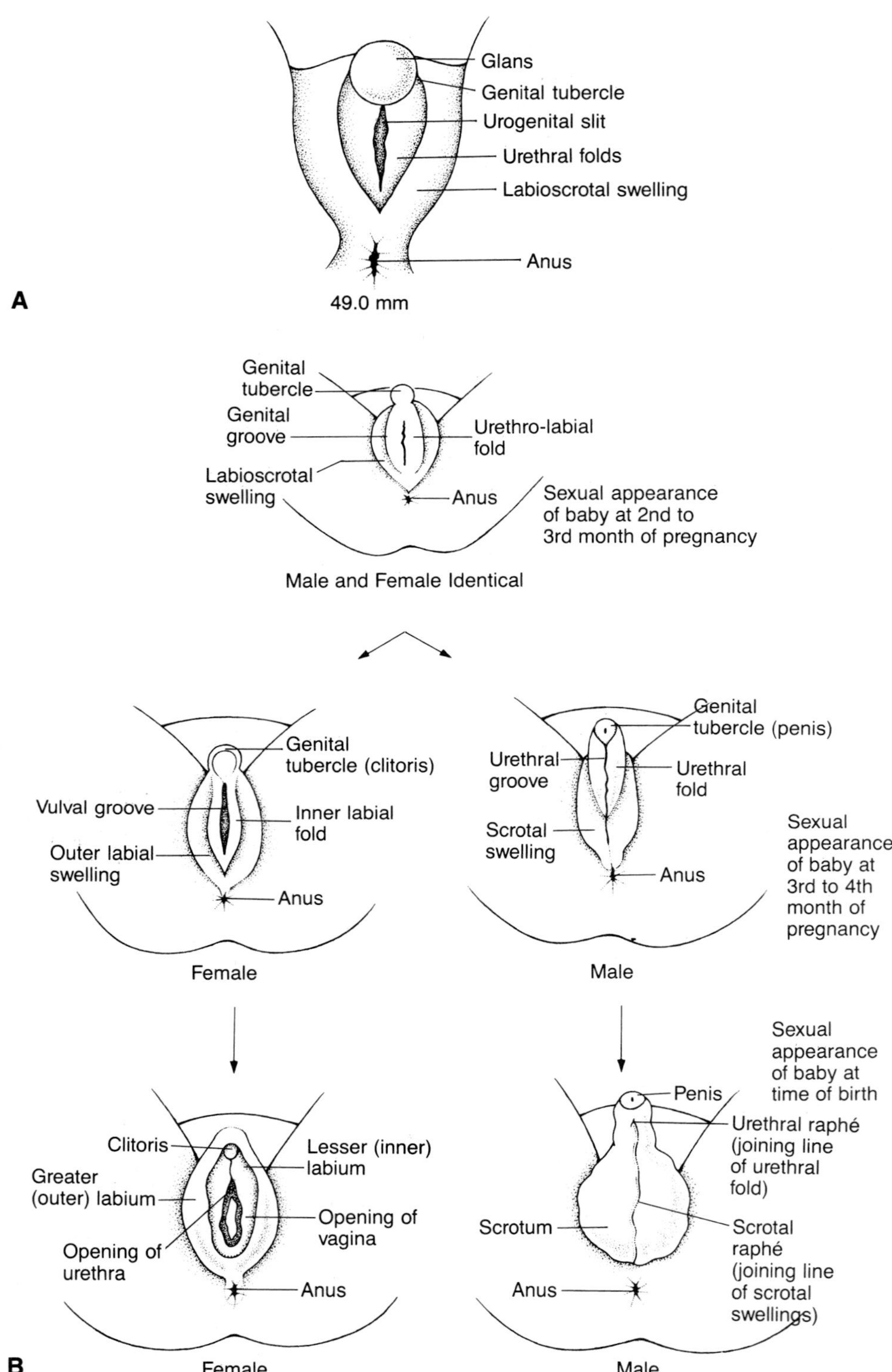

Figure 9-4.

Fetal genital differentiation. *(A)* Undifferentiated external genitalia of 7-week embryo. Male and female appear the same; sex can be determined only by the Barr body chromosome test. *(B)* Differentiation of external genitalia into male and female in the fetus. *(C)* Differentiation of internal sex organs into male and female in the fetus.

testes stimulate development of the wolffian ducts, which give rise to most of the male reproductive system. The müllerian ducts produce the female reproductive system and are probably suppressed in the male embryo. Even though the female embryo's ovaries secrete estrogen, this is not necessary for female sexual differentiation. If fetal gonads do not secrete hormones, and even if embryonic reproductive tracts (without gonads) are removed in experiments and kept alive, the genital structures continue to develop in the female pattern. Androgens must be added to produce male sexual differentiation, while their absence leads to female differentiation. This implies that nature's basic propensity, at least in mammals, is to produce a female.[6]

The embryonic glans and genital tubercle develops into the clitoral system in the female and the penis in the male. The labioscrotal swelling becomes the female labia or male scrotum, and the urogenital slit and urethral folds form the different urethral systems

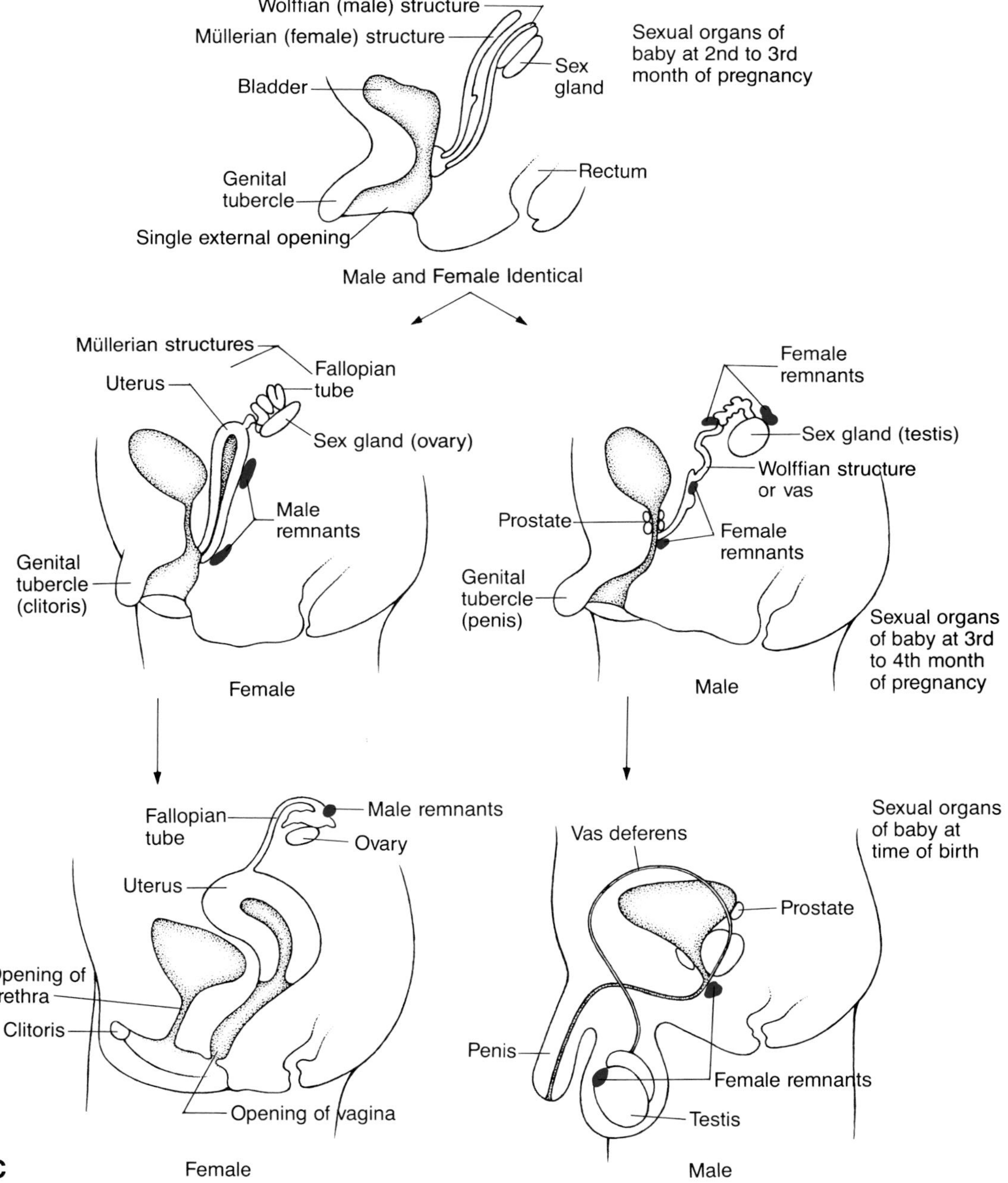

in males and females. Internally, the müllerian structures become the female fallopian tubes, uterus, and vagina, and the wolffian structures become the male vas deferens, prostate, and, seminal vesicles (Fig. 9-4).

Anatomy and Physiology of Sexual Response

Male and female sexual and reproductive anatomy and physiology have been presented in Chapters 7 and 8. A brief review of the most pertinent structures is included in this section, with a more detailed discussion of sexual physiology.

Female Sexual Response

The *labia majora,* which are well endowed with fat, hair, sweat glands, blood vessels, lymphatic vessels, and nerves, respond to vasocongestion with sexual excitation by spreading apart, becoming more flattened and elongating anteroposteriorally. The *labia minora,* which are continuous with the prepuce (clitoral hood), are well supplied with blood vessels, nerves, and lymphatics. The labial skin has a pink pigmentation that deepens in color with arousal, becoming bright red or purplish-red with high levels of sexual excitement. The labia minora increase in size and extend outward with vasocongestion, protruding past the labia majora and functionally elongating the vagina. Often called the "sex skin," the labia minora are highly sensitive to touch and play a major role in arousal and orgasm through their draping over the clitoris, providing continual clitoral stimulation as tension is increased and decreased with penile thrusting (see Fig. 9-6).

The *clitoris* is a complex anatomical structure with both external and cryptic, or hidden, parts. Its role in arousal and orgasm is central, and it appears the sole purpose of the clitoral structure is to enhance female sexual pleasure. There are four parts to the clitoris—the glans, shaft, crus, and vestibular bulbs. The glans and shaft are the most external and smallest portions, and are largely hidden under the prepuce. Comprising only one tenth of the volume of the clitoris in its resting state, the glans and shaft represent even a smaller proportion during sexual arousal when the cryptic structures may increase in size up to three times. The clitoral shaft contains two small erectile cavernous bodies enclosed in a dense fibrous membrane, similar to the male penis. The length of the shaft is about 1/4 inch to 3/4 inch, although there are marked variations. The glans is on average 4 mm to 5 mm in diameter, though normal range encompasses 2 mm to 1 cm.

The clitoral glans is the most sensitive female erogenous area, with its mucous membrane so densely packed with nerve endings that there is little room for blood vessels. The entire female sexual cycle can be initiated and maintained to orgasm by stimulation of only the glans. At rest, the shaft is sharply retroflexed posteriorly. With sexual stimulation, it becomes congested leading to erection, moving the tip through an 180-degree arc in a forward elliptical curve. As arousal proceeds, it is retracted under the prepuce and appears shorter because of the actions of muscles and the cryptic structures pulling it inward.

The cryptic structures of the clitoris include the crus and vestibular bulbs. At the end of the shaft, the clitoris bifurcates and branches into two crura, which extend inward bilaterally following the inferior rami of the symphysis pubis downward. The crura lie below the ischiocavernous muscles and bodies, with a tough, tendinous lower portion that anchors the clitoris to the inner surface of the ischium. The clitoral crus is homologous to the corpus cavernosum in the male, which becomes the crus of the penis. The crura play a lesser role in distention during arousal in the female than the vestibular bulbs because of their tendinous nature (Fig. 9-5).

The vestibular bulbs also divide and descend into the pelvis from the clitoral shaft. Extending outward bilaterally, they wrap fully three quarters of the way around the lower portion of the vagina. Each bulb presses closely against the lower third of the vagina, just above the vaginal opening. The vestibular bulbs are erectile and highly distensible and are covered with a mass of coiled blood vessels *(commissure of the bulbs).* These blood vessels also become distended during arousal and convey blood between the bulbs and the clitoral shaft. The greater vestibular glands (Bartholin's glands) are located at the bottom of the bulbs. The vestibular bulbs become greatly distended during arousal, contributing to the buildup of the orgasmic platform in the lower third of the vagina. The homologous structure in the male is the corpus spongiosum, which becomes the bulb of the penis.

The female *pelvic muscles* participate in engorgement during sexual arousal and have an important function in orgasm. The *ischiocavernous muscles* envelop the clitoral crura, and the *bulbocavernous muscles* surround the vestibular bulbs and the lower third of the vagina. Ascending from the vagina, the bulbocavernous terminates in fibrous tissue dorsal of the clitoris and overlies the crura, and joins the ischiocavernous to form the striated sphincter of the urethra. The *transverse perineal muscles* and *levator ani muscles* converge on the lateral walls of the lower third of the vagina and unite behind the vaginal opening to form the perineal body. These pelvic muscles

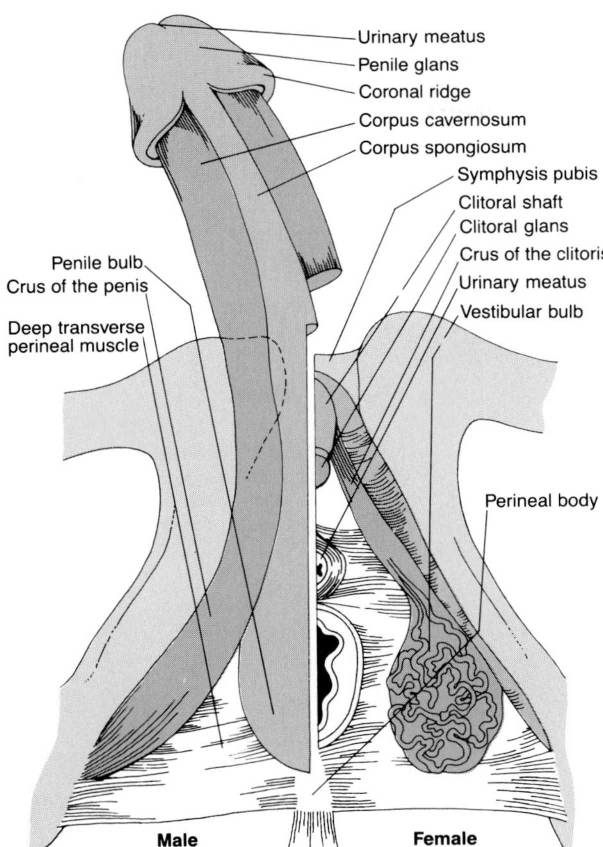

Figure 9-5.
Comparison of female and male cryptic structures.

become congested during arousal, and many women are aware that voluntary contractions of perineal muscles can heighten arousal. The muscles press on distended clitoral and vaginal structures, and when a critical point is reached in this distention, a reflex stretch mechanism is set off in the muscles and the contractions pressing on the distended clitoral crura, vestibular bulbs, and lower vaginal area cause orgasm.

The *vagina* is a muscular tube that is lined with mucous membranes and is richly supplied with blood vessels, glands, and lymphatics. The lower third of the vagina has many nerve endings, but the upper portion is not as well endowed and may be distended considerably laterally and posteriorly without discomfort. The circumvaginal venous plexus is a dense grouping of blood vessels surrounding the lower third of the vagina, and these vessels provide the blood supply for the massive congestion which produces vaginal lubrication during sexual arousal. They also contribute to building the orgasmic platform in later stages of excitement.

With effective sexual stimulation, pelvic venous dilatation and congestion occur quickly, and fluid from these venous networks passes into tissue spaces and causes edema. Within 10 seconds to 30 seconds, droplets of clear fluid called transudate appear on the vaginal walls, coalesce, and produce vaginal lubrication. Concurrently, the upper two thirds of the vagina begins to lengthen and distend. As excitement progresses, the upper vagina balloons outward as the uterus and cervix are pulled upward into the false pelvis. In the lower pelvis, a broad platform of distended tissues forms as pelvic congestion and edema reach a peak. The vestibular bulbs and labia minora are also highly distended and congested at peak excitement. The thickened area of congested tissue surrounding the lower vagina and vaginal opening is called the *orgasmic platform* (Fig. 9-6).

When this vasocongestive distention reaches a critical point, orgasm is triggered in a mechanism involving the clitoral shaft and glans, clitoral cryptic structures, vaginal platform, and pelvic muscles. The muscles contract vigorously at intervals of 0.8 seconds, expelling the blood and fluid trapped in the tissues and venous plexi, and create the sensations of orgasm. Orgasm usually consists of 8 to 15 contractions; the first five or six are the most intense. Mild orgasms may only have three to five contractions. Because of the extent of pelvic congestion and the capacity for distention of pelvic structures, much of the blood and edema cannot be removed and may flow back into the distended structures. As a result of this, many women are capable of restimulation seconds after orgasm and may have repeated orgasms.

The *cervix* and *uterus* have less dramatic roles in female sexual response. The uterus enlarges owing to vascular engorgement and rises gradually with increasing excitement until it is out of the true pelvis. It also pulls the upper vagina upward. Uterine contractions occur during orgasm; they are usually pleasurable, but sometimes they are not consciously perceived. For some women, however, these contractions may be painful owing to prolonged spasm; most often this occurs during menopause, pregnancy, or with dysmenorrhea or when an intrauterine device is used.[7] The cervix may undergo some congestion, but there is no significant response until the cervical os opens slightly after orgasm. During the final, resolution phase of the sexual cycle, the uterus drops back down into its usual position. The cervical os opens more widely during this time and is positioned in the seminal pool in the upper vagina; this is believed to be an aid to sperm entry into the cervix and ultimately to conception (see Fig. 9-6).

The breasts and other nongenital areas are also involved in sexual response. During sexual excitement, the *breasts* become enlarged and the nipple becomes erect owing to congestion. Both of these are erotic areas for women. Some women are able to reach orgasm by breast stimulation alone. The *skin* in some women may show the "sex flush," a mottled pinkish discoloration that is most prominant on the chest and trunk. Spasms of the abdomen, buttocks, and thighs may also occur with high levels of excitement.

Recently, interest has surfaced in a phenomenon called *female ejaculation,* the emission of fluid during orgasm by women. It has been thought that orgasmic muscle contractions squeezed out some vaginal lubrication to cause this sensation. It is now postulated that a homologous female structure to the male prostate secretes the jet of fluid from the vulval area during orgasm. The paraurethral ducts (Skene's ducts) develop from the same primitive tissue as the male prostate and consist of two small glands and their ducts which are located on either side of the urethra. It is possible that the Skene's ducts emit fluid during orgasm like the male prostate. Not all women

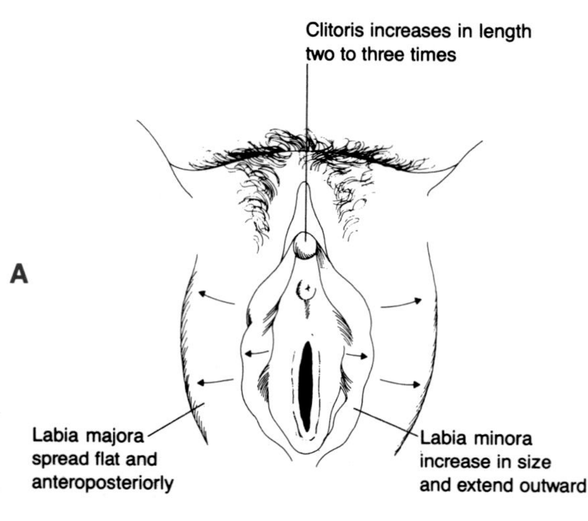

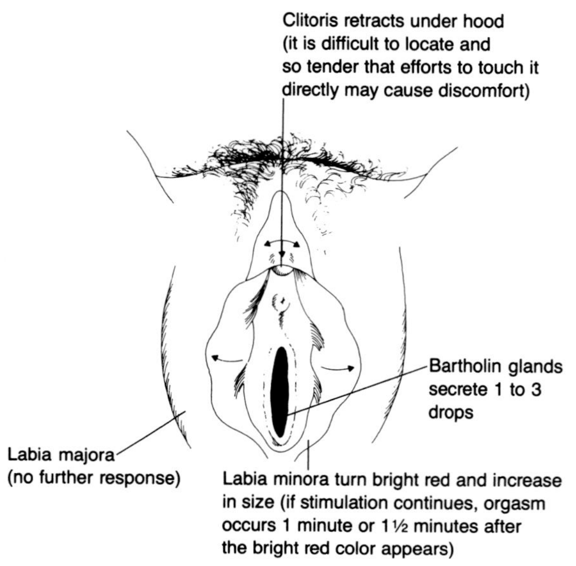

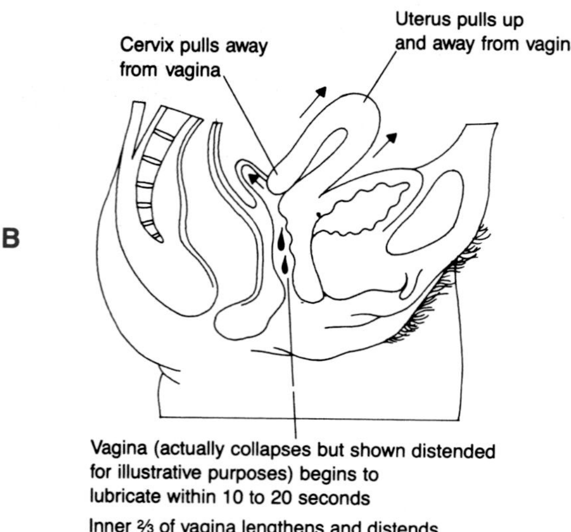

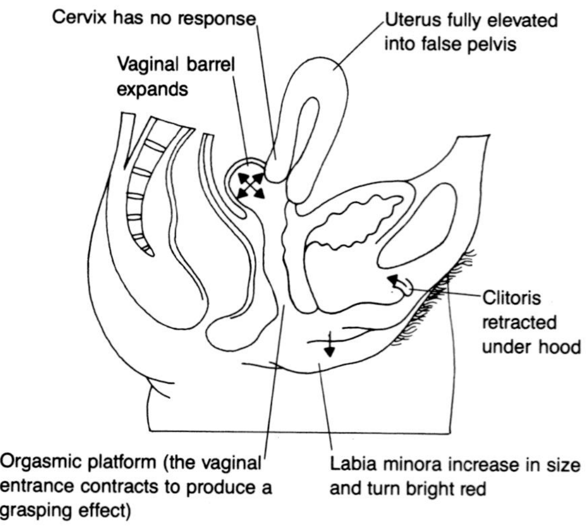

Figure 9-6.
Female sexual response cycle. *(A)* changes in external genitalia, *(B)* changes in internal genitalia.

experience fluid ejection with orgasm, and there is a great deal of variability in the amount and location of this tissue among women.[5]

Male Sexual Response

The *penis* consists of three long cylinders of erectile tissue that are surrounded by an elastic sheath. Each cylinder contains blood vessels and spaces that fill up with blood during sexual arousal. The two upper cylinders, the corpora cavernosa, are responsible for the rigidity and the increase in length and width of the penis with erection (Fig. 9-7). At the base of the penile shaft, where it joins the body, the corpora cavernosa diverge into the crura, which become tough tendinous fibers that attach to the pelvic bones. These are homologous to the clitoral crura in the female. On the underside of the penis is the third cylinder, the corpus spongiosum. On the external end it terminates in the glans, and on the internal end it terminates in the bulb. The urethra runs through the corpus spongiosum. During erection, the spongy body remains softer than the corpora cavernosa. The glans enlarges when

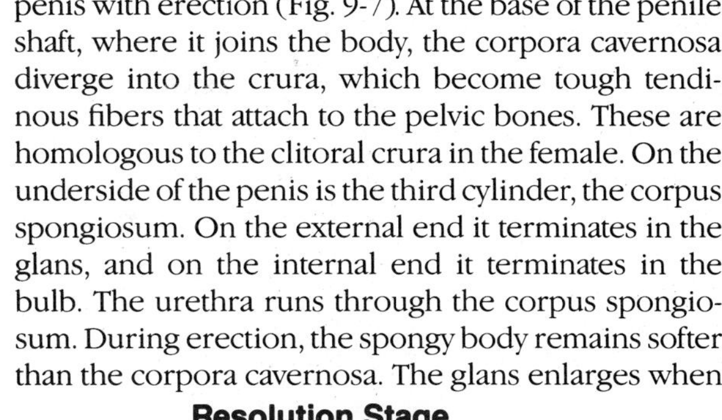

Orgasm Stage

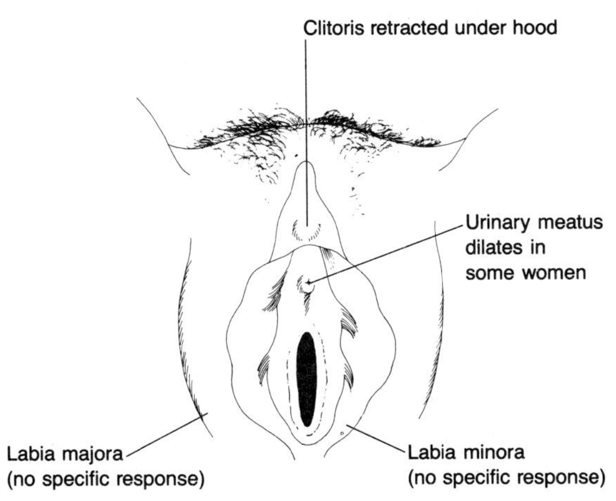

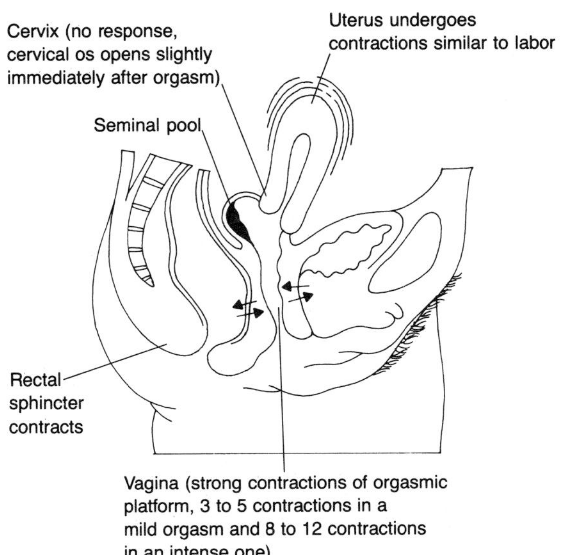

Resolution Stage

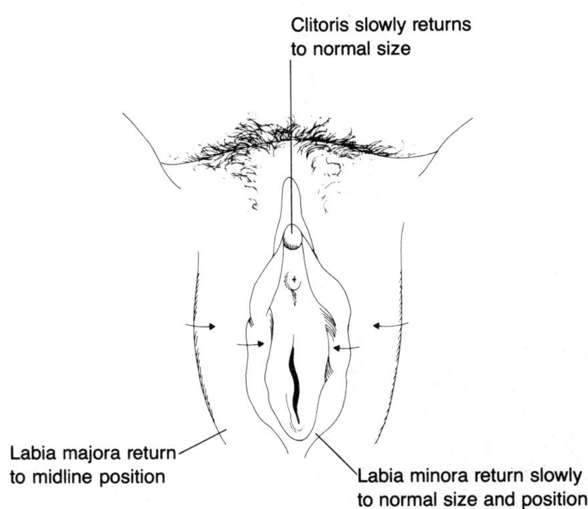

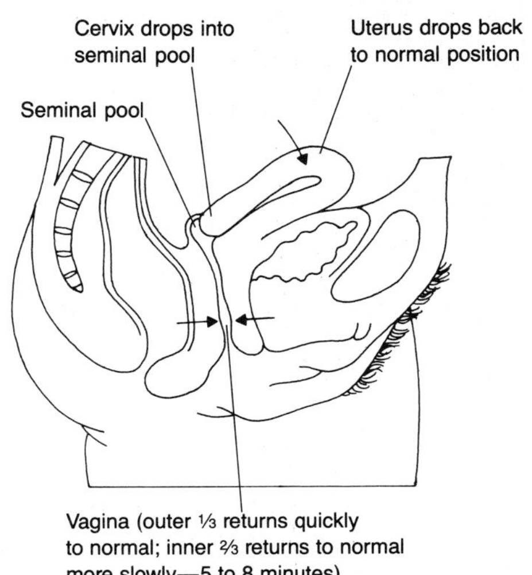

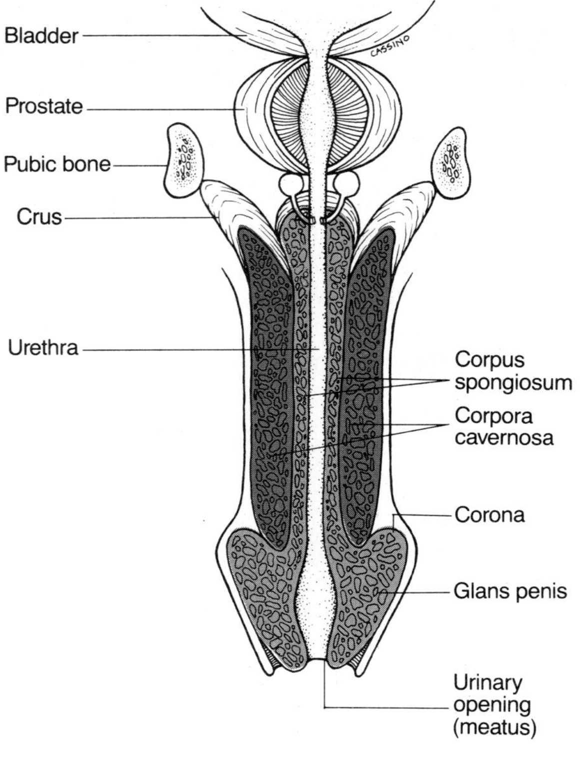

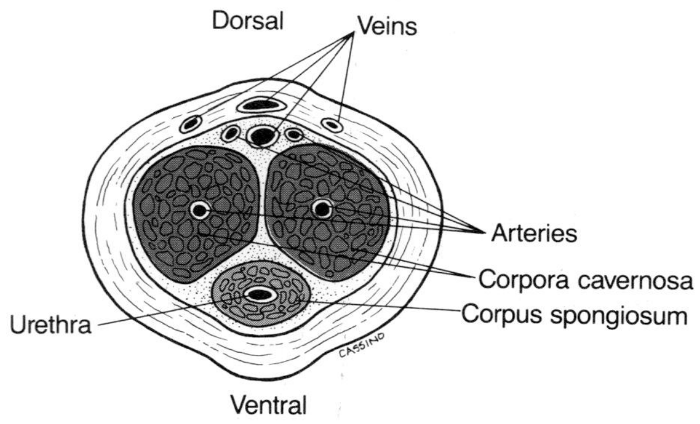

Figure 9-7.
Internal structures of erect penis.

it is excited to almost twice its quiescent size, and provides a soft protective cushion for the rigid corpora cavernosa (Fig. 9-8). The glans is highly endowed with nerve endings, and it is the male's area of maximum erotic sensation.

The penile bulb becomes very rigid and distended during sexual arousal, lengthens, and increases markedly in diameter. It nearly fills the space between the pubic rami and presses downward on the testicles. The bulb of the penis is homologous to the female vestibular bulbs, but is not as large. The penile structures continue to distend and enlarge until the peak of excitement is reached. Clear mucoid fluid is secreted from the urethra, probably from Cowper's glands or the prostate. At the critical point of vasocongestive distention, the reflex stretch mechanism is set off in the muscles and orgasm occurs. The same muscles are involved in the male as in the female—primarily the bulbocavernous, the ischiocavernous, the levator ani, and the transverse perineum.

As muscle contractions beginning around the seminal vesicles and prostate cause emission of the semen into the upper urethra, the man feels the sensation of "ejaculatory inevitability," immediately followed by the propulsive orgasmic contractions. Semen spurts out of the urethra at 0.8 second intervals in 3 to 7 ejaculatory spurts. Contractions of the penis and urethra are felt with each spurt of semen.

The skin of the *scrotum* begins to thicken and wrinkle with sexual excitement, and the *testes* begin to elevate closer to the perineum. The cremaster muscle elevates the testes and it also helps to heat and to cool the testes by bringing them closer to or further away from the body, maintaining an even temperature for effective sperm production. As excitement progresses, the scrotum thickens more and the testes increase up to 50% in size and rotate anteriorly. Vasocongestion causes increase in testicular size. At the time of orgasm, the testes are elevated closely against the perineum and maximally engorged. Following orgasm, the testes descend and decrease in size, and the scrotal skin thins and returns to its former texture (see Fig. 9-8).

The *prostate* is located just below the bladder and surrounds the urethra, and it contains an intricate series of ducts that secrete prostatic fluid. This fluid contains prostaglandins, a hormonal substance that causes contractions of the uterus and is thought to aid fertilization, and other biochemical substances including fibrinogenase, which causes temporary coagulation of semen in the vagina to prevent its dripping out. Prostatic fluid is alkaline and buffers the acidity of the vagina, allowing sperm to survive longer. It provides a vehicle for sperm transportation through the urethra and is secreted during orgasm to make up the largest part of the semen.

The *seminal vesicles* are coiled tubal structures that join the vas deferens with the ejaculatory ducts which enter the prostate. Sperm from the vas deferens mix with secretions, which are triggered by orgasm, from the seminal vesicles and pass through the prostate by way of the ejaculatory ducts. These secretions are high in fructose, a natural sugar that aids sperm motility.

The two *Cowper's glands* are the size of a pea and are located between the prostate and urethra. They produce an alkaline secretion that neutralizes the acidity of the urethra, which is caused by transporting

Excitement Stage

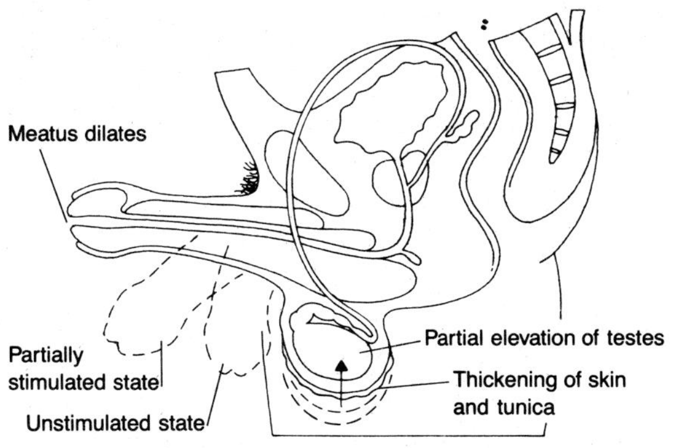

The smaller flaccid penis tends to enlarge proportionately more in erection, thus decreasing the difference between the larger and the smaller flaccid penis.

Plateau Stage

As seminal fluid collects in prostatic urethra, there is a feeling of ejaculatory inevitability. Larger fluid volume is experienced as more plea: .ırable.

Cowper's gland secretion
Color deepens
Final engorgement causes increase in diameter of glans
Testes rotate anteriorly
Scrotum thickens
Cowper's gland
Two-fold size increase in urethral bulb
Marked increase in size of testicles (up to 50%)

Testes fully elevated (orgasm never occurs without elevated testes, though they may be less elevated in men over 50 years of age.

Orgasmic Stage

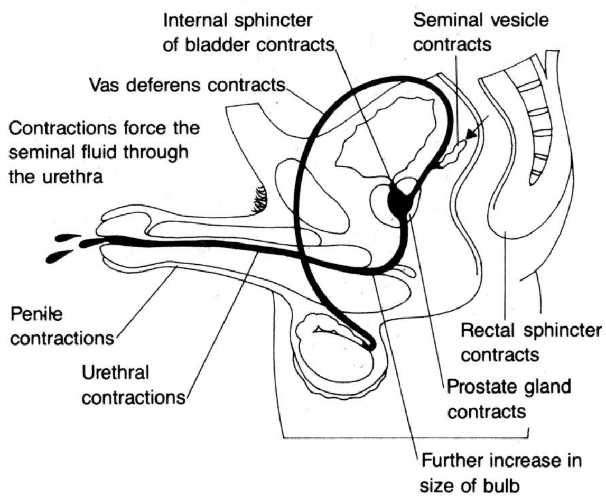

Resolution Stage

Duration of this stage varies proportionately with length of excitement and plateau stages

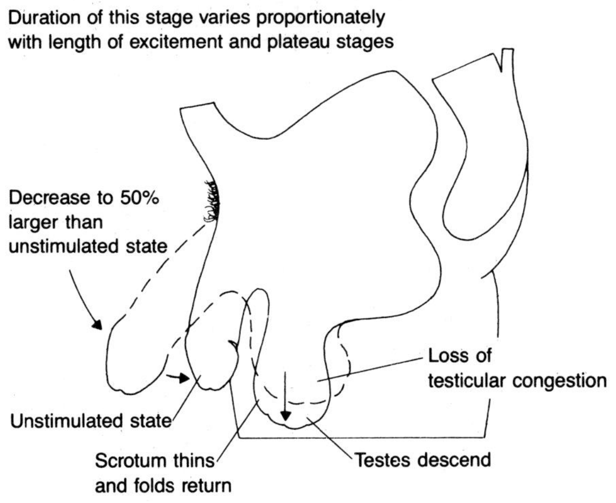

Figure 9-8.
Male sexual response cycle.

urine. It is important to neutralize this acidity before sperm are transported through the urethra because the acidity can damage sperm. The Cowper's glands usually secrete a drop or two of fluid, but the amount varies considerably. This fluid appears as preejaculate, and it is possible that sperm secreted into the urethra from the ejaculatory ducts might be carried along in the Cowper's gland fluid prior to orgasm. This accounts for the risk in using withdrawal for contraception, as sperm may be present in the fluid secreted before orgasm. The secretions from Cowper's glands usually appear during the plateau phase of sexual arousal, just before orgasm.

Men also experience nipple erection during sexual arousal, and they may have the "sex flush", as well as spasms of the buttocks and thighs. Although no muscles play an important role in initial erection of the penile shaft, pelvic muscles are the key to the final surge to orgasm in the male. The penile bulb and corpora cavernosa are enclosed in a muscular coat, which, along with almost all other muscles in the area, are responsible for complete erection and ejaculation. Contracting in a coordinated, downward rhythm, these muscles compress the prostate, seminal vesicles, and the internal structures (penile bulb and corpora cavernosa), which in turn compress the urethra and force semen forward with considerable pressure. Blood is also forced out of the distended cavernous spaces, leading to detumescence of the penis. The penis gradually becomes flaccid and returns to its original size after orgasm; the length of time varies for different occasions in the same man.

Patterns of Sexual Response

The sexual response cycle in men and women can be divided into several stages. The most popular model was introduced by Masters and Johnson in *Human Sexual Response*.[1] An orderly sequence of psychophysiologic events takes place and brings about marked changes in the shape and function of the genital organs, as described in the preceding section. Regardless of whether sexual stimulation is reflexogenic or psychogenic, reactions in the neurologic, vascular, muscular, and hormonal systems occur that affect many parts of the body.

Masters and Johnson developed a four-stage model, which progresses from excitement to plateau, to orgasm, and finally to resolution. The *excitement stage* begins with the onset of erotic feelings and sensations. This produces an immediate and intense vasocongestion and increased myotonia if stimulation is effective. Excitement in the man is signalled by erection, with scrotal thickening and elevation of the testes. In the woman, vaginal lubrication occurs rapidly, the clitoris enlarges and becomes erect, the uterus enlarges and begins to rise, and the vagina begins to enlarge and balloon in the upper portion.

As excitement progresses the *plateau stage* is reached; this is the stage immediately preceding orgasm. In men, the penis is fully distended and erect at its maximum size; the testes are enlarged and elevated closely against the perineum; and drops of fluid from the Cowper's glands appear at the urethral meatus. In women, pelvic congestion and edema are at a peak with maximum distention of the vestibular bulbs, labia minora, lower third of the vagina, and uterus. The orgasmic platform builds up in the lower vagina, and the uterus ascends from the true pelvis while the upper vagina widely balloons. The clitoris is completely retracted under the prepuce, enlarged, and has completed its upward arc.

The *stage of orgasm* is reached when vasocongestion passes a critical point and a reflex stretch mechanism is set off in the pelvic muscles of both sexes. The muscles contract vigorously, pressing on distended structures and expelling blood that is trapped in tissues and vessels, and then creates the sensation of orgasm. Ejaculation occurs in the man, with spurts of semen from the urethral meatus and contractions of the penis and urethra. In the woman, contractions occur at the same time interval (0.8 sec) as blood and fluid moves out of distended pelvic tissues and veins. The main sites of orgasmic sensation involve the clitoris and lower part of the vagina.

Resolution is the final stage of the sexual response cycle. The changes in genitals and other organs and structures are reversed. The testes decrease in size and descend immediately and the scrotum relaxes and returns to its usual position. The penis becomes flaccid, usually in two stages. It reduces to half the erect size soon after orgasm, and completes detumescence in 30 minutes or less. In the woman, the clitoris returns to its original position rapidly and the orgasmic platform undergoes detumescence. The vagina returns to a relaxed state in about 15 minutes, the uterus descends, and the cervical os gaps for about 30 minutes. The labia minora loses its deep coloration rapidly, but its edema takes longer to resolve. Genital swelling persists in most women for variable periods of time.

Some men and women perspire heavily and have a thin film of sweat over much of the body. There is often a feeling of calm and relaxation as muscle tension ceases; laughing or crying also happen frequently. Some people feel exhausted after orgasm, and rapidly fall asleep, while others feel invigorated and refreshed. Some may feel mildly depressed or have a sense of letdown; others feel elated or euphoric. There do not seem to be any consistent differences in postorgasmic responses between men and women.

If orgasm does not occur, resolution follows the same physiologic processes but takes considerably longer. Muscle tension and vasocongestion recede more gradually, and the pelvic area may remain congested for several hours. Responses to sexual experiences without orgasm vary by occasion and individual. In some instances, it may be desirable to avoid orgasmic release; and even if not sought, occasional occurrences will probably not be problematic. Consistent absence of orgasm, however, often leads to frustration, resentment, feelings of inadequacy, and unhappiness. There are cultural differences between the male and female responses to nonorgasm; a man generally is not satisfied with sex unless he has ejaculated, while women do not find it unusual to have some percentage of nonorgasmic sexual encounters. However, a chronic, high proportion of encounters without orgasm in women gradually leads to less interest in sex.[8]

The Male Sexual Pattern

There appears to be less variability in the man's pattern of sexual response than the woman's. Generally, excitement progresses continuously in the man unless prolonged by deliberate use of delaying tactics, until the plateau stage is reached. Plateau lasts for a relatively short period of time, then peaks in one definitive, usually strong orgasm. Resolution occurs rather rapidly, with a supposed refractory period during which restimulation of the penis is not possible.

This refractory period is much shorter in younger men, who may have another erection in a few minutes, and is longer in older men. Some have questioned the concept of a time during which the man cannot respond to sexual stimuli (Fig. 9-9). Men report experiencing orgasms of different intensity.

The Female Sexual Patterns

There are three basic types of sexual response patterns in women. One pattern resembles the male pattern, in that excitement builds rapidly to plateau, with some peaks and dips along the way, leading to one intense orgasm and a rapid resolution stage (Pattern C, Fig. 9-9). A second pattern among women involves a slower progression of excitement and a longer plateau stage. An intense and definite orgasm is then experienced, followed by a slower resolution stage. Or, after orgasm the woman may return to plateau for a while, then have another orgasm which may be either more or less intense. Some women can have multiple orgasms while rising and falling into plateau levels of arousal, followed by slower resolution (Pattern A, Fig. 9-9). In the third pattern, excitement progresses more slowly until plateau is reached, then there are minor surges toward orgasm causing repeated and prolonged pleasurable and tingly sensations without a definite orgasm. Resolution tends to be longest with this pattern.[1] (See Pattern B, Fig. 9-9).

Although this model is widely used, there is both subjectively and physiologically little difference between excitement and plateau. These tend to be continuous as most of the physiologic changes that

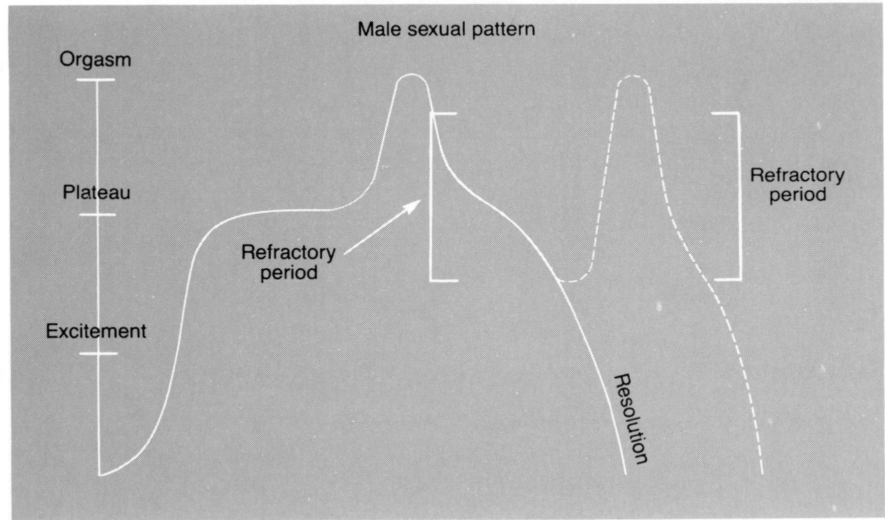

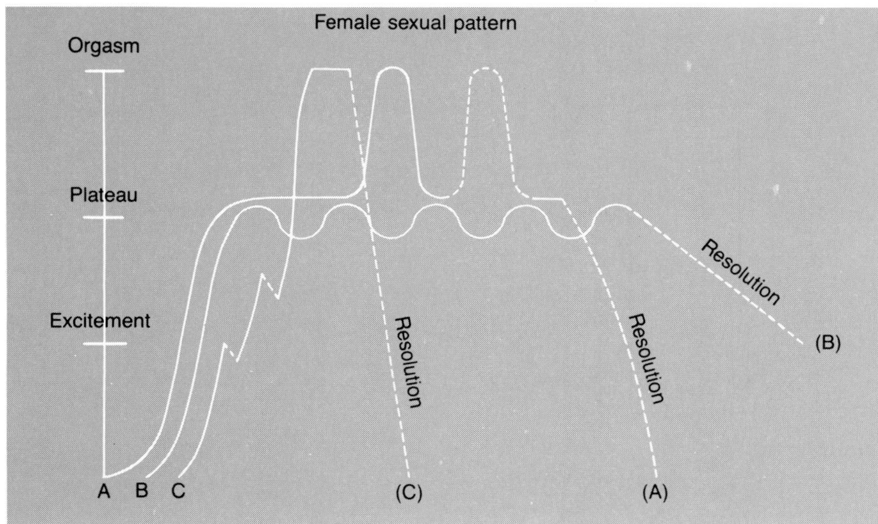

Figure 9-9.
Male and female sexual response patterns. Female Sexual Patterns—*(A)* Steady progression to plateau stage is followed by intense orgasm; subsequent orgasms may occur; resolution is slower. *(B)* Slower progression to plateau stage is followed by minor surges toward orgasm causing prolonged pleasurable feelings without definitive orgasm; resolution is slowest. *(C)* Rapid progression to plateau stage with some peaks and dips; one intense orgasm follows with rapid resolution. This most closely resembles male pattern.

occur during excitement continue into the plateau stage. However, it is still a useful abstraction for studying human sexual response.

There are a few other differences between the male and female sexual response that warrant discussion. Erection is attained within 3 to 5 seconds, while vaginal lubrication takes about 30 seconds. It takes longer for the woman to fill the much larger structures in her pelvic area, and greater amounts of vasocongestion and edema are required. The man has three erectile bodies to fill (two corpora cavernosi and one corpus spongiosum with its bulb), while the woman has five bodies to fill (two corpora cavernosi, two vestibular bulbs, and a large circumvaginal plexus). With all the bulbs and venous plexi maximally distended, the blood volume that a woman has to remove during orgasm is considerably greater than that of a man. Women need longer pelvic muscles to do this because the female pelvic outlet is greater in diameter. In the man, the greatest strength of muscle contractions occurs in the first three to four orgasmic contractions. This strong, concentrated muscular activity assures deposition of semen deep within the vaginal barrel. This results in a short, intense orgasm which enhances conception. The woman's orgasmic contractions generally last twice as long as the man's, and their strength is not as markedly concentrated in the first few contractions. These types of contractions remove a greater amount of the woman's more widespread pelvic congestion. However, as discussed previously, there is wide variation in a woman's orgasmic response with a generally greater range in intensity and duration than a man's.

Orgasm and Changes in Brain Waves

Because sexual response and orgasm are both a physical and a mental experience, it is not surprising that some striking changes in brain function have been found to parallel the physiological changes. A unique pattern in brain waves occurred in both men and women who participated in an experiment using an electroencephalogram (EEG) and physiological measures to check for changes during sexual response. The data revealed a typical pattern of brain waves through EEG recording before, during, and after orgasm. These patterns were the same for men and women (Fig. 9-10). There was a clear distinction between the left and right hemispheres of the brain just before and during orgasm. Frequency decreased in the right hemisphere to about four cycles per second, while in the left hemisphere it remained at

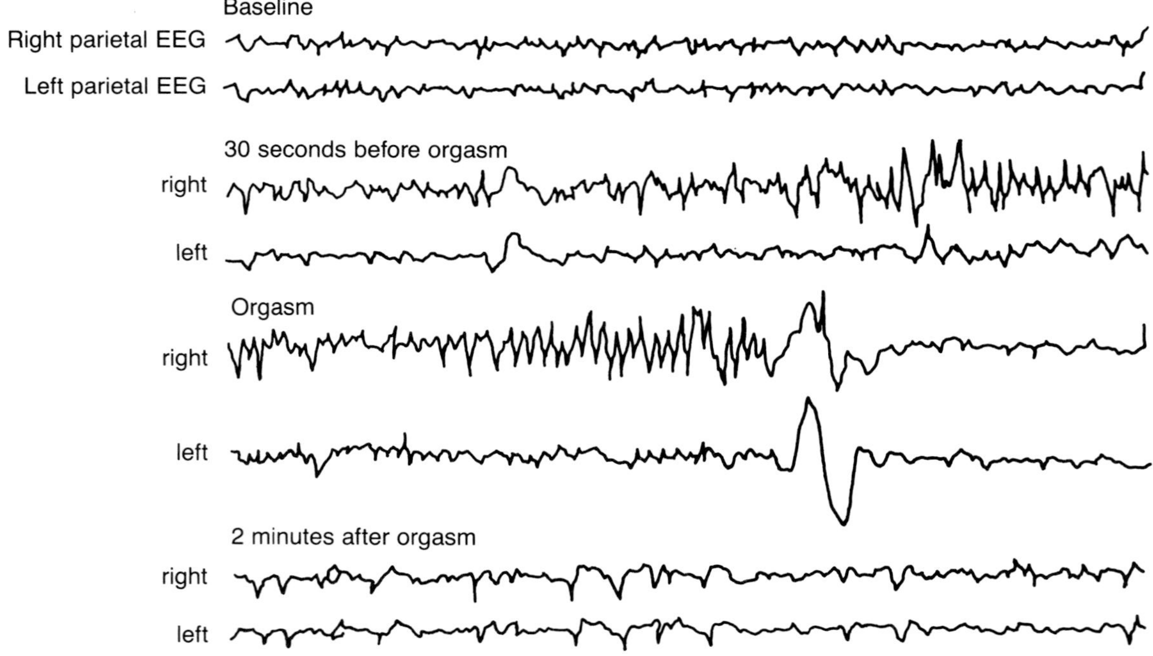

Figure 9-10.
Brain wave changes associated with orgasm.

about ten cycles per second. The amplitude response was also found much greater in the right hemisphere than in the left hemisphere.

The two hemispheres have been connected with different types of mental functions and cognitive activities. The left hemisphere is associated with verbal, logical, and rational thought processes. The right hemisphere has a larger role in spatial, intuitive, and emotional thought processes; it is considered the source of artistic and creative abilities. The slowing of brain wave cycles and increases in amplitude that occur in the right hemisphere with orgasm indicate its emotional-intuitive character. These brain wave patterns are unique to orgasm, and do not occur with other types of activities studied in laboratories. It seems likely that the experience of orgasm is a unique state of consciousness. This may be one reason why people find the orgasmic experience difficult to describe.[9]

References

1. Masters W, Johnson VE: Human Sexual Response. Boston, Little, Brown & Co, 1966

2. Green R: Sexual Identity Conflict in Children and Adults. New York, Basic Books, 1974

3. Money J, Ehrhardt AA: Man & Woman, Boy & Girl. Baltimore, The Johns Hopkins University Press, 1972

4. Nass GD, Libby RW, Fisher MP: Sexual Choices. Monterey, CA, Wadsworth Health Sciences Division, 1981

5. Rosen R, Rosen LR: Human Sexuality. New York, Alfred A. Knopf, Inc., 1981

6. Sherfey MJ: The Nature & Evolution of Female Sexuality. New York, Random House, 1972

7. Bragonier JR: Uterine spasms elicited by orgasm. Medical Aspects of Human Sexuality 14,11:99–103, 1980

8. Kaplan HS: The New Sex Therapy. New York, Brunner/Maxel, 1974

9. Cohen H, Rosen RC, Goldstein L: Electroencephalographic laterality changes during human sexual orgasm. Arch Sex Behav 5:189–199, 1976

CHAPTER

10

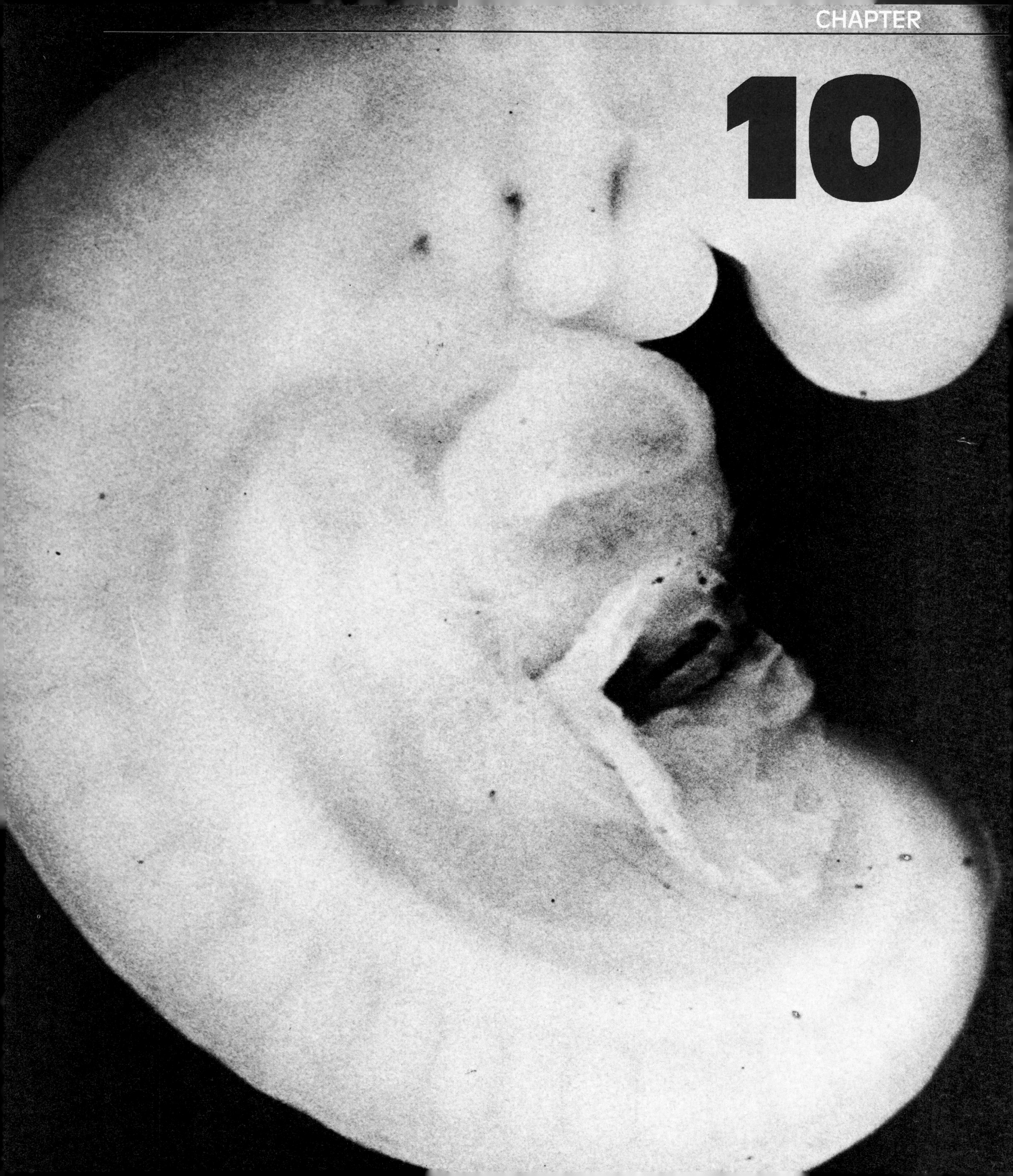

CHAPTER 10

Conception and Ovum Development

In all of nature's wide universe, there is no process more wondrous and no mechanism more fantastic than the one by which a tiny speck of tissue, the human egg, develops into a 7-pound baby. Primitive peoples consider this phenomenon so miraculous that they frequently ascribed it to superhuman intervention and overlooked the fact that sexual intercourse was a necessary precursor. Throughout unremembered ages, our own primitive ancestors doubtlessly held similar beliefs, but now we know that pregnancy comes about in only one way: from the union of a female germ cell, the egg, or ovum, with a male germ cell, the spermatozoon. These two germ cells, or *gametes* become fused into one cell, or *zygote,* which contains the characteristics of both the female and the male.

Maturation of Ovum and Sperm Cells

The ovum remains in a resting stage of development until about two days before ovulation. Its nucleus is large and round and has been described as vesicular, because it resembles a bleb or vesicle. The ovum undergoes the process of *meiosis,* the special method for cell division, while still in the follicle. Through meiosis the ovum matures and its genetic material (chromosomes) prepares for fertilization.

The spermatozoon is fully matured when it is discharged in the ejaculate. It has undergone a meiotic process in preparation for fertilization before it leaves the testis.

In all human cells, with the exception of the mature sex cells, there are normally 46 chromosomes (chroma, color; soma, body). Normally, the chromosomes within each somatic cell are paired. Thus, each cell contains 22 pairs of autosomes (auto, self) and one pair of sex chromosomes. Female cells normally contain two X chromosomes, and male cells normally contain one X and one Y chromosome. The sex chromosome of the mature ovum is always of the X type. The mature spermatozoon may have either an X chromosome or a Y chromosome (Fig. 10-1). When fertilization occurs with a spermatozoon containing the X chromosome, a female is produced. When an ovum is fertilized by a spermatozoon containing a Y chromosome, a male is produced.

Thus, in the human being, age, state of health, and physical strength have nothing to do with the determination of the sex of the offspring. The sex is determined at the time of fertilization by the spermatozoon, not by the ovum. At the completion of the fertilization process, the fertilized ovum contains 46 chromosomes, the number normally present in all somatic cells.

Prior to fertilization, each gamete undergoes a reduction in its total number of chromosomes to one half of the usual number, the *haploid number.* This reduction occurs through the process of meiosis (see Fig. 19-1). In the meiotic process, each gamete normally received only one chromosome of each pair. Thus, each mature spermatozoon has 23 chromosomes in its nucleus, and each mature ovum also contains 23 chromosomes, the haploid number.

The cells that will eventually produce mature spermatozoa within the seminiferous tubules are called

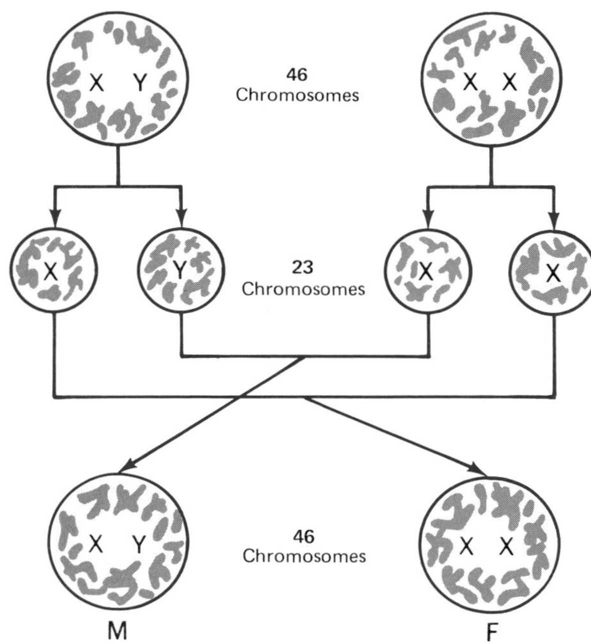

Figure 10-1.
The sex of the offspring is determined at the time of fertilization by the combination of the sex chromosomes of the spermatozoon (either X or Y) and that of the ovum (X). The ovum fertilized by a sperm cell containing the X chromosome produces a female (44 regular chromosomes + 2 X chromosomes). If it is fertilized by a spermatozoon containing the Y chromosome, the union produces a male (44 regular chromosomes + X + Y). Note that the structures depicted as chromosomes are diagrammatic only. In this illustration it was not possible to include the totai correct number.

spermatogonia. These are located at the periphery of the seminiferous tubules (Fig. 10-2). They divide by mitosis, forming a new generation of germ cells, the primary spermatocytes. In time these cells undergo a reduction division through the process of meiosis (see Fig. 10-2). Although their cytoplasm divides, the chromosomes do not split, instead, they are divided between each of two new cells, each now containing 23 chromosomes, the haploid number. These new haploid cells are called *secondary spermatocytes.* One contains 22 regular chromosomes *(autosomes)* and an X chromosome. In the other, there are 22 autosomal chromosomes and a Y chromosome. These cells divide again and form four spermatids, each with 22 autosomal chromosomes, two with X and two with Y sex chromosomes. Each spermatid develops a tail and eventually becomes a mature spermatozoon.

The reduction division of the oocyte begins as the follicle is being prepared for ovulation (see Fig. 10-2). While the primary oocyte is still within the follicle, it divides through meiosis into two cells, a secondary oocyte and a first polar body, so called because it is observed at one pole of the developing ovum. A second polar body is released upon penetration by the spermatozoon and, as a result of its release, the number of chromosomes is halved. The final product, the fertilized ovum, once again contains a set of 46 chromosomes, 23 from the ovum and 23 from the spermatozoon.

The individual chromosomes differ in form and size, ranging from small, spherical masses to long rods. By the use of cell culture techniques, it is possible to photograph the individual chromosomes in a given cell. (Techniques for chromosome analysis are discussed in Chapter 16.)

The Ovum

As described in Chapter 8, one ovum per month is normally discharged from the human ovary. Under the influence of the gonadotropins, the graafian follicle, which is destined to release an ovum, has matured. The ovum itself has been pushed to one side of the fluid-filled cavity of the follicle. It is surrounded by a translucent coat, the *zona pellucida.* Immediately adjacent to and connected to the zona pellucida is a layer of follicular cells, the *corona radiata,* which are arranged in a radial pattern. The *cumulus oophorus* is a more loosely structured layer of cells peripheral to the corona radiata. The ovum, surrounded by this

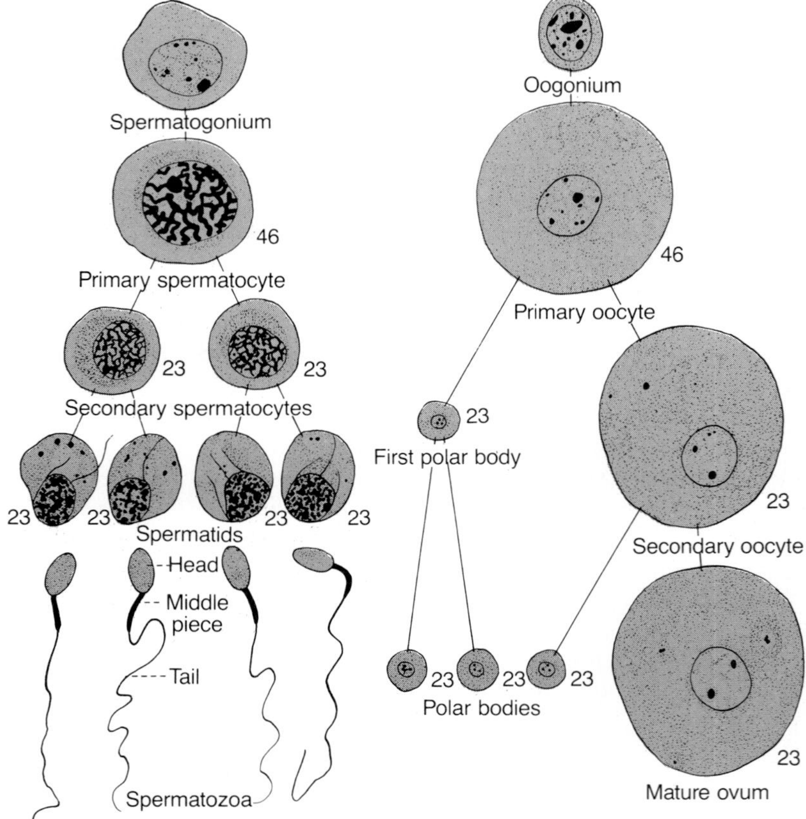

Figure 10-2.
Diagram of gametogenesis. The various stages of spermatogenesis are indicated on the left; one spermatogonium gives rise to four spermatozoa. On the right, oogenesis is indicated; from each oogonium, one mature ovum and three abortive cells are produced. The chromosomes are reduced to one half the number characteristic for the general body cells of the species. In man, the number in the body cells is 46, and that in the mature spermatozoon and secondary oocyte is 23.

entourage of cells, having matured through release of its first polar body, is released through the process of ovulation. The ovum, within its sticky cumulus mass, rapidly and efficiently is transported into the fallopian tube, the site of fertilization. The ovum is now about 0.2 mm (1/25 of an in) and is barely visible to the naked eye.

Transport Through the Fallopian Tube

The fallopian, or uterine, tube is an important structure that serves a number of functions in reproduction (Fig. 10-3). It is responsible for transferring the ovum into its lumen from the rupturing follicle and for providing a temporary environment for the ovum and the spermatozoon. It is also where fertilization occurs, and where the ovum passes through several cell divisions during the early stages of human life. Finally, this tube is responsible for transporting the fertilized, cleaving ovum into the uterus after a three-day interval.

The tube is uniquely designed anatomically for its various functions. The ovarian end is endowed with *fimbriae.* These are arranged in fronds and are lined with hairlike projections called *cilia,* which beat to direct any overlying fluid, as well as any particles contained therein, in the direction of the uterine cavity. The rest of the fallopian tube is also lined with cilia, which are important in transporting the newly released ovum along the tube (Fig. 10-4). The cilia create a current that courses along the tube. They are partially responsible for transporting particles through the tube.

The anatomical arrangement at the fimbriated end of the tube is important in ovum pickup mechanisms.

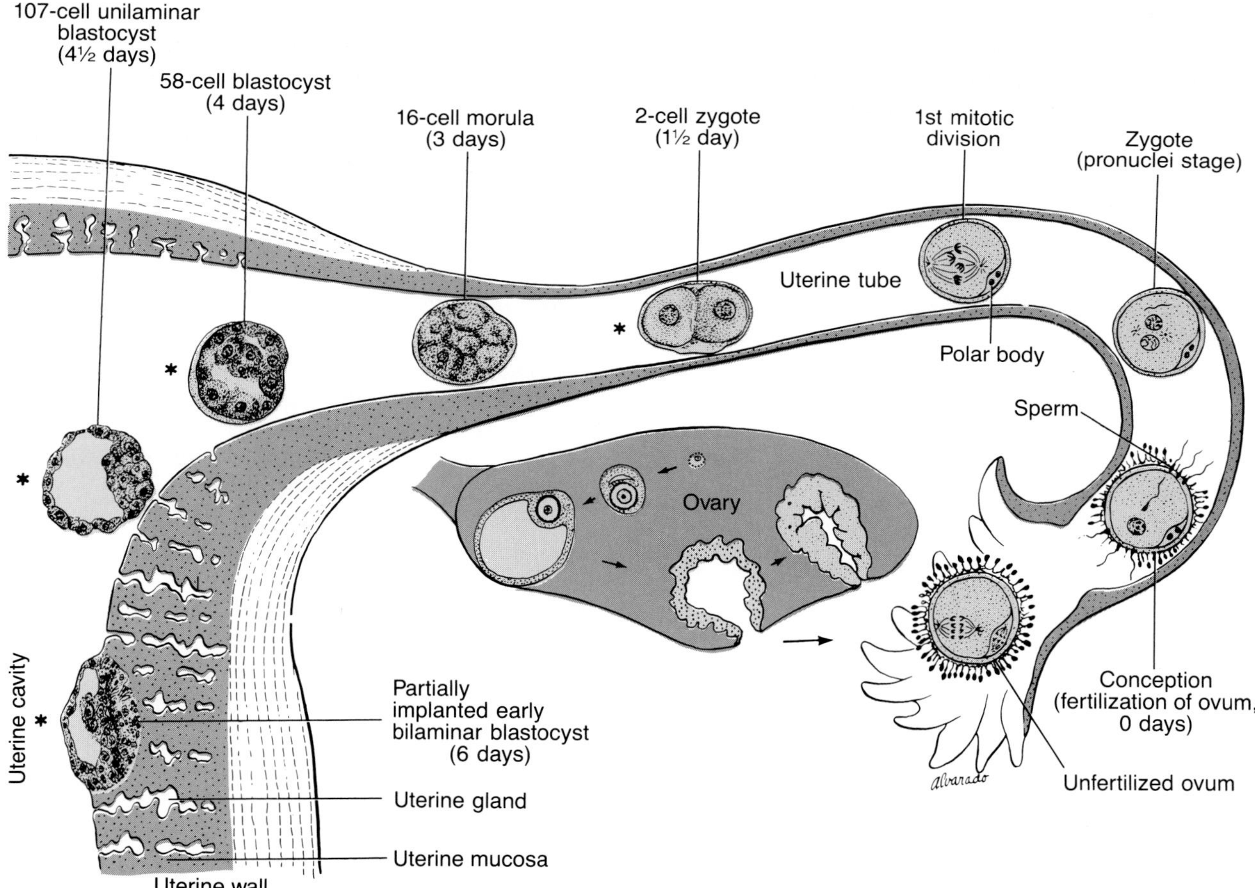

Figure 10-3.
Transport of the ovum into the fallopian tube, and fertilization within the tube followed by cleavage (cell division) to the 8- to 16-cell stage. The product, now referred to as a morula, is delivered into the uterus where it develops into a blastocyst and implants in the endometrium on the sixth to seventh postfertilization day. (Modified from Gasser RF: Atlas of Human Embryos. Hagerstown, Harper & Row, 1975)

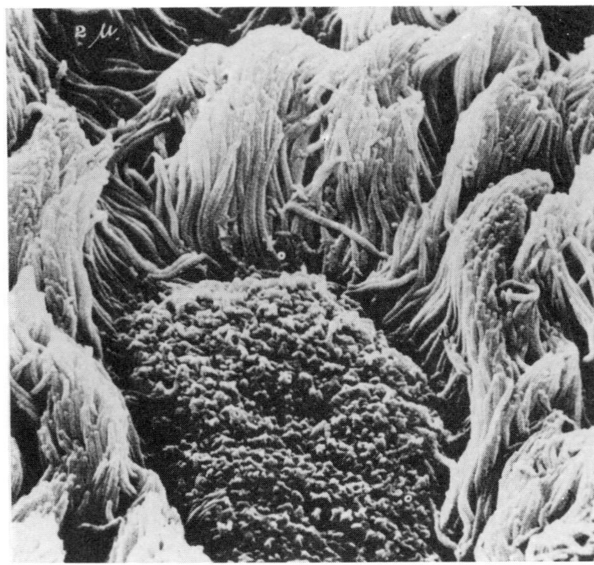

Figure 10-4.
Scanning electron micrograph of the human fallopian tube showing ciliated cells surrounding a nonciliated cell in the midproliferative phase of the menstrual cycle. (Patek E, Nilsson L, Johannisson E: Scanning electron microscopic study of the human fallopian tube: The proliferative and secretory stages. Fertil steril 23:459,1972)

A separate strand of fimbriae, the *fimbria ovarica,* extends from the tube to the ovary to which it is attached. This contains a separate bundle of smooth muscle. During ovulation this muscle contracts and pulls the ovary in the direction of the tubal opening. The remainder of the fimbriae are thought to embrace the ovary near or over the point of ovulation. They exercise muscular movement which moves them to and fro over the rupturing follicle. Thus, the cilia lining the fimbriae soon come into contact with the cumulus oophorus surrounding the ovum, and as they beat in the direction of the tubal lumen, they carry the sticky cumulus mass past the tubal ostium to a point well within the fallopian tube. An efficient process of ovum transfer is arranged through these mechanisms and ovum pickup is practically assured, despite the fact that the ovum is miniscule in size.

Once the ovum is safely past the tubal ostium, it is rapidly transported to a point well within the fallopian tube. Fertilization occurs there. The fertilizing spermatozoon has been previously conditioned in the female reproductive tract so that it has acquired the ability to fertilize an ovum.

After fertilization, the ovum passes through several cell divisions, during which it is retained in the fallopian tube for approximately three days. Eventually it develops into a solid mass of cells, a *morula.* It is finally transferred into the uterus at the 8 to 16 cell stage.

In the human, the mechanism by which the ovum is retained in the tube is not as yet clear. However, the importance of the three-day residence within the tube can be extrapolated from experiments in other mammals. In the rabbit, for example, if the ovum is removed from the tube and placed in the uterus prematurely, it degenerates and fails to implant. Although for obvious reasons, this experiment has not been carried out on humans, it is generally accepted that the three-day residence within the human tube is important. Premature expulsion of the ovum from the tube could result in failure of implantation. Prolonged retention could result in ectopic pregnancy, causing tubal rupture and hemorrhage. The latter condition constitutes a serious obstetrical emergency. The importance of the fallopian tube, a once-neglected organ that bridges the space between the ovary and the uterus, is now quite evident.

Spermatozoa

The minute, wriggling *spermatozoa* are in some respects even more remarkable than the ova that they fertilize. They resemble microscopic tadpoles, with oval heads and long, lashing tails about ten times the length of the head. The human spermatozoon consists of three parts—the head, the middle piece (neck), and the tail (Fig. 10-5). The head of the spermatozoon is covered by the acrosome. This acrosomal cap is an envelope in which enzymes that play an important role in sperm penetration are contained. The nucleus, and consequently the chromatin material, is in the head; the tail serves as a propeller.

Spermatozoa are much smaller than ova, their overall length measures about one quarter the diameter of the egg, and it has been estimated that the heads of 2 billion of them—enough to regenerate the entire population of the world—could be placed, with room to spare, in the hull of a grain of rice.

The wriggling motion of the tails allow spermatozoa to swim with a quick vibratory motion, as fast as 3 mm a minute. To ascend the uterus and the fallopian tube they must swim against the same currents that waft the ovum downward; they are assisted by the muscular action of the uterus, which propels them upward in the direction of the tube. Spermatozoa have been observed in the fallopian tube within minutes of insemination.

The most amazing feature of spermatozoa is the huge number of them. At each ejaculation, during intercourse, about 300 million are discharged into the vagina. If each of these could be united with an ovum,

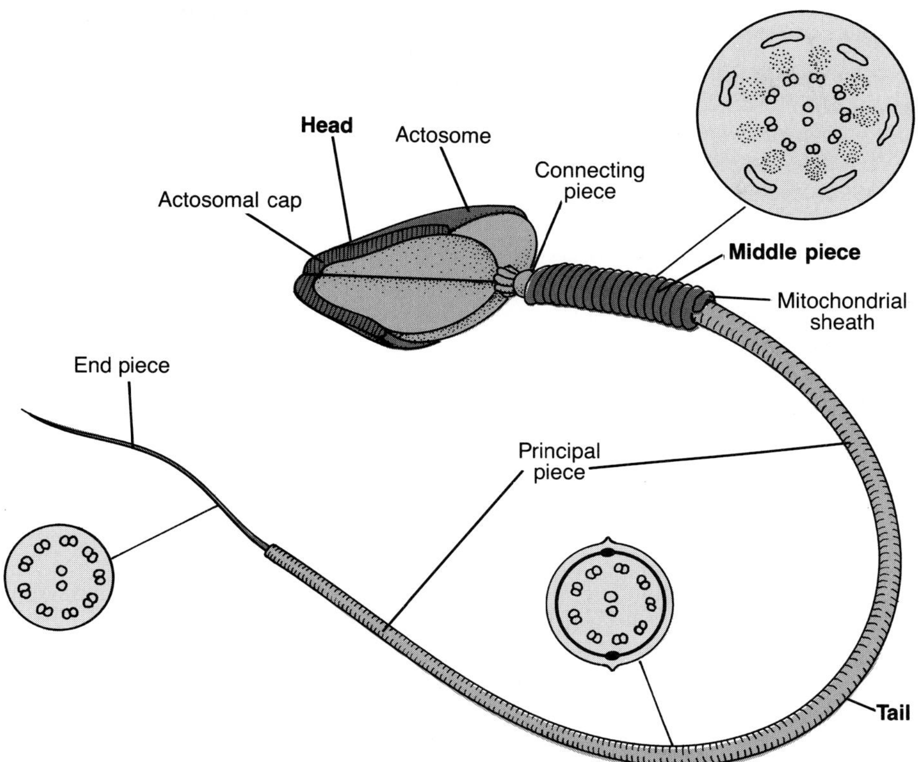

Figure 10-5.
Drawing of a mammalian spermatozoon with the cell membrane removed to show the arrangement of the underlying structural components. The appearance of cross sections as seen in electron micrographs at various levels is also depicted.

the babies that would be created would exceed the total number born in the United States during the past 100 years.

Of the millions of spermatozoa deposited in the vagina during coitus, many are expelled immediately and some remain in the vagina for an interval and are later extruded. Those retained in the vagina lose their motility in about an hour because of the acidic environment provided by the vagina.

Some spermatozoa reach the cervix almost immediately after ejaculation. Those transferred into the secretions of the cervix find a more favorable environment and may remain motile for as long as several days, especially in the preovulatory phase of the cycle.

Thousands of spermatozoa find their way into the cavity of the uterus; fewer still reach the lumen of the fallopian tube. Only one is afforded the privilege of continued biological life through fertilization and, at that, only occasionally. The remainder are disposed of in the reproductive tract, and as they degenerate they are phagocytized by the white blood cells in that region. However, once the spermatozoon is in the female reproductive tract it may retain its motility, and, therefore, its potential ability to fertilize for hours or days. Spermatozoa are conditioned to fertilize an ovum after they are exposed to the female reproductive tract, a process called *capacitation.*

Fertilization and Changes Following Fertilization

After the ovum is well within the fallopian tube, the cumulus oophorus disperses. These cells begin to separate, partly as a result of the influence of the enzyme hyaluronidase that is contained in the acrosome surrounding the head of the spermatozoon. The spermatozoon makes its way through this peripheral layer of cells; meanwhile the densely packed corona radiata has undergone certain changes. These cells become looser under the influence of tubal fluid, and the spermatozoon then finds its way through this layer to the zona pellucida. It is now thought that the zona pellucida is penetrated by the spermatozoon because of a trypsinlike enzyme that is present in the sperm acrosome. Prior to penetration, openings are created in the outer membrane of the acrosome through which the enzyme-rich contents of the acrosome escape. This process, called the *acrosome reaction,* leads to a loss of the membrane over the anterior half of the sperm head. The spermatozoon makes a channel through the zona pellucida as the trypsinlike enzyme, referred to as acrosin, dissolves the protein containing zona with which it comes into contact. After the spermatozoon traverses the zona pellucida, it is in a position to penetrate the membrane of the ovum. As the spermatozoon penetrates the ovum, it brings its tail with it.

Once penetration is complete, a physiological barrier occurs and penetration of the ovum by other spermatozoa is prevented. Soon after penetration, the nucleus of the spermatozoon and the nucleus of the ovum undergo characteristic changes. They become pronuclei—distinct, clearly identifiable bodies of chromatin, each contained in a membrane. The male pronucleus and the female pronucleus then fuse. The process of fertilization is now biologically complete. The new cell presents the full complement, or *diploid number* of chromosomes, one half from the spermatozoon and one half from the ovum. Soon thereafter the first cell division occurs. In this process, the male and female chromosomes and their genes are mingled and finally split, forming two sets of 46 chromosomes, one set of 46 going to each of the two new cells. This process is repeated again and again until masses containing 8, 16, 32, and 64 cells are produced successively. These early cell divisions produce a morula. At the 8 to 16 cell stage, the dividing ovum is delivered into the uterus.

The ovum remains in the fallopian tube for about three days. The fertilized ovum then spends about four days in the uterine cavity before actual embedding takes place. Thus, a total interval of some seven days elapses between ovulation and implantation.

Meanwhile, important changes are taking place in the internal structure of the fertilized ovum. Fluid appears in the center of the mulberry mass that pushes cells to the periphery of the sphere. At the same time it becomes apparent that this external envelope of cells is actually made up of two different layers, an inner and an outer. After some 260 days a specialized portion of the inner layer will have developed into the long-awaited baby. The outer layer is a sort of

Figure 10-6.
Early stages of development. *(Top, left* and *center)* The cells are separated into a peripheral layer and an inner cell mass; the peripheral layer is called the trophoblast, or trophectoderm; the entire structure is called a blastodermic vesicle. *(Top, right)* The formation of the amniotic cavity and yolk sac is indicated. The former is lined with ectoderm, the latter with entoderm. *(Bottom, left)* The location of the embryonic disk and the three germ layers is shown, together with the beginning of the chorionic villi. *(Bottom right)* The external appearance of the developing mass is shown; the chorionic villi are abundant.

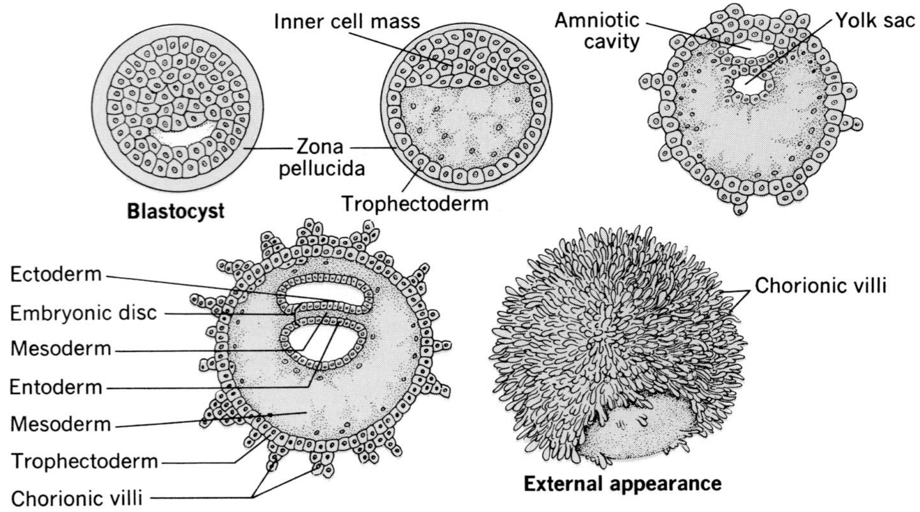

foraging unit called the *trophoblast* which means "feeding" layer; it is the principal function of these cells to secure food for the embryo (Fig. 10-6).

While the ovum is undergoing these changes, the lining of the uterus is preparing for its reception. Considering that ovulation took place on the fourteenth day of the menstrual cycle and that the tubal journey and the uterine sojourn required 7 days, 21 days of the cycle will have passed before the ovum has developed its trophoblastic layer of cells. This is the period when the lining of the uterus reaches its greatest thickness and succulence.

Implantation of the Ovum

The *trophoblast* is responsible for embedding the ovum. This process is carried out by means of enzymes. In this manner these cells not only burrow into the uterine lining and eat out a nest for the ovum, but they can also digest the walls of the many small blood vessels that they encounter beneath the surface. The mother's bloodstream is thus tapped and the ovum finds itself deeply sunk in the lining epithelium of the uterus, with tiny pools of blood around it. Finger-like projections or chorionic villi, now develop out of the trophoblastic layer and extend greedily into the blood-filled spaces. Another name for the trophoblast, and one more commonly used as pregnancy progresses, is the *chorion*. These chorionic villi contain blood vessels that are connected to the fetus and are extremely important because they are the sole means by which oxygen and nourishment are received from the mother. The entire ovum becomes covered with villi, which grow out radially and convert the chorion into a shaggy sac.

The cells of the chorionic villi begin to produce HCG. This hormone maintains progesterone production by the corpus luteum. In turn, progesterone stimulates and supports endometrial growth by providing a suitable environment for continued development of the conceptus.

Suggested Reading

Greep RO, Koblinsky MA: Frontiers in Reproduction and Fertility Control. Cambridge, MA, The MIT Press, 1977

Greep RO, Koblinsky MA, Jaffe F: Reproduction and Human Welfare: A Challenge to Research. Cambridge, MA, The MIT Press, 1977

Gwatkin RBL: Fertilization Mechanisms in Man and Mammals. New York, Plenum Press, 1977

Mastroianni L, Biggers J, Sadler W: Fertilization and Embryonic Development in Vitro. New York, Plenum Press, 1981

Seitz HM, Brackett BG, Mastroianni L: Fertilization. In Hafez ESE, Evans TN (eds): Human Reproduction: Conception and Contraception, pp 119–131. Hagerstown, MD, Harper and Row, 1973

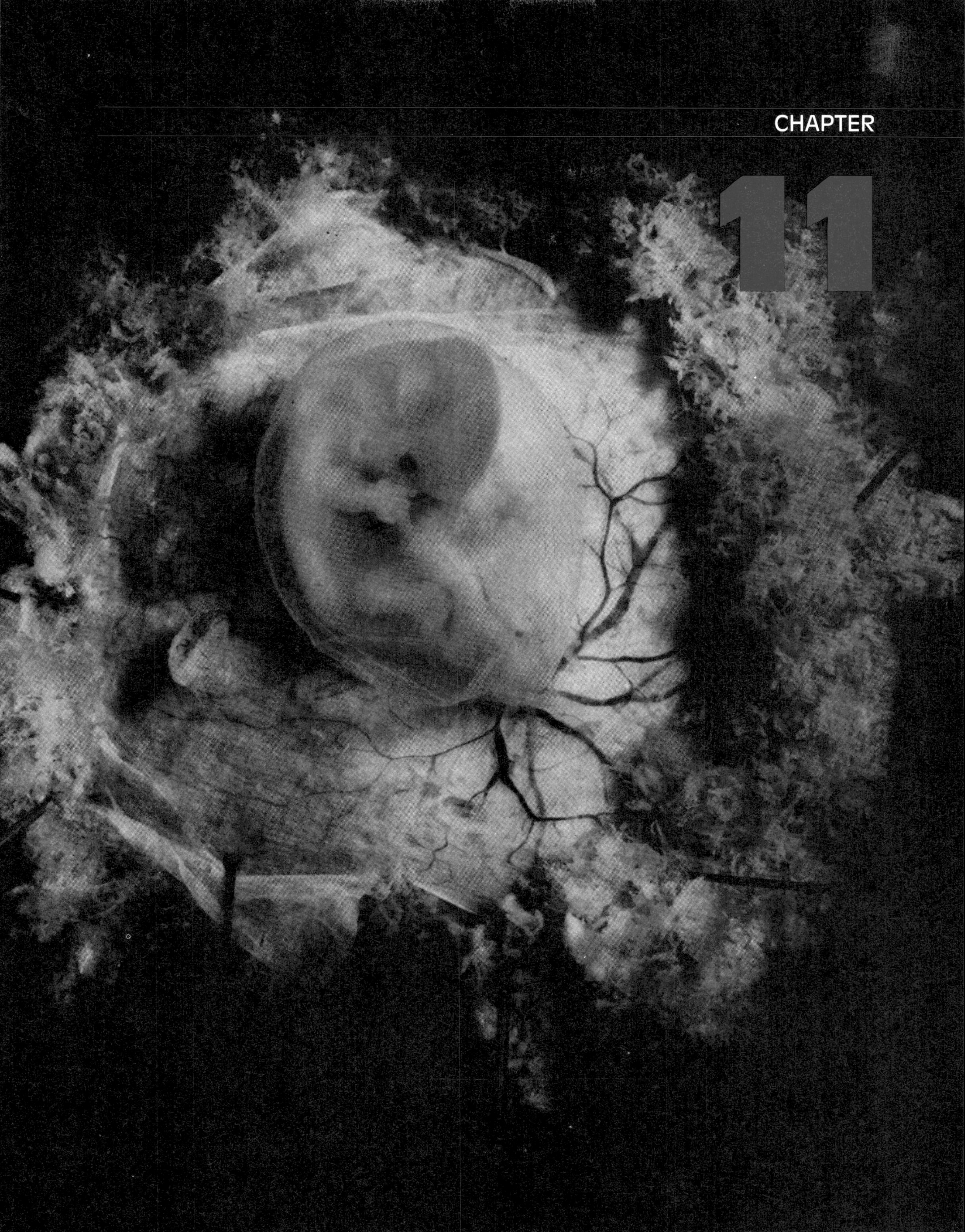
CHAPTER
11

CHAPTER 11

Development and Physiology of the Embryo and Fetus

Physiological Overview

By the time of implantation, the fertilized ovum has survived a series of delicately programmed events. It has been released from its ovarian follicle after resumption of the meiotic process. Following ovulation the ovum has been transported successfully into the lumen of the fallopian tube. There a single, properly conditioned spermatozoon has traversed the barriers surrounding the ovum to initiate the fertilization process. Ovum meiosis is completed and there is fusion of the male and female genetic components, followed by a series of mitotic divisions. Three days later the multicellular ovum is ushered out of the fallopian tube into the uterus. It lingers freely in the uterine cavity and bathes in uterine fluid while it develops further into a blastocyst. Implantation occurs on about the seventh postfertilization day and the conceptus begins to derive its nourishment from the blood and tissue juices of the endometrium.

As development continues, the conceptus begins to produce human chorionic gonadotropin (hCG) which maintains production of progesterone by the corpus luteum. Thus, the newly formed pregnancy is now essentially self-sufficient and is in control of its own environment. Support of the corpus luteum by hCG results in continued maintenance of the endometrium by progesterone and the next expected menstrual period is missed. At this point the conceptus is traditionally referred to as an *embryo*.

Throughout this two-week interval, there is a substantial incidence of pregnancy loss. It is estimated that 35% of fertilized ova develop abnormally and fail to progress beyond two weeks. Such a pregnancy loss is not surprising when one considers the complicated series of events that culminate in a successfully implanted pregnancy.

From the second week on, development occurs relatively rapidly. The mechanisms that support pregnancy as the now nearly self-sufficient embryo develops will be considered in this chapter.

The Decidua

The thickening of endometrium, which occurs during the premenstrual phase of menstruation, was described in Chapter 8. If pregnancy ensues, this endometrium becomes even more thickened, the cells enlarge, and the structure becomes known as the *decidua*. It is a direct continuation, in exaggerated form, of the already modified premenstrual endometrium.

For descriptive purposes, the decidua is divided into three portions. The part which lies directly under the embedded ovum is the *decidua basalis* (Fig. 11-1). The portion that is pushed out by the embedded and growing ovum is the *decidua capsularis*. The remaining portion, which is not in immediate contact with the ovum, is the *decidua vera*. As pregnancy advances, the decidua capsularis expands rapidly over the growing embryo and at about the fourth month lies in intimate contact with the decidua vera.

Amnion, Chorion, and Placenta (Fig. 11-1)

Amnion

Even before the previously noted structures become evident, a fluid-filled space develops around the embryo. This space, the amniotic cavity, is lined with a smooth, slippery, glistening membrane, the *amnion*. Because it is filled with fluid, it is often called the bag of waters; the fetus floats and moves in the amniotic cavity. At full term this cavity normally contains from 500 ml to 1000 ml of liquor amnii, or the "waters."

The amniotic fluid has a number of important functions—it keeps the fetus at an even temperature, cushions the fetus against possible injury, and it provides a medium in which the fetus can easily move; furthermore, the fetus drinks this fluid.

At the end of the fourth month of pregnancy, the amniotic cavity has enlarged to the size of a large orange and, with the fetus, occupies the entire interior of the uterus. At this point, the amniotic fluid, which contains viable cells that are cast off by the fetus, can be sampled by amniocentesis and the chromosomal makeup of the fetal cells evaluated in culture for prenatal diagnosis of genetic abnormalities (see Chap. 39).

Chorion

As explained in Chapter 10, the early ovum is covered on all sides by shaggy chorionic villi, but in a short period of time the villi that invade the decidua basalis enlarge and multiply rapidly. This portion of the trophoblast is the *chorion frondosum* (leafy chorion). Conversely, the chorionic villi covering the remainder of the fetal envelope degenerate and almost disappear, leaving only a slightly roughened membrane, the *chorion laeve* (bald chorion). The chorion laeve

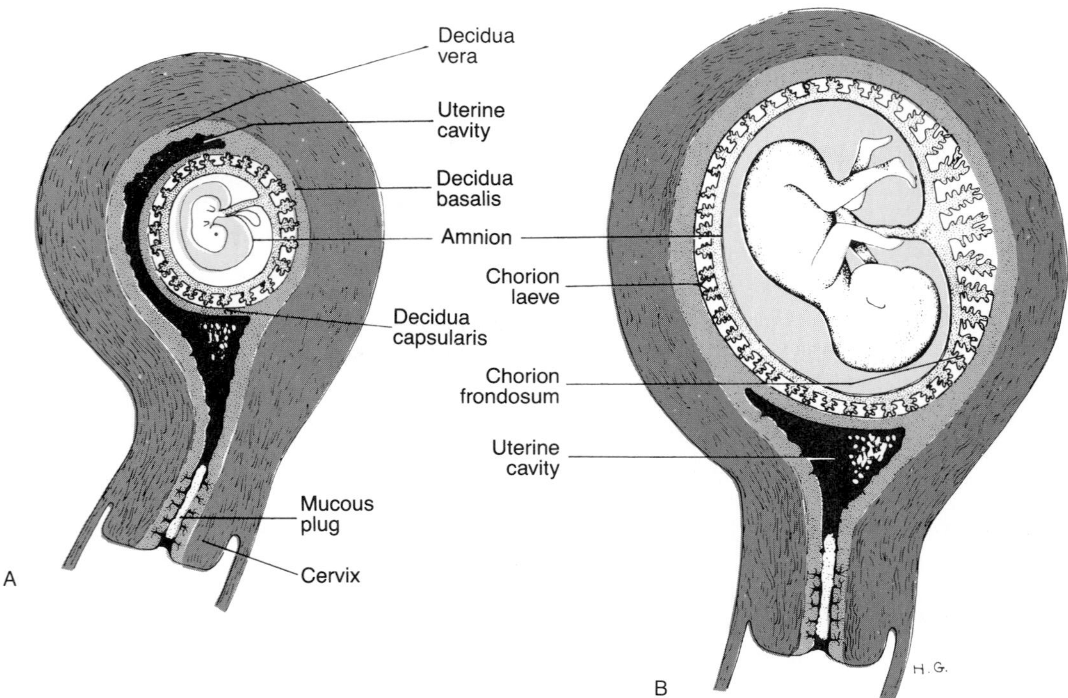

Figure 11-1.
Diagrams illustrating enlargement of the chorionic vesicle and progressive obliteration of the uterine cavity. *(A)* 6 weeks after fertilization, *(B)* 16 weeks after fertilization. (Modified from Fitzgerald MJT: Human Embryology: A Regional Approach. Hagerstown, MD, Harper & Row, 1978)

lies outside the amnion and has contact with its outer surface. The outer surface of the chorion laeve lies against the decidua vera. The fetus is thus surrounded by two membranes, the amnion and the chorion.

Placenta

By the third month the placenta ("flat cake" in Latin) has formed. This is a fleshy, disklike organ that measures about 20 cm in diameter and 2 cm in thickness late in pregnancy.

The placenta is formed by the union of the chorionic villi and the decidua basalis (see Fig. 11-1). A thin layer of the uterine bed clings to the branching projections of chorionic villi, and together they make up the organ that supplies food to the fetus, like the roots and the earth provide nourishment for a plant.

At term the placenta weighs about 500 grams. The fetal surface is smooth and glistening, and is covered by amnion. Beneath this membrane a number of large blood vessels may be seen. The maternal surface is red and fleshlike and is divided into a number of segments, or *cotyledons,* about 2.5 cm in diameter (Fig. 11-2).

The placenta is connected to the fetus by the *umbilical cord,* which is usually about 45 cm in length and about 1.5 cm in diameter. The cord usually leaves the placenta near the center and enters the abdominal wall of the fetus at the umbilicus, just below the middle of the median line in front. It contains two arteries and one large vein, which are twisted upon each other and are protected from pressure by a transparent, bluish white, gelatinous substance called *Wharton's jelly.*

The Three Germ Layers

The cells that are destined to form the baby grow rapidly with nutritional facilities provided. At first they all look alike, but soon after embedding, certain groups of cells assume distinctive characteristics and differentiate into three main groups—an outer covering layer *(ectoderm),* a middle layer *(mesoderm),* and in internal layer *(entoderm).*

The epithelium of the skin, hair, nails, sebaceous glands, and sweat glands; the epithelium of the nasal and oral passages; salivary glands and mucous mem-

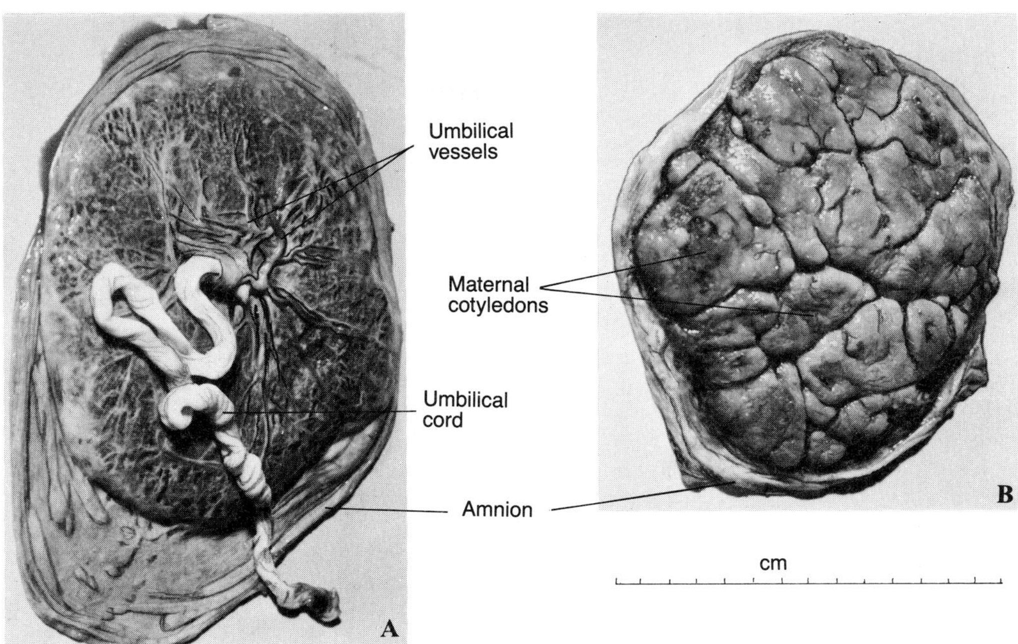

Figure 11-2.
Full-term placenta. *(A)* fetal surface, *(B)* maternal surface. (Fitzgerald MJT: Human Embryology: A Regional Approach. Hagerstown, MD, Harper & Row, 1978.

branes of the mouth and nose; the enamel of the teeth; and the nervous system are all derived from the *ectoderm.*

Muscles; bone; cartilage; the dentin of the teeth; ligaments; tendons; areolar tissue; kidneys; ureters; ovaries; testes; the heart; blood; lymph and blood vessels; and the lining of the pericardial, pleural, and peritoneal cavities are formed from the *mesoderm.*

The *entoderm* structures the epithelium of the digestive tract and the glands that pour secretion into this tract, the epithelium of the respiratory tract (except for the nose) and the bladder, the urethra, the thyroid, and the thymus.

Size and Development of the Fetus

Size of Fetus at Various Months

The physician, as well as the nurse, is sometimes called upon to estimate the intrauterine age of a fetus that has been expelled prematurely.

In general, length is a more accurate criterion of the age of the fetus than weight. Hasse's rule suggests that for clinical purposes, the length of the embryo in centimeters may be approximated during the first five months by squaring the number of the month of pregnancy; in the second half of pregnancy, the month may be multiplied by five to estimate the length of the fetus. Conversely, the approximate age of the fetus may be obtained by taking the square root of its length in centimeters during the first five months and thereafter by dividing its length in centimeters by five. For instance, a fetus that is 16 cm long is about four months old; a fetus that is 35 cm long is about seven months old.

Development of Fetus from Month to Month

Most women consider themselves one month pregnant at the time of the first missed menstrual period, two months pregnant at the second missed period, and so on. Since conception does not take place until ovulation, 14 days after the onset of menstruation in a 28-day cycle, it is obvious that an embryo does not attain the age of one month until about a fortnight after the first missed period (assuming a 28-day cycle),

Fetal Development

1st Lunar Month

The fetus is 0.75 cm to 1 cm in length.
Trophoblasts imbed in decidua.
Chorionic villi form.
Foundations for nervous system, genitourinary system, skin, bones, and lungs are formed.
Buds of arms and legs begin to form.
Rudiments of eyes, ears, and nose appear.

2nd Lunar Month

The fetus is 2.5 cm in length and weighs 4 g.
Fetus is markedly bent.
Head is disproportionately large, owing to brain development.
Sex differentiation begins.
Centers of bone begin to ossify.

3rd Lunar Month

The fetus is 7 cm to 9 cm in length and weighs 28 g.
Fingers and toes are distinct.
Placenta is complete.
Fetal circulation is complete.

4th Lunar Month

The fetus is 10 cm to 17 cm in length and weighs 55 g to 120 g.
Sex is differentiated.
Rudimentary kidneys secrete urine.
Heart beat is present.
Nasal septum and palate close.

5th Lunar Month

The fetus is 25 cm in length and weighs 223 g.
Lanugo covers entire body.
Fetal movements are felt by mother.
Heart sounds are perceptible by auscultation.

4 weeks

8 weeks

3 months

4 months

5 months

and its "birthday" by months regularly falls two weeks or so after any numerically specified missed period (Fig. 11-3). If the cycle is longer than 28 days, or if ovulation was delayed in the conceptive cycle, the duration of actual pregnancy, relative to the last menstrual period, will be shorter. This should be remembered in evaluating the month-by-month development of the fetus.

Physicians refer to the age of a pregnancy as *lunar months,* that is, periods of four weeks. Since a lunar month corresponds to the usual length of the menstrual cycle, it's easier to calculate this way (see Fig. 11-3).

End of First Lunar Month

The embryo is about 7 mm long if measured in a straight line from head to tail and recognizable traces of all organs are differentiated. The backbone is apparent but is so bent upon itself that the head almost touches the tip of the tail. The head is extremely prominent, representing almost one third of the entire embryo. The head is very large in proportion to the body throughout intrauterine life. This is still true at birth but to a lesser degree.

The rudiments of the eyes, the ears, and the nose now make their appearance (Fig. 11-4). The tube that will eventually form the heart has been formed, producing a large, rounded bulge on the body wall; even at this early age, this structure is pulsating regularly and propelling blood through microscopic arteries. The rudiments of the future digestive tract are also discernible. A long, slender tube leading from the mouth to an expansion becomes the stomach; connected with the latter, the beginnings of the intestines may be seen. The incipient arms and legs resemble buds.

End of Second Lunar Month

The fetus, the term used for the product of conception after the fifth week of gestation, now begins to assume human form (Fig. 11-5). As the brain develops, the head becomes disproportionately large so that the

6th Lunar Month

The fetus is 28 cm to 36 cm in length and weighs 680 g.
Skin appears wrinkled.
Vernix caseosa appears.
Eyebrows and fingernails develop.

6 months

7th Lunar Month

The fetus is 35 cm to 38 cm in length and weighs 1200 g.
Skin is red.
Pupillary membrane disappears from eyes.
The fetus has an excellent chance of survival.

7 months

8th Lunar Month

The fetus is 38 cm to 43 cm in length and weighs 2.7 kg.
Fetus is viable.
Eyelids open.
Fingerprints are set.
Vigorous fetal movement occurs.

8 months

9th Lunar Month

The fetus is 42 cm to 49 cm in length and weighs 1900 g to 2700 g.
Face and body have a loose wrinkled appearance because of subcutaneous fat deposit.
Lanugo disappears.
Amniotic fluid decreases.

9 months

10th Lunar Month

The fetus is 48 cm to 52 cm in length and weighs 3000 g.
Skin is smooth.
Eyes are uniformly slate colored.
Bones of skull are ossified and nearly together at sutures.

nose, the mouth, and the ears become relatively less prominent. It has an unmistakably human face, as well as arms and legs, with fingers, toes, elbows, and knees (Fig. 11-6). During the past four weeks it has quadrupled in length and measures about 2.2 cm from head to buttocks. It is during this period that the external genitalia become apparent, but it is difficult to distinguish between male and female.

End of Third Lunar Month

The fetus is over 7.5 cm long and weighs almost 28 g. The sex can now be distinguished because the external genitalia are beginning to show definite signs of sex. Centers of ossification have appeared in most bones; the fingers and the toes have become differentiated, and the fingernails and the toenails appear as fine membranes. Early in this month, buds for all the temporary "baby" teeth are present, and sockets for these develop in the jawbone. Rudimentary kidneys have developed and secrete small amounts of urine into the bladder, which probably escape later into the amniotic fluid. Movements of the fetus are known to occur at this time, but they are too weak to be felt by the mother.

End of Fourth Lunar Month

The fetus is now 16 cm long from head to toe and weighs about 110 g (Fig. 11-7). The sex, as evidenced by the external genital organs, is now quite obvious.

End of Fifth Lunar Month

The length of the fetus now approximates 25 cm and it weighs about 223 g. A fine, downy growth of hair, *lanugo*, appears on the skin over the entire body. Usually, the mother now becomes conscious of slight fluttering movements in her abdomen, as a result of fetal movement. Their first appearance is called *quickening*, or the perception of life. Fetal heart tones can easily be detected by auscultation at the end of the fifth lunar month. If a fetus is born now, it may make a few efforts to breathe, but its lungs are insufficiently developed to cope with conditions outside the uterus, and it invariably succumbs within a few hours at most.

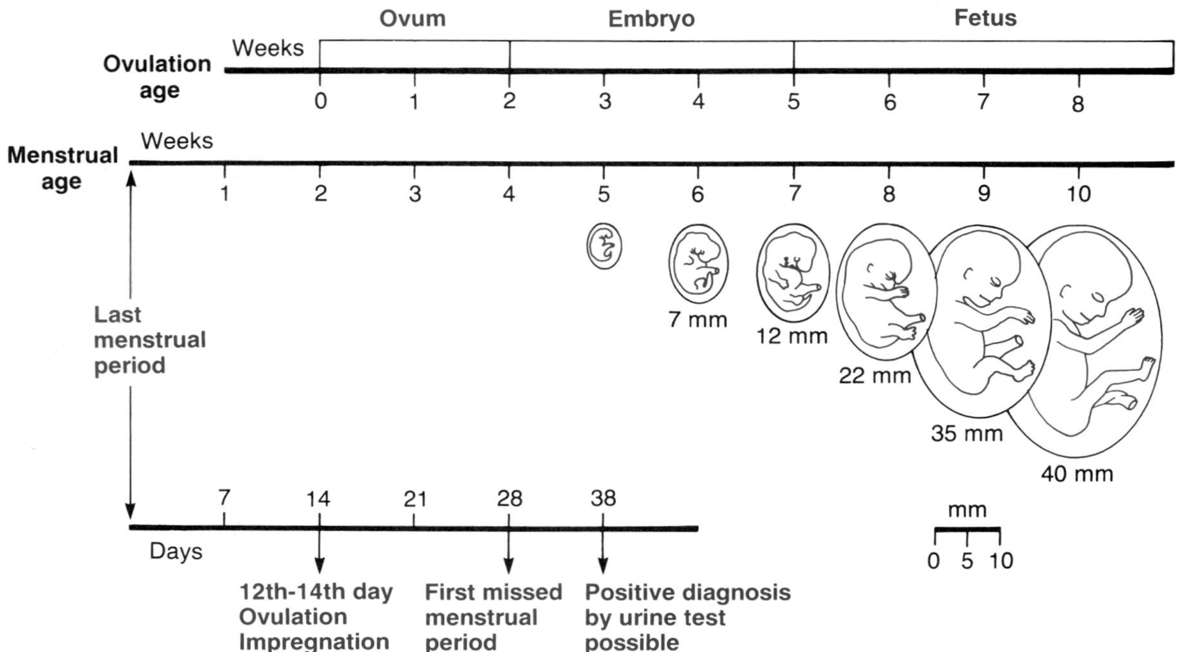

Figure 11-3.
Growth of ovum, embryo, and fetus during the early weeks of pregnancy.

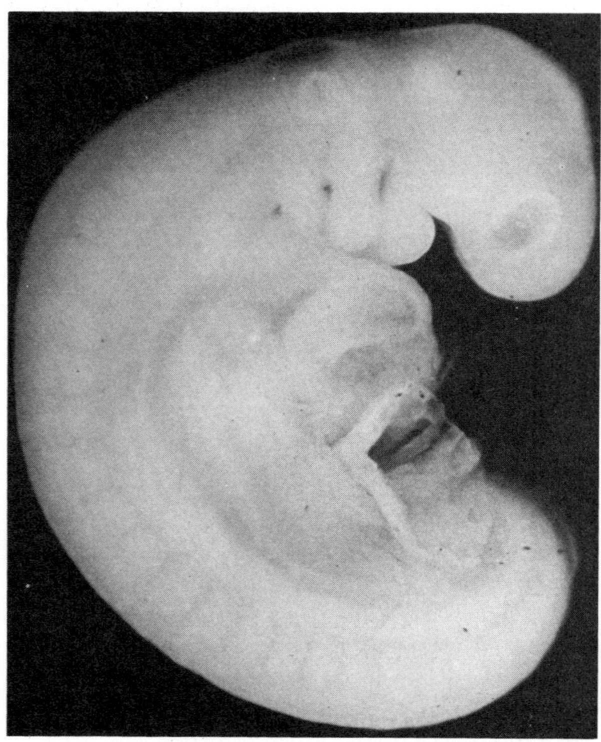

Figure 11-4.
Human embryo in the first lunar month of development. (Carnegie Institution, Washington, D.C.)

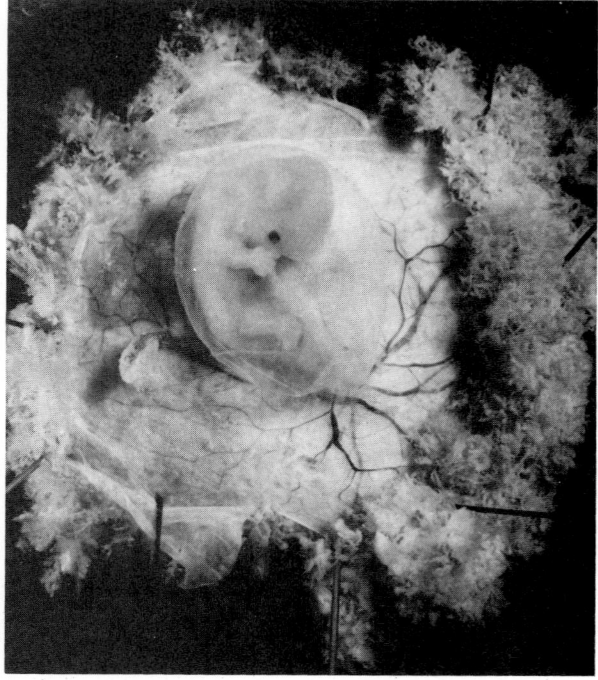

Figure 11-5.
Human embryo photographed by Chester F. Reather. This specimen represents about 40 days of development and is shown in the opened chorion. Original magnification × 1.7. (Carnegie Institution, Washington, D.C.)

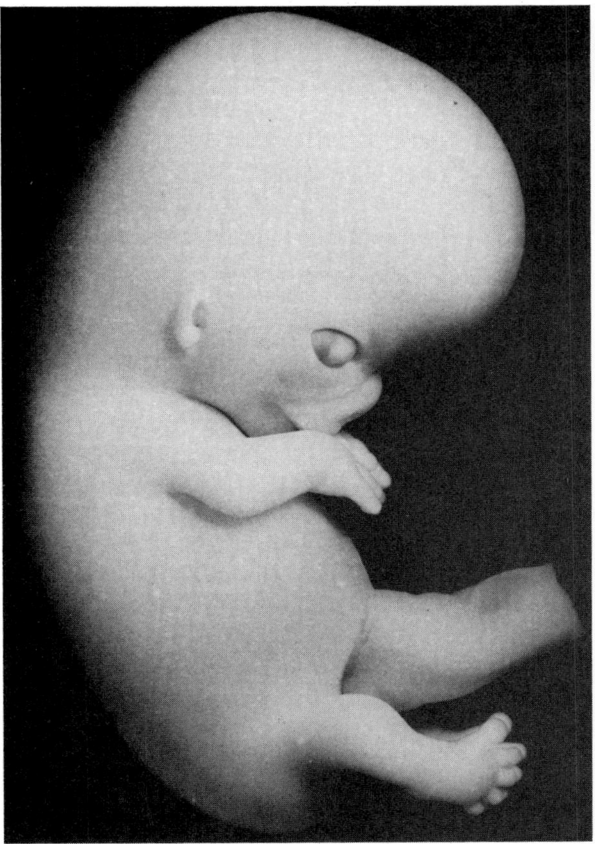

Figure 11-6.
Human fetus at about eight weeks development. Note the prominence of the head and the continuing development of the extremities. (Carnegie Institution, Washington, D.C.)

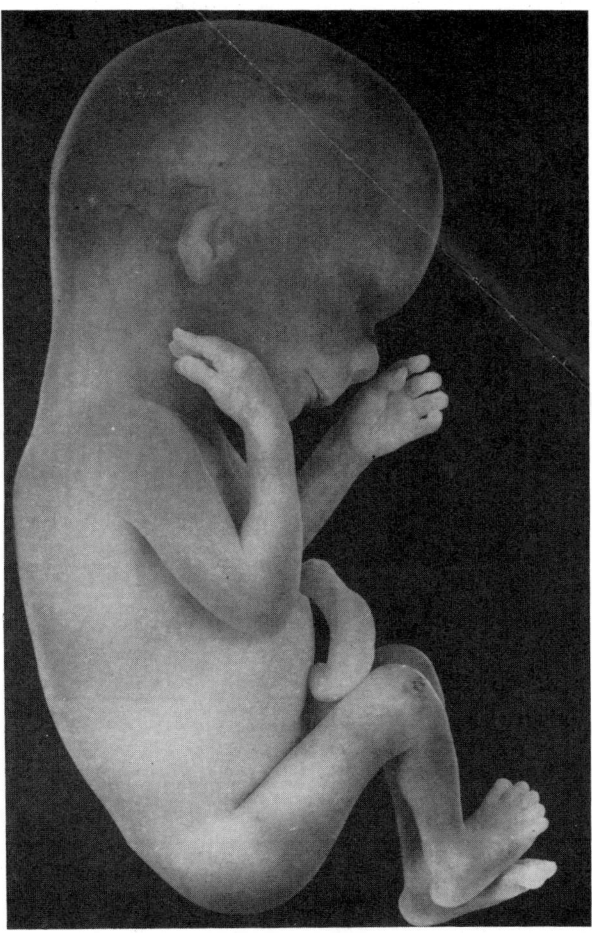

Figure 11-7.
At about 4 months external features are easily identified. Most organ systems have been formed and will continue to grow and mature. (Carnegie Institution, Washington, D.C.)

End of Sixth Lunar Month

The length of the fetus is 36 cm and its weight is 680 g. It now resembles a miniature baby, with the exception of the skin, which is wrinkled and red with practically no fat beneath it. At this time, however, the skin begins to develop a protective covering, *vernix caseosa,* which means cheesy varnish. This fatty, cheesy substance adheres to the skin of the fetus and at term may be 0.3 cm thick. Increasing numbers of fetuses of this size now survive in intensive care nurseries.

End of Seventh Lunar Month

The fetus measures about 37 cm in length and weighs approximately 1 kg. If it is born at this time, it has an excellent chance of survival.

End of Eighth Lunar Month

The fetus measures about 40 cm and weighs approximately 1.8 kg. Its skin is still red and wrinkled and vernix caseosa and lanugo are still present. The fetus resembles a little old man. With proper incubator and good nursing care, infants born at the end of the eighth month have a better than 90% chance of survival in many nurseries in the United States.

End of Ninth Lunar Month

For all practical purposes the fetus is now a mature infant. It measures some 47 cm and weighs approximately 2.7 kg. Because of the deposition of subcutaneous fat, the body has become more rotund and the skin less wrinkled and red. The fetus devotes the last two months in the uterus to putting on weight; during this period it gains 220 g a week. Its chances of survival are now as good as though it was born at full term.

Middle of Tenth Lunar Month

Full term has now been reached and the fetus weighs on an average 3 kg if it's a girl and 3.4 kg if it's a boy, and it is about 50 cm long. Its skin is now white or pink and thickly coated with the cheesy vernix. The fine, downy hair that previously covered its body has largely disappeared. The fingernails are firm and protrude beyond the end of the fingers.

Duration of Pregnancy

The length of pregnancy varies greatly; it may range between 240 days and 300 days and yet be entirely normal in every respect. The average duration from the time of conception is nine and one half lunar months, that is, 38 weeks or 266 days. From the first day of the last menstrual period its average length is 10 lunar months, that is, 40 weeks or 280 days. However, scarcely one pregnancy in ten terminates exactly 280 days after the beginning of the last period. Less than one half terminate within one week of day 280. In 10% of all pregnancies, birth occurs a week or more before the theoretical end of pregnancy, and in another 10%, it takes place more than two weeks later than expected. Indeed, it does appear that some fetuses require a longer time and others a shorter time, in the uterus for full development.

Calculation of the Expected Date of Confinement

In view of the wide variation in the length of pregnancy, it is obviously impossible to predict the expected day of confinement (EDC) with any degree of precision. The time-honored method, based on the average duration of pregnancy, is simple. Count back three calendar months from the first day of the last menstrual period and add seven days (Nägele's rule). For instance, if the last menstrual period began on June 10, we would count back three months to March and, adding seven days, arrive at the date of March 17. An easier way to calculate this is to substitute numbers for months. Then, this example becomes as follows: 6/10 − 3 months = 3/10 + 7 days = 3/17. Although it may be satisfying to the curiosity to have this date in mind, it must be understood that less than 5% of all pregnant women go into labor on the estimated date of confinement, and in 35% a deviation of one to five days before or after this date may be expected (Table 11-1).

Yet, whether pregnancy terminates one week before or two weeks later than the day calculated, the outlook for mother and baby is usually as good as though it had ended on the exact due date.

Actually, women seldom go overterm; in most of these cases it is the system of calculation and not nature that has erred. For example, ovulation and therefore, conception may have occurred days later than calculated; this error would make the beginning and the end of pregnancy that many days later. If, in addition to this circumstance, we were dealing with a fetus that required a slightly longer stay in the uterus for complete development, it would be clear that the apparent delay was quite normal and for the best.

Calculation of Expected Date of Confinement (Nägele's rule)

1. Count back three months from last menstrual period.
2. Add 7 days.

Table 11-1
Deviation from Calculated Date of Confinement, According to Nägele's Rule, of 4656 Births of Mature Infants

Deviation in Days	Early Delivery	Delivery on Calculated Date	Late Delivery
0		189(4.1)*	—
1–5	860(18.5)*	—	773(16.6)*
6–10	610(13.1)	—	570(12.2)
11–20	733(15.7)	—	459(9.9)
21–30	211(4.5)	—	134(2.9)
31 and over	75(1.6)	—	42(0.9)

The menstrual cycles of the mothers were 28 ± 5 days. The infants were at least 47 cm in length and 2600 g in weight (Burger and Korompai, Zentralbl. Gynäk 63:1290, 1939)

* Numbers in parentheses represent percent of cases considered

Physiology of the Fetus and Placenta

During the period when the ovum lies unattached in the uterine cavity, its nutriment is provided by an endometrial secretion, often called *uterine milk,* which is rich in glycogen. The ovum lies in a lake of fluid that represents the broken-down product of endometrial cells and obtains nourishment from this source.

Very early in pregnancy, by the third or the fourth week, the chorionic villi develop blood vessels within them (connected with the fetal bloodstream). Since these villi have already opened up the maternal blood vessels, nourishment is available from the maternal blood through the placenta.

Placental Function

The human placenta is a truly versatile organ. It functions as a lung in the transfer of gases, as a gastrointestinal tract in the transport of nutrients, as a kidney in the excretion of wastes, as skin in the transfer of heat, much like a liver in its conjugation of drugs and hormones, and as an endocrine gland through production of various protein and steroid hormones. The normal weight of a full-term human placenta is approximately 500 g and it covers about one quarter of the uterine wall. During the course of pregnancy its weight and mass increase in proportion with that of the fetus. The normal fetal to placental weight ratio at term is 6:1.

The structure and function of the placenta differ among mammalian species. Homo sapiens has a villous hemochorial placenta because the fetal vessels are contained within fingerlike villi that extend into an intervillous space (Fig. 11-8). There they are bathed by maternal blood (hemo), which transfers nutrients from across the chorionic membrane (chorial), which constitutes the outer surface of the villi. Nutrient-rich and well-oxygenated blood enters the intervillous space by way of the maternal spiral arteries. This blood surrounds the villi that contain fetal blood which has been delivered to them by the umbilical arteries, and therefore has been depleted of both nutrients and oxygen. Oxygen and nutrients from the blood in the intervillous space are delivered into the blood that is contained in the villous capillaries. The newly restored blood is then returned to the fetus along the veins contained within the villi, which converge into the umbilical vein.

Functions of Placenta

- Transfer of gases
- Transport of nutrients
- Excretion of wastes
- Transfer of heat
- Hormone production

Fetoplacental Oxygen Exchange

The partial pressure of oxygen (PO_2) in the intervillous space is approximately 40 mm of mercury. This is the highest oxygen tension that the fetal circulation

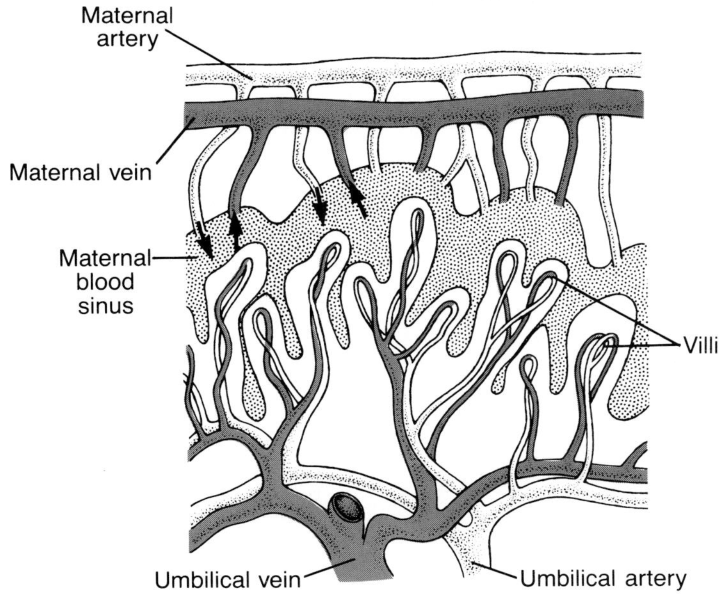

Figure 11-8.
Diagram of placental circulation. Note that maternal and fetal circulations are completely separate.

is exposed to. At any given time, the oxygen that is contained in the intervillous space is capable of satisfying fetal oxygen consumption for approximately one and a half minutes. On their way to the intervillous space, the spiral arteries traverse the muscular wall of the myometrium. The spiral arteries are compressed by the myometrium and blood flow through these vessels is interrupted with each uterine contraction. Thus, delivery of oxygen to the intervillous space is interrupted. The normal fetus can tolerate this brief period of oxygen deprivation without damage. In certain cases of abnormal labor, when the contractions are unusually prolonged, the resulting anoxia could cause fetal damage.

The umbilical cord is the other vulnerable link in the system for maternal-fetal exchange of oxygen. Under certain conditions of labor the umbilical cord can be compressed, for example, between the fetal head and the pelvis, or entangled above the fetus. Prolonged interference with cord circulation can seriously affect fetal oxygenation.

On gross examination of the maternal side of the placenta, one can usually see approximately 20 cotyledons or lobes. These are further divided into approximately 200 lobules, each of which is a circulatory unit containing a single spiral artery. When a spiral artery becomes obstructed, as when there has been a thrombosis or development of a clot within its lumen, the blood supply to that circulatory unit is interfered with, and results in tissue destruction or infarction of the area. Many term placentas contain an area of infarction. Fortunately, the placenta is endowed with a substantial reserve. It has been estimated that only half of the placental surface is required for maintaining a normal maternal-fetal exchange.

At the microscopic level, three layers of tissue separate the fetal circulation from the maternal blood. A molecule passing from the fetus to the mother must traverse these tissues. The outermost layer is the fetal trophoblast, which contains an outer syncytiotrophoblast and inner cytotrophoblast. Immediately beneath the trophoblast is a connective tissue layer. The innermost layer is the endothelial layer of the fetal capillary. As pregnancy progresses, the fetal capillaries are brought closer and closer to the surface of the villi and exchange is facilitated. At term, the diffusion distance for a molecule is approximately 3.5 microns, as compared to 0.5 microns in the adult lung.

Nutrition Placental Transmission

There are six well documented mechanisms for the transport of nutrients from the mother to the fetus—diffusion, facilitated diffusion, active transport, bulk flow, pinocytosis, and defects in placental membrane.

1. *Diffusion* is the passage of a substance from one area to another on the basis of its concentration gradient. Materials that are transported by diffusion include the respiratory gases, oxygen and carbon dioxide; the electrolytes, sodium and chloride; and some lipid soluble vitamins. The transport of gases depends on their partial pressures. The mechanism of diffusion is important because it is clinically evident that placental failure is generally the result of a limitation in substances exchanged by diffusion.
2. *Facilitated diffusion* involves passage along a concentration gradient that occurs when the concentration of material on the maternal side is greater than that on the fetal side. This kind of transfer occurs without the use of energy, but at a faster rate than can be explained on the basis of the concentration gradient alone. This mechanism is carrier mediated, that is, it is transferred by cellular elements which carry it into and through the membrane. Glucose, a most impor-

Placental Transport

Mechanism	Key Substances Exchanged
Simple diffusion	O_2, CO_2, sodium, chloride, vitamins (lipid soluble)
Facilitated diffusion	Glucose
Active transport	Amino acids, iron, calcium, iodine, water soluble vitamins
Bulk flow	Water
Pinocytosis	Immunoglobulins
Membrane breaks	Red blood cells

tant fetal fuel, is transported by facilitated diffusion.

3. *Active transport* requires the passage of substances from one area to another against a concentration gradient, and it is energy dependent. This mechanism requires the expenditure of energy by the cells. Amino acids are transported against a 2 to 1 concentration gradient from mother to fetus. Iron, calcium, iodine, and water soluble vitamins are transported by the mechanism of active transport.
4. *Bulk flow* involves the transfer of substances by hydrostatic or osmotic gradients through micropores in the membrane. This mechanism is important in maintaining maternal-fetal exchange of water.
5. *Pinocytosis* involves the transfer across a cell of materials contained in small vessels located at or near the cell membrane. Microdrops of plasma are taken up by the trophoblasts which transport immunoglobulins to the fetus.
6. *Breaks in the placental membrane* is the final mechanism by which substances are transported from mother to fetus. Defects in the placental membrane can allow the transfer of very large materials, such as red blood cells. This process is responsible for sensitization of the Rh negative woman carrying an Rh positive fetus. Rh positive fetal red blood cells are carried into the maternal circulation and produce antibodies. This most frequently occurs at delivery, when the incidence of breaks in the placental membrane is greatest.

Placental Permeability

Diffusion is the most important mechanism regulating the transfer of substances between mother and fetus. Thus impaired diffusion is often the cause of clinically evident placental dysfunction. Diffusion depends upon the characteristics of the placental membrane. It is purely a physical process and requires no energy. The process is governed by certain principles, which, in combination, are described in Fick's law. Fick's law states that the rate of transfer of materials is directly proportional to the permeability of the membrane and to the actual area of the membrane, but inversely proportional to the thickness of the membrane. This means that the more permeable the membrane and the greater the area presented by the membrane, the greater the rate of transfer. Conversely, the thicker the membrane, the slower the rate of transfer.

Other determinants of permeability for any molecule include the size of the molecule, as well as its molecular charge and lipid solubility properties. In general, molecules with a molecular weight greater than 1000 do not cross the placental membrane. For example, the anticoagulant heparin is a large molecule which, because of its size, will not traverse the placental membrane, hence, heparin treatment can be used safely in pregnancy. In contrast, the anticoagulant, dicoumeral is a much smaller molecule which readily crosses the placenta and, when used in pregnancy, may affect the fetus.

Lipid solubility is an extremely important characteristic in the transport of drugs from mother to fetus, as is the electrostatic charge on the molecules themselves. Many of the narcotic agents and analgesics used in labor and delivery are designed to reach the maternal brain quickly in order to provide rapid pain relief. The characteristics that allow this rapid transport to the brain also allow them to rapidly cross the placental membrane, and thus they can equally quickly affect the fetal central nervous system.

Factors Influencing Placental Exchange

Blood Flow to Uteroplacental Circulation

In general, impaired exchange of carbon dioxide and oxygen is not usually related to problems of diffusion. There is little, if any, resistance to the diffusion of these molecules. Their transfer is most often affected by interference with blood flow into the intervillous space and back to the fetus. Oxygen is brought to the intervillous space by the maternal uterine circulation. Uterine blood flow is approximately 600 ml per minute to 700 ml per minute, representing 10% of the total maternal cardiac output at term. Almost 90% of the total uterine blood flow goes into the intervillous space, while 10% supplies the myometrium. The amount of blood that flows into the intervillous space is directly affected by the perfusion pressure within the uterine arteries. Uteroplacental circulation is widely dilated at rest and therefore has little capacity to expand further. This circulation is, however, capable of marked vasoconstriction, which occurs through hormonal or neural mechanisms. Hence, uterine blood flow during pregnancy can be increased significantly by only one mechanism—maternal bedrest. At rest, blood flow to other organs and tissues, such as muscle and fat, is diminished and the supply of blood to the placenta and fetus is enhanced.

Many mechanisms exist by which blood flow to the uteroplacental circulation may be diminished. Each uterine contraction interrupts the supply of blood into the intervillous space. A contraction that lasts 45 seconds stops the blood flow for approximately 30 seconds. During this interval, the fetus must exist on stored nutrients or on those present in the stagnant blood of the intervillous space. This stress is well tolerated by the normal fetus. Abnormally prolonged uterine contractions or a decrease in maternal blood pressure can diminish blood flow to the uteroplacental circulation. For example, the large term uterus may compress the inferior vena cava, interfering with the return of blood to the right heart. Cardiac output and, therefore, delivery of blood to the uteroplacental unit are decreased. Diminished uterine blood flow can also result from chronic hypertension and pregnancy-induced hypertension owing to vasoconstriction. Various pharmacologic agents, such as vasopressers, may also cause constriction of these vessels. Finally, vigorous maternal exercise will increase blood flow to the muscles and may divert blood from the uteroplacental circulation.

Fetal Blood, Fetal Hemoglobin, Bohr Effect

Several other important determinants of oxygen transfer from mother to fetus should be considered. These include the actual affinity of fetal blood for oxygen, the concentration of fetal hemoglobin within the fetal blood, and the Bohr effect (to be discussed). *Fetal hemoglobin,* because of its special characteristics, has a greater affinity for oxygen than does maternal blood. By virtue of certain biochemical constituents, maternal hemoglobin has a greater capacity to unload oxygen, while fetal hemoglobin is endowed with a greater ability to accept oxygen. The actual concentration of hemoglobin in fetal blood is also greater than in maternal blood. Fetal blood contains 15 g of hemoglobin per 100 ml and adult blood contains approximately 12 g per 100 ml. Since hemoglobin is the agent which actually carries the oxygen, and since the fetus has more hemoglobin, a given unit of fetal blood can carry much more oxygen than can maternal blood.

The *Bohr effect* is the effect of *p*H on the ability of hemoglobin to accept or unload oxygen. A more acidic *p*H is associated with an increased ability of hemoglobin to unload oxygen, while a more alkaline *p*H will increase the ability to accept oxygen. Blood returning from the fetal circulation in the umbilical artery is more acidic, and therefore has a greater capacity to unload oxygen. It reaches the intervillous space, where it gives up its hydrogen ions and carbon dioxide, and its *p*H rises. Concomitantly, these hydrogen ions and carbon dioxide are accepted by the maternal circulation, and the *p*H of the maternal blood decreases. The increased fetal *p*H results in a greater capacity to accept oxygen, and the decreased maternal blood *p*H results in a greater capacity to deliver oxygen.

Adjustments in Fetal Blood Flow

Fetal blood flow is redistributed during periods of oxygen deprivation. Increased amounts of blood are supplied to the fetal brain and heart, while blood flow to the fetal gastrointestinal tract is diminished. This helps to ensure survival of the most vital fetal organs during a time of temporary oxygen lack. Nature has endowed the fetoplacental unit with a unique system of checks and balances whose purpose is to preserve the fetal well-being throughout pregnancy.

The Placenta as an Endocrine Organ

From very early pregnancy the cells that eventually form the placenta are hormonally active. Even before the skipped menstrual period the trophoblastic cells which have been responsible for allowing the embryo to invade into the endometrium have begun to secrete HCG.

Human Chorionic Gonadotropin (HCG)

This hormone is produced by the syncytial cells of the trophoblast. It is a glycoprotein with a very large molecular weight of 36,000 to 40,000. It is similar to pituitary LH in both structure and activity, but it differs physiologically in that its levels are maintained in the circulation for longer periods of time. It is composed of two subunits—an alpha subunit, which is similar to the alpha subunit of pituitary glycoprotein hormones, and a beta subunit, which is specific and unique to human chorionic gonadotropin. The beta subunit has recently been used to make antibodies for a pregnancy test, which is specific for human chorionic gonadotropin levels.

HCG appears in maternal blood by the eighth day after ovulation in the fertile cycle. Its levels increase steadily in early pregnancy, reaching a maximum in 60 to 90 days, and then the levels in the blood begin to fall. Very little HCG is secreted into the fetal compartment in comparison to the large quantities that are released in the maternal circulation. It is the circulating HCG that has served as the basis for all of the commonly used pregnancy tests.

Human Placental Lactogen (HPL) or Human Chorionic Somatomammotropin (HCS)

The placenta produces a second protein hormone, human placental lactogen (HPL), also called human chorionic somatomamotropin (HCS). This hormone is also formed in syncytial cells within the trophoblast of the placenta. Its production increases progressively during pregnancy, with a very marked increase after the 20th week. Very little HCS reaches fetal circulation. There is a distinct correlation between HCS levels and placental weight. For example, maternal

HCS levels are higher in multiple gestations. This hormone has an action similar to human growth hormone, and its purpose is to regulate maternal metabolism in order to maintain a supply of nutrients for the fetus. Specifically, HCS facilitates transport of glucose across the placenta by the process of facilitated diffusion. As its name implies, HCS also has a mammotropic effect.

Progesterone and Estrogen

The placenta also produces the steroid hormones progesterone and estrogen. Throughout pregnancy there is a steady increase in *progesterone* levels which reach maximum just prior to delivery. This progesterone maintains the endometrium and endometrial blood supply, brings about uterine growth, inhibits the activity of the uterine muscle, and stimulates alveolar development in the maternal breast. It also has significant effects on the mother's metabolism.

The *estrogens,* estriol, 17β-estradiol, and estrone, are products of the placenta. Estriol is biologically the weakest of the three major estrogens, but it is produced in greatest quantity. Its production by the placenta involves a unique interplay between the fetal adrenals, fetal liver, and placenta. Estriol is produced by a weak androgen, dehydroepiandrosterone (DHA) sulfate, which comes from the fetal adrenal gland. Ninety percent of all the estriol that is seen in pregnancy is derived from fetal adrenal DHA-sulfate. The fetal liver further modifies DHA-sulfate and converts it to a hormone, which the placenta can then use in estriol production. Thus, the requisites for the placenta to produce significant quantities of estriol are an intact fetal adrenal gland and a normally functioning fetal liver.

The placenta itself converts the modified DHA-sulfate into estriol. The estriol levels in the blood rise steadily during pregnancy. There is a positive correlation between urinary estriol excretion and fetal weight. The levels of the other two hormones, estradiol and estrone, parallel the estriol levels in maternal blood.

The physiological functions of the estrogens during pregnancy are multifold. They stimulate the growth of the uterus and uterine placental blood flow, and they stimulate contractile activity of the myometrium and growth of mammary tissue. The estrogens also have significant effects on maternal metabolism.

Clinically, it is important to understand the mechanism behind estrogen production by the placenta because estrogen levels can be used to detect certain deficiencies in the fetoplacental unit. If, for example, the placenta is not functioning properly (as in diabetes), the estrogens are not produced in normal amounts. Periodic determination of estrogen levels, either in the urine or in the blood, can be clinically useful in assessing the progress of such affected pregnancies.

Effects on the Newborn. Maternal estrogen is transmitted to the fetus and produces very striking effects in the newborn. First, as the result of the action of this hormone, the breasts of both boy and girl babies may become markedly enlarged during the first few days of life and even secrete milk—the so-called witch's milk (see Chap. 29, Breast Engorgement). Second, estrogen causes hypertrophy of the endometrium of the female fetus as it does in an adult woman. When this hormone is suddenly withdrawn after birth, the endometrium breaks down and bleeding sometimes occurs. For this reason, perhaps one girl baby in every fifteen manifests a little spotting on the diaper during the first week of life. This is entirely normal and clears up by itself within a few days.

Fetal Circulation

As the placenta acts as the intermediary organ of transfer between mother and fetus, the fetal circulation differs from that required for extrauterine existence. The fetus receives oxygen through the placenta because the lungs do not function as organs of respiration in the uterus. To meet this situation, the fetal circulation contains certain special vessels ("bypasses" or "detours") that shunt the blood around the lungs, with only a small amount circulating through them for nutrition.

The oxygenated blood flows up the cord through the umbilical vein and passes into the inferior vena cava; on the way to the inferior vena cava, part of the oxygenated blood goes through the liver, but most of it passes through a special fetal structure, the *ductus venosus,* which connects the umbilical vein and the inferior vena cava. The liver is proportionately large in a newborn infant because it receives a considerable supply of freshly vitalized blood directly from the umbilical vein.

From the inferior vena cava, the current flows into the right auricle and goes directly on to the left auricle through a special fetal structure, the *foramen ovale.* It then flows into the left ventricle and out through the aorta. The blood that circulates up the arms and the head returns through the superior vena cava to the right auricle again, but instead of passing through the foramen ovale as before, the current is deflected downward into the right ventricle and out through the pulmonary arteries. Part of it goes to the lungs (for purposes of nutrition only), but most of it goes into the aorta through the *ductus arteriosus*.

The blood in the aorta, with the exception of that which goes to the head and the upper extremities (this blood has been accounted for), passes downward to supply the trunk and the lower extremities (Fig. 11-9). Most of this blood finds its way through the internal iliac, or hypogastric arteries, and back through the cord to the placenta, where it is again oxygenated, but a small amount passes back into the ascending vena cava to mingle with fresh blood from the umbilical vein and again makes the circuit of the entire body.

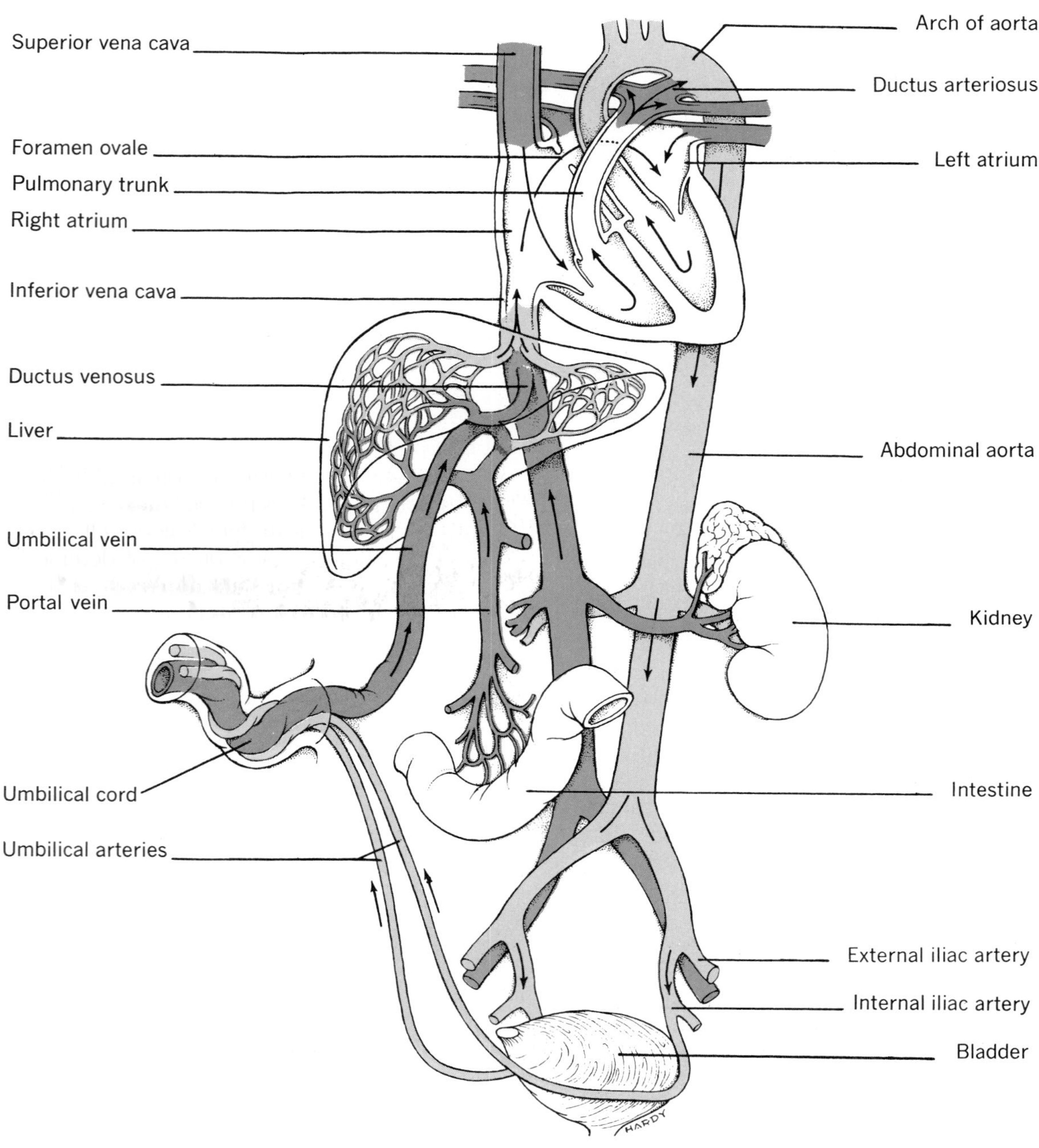

Figure 11-9.
Diagram of the fetal circulation shortly before birth. Course of blood is indicated by arrows.

Circulation Change at Birth

The fetal circulation is so arranged that the passage of blood to the placenta through the umbilical arteries and back through the umbilical vein is possible up to the time of birth, but it ceases entirely the moment the baby breathes and begins to take oxygen directly from its own lungs. During intrauterine life the circulation of blood through the lungs is for the nourishment of the lungs and not for the purpose of securing oxygen.

In order to understand, even in a general way, the course of the blood current and how it differs from the circulation after birth, it must be remembered that in infants after birth, as in the adult, the venous blood passes from the two venae cavae into the right auricle of the heart, then to the right ventricle and through the pulmonary arteries to the lungs, where it gives up its waste products and takes up a fresh supply of oxygen. After oxygenation, the arterial blood flows from the lungs, through the pulmonary veins to the left auricle, then to the left ventricle and out through the aorta, to be distributed through the capillaries to all parts of the body and eventually collected, as venous blood, in the venae cavae and discharged again into the right auricle.

Circulation Path After Birth

As soon as the baby is born and breathes, the lungs begin to function and the placental circulation ceases. This change not only alters the character of the blood in many vessels, but it also makes many of these vessels useless. The umbilical arteries within the baby's body become filled with clotted blood and are ultimately converted into fibrous cords, and after occlusion of the vessel, the umbilical vein within the body becomes the round ligament of the liver. After the umbilical cord is tied and separated, the large amount of blood returned to the heart and the lungs, which are now functioning, causes equal pressure in both of the auricles. This pressure causes the foramen ovale to close. The foramen ovale remains closed and eventually disappears, and the ductus arteriosus and the ductus venosus finally shrivel up and are converted into fibrous cords or ligaments in the course of two or three months. The instantaneous closure of the foramen ovale changes the entire course of the blood current and converts the fetal circulation into the adult type. The changes in the fetal circulation after birth are shown in Table 11-2.

Periods of Development

For the purposes of classification, human life has been arbitrarily divided into periods.

The *period of the ovum* extends from fertilization through the first two weeks of prenatal life. (The term ovum is also used to denote the female germ cell prior to fertilization). The successive phases of development during this interval include formation of the morula and blastocyst and implantation.

Table 11-2
Changes in Fetal Circulation After Birth

Structure	Before Birth	After Birth
Umbilical vein	Brings arterial blood to liver and heart	Obliterated; becomes the round ligament of liver
Umbilical arteries	Brings arteriovenous blood to the placenta	Obliterated; become vesical ligaments on anterior abdominal wall
Ductus venosus	Shunts arterial blood into inferior vena cava	Obliterated; becomes ligamentum venosum
Ductus arteriosus	Shunts arterial and some venous blood from the pulmonary artery to the aorta	Obliterated; becomes ligamentum arteriosum
Foramen ovale	Connects right and left auricles (atria)	Obliterated usually; at times open
Lungs	Contain no air and very little blood	Filled with air and well supplied with blood
Pulmonary arteries	Bring little blood to lungs	Bring much blood to lungs
Aorta	Receives blood from both ventricles	Receives blood only from left ventricle
Inferior vena cava	Brings venous blood from body and arterial blood from placenta	Brings venous blood only to right auricle

Williams JF: Anatomy and Physiology, 7th ed. Philadelphia, WB Saunders

The *period of the embryo* extends from the second week to the fifth week of gestation, during which time the various organs are developed and a definite form is assumed. The *period of the fetus* extends from after the fifth week to the time of birth. The *period of the newborn (neonatal)* extends from birth to the close of the first month of postnatal life. The *period of infancy* extends from the close of the first month to the close of the second year of life.

The *period of childhood* extends from the close of the second year to about the fourteenth year in females and to about the sixteenth year in males. Puberty ends the period of chidhood.

The *period of adolescènce* extends from puberty to the last years of the second decade (late teens) in females and to the first years of the third decade (early 20s) in males.

The *period of maturity* extends from the end of the adolescent period to old age.

Suggested Reading

Gruenwald P: The Placenta. Baltimore, University Park Press, 1975

Klopper A, Genazzani A, Crosignari PG (eds): The Human Placenta. Serono Symposium No. 35, New York, Academic Press, 1980

Moore KL: The Developing Human. Philadelphia, WB Saunders, 1973

Torpin R: The Human Placenta: Its Shape, Form, Origin and Development. Springfield, IL, Charles C Thomas, 1969

Study Aids for Unit II: Biophysical Aspects of Human Reproduction

Conference Material

1. Discuss the internal and external parts of the clitoral system in women and the penile system in men, and their significance in the sexual response cycle. Include their role in initiating sexual arousal, in developing vasocongestion, and in producing orgasm in the discussion. Describe how the male and female systems are homologues of each other, and their homologous origins in embryonic development. Include a discussion of the critical factors for male and female embryologic sexual differentiation.

2. Describe the various patterns of male and female sexual response cycles according to the four-stage model of Masters and Johnson. What are the main differences between the male and female patterns? What are the main similarities? What anatomic and physiologic explanations can you find for the differences in male and female patterns?

Multiple Choice

Read through the entire question and place your answer on the line to the right.

1. A patient who was in the latter part of her pregnancy reported to the nurse that she was suffering from backache and wanted to know the cause. What is the most likely reason that the nurse could give her?
   A. The larger size of the fetus tires her more easily.
   B. Increased mobility of joints throws greater weight on surrounding muscles.
   C. She must have some abnormality in pelvic structures.
   D. The descent of the presenting part into the pelvic cavity prior to labor increases pressure against the sacrum. ____

2. In each of the following write the term or the phrase by which the pelvic measurement described is commonly called.
   A. From the lower margin of the symphysis pubis to the sacral promontory ____
   B. The posterior portion of the symphysis pubis to the promontory of the sacrum ____
   C. From the inner aspects of the ischial tuberosities ____

3. By using the letter of the measurements described in question 2 indicate the following:
   A. The one which must be estimated rather than measured directly ____
   B. The one which represents the most important measurement ____
   C. The one which represents a transverse diameter ____

4. A patient's chart shows pelvic measurements of 10.5 cm for the diagonal conjugate and 9 cm for the true conjugate; therefore, the nurse caring for the patient in the labor room should anticipate that the patient might have which of the following:
   A. An easy, rapid delivery
   B. A labor and delivery of reasonable duration
   C. A protracted labor with difficult delivery ____

Multiple Choice
(continued)

5. To give adequate care to the patient during and after delivery, the nurse should fully understand the structure of the uterus. Which of the following are true of the uterus?

A. Its muscular tissue is
  1. Chiefly striated
  2. Chiefly nonstriated
  3. Entirely striated
  4. Entirely nonstriated ____

B. Its muscle fibers are arranged to run
  1. Circularly
  2. Longitudinally
  3. In all directions
  4. In three layers, the inner and the outer circularly, the other longitudinally ____

C. Its blood is supplied directly from
  1. Ovarian and uterine arteries
  2. Abdominal aorta and uterine arteries
  3. Internal iliac and ovarian arteries
  4. Internal iliac and uterine arteries ____

D. Normally, the uterus is
  1. Attached anteriorly to the bladder wall
  2. Suspended and freely movable in the pelvic cavity
  3. Suspended between the bladder and the rectum
  4. Attached posteriorly to the anterior wall of the sacrum ____

6. The perineum lies between the vagina and the rectum. This structure has

A. A single, strong elastic muscle
B. A strong elastic tendon
C. A tendon to which muscles are attached
D. Two strong muscles, the anal and the transverse perineal ____

7. A patient with small breasts in her first pregnancy is worried about her ability to feed her baby.

A. The nurse could respond correctly to the patient by telling her that:
  1. She probably would be unable to feed her baby
  2. The size of the breasts does not influence the amount of lactation possible
  3. Mothers with small breasts usually have less difficulty feeding their babies
  4. Her baby would be fed better by means of a formula ____

B. The structure most directly involved in milk production is
  1. Papillae
  2. Glands of Montgomery
  3. Acini cells
  4. Areola
  5. Lactiferous ducts ____

8. The structures in the testes that are responsible for spermatogenesis are
   A. The Sertoli cells
   B. The seminiferous tubules
   C. The interstitial cells of Leydig
   D. The tunica albuginea ____

9. Seminal plasma is made up of secretions derived from
   A. The seminal vesicles
   B. The prostate gland
   C. The bulbourethral glands
   D. All of the above ____

10. The time sequence of changes that occur at puberty in the female are:
   A. Appearance of axillary and pubic hair, breast development, and menarche
   B. Menarche, breast development, and appearance of axillary and pubic hair
   C. Breast development, menarche, and appearance of axillary and pubic hair
   D. Breast development, appearance of axillary and pubic hair, and menarche ____

11. The interval between ovulation and menstruation is normally:
   A. Extremely variable
   B. 14 ± 2 days
   C. 28 ± 2 days
   D. 10 ± 2 days

12. What are the ovarian hormones produced by the graafian follicle and the cells of the corpus luteum?
   A. Progesterone and gonadotropin
   B. Estrogen and progesterone
   C. Gonadotropin and FSH
   D. FSH and estrogen ____

13. The release of gonadotropins from the pituitary gland is directly regulated by
   A. GNRH
   B. HGH
   C. Insulin
   D. Androgens ____

14. The post ovulatory increase in basal body temperature is brought about by:
   A. Gonadotropins
   B. Estrogen
   C. Progesterone
   D. GNRH ____

Multiple Choice
(continued)

15. Spermatozoa are delivered into the lumen of the seminiferous tubules by:
A. Action of the Sertoli cells
B. Their own motility
C. Contraction of Leydig cells
D. Effect of testosterone ____

16. A young mother-to-be told a nurse that she was sure that she would have a boy because her husband was such a strong, physically well-developed man. The nurse could respond correctly by saying:
A. "It is the female cell which determines the sex of the child."
B. "It is unlikely because there are more girls born than boys."
C. "Physical strength does not influence the sex of the child."
D. "You are probably right." ____

17. Fertilization normally occurs in
A. The uterus
B. The ovarian follicle
C. The fallopian tube
D. The cervix ____

18. Following fertilization the ovum is
A. Transported into the uterus immediately
B. Retained in the tube for three days and then transferred to the uterus
C. Retained at the uterotubal junction for six days
D. Transferred to the abdominal cavity ____

19. Human chorionic gonadotropin (hCG) is produced by
A. The uterus
B. The ovarian follicle
C. The trophoblastic cells of the embryo
D. The uterine decidua ____

20. A patient expelled a 16-cm fetus prematurely. What would be the approximate age of the fetus?
A. 2 months
B. 3 months
C. 4 months
D. 5 months ____

21. Although the exact date of delivery cannot be predetermined, if a pregnant woman's last menstrual period began on September 10, the estimated due date would be nearest:
A. May 6
B. May 10
C. June 10
D. June 17 ____

22. The only direct connection between the fetus and any other structure is through the umbilical cord. The umbilical cord contains which of these important structures?
A. Umbilical artery
B. Umbilical arteries
C. Umbilical vein
D. Umbilical veins
E. Umbilical nerves
F. Umbilical lymphatic duct
G. Wharton's jelly
Select the number corresponding to the correct letters.
1. A, D, and F
2. B, C, and G
3. C, E, and G
4. All of the above ____

23. The placenta is formed by the union of
A. The chorion frondosum and the decidua basalis
B. The chorion laeve and the decidua capsularis
C. The amnion and the chorionic cavity
D. The decidua basalis and the chorion laeve ____

24. During a uterine contraction the blood flow to the uteroplacental circulation is
A. Unchanged
B. Increased
C. Decreased ____

25. When genetic, gonadal, and hormonal components of sexuality are incongruent with behavioral sex and sexual partner preference, yet the person has appropriate gender identity, the condition is
A. Transvestism
B. Homosexuality
C. Transsexualism ____

26. Core gender identity has been established by age
A. 1½ years
B. 2½ years
C. 3½ years
D. 4½ years ____

27. Sexual partner preference is believed influenced by all but which of the following
A. Early sexual experiences
B. Prenatal hormonal environment
C. Early mother-infant interactions
D. Values assigned to social sex roles ____

Multiple Choice
(continued)

28. Stimuli leading to sexual arousal which include thoughts, fantasies, sights, or sounds are classified as
   A. Reflexogenic stimuli
   B. Psychogenic stimuli ____

29. Which branch of the nervous system is most immediately responsible for the sexual responses of erection in the man and vaginal lubrication in the woman?
   A. Parasympathetic nervous system
   B. Sympathetic nervous system ____

30. Which biochemical substance triggers orgasm?
   A. Noradrenaline
   B. Acetylcholine
   C. Androgen
   D. Adrenaline ____

31. Which psychological mediator of sexual response invokes erotic images and fantasies?
   A. Informational responses
   B. Emotional reactions
   C. Imaginative capacity
   D. Attention ____

32. In order for an embryo to differentiate as male, what hormonal event must occur?
   A. Decrease in maternal estrogen secretion
   B. Secretion of androgen by the fetal gonad
   C. Secretion of estrogen by the fetal gonad
   D. Increase in maternal androgen secretion ____

33. The cryptic structures of the clitoris include
   A. Glans
   B. Shaft
   C. Crura
   D. Vestibular bulbs

   Select the number corresponding to the correct letters.
   1. A and B
   2. B and C
   3. C and D
   4. A and C
   5. B and D ____

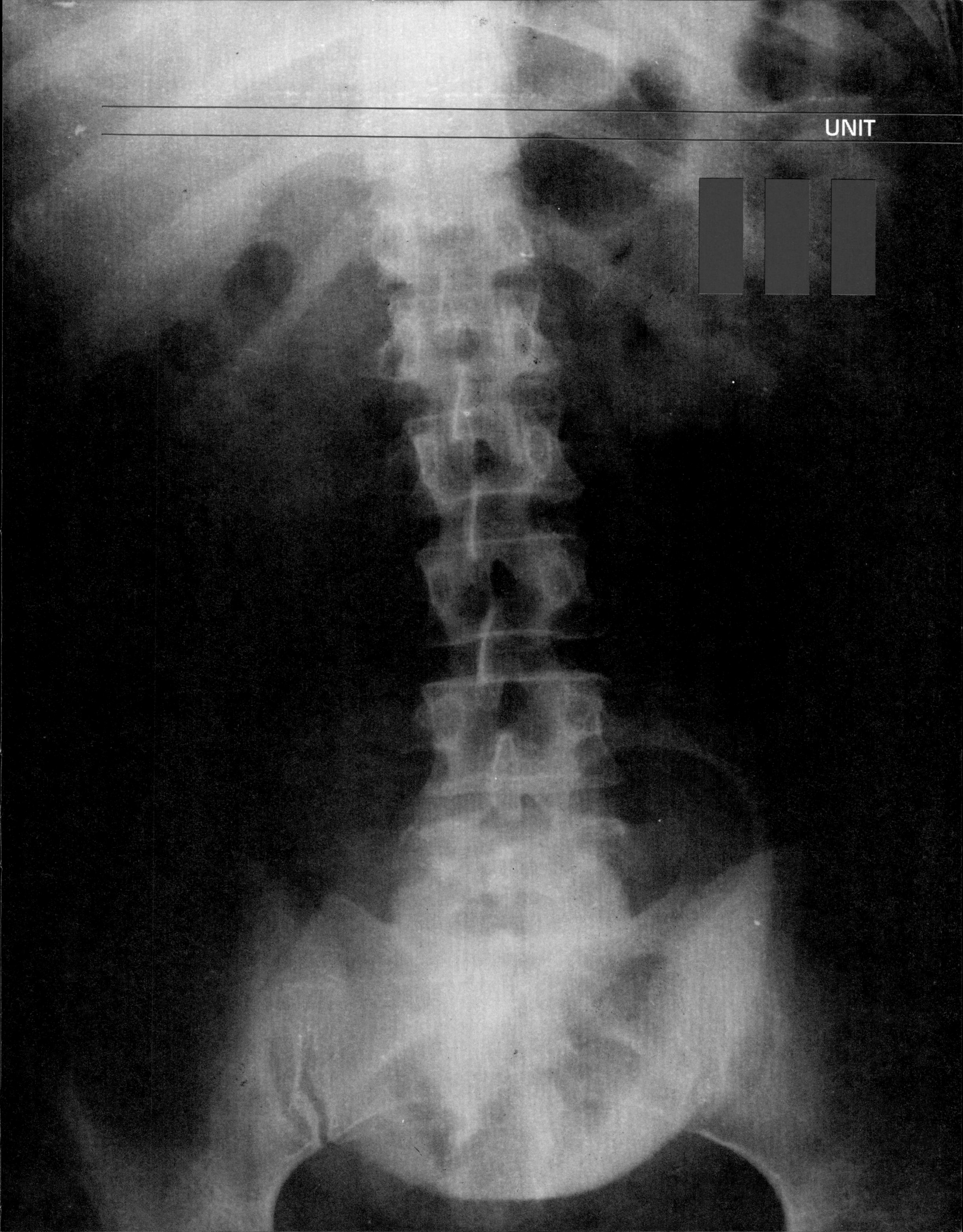
UNIT

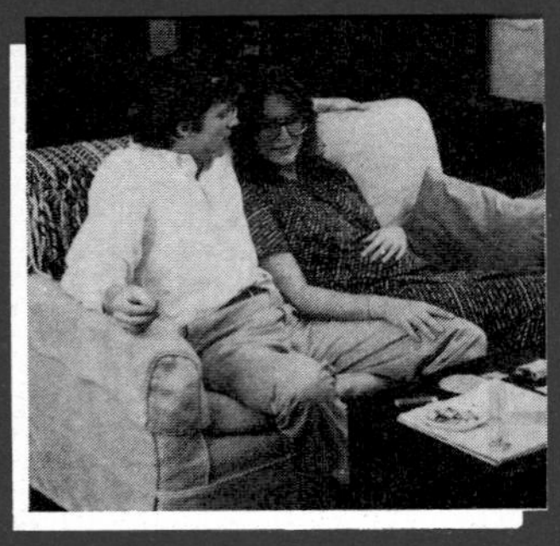

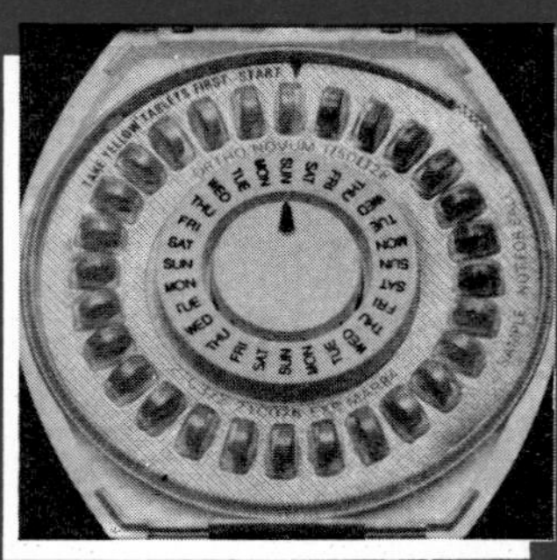

Reproduction Control and Sexuality: Assessment and Management

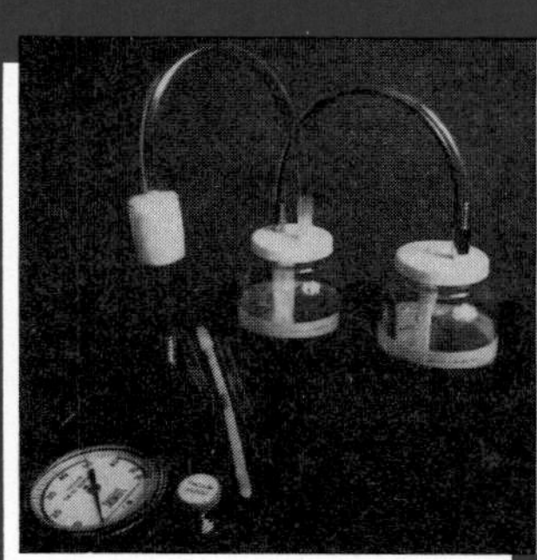

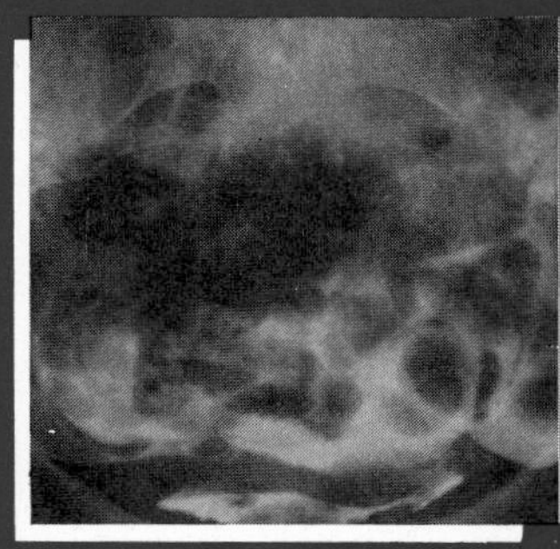

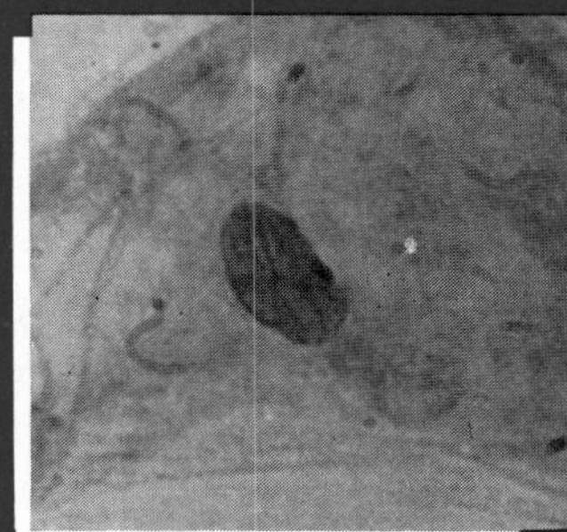

CHAPTER

12

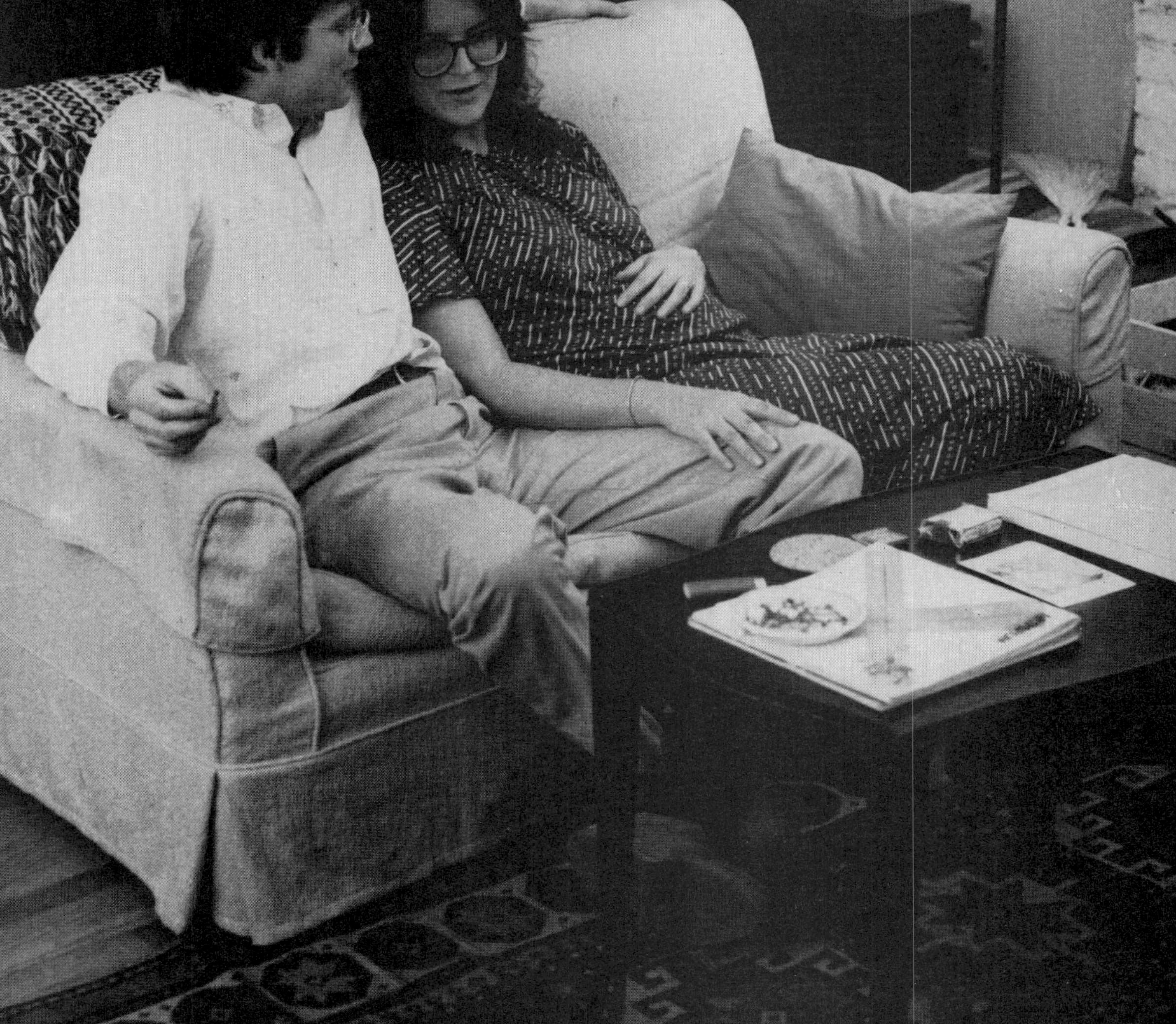

CHAPTER 12

Common Concerns Related to Sexuality

Most nurses believe they have a responsibility in promoting sexual health. The integration of sexuality into the practice of nursing, assessment of sexual health and concerns of patients, and nursing intervention to promote health or alleviate problems are all part of this nursing responsibility. Assembling a data base by taking a sexual history has become integrated into the nursing role.

The area of human sexuality has become a specialty within the health care field. Professionals from various disciplines have undergone preparation with all degrees of formality to become equipped to handle sexual problems. As more professionals participate in sex therapy, more research and empirical data are generated to expand the knowledge of sexuality. Across the country "institutes of human sexuality" are being formed by groups interested in this new branch of health care. They offer services ranging from sex education to intensive therapy. Groups and individuals in private practice or associated with health care institutions are providing many other opportunities for diagnosis and treatment of sexual problems. Many resources are available with prepared specialists, although their therapeutic approaches often vary significantly.

Although the field of sexual therapy has become a sophisticated and complex specialty in certain ways, there are actually different levels of practice within the field related to the nature of sexual problems. Because of changing public attitudes toward sex and a great increase in openness about sexuality in many channels of public communication and media, there is a greater expectation on the part of patients that health professionals will respond to sexual problems and concerns.

The nurse is an ideal member of the health-care team to assume responsibility for counseling patients about sexuality because of a background in the social, behavioral, and physical sciences as well as knowledge of counseling techniques. A comprehensive view of nursing care requires nurses to understand the relationship of sexuality to the particular patient's health needs or illness and the context of current living situations and sexual-affectional relationships in order to access and utilize support systems. Patients need adequate sex information whether they are coping with an illness or striving to attain a higher level of health. The importance of a positive integration of one's sexuality has been repeatedly demonstrated.

> Few authorities in human behavior would deny that sexual adjustment is prerequisite to an individual's maturation and successful adaptation to his environment. Indeed, history has demonstrated that the mental health of whole nations has been markedly influenced by the sexual attitudes

Developing Comfort With Sexuality

The nurse must be personally comfortable with the topic of sexuality to counsel effectively. Some approaches to developing this comfort include the following:

Information and Knowledge

Read books and articles.
View educational films.
Attend workshops.
Enroll in classes.
Join discussion groups.
Read popular books (source of the public's information).

Attitudes and Values

Join discussion groups (as part of classes, workshops, community activities) that cover topics such as human sexuality or values clarification.
Take self-administered questionnaires, inventories, or tests related to sexual values and attitudes found in textbooks and journals.*

*Examples of these are found in each issue of the journal Medical Aspects of Human Sexuality, and appendices of textbooks such as "Inventory for Self-Evaluation", Appendix A, in Nass GD, Libby RW, and Fisher MP: Sexual Choices: An Introduction to Human Sexuality. Monterey, CA, Wadsworth Health Sciences Division, 1981 and behavior of their citizenry—young and old, male and female alike. Scientific investigations and clinical observations have confirmed the premise that sexual adjustment is positively correlated with well-timed, ongoing, accurate sex education presented in a wholesome, guilt-free manner.[1]

The Maternity Nurse as Sexual Counselor

The care of the reproductive family is concerned with events intimately associated with sexual functioning and expression. This special area of nursing practice embraces a wide spectrum within the sexual-affectional system, although older concepts of "maternity care" viewed the processes largely in asexual terms. Pregnancy is a time of unusual sensuousness, with increased feelings of masculine and feminine potency, voluptuous sexual expression in fantasy and behavior, and profound primitive satisfactions in bearing, nursing, and nurturing children. Nurses have often sensed that the essence of the childbearing experience involves the mystery of life, as it springs forth in a sexual expression of creativity. Sexuality is undeniably an integral part of maternity nursing, and the nurse's view must expand to recognize that sexuality is more than reproduction; self-concept, roles, and interpersonal relations are modes of expressing sexuality in all phases of childbearing and parenting.

Maternity nurses can easily provide sexual counseling as they work in prenatal, postnatal, and family planning clinics; physician's offices; hospital maternity units, and public health agencies. Nurses frequently conduct classes for expectant parents and classes in parenting and contraception. In any of these areas, concerns related to sexuality are likely to surface if the atmosphere is comfortable and accepting. The nurse who is prepared to deal with both information and feelings about sex has much opportunity to assist patients in a wide variety of settings.

The Nurse's Comfort with Sexuality

Although it is always important for the nurse to be aware of his or her own feelings and attitudes toward a particular area of practice, human sexuality requires a level of self-understanding beyond that of most other areas. Nurses bring their personal experiences, values, and attitudes to the professional relationship, which may either facilitate or obstruct the process of caring for patients with sexual concerns and problems. A nurse who plans to provide sexual counseling must become comfortable with sexuality both generally and personally.

The first step in becoming comfortable with sexuality involves gathering information through reading books and articles, viewing films, and attending workshops and symposia. It is a good idea to read popular as well as professional books, because this is where the public gets its information. Knowing the facts about sex enables the nurse to provide accurate information, teach with authority, and refute commonly held myths and misconceptions.

Examination and reexamination of personal attitudes is an ongoing part of becoming comfortable with sexuality. The nurse must identify prejudices and blind spots as well as positive and healthy feelings about different sexual practices. Personal definitions of normal and acceptable sexual expression must be carefully identified, and the extent to which these may affect the ability to assist patients in these areas assessed.[2]

The nurse–patient encounter is a constant feedback loop, and how the nurse is perceived by the patient when sexual matters come up is an important part of the nurse's effectiveness. Attitudes are communicated in verbal and nonverbal ways and people are always reading each other's subtle behavioral cues and responding accordingly. The nurse who is aware of her or his own attitudes and feelings, and is comfortable with sexuality, will be less likely to react with shock, ambivalence, or discomfort when patients reveal unusual or unexpected sexual information. The ability to be accepting and understanding and to avoid passing judgment on others' sexual behaviors or concerns enables the nurse to provide more effective care.

A Framework for Sexual Counseling

Sexual counseling is basically talking to people about their sex-related problems and concerns. This can occur at various levels of depth and complexity and may involve problems of differing severity and character. The role of the maternity nurse in providing sexual counseling is determined by the individual nurse's background and expertise, as well as the origin and severity of the sexual problem of the patient. Sexual problems range from those involving gender identity, such as hermaphroditism and transsexualism, to those resulting from misinformation, confusion about the normal sexual response cycle, and minor sexual dysfunctions. The different levels of sexual problems can be approached by dividing them into three (often overlapping) categories—problems of knowledge, relationship, and attitudes.

Problems of Knowledge

Problems of knowledge are the most common and simple types of sexual problems, and usually arise out of misinformation or ignorance. A couple may fail to appreciate the erotic significance of the clitoris, be unaware of differing tempos of sexual arousal, have the idea that sex during pregnancy might injure or mark the baby, think that oral sex indicates latent homosexuality, expect the woman's sex drive to be decreased during pregnancy and be worried when it increases, and so forth. Lack of knowledge about changes in sexual drive and eroticism during pregnancy, which often happen to both partners, can be a cause of misunderstanding and conflict.

Fears created by minor unpleasant symptoms may lead to avoidance of sex when there is no understanding of the physiology or of what can be done about them. For the woman, the common symptom of painful intercourse during pregnancy can be related to a number of factors—vaginitis causing perineal or vulval irritation, insufficient vaginal lubrication due to inadequate foreplay, normal uterine contractions during orgasm setting off Braxton Hicks contractions, or increased pelvic pressure due to the presenting part deep in the pelvis. These can be alleviated with proper medical treatment, explanation of physiological causes of the pain, and teaching of techniques to heighten arousal or increase comfort. In this way, a potential stressor to the relationship and the couple's adaptation to pregnancy can be removed.

Couples need specific information about practical matters regarding sex and pregnancy. For instance, there is no reason in the absence of complications to avoid sex during late pregnancy or postpartum once lochia has ceased. The couple's own comfort and desires are their best guide when there is no physical pathology. However, understanding the vagaries of sexual drive during this time could prevent development of conflicts which might set up negative patterns as the couple tries to cope with the many demands of impending or new parenthood.

Nurses working with adolescents and young adults, as in family planning clinics, will find innumerable problems of knowledge related to sexuality. This is a setting in which provision of information can have an enormous impact on developing sexual practices and adjustments and can prevent many potential future problems involving unwanted pregnancy and sexual dysfunctions. Problems of knowledge related to sexuality are clearly within the scope of maternity nursing practice, and with the addition of specific factual content and a sense of comfort with sexuality to the nurse's repertory, this kind of sexual counseling can be readily carried out.

Problems of Relationship

A second level of sexual problems involves relationships between partners, and these may or may not fall within the scope of maternity nursing practice. This would depend largely on the nature of the given problem and the individual nurse's counseling skills. Communication problems between the partners are the most common types of relationship problems. The sending and receiving of messages between people is a highly complex symbolic process, with many variations of style and receptivity. Both sender and recipient must be attuned and ready for clear communication to take place; consequently, there are often garbled messages and lack of communication.

Good communication regarding sexual needs and preferences is even more difficult than in most interpersonal situations. Some people find it hard to talk about their own sexual feelings or to accept criticism or suggestions regarding sexual performance. Communication concerning sexual practices which one partner may dislike but is embarrassed to discuss or may desire but is unable to ask for is often faulty. Open and candid discussion of sexual preferences between partners can often dramatically improve satisfaction; but many fears about propriety, hurting the other's feelings, not knowing how to say it, or being embarrassed prevent this communication from occurring.

A first step, and one that the maternity nurse could take in dealing with common sexual problems such as painful intercourse, lack of interest in sex, early ejaculation, and nonorgasm, is to encourage the couple to talk with each other about what they like and do not like in sex. If they can settle on practices which are comfortable and enjoyable to both of them, often the problem will be resolved.

However, many other factors complicate communication. The bedroom as a battlefield and sex with a hidden agenda are familiar syndromes to those involved in marital counseling. Perceptions of male and female roles may hamper communication *(e.g.,* the notion that the woman is there to serve the man sexually and that her enjoyment of sex is secondary and her sexual needs do not deserve much attention.) Some couples may be in a struggle for power, attempting to frustrate the other sexually or doling out sex as a reward for compliance. Anger over real or imagined wrongs may interfere with giving oneself freely to the sexual experience or may be expressed in a desire to hurt the other partner, either mentally or physically.

Such situations create barriers to clear communication about sexual needs and preferences. They represent problems in the couple's relationship that must be worked out before the sexual problem itself can be resolved. If the maternity nurse is skilled in

Framework for Sexual Counseling

	Knowledge Problems	Relationship Problems	Attitudinal Problems
Occurrence	Most common Most simple	Quite common Intermediate complexity	Quite common Most complex
Origins	Misinformation Ignorance	Communication patterns Goals or intent in relationships and interactions	Internalized beliefs and values Psychological conflicts
Typical Problems	Concern over normalcy of sexual practices Labeling activities as abnormal or dangerous Worry over changes in sexual response patterns (*i.e.*,during pregnancy) Avoidance of certain practices or sexual activity under different circumstances (*i.e.*, in late pregnancy) Fears about effects of birth control Ineffective arousal owing to lack of proper stimulation Unsatisfying sex owing to mis-timing of arousal or orgasm	Painful intercourse Lack of interest in sex Early ejaculation Nonorgasm in women Ineffective arousal Unsatisfying sex	Impotence Premature ejaculation Nonorgasm in women Vaginismus Lack of arousal
Type of Counseling	Information, clarification Reassurance of normalcy Discussion of feelings	Encourage discussion between partners Information, clarification Family or marital counseling Sex therapy	Sex therapy Psychotherapy
Level of Nurse's Involvement	Major responsibility Provide entire counseling	Initial identification and discussion; marital or family therapy if nurse is a trained therapist	Initial identification Must be trained sex therapist or psychologist to undertake therapy

family or marital counseling, then she or he is able to deal with these relationship problems. Because sexual difficulties are part of the symptomatology, it is frequently necessary for the counselor to have an understanding of sexual physiology and to be familiar with basic sex therapy techniques in order to provide effective care.

Problems of Attitudes

Attitudes toward sexuality and the sexual self are established through internalized beliefs and values, originating from earliest childhood and often rooted in the unconscious levels of the psyche. This represents the third and most complex level of sexual problems. Arising from the individual's psychological conflicts, the more common of these sexual problems include impotence, premature ejaculation, nonorgasm, vaginismus, and lack of arousal. The underlying mechanism in the great majority of these sexual dysfunctions is fear. Whether this fear has its origins in sociocultural values, religious inhibitions and guilt, negative early experiences, familial patterns of dominance and discipline, or temporary functional failures of performance, it is the catalyst which sets into motion the psychodynamics that produce the sexual problem. This fear of inadequacy in sexual performance is the most significant deterrent to effective sexual functioning because it completely distracts the individual from her or his natural responsiveness by blocking reception of sexual stimuli. Both partners eventually become self-conscious, worrying about their own and each other's sexual performance. Crippling tensions can develop in the relationship as frustrations and dissatisfactions mount. Obviously, problems of attitudes and relationship often overlap. It is unlikely that the partner can remain uninvolved when a sexual problem occurs.

Numerous therapeutic approaches have been developed to help people with such sexual problems. These range from intensive residential sexual therapy to short-term behavior modification. Frequently a process of reeducation is used to modify negative attitudes and counteract inhibitive beliefs. These approaches combined with teaching effective techniques for sexual stimulation have a reasonably good success rate.

When deep anxieties, unresolved guilt or conflict, or other psychopathology are present, the person usually receives some kind of psychotherapy aimed at the specific problem. Many sex therapists prefer not to delve into old conflicts, but focus on changing the problematic behavior with a variety of sexual techniques. Whatever the cause, they reason, removal of the symptom will bring immediate relief and perhaps result in satisfactory long-term functioning without the need for extensive insight therapy.

Nurses have become involved in this type of sex therapy after undergoing additional education in human sexuality and training in specific techniques for treating sexual problems. This level of sexual counseling is specialty practice and is often provided by a team, using the cotherapist approach (one therapist of each sex) in an extensive program involving education, attitude change, setting a permissive environment for sexual experiencing, marital counseling or psychotherapy, and application of appropriate techniques of sex therapy. The scope of maternity nursing practice usually does not include this kind of sexual therapy, unless the nurse has been specially trained and works in a setting that provides these services.

Approaches to Sexual Counseling

Sexual counseling fits well into the nursing process, and the same principles and approaches apply to this area of nursing care as apply to others. The assessment phase concerns gathering information about the patient's past and current experiences with sex, how sexual knowledge was obtained, key attitudes toward sexuality, and difficulties. The person's sexual self-concept, relationship with sexual partner(s), and health status of both partners are also explored in the history. From the assessment phase the nurse is able to form conclusions about the nature of sexual concerns or problems and to diagnose the problem. Identifying the problem is the basis for planning care or intervention.

Nursing intervention is directed at assisting the patient or couple to find methods of alleviating their sexual difficulties. Many approaches may be used in this process, including the nurse providing facts about the sexual response cycle and the ranges of normal sexual experiences, teaching techniques to heighten sexual arousal or delay orgasm, facilitating better communication between partners, or assisting the couple to find sources of in-depth sexual therapy or marital counseling through referral. When illness or physical problems are involved, consultation with a physician is often necessary. A wide range of resources can be used to deal with problems from economic relief to child care, as any of these may adversely affect sexual functioning.

Evaluation of the effectiveness of care is an essential component of the nursing process. This is accomplished through return visits in which progress is assessed. It is often necessary to alter approaches, try new approaches, or examine what factors are interfering with satisfactory resolution of the problem, which in itself is frequently therapeutic. Simple sexual problems may resolve surprisingly rapidly through the reassurance of accurate information and by altering the context in which sexual activity occurs. However, there may be many layers of difficulty, and dealing with an apparently simple problem may reveal more deep-seated conflicts that require specialty referral.

The Sexual History

A sexual history can be incorporated into the usual health history, such as the menstrual and contraceptive history, pregnancy history, and gynecologic history. It flows nicely when included in assessment of the reproductive system; in fact, it should be a standard part of data gathering regardless of setting or area of practice. In clinics dealing specifically with sexual problems, the sexual history will, of course, be more detailed and the center of focus. But, even in the absence of indications of sexual problems, the information gathered serves a number of purposes which enhance the nurse–patient relationship and provide a broader base for nursing care.

Taking a sexual history provides a base for identifying present or potential sexual problems, from which nursing intervention can be planned, either therapeutic or preventive. Additionally, gathering information about the couple's sexual experiences and attitudes demonstrates that the nurse is comfortable talking about sex. By taking the initiative in bringing up the subject, the nurse implicitly gives them permission to discuss sexual concerns. This legitimizes sexuality as an important component of health and an integral part of care for reproductive families and indicates that sexual counseling is an appropriate part of care they can expect to receive from health providers.[3]

Varying degrees of formality may be used in taking a sexual history, although it is generally best to have a flexible structure so the discussion can go in the direction the patient wants it to go. If forms are used, they should be relatively short and simple to keep writing at a minimum and allow the nurse to focus attention on the interaction. A sexual history should proceed from more general to specific areas, from common to unusual, from simple to complex. Conditional statements which assume a range of behavior should be used.

The sexual history generally begins with a conditional or universal statement about why sexual health is included in the health history. The nurse might use a statement such as the following:

> "Sexual health is an important part of people's lives. A person's physical health sometimes affects sexual experiences, and sexual health can have effects on physical well-being. As part of your health history, I'd like to ask some questions about your sexual health that will help me to better understand your health status."

It is important to have a quiet, private place to talk and enough time for discussion and patient education to conduct a history. Confidentiality must be stressed. The patient should be assured that all questions are optional, and the nurse must continually assess the patient's readiness as the history taking progresses. The acceptability of declining to answer must be clearly communicated. A short form for a sexual history of an adult is shown below.

The advanced sexual history is taken in conjunction with beginning of sex therapy. The guidelines for taking a sexual history prior to brief sex therapy for a specific sexual problem include the following:

1. Description of current problem
2. Onset and course of problem
   a. Onset (age, gradual or sudden, precipitating events, contingencies)
   b. Course (change over time—increase, decrease, or fluctuation in severity, frequency, or intensity; any functional relationships)
3. Patient's concept of cause and maintenance of problem

Taking an Adult Sexual History

As part of the general health history, these questions about sexual experiences and concerns can be included.

1. When you were a child, how were your questions about sex answered (where did your sexual information come from)?
2. When you were a teenager, how were your questions about sex answered?
3. How did you first find out about sexual intercourse (how babies are made)?
4. How would you describe your current sexual activity?
5. What, if anything, would you change about your current sexual activity?
6. At this time in your life, how important is a sexual relationship to you?
7. Do you have any concerns about birth control?
8. Do you have any health problems that, in your opinion, affect your sexual health or happiness?
9. Are you taking any medicines that, in your opinion, affect your sexual health or happiness?
10. Is there anything about these questions that you would like clarified or explained?

Mims FH, Swenson M: Sexuality: A Nursing Perspective. New York, McGraw-Hill, 1980

4. Past treatment and outcome
   a. Medical evaluation (specialty, date, form of treatment, results, medication taken)
   b. Professional help (type and results)
   c. Self-treatment (type and results)
5. Current expectancies and goals of treatment (concrete or ideal)[4]

Sexual History During Pregnancy

Sexual expression during pregnancy is influenced by the physical and emotional changes that happen at this time, as well as attitudes and beliefs about sex during pregnancy. Difficulties can arise as a result of myths, misconceptions, and a lack of understanding of the physiology and emotional dynamics of couples during pregnancy. Questions related to the sexual self-concept, relationship, physical status, and attitudes are included in the sexual history as shown below.

Even if there are no significant sexual problems associated with the pregnancy, most couples have many questions about sexual activities and their sexual responses during this time and appreciate the opportunity to discuss them. Openly discussing the many changes during pregnancy with implications for sexuality can prepare the couple for potential reactions and prevent the development of conflicts and tensions in their relationship stemming from misunderstandings of physiological changes and psychodynamics.

Common Sexual Problems During Pregnancy and Postpartum

There is a wide range of sexual problems which couples may encounter during pregnancy. Sexual problems of a dysfunctional nature include dyspareunia (painful intercourse), changing and conflicting sexual drives, and impotence.[3] These problems may be specifically related to the pregnancy and a function of the couple's psychobiological responses, or they may represent deeper-seated difficulties brought to the surface by the psychological effects of pregnancy. Other common problems include the avoidance of intercourse, breast feeding and erotic response, and lack of arousal or dyspareunia during the postpartal period.

Changes in Sex Drive

Alterations in the woman's level of sensuousness and sexual responsiveness are undoubtedly very widespread during pregnancy. These may be a problem for some couples and rather insignificant for others. In early pregnancy, some women experience a heightened sexuality, enjoy sex more, and seek it frequently. Their general level of sensuousness may increase, with heightened awareness and responsiveness to stimuli. Other women have decreased sex drive during the first two to three months of gestation, often

Sexual History During Pregnancy

As part of the prenatal health history, these questions about sexual experiences and concerns can be included. Most questions are appropriate for both partners, and a joint history-taking session is recommended.

1. How does the pregnancy make you feel? (asked of both)
2. How do you feel about changes in appearance and emotions?
3. How do you feel about each other's experience of the pregnancy?
4. What are your feelings about sex during pregnancy?
5. Has the pregnancy made many changes in your life and sexual relationship?
6. How do you think having a baby will change your life? How do you plan to manage these changes?
7. What have you heard about what you should or should not do sexually during pregnancy?
8. How do you feel physically? What medications do you take? Have you had any recent changes in your health?
9. Are there any concerns or worries about your sexual relationship during pregnancy or afterwards?

NC Nursing Care: Sexual Problems in Pregnancy and Postpartum

Assessment	Intervention	Evaluation
Changes in sex drive		
Stage of pregnancy and associated physical and emotional symptoms Level of couple's understanding of psychophysiology of pregnancy Attitudes toward sex in pregnancy Communication patterns	Reinforce accurate knowledge Teach correct information, clear misconceptions Reassure about normality of fluctuating sex drives Support clear communication	Concern decreased Couple feels comfortable with changing sex drives
Dyspareunia in pregnancy		
When this occurs, associated factors and symptoms Techniques of intercourse Adequacy of stimulation Perineal irritation due to vaginitis	Instruct on alternate techniques and positions Discuss arousal patterns Refer for treatment of vaginitis Teach normal variations of pregnancy (Braxton Hicks contractions with orgasm, backache)	Comfortable intercourse attained or acceptable alternative found
Avoidance of sex		
Reasons why sex is avoided (fears, misconceptions, told by physician) Difficulties this poses for the couple Attitudes toward sex in pregnancy	Correct misinformation and teach normal fetal-maternal development Inform when sex should be avoided and reasons why Discuss alternatives to intercourse	Fears and misinformation cleared, no longer avoid sex when not medically necessary Use acceptable alternatives if indicated

(Continued)

because of nausea, bloating, breast soreness, fatigue, and the many other physical changes women experience at this time. As pregnancy reaches its midpoint, heightened sexuality becomes more common. Many women report an increase in erotic feelings, more interest in sex, actively seeking sexual encounters with partners, and, not uncommonly, occurrence of first orgasms. The physiological changes of pregnancy, including increased pelvic vascularity and vasocongestion, contribute to this phenomenon.[5]

During the first trimester, the pregnant woman is very aware of her pelvis. The feeling of fullness, the sharpened sensations, and the round ligament twinges that may occur deep in the groin with sudden movement all give rise to some anxiety. Even though she may have had previous successful pregnancies and enjoyed sexual relations, she still tends to view these symptoms as possible threats to the pregnancy. If there is occasional (common) spotting, there is all the more reason for her to believe (however mis-

Assessment	Intervention	Evaluation
Impotence		
Extent of the problem, how often this occurs Level of couple's concern Level of understanding of the man's psychophysiology in pregnancy	Teach about normal male reactions and psychological processes Reassure normality of occasional inability to maintain or attain erection Refer to specialist if problem is extensive	Concern decreased Able to have intercourse often enough to satisfy both partners
Breast feeding and erotic response		
Loss of milk with arousal or orgasm Extent to which this poses problem to the couple Arousal or orgasm with nursing, level of concern about this	Advise regarding normality of milk loss Suggest wearing bra with absorbent pads if a problem Avoid pressure or stimulation of breasts Advise of normality of arousal during nursing Discuss discomfort and concern, and meaning of this to woman	Comfortable with methods to prevent milk loss from interfering with sex Able to accept erotic feelings and continue nursing
Postpartum dyspareunia and lack of arousal		
When symptoms occur, how often, associated with what factors Weeks or months postpartum and stage of involution Contraceptive use Techniques of arousal and intercourse Level of understanding of postpartal physiology Perineal irritation due to vaginitis	Teach normal postpartal physiology and hormonal effects Reinforce that arousal levels are often lower at this time Discuss techniques of arousal, advise lubricants if needed Refer for treatment of vaginitis Discuss approaches to managing home and family demands to provide the couple with private time	Concern decreased Comfortable with level of sexual arousal Comfortable intercourse attained or acceptable alternative found

takenly) that the pregnancy is in danger. Very different sensations from those usually experienced occur with deep penile penetration when the woman has an enlarging soft uterus, although the uterus is still entirely in the pelvis. This does not imply that intercourse should not take place or that thrusting or movement need be curtailed. However, it does have implications for the woman's immersing herself in the pleasures of sexual stimulation, as she may be preoccupied with these other thoughts and sensations. Hence, she may not be orgasmic on all occasions or as often as is usual for her. This preoccupation may also give rise to unpredictableness in her general sexual desire. If there appear to be large changes from what is usual, concern may be generated in both partners. It is important for them to understand that the time of pregnancy can be one of the most anxiety-free, spontaneous sexual interludes of a couple's life. They can be counseled that intercourse poses no threat to pregnancy under normal circumstances. If they have been reasonably comfortable with their sexuality before the pregnancy, and there are no unusual problems, there is no reason to anticipate that their sexual activity need be curtailed.

If there are times when intercourse is not the desired sexual mode, there need be no limitation of any of the other variations of sexual stimulation and orgasmic release for either the man or the woman. Sexual techniques may need modification because of increased sensitivity of the breasts and genitals. As the secretions increase and change in character, there may be an accompanying odor which is not unpleasant if standards of hygiene are maintained daily. Candida vaginal infections which are common to pregnancy can cause irritation and odor. The physician will prescribe treatment as needed and the nurse can be helpful in eliciting the needed information about the existence of such problems.

In the second trimester, early in the fourth month, the uterus enlarges rather rapidly and becomes an abdominal organ rather than a pelvic organ. The expectant mother has usually adapted to increased pelvic awareness and is comfortable with intercourse. However, with the rapidly enlarging abdomen, new concerns are engendered regarding crushing the fetus. While there is no danger that this will happen, such concern is very real to both partners. The fetus is very well protected by the uterus and the abdominal wall, but the enlarging uterus can get in the way about the fifth month if the partners assume face to face, prone and supine positions for intercourse. Hence, modifications in positioning may be needed. Since the uterus is not pressing down in the vagina, there is not the feeling of hitting an immovable object with penetration.

Vaginal bleeding during the second trimester is very unusual. Even abortions and premature deliveries during this period are not generally preceded by bleeding, but by cramping and a gush of amniotic fluid. Stress incontinence of urine (losing urine with coughing, sneezing, or orgasm) may occur because the uterus is pressing on the bladder even though it is out of the pelvis. This incontinence is sometimes confused with loss of amniotic fluid and can be frightening during intercourse.

Intercourse using the side position may be preferred as the uterus enlarges. From a purely mechanical point of view, it is necessarily gentle. As the uterus grows larger, the expectant mother is usually much more comfortable lying on her side, with her uterus supported by a pillow (Fig. 12-1). If she is on her back for any length of time, with the enlarged uterus pressing on the abdominal aorta and the vena cava, there may be problems with hypotension and lightheadedness. Using a pillow under the hips during intercourse can be helpful in avoiding hypotension.

It is well to remember that sexual activity does not have to include intercourse per se, and often the female genitalia are so sensitive that the woman is not interested in intercourse and many prefer alternate practices or caressing.

As the woman's abdomen increases in size, giving evidence of the pregnancy, the couple may respond with feelings of shame or pride. For some women, the change in body image is an unwelcome development, making them feel unattractive; others take pleasure in this evidence of the growing fetus and feel a sense of heightened potency. These feelings also affect sexual response. Men react to the woman's changing shape too; some feel that their partner is more beautiful and sexy, others are turned off by the perceived distortion of the woman's body. Such feelings have a significant

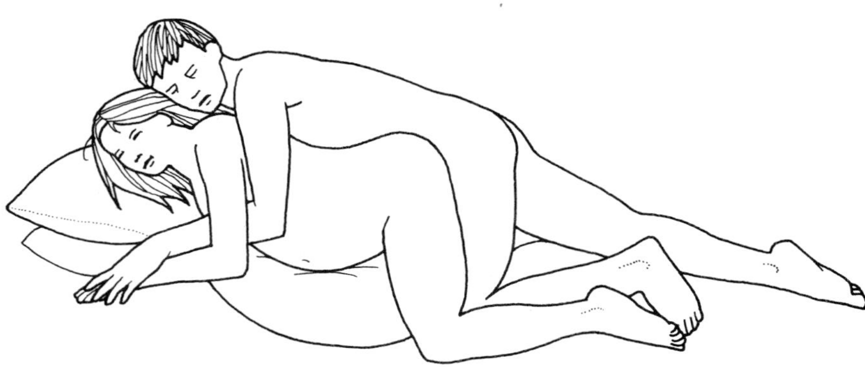

Figure 12-1.
Intercourse using the side position, supporting the uterus with a pillow, is often preferred in later pregnancy. It is gentle and avoids pressure on the enlarged uterus.

impact upon the man's sexual responsiveness, and naturally upon the woman's response to him. The woman's emotional lability and fluctuating sexual drives are often confusing for both the expectant father and mother. Fathers undergo psychological processes in pregnancy resembling those of the mother and may have symptoms and alternating periods of emotional stability and well-being and times of anxiety, unexplained fears, and compulsions.[6]

Communication between the expectant parents is very important if they are to understand their own and each other's responses to this time of emotional change and uncertainty. There is a tendency for women to withdraw as they become preoccupied with their physical and emotional changes and the psychological tasks related to incorporating and differentiating the baby, as well as preparations for motherhood. The father may at times feel excluded and seek other sources of understanding, support, and companionship.

Dyspareunia During Pregnancy

Painful intercourse during pregnancy can be caused by a number of things. Pressure on the pregnant abdomen may cause a generalized discomfort. Deep penile thrusting may be painful when there is pelvic congestion, when the presenting part is deep in the pelvis, or when certain positions are assumed that exaggerate pressure. Although vaginal secretions are increased during pregnancy, in some instances there may be a relative lack of lubrication due to inadequate stimulation, which leads to discomfort with intercourse. Irritation of the perineum or introitus, secondary to vaginitis, causes burning or pain on penetration and during intercourse. Cramps and backache may occur following coitus due to increased vasocongestion of sexual arousal combined with that of pregnancy. Orgasm may initiate Braxton Hicks contractions, which may continue and cause considerable pain. Aching postcoital pain may result from lack of orgasm to assist removal of the pelvic congestion associated with plateau levels of sexual arousal. If the woman experiences conflicts about having intercourse while pregnant, there may be a psychological overlay with the dyspareunia.

Avoidance of Sex

Misinformation and fears about the effects of intercourse during pregnancy on the mother and the fetus can prompt couples to avoid or abstain from intercourse. Common fears are that the baby will be injured or marked in some way or be aware of the parents having sex. If a previous baby was born with some kind of physical or mental impairment, this fear may be strong though rarely expressed. Some couples also fear injury to the mother, particularly if she experiences painful intercourse. The widespread practice of advising sexual abstinence during the last part of pregnancy may reinforce these fears of injury. For couples accustomed to frequent, regular intercourse, prolonged abstinence can be a real hardship and may encourage extramarital relations. It is now generally accepted that intercourse poses no problems in late pregnancy if there are no complications. Once membranes have ruptured or labor has begun, or if there is vaginal bleeding, intercourse should be avoided. When premature labor threatens and intercourse is proscribed because orgasm can initiate uterine contractions, the couple must also be advised against oral or manual stimulation which can produce orgasm.

Impotence During Pregnancy

Occasionally men find themselves unable to attain or maintain an erection during their partner's pregnancy. This is a type of secondary impotence; it may be a situational phenomenon with no long-term repercussions, or it may indicate a more significant psychological problem with sexual dysfunction. Almost all men, at one time or another, will fail to have an erection during a sexual encounter for a vast complex of reasons. This does not signify impotence and is usually connected with being upset, tired, preoccupied, or having too much alcohol. As men experience emotional upheavals during pregnancy, they may at certain times be disinterested in sex because of other psychological processes. For some men, a reawakening of maternal relationships and the projection of this relationship onto their pregnant wife create conflicts interfering with erotic response. If the woman's body is perceived as unattractive, sexual arousal may be blocked. This may also occur when the man fears injuring the mother or fetus, or if he is feeling a close identification with his partner in vicariously experiencing the pregnancy.

Inability to attain erection on occasion during pregnancy, as at other times, does not constitute a true sexual problem unless the couple perceives it as such. Expectations of male performance create enormous pressures on men and often exaggerate fears of inadequacy which further interfere with sexual arousal, perpetuating the difficulty in having or maintaining erections. A man is only considered impotent when he cannot achieve penile erection in 25% of his sexual attempts.[7]

Breast-Feeding and Erotic Response

The physiology of sexual responses includes changes in the breasts, which have characteristic variations during lactation. The contractile tissues surrounding the milk ducts contract during orgasm and may result in milk spurting out during sexual arousal and orgasm. Sexual stimulation may produce a "let down" reflex, causing milk to leak or spurt. If this is a concern to the couple, the woman can wear a bra with absorbent pads, and avoid pressure on the breasts. Breast tenderness can also present a problem during the postpartal period, but this is a temporary condition and the couple can avoid breast stimulation until the soreness subsides.

Another relatively common occurrence is sexual arousal in response to the baby's suckling. This may range from pleasant, mild excitation to orgasm. If women are aware that this is a normal response and does not indicate they are somehow perverted, they may become comfortable with this experience. Some women discontinue breast feeding, however, because they cannot accept these responses. Women who breast-feed also tend to resume intercourse sooner postpartally than those who do not, presumably because of increased eroticism associated with breast-feeding.

Postpartal Dyspareunia or Lack of Arousal

During the first six months following delivery, the vagina does not lubricate well because of relatively low levels of steroid hormones, which inhibit the vasocongestive response to sexual stimulation. There is also a time period of three to six weeks needed for healing to occur after childbirth, including the episiotomy, cervical, vaginal or perineal lacerations, and the site of placental attachment. Couples are usually advised to resume intercourse by the third or fourth postpartal week, if the bleeding has stopped and if the episiotomy is not painful. Their own comfort and sexual desires are used as the guide for resumption of intercourse if there are no contraindications.

However, women are at times concerned with their lack of sexual response in the months following childbirth. Taking their mothering responsibilities into consideration, with the lack of sleep, fatigue, and juggling of activities this usually requires, it is not surprising that their sexual interest might be low even without the additional factor contributed by their sexual physiology after delivery. Understanding this may alleviate fears and enable women to await full restoration of their hormonal and physical status. Residual tenderness of the perineum or vagina can also contribute to painful intercourse as well as to a lack of interest in sex. Vaginitis can result from low estrogen levels, further creating problems with dyspareunia. Fears that intercourse may be permanently affected by pregnancy, labor, and delivery grow out of the belief that these cause damage to the woman's genitalia. Painful intercourse and lack of arousal during the postpartal period can be taken as evidence that these fears have been realized unless the couple can be assisted in understanding the physiological processes of childbirth and of the postpartal period and their true effects on sexual functioning.

Educating Children About Sex

Parents are often concerned about sex education for their children, and a wide range of values are connected with where sex education occurs and who is responsible for this. Developing positive attitudes toward sexuality is very important, but so is conducting sexual activities responsibly. Guilt or conflicts arising from inadequate sex knowledge interfere with learning and schoolwork, happy relationships, and future adjustments with sexual partners. Anxiety owing to lack of understanding and confusion about sexual feelings inhibits the freedom of the sexual response, which can lead to various types of sexual dysfunctions. The greater the amount of accurate sex information, the less the anxiety; therefore, sex education is an important method of preventing sexual problems.

Sex Education in the Schools

Public schools are assuming increasing responsibility for sex education, and about 71% of parents do favor this as part of school curricula.[1] However, parents are often concerned about the quality of sex education in the schools. Some feel the information is presented in a dry, dehumanized way that does not assist children in understanding the emotional components of sexuality. Others fear that too much will be presented too rapidly, and that the children will not be well assisted to process this information or that the ethical issues will not be addressed. Valid concerns over the qualifications of those teaching sex education are voiced because few schools specifically train teachers for this sensitive subject. Teachers who are embarrassed, uncomfortable, and ill-informed, or who conduct their classes in a strained, mechanical manner will not enhance the development of healthy, positive attitudes toward sexuality.

Parental Responsibility

Parents need to assume a major responsibility in teaching their children about sex, recognizing that inevitably much information will come from other sources such as peers, older children, pornography, and mass media. One of the best ways of teaching is by the example of a caring, committed relationship between parents and the parents' comfort in answering sexual questions as they arise. Touching and physical expression of love among family members helps create a climate of acceptance of one's sexuality and body. Flexibility in habit training and weaning also prevents conflicts from developing over these primitive levels of sexuality and allows the young child's emotional and physical needs to unfold naturally.

Genital Exploration

Infants and small children touch their genitals as part of necessary exploration of the body, and parents need not discourage this activity. When the child is about three years old, parents can advise him or her that handling genitals in public is not polite. Children usually will not spend an inordinate amount of time with this self-stimulation if they are comfortable in their family environment. Any compulsive behavior that preoccupies a child can signify an emotional conflict, however, whether the behavior is masturbation, scratching, eating, talking, or something else. Giving the child the message that any part of his or her body or normal functions is bad or dirty can create guilt and conflicts later.

"Playing doctor" and other games involving genital exploration among children are very common. Parents occasionally find children at such games. Most feel the need to intervene in some way to assist children in learning the socially acceptable modes of sexual expression, but want to avoid causing a negative conditioning toward sexuality. Letting the children know this is not the time or place for such activities, without making them feel they are doing something terrible, can accomplish this goal.

Nudity in the home may be one way to dignify sexuality and body comfort. However, parents should be comfortable with nudity if they want to use this method, or else a negative or strained attitude might be communicated, which can confuse the child. Also, parents need to be ready to deal with the child touching breasts or genitals, which is a natural way children explore and learn. If parents act shocked or slap the child's hand, another double message is communicated; parents can limit touching with gentle expression of personal preferences and privacy needs.

Basic Explanations

When children encounter objects they do not recognize, their natural curiosity leads them to ask what these are for, as with sanitary napkins, tampons, or contraceptives. Simple explanations about normal body functions in a matter-of-fact tone are readily accepted by children. Usually short answers are enough, but if parents discuss more than they think the child can absorb, the child will not be dismayed as long as there is no sense of fear, embarrassment, or discomfort. Children will ask additional questions later to clarify what they have not fully understood.

Accurate explanations of the processes of menstruation, childbirth, erection and nocturnal ejaculations, development of secondary sexual characteristics, and sexual intercourse will enable children to attain comfortable sexual feelings. These explanations usually occur over many years, may be repeated several times at various levels of sophistication, and can occur spontaneously following the child's questions or be deliberately planned by parents. Actually, the process involves a combination of both, with reinforcements and clarifications as the child processes the information. The basic sex education should probably be completed by about age nine, as girls may menstruate around ten to eleven and boys begin having wet dreams at this age also. More discussion of intercourse, sexual expression, and contraception is needed during the early adolescent years.

Sexual Terminology

Using correct anatomic and physiologic terms when discussing genitals or sexual matters aids understanding and prevents problems in communicating. It is no more difficult for a child to learn to say penis or vagina than such slang terms as pee-pee and ding-dong, and it gives more dignity and acceptability to the sexual parts of the body.

Children pick up sexual words from many sources and usually sense when such terms or expressions are provocative or inappropriate. They may test parents' responses by suddenly saying the word with a straight face. Again, a calm reply with a straightforward explanation of the meaning of the obscene or sexual term is best. Then the child can be advised as to how the family feels about the use of the word or expression. By repeating the word, parents demonstrate that they are not upset or hurt by its usage or by other expressions, such as swear words or obscenities, and that it is useless to use them as a weapon or an attention-getting device. Children also learn that parents are willing to respond to sensitive areas of sexuality in a comfortable manner.

Teenage Sex

Parents find teenage sex a thorny issue and one they are often uncomfortable with. For many good reasons, they desire children to postpone intensive sexual involvements until they are emotionally mature enough to handle the powerful feelings associated with these kinds of relationships. Helping teenagers to recognize that there are many types of sexual expression not involving intercourse may be one approach, as is teaching sexual ethics about respecting the other person and relating with concern and caring. Teenagers can find a wide range of expression through masturbation, close physical contact without intercourse, dating and doing activities together, kissing, daydreaming, and having caring friendships with each other. Postponing intercourse until they feel ready can do much to prevent conflicts and tensions or the establishment of dysfunctional sexual patterns that can later plague the individual's expression of sexuality. Parents need to communicate the idea of responsible sex to adolescents in terms of avoidance of pregnancy, venereal disease, and emotional exploitation or injury to others.[8]

The intercourse decision among teenagers is affected by such factors as fear of pregnancy, cultural and peer group influence, religious and moral values, suitability of partner, access to an appropriate place, and respect and concern for oneself and others. Individual sexual needs and psychological pressures toward developing a comfortable sexual identity are also important. Nurses can help adolescents clarify values and make the best long-range decisions. In high school education programs or in contacts in health-care settings, nurses can emphasize that no one need enter a sexual relationship if it causes emotional discomfort.

A teenager has the right to be a virgin without harassment, and may need to be reminded that abstinence is normal and healthy. The majority of teenagers, in fact, are not sexually active in high school. They need to know that no method of contraception is perfect, that there are always some risks, but that birth control is essential to prevent pregnancy if their decision is to have sexual intercourse. Assisting adolescents in this decision-making process and guiding them toward acceptable and effective contraception during sexual activity is a primary responsibility of the nurse.

Objectives of Sex Education

To provide the individual with an adequate knowledge of his or her own physical, mental, and emotional maturational functions as they relate to sex.

To eliminate fears and anxieties regarding the individual's sexual development and adjustments.

To develop objective and understanding attitudes in the individual toward the self and toward others, regarding sex in all of its various manifestations.

To give the individual insight concerning relationships with members of both sexes, and to help him or her understand obligations and responsibilities to others.

To provide an appreciation of the positive good that wholesome human relations can bring to both the individual and the family group.

To build an understanding of the fact that ethical and moral values form the only rational basis for making decisions regarding one's behavior.

To provide enough knowledge about sexual abuse and aberration so that the individual can protect him or herself against exploitation and damage to physical and mental health.

To provide an incentive to work for a society in which prostitution, illegitimacy, archaic sex laws, irrational sex-related fears, and sexual exploitation are nonexistent.

To provide the insight and the climate conducive to the individual's eventually utilizing his or her sexuality effectively and creatively in the roles of spouse, parent, community member, and citizen.

(Sex Information and Education Council of the U.S.)

Objectives of Sex Education

Given that there are differences in religious traditions, philosophies, and personal-familial values related to sexual information and expression, the objectives for sex education set forth by the Sex Information and Education Council of the United States (SIECUS) provide an excellent framework for approaching this sensitive area. (See Objectives of Sex Education Chart.)

Sources of Information and Media Related to Sexuality

Professional Associations

Association of Sexologists
1523 Franklin Street
San Francisco, CA 94109

Sex Information and Education Council of the United States (SIECUS)
84 Fifth Avenue
New York, NY 10011

American Association of Sex Educators, Counselors, and Therapists
One East Wacker Drive, Suite 2700
Chicago, IL 60601

Society for the Scientific Study of Sex
310 East 46th Street
New York, NY 10017

International Academy of Sex Research
c/o Dr. Heinz Meyer–Bahlburg
722 West 168th Street
New York, NY 10032

Society for the Study of Alternative Lifestyles
2742 Orangethorpe, Suite A
Fullerton, CA 92633

Media and Printed Materials

Multi-Media Resource Center
1525 Franklin Street
San Francisco, CA 94109

Focus International Inc.
1776 Broadway
New York, NY 10019

Ed-U-Press
PO Box 583
Fayetteville, NY 13066

Sexual Abuse and Harassment of Women—Information, Research, and Programs

National Organization for Women
425 Thirteenth Street, NW, Suite 1048
Washington, DC 20004

Working Women's Institute
593 Park Avenue
New York, NY 10021

National Center for the Prevention and Control of Rape
5600 Fishers Lane
Rockville, MD 20857

References

1. McCary JL: Human Sexuality. New York, D Van Nostrand Company, 1973

2. Tanner LM: The Maternity nurse as counselor in human sexuality. In Anderson EH (ed): Current Concepts in Clinical Nursing, Vol. IV pp 169–178. St Louis, CV Mosby Company, 1973

3. Zalar MK: Sexual counseling for pregnant couples, MCN—The American Journal of Maternal-Child Nursing, 1:3, 176–181, May/June 1976

4. Mims FH, Swenson M: Sexuality: A Nursing Perspective. McGraw–Hill, New York, 1980

5. Martin LL: Health Care of Women. Philadelphia, JB Lippincott, 1978

6. Coleman AD, Coleman LL: Pregnancy: The Psychological Experience. New York, Herder and Herder, 1971

7. Masters WH, Johnson VE: Human Sexual Inadequacy. New York, Little, Brown & Co., 1970

8. Gordon S: Let's Make Sex a Household Word: A Guide for Parents and Children. New York, John Day Company, 1975

CHAPTER 13

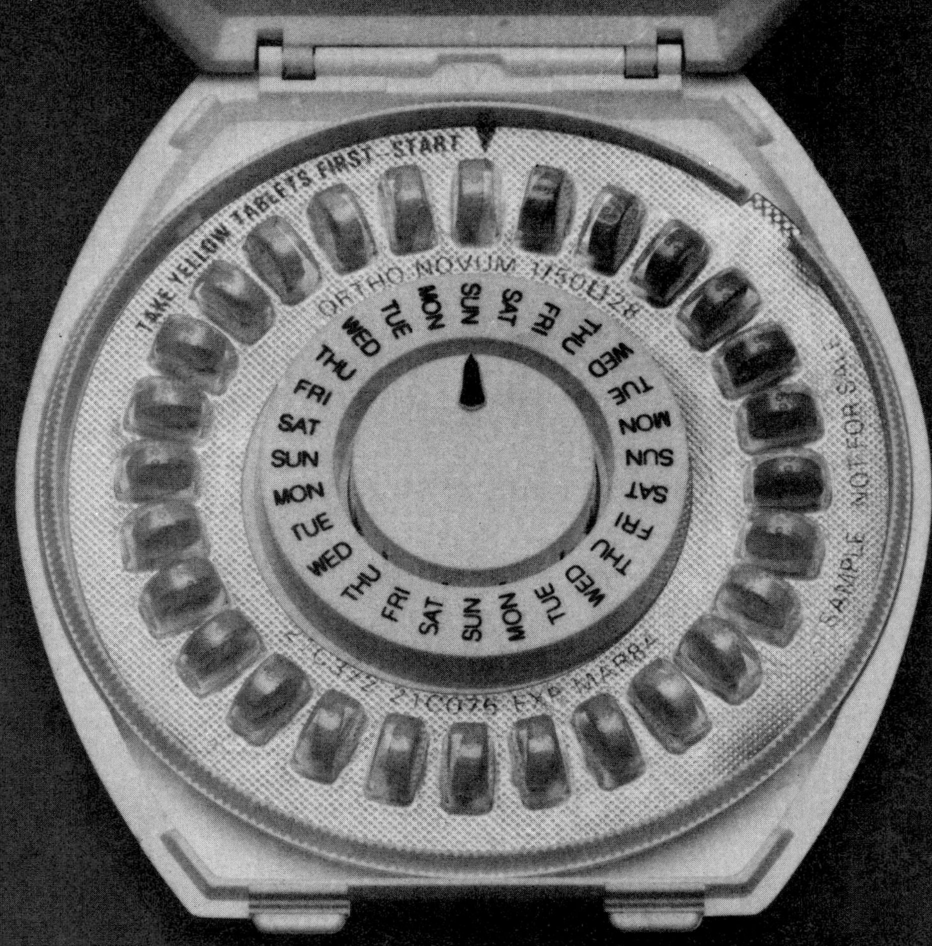

CHAPTER 13

Contraception

Changing attitudes and technological advances have given the majority of people in advanced societies the option of controlling reproduction. Contraceptive methods are widely used throughout most of the world, ranging from the ancient practice of coitus interruptus (withdrawal) to the use of chemical (hormonal) oral contraceptives by an estimated 150 million women around the world. Although governments may support a policy of limited population growth by encouraging use of contraceptives, decisions to control reproduction are based on individual choice and are made for highly personal reasons. The right of individual choice in fertility control has been emphasized by international bodies, as seen in the following statement made by the General Assembly of the United Nations in 1966: "The size of the family should be the free choice of each individual family."

The individual's right to choose freely has been expanded to include the right to have access to the means by which births may be safely and effectively limited or spaced. While highly effective contraceptive methods are available, their effectiveness is often lowered by inappropriate use. In addition, their safety has not yet reached levels at which risk is truly minimal. The ideal contraceptive would be a method that is 100% safe and 100% effective, inexpensive, simple to use and understand, not directly connected to intercourse, totally reversible at any time, and readily available. No currently available contraceptive method meets all these criteria, nor does it seem probable that research will find such a method in the near future. Despite the risks involved, people desire the benefits of reproductive choice, and must therefore make decisions about methods based on personal values and a full understanding of the risks and benefits involved.

In the United States, there is a trend toward smaller families, with women in the childbearing years expressing increased support for the concept of the two-child family.[1] The United States fertility rate (number of children/woman), which has dropped below replacement level, declined from a high of 3.68 in 1957 to 1.83 in 1977.[2] In 1981 the Social Security Administration's population projection foresaw continuing fertility rates of 1.7 to 2.4 until the year 2000. A number of factors are involved in the growing openness and acceptance of contraception, including social values, life styles, economics, and technology. Improved methods of mass communication have aided health professionals in making contraceptive information and methods available on a wider and more equitable basis. A better informed public, supported by changing social values that encourage individual choice and smaller family sizes, has demanded access to professional advice and contraceptive techniques as an integral part of health care services. Changes in family structures have placed greater emphasis on companionship and mutual growth and less on economic necessity, which in the past locked family members into separate role identities and stressed the importance of children as family workers. Traditional norms regarding children as an unquestioned duty to past or future generations have given way to the belief that children should be wanted and parenthood should be the result of deliberate choice. Modern urban life styles make large families an economic liability, and increasingly two-income families are needed to maintain high standards of living in an inflationary economy. The feminist movement and increasing numbers of women who work or pursue careers also significantly affect attitudes toward contraception.

The majority of American women, regardless of religious affiliation, approve of and use contraception. For the poor, having fewer children puts less strain on the family's resources and enhances the family's opportunities for economic and personal betterment. Black women have continued to use family planning clinics to meet their personal needs, despite accusations that this may constitute a form of genocide.[3] Although predominantly Catholic, Mexican-American women use family planning clinics and a range of contraceptive methods. Motives for contraceptive use are unique, and the choice of method and its meaning are highly individual. Therefore, differences must be respected by the nurse, without presumption based on external characteristics, and the full range of contraceptive possibilities needs to be discussed with each individual or couple so a fully informed and satisfactory choice can be made.

Contraceptive Counseling

Both the maternity and the community health nurse play an important role in the care of the patient seeking contraceptive advice. While not advocating any particular method of contraception, the professional nurse has a responsibility to see that help, understanding, and guidance in family planning are available to all patients. If the nurse is unable to give general contraceptive advice, he or she should state this to the patient and provide referral to another source for the information which is sought.

Certainly, every nurse who gives contraceptive advice needs to be aware of all the available methods of birth control and should be conversant with the advantages and disadvantages of each method, both at the functional and the psychological levels. The choice of a suitable contraceptive depends on many factors which vary even from year to year in any couple's contraceptive life span. These factors include expense, bathroom facilities, frequency of intercourse, number of children, the risk of pregnancy the couple wishes to accept, illness, and physical problems.

The nurse should also be acquainted with the increasing availability and acceptability of vasectomy and tubal ligation. Studies indicate that one fourth to one third of all couples look to this permanent method of contraception when their families are completed. Currently available methods of contraception are listed in Table 13-1.

General Approach to the Patient

A number of important principles should be observed when assisting couples in selecting a suitable means of contraception. Unlike other health measures, pregnancy prevention ideally involves the participation of both male and female partners. Good family planning programs should encourage participation of the male and provide an opportunity for him to share responsibility for fertility control. A discussion of some of the methods of male contraception, such as withdrawal, the use of condoms, vasectomy, or even rhythm when it is the method of choice should be included in the program.

Since family planning deals with the patient's sexuality, a private setting should be arranged whenever possible. The patient's feelings about contraception should be explored in a nonjudgmental way and the variety of choices summarized to allow selection of a method that fits the individual circumstance of the couple. There is no "best method" of contraception, but there is always a method which can work best in the circumstances at hand.

It should also be recognized that some patients appearing in a family planning clinic may be there because they may have an infertility problem or because they wish to have a Pap smear, a breast examination, or an evaluation for venereal disease. Family planning clinics often serve as a patient's initial introduction to the health-care system and offer opportunities for general health maintenance.

The postpartal period is an optimal time for exploring methods of family planning. Choices can conveniently be reviewed with the patient at that time so that knowledgeable selection of a method can be made. It has been shown that availability of contraceptive advice has resulted in a marked increase in the number of patients returning for postpartal care.

Table 13-1.
Methods of Contraception Currently Available

Male and Female	Male	Female
Abstinence	Withdrawal	Spermicides*
Total	Condoms	Foam, Cream, Gels
Periodic	Vasectomy	Diaphragm with Gel or Cream
Rhythm		Ovulation prevention†
Basal Body Temperature (BBT)		Oral
		Injectable
Nonvaginal variations		Implanted
Masturbation		Unknown action
Solitary		Minipill
Mutual		Morning-after pill
Oral-genital		Intrauterine device
Anal Intercourse		Mechanical
		Chemical
		Hormonal
		Heavy metals (copper)
		Tubal Sterilization‡

* Douching is not a contraceptive method.
† Breast feeding is not a contraceptive method.
‡ Abortion is not a contraceptive method.
(Pierson EC: Sex is Never an Emergency, 3rd ed. p 5. Philadelphia, JB Lippincott, 1973)

Contraceptive Effectiveness

The effectiveness of a contraceptive method is of primary concern to both patients and professionals. When counseling patients on effectiveness, professionals must be familiar with the two types of effectiveness rates—theoretical effectiveness and use effectiveness. *Theoretical effectiveness* is the method's effectiveness in preventing pregnancy under ideal conditions, that is, when it is completely understood and used perfectly. This is the method's maximum effectiveness; if a pregnancy occurs it is due to a failure of the method itself, not how it is being used. *Use effectiveness* takes into consideration the method's effectiveness under actual use, in which some people use the method correctly and others use it carelessly or incorrectly. Effectiveness rates are lower, naturally, because the human error factor is included.

In answering questions about effectiveness, the counselor may allow his or her bias to show by quoting theoretical effectiveness figures for preferred contraceptive methods, and use effectiveness figures for those methods not favored. This provides misleading data to the patient and is an attempt to influence choice according to the counselor's preference. Ethical counseling requires consistency in presenting effectiveness data to patients, either theoretical or use effectiveness for every contraceptive method discussed. Some contend that the patient deserves both sets of figures, so the potential for error in use can be clearly assessed. Table 13-2 shows figures for theoretical and use effectiveness of common contraceptive methods. When assisting patients to select a contraceptive method, it is good to keep in mind that the "best method" of contraception is one that a couple will use most consistently and correctly, and this is often the one that makes them feel most natural and comfortable. Questions in Factors That Lower Use Effectiveness provide a guide to factors which might lower effectiveness in contraceptive use. Any "yes" response indicates potential problems, and most people will have several "yes" answers for any contraceptive method. The one with the fewest "yes" responses would be best for that couple.

Informed Consent and Contraceptive Risk

There is a certain amount of risk in every contraceptive method, either the method itself or the risk of pregnancy due to contraceptive failure or misuse. It should be noted that the mortality associated with pregnancy is greater than that of any commonly used contraceptive method. Often the risk a given method poses for the individual cannot be completely determined in advance, although in many instances contraindications can be identified for known health

Table 13-2.
Effectiveness and Risks of Contraceptives and Pregnancies per 100 Women per Year

Method	Theoretical Effectiveness	Use Effectiveness	Continuing Pregnancies	Deaths due to Pregnancy	Deaths due to Contraception	Major Morbidity (%)	Minor Morbidity (%)
No contraception	—	—	80	0.016	0	—	—
Oral contraceptives (combined)	0.34	4–10	0.5	0	0.003	1	40
Low-dose oral progestin	1–1.5	5–10	—	—	—	—	—
IUD	2	5	3	0.001	0.001	1	40
Diaphragm	3	13–17	12	0.002	0	—	—
Rhythm (calendar)	14	21	25	0.005	0	—	—
Basal body temperature only	7	21	—	—	—	—	—
Cervical mucus only	2	25	—	—	—	—	—
Early abortion*	0	0	0	0	0.003	1	8
Laparoscopic tubal ligation	0	0.04	0.15	0	0.03	0.6	1
Vasectomy	0	0.15	0.15	0	0	1	5
Condom†	3	10–15	—	—	—	—	—
Spermicides†	3	13–22	—	—	—	—	—
Condom + spermicide	< 1	5	—	—	—	—	—
Coitus interruptus†	3	15–25	—	—	—	—	—

* Abortion is not a method of contraception, but is included here for comparison.

† Data on continuing pregnancies and deaths due to pregnancy are not available, but use effectiveness figures indicate these would be in the range found for the diaphragm.

After Hatcher RA, Stewart GK, Stewart F, Guest F et al: Contraceptive Technology 1980–1981, p. 4. New York, Irvington Publishers, Inc, 1980, and Romney SL et al, Gynecology and Obstetrics: The Health Care of Women pp. 551, 552. New York, McGraw–Hill, Blakiston, 1975

Factors That Lower Use Effectiveness

Every "yes" response indicates a potential problem with this method of contraception. You will probably be most comfortable with the method getting the fewest "yes" responses.

1. Am I afraid of using this method of birth control?
2. Would I really rather not use this method?
3. Will I have trouble remembering to use this method?
4. Have I ever become pregnant while using this method?
5. Are there reasons why I will be unable to use this method as prescribed?
6. Do I still have unanswered questions about this method?
7. Has my mother, father, sister, brother, or a close friend strongly discouraged me from using this method?
8. Will this method make my periods longer or more painful?
9. Will prolonged use of this method cost me more than I can afford?
10. Is this method known to have serious complications?
11. Am I opposed to this method because of my religious beliefs?
12. Have I already experienced complications from this method?
13. Has a nurse or doctor already told me not to use this method?
14. Is my partner opposed to my using this method?
15. Am I using this method without my partner's knowledge?
16. Will the use of this method embarrass me?
17. Will the use of this method embarrass my partner?
18. Will my partner or I enjoy sexual activity less because of this method?
19. Will this method interrupt lovemaking?[4]

problems or personal characteristics. Still, an apparently healthy woman with no major contraindications to a given method can develop serious complications, some of which are life threatening. Although the incidence of such complications is low, it is the patient's right to be well informed about the risks, benefits, and effectiveness of all contraceptive methods (Table 13-2).

The issue of informed consent is particularly critical in the field of contraception, because the services are not "therapeutic" in the traditional medical sense. Healthy patients request family planning methods, which are initiated without health indications in most instances. In evaluating possible malpractice considerations, the legal approach uses the "reasonable person" standard. Did the patient receive all the information a reasonable person would need in order to make a sound decision and give a truly informed consent to care? The professional counselor has the responsibility of ascertaining that the patient has sufficient information about the proposed method (treatment), and that the patient is competent to consent on his or her own behalf.

The key factors to sufficient information include discussion of the benefits and risks (all major and all minor) of the method, alternatives (including abstinence and no method), that the patient has a right and responsibility to ask questions about the method, that the patient may decide to withdraw or not use the method at any time without penalty, and an explanation of the use and results of the method. All the above information must be documented; a written consent form and signature alone are not enough. Legally, the professional must enter a record of the information covered in the patient's chart, and make some notation to document patient understanding. Often, patients are asked to sign a statement at the end of the record of information, such as, "I have read and discussed the above information about contraception (or the specific method) and I fully understand these points." The importance of a voluntary decision by the patient, without coercion or professional bias, is clearly evident.

The basic criteria for competence to consent are that the patient is capable of understanding the proposed treatment (method) and its alternatives and risks, and is capable of rational decision making. Competence to consent may be difficult to evaluate in some instances, such as the very young teenager, the mentally ill, or mentally retarded person. Legal consultation is recommended when there is doubt about a patient's ability to give consent to care. Documentation of such consultation is critical.

Informed consent is both a safeguard for the patient and a way of increasing proper contraceptive use. When the woman or couple fully understand the technique, have weighed the possible adverse effects against the convenience and acceptability of the method for them, and have made a choice based on which method best meets their needs, the likelihood of discontinuation and misuse is reduced. Guidelines for informed consent suggested by the United States Department of Health and Human Services are indicated in the Guidelines for Contraceptive Teaching chart.

Guidelines for Contraceptive Teaching

Informed consent is the voluntary, knowing assent from the individual on whom any procedure is to be performed after she or he has been given the following:

1. A fair explanation of the procedures or method;
2. A description of attendant discomforts and risks, including all major (life-threatening) and all common minor risks;
3. A description of the benefits to be expected;
4. An explanation of alternative methods and effectiveness rates with indication that nothing is 100%, and that sterilization is permanent;
5. An offer to answer any questions about procedures or method;
6. An instruction that the individual is free to withdraw consent to the procedure or method at any time prior to the procedure, or to discontinue the method, without affecting future care or loss of benefits;
7. A written consent document detailing the basic elements of informed consent and the information provided; this should be signed by the patient, an auditor–witness of the patient's choice, and by the person obtaining the consent.[5]

Teenagers, Family Planning, and the Law

The legal rights of teenagers to obtain contraceptive services without parental consent constitute an area of concern to many professionals involved in family planning. The laws related to minors' rights to contraceptive services, sterilization, and nonprescription contraceptives vary from state to state. In all 50 states, minors can consent to treatment for venereal disease, and in many they can consent to contraception and pregnancy-related care. In 1977 the United States Supreme Court ruled that minors have a constitutional right to contraceptives. Although there are no rulings on the rights of minors to prescription contraceptives, Planned Parenthood Federation of America reports no record of a suit being won against a physician or health service for providing contraceptive services to minors without parental consent.

Oral Contraception

Oral contraceptives ("the pill") are hormonal agents consisting most commonly of a combination of estrogen and a synthetic progestational agent. They act principally at the central nervous system level to inhibit ovulation through suppression of FSH and LH. There are secondary effects on endometrial development, tubal motility, and cervical mucus. Under the influence of the progestational agent, the cervical mucus becomes thick, viscous, and unreceptive to spermatozoa. However, the most important effect of standard dose combination pills is the inhibition of ovulation, which means that there is no ova to be fertilized.

Oral contraceptives are available in 21- and 28-day packages; in the 21-day packs a pill is taken each day for three weeks, followed by a week without any pills. In the 28-day pack, a pill is taken every day for four weeks, but only those taken during the first three weeks will have active hormonal ingredients; those pills taken during the last week consist of lactose or ferrous sulfate, but no hormones. The purpose of a week of nonhormonal pills is to keep the woman in the habit of taking a pill a day, and in some instances to provide an iron supplement for prevention of anemia. When the 21-day approach is used, the pill is taken daily beginning on the fifth day of the menstrual cycle through day 25. Two or three days after the last pill is taken there is usually a "withdrawal" menstrual flow.

There is a large number of oral contraceptives available, with differing combinations of estrogen or progestin doses (see Table 13-3). Basically there are two types—the combination pills which contain estrogen and progestin and are available at the standard or low (micro) dosage levels, and the progestin-

Table 13-3.
Most Currently Available Combination Microdose and Progestin Oral Contraceptives

Product/manufacturer	Type	Estrogen	Progestin
Envoid-E/Searle	Combination	100 mcg mestranol	2.5 mg norethynodrel
Ortho-Novum/Ortho	Combination	100 mcg mestranol	2 mg norethindrone
Norinyl/Syntex	Combination	100 mcg mestranol	2 mg norethindrone
Ovulen/Searle	Combination	100 mcg mestranol	1 mg ethynodiol diacetate
Ortho-Novum 1+80	Combination	80 mcg mestranol	1 mg norethindrone
Norinyl 1+80/Syntex	Combination	80 mcg mestranol	1 mg norethindrone
Norlestrin/Parke–Davis	Combination	50 mcg ethinyl estradiol	2.5 mg norethindrone acetate
Norinyl 1+50/Syntex	Combination	50 mcg mestranol	1 mg norethindrone
Ortho-Novum 1 + 50/Ortho	Combination	50 mcg mestranol	1 mg norethindrone
Norlestrin/Parke–Davis	Combination	50 mcg ethinyl estradiol	1 mg norethindrone acetate
Ovral/Wyeth	Combination	50 mcg ethinyl estradiol	0.5 mg norgestrel
Demulen/Searle	Combination	50 mcg ethinyl estradiol	1 mg ethynodiol diacetate
Ovcon-50/Mead Johnson	Combination	50 mcg ethinyl estradiol	1 mg norethindrone
Zorane 1+50/Lederle	Combination	50 mcg ethinyl estradiol	1 mg norethindrone acetate
Brevicon/Syntex	Combination	35 mcg ethinyl estradiol	0.5 mg norethindrone
Ovcon-35/Mead Johnson	Combination	35 mcg ethinyl estradiol	0.4 mg norethindrone
Modicon/Ortho	Combination	35 mcg ethinyl estradiol	0.5 mg norethindrone
Loestrin 1.5+30/Parke–Davis	Combination	30 mcg ethinyl estradiol	1.5 mg norethindrone acetate
Zorane 1.5+30/Lederle	Combination	30 mcg ethinyl estradiol	1.5 mg norethindrone acetate
Lo/Ovral/Wyeth	Combination	30 mcg ethinyl estradiol	0.3 mg norgestrel
Loestrin 1+20/Parke–Davis	Combination	20 mcg ethinyl estradiol	1 mg norethindrone acetate
Zorane 1+20/Lederle	Combination	20 mcg ethinyl estradiol	1 mg norethindrone acetate
Micronor/Ortho	Progestin		0.35 mg norethindrone
Nor-QD/Syntex	Progestin		0.35 mg norethindrone
Ovrette/Wyeth	Progestin		0.075 mg norgestrel

only type (minipills). As the majority of serious side-effects are due to estrogen, the trend has been toward reducing this hormonal agent from the original dosage of 80 mcg to 100 mcg to doses ranging from 50 mcg to 20 mcg. However, use of 20 mcg or 30 mcg pills is associated with high rates of breakthrough bleeding and unpredictable menses, making them less acceptable to many women. Similar problems are encountered with progestin-only pills, and increased amenorrhea, spotting, and irregularity of menses has discouraged their widespread use.

The theoretical effectiveness of the combined formulation pill approaches 100%. In fact, the method failure rate—failure when properly used—is negligible. When patient error is included (patient failures to take the pill for one or more days during the cycle), effectiveness falls to approximately 90% to 95%. The discontinuation rate has been reported to be from 20% to as high as 50%. Appearance of side-effects and untoward symptoms, as well as variations in motivational factors in the populations studied are often reasons for discontinuation of oral contraceptives.

Contraindications and Side-Effects

Generally accepted, absolute contraindications to oral contraception include a history of thrombophlebitis, thromboembolic disorders, cerebral vascular accident, the presence of marked impairment of liver function, hepatic adenoma, malignancy of the breast or of the reproductive tract, and, of course, pregnancy. Strong relative contraindications include migraine, hypertension, diabetes, gallbladder disease, sickle cell disease, undiagnosed vaginal bleeding, over age 35, abortion within the past 10 to 14 days, fibrocystic breast disease, and less than four weeks postpartum.

Common side-effects of the pill include accentuation of premenstrual symptoms, such as mastalgia, irritability, edema, nausea; spotting, weight gain, missed periods, and increased yeast vaginal infections. The major life-threatening side-effects include blood clots in the legs, pelvis, lungs, heart, or brain. The risk of heart attack is increased in women over 40, especially if they smoke. Liver tumors (adenomas), gallbladder disease, and hypertension are also serious complications.

The side-effects of oral contraceptives, according to the excess or deficiency of hormone responsible for the symptom or condition, are shown in Table 13-4.

Systemic Effects of Synthetic Hormones

Initially oral contraceptives were believed to affect only the reproductive system through suppression of ovulation and alteration of menstrual flow. However, there is increasing recognition that these powerful synthetic hormones affect many systems of the body, causing metabolic and endocrine changes with far-reaching impact. The possible long-term consequences and risks of taking the pill are creating a climate of true concern among women and health professionals and have led to a call for a more conservative and cautious approach involving careful selection and frequent monitoring.

Thrombotic Effects

Several factors seem to be involved in the increased risk of death or disability due to clotting disorders (*e.g.,* stroke, pulmonary embolism, retinal vein thrombosis, myocardial infarction, thrombophlebitis) in women taking the pill. There is more rapid fibrin formation with increased clot firmness among pill users than among nonusers, as well as an increase in certain blood factors associated with coagulation, an increase in platelet count with changes in electrophoretic mobility of platelets, and an increase in vascular lesions and venous stasis.[6,7] Women who use the pill have a seven to eight times greater risk of death from thromboembolic disease than nonusers. The incidence of complications is dosage related. There is a significant difference between women taking pills with less than 50 mcg of estrogen per day as compared to those taking dosages above 50 mcg of estrogen per day. The risk of death from clotting disorders secondary to oral contraceptives is age related, the risk increasing after age 35.

Effects of Cigarette Smoking

Evidence indicates that there is an increased death rate from cardiovascular complications among women over 35 who use oral contraceptives and smoke. Studies have shown that women over age 30 who both smoke and use oral contraceptives have a greater risk of fatal heart attack than younger women who use the pill and women over 30 who do not smoke. While other risk factors such as hypertension and high cholesterol are also associated with higher incidence of myocardial infarction, cigarette smoking was considered the most important factor. Women who smoke heavily and use the pill have 39 times the risk of cardiovascular disease, including heart attack, stroke, and thromboembolism, compared to women who neither smoke nor use the pill. Half of all the deaths associated with oral contraceptive use would be avoided if women who take birth control pills would not smoke.[8] Apparently women without these risk factors can continue taking oral contraceptives with relative safety during the years of 30 to 44.[9] The Federal Drug Administration has required the following antismoking warning be added to package inserts accompanying oral contraceptives:

> Cigarette smoking increases the risk of serious cardiovascular side-effects from oral contraceptive use. The risk increases with age and with heavy smoking (15 or more cigarettes per day) and is quite marked in women over 35 years of age. Women who use oral contraceptives should be strongly advised not to smoke.[10]

Hypertensive Effects

Blood pressure increases in some women who take oral contraceptives. Usually this is rapidly reversible once the pill is discontinued, but it can lead to permanent complications if the blood pressure elevation is high enough or persists for some time. In normotensive women, it is difficult to predict who will develop hypertension, so blood pressure monitoring is essential for all pill users. One study based on a sample of 2700 black women found that black women are less prone to develop clinical hypertension than white women. However, all the women in the study were less than age 35, most had higher baseline blood pressures than white women of similar ages, and almost all were taking pills with 50 mcg of estrogen. Those women in both the study and control groups who did have significant blood pressure elevations (20 mm or more increase in diastolic pressure) were those who had gained the most weight in the two-year study period.[11]

Liver and Gallbladder Effects

Changes in liver function due to oral contraceptives are related to estrogen dosage levels and apparently are reversible. An increased risk of liver adenomas develops after five years of pill use; it is predominately associated with mestranol (an estrogen).[12] The incidence of these benign tumors is about 3 to 4 per 100,000 long-term pill users; death, which is rare, is caused by internal bleeding.[13] An increase in gallbladder disease among pill users was reported in the early 1970s, but the Walnut Creek Contraceptive Drug Study, a prospective study by the federal government, has not yet confirmed this association.[8]

Table 13-4.
Hormonal Basis of Side-Effects of Oral Contraceptives

Estrogen		Progestin		Androgen
Excess	**Deficiency**	**Excess**	**Deficiency**	**Excess**
Nausea, vomiting Fluid retention (premenstrual tension, irritability, breast tenderness, corneal swelling, cramping, edema) Increased vaginal discharge Chloasma Headaches Increased breast size Weight gain Increased cervical ectropion Increased size of fibroids Telangiectasia Thromboembolic disorders Reduction of lactation Possible hypertension Hepatic adenoma	Amenorrhea Oligomenorrhea Early or midcycle spotting Loss of pelvic tone Hot flashes Nervousness, irritability Decreased interest in sex	Acne, oily scalp Increased appetite Weight gain Fatigue Depression Hair loss Headaches when not taking pills Increased breast size Increased muscle mass Increased monilial vaginitis (Candida) Breast tenderness not related to fluid retention Short menses Relative endometrial atrophy Decreased interest in sex Cholestatic jaundice Decreased carbohydrate tolerance Dilated leg veins	Hypermenorrhea with clotting Late cycle spotting Delayed onset of menses Dysmenorrhea Weight loss	Acne Oily skin Rashes Increased hair growth in male pattern Increased interest in sex Cholestatic jaundice Increased appetite Pruritus

Carbohydrate Metabolism

About 20% to 25% of women taking oral contraceptives have elevated fasting blood sugar, and an additional 20% show abnormal glucose tolerance test curves. Human growth hormone is significantly increased with a compensatory increase in insulin, which usually allows women to maintain a normal glucose tolerance test even though blood sugar levels are increased. A history of diabetes or the presence of obesity places women at a greater risk for abnormalities of carbohydrate metabolism with pill use. Although short-term studies show reversal of these changes after discontinuation of oral contraceptives, the long-term effects have not been established.

Lipids

Increases in plasma triglycerides and phospholipids among women taking the pill are related to dosage levels of estrogen. Increased hepatic production of lipids may possibly be involved, and although the long-term effects are not yet known, it is speculated that these changes may be associated with cardiovascular disease and acute vascular accidents.[14]

Fetal Abnormalities

Although there appears to be no increase in fetal abnormalities among women who have used oral contraceptives prior to conception, studies have indicated an association between use of progestins in the first four months of pregnancy and congenital heart and limb reduction defects. There was a 4.7-fold increase in the risk of limb reduction defects in infants exposed to sex hormones in utero, including oral contraceptives, hormone withdrawal tests for pregnancy, or treatment for threatened abortion.[15] Cardiovascular malformations occurred at an increased rate of 8.6 per 1000 among infants of women receiving progestins only during pregnancy.[16] These concerns are reflected in physician labeling and patient warnings that are now required by the FDA when progestational drugs are used during pregnancy.

A recent long-term, prospective British study found that pill users have no higher risk than other women of bearing a low-birth weight or malformed infant, or of having a stillbirth, miscarriage, or ectopic pregnancy.[17]

Cancer

There is still much question about the relationship between oral contraceptives and cervical, endometrial, and breast cancer. Because women taking the pill tend to have more frequent visits to clinics or physicians' offices, frequency of incidence data is confounded by greater diagnostic opportunity. However, a relationship has been established between prolonged unopposed estrogen stimulation of the endometrium and endometrial hyperplasia and adenocarcinoma. Certain types of breast cancer are known to grow more rapidly under higher levels of estrogen stimulation, and studies show that oral contraceptives cause breast cancer in animals. Because combination pills cause a hyperestrogenic state, there is concern about long-term effects on the breasts and endometrium.

Initiation of Therapy and Follow-Up

Patients on the pill should undergo regular checkups every 6 months. The initial visit should include assessment of the patient for contraindications to the pill, a blood pressure determination, Pap smear, hematocrit or hemoglobin, urinalysis, and, when circumstances dictate, a culture for gonorrhea, and a serologic test for syphilis. An alternate method of birth control should be reviewed thoroughly, in case the patient discontinues the pill without consulting the physician.

In many family planning centers, an early follow-up visit after six to twelve weeks is suggested. At that time, evidence of side-effects and the patient's general attitude are reviewed with specific questions about headaches, blurred vision, chest pain, leg pain, as well as a blood pressure check, and an evaluation to be sure the pills are being taken correctly.

When the pill is discontinued, ovulation and menstruation will usually return by the next monthly cycle. Some women, however, may experience a delay in ovulation and, therefore, of menstruation for several months. There is no evidence that future pregnancies are affected by the prior use of oral contraceptives.

Intrauterine Device (IUD)

This technique (actually an ancient practice but only recently validated scientifically) involves inserting a small, usually flexible appliance into the uterine cavity (Fig. 13-1) that remains in the uterus for as long as contraception is desired. Devices have been made in various shapes (spirals, loops, rings) and of various materials (plastic tubing, nylon thread, stainless steel). The most commonly used are the Lippes loop, Saf-T-Coil, Copper 7, Copper T, and Progesterone T. Although the mechanism by which these appliances prevent conception is not completely understood, there appears to be a local inflammatory effect on the endometrium making it unfavorable to implantation

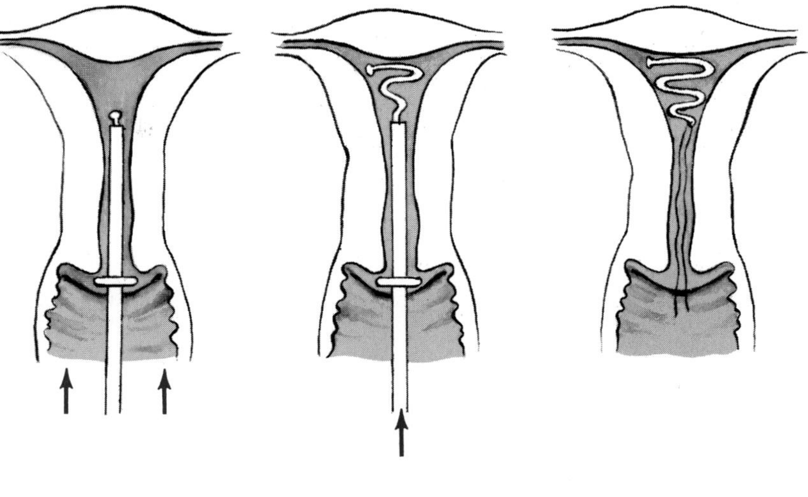

Figure 13-1A.
Insertion of a Lippes loop. *(a)* Inserter in position with stopcock at external cervical os. *(b)* Plunger advances and releases IUD into uterine cavity. *(c)* Inserter is removed when IUD is in place in uterine cavity with strings protruding from external cervical os. (Whitley N: A Manual of Clinical Obstetrics. Philadelphia, JB Lippincott. In preparation.)

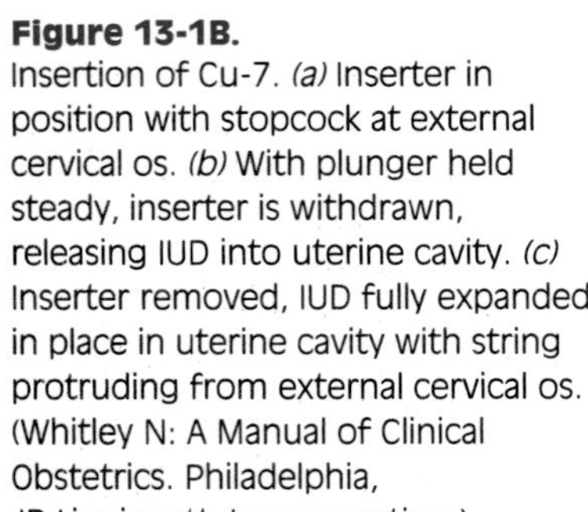

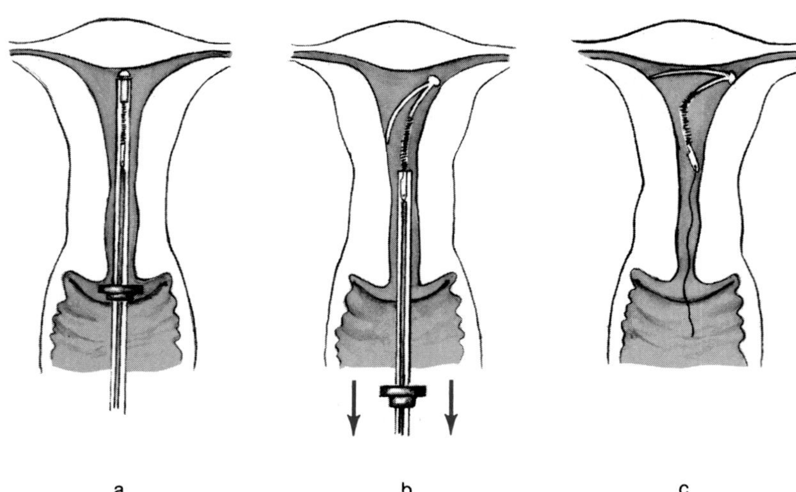

Figure 13-1B.
Insertion of Cu-7. *(a)* Inserter in position with stopcock at external cervical os. *(b)* With plunger held steady, inserter is withdrawn, releasing IUD into uterine cavity. *(c)* Inserter removed, IUD fully expanded in place in uterine cavity with string protruding from external cervical os. (Whitley N: A Manual of Clinical Obstetrics. Philadelphia, JB Lippincott. In preparation.)

or causing cytolysis. An immunologic antifertility mechanism may also be operating, or a dislodging effect may occur mechanically.

IUDs are about 97% effective (three pregnancies in 100 users with the IUD in place). They rank second only to the oral contraceptives and probably equal to the properly used diaphragm in the protection they afford. The advantages of intrauterine devices are that they are inexpensive and, once inserted, require no further attention, provided they remain in place. The main drawback of the appliances is that they are frequently expelled, and at times cause bleeding and cramps requiring that they be removed. Spontaneous expulsion or necessary removal occurs in 15% to 20% of patients.

Many commonly used IUDs have a nylon string attached. This serves two purposes—it aids in removal, and it allows the patient to check for its presence by palpating the strings at the cervix. The nurse should emphasize to the patient that it is important to check for the presence of the IUD before each sexual exposure during the first several months of use. Beyond this time the chance of spontaneous expulsion without the patient's knowledge is reduced, and it is at this time that the quoted 97% rate of effectiveness is valid.

The metallic copper in some IUDs appears to be associated with a lower expulsion rate and an increased effectiveness. The copper is slowly delivered from the device into the uterine fluid. For this reason, it is recommended that the copper device be replaced every two to four years. IUDs that contain progesterone slowly release the hormone from the device to provide a local effect on the endometrium; this is also reported to increase effectiveness. However, these types have to be replaced at intervals because the progesterone gradually disperses.

Contraindications and Side-Effects

The major contraindications to IUDs include active pelvic infection, recent or chronic pelvic infection, postpartum endometritis or septic abortion, pregnancy, endometrial hyperplasia or carcinoma, and abnormalities of the uterus such as myomatosis, polyps, or bicornate uterus making insertion problematic. In women with a small uterus (sounding to less than 6 cm) or with marked anteflexion or retroflexion, insertion is more difficult but may be accomplished with the smaller devices.

Commonly reported side-effects of the IUD include increased menstrual flow, dysmenorrhea, and intermenstrual spotting. Since flow is sometimes excessive, patients should be checked routinely for anemia. They should be instructed to report any fever, pelvic pain or tenderness, or unusual vaginal bleeding because these may be signs of pelvic infection. If pregnancy occurs when the IUD is in place, removal is recommended. An increased danger of intrapartum infection and deaths from sepsis have been reported among patients whose IUD was allowed to remain in place during pregnancy. The risk of spontaneous abortion is somewhat higher when the IUD remains in place (about 50%) than when it is removed at the time pregnancy is discovered (25%). Another major complication is uterine perforation which usually occurs at the time the IUD is inserted. When perforation through the uterine wall into the abdomen occurs, it is generally recommended that the IUD be removed. This can be done with the use of a laparoscope, avoiding an exploratory laparotomy.

Occasionally on insertion, the IUD may produce enough pain and stimulation to result in syncope. The nurse should be aware of this complication and should be ready to place the patient in a recumbent position if there are any signs of lightheadedness, sweating, or nausea.

Ectopic pregnancy may also be related to the use of an IUD. The incidence of ectopic pregnancy is considerably higher with the Progesterone T (Progestasert) IUD than with unmedicated or copper-containing IUDs. About 3% to 4% of women with unmedicated or copper IUDs who become pregnant have ectopic pregnancies, as compared to about 16% ectopic pregnancies with the progesterone IUD or no contraception. The FDA has alerted health professionals to carefully evaluate patients who become pregnant with progesterone IUDs in place to determine if the pregnancies are ectopic.[18]

The Diaphragm

The diaphragm, a dome-shaped rubber cap ranging in diameter from 7 cm to 10 cm, is inserted into the vagina and over the anterior vaginal wall and cervix prior to intercourse (Fig. 13-2). The diaphragm, by itself, is not a contraceptive device; it must be used with a spermicidal jelly or cream which is placed in the diaphragm between it and the cervix. The use of the diaphragm insures the placement of spermicidal jelly over the cervix (Fig. 13-3).

When the diaphragm is properly used—each time intercourse occurs, without exception—it is associ-

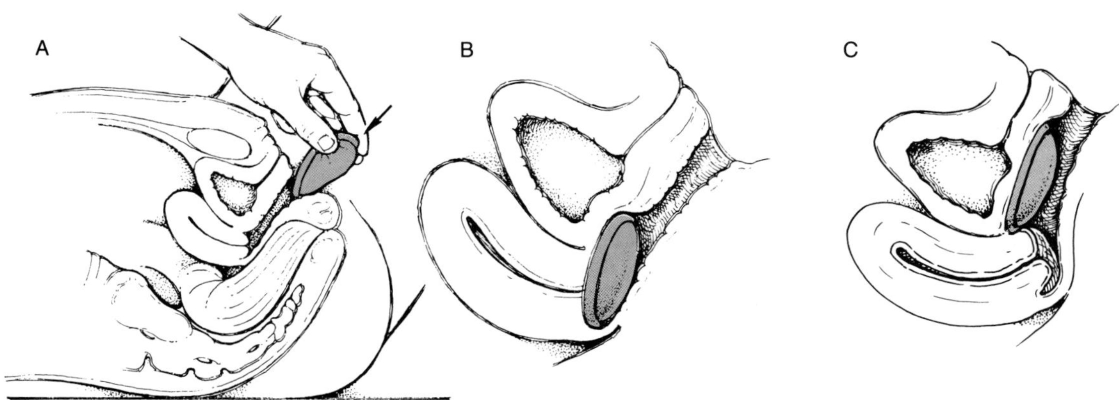

Figure 13-2.
(A) Method of manual insertion of diaphragm. Prior to insertion, contraceptive cream or jelly is placed over the dome around the edges of the diaphragm. Plastic inserters are also available for ease of insertion of the diaphragm. *(B)* Diaphragm proper position. *(C)* Diaphragm positioned improperly.

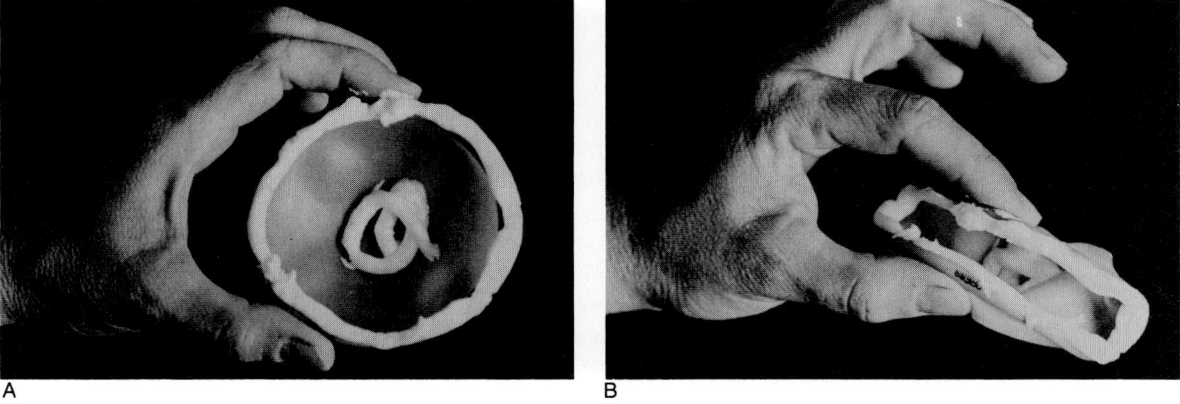

Figure 13-3.
(A) Diaphragm with spermicidal cream applied. *(B)* Compressed diaphragm that is ready for manual insertion.

ated with a failure rate of three pregnancies per 100 woman-years which is a very acceptable rate. In practice, however, the overall failure rate varies from 13 to 17 pregnancies per 100 women years of use. This may be a result of inconsistent use. A diaphragm requires motivation and premeditation, but despite these drawbacks it has again gained favor as some of the disadvantages of the pill and IUD are weighed.

Advantages of the diaphragm include safety, lack of side-effects, and flexibility according to frequency of intercourse. Since it can be inserted up to 2 hours before sex, it is relatively separated from coitus. Once in place it is unobtrusive, as its presence cannot be felt by either partner if properly fitted, and less cream or jelly is left in the vagina than with a spermicide alone. Well-motivated women have used the diaphragm effectively to limit pregnancies since the end of the 19th century.

A common objection to the diaphragm is the vaginal manipulation necessary for insertion, a procedure which is repugnant to some women. This problem is easily solved if the patient is fitted with a flat or coil-spring diaphragm (in contrast to the arc flex diaphragm). These diaphragms may be used with an "inserter" which allows the patient to insert it like a tampon, without touching the genital area (Fig. 13-4). The arc flex diaphragm cannot be used with an inserter. It was designed for ease of manual insertion and may, in some cases, give a better fit in the presence of a mild cystocele. Some women, after one or more pregnancies cannot be fitted with a diaphragm.

One of the stated disadvantages of prescribing a diaphragm is the office time consumed during fitting and instruction on its use. Increasingly, the nurse is called upon to play an active role in both. Sample diaphragms or rings of known size are inserted until a size is found that will cover the cervix and fit snugly behind the symphysis pubis (Fig. 13-5). The patient is then asked to remove the diaphragm by hooking a finger over it just beneath the symphysis and then to reinsert it (Fig. 13-6). Before the patient leaves the office, she should be able to insert and remove the

PE Instructions for Inserting and Removing Diaphragm

1. When being fitted for a diaphragm, practice insertion and removal several times before leaving the physician's office or clinic, and have the provider check your placement of the diaphragm after practice. If the diaphragm feels uncomfortable, or if you think it may be too small or too large, return to the office with it in place for a reexamination.
2. Apply contraceptive jelly or cream by holding the diaphragm with the dome down, like a cup. Place about one tablespoon of cream or jelly into the dome, and spread a thin layer around the rim also. The cream or jelly remains an active spermicide for up to six hours, so the diaphragm can be inserted well before intercourse.
3. With the dome down, insert the diaphragm by squeezing the opposite sides of the rim together. Spread the lips of the labia with one hand and insert the folded diaphragm with the other. The best positions for insertion are standing with one foot propped up, squatting, or lying down. Push the diaphragm downward into the vagina as far back as it will go, then tuck the front rim up behind the pubic bone inside the vagina. Check for proper placement by feeling for the cervix, which should be covered by the rubber dome of the diaphragm.
4. If you have intercourse more than once, you must apply more spermicidal cream or jelly with an applicator before each act of intercourse. Do not remove the diaphragm, but place the cream or jelly in front of it. You may use condoms for subsequent intercourse instead of more applications of spermicide.
5. After intercourse, the diaphragm must be left in place for six to eight hours. Do not douche during this time.
6. Remove the diaphragm by placing your index finger behind the front rim and pulling down and out. If the suction is tight, insert a finger between the diaphragm and the pubic bone to break suction. If the rim is hard to reach, bear down to bring it forward. Be careful not to puncture the diaphragm with long fingernails.
7. After use, clean the diaphragm with soap and water, rinse thoroughly, and dry with a towel. You may dust it with cornstarch, but do not use talcum or perfumed powder, as these damage the diaphragm and may irritate the vagina and cervix. Store the diaphragm in its plastic container in a cool, dry place.
8. Inspect the diaphragm each time you use it for tears or holes. Do not use Vaseline, as it can cause deterioration of the rubber of the diaphragm. Use K–Y Jelly or spermicidal jelly for additional lubrication. The diaphragm will become darker, mottled brown over time, but will last several years if properly cared for.
9. Have your diaphragm fitting checked if you gain or lose more than 10 to 20 pounds, have a pregnancy or abortion, have pelvic surgery, if the diaphragm causes discomfort or pain, or if you think it is too large or too small.

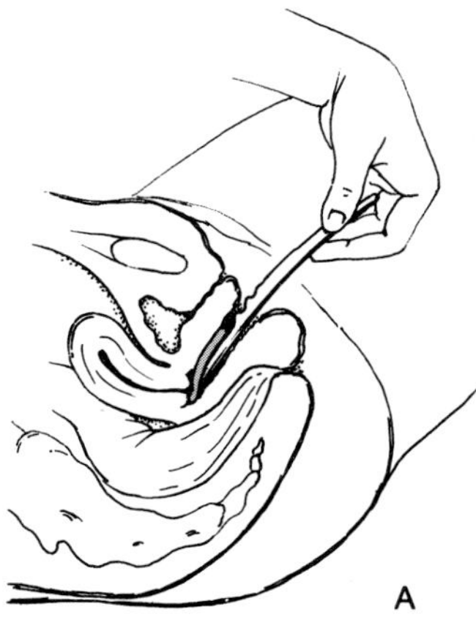

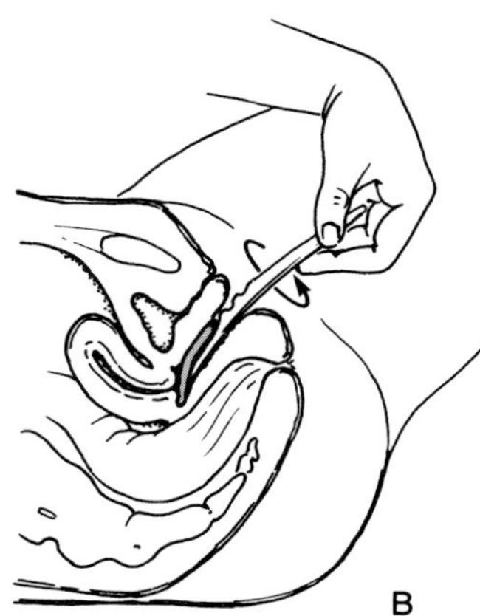

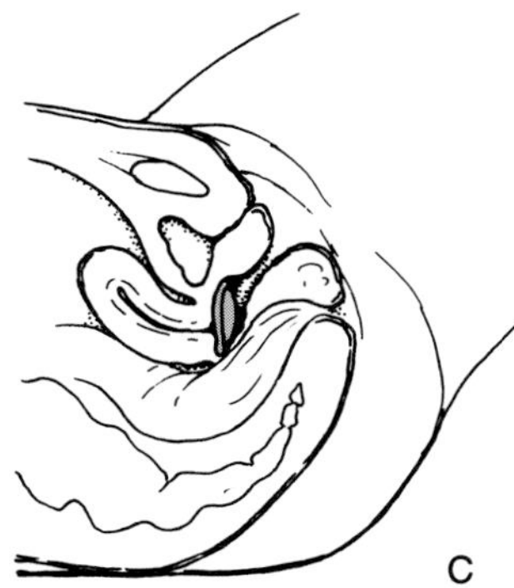

Figure 13-4.
Use of an inserter to position the diaphragm minimizes genital touching and may be easier for some women. *(A)* The inserter with diaphragm in place is positioned deep in the posterior fornix. *(B)* The inserter is twisted to release the diaphragm. *(C)* The diaphragm is pushed behind the symphysis pubis with a finger; here it is correctly positioned over the cervix. (Whitley N: A Manual of Clinical Obstetrics. Philadelphia, JB Lippincott. In preparation.)

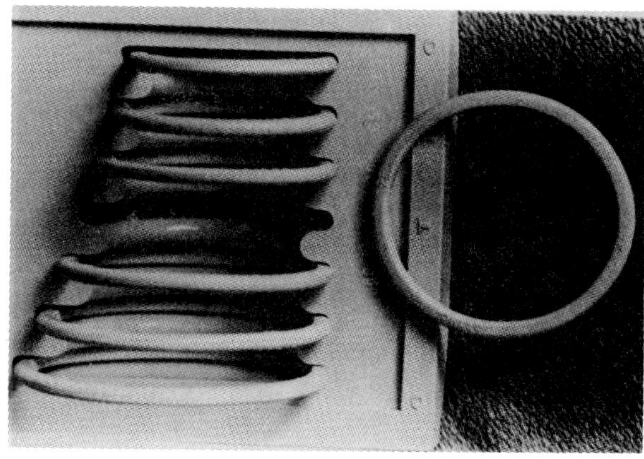

Figure 13-5.
Diaphragm fitting rings.

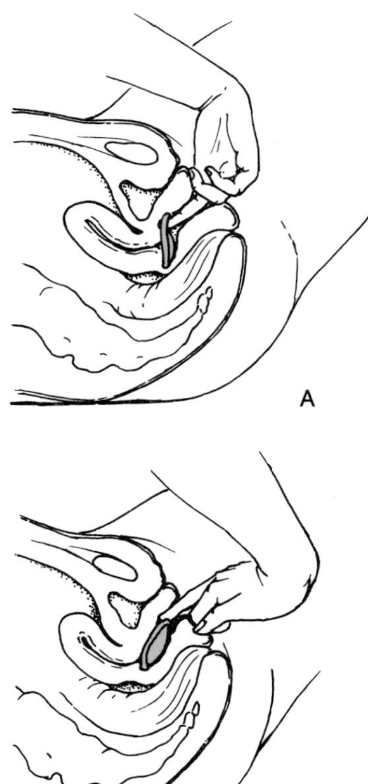

Figure 13-6.
Removal of diaphragm. *(A)* A finger is hooked around the diaphragm rim just below the symphysis pubis; diaphragm is pulled forward. *(B)* Alternate method in which a finger is slipped between the diaphragm rim and the symphysis pubis; diaphragm is pulled forward. (Whitley N: A Manual of Clinical Obstetrics. Philadelphia, JB Lippincott. In preparation.)

diaphragm with ease. She should be instructed to always use a spermicidal cream or jelly around the rim and in the dome of the diaphragm. If intercourse occurs a second or third time, additional spermicidal agent should be inserted for added protection. The diaphragm should be left in place for at least six hours following intercourse. A douche is recommended after removal to remove the remaining jelly or cream.

The diaphragm may be an excellent contraceptive for younger, nulliparous women who do not have intercourse with great regularity. In a study at the Sanger Bureau in New York, involving 2175 women over 2 years, an actual failure rate of two pregnancies per 100 users per year was documented. Significantly, most of the women in the study were under 30 (80%) and were unmarried (70%).[19] Proper fitting (a flat or coil-spring diaphragm is generally better for women with firm vaginal tone), thorough contraceptive counseling, and unhurried positive education and practice in insertion and removal are the key factors in the success of this method.

The Condom

Condoms ("rubbers") are thin sheaths of rubber or processed collagenous tissue that are placed over the penis to act as a mechanical barrier to prevent sperm from entering the vagina. Also effective in preventing venereal infections, condoms are a male method of contraception which has been used since ancient times. The condom is applied over the shaft of the penis after erection. Before withdrawal of the penis from the vagina, the condom should be held in place on the penis so that it does not slip off into the vagina. Some condoms are packaged with a lubricant and some have a small pouch at the tip to collect the ejaculate, which reduces the danger of tearing. In some cases, lubricants cause an irritation at the introitus and an unpleasant "stinging" sensation. In general, a lubricant should not be necessary if there is sufficient foreplay to produce the natural lubrication associated with female sexual arousal.

If it is used properly, the condom is an effective contraceptive. However, it must be applied before any penile-vaginal contact. Condoms are advantageous because they are available without a medical prescription, are easy to use, do not present any serious side-effects, are low in cost, and prevent transmission of sexual infections.

The major criticism of condoms is that they decrease sensation for both partners or, more commonly, for the man. In addition, the sex act must be interrupted to apply the condom; this may be distracting for some couples. There is also frequent worry that the condom might break.

The nurse might point out that no method of contraception is perfect (all have some disadvantages for one or both partners and have some anxiety-producing aspects). If they are used before any penetration, condoms are safe and rarely break. This information will help those couples who have anxiety over other forms of contraception.

Natural Methods and Fertility Awareness

The rationale underlying natural methods of birth control based on fertility awareness is that when there are regular periods, ovulation occurs at approximately the same time in each cycle (*i.e.,* 14 days prior to the beginning of the next cycle). The ovum is capable of being fertilized only for a period of 48 hours at the most after ovulation. Theoretically, therefore, abstinence from sexual intercourse on that day and for the two days before and after (a total of five days) should forestall conception.

In actual experience, however, even normal, regular cycles can be off by one or two days in either direction (*e.g.,* 28 ± 2 days). This puts the day of ovulation in the same four day range ± two days, and the period of abstinence must then be at least eight days. Because of the normal variability of menstrual cycles, however, the interval of fertility will often be as long as 15 or more days, or about half of the cycle.

There are three basic variations of natural methods of birth control. One is based on calendar calculations of ovulation, another on use of a record of the basal body temperature to determine ovulation, and the last on noting changes in the condition of cervical mucus for this purpose. Advantages of these methods are that they are devoid of any side-effects that may be caused by introduction of drugs or substances into or on the body; they are relatively inexpensive; they are acceptable to religious groups that oppose other contraceptive methods; and they are very helpful in planning pregnancy due to the familiarity with signs of fertility which result. Disadvantages of these methods include the need to keep records for several menstrual cycles before they can be used, the need for diligent record keeping to assure accuracy, the necessity for considerable initial and ongoing counseling in their use, a restriction of sexual spontaneity, and the need for abstinence or use of another contraceptive method for a considerable portion of the cycle. The inability of some women to recognize clear cervical mucus changes, and the problem of irregular cycles make cervical mucus, calendar and basal body temperature (BBT) methods difficult and unreliable.

Another consideration is the failure rates of these methods, which in actual use are in the range of 21 to 25 pregnancies per 100 women per year. Should pregnancy occur, there is increased risk that an "old" egg will be fertilized. When the ovum and sperm are at their outer limits of functioning, some deterioration has occurred and there are associated increases in fetal abnormalities from such fertilizations.[20] The longevity of sperm adds to this problem, as sperm have been found in cervical mucus as long as seven days after ejaculation.

Calendar Method

A menstrual calendar in which the woman records the length of each menstrual cycle over an eight month span must be kept. With the first day of bleeding counted as day one, the earliest fertile day is computed by subtracting 18 days from the length of the shortest cycle. Subtract 11 days from the length of the longest cycle to determine the latest day of fertility. These two numbers represent the beginning and end of the fertile period. During these days, intercourse must be avoided or another method of birth control used (Table 13-5).

This method is more effective if the woman has regular cycles, and if intercourse is avoided (or other forms of contraception are used) through the entire first part of the menstrual cycle until the last fertile day. Women who are younger, postpartum, postabortion, and premenopausal often have irregular menstrual cycles, so this method may be contraindicated unless it is the only acceptable method. In this case, it should be supplemented by the BBT or cervical mucus method to increase effectiveness.

Basal Body Temperature Method

The resting or BBT of a fertile woman normally rises each cycle just after ovulation. It will then remain higher until the next menstrual period begins. Most women can observe this temperature change if they take and record their temperature every day with a special thermometer before they get out of bed or begin any kind of activity, including smoking. The thermometer can be used orally or rectally, and should be left in place a full five minutes. It is recorded on a special BBT chart (see Chap. 8, Fig. 8-5).

There is usually a slight drop and then a rise of about 0.4 degrees to 0.8 degrees when ovulation has occurred. This rise should be sustained until the next menstrual period. However, some .women have no preliminary drop before the BBT rises. Because the woman cannot know that she has ovulated until after it has happened, it is best to use another method of contraception or to avoid intercourse the entire first part of the cycle, until the sustained rise in BBT is seen. The fertile period can be assumed to end after the BBT has remained elevated for three full days.

Many factors such as illness, nightmares, and changes in daily schedule can influence the BBT. When the pattern of rise is not clear or sustained, it is

Table 13-5.
Calculating the Interval of Fertility

No of Days Shortest Cycle	First Fertile Day	No of Days Longest Cycle	Last Fertile Day
21	3rd day	21	10th day
22	4th day	22	11th day
23	5th day	23	12th day
24	6th day	24	13th day
25	7th day	25	14th day
26	8th day	26	15th day
27	9th day	27	16th day
28	10th day	28	17th day
29	11th day	29	18th day
30	12th day	30	19th day
31	13th day	31	20th day
32	14th day	32	21st day
33	15th day	33	22nd day
34	16th day	34	23rd day
35	17th day	35	24th day

advisable to assume it is not safe to have intercourse. This method is more effective when combined with the calendar or mucus methods, which give earlier signs that ovulation is near.

Cervical Mucus Method

Many women can observe physiologic changes relating to ovulation which help determine when their fertile period begins. Changes in the character and appearance of cervical mucus occur just before ovulation in some women. In addition, ovulatory pain may be experienced. Characteristically, in the ovulatory cycle there is a rapid increase in the quantity of cervical mucus just prior to ovulation. At that time, the mucus becomes clear and stringy. The patient may observe the presence of such mucus at the introitus or may wipe the cervix to obtain a sample for observation. Subsequent to ovulation, mucus becomes more viscous. When this change is associated with a rise in temperature, it is assumed that ovulation has occurred.

The woman must be careful not to confuse other substances in the vagina, such as semen, lubricants, spermicides and discharges due to infections with cervical mucus at midcycle. Women who douche cannot observe changes because they wash the mucus away. This method is more effective when intercourse is restricted to the postovulatory phase of the cycle and when it is used in combination with the calendar or BBT methods.

Women need to observe their mucus changes for several cycles before relying upon this method. They need to check vaginal secretions several times a day and record the most fertile observation for that day. The peak of fertility occurs when the vagina feels very wet, mucus is abundant, clear, slippery, and very stretchable (can be stretched 3–4 in between the thumb and forefinger). When this type of mucus has decreased and is no longer detectable, there may be thick, cloudy sticky mucus or no mucus. When this change is observed, the woman is no longer fertile.

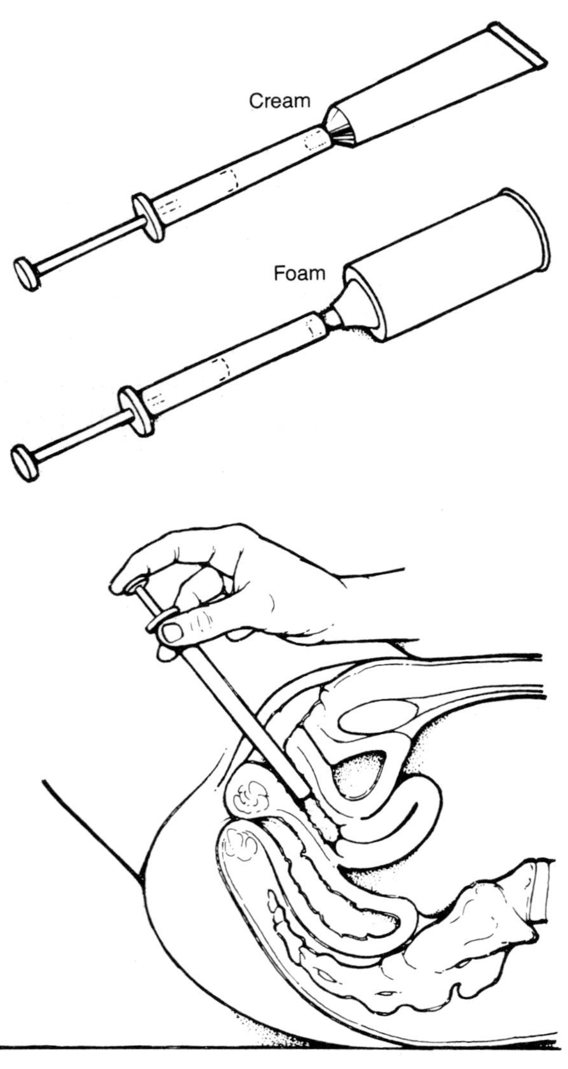

Figure 13-7.
Insertion of foam or cream near the cervix.

Jellies, Creams, Suppositories, and Foams

These contraceptives are inexpensive and available without consulting a physician. However, they are relatively ineffective, because the woman cannot be sure of the placement or the retention of the spermicidal agent (Fig. 13-7). For proper use, the spermicidal agent should be inserted vaginally no more than one half hour before intercourse; a separate application must be made for each act of intercourse. In addition, the woman should not douche for at least eight hours after intercourse. The aerosol foams expand rapidly when inserted, covering the vaginal folds and seeming to disappear. They also leave less vaginal residual than jellies or creams, which take longer to spread over the vaginal surface.

The major disadvantage of spermicides is their low effectiveness when used alone. Many couples find them aesthetically unpleasant, and there is limited usefulness for repeated acts of intercourse. However, these preparations are particularly useful as short-term contraceptives. During the postpartum period, spermicides are useful until the six-weeks checkup, when a more effective method can be instituted. They are frequently recommended for two weeks to one month after insertion of an IUD or initiation of an oral contraceptive regimen, as a precaution before these methods should be relied on alone. When the pill or IUD is discontinued, spermicides can be used for a few cycles until another method is begun or pregnancy is attempted.

Withdrawal

Withdrawal, or *coitus interruptus,* is an extensively used method of contraception and appears to be satisfactory for some couples. However, withdrawal as a method of contraception is a compromise at best. It requires concentration and willpower on the part of the male and trust on the part of the female. This trust is not always well founded and creates anxiety. Neither of these factors is conducive to relaxation and pleasure and may leave the couple with a distorted idea of what sexual pleasure is or can be. Also, preejaculatory secretion may contain motile spermatozoa, especially when there has been prolonged erection.

Withdrawal is one of the more ineffective contraceptive methods, with a failure rate of about 20 to 25 pregnancies per 100 woman years. However, it is always available and costs nothing. This method, often used by young people just beginning their sexual activities, can contribute to later sexual difficulties through a conditioning process. When intercourse occurs in circumstances associated with haste, fear, and guilt, and withdrawal is used in a way that interferes with communication and fulfillment, patterns of premature ejaculation in the male and orgasmic dysfunction in the female may be established.

Unreliable Approaches

Douching after intercourse is actually not a contraceptive method. Sperm enter the cervix within 20 seconds of ejaculation, and it is highly unlikely that douching could occur before this time. The douche must simply be considered a method of cleansing the vagina or a means of inserting a medicated solution to treat vaginal infections.

Lactation has been considered a method of postponing pregnancy by delaying ovulation. It is widely used in developing countries with some effectiveness for varying periods of months which is probably related to the nutritional status of the mother. However, in the United States, women generally have good nutrition, and the lactation period is shorter because infants are given formula supplements and solid foods at an earlier age. These factors contribute to an earlier and unpredictable return of fertility, making breast feeding an unreliable approach to contraception.

Postpartal Contraception

In the absence of complications, intercourse is commonly resumed 2 weeks to 3 weeks following delivery. The practice of advising couples to abstain from intercourse for 6 weeks has generally been discarded because there is no reason to avoid sex once lochia has ceased and the episiotomy is adequately healed. Although the incidence of ovulation within the first six weeks postpartum is small, fertility does occasionally return and women are well advised to use a contraceptive method during this time. The condom is probably the most practical method to use during this period because it does not involve introducing chemicals into the vagina. However, spermicidal foams and creams are frequently advised, either in combination with the condom or alone, if the condom is unacceptable. If foams and creams are not used too early in the postpartum period, there does not appear to be a problem with infection.

Insertion of an IUD within the first 6 weeks postpartum is generally not recommended, as the expulsion and infection rates are higher during this time. Oral contraceptives are contraindicated because of the increased incidence of thromboembolic complications associated with their use in the postpartum period. Nursing mothers are usually advised not to use oral contraceptives because lactation may be suppressed and because these synthetic hormones are excreted in breast milk.

Sterilization

Vasectomy in the male and tubal ligation in the female are being used with increasing frequency as a means of limiting family size. Since both are permanent methods of contraception, the decision to undergo these procedures must be very carefully considered. In many settings, the role of the nurse in the decision-making process is pivotal. The counselor is responsible for making sure that both husband and wife are aware that these methods are considered irreversible.

Total family circumstances which could influence the decision should be reviewed in depth and such factors as the number of children, stability of the marriage, age of marital partners, and ability to use nonpermanent methods should be considered.

In the United States, sterilization is the most commonly used method of contraception for married couples over 30 years of age. Approximately 11.5 million adults have been sterilized in the United States. The following laws and regulations are important in counseling couples about sterilization:

1. Strict adherence to informed consent procedures and voluntary choice are absolutely essential, both legally and practically.
2. There is no legal requirement for partner consent.
3. When federal funds are used, patients must be 21 years old and mentally competent.
4. Federal and some state regulations relating to use of Medicaid funds for sterilization require prescribed waiting periods of various lengths after counseling, and before the procedure can be performed.[4]

Vasectomy

The *vas deferens* is a tube that leads from the testis to the urethra in the male and carries spermatozoa from the testis to the urethra. It is a firm structure somewhat less than 0.5 cm in diameter that can be felt bilaterally in the scrotum, lateral to the base of the penis. *Vasectomy* involves surgical interruption and ligation of

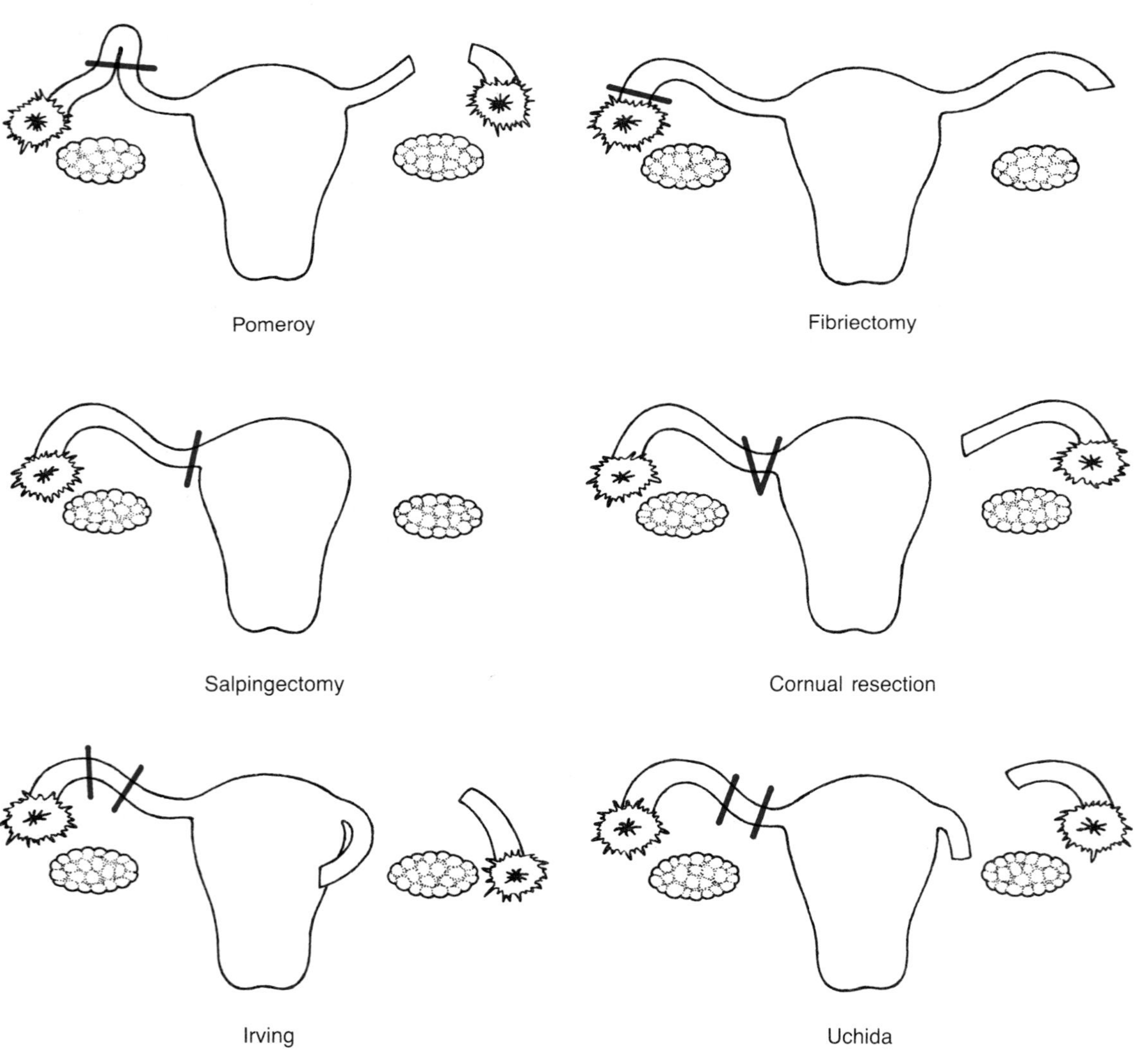

Figure 13-8.
Tubal ligation techniques. (Redrawn from Shain RN, Pauerstein CJ: Fertility Control. Hagerstown, MD, Harper & Row, 1980)

the vas and is a relatively minor operation. It can be carried out under local anesthesia and is associated with minimal risk and only slight morbidity. It is a simple procedure that takes about 15 minutes and can be done on an outpatient basis.

The major disadvantage is that it is permanent. Although surgical methods have been developed to reanastomose the ligated vas, the success rate is low. Even when a channel is recreated, the spermatozoa that subsequently appear in the ejaculate are not always normal, as they are affected by sperm antibodies which sometimes are produced after ligation.

Vasectomy failure is the result of recannulization of the ends of the ligated vas and occurs in 0.15 per 100 cases. Additional pregnancies occur following vasectomy when unprotected intercourse takes place before the male reproductive tract is cleared of spermatozoa. Couples must be advised that the first few postvasectomy ejaculates contain active spermatozoa. Except for the absence of spermatozoa, vas ligation does not affect the ejaculate itself, nor does it affect the ejaculatory process.

The fear of a reduction of potency or masculinity prevents many men from accepting vasectomy. However, the vast majority of men who have had vasectomies are satisfied with their decision and report that sexual performance is unchanged. Less than 2% report decreased sexual pleasure or other dissatisfaction with vasectomy.

Tubal Ligation

Tubal ligation is designed to eliminate the passage that spermatozoa and ova pass through. A number of approaches have been used to interrupt the continuity of the fallopian tubes (Fig. 13-8). The procedure may be carried out by way of an abdominal incision and is commonly done along with cesarean section or in the first few postpartal hours. Many workers in the family planning field now feel that patients should be encouraged not to accept a permanent form of contraception during emotionally charged intervals in their lives. An "on the spot" decision to have a tubal sterilization following an abortion or delivery should be explored with great care.

Coagulation and interruption of the fallopian tubes can be carried out using a *laparoscopic approach* (Fig. 13-9). In some centers this procedure is carried out under local anesthesia, but usually a general anesthetic is used. After the abdomen is distended with carbon dioxide, the laparoscopic trocar is introduced through a small incision in the umbilicus. The laparoscope is then passed into the peritoneal cavity. Visualization of the adnexa is usually complete. A coagulating instrument is used as the fallopian tubes are grasped, coagulated, and severed.

Because the procedure is relatively simple, it can be carried out on an outpatient basis. Although it is associated with a relatively low morbidity, the morbidity is considerably higher than for vas ligation.

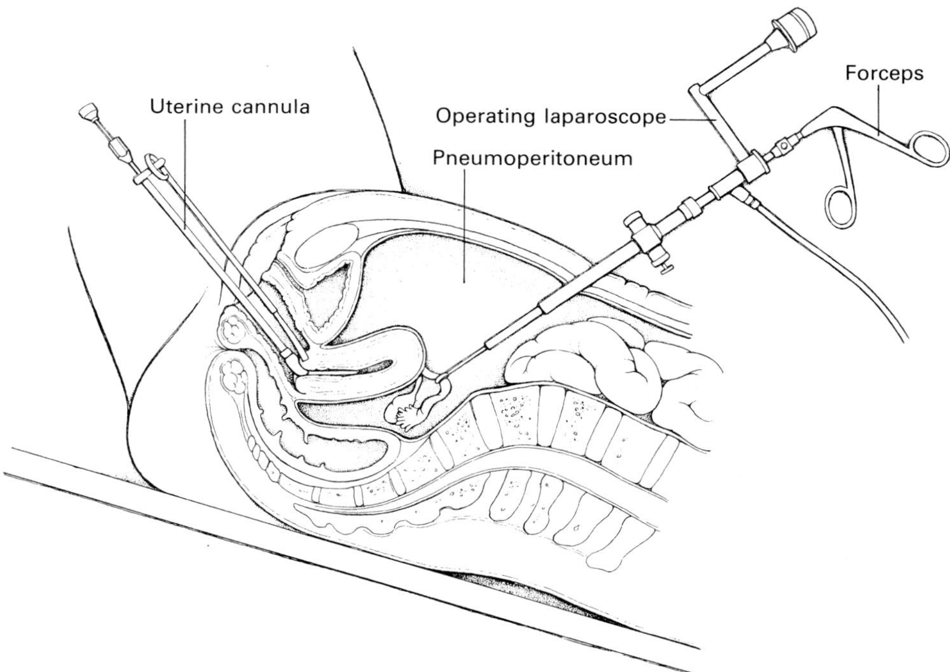

Figure 13-9.
One-incision technique using the operating laparoscope.

The *interval mini-laparotomy* is a sterilization technique in which a small suprapubic incision is usually made below the pubic hair line in order to enter the abdominal cavity. The fallopian tubes are isolated with grasping instruments and may be crushed, ligated, imbedded, clipped, or plugged as in other tubal ligation methods. About two days of hospitalization and a general anesthetic are required.

Most women who undergo tubal ligation are satisfied with their decision, but about 10% to 15% regret the termination of fertility or express other dissatisfactions, including diminished sexual enjoyment, dysmenorrhea, menorrhagia-metrorrhagia, and premenstrual tension. Although tubal interruption theoretically has no effects on hormone cycles, it is possible that interference with lymphatic and vascular drainage secondary to scar tissue formation could contribute to increased pelvic congestion.

Although tubal ligation must be considered a permanent method, surgical techniques have been developed to reunite the fallopian tubes. These are difficult procedures at best. The success rate is variable, depending upon the experience of the surgeon and the extent of the segment of tube which was damaged or removed. A decision to attempt reanastomosis is usually based on social circumstances—the death of a child, divorce and remarriage, or an agonizing reappraisal of an earlier decision which was made in haste.

New and Experimental Methods

Hormonal methods of contraception involving injections of a long-acting progesterone, medroxyprogesterone acetate, every three months are available and seem to be as effective as oral contraceptions. However, there are side-effects such as irregular bleeding, amenorrhea, and possible delayed fertility after discontinuation. Several other new methods are under study. Subdermal Silastic capsules containing progestins are being tested as a method of reversible long-term contraception, as are hormone impregnated Silastic endocervical devices and vaginal pessaries or rings. These devices are inserted each month after menstruation and left in place for 21 days, with dose-related effectiveness lower than that of combination pills. Major side-effects are irregular bleeding and amenorrhea. Tests are also being conducted on a long-acting estrogen, quinestrol, which is taken once a month, stored in body fat and gradually released. Effectiveness is comparable to that of minipills (progestin only), and nausea and amenorrhea are the major side-effects.

Luteinizing hormone releasing hormone (LHRH) is involved in the most promising research effort for contraception that is currently underway. Synthetic analogues of the LHRH with many times the potency of the natural molecule are undergoing clinical trials in two groups of women. Two modes of female contraception are possible with LHRH analogues—ovulation inhibition and luteolysis (interference with progesterone secretion by the corpus luteum, which prepares the uterine lining for implantation). In the first approach the analogues prevent normal maturation of the egg in the follicle by interfering with the buildup of LH and FSH in the early part of the cycle, and with the final gonadotropic surge that triggers the release of the ovum. In the second approach, the luteal phase of the second half of the menstrual cycle is disrupted, rendering the endometrium unfavorable to implantation. A major advantage of the LHRH analogues is that they are polypeptides rather than steroids, with more specific sites of action and remaining in the body for shorter periods of time than steroids. LHRH also holds possibilities as a male contraceptive, and is undergoing male clinical trials. Its promise is in differentiated LH and FSH responses in men; FSH must be depressed to suppress spermatogenesis, while LH must remain high enough to maintain secondary male sex characteristics and sex drive. Preliminary results indicate that LHRH does just that, and tests of two regimens of LHRH analogues in men seek further confirmation of its contraceptive potential.

Gossypol, a derivative of cottonseed oil which has been developed and used by the Chinese as a male contraceptive, is currently in preclinical testing in the United States. The drug suppresses sperm production and affects the structure and motility of sperm in the epididymis. It is excreted slowly and side-effects include weakness, gastric discomfort, nausea and reduced appetite, and decreases in sex drive. Fertility is reported in Chinese trials to return in about three months. Gossypol is currently being tested in animals in the United States, but species variability in response may make it difficult to obtain enough animal data for approval of human tests.

Other methods being investigated include testosterone as a male contraceptive to suppress spermatogenesis, a vaginal ring and IUD designed to provide controlled release of steroids into the female reproductive tract and inhibit sperm transport, several chemical agents as potential postcoital contraceptives and menses inducers, and two injectable contraceptives (a progestin-only product and Depo-

NC **Nursing Care: Contraception**

Method—Assessment	Intervention	Evaluation
All types		
Understanding of sexuality, characteristics of sexual activity (*i.e.,* regular or occasional intercourse, one or several partners) Knowledge of contraceptives and understanding of their use Satisfaction and dissatisfaction with previous contraceptive practices Menstrual and pregnancy history General health history Expectations of benefits from contraceptive method Concerns about various methods related to religious affiliation, life style, and values such as naturalism	Reinforce accurate knowledge Teach correct information, clear misconceptions Provide information about methods not well understood Provide feedback about effectiveness rates, reasons why method not effective Provide feedback about risks and contraindications of various methods Reinforce accurate expectations, clear misconceptions Discuss various methods, mechanisms of action, and implications	Affirms understanding, no further questions Able to select method and feel comfortable with it Effective contraceptive use (*i.e.,* no unwanted pregnancies)
Oral contraceptives		
Determine if contraindications are present from history and physical examination Explore understanding of requirements for this method to be effective (*i.e.,* regularity of pill taking)	Advise if contraindicated Discuss regular use of medication, need for periodic checkup, blood pressure, and Pap smears Explain how to begin and discontinue pills Discuss side-effects, serious complications, when to seek medical care, what to do if one or more pills are forgotten Discuss advantages and disadvantages	Finds method suitable and uses effectively
IUD		
Determine if contraindications are present from history and physical examination Explore understanding of requirements for this method to be effective (*i.e.,* checking IUD strings)	Advise if contraindicated Discuss techniques and experience of IUD insertion and removal, need for periodic checkup and Pap smears Explain method, discuss side-effects, serious complications, and when to seek medical care Note when IUD must be replaced if they contain copper or hormone Discuss advantages and disadvantages	Finds method suitable and uses effectively

(Continued)

NC Nursing Care: Contraception (continued)

Method—Assessment	Intervention	Evaluation
Diaphragm		
Determine if contraindications are present from history and physical examination Explore understanding of requirements for this method to be effective (*i.e.*, insertion/removal techniques, checking for tears, using with every act of intercourse)	Advise if contraindicated Discuss insertion/removal techniques, instruct and have patient practice until correctly done Explain method and necessity for constant use, applying more spermicide with additional acts of intercourse, and for leaving in 6–8 hours Advise that diaphragm must be refitted after each delivery and if substantial amount of weight is lost or gained Discuss advantages and disadvantages	Finds method suitable and uses effectively
Fertility Awareness		
Explore understanding of requirements for this method to be effective (*i.e.*, long periods of abstinence, regular menstrual periods, ancillary techniques to increase effectiveness)	Discuss methods to establish baseline menstrual patterns and identify ovulation Instruct on calculating fertile period Discuss advantages and disadvantages	Finds method suitable and uses effectively
Spermicides and condom		
Explore understanding of requirements for this method to be effective (*i.e.*, timing of application, regular use, precautions to avoid leakage or decreasing spermicide effectiveness)	Instruct on proper insertion of spermicides and application of condom Advise on repeated acts of intercourse and reapplications, care in condom removal, no douching for 6–8 hours when spermicides are used Discuss advantages and disadvantages	Finds method suitable and uses effectively
Sterilization		
Determine understanding of procedure as ending fertility and irreversible Obtain childbearing history, ages and health of children, marital situation, and values assigned to reproductive role	Discuss permanence of sterilization Explore meanings to couple Explain various procedures and required follow-up	Affirms understanding of permanence, desire to end childbearing; accepts requirements of procedure; satisfied with outcome

Provera) which are undergoing clinical trials sponsored by the WHO.[21]

Despite the promise of some of these methods, especially the LHRH analogues, no widely available contraceptive methods are likely to be developed until the end of the 1980s.

References

1. Birth expectation among U.S. wives. Fam Plann Perspec 7, 1:5–6, January/February 1975

2. Leridon H: Fertility and contraception in 12 developed countries. Fam Plann Perspect 13, 2:93–102, March/April 1981

3. Darity WA, Turner CB: Attitudes toward family planning: A comparison between northern and southern black Americans. Advances in Planned Parenthood 8:13, 1973

4. Hatcher RA, Stewart GK, Stewart F, Guest F et al: Contraceptive Technology 1980–1981, 10th ed. New York, Irvington Publishers, Inc., 1980

5. Hatcher RA et al: Contraceptive Technology 1976–1977, 8th ed. pp 131–132. New York, Halsted Press, Division of John Wiley & Sons, 1976

6. Fisch IR, Freedman SH: Oral contraceptives, ABO blood groups, and in vitro fibrin formation. Obstet Gynecol 46, 4:473–479, 1975

7. Romney SL, Gray MJ, Little AB, Merrill JA et al: Gynecology and Obstetrics: The Health Care of Women. New York, McGraw–Hill, Blakiston Division, 1975

8. Ory HW, Rosenfield A, Landman LC: The pill at 20: An assessment. Fam Plann Perspect 12, 6:278–283, November/December 1980

9. Digest: Cigarettes plus pill: Deadly for women 30 and over. Fam Plann Perspect 9, 1:36, January/February 1977

10. Drug data up-date. Am J Nurs 79, 1:137, January 1979

11. Digest: Black women, unlike white women, not prone to hypertension while using orals, study finds. Fam Plann Perspect 13, 1:40–42, January/February 1981

12. Edmondson HA, Henderson B, Benton B: Liver-cell adenomas associated with use of oral contraceptives. N Engl J Med 294, 9:470–472, February 26, 1976

13. Rooks JB, Ory HW, Ishak KG, Strauss LT et al: Epidemiology of hepatocellular adenoma: The role of oral contraceptive use. JAMA 242:644, 1979

14. Stern MP, Brown BW, Haskell WL, Farquhar JW et al: Cardiovascular risk and use of estrogens or estrogen–progestogen combinations, JAMA 235, 8:811–815, February 23, 1976

15. Janerich DT, Piper JM, Glebatis DM: Oral contraceptives and congenital limb-reduction defects. N Engl J Med 291:697, 1974

16. Heinonen OP, Slone D, Monson RR, Hook EB et al: Cardiovascular birth defects and antenatal exposure to female sex hormones. N Engl J Med 296:67, 1977

17. Vessey M, Meisler L, Flavel R, Yeates D: Outcome of pregnancy in women using different methods of contraception. Br J Obstet Gynecol 86:584, 1979

18. Progestasert IUD and ectopic pregnancy. FDA Bulletin, DHEW–PHS 8, 6:37, December 1978–January 1979

19. Lane M, Arleo R, Sobrero AJ: Successful use of the diaphragm and jelly in a young population: Report of a clinical study. Fam Plann Perspect 8, 2:81–86, March/April 1976

20. Jongbloet PH: Mental and physical handicaps in connection with overripeness ovopathy. Quoted in Ross MA, Pietrow PT: Birth control without contraceptives. Population Reports, Ser. 1 No. 1 June 1974 Washington DC, The George Washington Medical Center.

21. Benditt JM: Current contraceptive research. Fam Plann Perspect 12, 3:149–155, 1980

CHAPTER 14

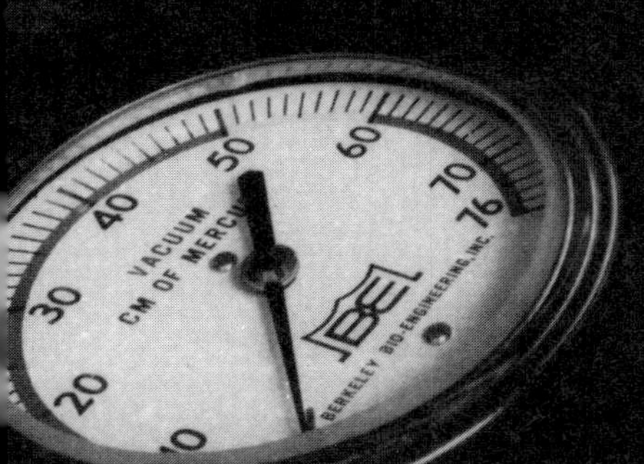
VACUUM
BERKELEY BIO-ENGINEERING, INC.
20
30
40
50
60
70
76

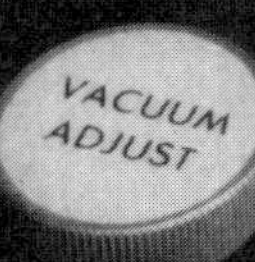
VACUUM
ADJUST

CHAPTER 14

Pregnancy Termination

The elective termination of pregnancy is sought by women for a variety of reasons including health, economics, marital status, family stability, the circumstances of conception, personal goals, age, and many other social and psychological factors. Most societies control or regulate abortion procedures in varying degrees. Whether the society's approach is permissive or restrictive depends on several factors—culture, economy, and ecology. For example, the existence of a predominant religion in a country can affect abortion laws and practices, as can the country's economic or sociopolitical system and its population trends, level of technology, and standard of living. In general, attitudes toward abortion and the availability of abortion procedures are strongly influenced by prevailing societal values.

Women have long sought abortion as a solution to unwanted pregnancy, regardless of whether their culture approved or disapproved of this practice. Although accurate abortion statistics are difficult to obtain, especially in countries where the procedure is illegal, it is estimated that from 30 to 55 million pregnancies are willfully terminated each year throughout the world. In the United States, the abortion ratio is reported at about 500 abortions per 1000 live births, although this varies with the area of the country.[1] Scandinavia, Japan, and Eastern European countries preceded the United States in liberalizing abortion laws and making legal abortion widely available. Prior to 1973, the United States had restrictive abortion laws which generally allowed "therapeutic" abortion only when the mother's life or health were threatened by the pregnancy, or when the pregnancy had resulted from felonious intercourse (rape, incest). Some states permitted the procedure when there was substantial risk that the child would be born with a serious physical or mental defect.

In 1973 a substantial change occurred in the legal status of pregnancy termination in the United States when the Supreme Court announced a decision to legalize abortion. This decision left the choice for abortion, before the end of the first trimester, to the judgment of the pregnant woman and her physician. During the second trimester, the state can regulate the circumstances of abortion to ensure safety, but cannot otherwise interfere with the decision. When pregnancy is advanced beyond the second trimester, state law determines what can and cannot be done. States can regulate and even proscribe abortion subsequent to viability, which is defined to be between 24 and 26 weeks gestation, except when necessary for the preservation of the life or health of the mother. As the result of the changed legal status, pregnancy terminations are now being sought and obtained in large numbers throughout the United States.

The number of abortions in the United States has been steadily increasing since 1973. Just under one million abortions were performed in 1975, and over 1.5 million abortions were performed in 1979. The rate of increase in abortions has been slowing down, however, since 1975 when it was 15% to 1979 when projections were for a 9% increase. Abortion services are highly concentrated in metropolitan areas, with only about 5% of abortions performed in nonmetropolitan counties, although 26% of women estimated in need of abortion services live in these more rural areas.[2] Table 14-1 presents statistics on the number of reported abortions in the United States.

Table 14-1
Abortion Rates and Ratios in the United States: 1973–1979

	1973	1974	1975	1976	1977	1978	1979
Abortion rates (Abortions per 1000 women between 15 and 44 years of age)	16.6	19.6	22.1	24.5	26.9	28.2	30.2
Abortion ratio (Abortions per 1000 live births 6 months later)	193	220	249	265	286	294	303

Henshaw S, Forrest JD, Sullivan E, Tietze C: Abortion in the United States, 1978-1979. Fam Plann Perspect, 13/1:6–18, 1981

Legal Status of Abortion

In 1973 the United States Supreme Court ruled that abortion was legal; a summary of the decision follows:

1. The abortion decision and its implementation must be left to the judgment of the woman and her physician when pregnancy is in the first trimester.
2. After the first trimester and before the end of the second trimester, the state, in promoting its interest in the health of the pregnant woman, may choose to regulate abortions in ways that are reasonably related to health.
3. After pregnancy has reached the time of viability (defined as 24 to 26 weeks gestation), the state, in promoting its interest in the potentiality of human life, may, if it chooses, regulate and even proscribe abortion except where it is necessary, in medical judgment, to preserve the life or health of the pregnant woman.

In 1976, the Supreme Court further ruled that the state cannot impose the requirement of consent by a third party on the woman's right to abortion, thus abortion cannot be denied if a spouse or parent objects.

In 1976 the United States Congress passed the Hyde Amendment, which forbids the expenditure of federal funds for abortion services except in cases where continuation of the pregnancy threatens the woman's life. Although the constitutionality of this law was challenged in courts, the United States Supreme Court declared the Hyde Amendment constitutional in 1980. The result has been a virtual withdrawal of federal funds to subsidize abortions for indigent women. Although some states have continued abortion payments for the poor, this federal restriction has had a significant impact on fertility regulation among poor women (further discussion follows in this chapter).

Availability of legal abortion has dramatically decreased the maternal mortality and morbidity previously associated with illegal, criminal abortion (see Chapter 24, Complications of Pregnancy).

Although abortion is now legal, it is still viewed with misgivings by many because of religious and personal attitudes toward pregnancy termination. Most agree that abortion is not a happy substitute for pregnancy prevention and that the procedures necessary for bringing about termination, though generally safe, are associated with a higher morbidity than are most contraceptive methods.

The nurse must recognize that attitudes toward abortion are varied and personal and that there are strong religious and moral influences in these attitudes. One is entitled to one's own conclusions on this matter but the opinions of others should be respected. Personal convictions of health professionals in this area are generally respected, and those who do not feel that abortion is ethically acceptable should make their views known so that arrangements can be made well in advance for substitute medical personnel.

Psychological Factors Affecting Abortion Decisions

Pregnancy is an event in a woman's life which is surrounded by many positive values, ranging from enhancement of the self-concept to social approval. The highest value placed on women in most societies is their role as mothers, and powerful systems of reinforcement operate to make motherhood central to women's lives. A decision to terminate a pregnancy is rarely taken without some conflict because of the complex meanings and values associated with reproduction and motherhood. Even if the outcome of pregnancy (a child) is consciously unwanted, the woman may on some level desire to be pregnant as a symbol of potency, vitality, or reconnection with primal inner forces. While pregnancy can be completely accidental, it is often used to affect relations with important people in the woman's life, such as parents, husband, or lover.

A teenage girl may become pregnant to demonstrate her maturity, prove her sexuality, or bolster her self-concept as a woman. She may become pregnant because her romantic ideals of motherhood and man–woman relations preclude the use of contraceptives which imply premeditated sexual activity. Or pregnancy may result from sexual experimentation when neither partner takes responsibility for avoiding unwanted consequences. A woman at any age may use pregnancy as a means of alleviating feelings of inadequacy or doubts about her femininity. A woman entering menopause may conceive to reinforce her sexual self-image or to avoid facing the loss of reproductive capacity. Although pregnancy per se may be desired in these instances, the woman may find she cannot face the responsibilities of caring for and raising a child, and so elects abortion as the most reasonable solution.

Marital status can also affect the decision to continue or terminate a pregnancy. Many unmarried women feel incapable of raising a child outside of marriage, although there are increasing numbers of single parents and more social acceptance of this situation. The critical factor is the quality of the man–woman relation and its meaning for the woman in terms of commitment and dependability. Pregnancy has historically been used to force a man into marriage but has proven to be a poor basis on which to build a lifetime relationship. In marriages that are in trouble and facing dissolution, pregnancy may be used as an attempt to prevent a break-up. A woman may also become pregnant, even though she does not truly desire a child, in order to meet her partner's expectation, for example, if the man's sense of masculinity or potency requires that "his woman" become pregnant. In many of these cases, however, the pregnancy does not produce the desired result, and the woman may seek abortion when she realizes that motives for pregnancy were not appropriate for her.

Poor physical or mental health can lead a woman to terminate her pregnancy if pregnancy poses a risk to her life or a drain on her already depleted energies. A life crisis or emotional upheaval may lead a women to feel incapable of coping with pregnancy and motherhood until her life becomes less chaotic.

Abortion may also be chosen when a pregnancy is untimely. Education or professional goals may have higher priority at the time, or pregnancy may occur too early in a marriage or too soon after the birth of a child. Or the couple may feel emotionally or economically unable to manage parenthood. Couples frequently seek abortion for economic reasons. They prefer to strive for a higher standard of living and greater social opportunity for themselves and their children and are unwilling to be subjected to increased material hardship.

Abortion may be sought for eugenic reasons, even if pregnancy and the child are desired. Patients are becoming better informed about the hereditary genetic defects that may be of risk to their offspring. They are taking advantage of screening programs to detect such conditions as Tay-Sachs disease, hemophilia, Down's syndrome, sickle cell disease, and other genetic abnormalities. Awareness of fetal anomalies caused by rubella, exposure to radiation, and teratogenic drugs may cause some women to elect abortion if they have been exposed during the first trimester.

Sociocultural factors play an important role in a decision to seek abortion. If abortion is illegal, the woman risks criminal persecution, and if social values condemn abortion she faces disapproval by peers, family, and community. When abortion is legal and there are generally accepting social values, deciding to have an abortion does not present such a traumatic experience and is usually emotionally well accepted. Studies have demonstrated that there are few negative psychological reactions to abortion when positive attitudes on the part of professional staff encourage acceptance.[3] It also has been shown that psychological sequelae are usually of short duration and reflect the circumstances surrounding abortion and attitudes conveyed by peer groups, family, and health providers.[4]

The rates of admission to psychiatric hospitals were found to be higher among postpartum and postabortion women who were separated, divorced, and widowed than among those currently or never married. Among this latter group, the admissions following abortion were considerably higher than those following delivery. The interaction of stress, lack of social support, and reversal of original intention for a previously desired pregnancy was felt to account for the higher rates among postabortion women.[5]

In a longitudinal study of children born to women who had been denied an abortion for that pregnancy, persistent and significant differences were found between children in the study group and those in control groups. When the children were nine years of age, the study group children had a higher incidence of illness despite the same biological start in life, had poorer grades in school despite the same levels of intelligence, and had worse integration in the peer group. At ages 14 to 16, more children in the study group did not continue into secondary education but began jobs without vocational training, and found their mothers inconsistent in emotional behavior toward them. In the latest report, when these children were 16 to 18 years of age, the boys in the study group more often reported that they felt neglected or rejected by their mothers than the controls; however, no difference could be found among the girls. These boys also felt that their parents' marriages were less happy, that they were insufficiently informed about sexual matters (especially contraception), and that they held more conservative views on such social issues as resolution of unplanned pregnancies, divorce, and coping with alcohol and drugs. The study concluded that "unwantedness" during early pregnancy constitutes a significant risk factor for the subsequent life of the child.[6]

Social Factors Affecting Abortion Decisions

Although the United States law places no restrictions on early abortions, and very few requirements for later abortions, this does not mean that every woman who desires to terminate a pregnancy can do so. The ability to obtain an abortion is greatly influenced by such factors as availability and accessibility of abortion facilities, methods of financing health-care services, and personal and economic resources. Other restrictions such as waiting periods between request for abortion and obtaining the procedure, parental consent and notification for minors, spousal consent and notification, residency requirements, hospital prohibitions, and requiring a second physician's certification all present barriers to obtaining abortions.

For women with health insurance or adequate means to pay for an abortion, the main problem may be a lack of abortion facilities. Eight out of every ten counties in the United States have no facility where legal abortions are performed. It is estimated that about one fourth of the women in need of abortion services reside in these counties, which have no physician, clinic or hospital that would perform abortions. Over one million women would need to travel to other counties to seek abortions, and it is likely that a large proportion of these women could not obtain abortion services at all. In 1978, 77% of all United States counties had no identified abortion facility, and 84% had no facility reporting more than two abortions per month. When services are so minimal, it is presumed that procedures are limited to physicians' regular patients or to medical emergencies. Approximately 434,000 women in need of abortion services live in such underserved counties.[2]

Abortion rates vary widely among the states, from highs of 173 abortions per 1000 women age 15 to 44 in the District of Columbia and 46 abortions per 1000 women in California and New York, to lows of 7 abortions per 1000 in West Virginia and Mississippi and 9 abortions per 1000 women in South Dakota and Idaho. In 1978, 113,000 women obtained abortions outside their home states (8% of total abortions performed in 1978). This has decreased from 21% needing to travel out of state in 1973, indicating a gradual increase in available services (Table 14-2). Those states with the lowest abortion rates also had the highest proportion of residents obtaining abortions in out-of-state facilities. See Table 14-3 for the abortion rates of all the states and the proportions obtained in and out of state.

Metropolitan areas contain most of the abortion facilities. In 1978 there were 2753 facilities where abortions were performed, representing a 2% increase over 1977. However, 2% of the women in need of abortion services could not get them in 1979. Of these, an estimated 641,000 women had unintended births. Based on surveys done by the Alan Guttmacher Institute and the Center for Disease Control, United States Department of Health and Human Services (DHHS), over 2 million women were in need of abortion services in 1978. Twenty-seven percent of these women lived in counties where abortion services were unavailable.[2]

The situation for poor women is made more difficult by the enactment of the Hyde Amendment which restricts the use of public funds to provide abortions for indigent women. As a result of this amendment, federal funding of Medicaid abortions fell by 99%. Many states adopted the Hyde restrictions, or narrower ones, instead of picking up the costs of abortions for poor women. Some of the more populous states, namely New York, California, Pennsylvania, Michigan and Illinois maintained more liberal standards for Medicaid abortions, however, and paid almost the entire cost from state monies. In fiscal year (FY) 1978, 99% of abortions were funded with state funds only, and 1% involved federal funding. The District of Columbia and 18 states spent over 51 million dollars in FY 1978 to provide 191,700 abortions for which federal funding was unavailable. Those states with liberal policies accounted for 98% of all public

Table 14-2
Percentage of Women Traveling Out of State to Obtain Abortions

Year	Percent
1973	21
1974	12
1975	10
1976	10
1977	9
1978	8

Table 14-3
Abortion Rates in All States in 1978

Abortion rate per 1,000 women aged 15–44 in 1978, by state of occurrence and of residence; and total number of abortions obtained by state residents in and outside of state of residence (and percentage performed out of state), according to state, 1978

State	Abortion rate		Abortions				
	Occurrence (1)	Residence (2)	By residence Total no. (3)	No. obtained in-state (4)	No. obtained out-of-state (5)	% obtained out-of-state (6)	Total no., by occurrence (7)
United States total	28.2	28.2	1,409,600	1,296,640	112,960	8	1,409,600
Ala.	17.6	19.3	16,510	13,770	2,740	17	15,120
Alaska	23.0	27.5	3,110	2,580	530	17	2,600
Ariz.	22.9	23.3	13,650	13,080	570	4	13,370
Ark.	10.4	14.0	6,930	4,930	2,000	29	5,150
Calif.	45.7	45.4	232,700	231,470	1,230	1	234,520
Colo.	28.5	26.6	18,480	18,020	460	2	19,800
Conn.	25.4	28.6	20,040	17,660	2,380	12	17,800
Del.	24.2	29.8	4,270	3,170	1,100	26	3,470
D.C.	173.4	82.5	14,680	14,280	400	3	30,850
Fla.	32.2	28.6	56,460	56,010	450	1	63,470
Ga.	29.2	28.2	34,950	31,570	3,380	10	36,080
Hawaii	33.0	31.9	6,870	6,850	20	*	7,090
Idaho	9.0	13.2	2,650	1,680	970	37	1,800
Ill.	27.6	27.6	70,250	65,220	5,030	7	70,280
Ind.	12.8	20.5	24,650	15,030	9,620	39	15,340
Iowa	12.1	14.3	8,920	6,220	2,700	30	7,530
Kans.	25.4	17.0	8,630	7,750	880	10	12,870
Ky.	15.6	16.1	12,910	10,350	2,560	20	12,470
La.	14.7	14.3	12,970	12,280	690	5	13,290
Maine	20.9	22.0	5,420	5,040	380	7	5,150
Md.	25.1	37.3	38,230	24,800	13,430	35	25,780
Mass.	31.7	30.4	40,760	39,840	920	2	42,610
Mich.	26.5	25.2	53,870	52,700	1,170	2	56,550
Minn.	19.5	17.0	15,300	14,820	480	3	17,580
Miss.	7.4	14.8	8,080	3,710	4,370	54	4,010
Mo.	14.5	18.8	20,180	13,190	6,990	35	15,570
Mont.	17.2	20.6	3,720	2,980	740	20	3,100
Nebr.	18.8	14.1	5,000	4,630	370	7	6,630
Nev.	38.1	38.9	6,180	5,210	970	16	6,060
N.H.	20.9	23.8	4,520	3,650	870	19	3,980
N.J.	29.1	35.0	57,640	46,650	10,990	19	48,040
N. Mex.	20.9	22.0	6,590	5,910	680	10	6,250
N.Y.	46.1	43.0	174,650	172,830	1,820	1	187,050
N.C.	22.6	22.9	30,510	28,580	1,930	6	30,120
N. Dak.	14.7	9.2	1,410	890	520	37	2,240
Ohio	23.5	23.1	56,170	54,170	2,000	4	57,140
Okla.	17.9	16.8	10,500	9,920	580	6	11,180
Oreg.	26.8	29.5	15,950	13,860	2,090	13	14,450
Pa.	25.3	24.3	62,650	58,640	4,010	6	65,150
R.I.	22.9	26.8	5,350	4,200	1,150	21	4,570
S.C.	18.6	21.8	15,340	12,700	2,640	17	13,050
S. Dak.	9.2	14.3	2,170	860	1,310	60	1,400
Tenn.	23.1	19.5	19,420	18,390	1,030	5	23,040
Tex.	27.4	27.3	82,790	82,030	760	1	83,280
Utah	10.5	12.1	3,650	2,970	680	19	3,150

(Continued)

Table 14-3
Abortion Rates in All States in 1978

Abortion rate per 1,000 women aged 15–44 in 1978, by state of occurrence and of residence; and total number of abortions obtained by state residents in and outside of state of residence (and percentage performed out of state), according to state, 1978

State	Abortion rate		Abortions				
	Occurrence (1)	Residence (2)	By residence Total no. (3)	No. obtained in-state (4)	No. obtained out-of-state (5)	% obtained out-of-state (6)	Total no., by occurrence (7)
Vt.	30.2	29.9	3,260	2,560	700	21	3,290
Va.	24.2	27.5	34,500	28,320	6,180	18	30,370
Wash.	42.1	38.4	31,440	30,870	570	2	34,490
W. Va.	7.1	15.4	6,170	2,400	3,770	61	2,840
Wis.	16.9	15.9	16,510	16,350	160	1	17,510
Wyo.	10.8	20.6	2,040	1,050	990	49	1,070

* Less than 0.5 percent
Henshaw S, Forrest JD, Sullivan, Tietze C: Abortion in the United States, 1978–1979. Fam Plann Perspect, 13, 1:6–18, 1981.

funds expended for abortion services during FY 1978. Ten states had no publically-funded abortions, and another 11 had ten or less publically-funded abortions.[7]

There was a 34% decrease in the number of publically-funded abortions from 1977 to 1978. This aggregate United States figure does not adequately represent the plight of poor women in those states which severely restricted payment from public funds, because it is raised by the efforts of those few states which continued to pay for abortions largely out of state monies. The Alan Guttmacher Institute estimated that nearly one third of the Medicaid-eligible women in need of publically-funded abortion services in 1977 were unable to obtain them. After the Hyde Amendment went into effect in 1978, this figure increased to over 54%[7] (See Table 14-4).

Although the restrictions on publically-funded abortions did not completely eliminate use of federal funds, they have had a major impact. The number of subsidized abortions decreased by more than one third, and in states with restrictive policies regarding use of state funds, abortions for poor women with public support were virtually eliminated. A large estimated unmet need for publically-funded abortions existed before these funding restrictions, and it has increased substantially following the institution of these restrictions.

The impact of this decrease in publically-funded abortions is felt in several ways. Indigent women intent to have abortions often had to delay their abortions while seeking the necessary funds. This leads to an increase in complications because the pregnancy is at a later gestational age and often may mean a more costly procedure for a second trimester abortion. Indigent women who are able to raise the money to pay for their own abortions often do so at the expense of their rent or utility bills, by pawning household goods, diverting food or clothing money, or possibly by fraudulent use of a relative's insurance policy. Some women have been driven to theft. It was found that the price Medicaid-eligible women were paying for abortions was almost the same as those not eligible; they paid the full price themselves. The distress and hardship involved in obtaining or foregoing an abortion is hardly reflected in the statistics; cases have been reported of indigent women attempting self-induced abortion or suicide after being denied publically-funded abortions.[8]

The several tactics used by states to discourage women from seeking abortions also present barriers to fully exercising fertility regulation. Laws vary from state to state and are changing as challenges to their constitutionality are made. Parental consent for minors can be a formidable restriction, leading to delays in the abortion procedure or unintended births to a high-risk teenage mother. Less states require spousal consent, and some make this a requirement only for later (postviability) abortions. States that require a second physician's opinion cause delays in the procedure and increase the cost. Mandatory waiting periods have been overturned in some states and upheld in others. In a survey done of the benefits and drawbacks of mandatory waiting periods, it was found that seven out of ten women required to go through a waiting period disapproved of the delay. They were unable to name a single benefit derived from waiting, and six out of ten women described problems they had including extra expense, missing work or school, inconveniences with transportation

Table 14-4
Publically-Funded Abortions and Unmet Need

	1977	1978	Change
Federal-state Medicaid abortions	294,600	193,800	34% decrease
Estimated need for publically-funded abortions	427,300	427,300	No change
Estimated number of women unable to obtain publically-funded abortions	132,700	233,500	23.6% increase

Gold RB: After the Hyde Amendment: Public funding for abortion FY 1978. Fam Plann Perspect, 12, 3:131–134, 1980

and child care, mental anguish, and entering the second trimester of pregnancy, as a result of the waiting period. Waiting periods raised the cost of the procedure by 48% for low-income women and 14% for higher income women. The women who did find benefits in waiting tended to be younger, to take longer to reach a decision to have an abortion, and did not incur extra transportation expenses. The benefits most often named were having time to reconsider the decision, to adjust psychologically, to learn about medical aspects, and to consider the effects of abortion on others.[9]

Abortion Counseling

The nurse is often a key professional in providing counseling to patients considering abortion. The need to weigh alternatives and make responsible decisions about an unwanted pregnancy may become apparent in the prenatal or family planning clinic or other health-care setting. As part of patient education and the supportive role, the nurse may offer initial discussion and assistance in problem solving to women or couples facing the problem of an undesired conception.

The approach to pregnancy termination varies according to gestational age. Prior to the twelfth week, abortion is generally a relatively uncomplicated vaginal procedure. Beyond the eleventh to twelfth week, termination requires more complex procedures, often involving amniocentesis, for which one to three days of hospitalization is often necessary and the complication rate is considerably higher. Many physicians or hospitals will not perform abortions beyond the 20th to 24th week of gestation.

First trimester abortion may be carried out as an outpatient procedure. Nonhospital facilities have been established, and many hospitals have designed facilities for outpatient procedures. Over 75% of abortions now take place in nonhospital facilities. Personnel in such units should include counselors, whose role is to help the patient evaluate the decision to terminate pregnancy, to review alternate possibilities (having the baby and placing it for adoption), and to provide contraception advice. Termination of a pregnancy is often an emotionally charged situation and must be handled with the greatest skill and delicacy.

Many women need help to think beyond their first reaction to the unwanted pregnancy. They need to be encouraged to consider other options available to them. Many women feel ambivalent and confused and are under pressure from family or their own social values. It is important that the nurse encourages the woman to make the decision for herself, because there is less regret and emotional sequelae when the choice is not perceived as being forced by other people. Exploring alternatives realistically helps clarify the situation and places manageable boundaries within which the decision can be made. Thinking through what each choice means not only for present feelings and relations but also for future circumstances, goals, and needs, both from a practical and emotional-values standpoint, encourages a carefully weighed choice. While the counseling is in progress, tests are carried out to confirm the pregnancy and determine the length of gestation, and the type of abortion procedure indicated is discussed. These factors alone in and of themselves may influence the decision. Simply knowing that the pregnancy has progressed beyond the time when simple curettage can be used and that the abortion may actually involve labor and expulsion of the fetus may cause a woman to decline abortion. In any event, understanding the nature of the procedure required is essential to informed decision making.

Abortion Procedures

The abortion procedure used will depend on the length of the pregnancy. Pregnancies up to 12 weeks gestation are usually terminated by dilatation and evacuation (D and E, suction curettage) or by standard dilatation and curretage (D and C). In the early stages of pregnancy, prostaglandins may be used in the form of vaginal suppositories, intramuscular injections, or transcervical instillation to induce abortion. Or a suctioning method for menstrual extraction or regulation may be carried out by means of a very small cannula (Fig. 14-1). This procedure is occasionally used during the first two weeks after a missed menstrual period, frequently before pregnancy is confirmed. When pregnancy has progressed to between 12 weeks to 14 weeks, termination becomes more difficult. Suction curettage can be used, but the complication rate increases, and intraamniotic instillations of solutions to induce labor are not yet effective. Serial intramuscular injections of prostaglandins (the 15 methyl analogues) have been quite successful in inducing abortion during this time, but with the usual side-effects, including temperature regulation and gastrointestinal symptoms. From 16 weeks to 20 weeks gestation, intraamniotic instillation of hypertonic saline, urea, and prostaglandins are effective.

Techniques Used Prior to 12 Weeks Gestation

Suction Curettage

Increasingly, the procedure of choice for the termination of early pregnancy is *suction curettage* (Figs. 14-2 and 14-3). A local anesthetic (paracervical block) or a light general anesthetic may be used. The cervix is dilated with graduated dilators and a suction curette is placed into the endometrial cavity to the fundus. Suction is applied, usually by an electric pump, and the products of conception are evacuated into a container. These are usually sent to the pathology laboratory for confirmation of the pregnancy and to rule out unusual conditions such as hydatidiform mole. Generally, recovery takes from 2 hours to 3 hours, during which time the patient is observed for excessive bleeding.

In some circumstances, the cervix is prepared for the abortion by the use of *laminaria.* These are lengths of sterile hydroscopic material derived from seaweed, which absorb moisture at a rapid rate. When placed in the cervical canal, they expand in 3 hours to 6 hours and cause cervical dilatation. Insertion of laminaria several hours prior to a first trimester abortion can reduce the need for mechanical cervical dilatation. Some feel that using them decreases the incidence of cervical lacerations. The most common complications of suction curettage are infection, hemorrhage, retained products or blood clots in the uterus, and cervical or uterine trauma.

Surgical (Sharp) Curettage

Standard dilatation and curettage, which are used for first trimester abortions, requires a general anesthetic and the usual preoperative precautions. The cervix must be dilated more than for suction curettage, and there is more danger of cervical laceration and blood loss. The advantage of this technique is that it is widely used and known by family physicians, general practitioners, and obstetrician–gynecologists.

Menstrual Extraction

Aspiration of the endometrium on an outpatient basis performed from 5 weeks to 7 weeks after the last menstrual period is called menstrual extraction, menstrual regulation, menstrual induction, minisuction, miniabortion, and interception. The procedure is simple and relatively atraumatic, little or no cervical

Figure 14-1.
A flexible plastic Karman cannula and a self-locking syringe for menstrual extraction (Rocket of London).

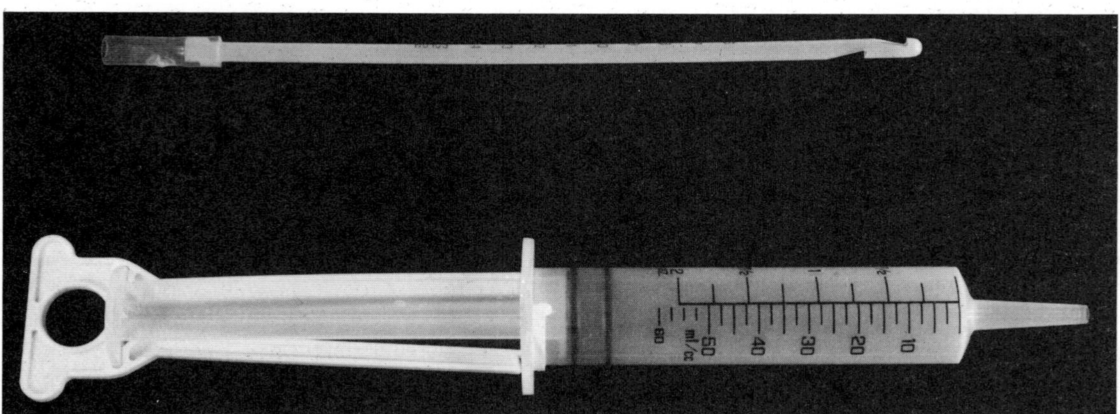

dilatation is required and usually no anesthetic is given. A 4 mm to 6 mm flexible plastic cannula and a syringe or other low pressure suction are used. The uterus does not need to be clinically enlarged, and often a pregnancy test is not required since one of the advantages of the procedure is that the woman need not know for certain if she is pregnant. Although this procedure has been taught and used among women's groups as a self-administered technique, it is not safe to use it this way because of the dangers of hemorrhage, retained products, and infection.

Prostaglandins

Prostaglandins, a group of fatty acids found in the semen, are very effective abortifacients at any stage of pregnancy. The exact mechanisms by which they work are not clearly understood. Oral administration is impractical because of the high incidence of side-effects, the most common being vomiting, diarrhea, fever, and shaking. Vaginal, intramuscular, and transcervical administration produce fewer side-effects and serious complications are rare. Prostaglandins will no doubt be used more frequently as preparations are refined and side-effects are minimized.[10]

Techniques Used after 12 Weeks Gestation

Hypertonic Saline

When pregnancy has progressed beyond the 12th week, termination is often carried out by instilling *hypertonic saline* into the amniotic cavity. This procedure is most easily carried out beyond the 14th week, when there is sufficient fluid in the amniotic cavity to be identified and aspirated. The bladder is emptied, and the patient is placed in the supine position. The skin is prepped and draped with sterile towels, and infiltrated with a local anesthetic over the injection site. An 18-gauge spinal needle is then inserted through the uterus into the amniotic cavity. When properly placed, clear amniotic fluid flows into the syringe attached to the needle. After a small amount of fluid is removed to verify proper placement of the needle, hypertonic saline is injected into the amniotic cavity. Initially, a small amount is placed, and if there is no reaction, the remainder is delivered over approximately 15 minutes.

Following a latent period of several hours, labor usually ensues and the fetus with part or all of the placenta is delivered within 24 hours to 72 hours. If the placenta cannot be extracted completely after delivery, a curettage must be carried out to complete the abortion. During the course of labor, the contractions can cause considerable discomfort. As the cervix dilates, the patient should be medicated at intervals and generally a substantial amount of emotional support is needed during this process. The previable fetus is usually dead at the time of delivery, but at this late stage of gestation it has human form.

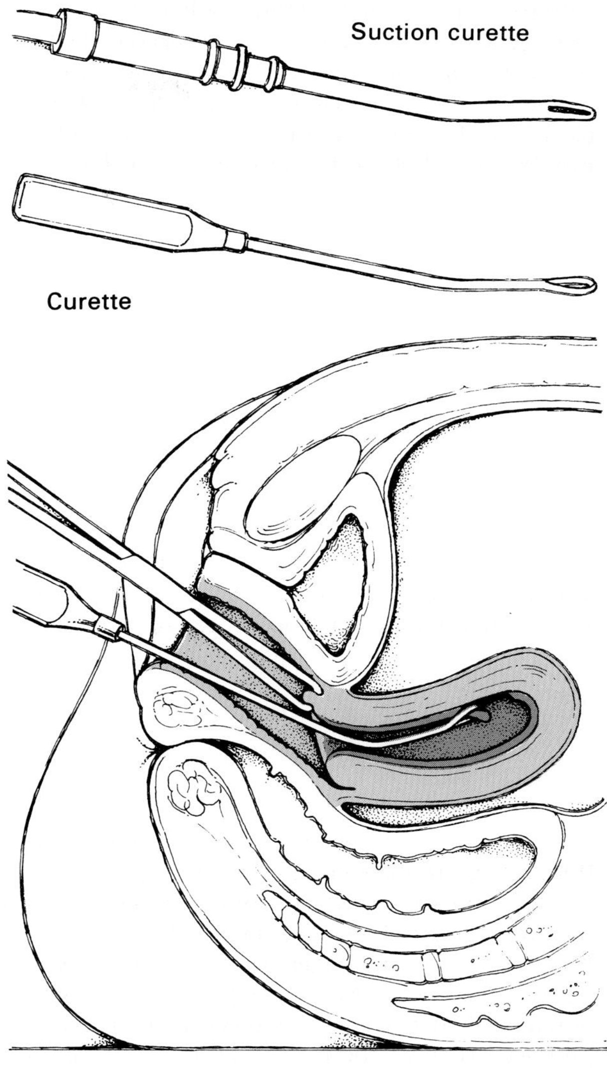

Figure 14-2.
Curettage or vacuum aspiration for first trimester abortion.

Oxytocin infusion is often used as an adjunct to saline abortion to decrease the time needed for completion of the process. Oxytocin is used in a manner similar to that employed for induction of labor (see Chap. 34), except that a more concentrated solution is used. The oxytocin drip is begun six hours to twelve hours after amino infusion of saline. Maximum time of

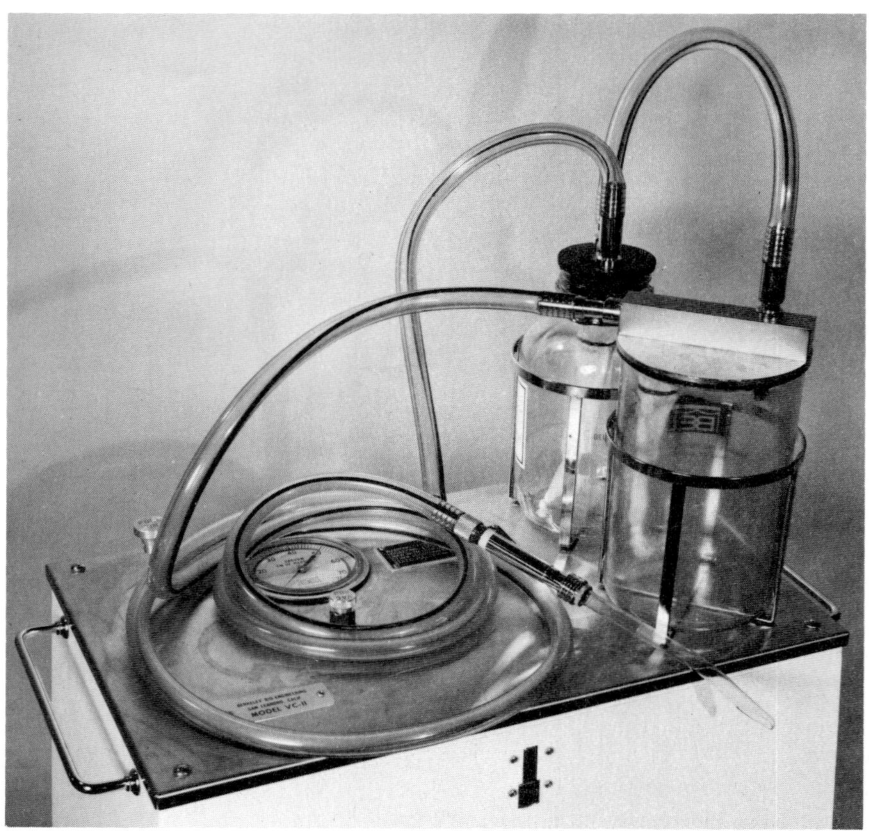

Figure 14-3.
An electric suction apparatus with a swivel handle and a curette. (Model V C II by Berkeley Bio-Engineering, Inc.)

oxytocin use should be limited to 24 hours. If it is used longer, there is an increased incidence of water retention which could lead to water intoxication.

In cases where the hypertonic saline fails to induce contractions, a repeat dose must be administered. In some circumstances, as in severe hypertension, infusion of hypertonic saline is contraindicated. Complications most often include hemorrhage, infection, and retained placenta. Occasionally more serious complications occur as a result of the intravenous injection of saline, including hypernatremia, amniotic fluid embolism, disseminated intravascular coagulation, and necrosis of the myometrium from saline entering the uterine musculature.

Intraamniotic Prostaglandins

Instillation of prostaglandins into the amniotic cavity by a similar amniocentesis technique has become the preferred method of inducing midtrimester abortions because its complication rate is lower than with saline and the onset of labor with subsequent expulsion is more rapid. Medication can be used to control the gastrointestinal side-effects. Women with asthma or pulmonary disease are at increased risk because the drug can cause marked bronchospasm. Other rare serious complications are arrhythmias, cardiovascular changes, and grand mal seizures. These complications are more frequent when the prostaglandins enter systemic circulation; therefore, careful placement in the uterine cavity reduces the incidence of such complications.

Over half of the women given intraamniotic prostaglandins abort within 24 hours, and 93% abort within 48 hours.[11] Although these drugs are more expensive than sodium chloride, this may be offset by shorter hospitalization and fewer complications.

Intramuscular Prostaglandins

Serial intramuscular injections of the 15 methyl analogues of prostaglandins are effective in terminating pregnancies of between 10 weeks and 17 weeks gestation. Contractions begin rapidly and are intense within 40 minutes. Abortion is completed within 12 hours in 76% of the patients and within 24 hours in 96%. One type of prostaglandin causes greater gastrointestinal symptoms, and the other type causes more temperature elevation, shaking, and chills. This method is managed as an inpatient procedure because repeated injections are necessary and labor must be carefully monitored.[12]

Table 14-5
Morbidity and Mortality Rates for Common Methods of Induced Abortion

Type of Complication	D and C	Suction	Saline	Hysterotomy
Hemorrhage	1	0.5	4	3.7
Infection	0.9	0.8	5.4	11
Perforation	1.9	1.3	0.2	5.1
Anesthesia	0.1	0.1	0.1	0.7
Shock	—	—	0.2	0.7
Retained products	0.5	0.5	14.7	1.5
Lacerated cervix	0.3	0.2	0.1	0.7
Other	0.3	0.3	1	4.4
Unspecified	0.1	—	0.2	—
Total morbidity*	5.1	3.7	28.3	27.8
Total mortality†	2.8	1.2	22.9	235.3

*Complications per 1000 abortions
†Deaths per 100,000 abortions
(Martin L: Health Care of Women. Philadelphia, JB Lippincott, 1978)

Hysterotomy

When other methods of midtrimester abortion fail, or saline or prostaglandins are contraindicated for various reasons, a hysterotomy or minicesarean section may be performed. The operation is major surgery and may be done abdominally or vaginally. This procedure requires the standard preoperative preparations and general or spinal anesthesia. The morbidity and mortality from this procedure are greater than for other techniques and a live fetus may be delivered. Advantages of this method include the opportunity for concomitant sterilization by tubal ligation or hysterec-

PE Instructions for Patients Following an Abortion

1. Bleeding and cramps are not unusual for the first 2 weeks following an abortion. Some spotting may occur for as long as 4 weeks after the procedure.
2. The patient should be instructed to seek medical attention if bleeding is severe or if she experiences bleeding that is heavier than the heaviest day of her normal menstrual period for 2 consecutive days.
3. The patient should be instructed to expect her next normal menstrual period to begin in about 4 to 6 weeks except when birth control pills have been prescribed. If birth control pills are used, the normal period should resume at the end of the first month on the pill. If the menstrual period does not resume within 8 weeks, the patient should seek medical attention.
4. The patient should be instructed to use sanitary pads, instead of tampons, for the first week after an abortion to help reduce the chance for infection.
5. The patient should be instructed not to douche during the first week following the abortion to help prevent infection.
6. The patient should be instructed to avoid sexual intercourse for at least the first week following the abortion to help prevent infection.
7. The patient should be instructed to take her temperature twice each day during the first week, preferably at noon and at bedtime. If her temperature reaches 100°F or more she should seek medical attention. Remind the patient that if she is taking aspirin or other pain medications, her temperature should be taken before she takes the medication.
8. The patient should be instructed to seek medical attention if she experiences severe pain, breaks out in a rash or hives, or if the symptoms of pregnancy such as breast tenderness or nausea persist for over a week after the abortion.
9. The patient should be instructed to obtain a follow-up exam 2 weeks after the procedure.

NC Nursing Care: Pregnancy Termination

Assessment	Intervention	Evaluation
Menstrual history and last menstrual period, use of contraceptives Assist in physical examination, collection of specimens, pregnancy tests to determine length of gestation Circumstances surrounding unwanted conception Understanding of physiology of conception and contraceptive methods Level of ambivalence or certainty about abortion decision Involvement of partner, family, parents and sources of support Consideration of alternatives to abortion Presence of crisis, need for further psychological counseling Pregnancy and health history to identify special needs and risks	Advise of length of gestation and what type of procedure this indicates; discuss various types of abortion procedures, time in hospital or if outpatient, techniques and what the experience entails, risks, and complications Explore alternate choices (*i.e.,* have abortion, continue pregnancy and either keep or give baby for adoption) and meanings these have for woman, partner and family Assist during procedures, provide support, clarification, and keep patient informed of process Advise of postabortion complications, when to seek medical care, preventive measures, and when to resume activities and sex Discuss contraception, follow-up visits, and emotional reactions Initiate referral to psychological counseling if indicated For midtrimester abortion, monitor during labor, provide pain relief and supportive care, and facilitate presence of companion if desired	Able to reach decision about pregnancy termination with which patient feels comfortable Accepts requirements of various procedures as indicated by gestational age Affirms understanding of process of conception and effective use of contraception Returns for follow-up visit and institutes contraceptive method Feels accepting of abortion if undertaken; no serious emotional problems Seeks prenatal care if abortion decided against Avoids future unwanted pregnancies. Initiates psychological counseling if emotionally distressed

tomy, and treatment of pelvic disease. Table 14-5 summarizes morbidity and mortality rates for the commonly used methods of pregnancy termination.

Follow-Up Care

After a first trimester abortion, the woman is instructed about signs and symptoms of complications and how to contact the clinic or physician if these occur. Fever and chills, foul-smelling discharge, heavy bleeding, severe abdominal pain, and nausea and vomiting can indicate complications. Abstinence from intercourse and avoidance of tampons and douching for two weeks are advised. Normal activity may be resumed in one or two days in most instances. Contraception is discussed and occasionally an IUD is inserted at the time of abortion, but perforation and expulsion rates are high. Oral contraceptives may be given with instructions that they be started one week after the abortion. It is standard to have a follow-up office visit in two weeks, at which time contraceptives are prescribed if not already begun. The patient's adjustment to termination of pregnancy, as well as her partner's or family's reactions, can be discussed and referral made if needed for psychological, social, or economic reasons.

Following midtrimester abortion, RhoGAM is administered to desensitized Rh negative women. Instructions about signs and symptoms of infection and hemorrhage are given, and patients are advised to avoid sex, tampons, and douches for two weeks. Women need to be prepared for frequently occurring depression, which is probably related to drastic hormonal changes. A return visit is scheduled for two weeks after the abortion, at which time uterine size should be normal and bleeding ceased. Contraception is usually initiated and reactions to the abortion discussed with referral as needed.

References

1. Tietze C: Incidence of legal abortion. IN Omran AR (ed): Liberalization of Abortion Laws: Implications, pp 1–4. Chapel Hill, University of North Carolina, Carolina Population Center, 1976

2. Henshaw S, Forrest JD, Sullivan E, Tietze C: Abortion in the United States, 1978–1979. Fam Plann Perspect 13, 1:6–18, January/February 1981

3. Osofsky JD, Osofky JH: The psychological reaction of patients to legalized abortion. Am J Orthopsychiatry 42, 1:48–60, 1972

4. Woods NF: Human Sexuality in Health and Illness. St Louis, CV Mosby, 1975

5. David HP, Rasmussen NK, Holst E: Postpartum and postabortion psychotic reactions. Fam Plann Perspect 13, 2:88–91, March/April 1981

6. David HP, Matéjćek Z: "Children born to women denied abortion: An update," Fam Plann Perspect 13, 1:32–34, January/February 1981

7. Gold RB: After the Hyde Amendment: Public funding for abortion in FY 1978. Fam Plann Perspect 12, 3:131–134, May/June 1980

8. Trussel J, Menken J, Lindheim B.L., Vaughan B: The impact of restricting Medicaid financing for abortion. Fam Plann Perspect 12, 3:120–130, May/June 1980

9. Lupfer M, Silber B.F.: How patients view mandatory waiting periods for abortion. Fam Plann Perspect 13, 2:75–79, March/April 1981

10. Bygdeman M, Martin JN, Eneroth P, Leader A: et al: Outpatient postconceptional fertility control with vaginally administered 15 (S) 15-methyl-PGF, a-methyl ester. Am J Obstet Gynecol 124, 5:495–498, March 1, 1976

11. Brenner WE: The current status of prostaglandins as abortifacients. Am J Obstet Gynecol 123, 3:306–328, October 1, 1975

12. Lauersen NH, Secher NJ, Wilson KH: Midtrimester abortion induced by serial intramuscular injections of 12 (s)-12-methyl-prostaglandin E_2-methyl ester. Am J Obstet Gynecol 123, 7:665–670, December 1, 1975

Suggested Readings

Bendel RP, Williams PP, Butler JC: Endometrial aspiration in fertility control. Am J Obstet Gynecol 125, 3:328–332 June 1, 1976

Brenner WE, Edelman DA, Davis JLR, Kassell E: Suction curettage for 'menstrual regulation:' advances in planned parenthood. Proceedings of the Annual Meeting of American Association of Planned Parenthood Physicians Excerpta Medica, Amsterdam. 9, 1:15–21, 1974

Burchell RC: Professional perspectives on abortion. Journal of Obstetric, Gynecologic and Neonatal Nursing 3:25–27, November/December 1974

Geden S: Abortion counseling with adolescents. Am J Nurs 74:1856–58, 1974

Irani KR, Henriques ES, Friedlander RL, Berlin LE et al: Menstrual induction: Its place in clinical practice. Obstet Gynecol 46, 5:596–598, November 1, 1975

Sarvis B, Rodman H: Social and cultural aspects of abortion: Class and race. In Ostheimer N, Ostheimer JM (eds): Life or Death—Who Controls?, pp 104–118. New York, Springer, 1976

Tanis JL: Recognizing the reasons for contraceptive non-use and abuse. The American Journal of Maternal Child Nursing, 2, 3:364–369, May/June 1977

Grimes DA, Cates WC, Selik RM: Abortion facilities and the risk of death. Fam Plann Perspect 13, 1:30–32, January/February 1981

Hatcher RA, Stewart GK, Stewart F, Guest F: Contraceptive technology 1980–1981. Chapter 17, Abortion, pp 139–156. New York, Irvington Publishers, Inc., 1980

Mims FH, Swenson M: Sexuality: A nursing perspective, Abortion, pp 195–207. New York, McGraw–Hill, 1980

CHAPTER 15

CHAPTER 15

Infertility

- **Counseling Considerations**
- **Infertility as a Life Crisis**
- **Standards for Infertility Studies**
- **The Infertile Couple**
- **The Seminal Factor**
- **The Postcoital Test—Evaluation of Insemination**
  - The Cervical Factor
  - Artificial Insemination
    - AIH
    - AID
- **The Ovarian Factor**
  - Treatment of Ovulatory Failure
- **Tubal Factors**
- **Surgical Treatment of Pelvic Disease**
- ***In Vitro* Fertilization and Embryo Transfer**
- **The Uterine Factor**

Technology has introduced an element of choice in reproduction. Yet, during the course of nursing practice, one will surely encounter patients who are pregnant when they do not wish to be or who are infertile when pregnancy is consummately desired.

Fertility regulation is most often expressed in demographic terms. Indeed, population pressures represent a major social force. For the practicing nurse or physician, however, the importance of understanding and controlling reproductive potential is more cogently expressed in individual terms. The right of choice of the individual has been emphasized by international bodies. The General Assembly of the United Nations has declared that, "The size of the family should be the free choice of each individual family." The concept was later expanded to include the right to the means to space and limit births.

At the other end of the spectrum, fertility is not always a matter of choice. The generally accepted estimate is that about 10% of couples are infertile. One can realistically project a rise in the incidence of infertility due to social causes. The increase in the prevalence of gonorrheal salpingitis, and recent changes in women's social orientation—with the concomitant trend toward postponement of childbearing until the late reproductive years—will materially influence reproductive potential. A shortage of children for adoption has created additional pressures.

Counseling Considerations

Often the nurse is called upon to act as counselor in what is an emotionally charged situation—as a couple faces the prospect of a barren marriage. Ideally, the nurse should be prepared to schedule and interpret the various tests used in an infertility investigation and to understand, in order to be able to explain the physiologic basis for treatment.

Basic reproductive mechanisms were discussed and events beginning with spermatogenesis and oogenesis and ending in the development of the term fetus were explored in preceding chapters. This information will now serve as a basis for understanding the clinical approach to problems of human reproduction.

When one considers the complexity of reproductive processes, it is not surprising that unprotected coitus at about the time of ovulation does not always result in a pregnancy. In fact, under normal circumstances an average of six cycles of exposure is required. It is generally felt that infertility should be explored after a year's exposure without contraception. However, it is unwise to insist on an interval of one year before investigation is initiated in each case. A reassuring consultation is often helpful, if only to dispel doubts concerning the existence of major abnormalities. Because fertility declines with age, it would seem justifiable for couples in their thirties to seek advice somewhat earlier. Even among younger couples, when the nurse or physician senses that there is anxiety over failure to conceive or when on cursory exploration there is an obvious reason for infertility, for example, amenorrhea, or a history of acute salpingitis or postabortal infection, early evaluation is in order.

Infertility as a Life Crisis

Professionals treating infertility should recognize that it invariably represents a life crisis situation. Infertility involves many feelings which must be recognized and dealt with; the infertile couple is often sensitive and extremely vulnerable. During the course of the diagnostic workup and treatment, it is important to acknowledge the pressures associated with infertility and to allow opportunities to review the sense of isolation, guilt, depression, and even anger which often accompany infertility. Emotional support is provided most effectively when the couple is approached as a unit, without singling out one of the partners for exclusive attention.

The need for addressing the emotional aspects of human infertility has prompted organization of a national support group, Resolve, Inc., which now has chapters in many cities in the United States. In her paper entitled *The Emotional Needs of Infertile Couples*, Barbara Eck Menning, Executive Director of Resolve, outlines the feelings of infertile couples that most frequently surface during support group meetings. The first reaction is commonly one of shock. Most couples have not considered the possibility that they will be infertile and are unaware of how common infertility is. The next reaction is usually denial—"this can't happen to me." Denial is a useful mechanism which allows time for adjustment to a threatening situation.

Medical help is not sought until after the couple comes to grips with the problem. Anger may occur in response to the discomfort and inconvenience of infertility testing or perhaps from social pressure from well intended friends and family members. Infertile people may direct their anger at the nurse or physician who is perceived as exercising an element of control over them. Allowing an opportunity to express rage is the most effective way to dissipate it. When faced with irrational anger the health-care professional should strive to avoid becoming defensive. Nonjudgmental acceptance of the patient's feelings and sincere empathy are essential in these circumstances.

People facing infertility commonly experience a sense of isolation. The infertile couple may find it difficult to share their problem with others, even with those close to them. For this reason they should be encouraged to discuss their feelings at every visit during the course of investigation and treatment. It is especially important to provide an opportunity to consider marital and sexual conflicts which may have arisen out of the infertility.

Infertility is often associated with a sense of guilt. This may be engendered by a completely unrelated past event such as an induced abortion, an extramarital affair, venereal disease, premarital sex, or homosexual acts or thoughts. When guilt feelings are intense, they are associated with a sense of worthlessness. During the sometimes prolonged interval of investigation and treatment, those health-care professionals involved must be aware of the emotional impact of infertility on the persons affected.

Standards for Infertility Studies

Before selecting a method of treatment, efforts should be made to identify the underlying cause of infertility. Appropriate therapy can be selected only after the cause for infertility is determined. Shotgun measures involving use of so-called fertility drugs are useless. There is no quick substitute for a carefully planned investigative program. Minimal standards that are suggested for a complete infertility investigation include evaluation of seminal, cervical, ovarian, tubal, peritoneal, and uterine factors. In addition, the frequency and technique of intercourse should be explored. The ultimate goal of infertility investigation is not solely that of a successful pregnancy. It is equally important to establish a prognosis and to help couples who, after careful evaluation, are finally adjudged hopelessly sterile, plan their lives realistically. Some of the outpatient procedures used in a standard infertility investigation are outlined in Table 15-1.

The Infertile Couple

Since infertility is usually caused by abnormalities in the anatomy and physiology of the male or female reproductive tract, management of the problem involves both marital partners. Male abnormalities are responsible in at least 35% of infertility in couples, and evaluation of the husband early in the course of the investigation is mandatory.

In the initial interview, sexual habits should be reviewed with both husband and wife. Although the frequency of coitus varies greatly from one couple to the next, patterns of intercourse do influence fertility. Only about 16% of couples who are having intercourse less than once a week will conceive in less than six months. Over 80% conceive in the same interval when exposure occurs four or more times weekly. When intercourse occurs infrequently the sexual adjustment in the marriage should be explored. There is no evidence to suggest a relationship between female orgasm and conception. Nevertheless, the frequency of coitus is influenced by sexual satisfaction; intercourse may be infrequent because it is associated with discomfort (dyspareunia) or because it is simply not a pleasurable experience for the wife.

Patients who make it a habit to arise from bed immediately after intercourse, spilling much of the ejaculate shortly after it is placed in the vagina, should be advised to remain in bed for at least 30 minutes following coitus. Occasionally, couples admit to using lubricants during intercourse or to douching postcoitally, which may interfere with sperm migration. Petroleum jelly and some of the water-soluble lubricants have been shown to be spermicidal. These factors may not cause infertility when the husband's fertility potential is normal, but may play a role when sperm production is marginal. In some patients, there is even anatomical evidence that normal intercourse is not occurring (*e.g.*, an intact hymenal ring or a rigid perineal body). Other sexual problems such as premature ejaculation may result in failure of proper placement of sperm. Sympathetic and knowledgeable advice in these areas is often useful not only in the treatment of infertility but also in bringing about a better sexual relationship.

Table 15-1
Standard Outpatient Procedures for Infertility

Test	Timing	Interpretation
Semen analysis	Suggested as initial procedure Repeated if questionable 2–3 days of abstinence prior to collection	Volume 2–5 ml Count >20 million/ml Motility >60% with good quality Morphology >60% normal
Postcoital test	1–2 days prior to ovulation (days 12–14 in a 28-day cycle)	10–20 sperm/h.p.f. in favorable mucus is considered normal
Plasma progesterone	Presumed postovulatory phase (last 10 days of cycle)	>4 ng/ml strongly suggests ovulation
Endometrial biopsy	Luteal (postovulatory) phase of cycle (days 21–24 of a 28-day cycle)	Secretory changes as interpreted in relation to onset of next menses
Hysterosalpingogram	Preovulatory (before day 12 in the 28-day cycle)	Contour of uterus and patency of tubes as seen on fluoroscopy and roentgenograms

The Seminal Factor

Because evaluation of the male is much less complicated than the series of tests required to explore female infertility, his reproductive potential should always be assessed first. The postcoital test—examination of cervical mucus for the presence of spermatozoa—is useful in this regard. Unless adequate numbers of spermatozoa are seen in the cervical mucus following coitus, the semen should be evaluated. This involves assessment of the fresh ejaculate obtained by masturbation after at least three days of abstinence. The ejaculate is collected in a clean, dry container and brought to the laboratory as soon after collection as practical. The patient should be cautioned not to lose the first few drops of the ejaculate because the majority of active spermatozoa are located in the first portion of the specimen. Normally, seminal fluid becomes coagulated immediately upon ejaculation. Liquefaction of the coagulum occurs within 20 minutes. Examination should be deferred until liquefaction is complete because the coagulum interferes with the distribution of spermatozoa in the counting chamber.

The volume of the specimen, sperm density, percentage of motile forms, quality of the motility, and the percentage of abnormal spermatozoa are determined. The volume of the normal ejaculate ranges from 2 ml to 5 ml. A sperm count of more than 20 million/ml is considered normal, provided the quality and percentage of motility in the specimen are also normal. The single most useful criterion is the actual quality of motility—the ability of spermatozoa to progress.

Because there is usually some variation in the quality of semen ejaculated at various times, assessment of the husband's fertility potential should never be based on a single analysis. Since maturation of spermatozoa within the testis occurs over a 60-day interval, the quality of semen could be influenced by an event, such as a viral infection, that took place many days before the spermatozoa appeared in the ejaculate.

If the postcoital test is abnormal, but the semen analysis is within normal limits, the possibility that semen is not being ejaculated deep in the vagina during intercourse should be considered. In such cases, further investigations of coital techniques and examination of the male genitalia is often helpful. Hypospadias, a condition in which the opening of the urethra is located along the shaft of the penis and not at the glans, may result in loss of the ejaculate high in the vagina. Discussion may uncover unsuspected sexual difficulties such as premature ejaculation or even impotence.

When the semen analysis or postcoital test is abnormal, the male partner should be evaluated further for anatomical, genetic, or endocrine abnormalities. These evaluations are usually carried out by urologists who specialize in infertility. A recently emerging subspecialty, *andrology,* the study of male reproductive problems, places major emphasis on the diagnosis and treatment of the infertile male.

The Postcoital Test—Evaluation of Insemination

A couple is instructed to have intercourse during the 12 hours preceding the examination. The test is timed for within a day or two before expected ovulation, that is, the 12th or 13th day in the 28-day menstrual cycle. At that time, the cervical mucus, under the influence of estrogen, is normally clear and abundant and is most receptive to spermatozoa. At other times in the cycle, the mucus is scanty, thick, turbid and generally unreceptive.

A sample of cervical mucus is obtained in the following manner. The cervix is exposed with vaginal speculum, and after secretions and debris are gently wiped from the exocervix, mucus is removed from well within the endocervical canal with fenestrated intestinal forceps or a nasal polyp forceps, or the mucus may be aspirated from the cervix into a polyethylene tube. Its gross characteristics, quantity and clarity are evaluated, and its ability to form a thin continuous thread (a quality referred to as *spinnbarkeit*) is assessed. *Spinnbarkeit* is determined by stretching the mucus between the tips of the forceps until the thread breaks. Normal preovulatory mucus can be stretched for a distance of up to 10 cm. The sample is then placed on a clean, dry slide and a cover slip is applied. The specimen is then examined microscopically for spermatozoa. The test is normal when there are more than 20 motile spermatozoa per high power field in areas of clear, abundant cervical mucus. In addition to assessing the placement of spermatozoa during coitus, the postcoital test permits evaluation of the quality of cervical secretions and their ability to support the life of the spermatozoon—the cervical factor.

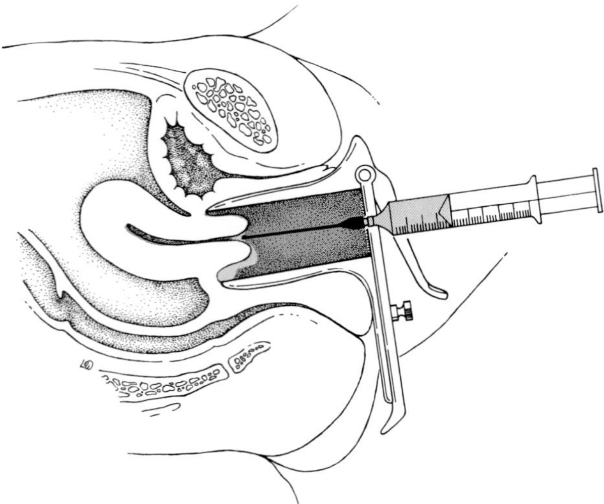

Figure 15-1.
Technique for artificial insemination.

The Cervical Factor

In order to assess the quality of the cervical secretions and to diagnose abnormalities at that level, the timing of the recovery of the mucus in the cycle is critical. The health-care professional should be aware of the normal variations in mucus quality in the menstrual cycle. If the mucus never demonstrates the characteristics of normal ovulatory mucus after serial evaluation on alternate days during the presumed ovulatory period, the possibility that mucus production is deficient should be seriously considered. Inability of spermatozoa to penetrate and survive in such mucus may reasonably be inferred to be a cause of infertility.

Because little is known about the physiology of cervical mucus production, treatment of the cervical factor has not been uniformly successful. Local treatment of the cervix when there is a cervicitis and the use of small doses of estrogen prior to ovulation have been suggested to produce a mucus more favorable to sperm migration, but success with such treatment has been limited.

Artificial Insemination

In selected cases, artificial placement of semen is an effective therapeutic modality. The technique involves insertion of a freshly ejaculated specimen at the cervical os with a cannula and syringe within a day or two of the estimated time of ovulation (Fig. 15-1). Alternatively, the specimen can be injected into a plastic cervical cap that is placed around the cervix. The cap retains the specimen at the cervix and is removed several hours later. In order to be sure that ovulation has been covered, insemination is repeated on alternate days until it has been determined by the temperature chart that ovulation has occurred.

AIH

Artificial insemination with the husband's specimen (AIH) is especially useful in cases in which the postcoital test consistently reveals few or absent spermatozoa in cervical mucus of good quality. In selected cases, the use of a "split ejaculate" is recommended. Here, the specimen is collected into two containers. By and large, the first portion of the ejaculate contains a significantly higher portion of normal motile spermatozoa and it is this first portion which is used for the insemination.

AID

In cases of azoospermia (absence of spermatozoa in the ejaculate) or severe oligospermia (markedly decreased numbers of spermatozoa in the ejaculate) which has failed to respond to treatment, insemination of a specimen from a donor (AID) may be employed. AID is sometimes called "semi-adoption" and has gained increasing popularity and acceptability in recent years. Willingness of a couple to consider AID has been influenced to a large degree in recent years by the lack of availability of children for adoption. AID is also used in cases in which the husband suffers from a genetic defect or in cases of RH sensitization. In the latter instance, an RH negative donor is used.

The physician who wishes to use donor insemination should settle on an organized approach and must be willing to give this procedure the necessary time and attention it demands. Selection of the donor must be carried out with great care, with attention to general state of health, genetic background, RH type, and physical characteristics which at least to some degree resemble those of the husband. Those advising patients on this matter should be aware of the social and ethical implications of the procedure and should allow adequate time to explore matters with the couple in depth before proceeding. On the positive side, when donor insemination is accepted by informed consenting partners, the end result is usually satisfactory. There is a remarkable marriage stability among properly selected couples who have been treated with AID. Recently, freeze-stored semen has been used to increase the rate of availability of specimens for donor insemination.

The Ovarian Factor

Clearly, conception cannot occur when there is failure of ovulation, and fertility is impaired when ovulation is infrequent. Thus, ovulation detection is an integral part of the infertility investigation. Clues as to the occurrence of ovulation are derived from menstrual history, evaluation of characteristic changes in cervical mucus, and by the basal body temperature chart. Additional parameters used to assess ovulation include histologic evaluation of a sample of endometrium obtained by biopsy and a plasma progesterone determination obtained late in the cycle.

Endometrial biopsy is a simple office procedure that offers the additional advantage of ruling out a chronic inflammatory condition in the endometrium (Fig. 15-2). It is usually scheduled 5 days to 7 days before the expected onset of the next menses or on days 21 to 24 of a 28-day cycle. Any one of the available specially designed biopsy curettes may be used.

After the position of the uterus is determined, a curette is gently introduced through the cervical canal to the level of the fundus and one or two samples of tissue are removed. The endometrial sample is then sent to the pathologist's laboratory for evaluation.

Following ovulation, the endometrium takes on "secretory" changes under the influence of progesterone. The changes after ovulation are progressive and predictable and timing of ovulation can be established retrospectively. Additional evidence of corpus luteum function and, therefore, indirect evidence of ovulation is obtained when plasma progesterone levels are greater than 4 ng per ml.

Treatment of Ovulatory Failure

Treatment of anovulatory infertility depends on the underlying cause. When failure of ovulation is suspected, a thorough endocrine evaluation is in order. The defect may occur at the level of the hypothalamus, the pituitary, or the ovaries themselves. Ovulation is also influenced by the patient's general state of health and thyroid and adrenal abnormalities.

Ovulatory failure can be caused by a pituitary adenoma, a space-occupying tumor within the pituitary gland. Such tumors produce the breast-stimulating hormone, prolactin, and thus are often associated with secretions from the breasts (galactorrhea). Patients with ovulatory failure should be screened for this condition by careful examination of the breasts

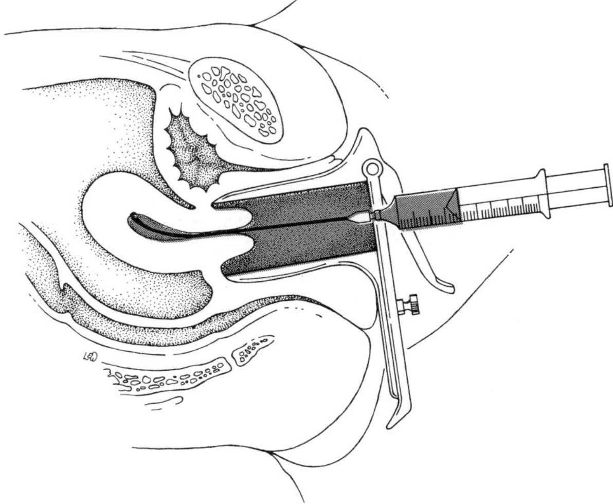

Figure 15-2.
Technique of office endometrial biopsy.

for secretions and if galactorrhea is present, a serum prolactin determination should be carried out. When prolactin levels are elevated, the pituitary must be evaluated further. Serial x-ray films or tomograms of the sella turcica, the bony structure in which the pituitary gland is located, are useful in this regard. Any patient exhibiting galactorrhea with elevated prolactin levels should be evaluated with tomography before treatment with ovulation-inducing methods is considered.

Recent availability of effective agents for the induction of ovulation has made careful evaluation of patients suspected of anovulatory infertility all the more important. In properly selected cases, mainly patients with clinical evidence of continued estrogen production, the use of an estrogen antagonist, *clomiphene citrate,* is associated with more than a 50% success rate. Patients with hyperprolactinemia may be candidates for treatment with bromocryptine, an agent capable of inducing ovulation by reducing prolactin levels. In patients whose ovulatory failure is the result of a defect at the hypothalamic-pituitary level, the use of *human menopausal gonadotropin (HMG),* which is derived from the urine of postmenopausal women, is associated with some success. Multiple pregnancies, which have received considerable attention from the press, are usually the result of HMG treatment. Even in expert hands, it is difficult to avoid overstimulation of the ovary with HMG and induction of more than one ovulation in a given cycle.

Tubal Factors

The clinical approach to tubal disease involves assessment of tubal and peritubal anatomy. Because the human tube is a conduit that provides a passage between the ovary and uterus, tubal obstruction, of course, results in infertility. In addition, since the fimbriated end of the tube is important in transferring the ovum from the rupturing follicle to the tubal lumen, when the relationship between it and the ovum is distorted by pelvic adhesions, fertility is also diminished.

Anatomic defects in and about the fallopian tubes are generally a result of a past infection or pelvic irritation. Acute gonorrheal salpingitis is a common offender. A ruptured appendix associated with pelvic peritonitis may also cause peritubal and periovarian adhesions.

Endometriosis, a condition in which the endometrium has been displaced into the peritoneal cavity around the tube and ovaries, may also result in pelvic adhesions and distortion of pelvic architecture. Anatomic tubal disease is treated surgically with lysis and excision of the adhesions and special techniques to reestablish the patency of the fallopian tubes.

The commonly used tests for evaluation of tubal function include uterotubal insufflation (the Rubin test), hysterosalpingography. and endoscopy.

Uterotubal insufflation involves the introduction of carbon dioxide into the uterus through a cannula. If one or both of the tubes are patent, the carbon dioxide flows along the uterus and tubes into the peritoneal cavity. When the patient sits up, the carbon dioxide rises to the diaphragm, causing pain in the shoulder referred there by way of the phrenic nerve. This test is useful only as a screening measure and, increasingly, physicians have substituted other methods for it.

Hysterosalpingography involves introduction of radiopaque material into the uterus and fallopian tubes (Fig. 15-3). This is usually done under fluoroscopic visualization, and x-ray films are taken at intervals to provide a permanent record. When the tubes are patent, the radiopaque material enters the peritoneal cavity and is evenly distributed there. When the tubes are closed, the peritoneal egress is prevented by the obstruction, and a diagnosis of tubal occlusion can be made without further delay.

Peritoneoscopy involves direct visualization of the tubes and ovaries with an endoscope. This may be carried out through the cul-de-sac (*culdoscopy*) or through the umbilicus (*laparoscopy*). The former is carried out under local anesthesia with the patient in the knee–chest position. In expert hands, visualization is usually satisfactory. It is a more difficult procedure, however, than laparoscopy which has become the procedure of choice.

Diagnostic laparoscopy is generally carried out under general anesthesia (Fig. 15-4). This is the same procedure that is used for tubal sterilization. In this case, however, tubal patency is evaluated by the introduction of a dilute solution of dye while the ends of the tubes are under visualization. Dye can be seen spilling from the ends of patent tubes. In addition, the area in and about the fallopian tubes can be evaluated directly for the presence of adhesions. When adhesions are present, the condition is called the peritoneal factor in infertility.

Surgical Treatment of Pelvic Disease

Surgical techniques have been developed for the treatment of pelvic adhesions and tubal occlusion. The postoperative prognosis depends on the extent of

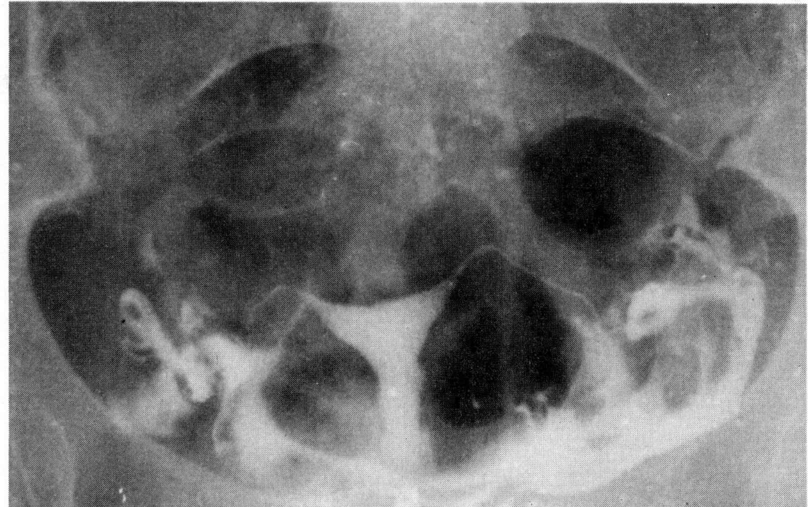

Figure 15-3A.
A normal hysterosalpingogram revealing bilateral tubal patency with spill of radiopague material into the peritoneal cavity. (Mastroianni L Jr: Variations of Fertility. In Romney SL, Gray MJ, Little AB (eds): Gynecology and Obstetrics: The Health Care of Women. New York, McGraw–Hill, 1975)

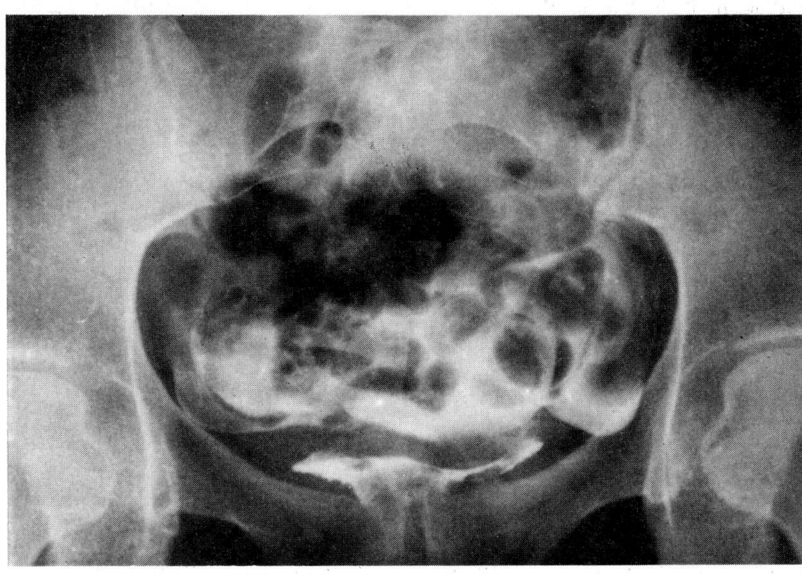

Figure 15-3B.
Pelvic (peritubal and periovarian) adhesions associated with infertility. Ruptured appendix occurred at age eight. (Mastroianni L Jr: Variations of Fertility. In Romney SL, Gray MJ, Little AB (eds): Gynecology and Obstetrics: The Health Care of Women. New York, McGraw–Hill, 1975)

the previous damage to adnexal structures. It is also greatly influenced by the skill of the surgeon and has been enhanced in recent years by using the principles of plastic surgery. Microsurgery, with the operating loup or an operating microscope has also been particularly helpful.

Laparotomy should not be considered until all of the other causes of reproductive failure have been conscientiously investigated. For example, an operation is not generally justifiable if the husband is severely oligospermic, or if the patient suffers from ovulatory failure that is refractory to treatment. In some cases, the tubes have been so extensively damaged and the ovaries so severely compromised by periovarian adhesions that pelvic reconstruction is illadvised. Prior to surgery for infertility, the couple should be given a realistic appraisal of the prognosis. In large measure, this is based on the appearance of the adnexa at the time of laparoscopy. Risks of this procedure should be thoroughly reviewed, and the mistaken impression that failure to accept treatment will affect general health later on should be dispelled. The decision to accept an operative procedure solely to enhance fertility is a serious matter deserving the most careful review.

The role of pelvic adhesions in infertility depends on their location in relation to the tubes and ovaries. When the tubes are patent, pelvic adhesions present the best prognosis, with postoperative pregnancy rates in the 40% to 50% range.

Tubal obstruction usually occurs in the proximal (uterine) or distal (fimbrial) segments. A diagnosis of nonpatency at the uterotubal junction should be made with extreme caution. Obstruction in this area may be

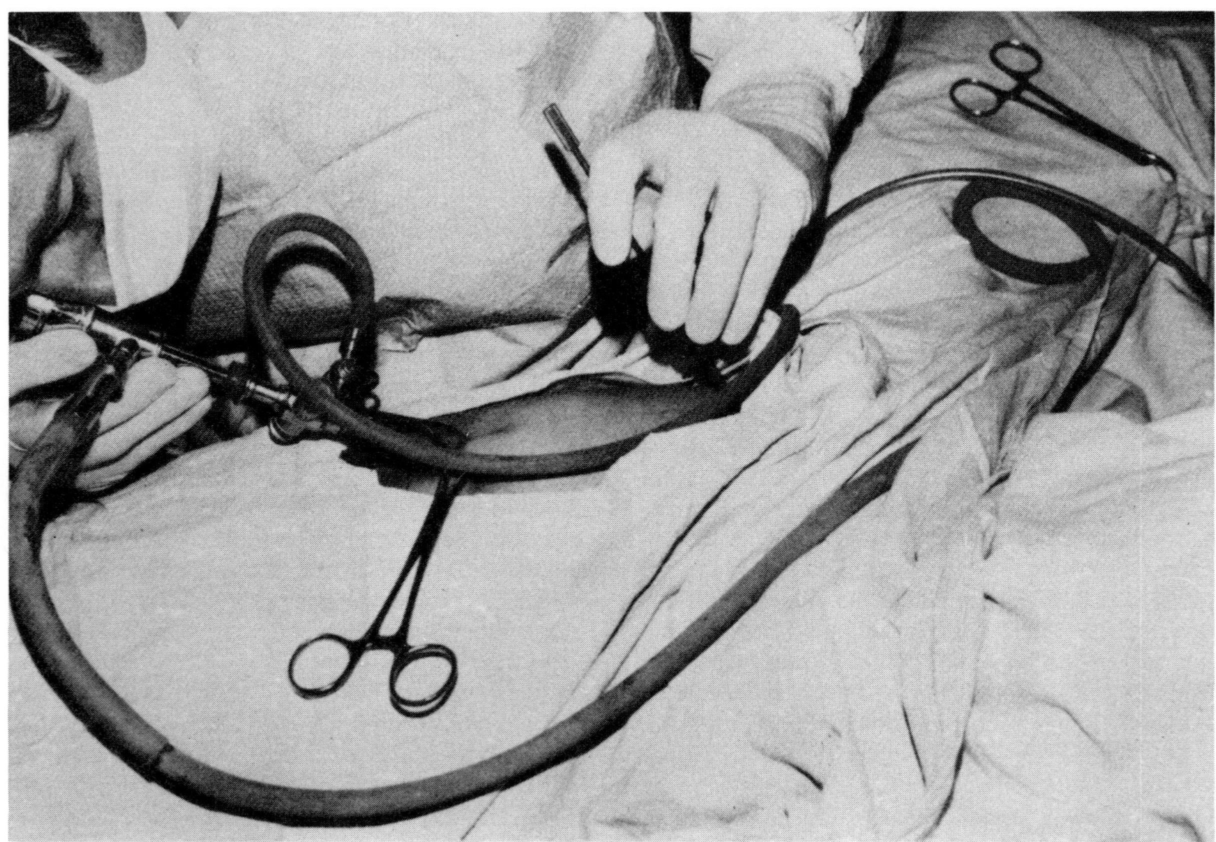

Figure 15-4.
The double-puncture laparoscopic technique utilizing the probe to position the pelvic structures for optimum visualization. (Seitz HM Jr, Rosenfeld RL: Endoscopy in the management of infertility. Clin Ob Gynecol 17:86, 1974)

caused by tubal spasm, and actual anatomical obstruction must be corroborated both by hysterosalpingogram and laparoscopy. With the use of the operating microscope, the point of obstruction near the uterus can be accurately identified, and a tubal anastomosis is carried out. When the intrauterine portion of the tube is completely occluded, reimplantation of the patent segment into the uterus can be carried out. The prognosis following these procedures is relatively poor, in the 10% to 30% range.

When the tube is occluded at its fimbriated extremity, efforts are made to salvage any remaining fimbriae and the distal end of the tube is reconstructed microsurgically. The prognosis depends on the extent of prior tubal damage, but in the hands of a skilled surgeon, it is in the 20% to 30% range. Subsequent to tubal surgery, the possibility of a tubal ectopic pregnancy must be seriously considered when conception occurs. The incidence of ectopic pregnancy is 5% to 10%.

In Vitro Fertilization and Embryo Transfer

One of the most dramatic events in the treatment of infertility was the birth of baby Louise in England, following successful *in vitro* fertilization and embryo transfer. This first recorded success was in a patient whose fallopian tubes had been previously surgically removed. This breakthrough offers hope for patients with extensive tubal disease or whose tubes are absent. A number of principles have been applied in the successful application of this approach to infertility. The development of multiple follicles is stimulated with ovulation inducing agents. At a precisely timed interval, a laparoscopy is carried out. The ovarian follicles, matured under the influence of ovarian stimulation, are aspirated and the oocytes received are then cultured *in vitro* with the husband's treated spermatozoa under carefully controlled laboratory conditions. If fertilization is successful, the oocyte divides and is transferred into the uterus at the four to eight cell stage. As techniques have been refined, there has been a gradual improvement in the success rate.

These procedures have engendered a great deal of controversy among those who feel for moral and ethical reasons, that the creation of new life *in vitro* is inappropriate. In 1982, the American Fertility Society drafted the following position on *in vitro* fertilization and embryo transfer, "In view of the current rate of success in programs of *in vitro* fertilization, it is the sense of the Board of Directors of the American Fertility Society that in appropriately staffed and equipped institutions that have demonstrated proficiency and success, *in vitro* fertilization must now be recognized as the acceptable treatment for achieving pregnancy for couples whose wives have absent or irreparably damaged fallopian tubes."

It is clear that this technology represents a significant advance in our ability to treat otherwise hopeless cases of infertility, and knowledge gained from this work has done much to improve our understanding of human reproductive processes.

The Uterine Factor

Pathologic conditions of the uterus associated with decreased fertility include uterine fibroids, congenital malformations, and intrauterine adhesions. Inflammatory lesions of the endometrium also occur.

Congenital defects of the uterus, as well as uterine fibroids are more often related to habitual abortion than to infertility. Fibroids may distort the endometrial cavity, and if they are strategically located and large enough, they presumably could interfere with implantation. If located adjacent to the tube, they may cause tubal obstruction. When a causal relationship is thought to exist, *myomectomies* (removal of the fibroids), with preservation of the uterus are usually technically possible. Treatment of congenital abnormalities, more commonly associated with habitual abortion than infertility, is also surgical.

Asherman's syndrome, or adhesions within the uterine cavity, are usually the result of a postpartal or postabortal infection or pelvic tuberculosis. There is often a history of a previous dilatation and curettage followed by a stormy postoperative course. Increasing use of abortion as a backup for contraceptive failure may be associated with an increased incidence of this uncommon but potential fertility-impairing lesion. Intrauterine adhesions are treated with surgery plus steroid and estrogen therapy to decrease the incidence of repeat formation of adhesions.

Some patients, for reasons that are not understood, conceive during the course of the diagnostic evaluation for infertility. Occasionally, conception occurs after not more than a preliminary examination and discussion of the diagnostic approach to follow. It is tempting to conjecture that, in some cases, the decision to seek aid for infertility is associated with a release of emotional tension followed, somehow, by improved reproductive performance. With the exception of ovulatory failure, which may have a psychological basis, and decreased frequency of intercourse, which sometimes has a psychological basis, there is as yet no proved somatic basis for psychologically-induced infertility. The general impression that adoption is often followed by conception has not been substantiated. Nevertheless, throughout the infertility investigation, the emotional support provided by those involved in patient management is especially important. Infertility is a threatening condition, and both husband and wife inevitably display anxiety. The role of the nurse in such situations is to understand the purpose of the various diagnostic procedures for infertility and to provide the couple with information so that both partners can cope with the problem knowledgeably.

Suggested Readings

Amelar RD, Dublin L, Walsh P: Male Infertility. Philadelphia, WB Saunders, 1977

Beck W: Critical look at the legal, ethical and technical aspects of artificial insemination by donor. Fertil Steril 27:1–8, 1976

Garcia CR, David S: Pelvic endometriosis: Infertility and pelvic pain. Am J Obstet Gynecol 129:740–747, 1977

Mastroianni L Jr, Biggers JD: Fertilization and Embryonic Development *in Vitro*. New York, Plenum Press, 1981

Menning BE: The emotional needs of infertile couples. Fertil Steril 34:313, 1980

Speroff L, Glass RH, Kase HG: Clinical Gynecologic Endocrinology and Infertility, 2nd ed. Baltimore, Williams & Wilkins, 1979

Wallach E, Kempers RD (eds): Modern Trends in Infertility and Conception Control, Vol 10. Baltimore, Williams & Wilkins, 1979

Wallach E, Kempers RD (eds): Modern Trends in Infertility and Conception Control, Vol 1. Baltimore, Williams & Wilkins, 1979

Wallach E, Kempers RD (eds): Modern Trends in Infertility and Conception Control, Vol 2. Philadelphia, JB Lippincott, 1982

Wheeler J, Mastroianni L Jr: Pathology of the fallopian tube, In Blaustein A (ed): Pathology of Female Genital Tract, pp 341–365. New York, Springer, 1977

CHAPTER

16

CHAPTER 16

Genetic Counseling and Diagnosis During Pregnancy

Since 1956, when it was determined that human cells contain 46 chromosomes, the knowledge gained from research in human genetics has expanded rapidly. During that time, clinical genetics has developed as a medical discipline, which uses and integrates expertise from all other medical fields. Genetic information has been disseminated beyond the academic community and research laboratory to the practicing physician. The amount of genetic information available to the lay public has also increased markedly in the last few years. Magazine and newspaper articles and television programs frequently discuss genetic disease, often focusing on dramatic new advances in diagnostic methods or therapy. As a result, patients, as health-care consumers, expect providers to respond to their increasing sophistication and needs in this area. Many more patients are requesting genetic counseling and are willing to make decisions about their health care. These changes in information and attitudes facilitate the counseling process. Nurses are an integral part of the health-care team and should recognize of the need for, and content of, genetic services.

As a necessity, comprehensive genetic service programs employ a multidisciplinary approach to the care of patients and their families. A team composed of physicians (geneticists with specialty backgrounds in obstetrics, pediatrics, and internal medicine), nurses, genetics associates, laboratory personnel, and other support services is required.

Patients invariably feel anxious as they approach genetic counseling. Many have only a limited understanding of the inheritance of diseases and what the couseling process will involve. Often these patients are in the process of grieving over the birth of a malformed child or a serious illness of a family member. Guilt frequently compounds this anxiety. One or both parents may feel that there is something inherently wrong with themselves because a "defective" child has been born. On the other hand, they may blame the child's problems on the other partner or his or her "side of the family." The anxiety associated with counseling is easily exaggerated during pregnancy; therefore, it is important that genetic counselors be particularly sensitive to the pregnant patient's concerns and family dynamics, so that disruption of the marriage or other family relationships may be avoided.

The field of prenatal genetic diagnosis has developed rapidly over the past ten years. The number of genetic disorders and birth defects which can be diagnosed continues to increase dramatically. Public education has resulted in a large number of patients who consider having these studies performed. Nurses involved with the health care of women should also be aware of these services and be able to identify patients who might benefit from them. In an extended role of the maternal-child health nurse, the nurse-counselor is ideally suited to coordinate and deliver essential elements of this care.

The Nurse's Role

The nurse's role in genetic counseling often parallels that of the genetics associate with a master's degree in human genetics and counseling. Both are involved in the initial patient contact, assessing patients for referral, and taking family histories. They perform preliminary counseling and coordinate appointments with physicians for evaluation and extended counseling. Throughout the counseling, the rapport which has been established permits them to serve as a patient advocate. Through continued contact after counseling, they are able to evaluate the patient's understanding of the information presented to them and their response to it. The nurse works with the patient during the decision-making process and identifies resources for implementation of decisions.

A nurse–counselor or coordinator is especially suited to the prenatal genetic diagnostic team. In addition to having a basic knowledge of human genetics, the educational preparation of the nurse in reproduction and in obstetrical procedures makes her invaluable for both patient education and emotional support during prenatal diagnosis. The nurse's role is easily adapted to these services because nursing has traditionally espoused the philosophy of treating the whole patient, including family members in patient care, rather than focusing on the disease process or therapeutic regimen in itself. Additionally, in other areas of health-care delivery, nurses often assume the role of coordinating total patient care.

Genetic Counseling

Individuals and families are given information that is needed to understand a hereditary disorder through genetic counseling. This information may deal with a genetic disease in the individual, a family member, or future offspring. While the basic approach and principles are the same as those used at other times, certain situations, such as critical time limitations for decision making, occur more frequently in pregnancy. The aspects discussed during the counseling process include medical considerations, genetic mechanisms, and the options available. Medical considerations include a description of the disease or defect, the clinical manifestations, therapy, and prognosis. The burden of the disease for the affected person, as well as the family, should be presented during the counseling process. For example, in the case of maternal age, it is important that the patient understands not only the risks of having a child with Down's syndrome, but also the burden associated with it. Only with this understanding can the couple make a fully informed decision regarding prenatal diagnosis.

The genetic mechanism by which the disorder occurs and the risk of occurrence or recurrence should be explained to the patient in terms that can be readily understood. It may be necessary to review and summarize the information several times. Having the patient relate the information back to the counselor is a useful way of assessing the effectiveness of the counseling.

During counseling any alternatives that may reduce the risk for or alter the course of the genetic disease are discussed. It may also be important to discuss new or anticipated developments in therapy when they are relevant.

Counseling should enable patients to make decisions regarding a genetic disease in their present family or in future generations. These decisions may involve selecting reproductive options (*e.g.*, childless marriage, selective abortion of affected fetus, AID, or sterilization). The impact of how genetic counseling and testing may alter their views of themselves and family members in terms of health and disease is significant.

Identification of Risk

An important aspect of primary obstetrical care is identifying families who have an increased risk of having a child with a genetic disorder or birth defect. Ideally, these factors should be recognized prior to pregnancy; however, it cannot be assumed that couples are aware of a specific risk, no matter how obvious it may seem.

The nurse's interview during the first obstetrical visit can identify patients who might benefit from genetic counseling. A brief screening questionnaire may be used effectively to identify the majority of patients who might wish to consider prenatal diagnosis (See sample questionnaire). The following aspects should be reviewed with the patient:

1. Maternal age—The risk of having a child with Down's syndrome increases significantly when the mother is over 35.
2. Ethnic background—A number of rare genetic disorders occur with higher frequency in certain ethnic groups. For example, Eastern European Jews have a ten times greater chance of carrying the Tay-Sachs gene than the general population in the United States; descendants of Mediterranean forebears have a greater chance of carrying the gene for thalassemia; and blacks have a much greater chance of carrying the sickle-cell trait.
3. Family history—Specific diseases (*e.g.*, Huntington's chorea and hemophilia), birth defects (*e.g.*, neural tube defects), or mental retardation may be hereditary.
4. Reproductive history—Spontaneous abortions, stillborns, and previous liveborn children with birth defects, slow development, or mental retardation may indicate an increased risk.
5. Maternal disease—Several maternal disorders are associated with higher frequency of birth defects (*e.g.*, diabetes mellitus and seizure disorder) or with mental retardation (*e.g.*, maternal phenylketonuria).

Referral Considerations

Although any patient who requests genetic information should be referred for counseling, initiation of the referral by the health-care provider is most appropriate for patients with more than one course of action available to them. Many patients who suspect that their child might have an increased risk for a birth defect use denial effectively until a pregnancy occurs. The reality of the pregnancy and concern for the fetus motivate them to seek information for the first time during early pregnancy. It is also important to recognize that patients may presume that a risk is not significant if it is not specifically mentioned by the nurse or physician. Occasionally, patients with the greatest anxiety are identified among those seeking pregnancy terminations. Their concerns for having a malformed child may be based on misinformation. Genetic counseling in these circumstances should allow the patients to make an informed and appropriate decision. Moreover, counseling may provide reassuring information by clarifying the actual risk. The gestational age of the pregnancy, the availability of preg-

AT **Prenatal Diagnosis Screening Questionnaire**

1. Will you be age 35 or older when the baby is due? ______YES ______NO
   Age when due?__________
2. Have you or the baby's father or anyone in either of your families ever had:
   a. Down's syndrome or mongolism? ______YES ______NO
   b. Spina bifida or meningomyelocele (open spine)? ______YES ______NO
   c. Hemophilia? ______YES ______NO
   d. Muscular dystrophy? ______YES ______NO
3. Have you or the baby's father had a child born dead or alive with a birth defect not listed in question 2? ______YES ______NO
   If yes, describe:__________
4. Do you or the baby's father have any close relatives who are mentally retarded? ______YES ______NO
   If yes, list cause if known:__________
5. Do you or the baby's father or close relatives in either of your families have any inherited genetic or chromosomal disease or birth defect not listed above? ______YES ______NO
   If yes, describe:__________
6. Have you, or the spouse of this baby's father in a previous marriage, had 3 or more spontaneous pregnancy losses? ______YES ______NO
7. Do you or the baby's father have any close relatives descended from Jewish people who lived in Eastern Europe (Ashkenazic Jews)? ______YES ______NO
   If yes, have either you or the baby's father been screened for Tay-Sachs disease? ______YES ______NO
   If yes, indicate results and who was screened:__________
8. If patient or her spouse is black:
   Have you or the baby's father, or any close relative ever been screened for sickle-cell trait and found to be positive? ______YES ______NO
9. If patient or her spouse is of Mediterranean ancestry:
   Have you or the baby's father or any close relative ever been screened for or found to have a trait for Thalassemia or Cooley's anemia? ______YES ______NO

nancy termination, and the patient's attitude regarding this option should be assessed very early in the course of genetic referral or counseling.

Considerations in Prenatal Diagnosis

If prenatal diagnosis and selective abortion of the affected fetus are to be considered, several prerequisites as listed below should be met.

1. *Gestational age*—Counseling should be offered as early as possible during pregnancy. Restrictions on pregnancy termination limit the gestational age at which prenatal diagnosis can be initiated. Most often, procedures for genetic diagnosis are performed between 14 weeks and 20 weeks gestation. The time required for the counseling, decision-making process, and the completion of a genetic study of a pregnancy may be limited and frequently makes the situation an urgent one.
2. *Reliability and Safety*—There must be a reasonably reliable and safe method for diagnosis of the particular disorder. The testing, including its safety, limitations, and accuracy, should be explained in detail, and they must be accepted by the patient. In discussing risk, it may be helpful to

contrast the patient's individual risk to the risk in the general population for the defect in question and for birth defects in general.

3. *Value of the test results*—This must be established early in the course of counseling. While negative test results will provide reassurance, the patients must consider in advance their options if a positive diagnosis is made. After counseling, the couple is given the time necessary for reaching a decision regarding testing. This may be difficult because of the time limitations imposed by pregnancy. Specific time limits are set when necessary. Many centers provide written information as an adjunct to counseling. This may be in the form of a letter from the counselor, a booklet, or an article.

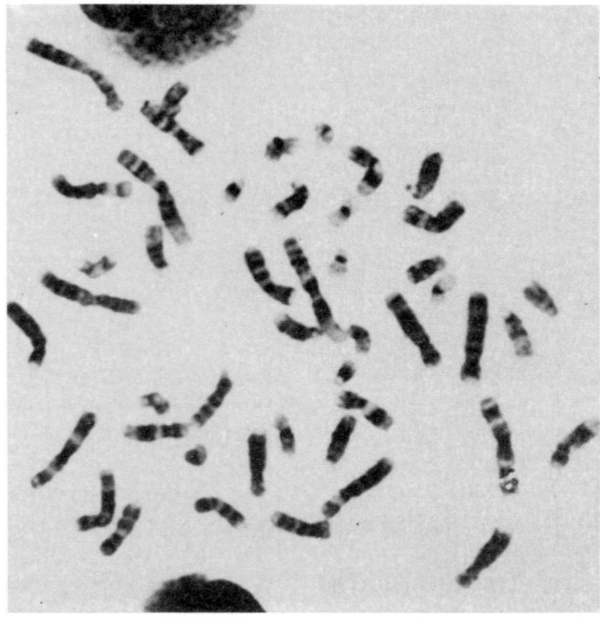

Figure 16-1.
G-banded chromosome spread shown. Karyotype of same spread above.

Disorders Amenable to Prenatal Diagnosis

Chromosome Disorders

The nucleus of a normal human cell contains 46 chromosomes (diploid number of 2N), which includes 22 pairs of autosomes and one pair of sex chromosomes (XX in females and XY in males). Each chromosome is composed of DNA strands containing thousands of genes and a supporting protein structure. The mature gamete contains only 23 chromosomes (haploid number of N), one member of each chromosome pair and one sex chromosome (an X in the ova and either an X or a Y in the sperm) as a result of meiosis (Fig. 16-2A). At the time of fertilization, the diploid number is restored, and one member of each chromosome pair is inherited from each parent.

The chromosomes of an individual may be examined by arresting the metaphase of dividing cells with colchicine or related agents. This can be done with lymphocytes, cultured skin fibroblasts, or amniotic fluid cells. After appropriate preparation, the chromosome content of the cell is analyzed microscopically, photographed, and karyotyped (Fig. 16-1). Pretreatment of the chromosomes with a number of different chemical agents will cause distinctive staining patterns (banding) which allows the identification of each chromosome pair and definition of small subsegments of the chromosomes. The successful culture and cytogenetic study of human amniotic fluid cells was first reported in 1966. Since that time, cytogenetic analysis of cultured amniotic fluid cells has been the most frequently used method for prenatal diagnosis of genetic disorders.

Numerical Chromosome Errors

An abnormal number of chromosomes (*aneuploidy*) in conception results in major developmental defects. When there is an extra chromosome in each cell, the

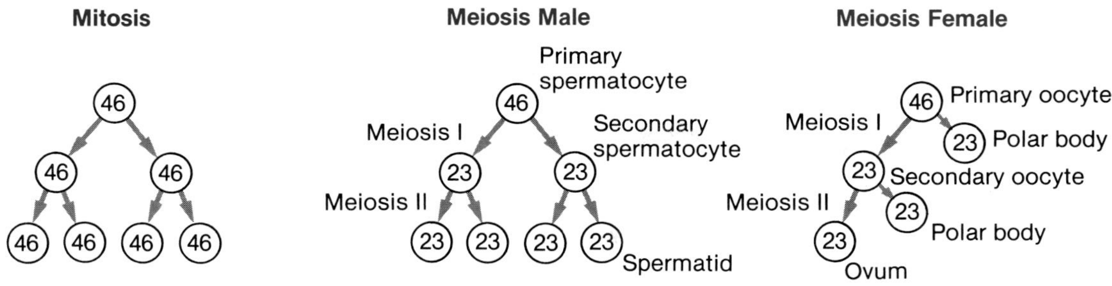

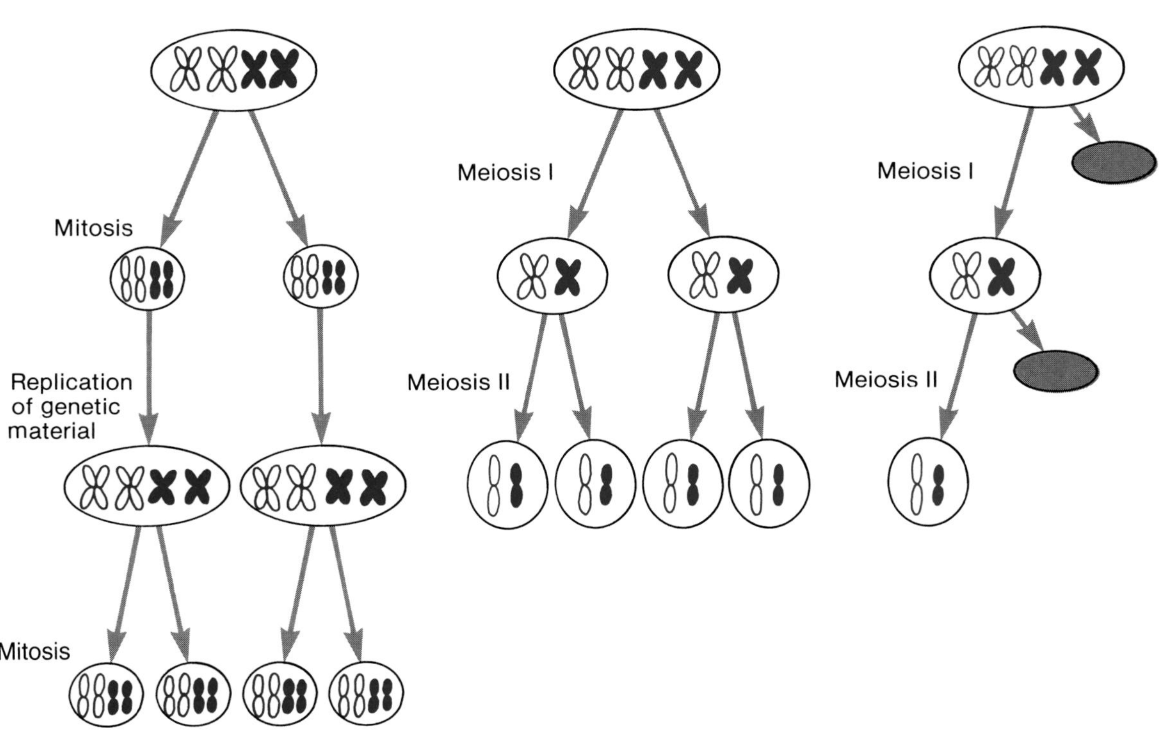

Figure 16-2A.
Normal mitosis and meiosis. Upper portion demonstrates the segregation of chromosomes numerically and lower portion depicts the segregation of two of the 23 chromosome pairs. *(Left)* two normal mitotic divisions, *(center)* normal meiosis in the male, *(right)* normal meiosis in the female.

disorder is termed a *trisomy* and when there is a missing chromosome in each cell, the disorder is termed a *monosomy*. These disorders may originate at conception because the egg or sperm had an abnormal chromosome content, or after fertilization as a result of misdivision of the chromosomes to daughter cells during mitosis. *Nondisjunction,* meaning that there is unequal distribution of chromosomes to daughter cells during either meiotic or mitotic division, accounts for the majority of numerical chromosome abnormalities (Fig. 16-2B). Trisomic conceptions are most often lost during the first trimester of pregnancy. Nevertheless, conceptions with certain abnormalities may be live born.

The cells of a conception may contain 69 (3N or triploid) or even 92 (4N or tetraploid) chromosomes. These conditions, known as *polyploidy,* can be caused by an error in fertilization, for example, two sperm *(dispermy)* penetrating an egg, resulting in a triploid (3N) conception. Polyploid conceptions usually abort, although occasional cases of the prenatal diagnosis or live birth of triploid fetuses are reported.

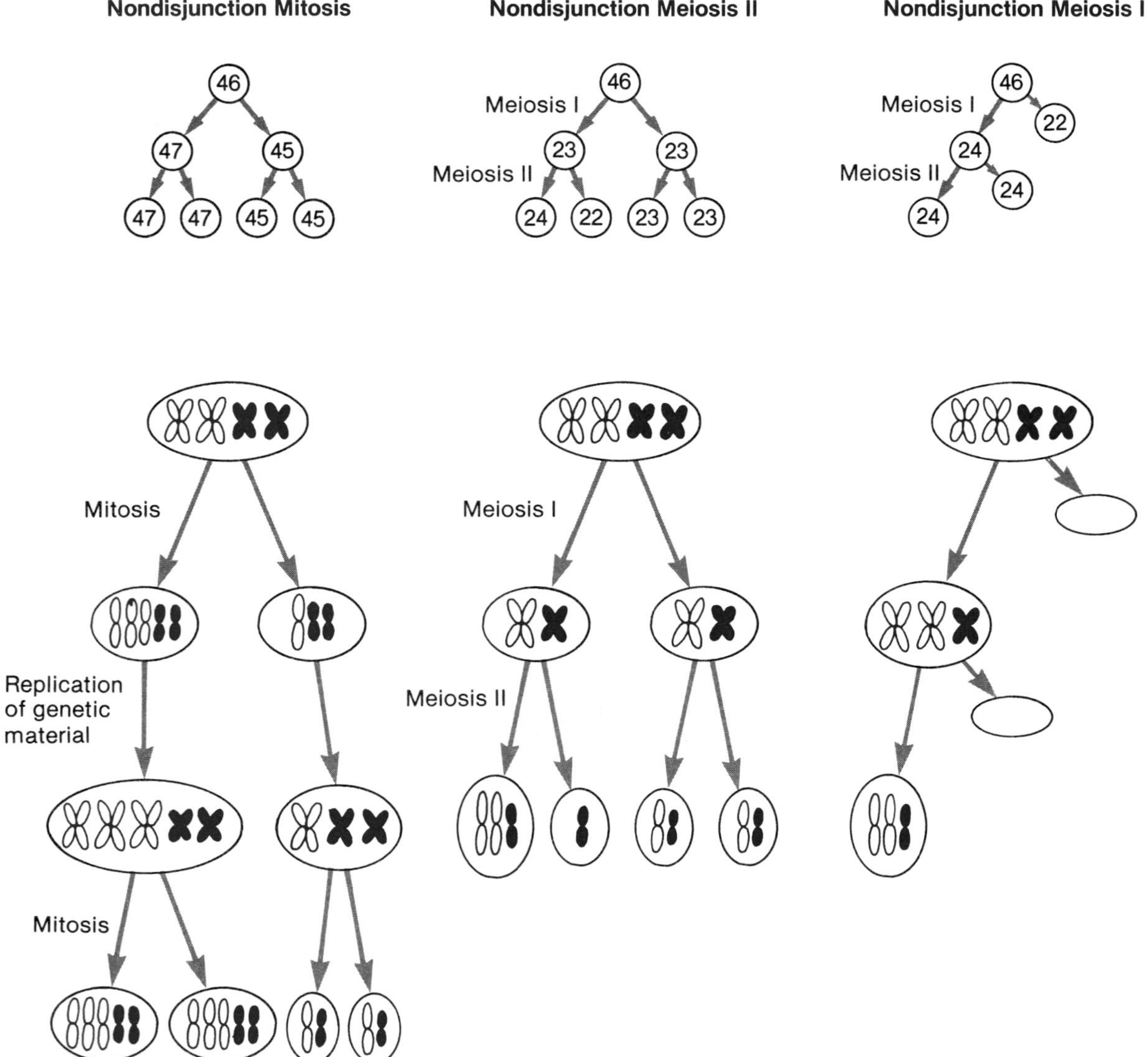

Figure 16-2B.
Nondisjunction in mitosis and meiosis. Upper portion demonstrates the segregation of chromosomes numerically, and lower portion depicts the segregation of two of the 23 chromosome pairs. *(Left)* mitosis, two mitotic divisions with nondisjunction occurring in the first and the error passed through the subsequent division; *(center)* meiosis in male, with nondisjunction occurring in the second division of meiosis resulting in normal and abnormal spermatids; *(right)* meiosis in female, nondisjunction occurring in the first meotic division resulting in abnormal ovum.

Anaphase Lag

Anaphase lag occurs when homologous chromosomes fail to attach or separate correctly on the spindle during cell division, resulting in the loss of one member of the pair. This results in monosomy and is believed to be the mechanism responsible for the majority of X chromosome monosomy (45, X) in human conceptions.

Frequency of Occurrence

The frequency of numerical chromosome errors in human conceptions is much higher than previously suspected, but the vast majority of these pregnancies are lost by spontaneous abortion. It is estimated that in 50% of early spontaneous abortions there is an abnormal number of chromosomes. Autosomal trisomies, 45, X (Turner's syndrome), and polyploidy are the most common abnormalities detected in early abortuses. Surveys of late pregnancy loss, including stillbirth and neonatal deaths, have shown chromosome abnormality in 5% to 10% of these infants. An abnormal chromosome constitution occurs in approximately one in every 200 live births (Table 16-1). The most common numerical abnormalities encountered in newborn surveys are autosomal trisomies (trisomy 21, 18, 13) and sex chromosome aneuploidy (45, X; 47, XXY; 47, XYY; 47, XXX).

Age Factor

The frequency of meiotic nondisjunction resulting in trisomic conceptions increases with maternal age. This is exemplified by the well-defined association between age of the mother and the birth of children with Down's syndrome (trisomy 21). The increased frequency of Down's syndrome births is most dramatic in pregnancies of women over the age of 35 years (see Table 16-2). For this reason, it has become generally accepted that pregnant women in the later reproductive years should have the opportunity to consider amniocentesis. Analysis of the frequency of chromosome abnormality by maternal age in women having prenatal diagnosis has uniformly indicated a higher incidence of Down's syndrome than that observed in newborn studies. Mothers between 35 years of age and 40 years of age had approximately 1.5% rate of positive diagnosis; mothers over 40 years of age had a rate of approximately 5%. The marked discrepancy between newborn and amniocentesis data is probably largely due to the natural loss of chromosomally abnormal fetuses after 16 weeks gestation.

It had been believed that nondisjunction in female meiosis accounted for the majority of trisomic conceptions. Recently, banding techniques have enabled identification of the parental origin of the extra chromosome in some cases. The paternal contribution to Down's syndrome births is more substantial than previously estimated. Currently, there is controversy surrounding a paternal age effect and the clinical counseling which should be given for this.

Although the likelihood of bearing children having different autosomal trisomies (*i.e.,* trisomy 13 or trisomy 18) increases with age, these are much less common abnormalities and the numerical risk is not as well defined as that for trisomy 21. Children with trisomy 18 and trisomy 13 most often do not survive the first year of life. Thus, the burden of these disorders differs from that of Down's syndrome, which is compatible with prolonged survival. Younger women who have had a child with trisomy 21 have a recurrence risk of 1% to 2%, irrespective of their age. These patients, as well as those who have had children with other trisomies, often request amniocentesis.

Table 16-1
Incidence of Chromosome Abnormalities Newborns

Type	Incidence
Sex chromosome	
Males	1:400
47XYY	1:1100
47XXY	1:1100
Other	1:1300
Females	1:700
45X	1:9500
47XXX	1:950
Other	1:2700
Autosome	
Trisomies	1:700
Trisomy 13	1:19,000
Trisomy 18	1:8000
Trisomy 21	1:800
Other	1:5500
Autosomal structural abnormalities	
Unbalanced	1:1700
Balanced	1:500

Table 16-2
Incidence of Down's Syndrome Births Related to Maternal Age

Age	Ratio	Age	Ratio
<20	1:2300	34	1:527
20–25	1:1600	35	1:413
25–30	1:1200	36	1:333
		37	1:266
30–35	1:880	38	1:183
35–40	1:290	39	1:135
		40	1:106
40–45	1:100	41	1:83
>45	1:46		

Retrospective data for maternal age related risk of Down's syndrome taken from: Collman, R.D., Stoller, A.: "A Survey of Mongoloid Births in Victoria, Australia 1942–1957." *American Journal of Public Health* 52:813, 1962; Hook, E. B.: "Estimates of Maternal Age—Specific Risks of a Down's-Syndrome Birth in Women Aged 34—41." *Lancet* 2:33, 1976.

Structural Chromosome Abnormalities

Structural chromosome abnormalities occur as a result of breakage and reunion of chromosomes. Exchange of material between chromosomes of different pairs is known as a *translocation* (Fig. 16-3A). If all the genetic material is conserved, the individual is unaffected by this and is designated a balanced carrier of the rearrangement. There are no phenotypic consequences for the balanced carrier except the reproductive problems associated with the conceptions of pregnancies with an unbalanced chromosome constitution. The gametes that are produced by a balanced translocation carrier may contain a normal chromosome constitution, the balanced rearranged chromosomes, or a combination of the two chromosome pairs which would result in deleted or duplicated chromosome segments (Fig. 16-3B). In the latter case, spontaneous abortion may occur; however, if

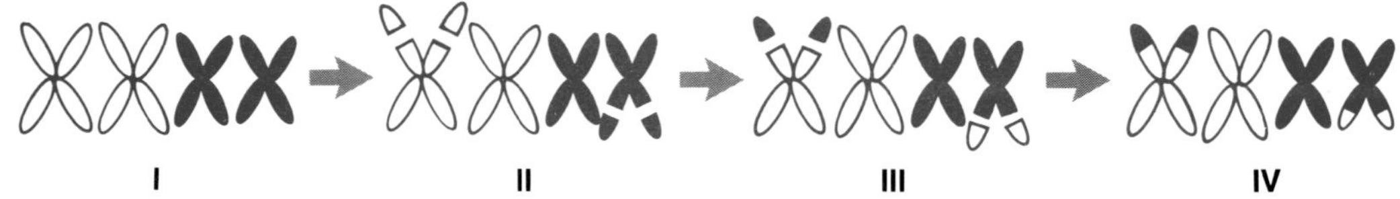

Figure 16-3A.
Mechanism of reciprocal translocation. I. two normal chromosome pairs; II. breakage of one member of each pair; III. exchange of broken segments; IV. reunion to form balanced rearrangement (translocation).

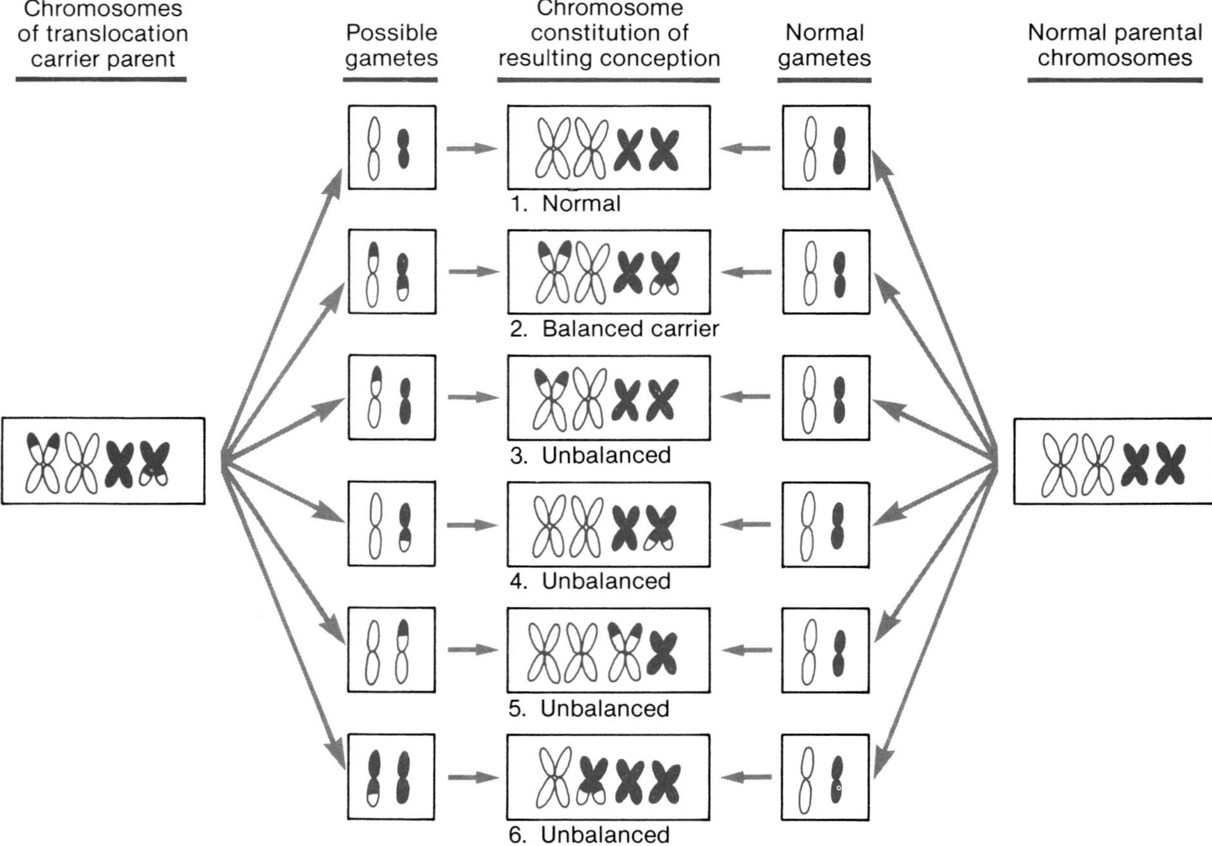

Figure 16-3B.
Depicts gametes formed by parent with translocation shown in part A and resulting conceptions after fertilization with normal gametes. 1. normal; 2. balanced translocation carrier; 3. 4. 5. and 6. conceptions with unbalanced chromosomal segments.

there are live-born infants with missing or extra chromosome segments they are likely to have serious physical and mental defects.

Since the development of banding, which helps to identify chromosome regions, many more children are being diagnosed as having structural chromosome abnormalities. This may occur *de novo* (as a new event) or it may be secondary to a balanced translocation or other structural rearrangement in one parent. Persons with translocations are usually detected by a history of habitual abortion or the birth of a child with an abnormal chromosome constitution. The majority of balanced structural rearrangements detected in humans are familial.

Translocations involving the number 21 chromosomes may result in children born with Down's syndrome due to additional chromosome material. Because a balanced translocation may be passed from one generation to another, a family history of Down's syndrome should be investigated. Chromosome analysis of the affected child will indicate whether the abnormality is due to nondisjunction (sporadic) or if it is secondary to a familial translocation. If an unbalanced translocation is found, chromosome studies to identify relatives who are translocation carriers are indicated. The reproductive risk when a parent carries a translocation varies with the sex of the carrier and the particular rearrangement. In these cases the parents may elect amniocentesis to determine if the fetus has an unbalanced chromosome constitution. If the family member with Down's syndrome is unavailable for study, chromosome analysis performed on the patient's blood will readily determine if he or she is a carrier of a translocation involving the number 21 chromosome.

On occasion, patients without the usual indications request cytogenetic testing of a pregnancy by amniocentesis. In many instances, the motivation for this request is previous experience with Down's syndrome. Often this contact is with a family member who has the disorder or occupational, as with nurses, physicians, or educators. Counseling is given based on the patient's particular age-related risk. The risks and accuracy of the testing are presented. It is explained to the patient that she and her partner are the only ones who can decide whether the benefit of the reassurance gained by the testing justifies the risk involved (See the chart for Indications for Prenatal Cytogenetic Testing).

Mendelian Disorders

A large number of genetic disorders that follow the inheritance patterns described by Mendel (*i.e.,* dominant gene, recessive gene, X-linked gene) have been delineated. For some of these diseases, the expression of the gene in cultured cells can be studied, permitting fetal diagnosis by amniotic cell culture (Table 16-3).

Dominant Disorders

Dominant disorders are those in which the presence of a single abnormal gene results in important phenotypic changes or disease, even though the other member of the gene pair is normal. Dominant disorders may occur as a result of a new mutation of a gene or by transmission of an abnormal gene from one of the parents. When one parent has a dominant disorder, the chance that he or she will contribute the abnormal member of the gene pair to a fetus is one in two, or 50%. Because the penetrance and expression of some dominant genes vary greatly, the diagnosis of the disorder in a parent may only be made after the birth of an affected child. It is important that the counselor be familiar with the frequency of penetrance and the variability of expression of the gene for a disease when discussing the concepts of risk and burden with the family.

The biochemical expression of the gene for many dominant disorders is not known at the cellular level, and they are not detectable by amniocentesis. In some instances, anatomic defects associated with the disorder may be diagnosed by methods that define fetal anatomy. Prenatal diagnosis may be possible when the gene for a dominant disorder is linked (*i.e.,* in close proximity) on the chromosome to other traits that can be studied. The risk of the disease in this instance is defined by studying the linked gene rather than the gene for the disease. The applicability of this approach is limited at present, but it may become considerably more useful in the future. Several requirements must be met before a linkage study may be used for prenatal diagnosis—close linkage of the

Text continued on page 273

Indications for Prenatal Cytogenetic Testing

- Advanced maternal age
- Previous trisomy
- Parent with balanced structural rearrangement (translocation)
- Mother carrier of X-linked recessive disorder
- Mother carrier of fragile X (X-linked mental retardation)
- Client request

Table 16-3
Prenatal Diagnosis of Metabolic Diseases

Disease	Diagnostic Test
Lipid Metabolism	
Tay-Sachs	Hexosaminidase A
Sandhoff	Hexosaminidase A and B
Gaucher	β-glucosidase
G_{M1}-gangliosidosis	β-galactosidase
Niemann–Pick	Sphingomyelinase
Fabry	α-galactosidase
Metachromatic leucodystrophy	Aryl sulphatase A
Krabbe	Galactosylceramide-galactosidase
Wolman	Acid esterase
Familial hypercholesterolemia	LDL cell-surface receptor
Mucopolysaccharidoses and Related Disorders	
Hurler (MPS IH)	α-iduronidase
Scheie (MPS IS)	α-iduronidase
Hunter (MPS II)	Sulphoiduronate sulphatase
Sanfilippo A (MPS IIIA)	Heparan sulphate sulphamidase
Sanfilippo B (MPS IIIB)	α-N-acetylglucosaminidase
Maroteaux-Lamy (MPS IV)	Arylsulphatase B
Mucolipidosis II (I-cell disease)	Lysosomal hydrolases
Mucolipidosis III	Lysosomal hydrolases
Mucolipidosis IV	EM ultrastructure
Fucosidosis	α-fucosidase
Mannosidosis	α-mannosidase
Sialidosis (variant)	Neuraminidase + β-galactosidase
Amino Acid Metabolism	
Argininosuccinicaciduria	Argininosuccinate
Cystinosis	^{35}S-cystine uptake
Citrullinaemia	Argininosuccinate synthetase
Homocystinuria	Cystathionine synthetase
Maple syrup urine	α-keto acid decarboxylase
Methylamalonic acidemia	
B_{12}-responsive	Deoxyadenosyl-B_{12} synthesis
B_{12}-nonresponsive	Methylmalonyl-CoA mutase
Propionic acidemia	Propionyl-CoA decarboxylase
Carbohydrate Metabolism	
Glycogen storage type II	α-glucosidase
Glycogen storage type IV	Amylo-(1, 4 $\rightarrow$ 1, 6) transglucosidase
Galactosaemia	Gal-1-P uridylyl transferase
Pyruvate decarboxylase deficiency	Pyruvate decarboxylase

(Continued)

Disease	Diagnostic Test
Blood	
Haemophilia A	Factor VIII/Factor VIII Antigen
Sickle-cell anemia	β-chain synthesis/restriction enzyme analysis
Homozygous β-thalassemia	β-chain synthesis/restriction enzyme analysis
Homozygous α-thalassemia	c-DNA hybridization
$\beta^{\circ}\delta^{\circ}$ - Thalassemia	c-DNA hybridization
Chronic granulomatous disease	NBT/superoxide formation
Miscellaneous	
Combined immunodeficiency	Adenosine deaminase
Lesch–Nyhan syndrome	HGPRT
Menke's disease	Copper uptake
Xeroderma pigmentosum	DNA repair
Hypophosphatasia	Alkaline phosphatase isoenzymes
Acute intermittent porphyria	Uroporphyrinogen I synthesis
Congenital adrenal hyperplasia (21-hydroxylase)	HLA-B linkage
Lysosomal acid phosphatase deficiency	Acid phosphatase
Congenital nephrosis	α-fetoprotein

genes for the disease and marker (*i.e.*, the linked trait being studied), assignment of the gene and marker in the family by studying affected and unaffected family members, and an information mating (*i.e.*, transmission of the abnormal gene can be determined or excluded with a high level of confidence by studying the linked markers in the fetus).

Recessive Disorders

Recessive disorders are those in which both members of the gene pair are abnormal or deficient. When only one member of the pair is abnormal, the individual is unaffected but is heterozygous for, or a carrrier of, the gene. Production of a child with recessive disorders can only occur when both parents are carriers of the same abnormal gene. In this instance there is a 50% chance (1:2) that the child will inherit the abnormal gene from either parent. The likelihood that the child will inherit the abnormal gene from both parents and, thus, have the disease (homozygous) is 25%. ($1/2 \times 1/2 = 1/4$). For prenatal diagnosis of a recessive disorder it is essential that the test be able to discriminate between the heterozygous (carrier) and the homozygous (affected) because two thirds of normal offspring will be carriers. (Fig. 16-4).

Everyone carries recessive genes for several rare disorders. Although these may be passed from generation to generation, the likelihood that a carrier will reproduce with another carrier of the same rare gene is quite low. In some instances, a couple are carriers of the same abnormal gene because they are closely related (consanguinity). The genes for some disorders that are otherwise quite rare have a relatively higher frequency in certain geographic areas or ethnic groups. Common examples of this were previously cited. Most often, couples in which both members are carriers of the gene for a rare recessive disorder are not identified until birth of an affected child. If laboratory testing can detect carriers for a recessive disorder, counseling and monitoring of pregnancies can be offered prior to the birth of an affected child. Screening programs for *Tay-Sachs disease* (hexosaminidase A deficiency) are examples of this approach. The carrier frequency for this disorder in United States population is about 1/300. Thus, the

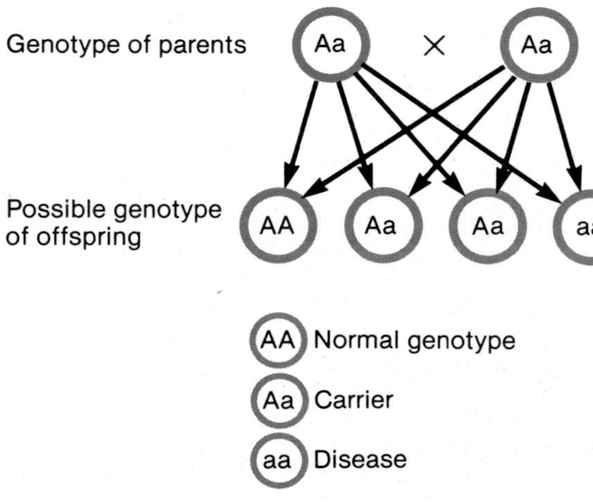

Figure 16-4.
Recessive inheritance. A-normal gene, a-abnormal gene, AA-normal genotype, Aa-carrier, aa-disease. Note that the frequency of aa children when both parents are Aa carriers is 1:4 or 25%.

chance that both members of any couple are carriers of the gene is 1/300 × 1/300 = 1/90,000. Because the risk to a "carrier couple" of having a child is one in four, the frequency of the disease is 1/90,000 × 1/4 = 1/360,000. The likelihood that a person of Eastern European Jewish origin carries this gene is one in 30. Thus, the frequency of a "carrier couple" is 1/30 × 1/30 = 1/900 and the frequency of the disease is 1/900 × 1/4 = 1/3600. Because reliable prenatal diagnosis is available for this lethal disease, many Jewish communities support voluntary screening programs for carrier detection.

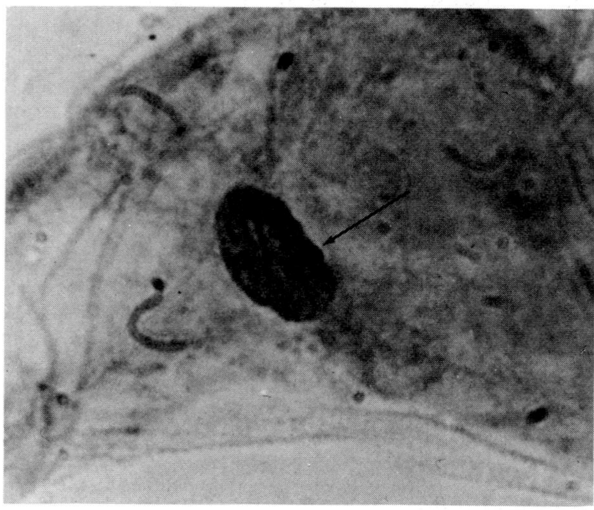

Figure 16-5.
Cell from buccal mucosa. Arrow points to Barr body.

More than 50 recessive disorders may be diagnosed by amniocentesis. For many of the disorders, the availability of diagnosis is limited to a few research laboratories.

X-Linked Recessive Disorders

The genes of X-linked recessive disorders are present on the X chromosome. In women, one X chromosome is inactivated in each cell. This inactivated X chromosome may be visualized as a chromatin mass in the periphery of the cell nucleus and is called a *Barr body* (Fig. 16-5). In women with Turner's syndrome (45, X), the single X chromosome is active in each cell and Barr bodies are absent. Individuals with more than two X chromosomes (47, XXX) maintain only one active X in each cell.

Inactivation of the X chromosome in normal women occurs randomly; that is, in some cells the maternally inherited X chromosome is active while in the other cells the paternally inherited X chromosome is active. Thus, when a woman has a gene for an X-linked recessive disorder on one of her two X chromosomes, it will be genetically active in only a portion of her cells. The woman is a carrier of the gene for the disorder and in some instances, the X chromosome with the abnormal gene will be active in enough cells to allow laboratory identification of the carrier state. Unless the normal X chromosome happens to be inactivated in the vast majority of cells, the disease will not be manifested.

The single X chromosome that is present in the male is active in each cell. When a gene for an X-linked recessive disorder is present on that chromosome, the male will manifest the disease. Commonly cited examples of X-linked recessive disorders are hemophilia (Factor VIII deficiency) and Duchenne type muscular dystrophy. In some instances, a male child will have the disorder by new mutation. When the gene is inherited in the family, there may be a history of the disease in the mother's brothers or her uncles. Half of the daughters born to a carrier mother will also be carriers of the gene. Likewise, half of the sons born to a carrier mother will inherit her X chromosome with the mutant gene and will have the disease.

Amniotic fluid studies can detect affected males for a few X-linked recessive disorders such as Lesch–Nyhan and Hunter's syndromes. Hemophilia A may be diagnosed by using fetal blood obtained by fetoscopy in male fetuses at risk. In the majority of cases when a woman is a carrier of an X-linked recessive disorder, the risk can only be refined by identifying the sex of the fetus. Sex identification of the fetus is most reliably performed by chromosome analysis.

A proportion of nonspecific mental retardation in males is due to X-linked recessive genes. Recently the expression of a fragile site on the X chromosome of some of these males using specific cell culture conditions has enabled diagnoses of one form of X-linked mental retardation. A fragile site on a chromosome is a specific segment or band of the chromosome that demonstrates breakage with a higher frequency than expected as a random phenomenon. Methods for carrier identification and prenatal diagnosis of the fragile X chromosome associated with mental retardation are being actively investigated and will probably be clinically applied in the very near future.

When the fetus of a mother who is a carrier for an X-linked recessive disorder is male, there is a 50% risk that the child will have the disease. If the disorder cannot be specifically diagnosed by other methods, the patient and her husband face the dilemma of selective termination based on the sex of the fetus.

Multifactorial Defects

Multifactorial defects occur when several genes predispose the fetus to or lower the threshold for an abnormality in development. In addition to the genetic constitution, environmental factors are thought to play a part in the development of these defects. Many of the most common birth defects are multifactorial in origin. Most often, these are single defects such as cleft palate, pyloric stenosis, congenital heart disease, or neural tube defects (*e.g.,* anencephaly and myelomeningocele).

The occurrence risks in close relatives are based on empiric studies of families in which the defect has occurred. The risk for siblings is frequently in the range of 2% to 7% and increases with each affected child. The risk to other close relatives (*e.g.,* nieces, nephews, and first cousins), although low, is often higher than that of the general population. More distantly related persons (*e.g.,* second cousins) are usually not at a substantially increased risk compared to the population. Advances in the methods used to detect structural abnormalities in the fetus, especially ultrasound and fetoscopy, may be useful for the diagnosis of some of these defects.

Neural-Tube Defects

The only group of the more common multifactorial disorders that can be reliably diagnosed by amniocentesis at present are neural-tube defects (NTDs). These defects arise during early fetal development due to a failure of fusion or disruption of the neural tube, which will form the central nervous system. Although they may be associated with chromosome abnormalities or certain recessive disorders, the majority of NTDs are multifactorial in origin. The frequency of NTDs in the United States population is one per 1000 live births to two per 1000 live births. The risk of recurrence when there has been an affected child is 3% to 5%. Following two affected pregnancies, this risk increases to 10% to 12%.

Neural-tube defects are described according to their location and anatomic structure. *Anencephaly,* a failure of development of the brain and skull, is the most severe NTD and is incompatible with survival. *Myelomeningocele* (spina bifida), in which there is a defect in formation of the spinal cord, surrounding tissues, and spinal column, is the other most common NTD. Neural tube defects are also seen in children with other malformations. In some situations these may be sporadic or chromosomal. In other cases, the defect is caused by a single mutant gene (*e.g.,* Meckel's syndrome, which is autosomal recessive and may be confused with trisomy 13). Because of the heterogeneity of these defects, accurate diagnosis before counseling is essential in order to present accurate information.

Advances in neurosurgical techniques and aggressive medical management have improved the survival and quality of life for children with NTDs. Nevertheless, the likelihood of serious handicaps remains quite high for most of these children.

The prenatal diagnosis of NTDs by amniotic fluid analysis is based primarily on measure of the *alpha fetoprotein* (AFP) concentration in the amniotic fluid. Alpha fetoprotein is produced in large quantities by the fetal yolk sac and liver during early fetal life, resulting in high concentrations in the fetal blood. A substantially lower concentration of AFP is normally present in amniotic fluid. When a highly vascularized, nonskin-covered defect such as a meningomyelocele is present, the leakage of AFP from the fetal circulation into the amniotic fluid will elevate the levels of AFP in the amniotic fluid. Other abnormalities in which there are skin defects, such as omphalocele, may also be associated with elevated AFP levels in the amniotic fluid. To enhance the accuracy of this testing, confirmatory amniotic fluid tests and definition of the anatomic defect by ultrasound or amniography have been developed.

Very low concentrations of AFP are measurable in maternal blood by sensitive radioimmunoassay techniques. Maternal serum AFP concentration increases during the second trimester and peaks at approximately 34 weeks gestation to 36 weeks gestation. Studies have shown that maternal serum testing is a reasonably reliable method of identifying a large percentage of fetuses with an open neural-tube defect. Because of the changing levels of maternal serum AFP as pregnancy advances, cut-off values for normal results must be established on a week by week basis and interpretation of results requires accurate gestational dating. The feasibility of large-scale maternal serum screening has been investigated in areas of the United Kingdom, where the frequency of these defects is several times higher than in the United States. It is possible that this type of screening may be offered in the United States on a voluntary basis, after the reliability and cost effectiveness are further evaluated in our lower risk population.

Methods Used in the Prenatal Detection of Birth Defects

Several techniques may be employed in the prenatal diagnosis of genetic disorders or birth defects. Ideally, these methods should define the genotype (genetic constitution) of the fetus; however, in some instances only techniques to delineate the phenotype (observable characteristics) of the fetus are available. The latter include fetal visualization by roentgenogram, ultrasound, and fetoscopy.

Roentgenograms

Roentgenograms performed as early as 20 weeks of pregnancy have been used to examine the fetus for skeletal manifestations of certain genetic disorders or birth defects. Because the fetal skeleton is rather poorly visualized at this gestational age, *amniography* is often employed. In this procedure, a water-soluble contrast material is injected into the amniotic fluid to provide a more distinctive outline of the fetus and improve the identification of skeletal structures (Fig. 16-6). The usefulness of radiographic procedures is limited to the diagnosis of severe disorders with major skeletal manifestations early in development or, occasionally, large soft tissue defects (*e.g.*, a bulging myelomeningocele). Unfortunately, many skeletal disorders can only be diagnosed so late in pregnancy that the option of termination is not feasible.

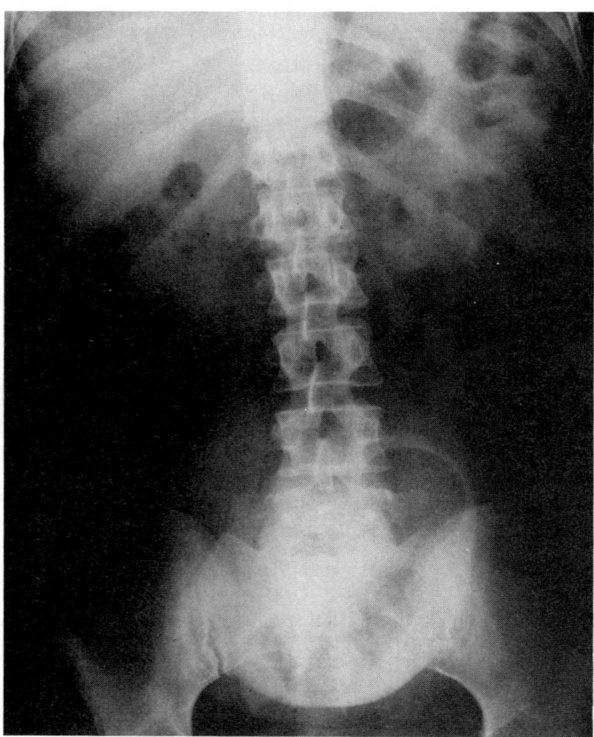

Figure 16-6.
Amniogram outlining 16-week fetus with normal skull.

Ultrasound

Rapid advances in *ultrasound* have enabled the definition of fetal anatomy to a degree not imagined ten years ago. Fetal organs may be evaluated and single organ defects can be detected with this technique. Additionally, the examination of one organ may permit the diagnosis or refine the risk of certain multiple malformation syndromes. Examination of the cerebral ventricles for dilation owing to hydrocephalus, renal evaluation for the diagnosis of renal agenesis (Potter's syndrome) or polycystic kidneys, and evaluation for short-limbed dwarfism are only a few examples.

Fetoscopy

Delineation of other defects will require more direct examination of the fetus by *fetoscopy*. Under local anesthesia, a fine caliber endoscope, about the thickness of a 14-gauge needle, is inserted percutaneously into the amniotic cavity to visualize the fetus (Fig. 16-7). Although it is easy to imagine the great potential of this instrument, wide scale use for direct visualization awaits improvement in the optics of the system and further experience for evaluation of its safety. Small amounts of fetal blood obtained from the placental vessels during fetoscopy have been used for fetal diagnosis of a number of diseases, particularly those with abnormality of blood elements, such as, Hemophilia A, hemoglobinopathies, and platelet or white blood cell disorders.

Amniocentesis

Prenatal genetic diagnosis is most often performed when the fetus is at risk of having a disorder which may be diagnosed by studying cells obtained by *amniocentesis*. This relatively simple and safe outpatient procedure may be performed as early as 14 weeks of pregnancy to 16 weeks of pregnancy (Fig. 16-8). Amniotic fluid contains desquamated fetal cells that are separated from the fluid by centrifugation. The supernatant fluid contains a number of hormones, proteins, and other elements that are useful for diagnosis, for example, AFP measurement for the prenatal diagnosis of neural-tube defects. Although the cells present in amniotic fluid come from a variety of sites—amnion, skin, and the gastrointestinal and the genitourinary tract—all are of fetal origin. Of these desquamated cells, a large proportion are dead or dying. Generally, enough viable cells are collected to permit cell culture. The cells are placed in plastic flasks or dishes containing a nutrient medium. The temperature, *p*H, and atmospheric conditions of the culture are adjusted and controlled in specially designed incubators. After a period of time, viable cells will attach to the flask and begin to multiply by cellular division. Chromosome analysis, detection of enzyme defects, and more recently, DNA isolation procedures can be performed following adequate cell growth. With the latter methods, the absence of a gene or a mutant gene may be detected by sophisticated molecular genetic techniques.

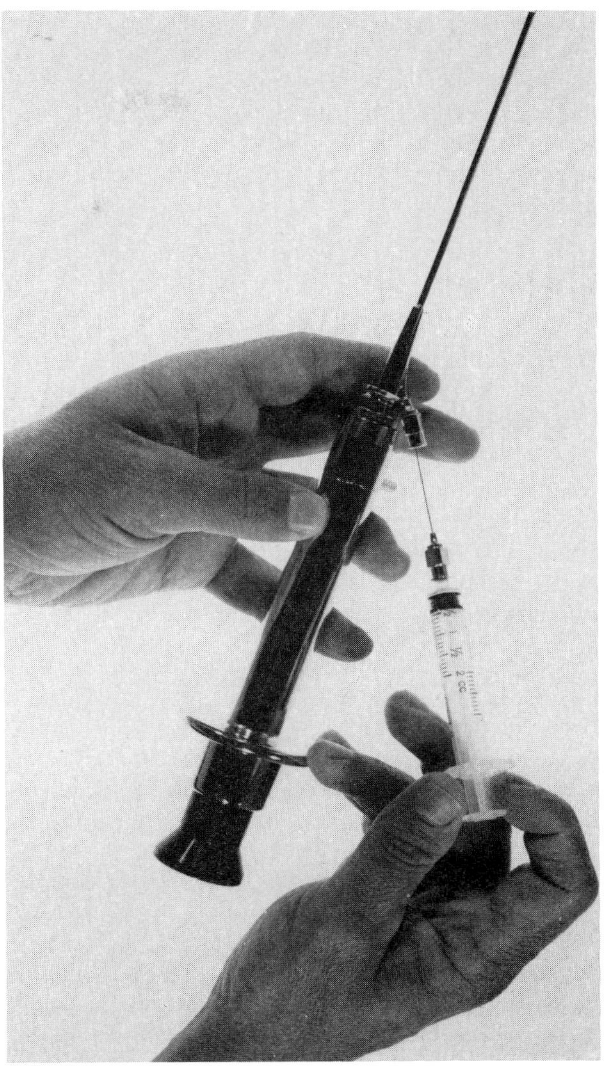

Figure 16-7.
Amnioscope. Endoscope for transabdominal amnioscopy with needle for aspiration.

Role of the Nurse in Prenatal Genetic Counseling and Diagnosis

While the majority of patients referred for genetic counseling and prenatal diagnosis are aware of the reason for referral, most are unsure of what to expect. Contact with the patient should be made as soon as possible after referral. Any delay can only serve to intensify the patient's anxiety, while the advancing gestational age may limit the options available to the patient.

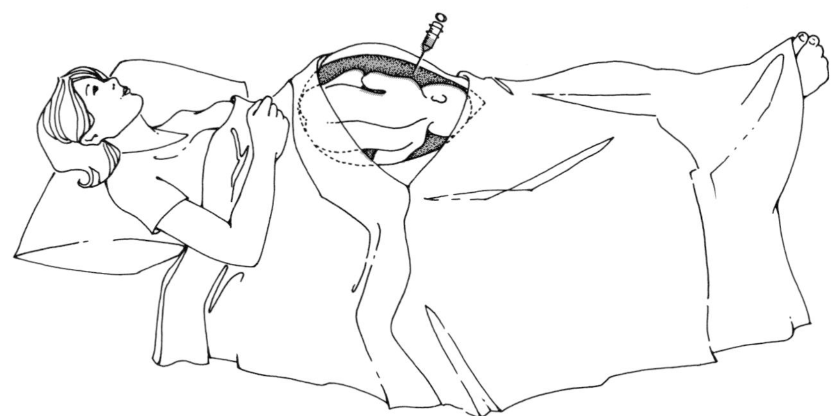

Figure 16-8.
Technique for amniocentesis (From Mennuti MT and Zackai E: Causes and Treatment for Genetic Disorders. An American College of Obstetricians and Gynecologists Patient Information Booklet. Chicago, The American College of Obstetricians and Gynecologists, 1977)

The nurse–counselor must assume an attitude of calm reassurance from the beginning to ensure good rapport. At the outset, the nurse–counselor should make it clear that the decision to have a study performed will rest with the couple and a nondirective approach should be maintained throughout the counseling.

History Taking

During the initial interview, it is useful to assess any factors that may alter the approach to counseling. First, determine how the referral was made and by whom (physician, nurse, advice of a friend or family member, or self-referred because of publicly available knowledge). The patient's response to the referral and her perception of prenatal diagnosis are then discussed. The gestational age of the pregnancy is determined, and the couple's feelings concerning the pregnancy are explored. The counselor should determine if the pregnancy was planned or if there is ambivalence about continuing the pregnancy. It is extremely important to allow the patient to express her ideas and anxieties prior to counseling. If the opportunity for this is not given, the focus during counseling may be diverted from the information presented and may be clouded by prior misinformation or denial.

To ensure comprehensive counseling, the nurse–coordinator obtains a detailed family history (pedigree) (Fig. 16-9). The outcome of all previous pregnancies and the health and development of liveborn children are reviewed. The health and reproductive histories of the couple's parents, their siblings, and both sets of grandparents are taken. In addition, the ethnic origin of the families and any possibility of consanguinity of families are noted.

If a family member is deceased, it is important to know the cause of death and approximate age at which death occurred. When there is a history of a birth defect or mental retardation, there may be a need to review medical records including autopsy reports, x-ray films, photographs, and pathologic slides. This permits the most precise definition of identifiable genetic risks for the couple. If a hereditary disorder in the family is ascertained, this may have great impact on the counseling. For example, if a woman is referred for prenatal cytogenetic diagnosis at age 35 with a one in 400 chance of having a child with Down's syndrome and it is learned from the pedigree that her father recently died from Huntington's chorea (a dominant disorder with late onset of neurologic deterioration), the entire focus of the counseling changes. In that instance, although the chance for a child with Down's syndrome is quite low, the chance that the child will develop Huntington's chorea is 25% (a 50%

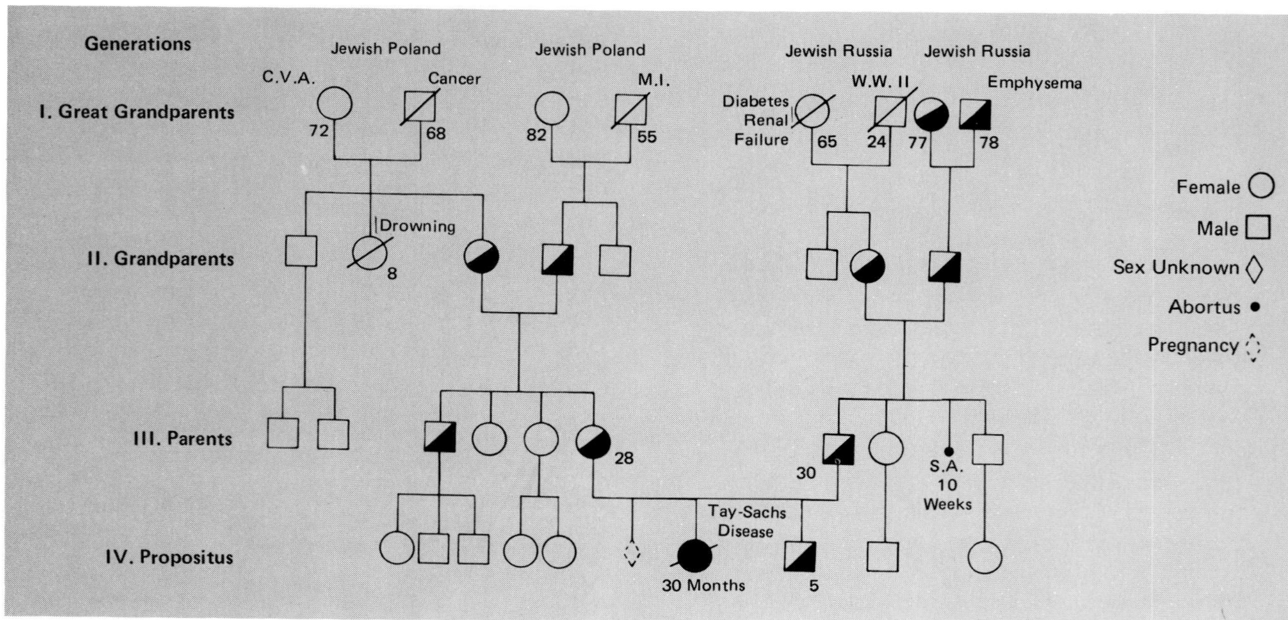

Figure 16-9.
Sample pedigree—demonstrates recessive inheritance of Tay-Sachs disease and the carrier state. Slanted line (/) through symbol represents deceased individual. Carriers are depicted by partially blackened symbol. Affected individual is depicted by totally blackened symbol.

chance that the patient herself has the gene and will develop the disease and a 50% chance if she has the gene that the fetus will inherit it from her). Although prenatal diagnosis of Down's syndrome is available through amniocentesis, there is no predictive study for Huntington's chorea. Thus, this new information may become the most important factor for this couple in selecting options.

When review of family medical records becomes important because of the medical history, it is essential that they are requested in a nonthreatening manner. Many families with malformed or retarded children are very protective of these individuals. Often, their diagnosis is not discussed outside the immediate family and a long-standing silence about their problem has prevailed. Since medical records are confidential, permission is required to obtain them. In order to obtain cooperation, the patient must understand the reason for and value of these records. The release forms are sent to the patient and forwarded to the relatives by her. While family members should not be contacted independently by the counselor, it is vital that the patient be assured that relatives should feel free to contact the counselor for any explanation or clarification. Through this approach, the counselor may create opportunities to offer services to the extended family, while maintaining the privacy of the individual.

A review of medical records may enable the nurse or the physician to determine that the health problems of other family members do not indicate an increased risk for the fetus. If there has been unspoken or denied anxieties about the medical problems of close relatives, the reassurance provided by the counselor is of great value to the couple and, frequently, to other family members.

Once the background information has been gathered and the scope of the counseling has been established, the counseling process begins. In most cases, prenatal counseling can be done by the nurse–counselor. In the usual situation (advanced maternal age without significant family history), an explanation of chromosomes, genes, and their functions is given. The mechanism for, and the numerical risk of, having a child with Down's syndrome at the patient's age are explained and contrasted with the risk at other ages. The couple's knowledge of Down's syndrome is assessed and their information is clarified and supplemented. Studies in genetics clinics have shown that, in addition to numerical risk, the perception of burden is of paramount importance in the decision-making process. The presentation of burden must not be biased by the opinion or experience of the counselor, but must be well founded in fact.

The medical procedures involved in prenatal diagnosis and the rationale for them are explained. It is vitally important to conduct the discussion in terms that the patient can readily understand. The vocabulary must be individualized for each patient. The risks and diagnostic limitations of the procedure are discussed in detail. For example, when ultrasonography is to be performed prior to amniocentesis, it is often necessary to distinguish this procedure from x-ray films. The reasons for performing this test are explained. Ultrasonography allows localization of the placenta. Placental puncture or injury during amniocentesis may be avoided when the implantation site is defined (Fig. 16-10). Measurement of the biparietal diameter of the fetal skull by ultrasound confirms the gestational age. The detection of multiple gestation is also a benefit of the procedure. It is also explained that ultrasound is not painful and requires no special preparation by the patient (*i.e.,* fasting); however, the bladder must be full during the study. The anatomic relationship of the bladder to the anterior lower segment provides a landmark for the evaluation of the uterus and its contents.

Counseling for Amniocentesis

Following a description of the technical aspects of the test, the patient must consider the limitations, safety, and the diagnostic accuracy of the procedure.

Limitations

The nurse–counselor should explain to the patient that amniocentesis is not invariably successful. If ultrasound or clinical examination indicates that the pregnancy is earlier than 14 weeks gestation to 16 weeks gestation, the procedure is postponed. If amniotic fluid is not obtained by the initial needle insertion, the physician may suggest another attempt or postponing the procedure for seven to ten days until a slightly more advanced gestational age. Once an adequate fluid sample is obtained, successful completion of the study depends upon the growth of cells in tissue culture. The patient is told that if culture failure occurs (less than 1% of cases) a repeat amniocentesis must be considered. Most important, the couple must understand that the study is not a general test for birth defects or mental retardation, but is designed to detect the specific disorder which has been discussed in the counseling. It should be explained that any pregnancy has a 2% to 3% chance of resulting in a child born with a birth defect or congenital malformation and that the vast majority of these defects will not be detected by amniocentesis. Chromosome analysis and AFP determination are usually offered even when

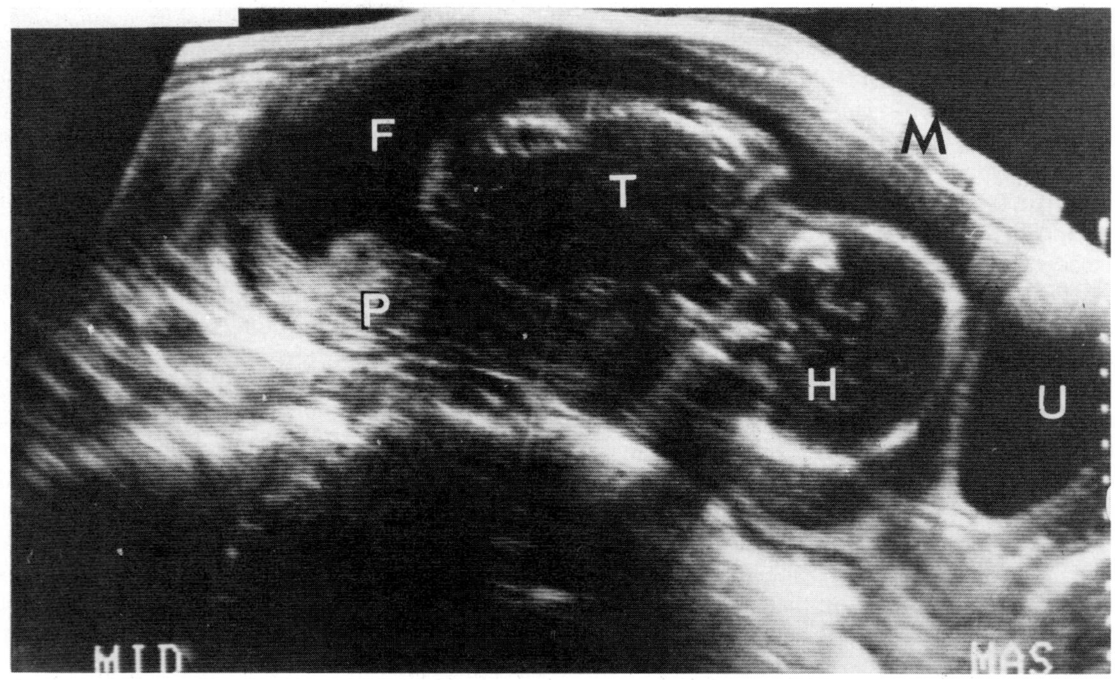

A

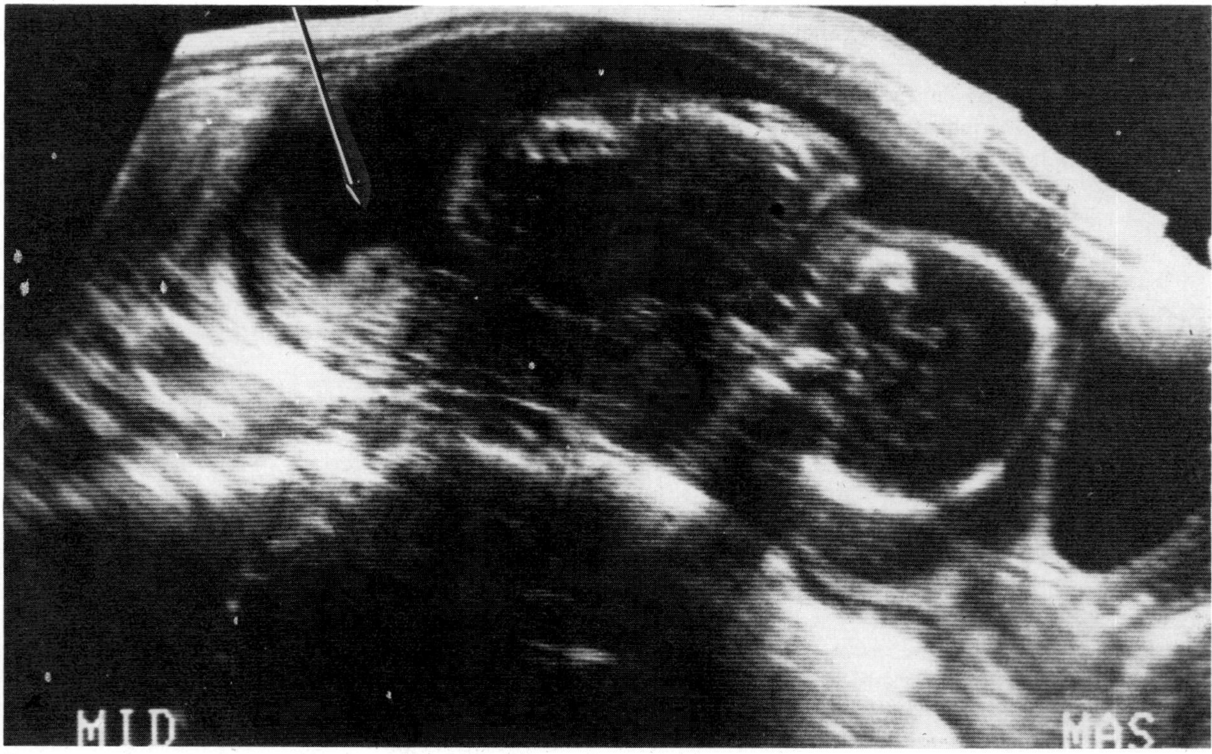

B

Figure 16-10.
(A) B-mode gray scale ultrasound of intrauterine pregnancy. M = maternal abdominal wall; H = fetal head; T = fetal trunk; P = posterior placenta; F = amniotic fluid; U = maternal urinary bladder. *(B)* Same ultrasound. Arrow shows site selected for amniocentesis.

these are not the primary studies being performed. The parents are told that if they wish to know the sex of the child when the chromosome studies are completed, the information will be available to them.

Risks

The risks of amniocentesis must be explained in detail. Concerns regarding spontaneous abortion related to the procedure prompted a collaborative controlled study by a number of centers in the United States. The frequency of pregnancy loss in approximately 1000 patients undergoing midtrimester amniocentesis and in the controls was not significantly different; the incidence of pregnancy loss in both groups was approximately 3.5%. The results were confirmed by a similar study performed in Canada. These studies indicate that the risk of pregnancy loss related to midtrimester amniocentesis is probably considerably less than 1%. More important, if pregnancy loss occurs following amniocentesis, it is most likely unrelated to the procedure. Instances of septic abortion due to chorioamnionitis following midtrimester amniocentesis have been reported. Most often, parents express a fear of fetal injury by the needle. Minor skin scars, secondary to midtrimester amniocentesis injury, occur infrequently and more significant injuries have rarely been reported. Because of the large number of studies being performed, it is reasonable to assume that the likelihood of serious fetal injury is exceedingly low.

Entry of fetal blood cells into the maternal circulation as a result of amniocentesis occurs in approximately 10% of cases. When the woman is Rh negative and the fetus is Rh positive, Rh sensitization may occur. Many centers administer Rh immunoglobulin prophylaxis to Rh negative women in conjunction with amniocentesis. When the potential for Rh sensitization is present, the rationale for this approach is explained.

Other complications following amniocentesis are spotting of blood or leakage of a small amount of fluid from the vagina. These occur in about 1% of cases and are generally limited to an isolated episode. Many patients will experience mild discomfort at the needle site for one to two days and few may have ecchymosis or more rarely, abdominal wall hematoma.

Accuracy

It is of paramount importance that prenatal genetic diagnosis be highly accurate. Nevertheless, every laboratory test has limitations. Every effort is taken to avoid human error, including independent duplicate analysis. When cultured amniotic fluid cells are used for testing, error owing to maternal cell contamination may be unavoidable. In less than 1% of cases, maternal cells are "picked up" by the needle as it penetrates the abdominal wall, and these cells grow in the tissue culture. When this occurs, the study may reflect the genotype of the mother rather than of the fetus.

During counseling, it is not unusual for the patient to ask for the nurse–counselor's opinion or advice regarding the testing. The counselor must emphasize that the decision to have prenatal diagnosis is one that belongs only to the couple. The same information is interpreted differently by each couple based on personal factors. For example, a 40-year-old primigravida with a long-standing infertility problem may view any risk of spontaneous abortion associated with a procedure as unacceptable, and her risk for having a child with Down's syndrome as low (99% chance that it will not occur). When patients ask for advice it should be explained that the opinion of the counselor may not be appropriate to their particular situation.

Postcounsel Follow-Up

After counseling, the couple needs time to discuss all of the information presented with each other and to explore their feelings about the diagnostic procedure. Ideally, the counseling is given at a time when they have several weeks to make a decision regarding the testing. Even when the initial contact is made late in gestation (16 weeks to 18 weeks), the couple should have at least several days to consider the procedure. It should be emphasized that both the husband and the wife must feel comfortable with the decision.

Several days after the counseling the nurse contacts the patient. Any questions that have arisen are answered. If there is a great deal of ambivalence, difficulty, or disagreement about the decision, additional counseling is offered. It may be suggested that the couple speak with the physician either individually or together. Some couples wish to discuss the decision with other family members or advisors as well.

Procedure for Amniocentesis

Shortly prior to amniocentesis, the obstetrician reviews the counseling and answers any additional questions from the couple. The patient is asked to sign a consent form, which includes statements regarding the risks and limitations of the procedure. Because of the rapport which has been established, the presence of the nurse–counselor during the procedure is invaluable in minimizing anxiety. The steps in the pro-

NC Nursing Care: Genetic Counseling

Problem	Intervention	Rationale
Physiological status of pregnancy	Take general health and obstetrical history	Identification of health problem, concurrent disease, and high risk factors. Identification of gestational age (especially important to ascertain ovulation pattern and specific dating information [*e.g.*, BBT, use of Clomid or Pergonal])
Psychological status of pregnancy	Obtain attitudes toward pregnancy, nuclear family composition, initiation of referral, general knowledge and attitude toward prenatal diagnosis	Identify anxieties and receptiveness to referral and counseling Establish rapport
Genetic history of extended family	Obtain multi-generation family pedigree (when necessary, request medical records, arrange appropriate consultations, and perform laboratory studies)	Identify families at risk and provide extended counseling and reevaluation of risks
Counseling for prenatal diagnosis and amniocentesis	Provide precise, detailed information (*e.g.*, ultrasonography and its purposes, length of time for procedures and results) in objective, nonjudgmental manner	Enable couple to weigh advantages and risks for their *individual* situation; alter vocabulary appropriately to meet needs of each couple; avoid giving *personal* opinion or advice
Greet couple and introduce to physician	Brief overview of initial counseling (by nurse–counselor and physician)	Provide opportunity for couple to ask additional questions or to clarify details
Prepare for ultrasound and amniocentesis	Assist patient to examination table; position and drape patient; direct father to best position to observe ultrasound	Make mother as comfortable and as much at ease as possible; father feels included in procedure; parents continue to develop rapport with nurse–counselor

cedure and possible sensations that the patient will feel are anticipated by the nurse and explained to the patient.

After emptying the bladder, the patient is instructed to rest on the examining table in a supine position with her legs extended. The site selected for needle insertion is determined by abdominal examination and the ultrasonic findings. The skin is prepared with antiseptic solution and a sterile field is established. Local anesthesia is injected into the skin and through the abdominal wall to the peritoneum. A stinging or burning sensation upon injection of the local anesthetic is usually the most uncomfortable aspect of amniocentesis. A number 18 gauge or a number 20 gauge spinal needle is inserted through the anesthetized area and uterine wall into the amniotic cavity. The patient may have a sensation of deep pelvic pressure during the procedure.

Amniotic fluid will often spill spontaneously after the amniotic sac is entered with a needle. One ml to two ml of fluid is discarded to help avoid contamination of the sample with cells from the maternal abdominal wall. If blood is obtained at first, the fluid may become clear again before the specimen is collected. The amount of fluid withdrawn varies with the studies performed, but generally it ranges from 5 ml

Problem	Intervention	Rationale
Post amniocentesis instructions	Review possible after effects and complications; provide couple with phone number for answering service (24 hour availability)	Reassure couple that anxiety is a normal response and that nurse–counselor will keep in close contact; encourage couple to call if there are any questions
Notification of normal results	Arrange per couple's preference (call directly, referring physician call with results, or arrange return visit to review results with nurse–counselor or physician)	Allow couple to exercise control in receiving information
Notification of abnormal results	Arrange appointment with couple to return for detailed objective discussion of findings; be prepared to answer any questions regarding diagnosis, prognosis, and pregnancy termination	Allow couple to feel secure that diagnosis is accurate; provide factual information to enable couple to evaluate options and to make decisions
Support during hospitalization	Discuss case history with primary care nurse prior to admission; frequent visits by nurse–counselor; when appropriate, have separate meeting with father	Maintain rapport; prevent father (partner) from feeling excluded or isolated in the hospital setting; allow couple to begin grieving process by expressing their feelings
Follow-up care; check progress in returning to normal lifestyle	Frequent telephone contact (or in-person visits) with couple; encourage expression of feelings (anger, depression, etc); arrange formal appointment with nurse–counselor or physician after several weeks to assess emotional adjustment and answer questions regarding future reproduction	Be alert for signs of severe depression or problems developing in couple's relationship; make referrals when appropriate for mental health care or marriage counseling; discourage couple from making hasty *permanent* decisions regarding future reproduction

to 30 ml. The fluid specimen is collected in two or more separate, sterile syringes which are capped and labeled immediately. The samples are transported to the laboratory in the same syringes to avoid the possibility of bacterial contamination during transfer to another container. The volume of fluid withdrawn rapidly reaccumulates.

Following the procedure, the needle puncture site is dressed with a bandage and the patient is asked to rest on the examining table for several minutes. There are usually no symptoms after the procedure. Although apprehension and anxiety levels are quite high prior to amniocentesis most patients state that the experience involves less discomfort than a dental appointment.

At the conclusion of the procedure, the patient is often shown the labeled sample before it is transported to the laboratory. This helps to alleviate concerns regarding mislabeling of samples, especially if a positive diagnosis occurs. Signs or symptoms of complication, such as bleeding, leakage of amniotic fluid, and fever, are reviewed and instructions for contacting the nurse or physician are given. The length of time required for completion of the studies, usually two to four weeks, is discussed again and the mechanism for notifying the patient of the results is decided.

Counseling after Amniocentesis

Prior to amniocentesis, much of the patient's anxiety is focused on the procedure. Following amniocentesis, the patient's concerns shift to possible complications and the test results. Several days later, the nurse may contact the patient to determine if there are any unusual symptoms related to the procedure. Most often there are none. If necessary, an examination may be arranged. The patient is aware that the successful completion of the study depends on the adequate growth of fetal cells in culture, and that delays or, rarely, failure of culture can occur. The success of the cell culture can usually be determined by the examination of the sample after seven to ten days, and the patient is notified immediately. If repeat amniocentesis is required, this should be discussed with the patient as soon as possible. The patient is reassured that failure or delays in establishing cell culture are not indicative of a problem with the pregnancy. If this occurs, or more commonly, if fluid is not obtained after the initial amniocentesis is attempted, the decision regarding a repeat amniocentesis must be made by the couple.

The anxiety during the interval between successful amniocentesis and final results is also accentuated by physiologic changes and social pressures. In some cases, the parents have not announced the pregnancy to relatives and friends and wish to wait until the diagnostic results are known. During the 16th week of gestation to the 20th week of gestation, the uterus grows and the pregnancy begins to "show" or be more apparent. The mother may feel fetal movement for the first time while awaiting the results of the studies. This will intensify her fears of an abnormal result and her ambivalence about termination. It is interesting that many patients ignore or deny fetal movement until after the studies are completed. A most important aspect of the nurse–counselor's role is giving emotional support to the parents during this waiting period. There should be ample telephone communication with the couple and they should feel free to call as frequently as necessary for reassurance.

Giving the parents the normal results following amniocentesis does not end the nurse–counselor's contact; follow-up is also important. The accuracy of prenatal diagnosis is not confirmed until the baby is born. After delivery, the nurse may also wish to discuss the patient's reactions to amniocentesis once again.

When a positive diagnosis occurs, the nurse–counselor and physician notify the parents, preferably in person. Prior to informing patients of positive results, all studies should be completed and verified; most patients will ask about the certainty of the results. After counseling, these patients often desire termination of the pregnancy as rapidly as possible. The method of termination is selected with maternal safety as the greatest priority. Confirmation of the diagnosis for scientific purposes and parental information are important but should be secondary. Because detailed information regarding pregnancy termination during the second trimester is not offered prior to the test results, this information must be presented to the patient at this time. The nurse–counselor maintains contact with the patient throughout the termination procedure and recovery.

Following selective abortion of an affected fetus, the parents experience grief. Observation of these patients has documented a high frequency of depression and marital discord. Because of the emotional stress following selective abortion of a wanted pregnancy, the couple is dissuaded from making permanent decisions about their future reproduction. Sterilization is not advisable at this time. Several weeks to months later, one or more visits are arranged for the couple to assess their resolution of grief, and if they wish, to discuss future reproduction. In the interval between these visits, the nurse–counselor maintains close contact with the patient. Often she may be the only person with whom the couple can freely discuss their feelings about the pregnancy and termination. Communication between the husband and wife is fostered, and psychiatric care or marriage counseling are offered when appropriate.

Suggested Readings

Harris H: Prenatal Diagnosis and Selective Abortion. Cambridge MA, Harvard University Press, 1975

Milunsky A: Genetic Disease and the Fetus: Diagnosis, Prevention and Treatment. New York, Plenum Press, 1979

NICHD National Registry for Amniocentesis Study Group: "Midtrimester amniocentesis for prenatal diagnosis: Safety and accuracy." JAMA 236, 1976

Simpson NE, et al: Prenatal diagnosis of genetic disease in Canada: Report of a collaborative study. Can Med Assoc J 115, 1976

Smith D: Recognizable Patterns of Human Malformation, 2nd ed., Vol VII. Philadelphia, WB Saunders, 1976

Thompson JS, Thompson MW: Genetics in Medicine, 2nd ed. Philadelphia, WB Saunders, 1973

Study Aids for Unit III:
Reproductive Control and Sexuality—Assessment and Management

Conference Material

1. Ruth W. is 24 years old, pregnant for the first time, and in the eighth month of pregnancy. She and her husband Tom report a generally satisfying sexual relationship during pregnancy. For the last week, however, intercourse has been quite painful on deep thrusting, and she notices continued uncomfortable contractions for one half hour after sex. Because of this, Ruth has been avoiding sex, which is creating tension in their relationship. What additional information would you need, and how would you assist this couple in understanding what is happening and finding approaches to alleviate this problem?

2. Sally and Bill S. are having their second child, and in early pregnancy they seek counseling about the changes in sex drive and responsiveness during pregnancy. They were worried and confused about these changes during the first pregnancy, and did not enjoy their childbearing experience as much as they wanted. Both usually have an intense, enjoyable sexual experience, and this is an important part of their lives. To counsel this couple effectively, what information do you need, and what specific knowledge about sexuality in pregnancy can you draw from?

3. Louise H. is a 34-year-old mother of three who has used oral contraceptives successfully for a total of seven years. Her weight and blood pressure are normal, and there is no history of thromboembolic disease in her family. She smokes a half pack of cigarettes per day and has smoked for 15 years. She is currently taking a combination pill with 50 mcg estrogen. Louise has a stable marriage, her husband is 38 years old, and they feel their family is complete. On this visit for her biannual examination, how would you counsel Louise concerning continuation of oral contraceptives and alternative methods of birth control?

4. Aurora and Saadi are in their early 20s, unmarried and have been living together for 2 years. She had an IUD in place, but became concerned about complications and had the IUD removed last week. They are now interested in a natural method of birth control, which would be more compatible with their life style and philosophy (includes avoiding the introduction of unnatural substances into the body). In discussing their options, what information do you need to know about Aurora's menstrual cycles, the pattern of their sexual relations, and their feelings about an accidental conception? Outline the benefits and risks of using one or a combination of natural contraceptive methods.

5. Vikki is 16, a high school sophomore who is active in student government and has a part-time job. She and her boyfriend Chris have been going steady for 3 months. Vikki has come to the family planning clinic requesting birth control pills, because she and Chris want to begin having sex, but strongly want to avoid pregnancy. In counseling

Conference Material (continued)

Vikki about contraception, what information about teenage sexuality will you draw upon? How would you present their options regarding intercourse and contraception to her? What would be the main considerations in their using the following contraceptive methods: the pill, the IUD, condom, spermicidal cream or foam, diaphragm, and withdrawal?

6. A 44-year-old woman has just been evaluated for a first trimester abortion. She has four children, ages 6 to 17, and had two miscarriages. Presently she is divorced and receiving both state welfare assistance and Aid to Dependent Children, and she has no job. The pregnancy is 10 weeks gestation, and she is definite about wanting an abortion. She desires no further children, and had been using foam and condom as contraception. Although receiving Medicaid, she lives in a state which does not provide funds for abortions. What factors will you take into consideration in discussing the patient's options with her? Since she feels strongly about wanting to have the abortion, what types of assistance can you provide her in carrying out this decision? (Her state of health is good.)

7. Marianne is 17, unmarried, and 12 weeks pregnant. No one but her boyfriend knows that she has come to the clinic for pregnancy evaluation. She is from a middle-class family, her parents have been divorced for 5 years, and she is the oldest of three children. A junior in high school, she is not very interested in her studies and has no clear career plans. Marianne and her boyfriend Jeff have talked about getting married, but he is reluctant as he wants to go to college. She is unhappy with her home situation as she feels she has too much responsibility for her younger siblings; her mother works. She has mixed feelings about the pregnancy, is confused about what she wants to do, and has little understanding about what her choices entail. How would you counsel Marianne and Jeff about their decision making and implementing their choice?

Multiple Choice

Read through the entire question and place your answer on the line to the right.

1. Cervical mucus is not receptive to spermatozoa when it is

A. Clear, abundant, and acellular
B. Turbid and thick
C. Under the influence of progesterone
D. Under the influence of estrogen

Select the number corresponding to the correct letters.

1. A and C
2. A and D
3. B and C
4. B and D ______

2. A pituitary tumor should be suspected and ruled out in the patient with amenorrhea who exhibits
   A. Elevated levels of FSH and LH
   B. Elevated prolactin levels
   C. Low estrogen levels
   D. Pregnanediol in the urine ____

3. A 35-year-old nulligravida has had unprotected intercourse for 10 months. She and her husband both want a pregnancy. She should be told
   A. Not to worry; it will happen in time
   B. To consider having a fertility investigation if pregnancy does not ensue soon
   C. Patients over 35 years of age have a higher incidence of children affected by Down's syndrome, and therefore, pregnancy is unwise ____

Discussion

4. What preparation is necessary for the maternity nurse to provide basic sexual counseling to pregnant families?

5. What areas should be covered in taking a sexual history? What areas should be covered in taking a sexual history during pregnancy?

6. What are the common dysfunctional sexual problems during pregnancy?

7. List three reasons why sexual responsiveness might be both increased and decreased during the first trimester.

8. Under what conditions should intercourse be avoided during pregnancy?

9. During the second and third trimesters, when the uterus is quite enlarged, what are some suggestions to increase the couple's comfort and enjoyment of sex?

10. How would you respond to couples who were afraid of harming the baby by having intercourse?

11. When should a couple resume sexual intercourse after delivery?

12. How would you counsel a couple in which the woman is having painful intercourse 8 weeks after delivery?

13. What general principles would you discuss with parents who are concerned about how to respond to their children's questions and activities related to sex?

Discussion
(continued)

14. What is the difference between theoretical effectiveness and use effectiveness of contraceptives, and what are the implications of this for contraceptive counseling?

15. What are the basic components of informed consent?

16. Name four absolute contraindications to use of oral contraceptives.

17. Name six common side-effects (not major life-threatening side-effects) of oral contraceptives.

18. What information is essential to know in counseling women who smoke about use of oral contraceptives?

19. Name four major contraindications to IUD insertion.

20. Name three common side-effects (not major life-threatening side-effects) of the IUD.

21. What are the key elements in successful use of the diaphragm?

22. What are the key elements in successful use of the condom?

23. What is the rationale underlying natural methods of birth control that rely on fertility awareness?

24. When might spermicidal creams, jellies, or foams be the contraceptive method of choice?

25. In counseling a couple about sterilization, what key factors must be included for a satisfactory long-term decision?

26. What are the major provisions of the 1973 United States Supreme Court decision which legalized elective abortions?

27. What did the 1976 Hyde Amendment contain that is relative to use of federal funds for abortion, and what have been some outcomes of this?

28. Discuss four reasons why a woman might want to terminate her pregnancy.

29. What have been three findings of studies on the psychological sequela of abortions?

30. Discuss the effects of three legal and regulatory restrictions placed on obtaining an abortion upon the woman and her family.

UNIT

IV

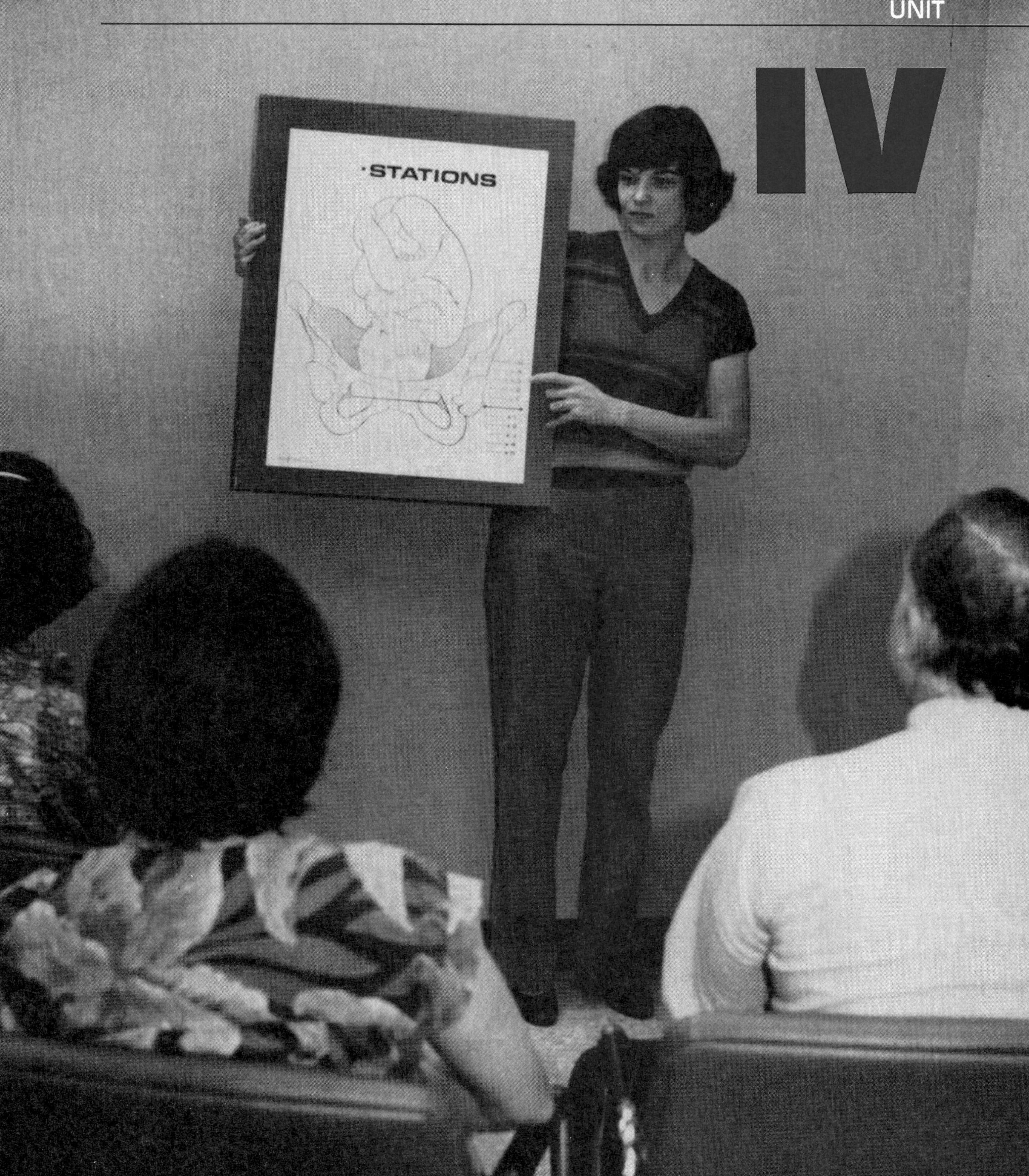

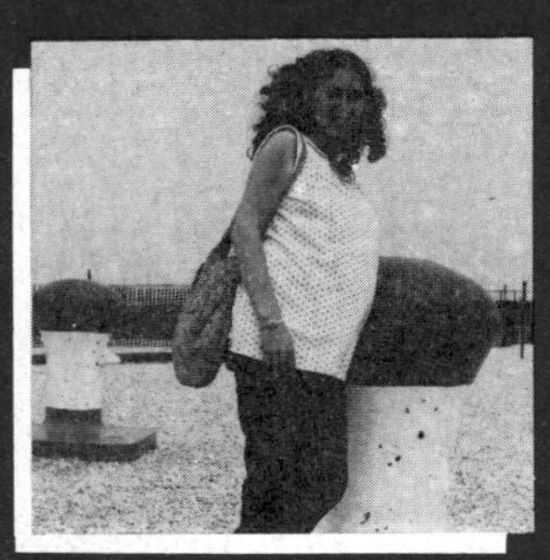

17
Biophysical Aspects of Normal Pregnancy

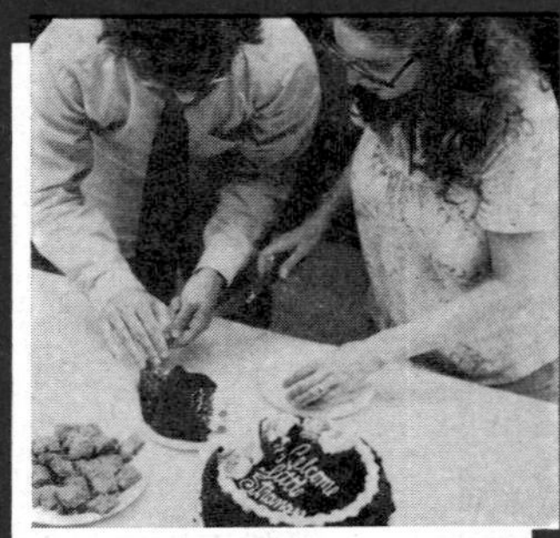

18
Psychosocial Aspects of Normal Pregnancy

UNIT IV

Antepartal Assessment and Management

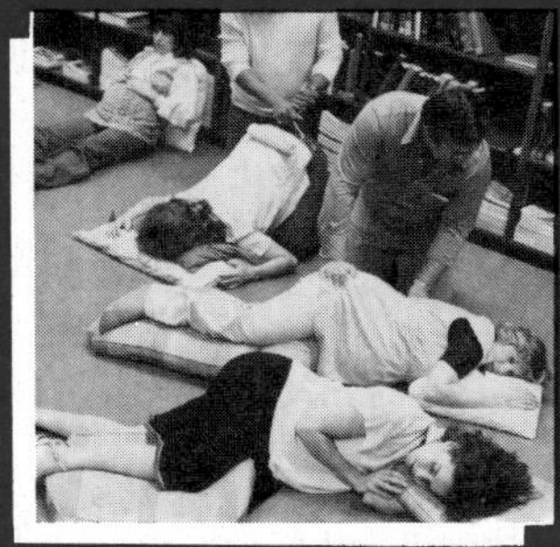

19 Parent Education

Factors in Parent Education

Types of Education for Childbearing

Guide for Preparing Parents for Childbirth and the Puerperium

Comfort During Pregnancy

Postpartum Teaching

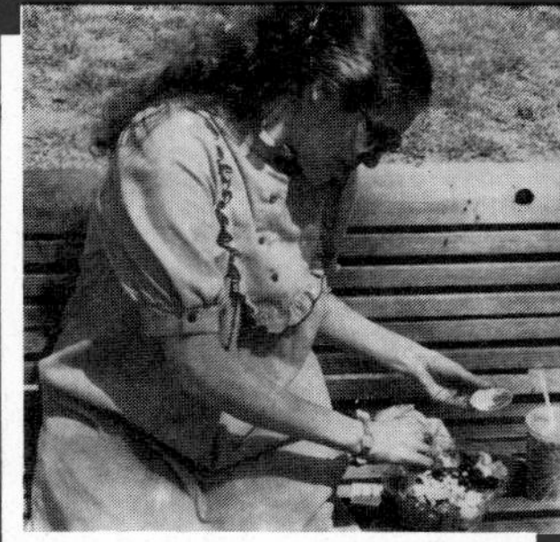

20 Nutrition in Pregnancy

Importance of Nutrition During Pregnancy

Nutritional Assessment

Factors in Planning the Diet

Dietary Counseling

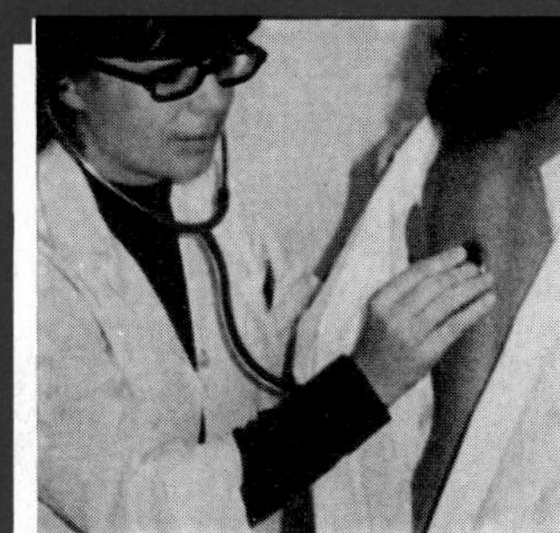

21 Antepartal Care

Concepts of Prevention and Early Detection

Antepartal Management

General Health Maintenance in Pregnancy

Minor Discomforts

Drugs During Pregnancy

Preparations for the Baby

Use of Community Resources

CHAPTER 17

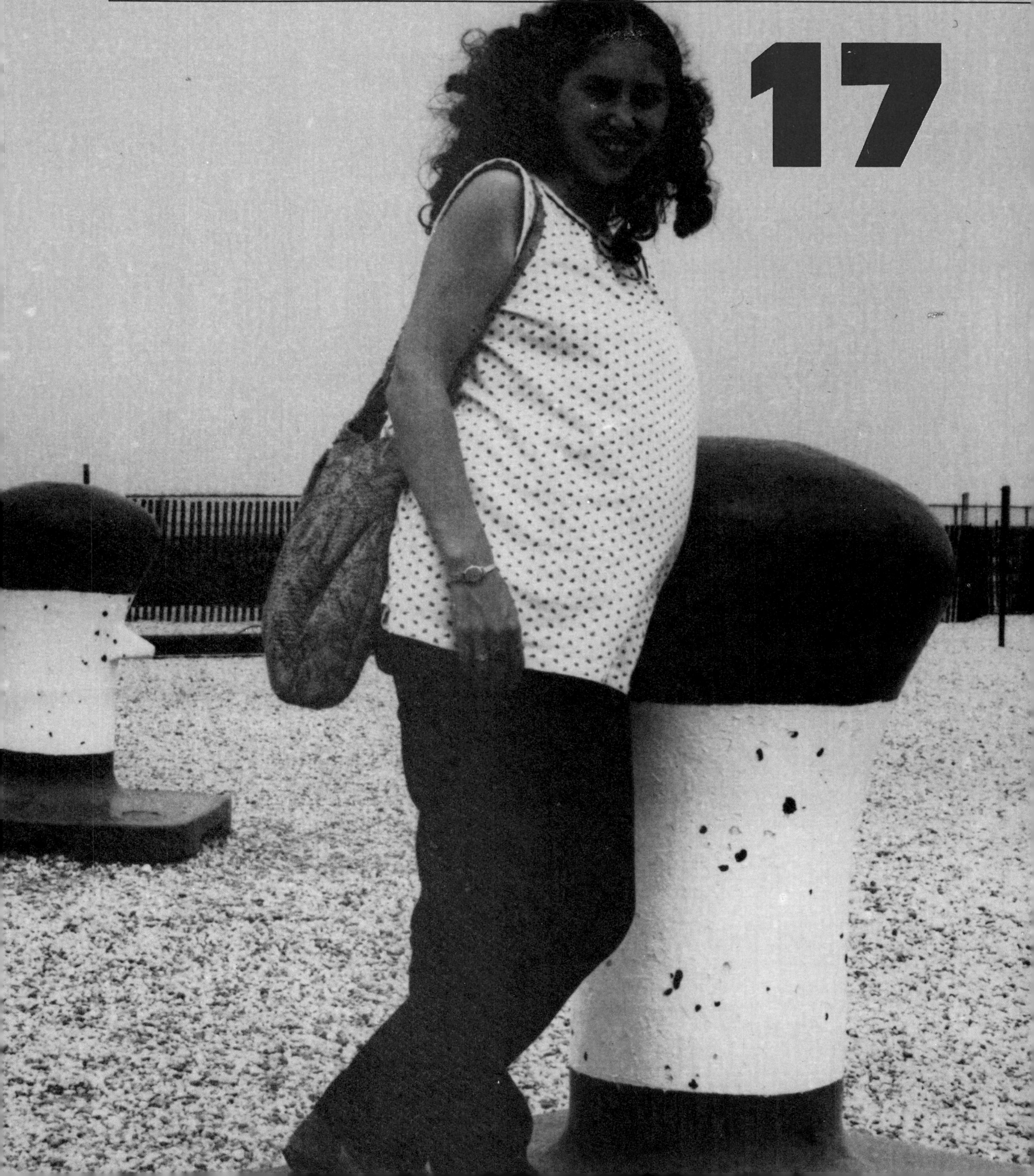

CHAPTER 17

Biophysical Aspects of Normal Pregnancy

This chapter is concerned with the anatomical and the physiological adaptations of the human organism to pregnancy. Knowledge of human reproduction, which was presented in the previous unit, is essential to the understanding of this phase of the reproductive process. From a biological point of view, pregnancy and labor represent the primary function of the female reproductive system and should be considered a normal process.

The length of human pregnancy varies greatly, but the average duration, counted from the time of conception, is approximately 267 days or 38 weeks (see Chap. 11).

Many changes in maternal physiology occur during pregnancy. These adaptations to pregnancy, although most apparent in the reproductive organs, involve other body systems as well. In addition to these physical changes, the expectant mother usually has many emotional adjustments to make—sometimes to fear, apprehension, worries (financial as well as physical), and family problems. The fact that delivery must be "faced," and that there is no turning back or "changing one's mind," can in itself sometimes create an overwhelming crisis (see Chap. 18). However, these are all temporary alterations, and are usually forgotten after the birth of the baby.

Signs and Symptoms of Pregnancy

The first visit of the expectant mother to her physician is usually prompted by the query, "Am I really pregnant?" Oddly enough, this is the one question which the physician may answer equivocally after an initial pelvic examination, because even the most careful of examinations will rarely reveal clear-cut evidence of pregnancy until two menstrual periods have been missed. The availability of rapid, accurate, and easy-to-perform pregnancy tests has markedly improved our ability to substantiate the diagnosis.

Certain signs are absolutely indicative of pregnancy, but even these may be absent if the fetus has died in the uterus. Some so-called positive signs are not present until about the middle of gestation, and at that time the diagnosis of pregnancy can be made without them by the "circumstantial evidence" of a combination of earlier and less significant symptoms. The signs of pregnancy are usually divided into three groups—presumptive, probable, and positive signs, as indicated by the chart.

Important Definitions

Gravida—A pregnant woman

Primigravida—A woman pregnant for the first time

Primipara—A woman who has given birth to her first child

Multipara—A woman who has had two or more children

Para I—A primipara

Para II—A woman who has had two children (and so on up numerically, para III, para IV, *etc*).

The plural of these words is usually formed by adding "e," as "primigravidae."

The term *gravida* refers to a pregnant woman, regardless of the duration of pregnancy. In reference it includes the present pregnancy. The term *para* refers to past pregnancies that have produced an infant of viable age, whether or not the infant is dead or alive at birth. The terms *gravida* and *para* refer to pregnancies, not to fetuses.

>28 wks. gestation

Signs and Symptoms in Pregnancy

A. Presumptive signs
   1. Menstrual suppression
   2. Nausea, vomiting, and "morning sickness"
   3. Frequency of micturition
   4. Tenderness and fullness of the breasts, breast pigmentation, and discharge
   5. "Quickening"
   6. Dark blue discoloration of the vaginal mucous membrane (Chadwick's sign)
   7. Pigmentation of the skin and abdominal striae

B. Probable signs
   1. Enlargement of the abdomen
   2. Changes in the size, shape, and consistency of the uterus (Hegar's sign)
   3. Fetal outline, distinguished by abdominal palpation and detection of a fetal part vaginally by ballottement
   4. Changes in the cervix
   5. Braxton Hicks contractions
   6. Positive pregnancy test

C. Positive signs
   1. Fetal heart sounds
   2. Fetal movements felt by examiner
   3. Roetgenogram—outline of fetal skeleton
   4. Ultrasonographic demonstration of the presence of a conceptus

Presumptive Signs

Menstrual Suppression

In a healthy woman who has previously menstruated regularly, cessation of menstruation strongly suggests that impregnation has occurred. However, not until the date of the expected period has been passed by ten days or more can any reliance be put on this symptom. When the second period is also missed, the probability naturally becomes stronger.

Although cessation of menstruation is the earliest and one of the most important symptoms of pregnancy, it should be noted that pregnancy may occur without prior menstruation and that occasionally menstrual periods may continue after conception. An example of the former circumstance is noted in certain cultures in which girls marry at a very early age; here pregnancy may occur before the menstrual periods are established. Nursing mothers, who usually do not menstruate during the period of lactation, may conceive at this time from the first postpartal ovulation. More rarely, women who think they have passed the menopause are startled to find themselves pregnant.

Conversely, it is not uncommon for a woman to have one or two periods after conception, but almost without exception, these are brief in duration and scant in amount. In such cases the first period ordinarily last two days instead of the usual five, and the next lasts only a few hours.

Although some women claim that they menstruated every month throughout pregnancy, these claims are of questionable authenticity and can probably be ascribed to some abnormality of the reproductive organs. Indeed, vaginal bleeding at any time during pregnancy should be regarded as abnormal and reported at once.

Absence of menstruation may result from a number of conditions other than pregnancy. Any condition that affects the function of the CNS–hypothalamic-pituitary-ovarian-endocrine axis may cause amenorrhea. Probably one of the most common causes of delay in the onset of the period is psychic influence. In addition, certain chronic systemic diseases, such as tuberculosis, advanced thyroid disease, chronic malnutrition, and the like may be associated with amenorrhea.

Nausea and Vomiting

About one half of pregnant women suffer no nausea whatsoever during the early part of pregnancy, and about 50% experience waves of nausea. Of these perhaps one third experience some vomiting. *Morning sickness* usually occurs in the early part of the day and subsides in a few hours, although it may persist longer or may occur at other times. When morning sickness occurs, it usually begins about two weeks after the first missed menstrual period and subsides spontaneously six or eight weeks later.

Since this symptom is present in many other conditions, such as ordinary indigestion, it is of no diagnostic value unless it is associated with other evidence of pregnancy. When the vomiting is excessive, lasts beyond the fourth month, begins in the later months, or affects the general health, it must be regarded as pathologic. Such conditions are termed *hyperemesis gravidarum,* or pernicious vomiting, and will be discussed with complications of pregnancy in Chapter 34.

Frequent Micturition

Irritability of the bladder with resultant frequency of urination may be one of the earliest symptoms of pregnancy. It is attributed to the fact that the growing uterus stretches the base of the bladder, so that a sensation results identical with that felt when the bladder wall is stretched with urine. As pregnancy progresses, the uterus rises out of the pelvis, and the frequent desire to urinate subsides. Later on, however, the symptom is likely to return, because during the last weeks of pregnancy the head of the fetus may press against the bladder and give rise to a similar condition.

Although frequency of urination may be somewhat bothersome, it should never constitute a reason for reducing the quantity of fluid consumed.

Breast Changes

Slight temporary enlargement of the breasts, causing sensations of weight and fullness, is noted by most women prior to their menstrual periods. The earliest breast changes of pregnancy are merely exaggerations of these changes. After the second month, the breasts begin to become larger, firmer, and more tender (Fig. 17-1). A sensation of stretching fullness, accompanied by tingling in the breasts and in the nipples, often develops, and in many instances a feeling of throbbing is experienced also. As time goes on, the nipple and the elevated, pigmented area immediately around it—the *areola*—become darker in color. The areola tends to become puffy, and its diameter, which in the nulligravida rarely exceeds 3 cm (1½ in), gradually widens to reach 5 cm or 6 cm (2 in or 3 in). Tiny sebaceous glands, which take on new growth with the advent of pregnancy and appear as little protuberances or follicles, are embedded in the areola.

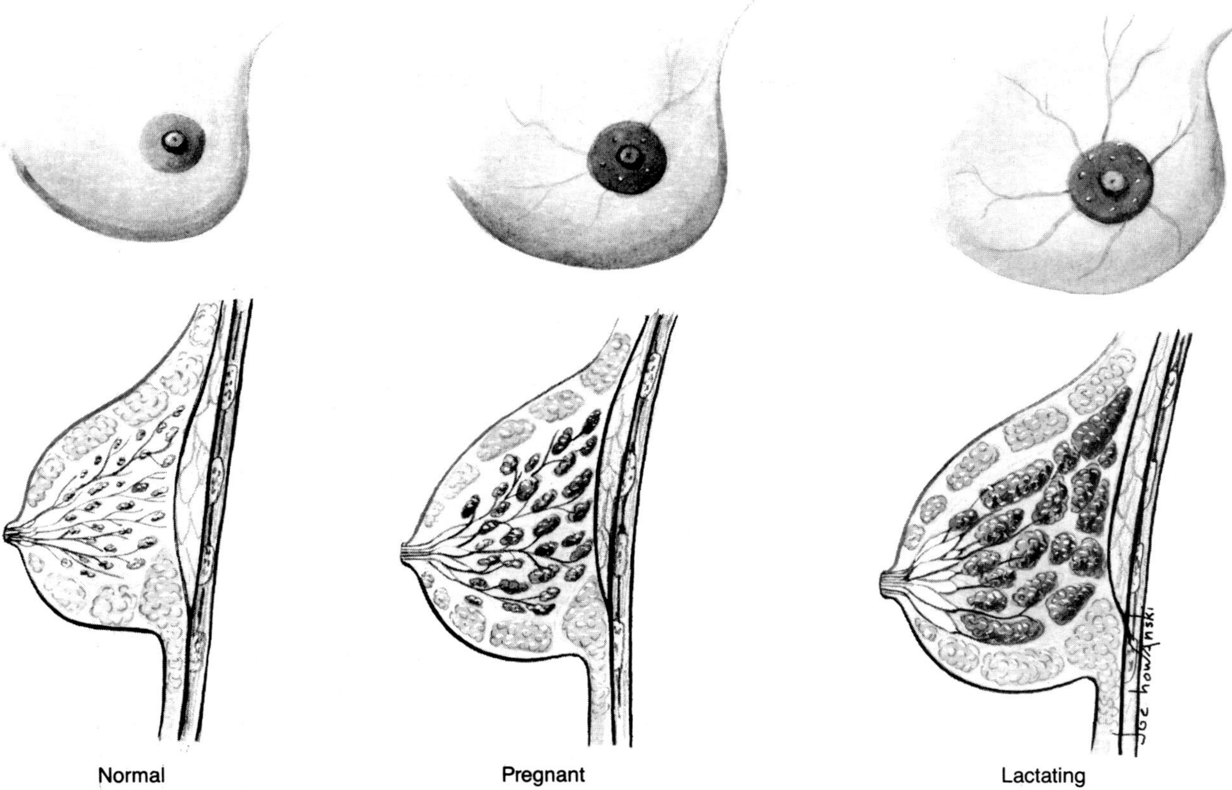

Figure 17-1.
Breast changes during pregnancy. (Whitley N: A Manual of Clinical Obstetrics. Philadelphia, JB Lippincott. In preparation.)

In a few cases, patches of brownish discoloration appear on the normal skin immediately surrounding the areola. This discoloration is known as the secondary areola and is a sign of pregnancy, provided the woman has never nursed an infant previously.

With the increasing growth and activity of the breasts, it is not surprising that a richer blood supply is needed; consequently, the blood vessels supplying the area enlarge. As a result, the veins beneath the skin of the breasts, which previously may have been scarcely visible, now become more prominent and occasionally exhibit intertwining patterns over the whole chest wall.

The alterations in the breasts during pregnancy are directed ultimately to the preparation for breast-feeding the baby. After the first few months, a thin viscous yellowish fluid may be expressed by gentle massage, or may appear spontaneously, from the nipples. This is a watery precursor of breast milk, *colostrum.*

In primigravidae breast changes are helpful adjuncts in the diagnosis of pregnancy, but in women who have already borne children, particularly if they have nursed an infant within the past year, these changes are much less significant.

"Quickening"

"Quickening" is an old term derived from an idea prevalent many years ago that at some particular moment of pregnancy, life is suddenly infused into the infant. At the time this notion was in vogue, the first tangible evidence of intrauterine life lay in the mother's feeling the baby move, and the conclusion was only natural that the infant "became alive" at the moment these movements were first felt. As is reflected in the biblical reference to "the quick and the dead," the word quick used to mean alive, and the word quickening meant becoming alive. Hence, our forebears were accustomed to saying that when fetal movements were first felt, the baby had quickened or come to life. The old term quickening is still used in obstetric terminology, whereas the common synonym among the laity is "feeling life." As used today, quickening refers only to the active movements of the fetus as first perceived by the mother.

Quickening is usually felt as a tremulous fluttering low in the abdomen toward the end of the fifth month. The first impulses caused by the stirring of the fetus may be quite faint; later on, however, they grow stronger and become clearly perceptible.

Many fetuses, although alive and healthy, seem to move about very little in the uterus, and, not infrequently, a day or so may pass without a movement being felt. Inability to feel the baby move for brief periods of time does not mean that it is dead or in any way a weakling but, in all probability, that it has assumed a position in which its movements are not felt so readily by the mother. If three or four days pass without movements, the nurse or physician should listen for the fetal heart sounds. If fetal heart sounds are heard, it means that beyond doubt the fetus is alive and presumably in good condition.

It might seem that the sensations produced by the baby's movements would be so characteristic as to make this a positive sign of pregnancy, but, oddly enough, women occasionally misinterpret movements of gas in the intestines as motions of a baby and, on this basis, imagine themselves to be pregnant. Therefore, the woman's statement that she feels the baby move cannot be regarded as absolute proof of pregnancy.

Vaginal Changes

On inspection of the vagina, one is able to observe discoloration of the vaginal mucous membrane due to the influence of pregnancy. The mucosa about the vaginal opening and the lower portion of the anterior wall frequently becomes thickened and of a dark bluish or purplish congested appearance because vascularity is greatly increased. This increase in the blood supply of the genital canal gives a dark violet hue to the tissues (Chadwick's sign), in contrast with the ordinary pink color of the parts, and is often described as a valuable sign of pregnancy. As a result of the succulence of the parts, the vaginal secretions may be considerably increased toward the end of gestation. The increased vascularity extends to the various structures in the vicinity (*i.e.,* tissues in the perineal region, skin, and muscle) and effects changes in preparation for labor.

Chadwick's sign is of no special value in women who have borne children; and, as it may be due to any condition leading to the congestion of the pelvic organs, it can be considered only a presumptive sign of pregnancy.

Skin Changes

Striae Gravidarum. The abdomen naturally enlarges to accommodate the increase in size of the uterus. The distention of the abdominal wall causes (in the later months of pregnancy) certain pink or slightly reddish streaks, or *striations,* to form in the skin covering the sides of the abdomen and the anterior and the outer aspects of the thighs. These streaks, or *striae gravidarum,* are caused by the stretching, rupture, and atrophy of the deep connective tissue of the skin. They grow lighter after labor has taken place and finally take on the silvery whiteness of scar or cicatricial tissue. In subsequent pregnancies new pink or reddish lines may be found mingled with old silvery-white striae. The number, size, and distribution of striae gravidarum vary, and some patients have no such markings whatever, even after repeated pregnancies.

Striae are not peculiar to pregnancy but may be found in other conditions which cause great abdominal distention, such as the accumulation of fat in the abdominal wall or the development of large tumors of rapid growth.

Striae gravidarum often develop in the breasts, the buttocks, and the thighs, presumably as the result of deposition of fat in those areas with consequent stretching of the skin.

Pigment Changes. Certain pigmentary changes are also common, particularly the development of a black line running from the umbilicus to the mons veneris, the so-called *linea nigra.*

The external genitalia and pigmented nevi also darken. In certain cases, irregular spots or blotches of a muddy brown color appear on the face. This condition is *chloasma,* or the "mask of pregnancy." Oral contraceptives may also cause chloasma in some women. These facial deposits of pigment often cause the woman considerable mental distress, but her mind may be relieved by the assurance that they will often disappear after delivery. However, the increased pigmentation of the breasts and the abdomen never disappears entirely, although it usually becomes much less pronounced.

All these pigmentary deposits vary exceedingly in size, shape, and distribution and usually are more marked in brunettes than in blondes.

Vascular Markings. Vascular spiders are minute, fiery-red blemishes on the skin with branching legs coming out from a central body. They develop more often in white women; however, they are of no clinical significance and will disappear.

Variations in Skin Changes. The changes in the skin which may accompany pregnancy (*i.e.,* striae gravidarum, linea nigra, chloasma, and pigmentation of the breasts) vary exceedingly in different women; often they are entirely absent. The pigmentation changes are frequently absent in blondes and exceptionally well marked in pronounced brunettes. As already mentioned, this pigmentation may remain from former pregnancies and cannot be depended on as a diagnostic sign in women who have borne children previously.

Sweat Glands. In addition to the aforementioned skin changes, there is a great increase in the activity of the sebaceous glands, the sweat glands, and the hair follicles. The augmented activity of the sweat glands produces an increase in perspiration, an alteration that is helpful in the elimination of waste material.

Probable Signs

Abdominal Changes

The size of the abdomen during pregnancy corresponds to the gradual increase in the size of the uterus, which at the end of the third month is at the level of the symphysis pubis. At the end of the fifth month it is at the level of the umbilicus, and toward the end of the ninth month it is at the ensiform cartilage (Fig. 17-2). Mere abdominal enlargement may be due to a number of causes, such as accumulation of fat in the abdominal wall, edema, or uterine or ovarian tumors. However, if the uterus can be distinctly felt to have enlarged progressively in the proportions stated above, pregnancy may properly be suspected.

Changes in the Uterus

Changes in shape, size, and consistency of the uterus that take place during the first three months of pregnancy are very important indications. These are noted in the bimanual examination which shows the uterus to be more anteflexed than normal, enlarged, and of a soft, spongy consistency. About the sixth week, the so-called Hegar's sign is perceptible (Fig. 17-3). At this time, the lower uterine segment, or lower part of the body of the uterus, becomes much softer than the cervix. It is so soft that in its empty state (for it has not yet become encroached upon by the growing embryo) it can be compressed almost to the thinness of paper. This is one of the most valuable signs in early pregnancy.

Figure 17-2.
Changes in abdominal contour in pregnancy.

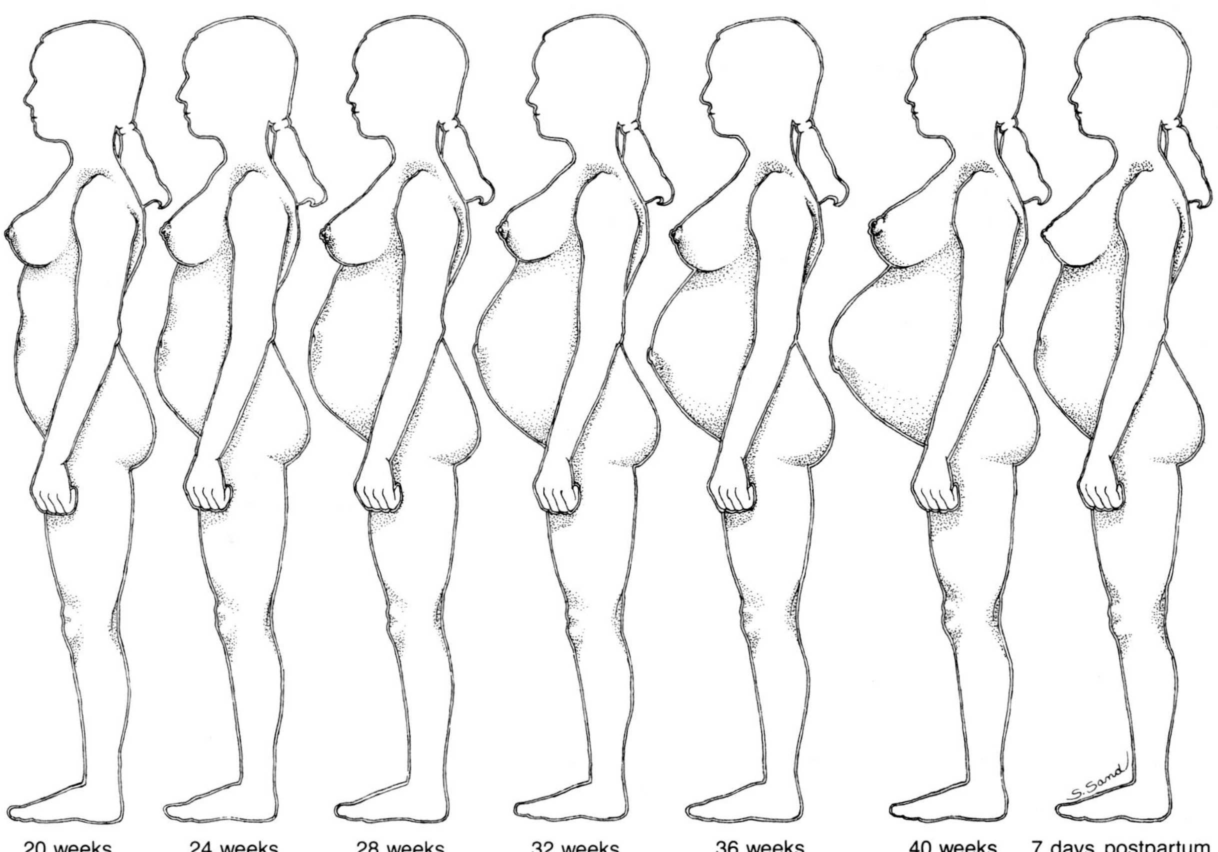

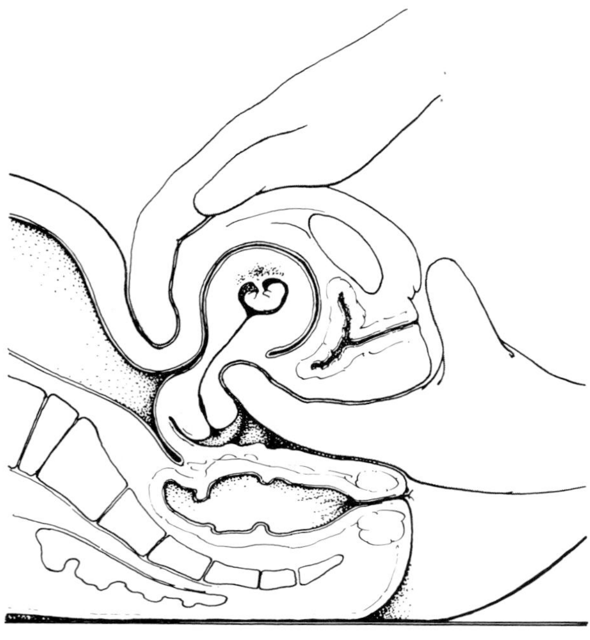

Figure 17-3.
Hegar's sign.

The uterus increases in size to make room for the growing fetus. It increases in size from approximately 6.5 cm long, 4 cm wide, and 2.5 cm deep to about 32 cm long, 24 cm wide, and 22 cm deep. The uterine wall thickens during the first few months of pregnancy from about 1 cm to almost 2 cm, but thereafter it thins to about 0.5 cm or less. By the end of pregnancy, the uterus becomes a soft-walled muscular sac which yields to the movements of the fetal extremities and permits the examiner to palpate the fetus easily. Its weight increases from 50 g to 1000 g. The small, almost solid organ which has a capacity of about 2 ml increases to become a thin-walled muscular sac capable of containing the fetus, the placenta, and over 1000 ml of amniotic fluid.

The tremendous growth is owing partly to the formation of new muscle fibers during the early months of pregnancy but principally to the enlargement of preexistent muscle fibers that are seven to eleven times longer and two to seven times wider than those observed in the nonpregnant uterus. Simultaneously, fibroelastic tissue develops between the muscle bands and forms a network around the various muscle bundles. This is of great importance in pregnancy and labor because it strengthens the uterine walls. During early pregnancy, the hypertrophy of the uterus is probably due to the stimulating action of estrogen on muscle fibers.

The muscle fibers are arranged in three layers—the external hoodlike layer which arches over the fundus, the internal layer of circular fibers around the orifices of the fallopian tubes and the internal os, and the figure-8 fibers in the middle layer which make an interlacing network through which the blood vessels pass. This last group plays an important role in childbearing and will be referred to particularly in the care of the mother during labor and after delivery. When these muscle fibers contract, they constrict the blood vessels.

Fetal Outline

After the sixth month, the outline of the fetus (head, back, knees, elbows, and so on) can usually be identified sufficiently well by abdominal palpation to justify a diagnosis of pregnancy. As pregnancy progresses, the outline of the fetus becomes more and more clearly defined. The ability to outline the fetus makes pregnancy extremely probable. In rare instances, however, tumors of the uterus may so mimic the fetal outline as to make this sign fallible.

Ballottement. Another valuable sign suggesting the presence of a fetus is ballottement (from the French *balloter,* to toss up like a ball). During the fourth and the fifth months of pregnancy, the fetus is small in relation to the amount of amniotic fluid present; during vaginal examination, a sudden tap on the presenting part makes it rise in the amniotic fluid and then rebound to its original position and, in turn, tap the examining finger. When elicited by an experienced examiner, this response is the most certain of the probable signs.

Cervical Changes

Softening of the cervix usually occurs about the time of the second missed menstrual period. In comparison with the usual firmness of the nonpregnant cervix (which has a consistency approximate to that of the cartilaginous tip of the nose), the pregnant cervix becomes softened, and on digital examination the external os feels like the lips or like the lobe of the ear (Goodell's sign).

Softening of the cervix may be apparent as early as a month after conception. The softening of the cervix in pregnancy is owing to increased vascularity, edema, and hyperplasia of the cervical glands.

As shown in Figure 17-4, the glands of the cervical mucosa undergo marked proliferation and distend with mucus. As a result they form a structure resembling honeycomb and make up about one half of the entire structure of the cervix. This is the so-called mucous plug and is of practical importance for a number of reasons. First, it seals the uterus from contamination by bacteria in the vagina. Second, it is expelled at the onset of labor and along with it a small amount of blood; this gives rise to the discharge of a small amount of blood-stained mucus, or *show*. Frequently, the onset of labor is heralded by the appearance of show.

Braxton Hicks Contractions

Uterine contractions begin during the early weeks of pregnancy and occur at intervals of from five to ten minutes throughout pregnancy. These contractions are painless, and the patient may or may not be conscious of them. They may be observed during the later months by placing the hand on the abdomen and during the bimanual examination. By means of these contractions, the uterine muscles contract and relax, thereby enlarging in size to accommodate the growing fetus. These contractions are called the Braxton Hicks sign, after a famous London obstetrician of the last century who first described them. They often account for false labor.

Pregnancy Tests

Since the dawn of civilization efforts have been made to devise a satisfactory test for pregnancy. In the earliest writings handed down to us the priest–physicians of ancient Egypt tell of a test that was based on the seeming ability of pregnancy urine to stimulate the growth of wheat and barley seeds. The itinerant physicians of classical Greece employed similar tests, and during the Middle Ages the omniscient physician merely gazed at the urine and claimed to be able to diagnose not only pregnancy but also many other conditions.

Today, interestingly enough, as in the tests of old, urine is used in a large number of tests for pregnancy. The tests are based on the fact that the early chorionic villi of the implanted ovum secrete HCG, which appears in the maternal blood and is excreted in the urine. This hormone may be detected in maternal serum or urine by biologic or immunologic methods. Some of the biologic tests which were used extensively in the past include the Aschheim–Zondek test (immature female mouse), the Friedman test (female rabbit), the Hogben test (Southern African toad), and the American male frog test.

Immunologic Pregnancy Tests. Numerous systems for immunologic pregnancy testing have been devised. Since HCG is an antigen capable of producing specific antibodies when injected into an animal such as the rabbit, the serum of the animal so injected will contain an antibody or antihormone specific for HCG. This serum then can be used by reliable

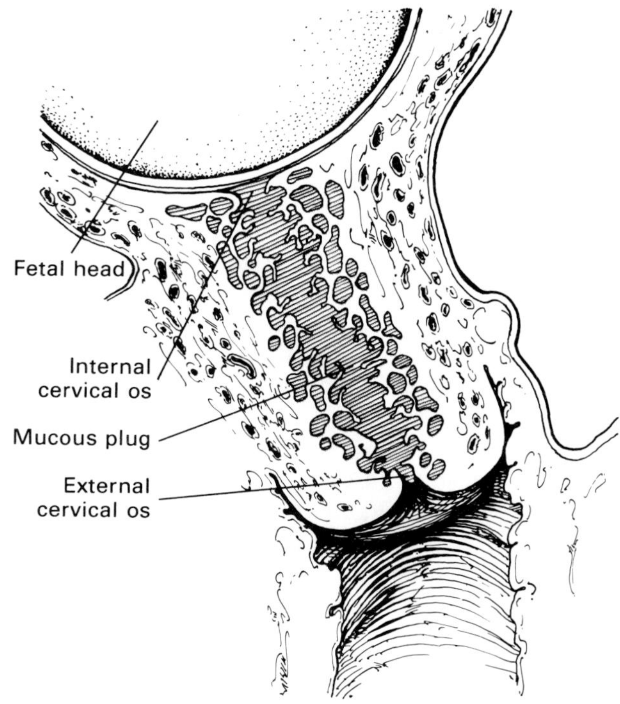

Figure 17-4.
Cervix with mucous plug.

immunologic methods to establish the presence or absence of HCG in maternal serum or pregnancy urine.

Kits for immunologic pregnancy testing are available and have been simplified so that with a little practice the test can be carried out within minutes. Immunologic tests have two main advantages over the older biologic ones—they provide an answer within a few minutes rather than many hours, and they eliminate the need for maintaining an animal colony. These tests are more accurate than the older biologic methods.

The great value of the endocrine tests is that they become positive very early in pregnancy. The standard office pregnancy tests are usually positive about ten days after the first missed menstrual period, sometimes even a few days earlier than this. If any of the tests have been carried out properly, the results are accurate in more than 95% of cases. They are not, therefore, absolutely positive signs of pregnancy, but very nearly so.

Radioimmunoassay Test. Recently, very accurate tests to detect HCG in maternal serum by radioimmunoassay have been developed. These methods are capable of detecting pregnancy from about the eighth postfertilization day on, and thus pregnancy can be diagnosed even before the skipped menstrual period. HCG is made up of an alpha and a beta subunit. The alpha subunit is common to the pituitary gonadotropic hormones. The beta subunit has molecular characteristics that are specific for HCG. Antibodies specific for this subunit have been produced. These antibodies are used in a radioimmunoassay for HCG. This assay system has the advantage of being specific for HCG, and it is capable of detecting minute amounts of HCG in blood. It is a much more elaborate assay than those used in the office to detect urinary HCG, and it must be carried out in the laboratory with radioisotope techniques (radioimmunoassay).

The radioreceptor assay is another radioimmunoassay test for HCG which is based on a slightly different principle. In this system, antibodies against the combination of HCG and the intracellular receptor for HCG (the constituent in the cell to which HCG attaches when it exerts its effects) are used. This method is also highly sensitive, but is not quite as specific as the beta subunit assay. As there is some crossreaction with pituitary LH, LH levels are also detected by this method. These tests have found increasing use for the early diagnosis of pregnancy and are especially useful clinically to diagnose abnormalities, such as ectopic pregnancy, as well as to follow the course of early pregnancy when abnormalities of embryonic development are suspected.

Positive Signs

Although some of the signs mentioned above, particularly the hormone tests, ballottement, and palpating the fetal outline are nearly positive evidences of pregnancy, they are not 100% certain; errors in technique occasionally invalidate the hormone tests, and on rare occasions the other signs may be simulated by nonpregnant pathologic states. If the term "positive" is used in the strict sense, there are only four positive means of detecting pregnancy, namely, the presence of fetal heart sounds, fetal movements felt by the examiner, the roentgenogram outline of the fetal skeleton, and delineation of a pregnancy by ultrasonography.

Fetal Heart Sounds

When fetal heart sounds are heard distinctly by an experienced examiner, there is no longer any doubt about the existence of pregnancy. Ordinarily, they become audible at about the middle of pregnancy, or approximately the 20th week. If the abdominal wall is thin and conditions are favorable, they may become audible as early as the 18th week, but obesity or an excessive quantity of amniotic fluid may render them inaudible until a much later date.

Although the usual rate of the fetal heart is approximately 140 beats per minute, it may vary under normal conditions between 120 beats per minute and 160 beats per minute. The use of the ordinary bell stethoscope, steadied by rubber bands, is entirely satisfactory, but in doubtful cases the head stethoscope is superior because the listener receives bone conduction of sound through the headpiece in addition to that transmitted to the eardrum (Fig. 17-5).

Office electronic fetal heart monitors which detect fetal heartbeat by ultrasound are now available. The heartbeat is transmitted to a monitor and amplified so that it can be heard by both the examiner and the patient (Fig. 17-5). The use of this instrument provides an exciting experience and can be appreciated by all, including the patient's mate who is present at the time.

Learning Technique. It is advantageous to determine the fetal position by abdominal palpation before attempting to listen to the fetal heart tones, since ordinarily the heart sounds are best heard through the fetus's back (see Chap. 22). One method to use while learning the characteristics of the fetal heart sounds is to place one hand on the maternal pulse and feel its rate at the same time that the fetal heart tones are heard through the stethoscope. Occasionally, the inexperienced attendant, particularly when listening high in the abdomen, may mistake the mother's heart sounds for those of the fetus. Since the two are not synchronous (fetal, 140 beats per min; maternal, 80 beats per min), the method suggested above will obviate this mistake; in other words, if the rate that comes to the ear through the stethoscope is the same as that of the maternal pulse, it is probably the mother's heartbeat. On the other hand, if the rates are different, it is undoubtedly the sound of the fetal heart.

Funic and Uterine Souffles. Two additional sounds may be heard in listening over the pregnant uterus—the funic souffle and the uterine souffle. Since the word *souffle* means a blowing murmur, or whizzing sound, the nature of these two sounds is similar, but their timing and causation are quite different.

The word *funis* is Latin for umbilical cord, and, accordingly, the term *funic souffle* refers to a soft blowing murmur caused by blood rushing through the umbilical cord. Since this blood is propelled by the fetal heart, the rate of funic souffle is synchronous to that of the fetal heart. It is heard only occasionally, perhaps in one case out of every six.

The funic souffle is a positive sign of pregnancy, but it is not usually so listed, because it is almost always heard in close association with the fetal heart sounds.

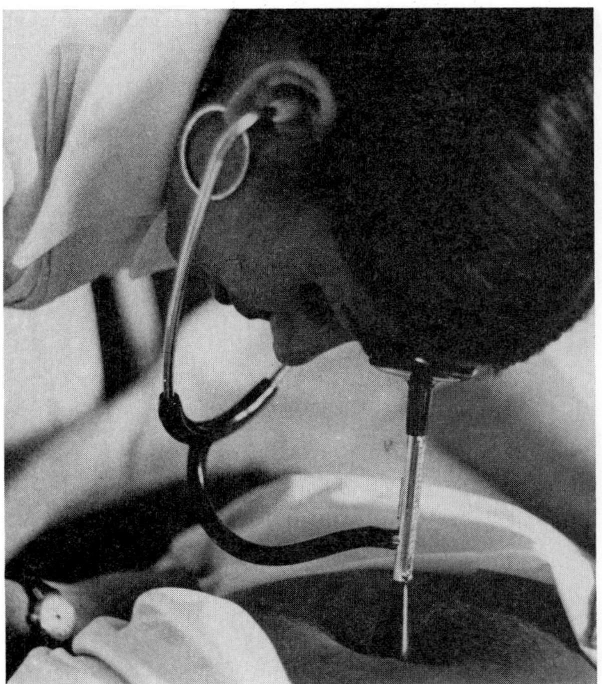

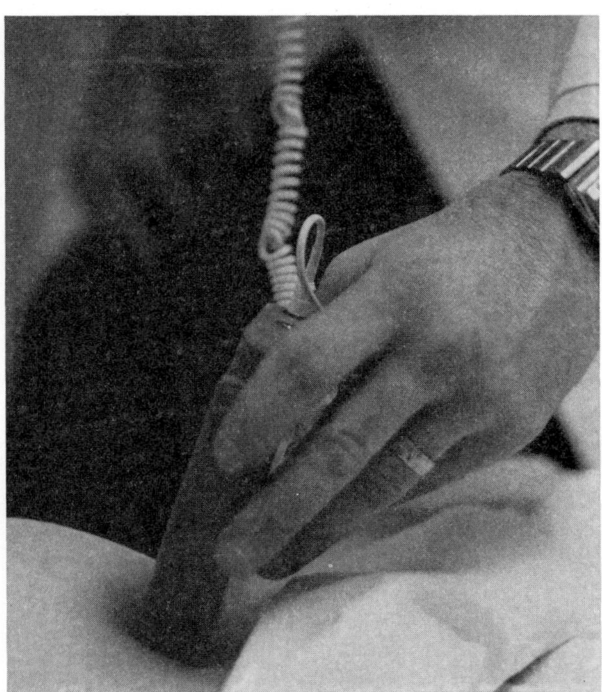

Figure 17-5.
Auscultation of fetal heart beat by means of head stethoscope *(left)* and by ultrasound *(right)*.

The *uterine souffle* is produced by blood rushing through the large vessels of the uterus. Since this is maternal blood, propelled by the maternal heart, it is synchronous to the rate of her heartbeat. In other words, the rate of the funic souffle is ordinarily around 140 beats per minute (or the same as that of the fetal heart rate); the rate of the uterine souffle is near 80 beats per minute (that of the maternal heart rate). The fetal heart may also be detected electronically or with ultrasound techniques described in detail in Chapter 40.

Fetal Movements Felt by Examiner

As already noted, fetal movements supposedly felt by the patient may be very misleading in the diagnosis of pregnancy. However, when an experienced examiner feels the characteristic thrust or kick of the fetus against the hand, this is positive evidence of pregnancy. Often this can be felt after the end of the fifth month.

Roentgenogram

A roentgenogram showing the outline of the fetal skeleton is, of course, undeniable proof of pregnancy. How early the fetal skeleton will show in the roentgenogram depends on the thickness of the abdominal wall, the x-ray equipment, and other factors. It has been demonstrated as early as the 14th week and is quite easily demonstrated as a rule after the 20th week (Figs. 17-6 and 17-7).

Ultrasonography

The presence of an early embryo can be detected by the use of ultrasound techniques. This test is most useful clinically when the diagnosis of intrauterine pregnancy is in question. A fetal sac within the uterus usually provides an unmistakable pattern on the ultrasonogram. Sonography is of great clinical use when tubal ectopic pregnancy is suspected. The test is increasingly accurate as pregnancy advances, and ultrasonographic outline of a fetus within the fetal sac constitutes a positive sign of pregnancy. This technique is described in greater detail in Chapter 39.

Physiological Changes of Pregnancy

The physiological changes of pregnancy are both local and general alterations that affect the maternal organism as a result of pregnancy but subside at or before the end of the puerperium. Such changes are to be regarded as normal, inevitable, and purely tem-

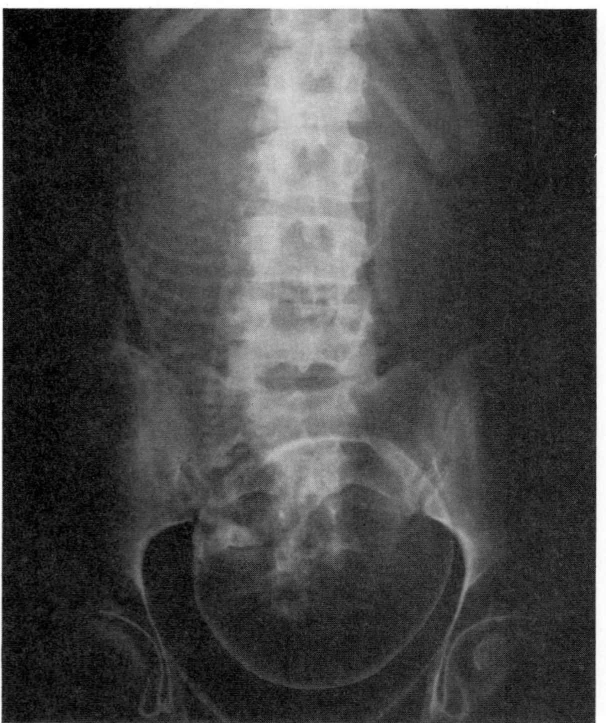

Figure 17-6.
Normal vertex position. (Bonner KP: Radiography and Clinical Photography. Rochester, NY, Eastman Kodak Company)

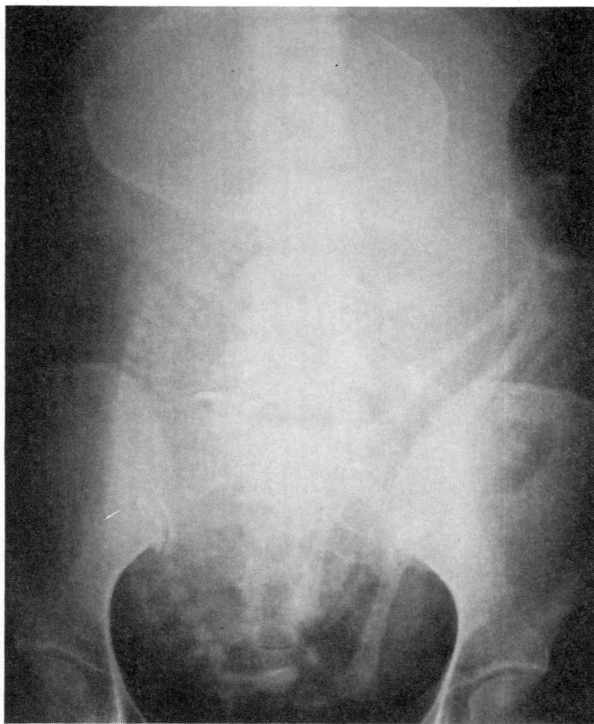

Figure 17-7.
Normal breech position. (Bonner KP: Radiography and Clinical Photography. Rochester, NY, Eastman Kodak Company)

porary. They are present in varying degrees in every instance, and in the case of a physically healthy woman there should be no significant traces of them after convalescence is complete. It must be remembered, however, that after pregnancy the uterus does not return to its normal nulliparous size, though it does return to a normal nonpregnant state. The adult parous uterus is slightly larger than that of a woman who has never borne a child.

Bodily Changes Associated With Uterine Growth

Between the third month and the fourth month of pregnancy, the growing uterus rises out of the pelvis and can be palpated above the symphysis pubis. It rises progressively to reach the umbilicus at approximately the sixth month and almost impinges on the xiphoid process at the ninth month (Fig. 17-8).

In the majority of pregnancies the uterus is rotated to the right as it rises out of the pelvis. This dextrorotation is probably caused by the presence of the rectosigmoid on the left.

As the uterus becomes larger, it comes in contact with the anterior abdominal wall and displaces the intestines to the sides of the abdomen.

Coincident with the uterine and abdominal enlargement, the umbilicus is pushed outward until about the seventh month when its depression is completely obliterated and it forms merely a darkened area in the smooth and tense abdominal wall. Later, it is raised above the surrounding integument and may project, becoming about the size of a hickory nut.

When the abdominal wall is unable to withstand the tension created by the enlarging uterus, the recti muscles become separated in the median line—so-called *diastasis recti.*

About two weeks before term, in most primigravidae, the fetal head descends into the pelvic cavity. As a result, the uterus sinks to a lower level and at the same time falls forward. Since this relieves the upward pressure on the diaphragm and makes breathing easier, this phenomenon of the descent of the head has been called *lightening.* These changes usually do not occur in multiparas until the onset of labor. By palpating the height of the fundus, experienced examiners can determine the approximate length of gestation.

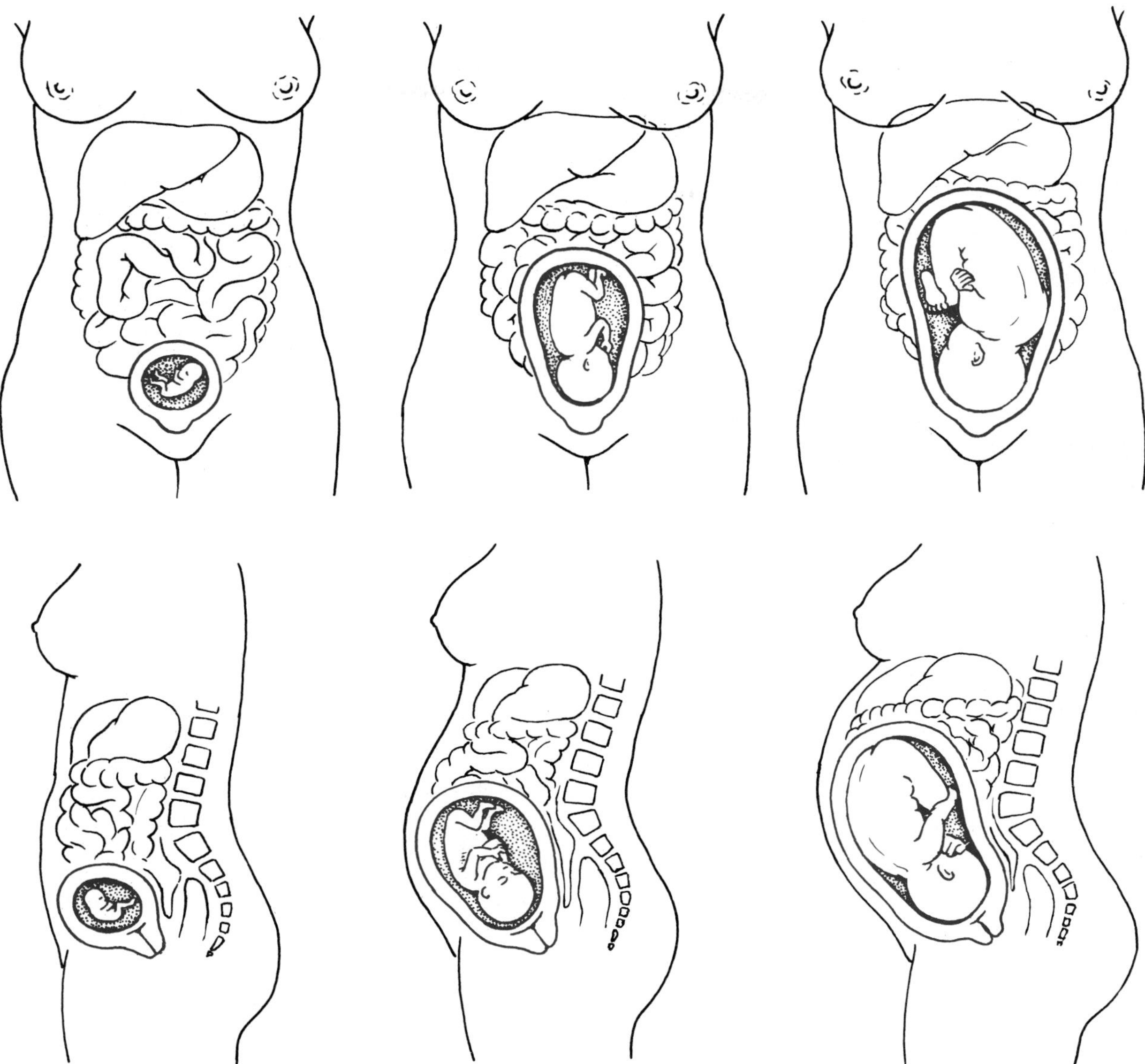

Figure 17-8.
Relative size of the growing uterus. *(Top)* front views, *(bottom)* lateral views, showing the fetus at four, six, and nine months of gestation. The fundus reaches a height between the symphysis pubis and the umbilicus by the fourth month, is about the level of the umbilicus at six months, and almost impinges on the xiphoid process at about the ninth month of gestation.

Effects on Posture

Since the full-term pregnant uterus and its contents weigh about 6000 g (12 lb), a gravid woman may be likened to a person carrying a heavy basket pressed against the abdomen. Such a person will instinctively lean backward to maintain equilibrium. This backward tilt of the torso is characteristic of pregnancy. From a practical viewpoint it is important to note that this posture imposes increased strain on the muscles and the ligaments of the back and the thighs, and in this way is responsible for many of the skeletomuscular aches and cramps so often experienced in late pregnancy.

An additional contributing factor is a relaxation of the ligaments which support the joints of the spinal column and pelvis. This feature is increasingly prominent as pregnancy progresses. Relaxation of the sacroiliac joints and the pubic symphysis creates a certain amount of pelvic instability, producing additional strain on the back muscles and thighs. These changes account for the waddling gait observed in late pregnancy and in the early postpartal period.

Changes in the Various Systems

Carbohydrate Metabolism

Pregnancy has a decided influence on carbohydrate metabolism. In general, the levels of fasting blood sugar are lower, and the secretion of insulin by the pancreas is increased. The stress of pregnancy may actually bring to light subclinical diabetes (see Chap. 35). In fact, diabetes is often detected for the first time during the course of prenatal care.

Blood

The total volume of blood in the body increases approximately 30% during pregnancy. The minimal hematologic values for both nonpregnant women and pregnant women is 12 g of hemoglobin, 3.75 million erythrocytes, and 35% hematocrit. If there are adequate iron reserves in the body, or if sufficient iron is supplied from the diet, the hemoglobin, the erythrocyte count, and the hematocrit values remain within normal limits during pregnancy.

During pregnancy, there is an increased production of red blood cells by the bone marrow. At the same time, the maternal blood volume, the total amount of fluid circulating in the vessels, increases. Thus, the actual concentration of red blood cells is more or less the same as under normal conditions.

Iron Needs

The marked increase in production of red blood cells places an inordinate demand on bodily iron stores. Iron stores in the female are often marginal anyway because of the normal loss at menstruation. Iron deficiency anemia is often present prior to pregnancy, especially when there has been inadequate dietary intake of iron, frequently the case among patients in poor socioeconomic circumstances. Iron deficiency is markedly aggravated by pregnancy because of the heavy demand for iron by the growing fetus, especially late in gestation. The increased demand for iron as a result of the changes associated with pregnancy should be kept in mind during the course of prenatal care, and the use of supplementary iron should be seriously considered.

Heart

An important aspect of this increase in blood volume relates to its effect on the heart. During pregnancy, the heart has about 50% more blood to pump through the aorta per minute. This augmented cardiac output attains a peak at the end of the second trimester, then declines to the nonpregnant level during the last weeks of gestation. Immediately following delivery there is a sharp rise again. In women with normal hearts this is of no particular concern. However, in women with heart disease this increase in the work that the heart has to do may add to the seriousness of the complication (see Chap. 35).

Palpitation of the heart is not uncommon; in the early months of pregnancy this is owing to sympathetic nervous disturbance, and toward the end of gestation to the intraabdominal pressure of the enlarged uterus.

Respiration

In the later months of pregnancy the lungs are subjected to pressure from the underlying uterus, and the diaphragm may be displaced upward. As a consequence, shortness of breath at that period is common. It might seem that this upward displacement of the diaphragm would decrease the capacity of the lungs, but a concomitant widening of the thoracic cage occurs which more than compensates for the other change. Actually, the pregnant woman breathes in much more air than the nonpregnant woman. This is necessary because the mother must oxygenate not only her own blood, but, by osmosis, that of the fetus too.

Digestion

The function of the digestive organs may be somewhat altered during pregnancy. During the early months the appetite may be diminished, particularly if nausea exists. Since the nutritional requirements to meet the needs of the mother's body and the growing fetus demand quality of the diet rather than an appreciable increase in the quantity of food ingested, this temporary manifestation should not produce injurious effects. As pregnancy advances, and the digestive apparatus seems to become accustomed to its new conditions, the appetite is increased and may be voracious. Heartburn and flatulence may occur at this time. Also, the pressure from the diaphragm and the diminished tone may delay the emptying time of the stomach.

Constipation is exceedingly common in pregnancy; at least one half of all gravid women suffer from this disorder. This suggests that the entire gastrointestinal tract is limited by diminished tone and pressure of the growing uterus during gestation.

Urinary System

The urine in pregnancy usually is increased in amount and has a lower specific gravity. Pregnant women show a tendency to excrete dextrose in the urine. Although a reduction in the renal threshold for sugar is often associated with pregnancy, the presence of any sugar in the urine should always be reported to the physician. Lactosuria may be observed at times, especially during the latter part of pregnancy and the puerperium. Lactosuria is associated with the presence of milk sugar which is from the mammary glands and is not of any significance.

The *ureters* become markedly dilated in pregnancy, particularly the right ureter. This change apparently is due in part to the pressure of the gravid uterus on the ureters as they cross the pelvic brim and in part to a certain softening which the ureteral walls undergo as the result of endocrine influences. These dilated ureters, the walls of which have now lost much of their muscular tone, are unable to propel the urine as satisfactorily as previously; consequently, stasis of urine is common. Following delivery, the ureters return to normal within four to six weeks. The stretching and the dilatation do not continue long enough to impair the ureter permanently unless infection has developed or pregnancies are repeated so rapidly that a subsequent pregnancy begins before the ureters can return to normal.

The *bladder* functions efficiently during pregnancy. The urinary frequency experienced in the first few months of pregnancy is caused by pressure exerted on the bladder by the enlarging uterus. This is observed again when lightening occurs prior to the onset of labor.

■ ■ ■

Endocrine Changes

Placenta

In Chapter 11 the placenta was considered as an organ designed to transmit nutritive substances from mother to fetus and waste products in the reverse direction. The role of the placenta as an important organ of internal secretion was also reviewed. As discussed previously, the early chorionic villi of the implanted ovum secrete HCG, which prolongs the life of the corpus luteum. The result is the continued production of estrogen and progesterone, which are so necessary for the maintenance of the endometrium. During pregnancy this hormone appears in maternal blood and is excreted in the mother's urine, which makes the standard urine tests for pregnancy possible.

The chorionic cells of the placenta produce yet another unique protein hormone, human chorionic somatomamotropin (HCS), which is also known as human placental lactogen (HPL). This hormone is detectable in placental cells as early as the third week after ovulation and is found in maternal serum by the sixth week. Its name suggests its actions. It influences somatic cell growth of the fetus and facilitates preparation of the breasts for lactation.

In addition to its function in the formation of HCG and HCS, the placenta takes over the production of estrogen and progesterone from the ovaries, and after the first two months of gestation becomes the major source of these two hormones. The increase in these hormones in the maternal organism is thought to be responsible for many important changes that take place during pregnancy, such as the growth of the uterus and the development of the breasts. In the breasts, the development of the duct system is promoted by estrogen, and the development of the lobule-alveolar system by progesterone.

Pituitary Body

The pituitary gland enlarges somewhat during pregnancy, but, as such, is not essential for the maintenance of pregnancy.

Anterior Lobe

The *anterior lobe* of this small gland, located at the base of the brain, has already been referred to as the "master clock," which, under the influence of the hypothalamus, controls the menstrual cycle (see Chap. 8). In addition to gonadotropins, the anterior lobe secretes hormones that act on the thyroid and adrenal glands, and yet another hormone which influences the growth process. Production of these hormones continues during the course of pregnancy. Gonadotropins, on the other hand, are no longer released cyclically. The estrogen and progesterone produced by the placenta inhibit their release from the pituitary gland.

Posterior Lobe

The *posterior lobe* of the pituitary secretes an oxytocic hormone, *oxytocin,* which has a very strong stimulating effect on the uterine muscle. The portion of the pituitary gland that contains oxytocin is widely employed in obstetrics to cause the uterus to contract after delivery, thereby diminishing postpartal hemorrhage. It is sometimes used to initiate labor and to stimulate contractions during labor when they are of poor quality. Oxytocin also has an influence on the breasts. It causes *milk let-down,* or ejection of milk from the nipples. This effect is of clinical use in the care of the nursing mother. Oxytocin is marketed under the names Pitocin and Syntocinon, the latter a synthetic product, and is administered either parenterally or, for milk let-down, by a nasal spray.

Other Endocrine Glands

It is quite clear that the placenta is the major endocrine gland in pregnancy. Other endocrine glands display alterations during normal pregnancy.

Thyroid

During the course of pregnancy, there is slight to moderate enlargement of the thyroid. It is now known that this hypertrophy of thyroid tissue is not associated with increased thyroid activity, although there is an elevation in the basal metabolic rate which increases throughout the course of pregnancy. This is merely a reflection of the increased oxygen consumption as a result of the metabolic activity of the products of conception.

Other parameters for the measurement of thyroid function also display changes. The serum protein-bound iodine (PBI), butyl extractable iodine (BEI) and thyroxine (T_4) levels increase, and the elevated levels are maintained until shortly after delivery. The increase is due not to increased thyroid activity as such but, rather, to an elevation in the level of thyroid-binding protein normally present in the blood. Thus, although there is an increase in the amount of circulating thyroid hormones and, therefore, the total concentration of hormone is elevated, the actual amount of unbound or available hormone remains within normal limits.

The triiodothyronine (T_3) uptake test displays decreased values in pregnancy, which indicates an increase in the binding of circulating triiodothyronine. A similar increase in the level of thyroid-binding proteins is seen in the nonpregnant patient following the administration of estrogen, and it is likely that in pregnancy the increase is a reflection of the high level of circulating estrogen.

Adrenals

The *adrenal cortex* hypertrophies during pregnancy, and it is believed that its activity increases. The actual secretion of cortisol by the adrenals is unchanged, although there are alterations in the metabolism of cortisol as a result of the influence of estrogen. There is clearly an increase in the production by the adrenal glands of aldosterone, the hormone responsible for the retention of sodium by the kidneys. This increase begins early in pregnancy and continues throughout. The net result of the increase is a decreased ability of the kidneys to handle salt during pregnancy. In the absence of proper dietary control of salt intake, there is often fluid retention, and either occult or overt edema.

Ovary

The *ovary,* except for the activity of the corpus luteum of pregnancy, remains relatively quiescent. Gonadotropin levels are low, inasmuch as their release is inhibited by the estrogen and progesterone produced by the placenta. Thus, follicular activity in the ovary remains in abeyance, and there is no further ovulation until after delivery.

Suggested Readings

Pritchard JA, Macdonald PC: Williams' Obstetrics, 16th ed. New York, Appleton–Century–Crofts, 1980

Quilligan EJ: Prenatal care. In Romney SL, Gray M, Little AB (eds): Gynecology and Obstetrics; The Health Care of Women, pp 579–594. New York, McGraw–Hill, 1980

CHAPTER 18

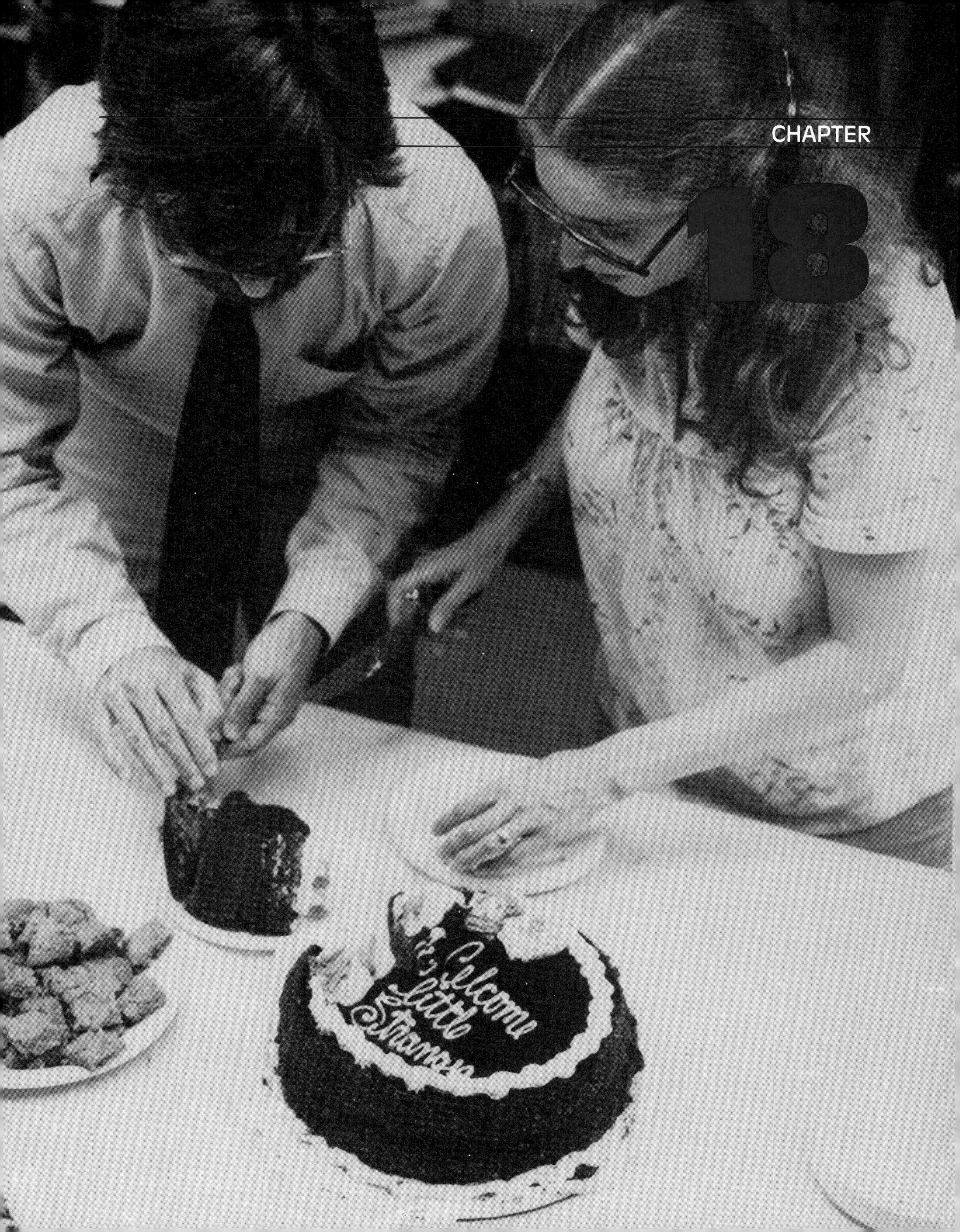

CHAPTER 18

Psychosocial Aspects of Normal Pregnancy

Cultural Influences on Perceptions of Pregnancy

As indicated previously, the family is society's most basic unit, surviving through the centuries as it has because it serves vital human needs. We have seen that there may be very different styles of family living and different ways of relating the family to the larger society. However, whatever the form, the family will no doubt continue to exist as long as humans continue to populate this planet.

In the family, as previously noted, each member assumes roles for which the culture dictates overt and covert behavioral expectations. Each member's perceptions of these roles also vary according to the manner of socialization and the kind of interaction he or she has had with others. As the society evolves and changes, so do the various role expectations. Each successive generation may hold different expectations as they adapt to changing times and needs, although there are always socially imposed limitations.

So it has been with childbearing. Pregnancy and birth are very important events in most cultures. However, attitudes toward these processes vary considerably among different cultures and even within one society. In some cultures, birth is a social event, with open attendance by all friends and family; in other cultures it is conducted in secrecy.[1] Similarly, pregnancy may be seen as a normal uneventful preparatory phase to a desired change in status connoting achievement; conversely, it may be viewed as mysterious, crisis ridden, and the harbinger of possible disaster. Again, it may be looked upon as atonement for simply being a lowly female.[2]

Pregnancy in the American Culture

There have been two competing views of pregnancy in our culture. One conceptualizes pregnancy and childbirth as a "crisis" situation, and the other regards them as more of a role transition experience. Each of these attitudes has quite different assumptions that if carried to their logical conclusions have very different implications for the delivery of health care. Unfortunately, assumptions and terminology have not always been clearly articulated and when the rhetoric has been uncritically accepted and applied to the health-care scene, some peculiar innovations and traditions have been incorporated into the delivery of care. In this chapter we will discuss these two orientations to pregnancy so that the implications of these attitudes for actual maternity care can be seen.

Pregnancy as Crisis

A couple's first pregnancy, in particular, constitutes a critical period in the evolution of a family. During the last three decades, there have been a variety of disciplines interested in this critical event. Psychologists and psychiatrists, notably Bibring, Hass, Larsen, Menninger, Caplan and Coleman and Coleman, have all written about the critical nature of this event and have at least alluded to the assumed crisis implications of such a stressful event.[3–8] Shainess, in fact, refers to this period as a "crucible tempering the self" and recognizes the possibility that the tempering process may go wrong, resulting in damage to the person and to the person's relationships with others.[9] Chertok speaks of pregnancy as a progressively developing crisis with the labor and delivery as the peak of the crisis since parturition results in separation of the mother and child and isolation from significant others.[10]

It is important to note that these writings are based largely on experiential or clinical impressions of individuals who have experienced difficulty. There have been no comparison studies with control groups.

Another tradition of research in the crisis vein has led to the formulation of the "normal crisis of parenthood." While the focus here is on parenthood, the time of pregnancy was often included rather by default and so has become intermingled with the general research in this area.

Some of the early studies of parenthood focused entirely on this event as a crisis or extremely disruptive event.[11–13] From these early studies with their small skewed samples, inferences were drawn which were often unfounded. The inferences included pregnancy in the whole process, although this aspect was not studied per se. Moreover, there was some confusion as to the connotation of "crisis" and "normal crisis." In many of the conceptual formulations, both psychological and sociological, a crisis appears to be considered a critical event but not necessarily one that is totally psychologically or interpersonally disruptive. However, the authors' true meaning is often subverted because they do not precisely define their terms.

In the original stress research on the family as exemplified by Hill and Hansen[14] and Hill,[15] the term crisis connoted a sharp change. Specifically, crisis was defined as any sharp, decisive change for which old patterns (of behavior) are inadequate.[15] Thus, a crisis was considered an interruption in the routine of the family's social system and was sharp enough to render former patterns of interaction inadequate. There was also the implication that resolution and reintegration were not only possible, but quite normal and well within the family's capabilities. In sum, then, there has been some confusion, both semantic and conceptual, over the way the term crisis has been applied to the events of pregnancy, childbirth, and parenthood. At times this has led to the acceptance of pregnancy as always being disruptive and potentially damaging.

Pregnancy as a Role Transition

Rossi suggested that the term "normal crisis" was a misnomer as applied to parenthood because the concepts of "normal" and "crisis" are basically incongruous since one implies natural successful resolution and the other plainly indicates the possibility of nonresolution.[16] She suggested that parenthood be viewed as a role transition and be based on a stage–task conceptual framework such as is found in the work of Erickson, Benedek and Hill.[15,17,18] This type of orientation puts parenthood and other phases of the reproductive cycle, including pregnancy, into a developmental task formulation and allows these phenomena to be seen as essentially normal or usual, but also respects the fact that deviation, stress, or disruption can occur depending on a variety of circumstances. In Chapter 29 we will discuss this concept as applied to the postpartum period when parenthood becomes very tangible. In this chapter we will limit the discussion to pregnancy.

If one views the total life span in terms of a developmental task interaction, then we can view individuals' life spans as having cycles composed of stages or phases, each with its unique tasks. As the various cycles occur, social roles develop out of interaction with others in our social network. By analogy, social roles may be said to have cycles and each stage in the cycle has its set of tasks and adjustments. Rossi has outlined four broad stages in the role cycle that have implications for pregnancy as well as parenthood.[16]

1. *Anticipatory stage*. Almost all social roles have some kind of formal or informal training, either through formal schooling, role modeling, or watching others. This stage serves to socialize or train the potential actor for the role he or she is to assume. As its name implies, this stage precedes the assumption of the role and may take place years ahead of the actual role assumption.
2. *Honeymoon stage*. This is the time period immediately following the full assumption of the role. Here intimacy and exploration occur as the person tries to adjust the "fit" of his or her personality to the role demands. Reality testing takes place rather than the fantasizing that often accompanies the anticipatory phase.
3. *Plateau stage*. This is the protracted middle period of a role cycle during which the role is fully exercised. In this phase, the individuals validate themselves as adequate or inadequate depending on how well they and others see themselves performing in the role.
4. *Disengagement–termination stage*. This period immediately precedes and includes the actual termination of the role. For some roles, this stage is quite tangible. The marital role, for instance, ends abruptly with death or divorce. For other roles, such as parenthood or pregnancy, the distinction is much less clear because there is little cultural prescription about when the authority and obligations end.[16]

The Meaning and Effect of Pregnancy on the Couple

As we discuss the impact of pregnancy on the potential father and mother, we will relate some of the psychosocial aspects to the stages of the role cycle. We can see that pregnancy is a unique experience in which a sexual union between a male and female leads to the creation of a new life. This new life in turn will result in the creation of many new and unprecedented relationships.

One example of the profound influence that pregnancy has on the couple lies in the realm of body image. Body image refers to the way one pictures his or her own body. It is a composite of attitudes, feelings and perceptions that each individual has regarding how his body appears.[19] Research indicates that it is not only the mother that experiences a change in body image perception as she literally grows during pregnancy, but her mate as well.[20] Fawcett found that both husbands and wives demonstrate statistically similar patterns of change in perceived body space from the eighth month of pregnancy through the twelfth postpartal month. The data also show that the couple's ability to identify with one another plays a mediating role in the process. Interestingly, marital adjustment did not.

Other studies have found that husbands have a variety of signs and symptoms that mimic or imitate the pregnancy signs and symptoms that their wives are experiencing. The British researchers, Trethowen and Conlon, for instance, found that the men in their study experienced symptoms of physical illness during their wives' pregnancies. These include increased and decreased appetite, gastrointestinal disorders, toothache, and backache. It was noted that these men did not ordinarily experience these conditions at other times.[21] Similarly, studies of American men found that they expressed concerns about body intactness and tended to demonstrate "sympathetic" pregnancy symptoms. These included nausea and vomiting, dizziness, fainting, weight gain, backache and leg cramps.[22,23] Coleman and Coleman have made the observation that was documented in Fawcett's study that the father's close proximity to the mother influences his response to the pregnancy. They also postulate that the more closely the man identifies with his mate, the more intensely he will experience changes in his own body during pregnancy.[24] Thus, we can see what a momentous physiological, psychological and emotional milestone pregnancy can be.

For the Mother

Though the normal female may love her partner greatly and desire a child very much, there still are major developmental changes that she must make to become a mother. In the process of childbearing, she is creating from the union of herself and her mate, another individual *inside* herself which must ultimately grow to become a separate person *outside* herself. Hence the coming child represents the synthesis of three distinct entities—the mother's relationship to her partner, the relationship of the mother to the child as a representative of herself, and the relationship to the unique individual which is the unborn child itself. As with puberty, when the individual can never again be a child, or with menopause when the individual can never again reproduce, with pregnancy the individual can never become a completely single unit again. As long as the child lives, it will never cease to exist as a representative of the woman, her mate, and itself.[25]

The Psychological Tasks of Pregnancy

Several psychological tasks that the pregnant woman must accomplish have been delineated. First, she must believe she is pregnant and incorporate the fetus into her body image.[26] Rubin has spoken of the two questions that the pregnant woman continues to ask during the course of her pregnancy—"Now?" and "Who, me?" The woman questions if this is the right time to have the infant and acknowledges the ever-present surprise she feels being in the pregnant state.[27] As the mother feels the fetus move and her body change in both subtle and very apparent ways, she begins to realize that the fetus inside her is a real and separate being complete with its own boundaries and identity.[25] With this comes a lessening of the surprise and gradual integration. This is not to say there is no turmoil; there is a great range of behavioral displays—mood swings, introspection, physical and psychological weariness. Hence, we have many descriptions of the emotional lability of pregnancy. We must note, however, that there is ample evidence that the physiological and hormonal changes play an additional role in this lability.

The mother's second task is to prepare for the physical separation—the birth of the infant. As with all aspects of pregnancy, there are various responses. Many women are eager to have the baby; they are "tired" of being pregnant. Some even state they are frightened to have this intrusive "invader" within them. However, others do not want to let the fetus go; they anticipate delivery as a loss of a loved object, and this anticipation may actually cause depression. Nevertheless, the task must ultimately be resolved, for every fetus lost is, in a moment, a baby gained.[26]

A third task is to resolve the identity confusions that accompany role transition and thus prepare for the smooth functioning of the family after birth. Coleman and Coleman suggest that, as the woman progresses in pregnancy, she becomes one with "mother"—the primitive memory of the omnipotent being who nurtured her. Moreover, she becomes increasingly prone to evaluate her partner with respect to his appropriateness as a father. She may criticize his current behavior patterns in order to bring them more into line with her idea of what constitutes an ideal father. Similarly, the pregnant father watches his partner become transformed into "mother" as her body changes, her behavior becomes more nesting and so on. He is simultaneously confronting his own feelings and aspirations as he metamorphoses into father. Pregnancy may be the first occasion in the relationship when the partners realize the extent to which they are interdependent psychologically, socially, and economically. On the one hand, this represents a physiological union which can be mystical; on the other hand, however, the merger may be experienced as a trap.[26] No wonder this resolution of identity confusions requires energy, commitment, and work.

Emotional Reactions to Pregnancy

As indicated previously, pregnancy is a time of physical and psychological change. Although the physiological changes are overt manifestations of pregnancy, the psychological changes are more subtle but just as important.

At various times throughout pregnancy, a woman's emotional reactions have been described as ambivalence/uncertainty, introversion/narcissism, passiveness/dependency, and fear/anxiety. These feelings predominate at different periods of pregnancy; others fade in and out as pregnancy progresses.

First Trimester. Ambivalence. At the outset, many women experience ambivalent feelings about being pregnant. Even those who have planned their pregnancy are plagued by doubts as to whether it is the "right time" to have a child. A woman who is pregnant for the first time may wonder if she is really ready for a child. A frequently heard question, asked by both parents, is "What kind of parent will I be?" "How will I be able to cope with the total responsibility of a child—24 hours a day, seven days a week?" Assuming that these women will carry to term, there is no going back for them. Whatever their life style, a drastic change is in the making, which may account for some of the ambivalence they feel as a result of a reluctance to let go of old and familiar ways. For a woman who has other children and has already made the transition to parenthood, doubts may exist as to whether the spacing between that last child and the expected child is suitable. These basic uncertainties may be compounded by other concerns related to the timing of the pregnancy, the impact on the other children (if there are other children), the economic considerations of providing for another family member, the possibility of giving up a job and losing a second income—all of these doubts and concerns can contribute to the unsettling prospects of pregnancy. Added physical discomforts such as nausea and vomiting that frequently accompany early pregnancy only serve to underscore the sense of ambivalence felt by so many women.

This is not to say that a woman does not feel positive about her pregnancy. At the same time that she is struggling with her doubts she may also be experiencing joy and excitement as well as happiness and anticipation. The point is that in all likelihood her feelings will fluctuate between doubts and joys, and she may need to be reassured that what she is feeling is not unnatural and that she need not feel guilty about her ambivalence.

Fears and Fantasies. The first trimester is a time of speculation and anticipation on the part of the mother as she works her way toward accepting the fact that she is pregnant and deals with the physical changes and possible discomforts that she is experiencing. Much time is spent fantasizing about her pregnancy and the impact it will have on her life and the lives of other family members. Mixed with the sense of anticipation is a sense of concern over whether the baby will be normal and healthy, especially if the mother has been recently exposed to a questionable infection.[27]

Shereshefsky and Yarrow noted that mothers who visualized themselves with confidence and clarity during the first trimester tended to make satisfactory adaptations during the entire pregnancy.[28]

If the fantasies become moribund or are characterized by fear and despair, professional intervention may be necessary. If concrete evidence for concern exists (*e.g.,* the presence of genetic defects in the mother's or father's family, the exposure to infection, or the use of drugs or alcohol), the mother should be encouraged to discuss these conditions with the nurse or physician. In some cases, counseling may be necessary if the nurse is not able to allay the mother's fear by simply listening and clarifying misconceptions.

In general, it is important for the nurse to be aware that pregnancy has been recognized as a source of anxiety, particularly for the mother, for the reasons discussed previously. Research has indicated for some time that emotions, although perceived and interpreted by the cerebral cortex, have physiological effects on the body. When the emotion is anxiety, there is motor tension, restlessness, tachycardia, sweating, and flushing. These symptoms are mediated by the sympathetic nervous system through the release of catecholamines and through changes in circulating levels of adrenocortical hormone and other hormones. Animal studies indicate that when catecholamines are released in pregnant animals, there is an increase in maternal blood pressure, a decrease in placental blood flow and more infant stress than is produced by the administration of oxytocin. Studies with humans indicate that anxiety, as measured by a variety of psychological tests, has been correlated with fetal/neonatal abnormalities, decreased infant birthweight, maternal obstetric complications, and parity.[29–34] It is important to note that these data are not definitive and conclusive as yet. However, there is enough evidence to warrant a very careful family assessment, particularly in terms of the mother experiencing undue anxiety during her pregnancy.

Sometimes, old wives' tales underlie the mother's concern. For example, some mothers believe that eating certain foods (*e.g.,* strawberries or watermelon) will cause the baby to have birthmarks. Other mothers believe that, if they are frightened during the pregnancy, their babies will be adversely affected. Assessing the mother's fears, beliefs, or notions provides the nurse with a framework from which to work. Adequate data collection allows the nurse to know what factors are likely to influence the mothers. This information allows the nurse to plan a more appropriate, individualized strategy for working with the expectant mother.

Second Trimester. The second trimester is often marked by a feeling of well-being as the body adjusts to the hormonal changes and some of the early discomforts of pregnancy (nausea and vomiting) subside. Usually, the woman has adjusted to the reality of the pregnancy and reconciled herself to whatever inconvenience it carries. Many of the fears regarding the health and well-being of the infant are forgotten temporarily. Feeling the baby move and hearing the heartbeat are immensely reinforcing and rewarding events for both the expectant mother and father. Allowing the father and the children to share in the experience of feeling fetal movement and hearing the fetal heart tone is a tangible way of incorporating the entire family into the pregnancy.

In the second trimester, mothers become particularly engrossed in fetal growth and development. Both parents become fascinated with pregnancy and the birth process and extremely conscious of the behavior of infants and children with whom they come in contact. At this time parents begin to plan for the actual birth of the baby. They may arrange to attend childbirth classes, read books on infant care, and prepare to face the issues of parenthood.

It is during the second trimester that the mother has been described as becoming narcissistic, passive, and introverted as she concentrates on her own needs and the needs of the fetus growing inside her. As she prepares for her transition to parenthood she may reflect upon her own childhood and her relationship with her mother from whom she may draw her sense of maternal identity.

Because of her preoccupation with her own thoughts and feelings, the mother may seem to be self-centered and egocentric to those around her. Her moods may change drastically from happy to sad for no apparent reason. At times she may seem romantic and preoccupied with daydreams.

Because her preoccupations may be somewhat troublesome to both her and those around her, people close to the mother should be alerted to her passiveness and dependency needs. In this way they can provide the extra love and attention she needs. This, in turn, will enable her to give more of herself to others. Family members should also be reassured that the mother's behavior and emotional lability are not abnormal but are part of the reaction to pregnancy.[35]

Third Trimester. The third trimester adds further psychosocial dimensions. As the woman's body changes, so does her self-image, reflected at times in a feeling of awkwardness and clumsiness. She may feel more unfeminine than at any point in pregnancy and worry about how her husband or mate perceives her.

The third trimester is a time of heightened introversion marked by periods of thinking back on her own childhood and projecting forward in thoughts of her yet-to-be-born child. New fears arise at this time concerning the health and well-being of the baby, as well as her own health and well-being as she contemplates the approach of labor. Mothers frequently distress family members by talking about the possibility of dying during labor. This may reinforce fears that the father is likely to have concerning the outcome of labor.

Furthermore, the mother is likely to wonder how she will "perform" during labor and will be interested in hearing about labor and what she can expect. She may wish to discuss the labor experience with other mothers or to read about it in books and pamphlets.

Regardless of the apprehension she may feel about labor, as the mother approaches the end of pregnancy, she wonders if "her time" will ever arrive. Many mothers cannot seem to wait for pregnancy to be over as they approach full-term. The obsession with delivery frequently finds expression in dreams about labor and the birth of the child. In conscious fantasies, the mother's thoughts center on the appearance of her infant. Toward the end of pregnancy, many expectant parents can clearly conceptualize what the baby will look like and imagine what characteristics he or she will have.[36]

As she contemplates her own labor, the mother may again wonder what kind of parent she will be. Because both father and mother may share the same feelings, some form of role playing may take place with the parents presenting each other with hypothetical situations in an effort to think out what their responses should be. Such "fantasies" seem to be useful to parents during the transition to parenthood. For the couple expecting their first child, the birth of the baby will signal the crossing of a one-way bridge—that of parenthood. No matter what happens, the new parents cannot go back developmentally to a time prior to the conception.

Pregnancy as a Social Role

Although there have been positive attempts to describe the various stages of pregnancy, emotional reactions together with the developmental tasks that need to be accomplished, we still do not have definite boundaries, expectations, and prescriptions for the pregnant role. How are the incumbents supposed to act? What kinds of behaviors are really expected? Does one act "ill," or is pregnancy essentially a well state? Is it "business as usual," or are there special restrictions or exemptions that may be claimed? There are several interesting explanations of the many and varied behaviors that we see in parents to be.

If we examine the stages we outlined in a role cycle transition, we find that being pregnant is, in fact, in itself, an *anticipatory* stage in a role transition to parenthood. This can cause confusion at the outset. As she enters the *anticipatory* stage of the pregnant role, the woman attempts to learn the role by observing others, both family and friends, and she recalls how other significant people in her life acted when they were pregnant. She also takes cues from her physician, who may overtly or covertly influence her thinking, even to the extent of regarding pregnancy as a "sick" or "well" state.[37,38] It is interesting that, in our culture, we do not have any socialization or role modeling for the pregnant role—little girls play at being mothers, but not at being pregnant. Thus, although there are certain behaviors that directly relate to women and their fetuses during pregnancy and are essential for the collective well-being of the entire family (to say nothing of the happiness), the prescriptions for these activities are very amorphous and vary considerably in different social classes. These include such behaviors as positive, personal health habits, prompt and consistent attendance to prenatal care, and adequate nutrition practices.

The *honeymoon* and *plateau* stages of the role cycle come quickly upon the anticipatory stage. The showers, coffee klatches, and conversations with mother and pregnant friends or new mothers help the woman adjust the "fit" of the pregnant state to her personality. Some women find that they adore being pregnant. They feel at one with the earth and sky and see themselves at the center of the universe. They find that they seem to bloom physically and emotionally. Others find the condition almost unbearable. They feel unwell, ugly and put upon and cannot wait to be "unpregnant." By far the more usual are those women who come to accept this condition and tolerate the discomforts and inconveniences. They see it as a necessary stepping stone to another larger role change.

With the infant's birth comes a relatively sudden *disengagement* stage. As we stated previously, there are few cultural norms concerning when the duties and privileges of pregnancy end and parenting begins. It is this role ambiguity that makes this condition difficult. The student is referred to the Suggested Reading for articles that examine this issue in depth.

For the Father

In our culture, being pregnant refers almost exclusively to the woman. In fact, if a man says "We're pregnant," he is still apt to raise eyebrows and be the target of some merriment. Men undergo far less social preparation than women do for parenthood and there is essentially nothing to prepare them for pregnancy per se. Experience with fathers who have actively involved themselves in pregnancy indicates that men, like women, go through various phases during the pregnancy.

The introduction comes with the confirmation of the diagnosis of pregnancy. This places fathers almost immediately into a honeymoon stage. As we know, the reactions are as many and varied as with the women. There may be very unclear feelings because the intellectual focus is on the impending fatherhood, rather than the immediate state of pregnancy.[1] Like his partner, he must assimilate the fact that the baby is his. He may not have the physiologic changes to help him in this as the woman does, although we have seen some men who do experience many of the same physical symptoms of early pregnancy.[2] How men accomplish this psychological task is still unclear and should be the topic of some fascinating research. We do know that there may be guilt reactions about getting the partner pregnant or causing her to be sick and uncomfortable. On a more positive note, there may be feelings of pride at his virility or mutual pride that "We did it!"[4] There may also be feelings of distance between him and his partner as she continues through her introverted first trimester. Jealousy, worry about the change in sexual relationships, and concern about his own competence as a man and provider may occur.[41]

The first perceptible movement of the fetus generally creates a profound feeling that the fetus is real; most men, when questioned, recall the time when "I first felt the baby move." In the second trimester, more thought is given to what it means to be a father and the plateau stage is entered. Men observe children and pregnant women more intently and become more acutely aware of their partners' growing uterus. A myriad of thoughts, concerns, and downright worries may sweep over the father just as with the mother. Often these center on his ability to provide for the expanding family. However, there is also concern and thought about how well he will be able to "father" the new progeny and meet the newly evolving expectations of the mother.[1]

As with pregnancy for the woman, there is a good deal of literature that describes this period as a crisis time for fathers. Yet there is evidence to indicate that psychologically healthy men cope without major problems.[1] What is clear, however, is that pregnancy requires as much adjustment for the father as it does for the mother.

As with the mother, labor and delivery mark the disengagement–termination stage of the role transition of pregnancy for the father. How these proceed can have a profound effect on the father. Most health providers who have had experience with pregnant couples believe that men who take an active part in the pregnancy by attending childbirth and parent education classes, participating in preparations for the infant, and so on, are more likely to participate in the birthing with positive psychological outcomes and this, in turn, strengthens the building of the parental bond.[35]

Implications for Health Providers

The nurse can function in collaboration with other members of the health team by providing emotional support together with counseling and teaching for the pregnant couple. As we have seen, regarding pregnancy as a role transition rather than a crisis helps us emphasize the normality of the condition and avoid a search for illness and other negative aspects. We can then structure our care to support the resources of the couple rather than looking for problems which may not exist until we create them. The key to appropriate intervention in this instance is *family* assessment.

Family Assessment

There are certain extrafamilial stressors, both developmental and situational, that must be taken into account. Pregnancy and parenthood are examples of developmental stressors. Death, divorce, natural catastrophes, and loss of a job are examples of situational stressors (Fig. 18-1). These extrafamilial stressors work in conjunction with the intrafamilial stressors (*e.g.,* inadequate communication, personal disorganization) to affect the role relationships within the family by producing varying amounts of difficulty in role transition. The amount of difficulty produced is related to how well the family roles are organized and how good their resources are.

The way the family is organized (their role structure) depends on each member's values, goals, and ability to put a meaning on events (definition of the situation). On the basis of these goals and definitions, roles are given to the members and certain behaviors become associated with each role (role differentiation and allocation). Strength is gathered from the family resources which can be material (finances) or interpersonal (integration, cohesiveness, good communication). Appropriately structured roles and a reservoir of family resources serve to buffer the family from the impact of the various stressors and make role transition easier (Fig. 18-1).

The following is a guide for the development of a family care plan. These questions are the type of questions the nurse would include during an assessment.

Assessment

A. Family Composition
   1. Who are the family members?
      a. What are their ages? What are their relationships to one another?
      b. Where do they live? Do they interact frequently?
      c. Are they "close" emotionally if not physically?
      d. What is the family's relationship to the larger community? Is the family involved in community affairs and religious activities? What is its community support structure?
      e. Does the family have additional members in its social network? Are there other relatives or friends available for support?

B. Family Functioning
   1. How are the roles allocated and differentiated?
      a. Who does what in the house? Is this mutually satisfactory?
      b. Who makes decisions? How are they made?
      c. What are the changes that members would like?
      d. How do the parents see their roles being changed with the new infant?
   2. How do members usually define situations that happen?
      a. Does the family generally consolidate in time of trouble?
      b. Do they tend to be optimistic, pessimistic, or do attitudes vary with situations?

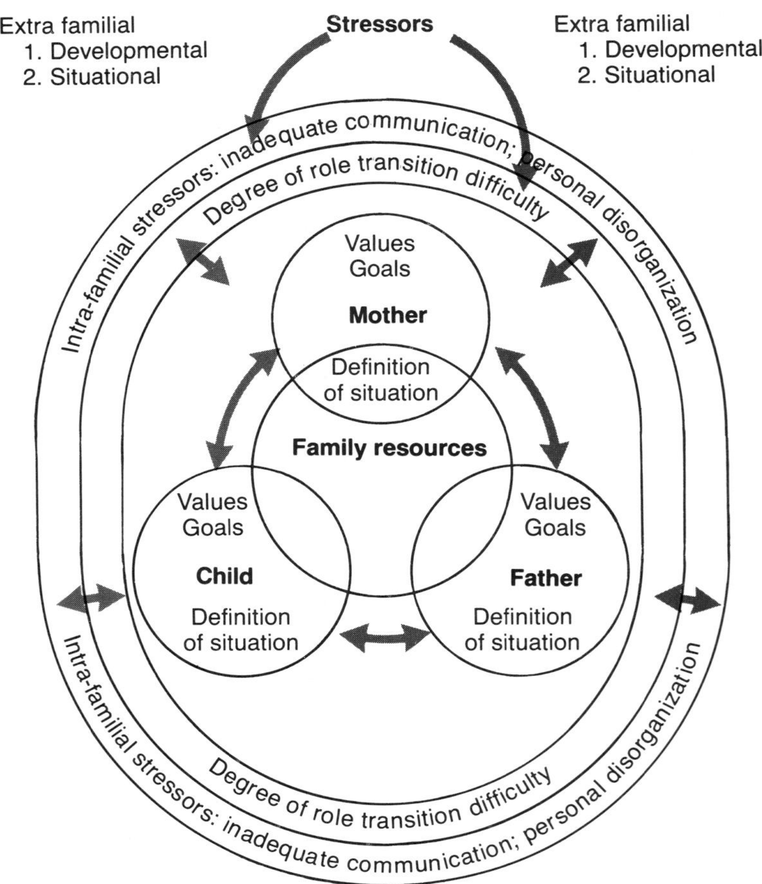

Figure 18-1.
Model of family interaction during role transition and components of assessment.

   c. What are the communication patterns? Who talks to whom? Do problems usually get solved with discussion?
3. What are the family's material and emotional resources?
   a. Who turns to whom for emotional support? Who is the mother's main support at this time? Who is the father's main support at this time?
   b. Are finances adequate? Who contributes? Will the pregnancy make a difference?
4. Are there interpersonal or intrapersonal difficulties?
   a. Are there long-term problems? What are the attempts to resolve them?
   b. Are there problems specific to this pregnancy?
   c. What alternatives for solution for the existing problems do the parents see?
5. What are the specific plans for the baby and for themselves during pregnancy?
   a. What are their plans for themselves as parents?
   b. What are their plans for the infant?
   c. Are siblings anticipated (if this is the first child)?
   d. What are plans for siblings?

Intervention and Evaluation

Intervention is aimed at helping the parents define possible stressors and resources within their family unit and developing strategies for coping with manifest or possible disruptive elements. By helping parents become aware of their resources and supporting them in their decision making, the nurse can minimize a great deal of stress associated with this role transition. Parents need to validate their impressions of what is happening to them, both physically and emotionally, with an outside person. Family, friends, and health professionals all can be useful in this way. The nurse will want to encourage the parents to use their network of family and friends if it is determined that this network can supply material and emotional support.

Intervention can be evaluated as effective if the

NC Nursing Care: Normal Pregnancy

Assessment	Intervention	Evaluation
Family Composition		
Ages; relationships to one another Where they live; frequency of interaction Emotional closeness Family's relationship to larger community; family's involvement in community affairs and, religious activities; community support structure Additional members in its social network; other relatives or friends available for support	Identify potential stressors and sources of support within family and between family and community Support family in their decision making Allow family to validate their impressions of what is happening to them Encourage family to utilize identified support systems	Family verbalizes understanding of stressors or potential stressors Family utilizes support systems appropriately
Family Functioning		
Role allocation and differentiation Who does what; mutually satisfactory Decision maker; how made Any changes members would like Parents' views of role changes with new infant	Identify potential stressors and sources of support within familial roles or decision making Encourage family to utilize identified support systems Identify family's realistic views of role changes	Family verbalizes understanding of stressors or potential stressors Family utilizes support systems appropriately Family has realistic perception that infant will change their lives and adjustment is possible
Member definitions of situations that happen Family consolidation in times of trouble Tone of attitudes—optimistic, pessimistic, or varying Communication patterns; who talks to whom; problem solving with discussions	Identify potential stressors and sources of support within family communication patterns Share with the family any communication patterns	Family verbalizes understanding of stressors or potential stressors Family utilizes support systems appropriately Family is perceived as drawing together by family and nurse
The family's material and emotional resources Who turns to whom for emotional support; mother's support; father's support Adequate finances; who contributes; differences with pregnancy	Identify stressors in support systems—emotional and financial Identify alternative support systems Refer family to financial services as necessary	Family shows adequate emotional and financial support systems Family utilizes support systems appropriately
Interpersonal or intrapersonal difficulties Long-term problems; resolution attempts Problems specific to this pregnancy Alternative solutions for existing problems	Identify any long-term problems or problems specific to this pregnancy Determine support systems and solutions best for this family	Family's long-term problems are resolved Family's problems specific to this pregnancy are resolved
Specific plans for baby and selves during pregnancy Plans for themselves as parents Plans for infants Siblings anticipated Plans for siblings	Identify whether plans are realistic or not Identify potential sibling rivalry situations Offer individualized family solutions	Family has realistic plans for the pregnancy Parents have realistic expectations of selves as parents Minimal sibling rivalry experienced

family unit is perceived as drawing together (by the family as well as the nurse), if there is open discussion of problems and experiences, and if concrete plans are made for the infant's arrival and the parents have a realistic perception that the infant will change their lives and that adjustment is possible for this momentous new role.

References

1. Phillips CR, Anzalone SJ: Fathering, Participating in Labor and Birth. St Louis, CV Mosby, 1978
2. Brown ML: A cross-cultural look at pregnancy, labor and delivery. JOGN Nurs 5, 5:35–38, September/October 1976
3. Bibring GL, et al: A study of the psychological processes in pregnancy and of the earliest mother–child relationship. Psychoanalytic Study of the Child, pp. 9–72. New York, International Universities Press, vol. 16
4. Haas S: Psychiatric implications in gynecology and obstetrics. In Ballak (ed): Psychology of Physical Illness. New York, Grune and Stratton, 1952
5. Larsen VL: Stresses of the childbearing years. Am J Public Health 56:32–36, 1966
6. Menninger WC: The emotional factors in pregnancy. Bull Menninger Clin 7:15–24, 1943
7. Caplan G: Patterns of parental response to the crisis of premature birth: A preliminary approach to modifying the mental health outcome. Psychiatry, 23:365–374, 1960
8. Coleman AP, Coleman L: Pregnancy: The Psychological Experience. New York, Herder and Herder, 1971
9. Shainess N: The structure of the mothering encounter. J Nerv Ment Dis 136:146–161, 1963
10. Chertok L: Motherhood and Personality. London, Tavistock, 1969
11. Le Masters EE: Parenthood as crisis. Marriage and Family Living 19:352–355, 1957
12. Dyer ED: Parenthood as crisis: A restudy. Marriage and Family Living 25:196–201, 1963
13. Hobbs DJ, Jr: Parenthood as crisis, a third study. Journal Marriage and the Family, 27:367–372, 1963
14. Hill R, Hansen DA: The identification of a conceptual framework utilized in family study. Marriage and Family Living, 22:299–311, 1960
15. Hill R: Generic features of families under stress. Social Casework, 39, 2–3:32–54, 1958
16. Rossi AS: Transition to parenthood. Journal Marriage and the Family, 30:26–39, February 1968
17. Erickson E: Identity and the life cycle: Selected papers. Psychol Issues, 1:1–171, 1959
18. Benedek T: Parenthood as a developmental phase. J Am Psychoanal Assoc 7, 8:389–417, 1959
19. Schilder P: The Image and Appearance of the Body. New York, International Universities Press, 1950
20. Fawcett J: Body image and the pregnant couple. MCN 227–233, July/August 1978
21. Trethowen WH, Conlon MF: The Couvade syndrome. Br J Psychiatry 111:57–66, January 1965
22. Liebenberg B: Expectant fathers. Child Family 8:265–278, Summer 1969
23. Munroe RL, Munroe RH: Male pregnancy symptoms and cross-sex identity in three societies. J Soc Psychol 89:147–158, February 1973
24. Coleman AD, Coleman LL: Pregnancy: the Psychological Experience. New York, Herder and Herder, 1971
25. Osofsky HJ: Psychological and sociological aspects of normal pregnancy. Medical Services Journal, Canada, 23, 4:512–521, 1967
26. Coleman AD, Coleman L: Pregnancy as an altered state of consciousness. Birth and the Family J 1, 1:7–11, 1974
27. Rubin R: Cognitive style in pregnancy. Am J Nurs 3:502–508, 1970
28. Shereshefsky P, Yarrow L (eds): Psychological Aspects of a First Pregnancy and Early Postnatal Adaptation. New York, Raven Press, 1973
29. Ascher BH: Maternal anxiety in pregnancy and fetal homeostasis. JOGN Nurs 7, 3:18–21, May/June 1978
30. Greiss FG, Gabble FL: Effect of sympathetic nerve stimulation on the uterine vascular bed. Am J Obstet Gynecol 21:295, 1967
31. Shabanah EH, Tricorni EV, Suarez J: Fetal environment and its influences on fetal development. Surg Gynecol Obstet 129:556, 1969
32. Adamson KE, Mueller–Heubach KE, Myers R: Production of fetal asphyxia in the rhesus monkey by administration of catecholamines to the mother. Am J Obstet Gynecol 109:248, 1971
33. Shaw JA, Wheeler JP, Morgan W: Mother–infant relationship and weight gain in the first month of life. J Am Acad Child Psychiatry 9:428, 1970
34. Davids A, DeVault AS, DeVault S: Maternal anxiety during pregnancy and childbirth anomalies. Psychosom Med 24:464, 1962
35. Stichler J, Bowden JM, Reimer E: Pregnancy, a shared emotional experience. MCN 153–157, May/June 1978
36. Pharis ME, Manosevitz M: Parental models: A means for evaluating different prenatal contexts. In Sawin DB, Hawkins RC II, Walker LO, Penticuff JH (eds): Exceptional Infant IV: Psychosocial Risks in Infant-Environment Transactions. New York, Brunner/Mazel 1980
37. Rosengren W: The sick role during pregnancy: A note on research in progress. Journal of Health & Human Behavior, 3, 3:213–218, Fall 1962
38. Rosengren W: Social instability and attitudes toward pregnancy as a social role. Social Problems 9, 4:371–378, Spring 1962
39. Antle K: Psychologic involvement in pregnancy by expectant fathers. JOGN Nurs 4, 4:40–42, July/August 1975

Suggested Reading

Antle K: Psychologic involvement in pregnancy by expectant fathers. JOGN Nurs 4, 4:40–42, July/August 1975

Brown MS: A cross-cultural look at pregnancy, labor and delivery. JOGN Nurs 4, 5:35–38, September/October 1976

Galloway KG: The uncertainty and stress of high risk pregnancy. Amer J Mat Child Nurs 294–299, September/October 1976

Hern WM: The illness parameters of pregnancy. Soc Sci Med 9:365–372, 1975

Antle MK: Active involvement of expectant fathers in pregnancy, some further considerations. JOGN Nurs 7, 2:7–12, March/April 1978

Rosengren WR: Social instability and attitudes toward pregnancy as a social role. Social Problems 9, 4:371–378, 1962

Rossi AS: Transition to parenthood. Journal Marriage and the Family 30:26–39, February 1968

Woolery L, Barkley N: Enhancing couple relationships during prenatal and postnatal classes. MCN 6:184–88, May/June 1981

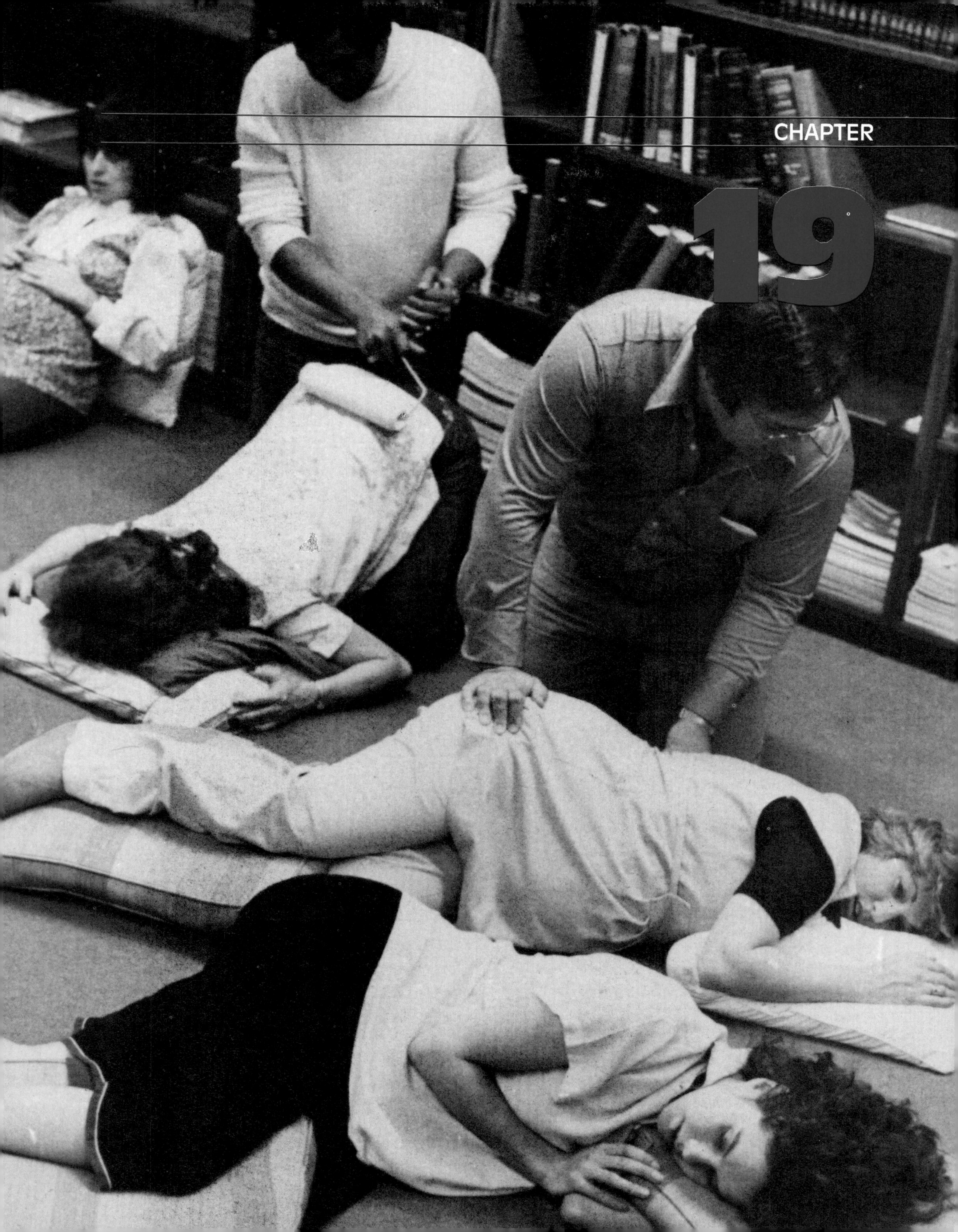

CHAPTER

19

CHAPTER 19

Parent Education

Education of the patient is a major component of the professional nurse's role. In this era of the consumer movement, greater emphasis must be placed on helping the patient and family to fully understand the body processes and the rationale for medical and nursing management of health problems. Particularly in the area of maternity, patients and families are not only very interested in learning but have come to view such knowledge as their right. They expect the nurse to be willing and able to assist them in acquiring knowledge and to take their individual wants and needs into consideration.

The increased involvement of childbearing couples in all phases of the reproductive cycle benefits not only the parents, as receivers of care but also nurses, as givers of care. A concerned and knowledgeable woman will follow a more healthful regimen during pregnancy, including nutrition, exercise and rest, physical care, and psychological processes. A prepared woman and an involved partner can cope positively with the stresses of labor, enriching their relationship and promoting psychological maturation. Parents who are informed and who actively seek understanding of their child's numerous needs for comfort, security, and stimulation during the early formative years can attain a happier, more satisfying parent–child relationship and foster optimal growth and development of the child.

When the childbearing couple desires to learn, and the health professional is ready to teach, their shared experiences can be most satisfying to all involved. The roles of teacher and learner are not rigid, however, because often the nurse learns much of value from the parents, and gains deeper understanding of the reproductive experience through appreciating their perspectives.

The cornerstone of patient education is recognition and respect of the learning needs of patients. The nurse may design content, but if it does not meet the patient's learning needs, it is pointless and ineffective. The nurse is responsible for developing the skill to assess these learning needs accurately.

Parent education encompasses an enormous body of knowledge, only a portion of which is included in this chapter. Throughout the text, additional information about teaching as a part of nursing intervention for specific parent/patient needs or problems will be found. Concepts related to the teaching-learning process, some approaches to group and individual teaching, and programs providing preparation for childbirth and parenting are discussed here.

"Teaching is an interactive process between a teacher and one or more learners."[1] The teaching-learning process is a complex entity composed of various interrelated parts—1) identifying the need or needs of the learner, 2) determining the motivation of the learner, 3) establishing the objectives of learning, and 4) evaluating the results in terms of desired learn-

Factors Affecting the Teaching-Learning Process

1. Learners and teachers bring with them to the classroom a cluster of understandings, skills, appreciations, attitudes, and feelings that have personal meaning to them and are in effect the sum of their reactions to previous stimuli.
2. Learners and teachers are individually different in many ways even when grouped according to ability.
3. Learners and teachers have developed concepts of self that directly affect their behavior.
4. Learning may be defined as a change in behavior.
5. Learning requires activity on the part of the learner. The learner should not be passive.
6. Learners ultimately learn what *they* actively desire to learn; they do not learn what they do not accept or come to accept.
7. Learning is enhanced when learners accept responsibility for their own learning.
8. Learning is directly influenced by physical and social environment.
9. Learning occurs on successively deeper levels.
10. Learning is deepened when the learning situation provides opportunity for applying learnings in as realistic a situation as is feasible.
11. Learners are motivated when they understand and accept the purposes of the learning situation.
12. Learners are motivated by successful experiences.
13. Learners are motivated by teacher acceptance.
14. Learners are motivated when they can associate new learnings with previous learnings.
15. Learners are motivated when they can see the usefulness of the learning in their own personal terms.[2]

ing. Learning may be defined as a desired change in behavior. Teaching is accomplished only when the learner learns, retains new knowledge, and is able to use it at the present or in the future.

Many factors affect the teaching-learning process, and the nurse must be aware of those which might either enhance or interfere with learning. The concepts treated in Factors Affecting the Teaching-Learning Process on the preceding page illustrate some of these influences.

The idea of educating women during pregnancy is probably very ancient. In Manchester, England, during the 18th century, Dr. Charles White wrote a book of instructions for the supervision of women during pregnancy and how to help them in labor and make them more comfortable. During the last few decades of this century, increased understanding of the psychodynamics of pregnancy and the puerperium has established a scientific basis for the content and structure of antepartal and postpartal education.

Factors in Parent Education

Psychological Tasks of Pregnancy and Women's Interests

Nurses have long observed that pregnant women ask different kinds of questions and express different concerns in early pregnancy than in later periods of gestation. The widely recognized receptiveness of women in the third trimester toward information about baby care and behavior led to the common practice of scheduling prenatal classes at this time. Women in the first or second trimester did not exhibit the same level of interest in parenting classes; thus, they were largely omitted from prenatal education.

Professional interest in the many behavior changes characteristic of pregnant women led to identification of the specific and unique psychological tasks which appear to be a universal phenomenon of pregnancy. Viewing pregnancy as a developmental process, involving profound endocrine and general somatic as well as psychological changes, it can be understood as a period of disequilibrium and a significant turning point in the woman's (and probably her partner's) life.[3] Certain specific psychological tasks are necessary to cope with the numerous changes, and these seem to occur at specific times during gestation.

1. The first task, incorporation and integration of the fetus, occurs during the first trimester and is not evident during later stages of pregnancy.
2. The second task, perception of the fetus as a separate object, seems to begin in the second trimester and is well established by the third trimester.
3. The third task, readiness to assume the care-taking relationship with the baby, increases from the second trimester to the third trimester and is not apparent in early pregnancy.
4. The fourth task concerns preparation for labor. The highest level of anxiety about labor is manifested during the second trimester, while women in the third trimester express more confidence about undergoing labor.[4]

This "time schedule" of involvement with different psychological tasks suggests that pregnant women's interests and needs for information will vary according to the stage of gestation. While research has not yet identified exactly what periods of time are involved in each psychological task, nurses can use these data to plan appropriate antepartal education.

During early pregnancy, when the woman is working through the idea of being pregnant, informational needs center on validating the pregnancy, understanding physical changes, and recognizing normal emotions and feelings. In midpregnancy, a woman begins to identify the baby as a unique individual and is receptive to information about fetal growth and development and about maintaining her own health and the baby's health. As pregnancy draws to an end, the woman becomes concerned about preparing for the baby's arrival and becomes interested in preparation for childbirth, infant behavior, and care-taking activities including feeding, handling, bathing, and so on. By tailoring the information presented to the different interests of each group and providing women with the opportunity to express their own learning needs, nurses can conduct meaningful antepartal educational programs.

Postpartum Processes and the Mother–Child Relationship

Although the experience of labor is undoubtedly significant for the woman's self-concept, maternal-infant bonding, and possibly the couple's relationship, few data are available to substantiate what impact nursing intervention during labor might have on these perceptions. Advocates of prepared childbirth believe that women move more rapidly into the care-taking role when they are awake and actively participating in their labor. There is some empirical evidence that fathers who act as labor coaches develop stronger and more recognizable paternal feelings toward the babies of these labors than toward their other children. The work of some neonatologists in the area of high-risk infants strongly suggests that early and prolonged contact between mother and baby following labor and delivery enhances the bonding process. As with other mammals, humans seem to have a critical time for optimal mother-infant bonding, and this time is probably the first several hours after delivery. There also appear to be certain species-specific maternal behaviors which initiate and carry out the attachment process.[5]

On first contact with their babies, mothers seek an *en face position* in which their eyes are in the same vertical plane as the baby's (Fig. 19-1). It has been suggested that this eye-to-eye contact may initiate or release maternal care-taking responses. Mothers then begin to explore the infant, first with fingertips touching the infant's extremities, then within a few minutes proceeding, with encompassing palm contact, to massage the infant's trunk. Some fathers have been observed going through these same steps. Kennell and Klaus described this process as taking only a few minutes.[6] Many years earlier, Rubin observed very similar behavior patterns in mothers as they moved from fingertip to palm touch, then encompassed their infants in their arms. However, this process took about three days according to Rubin's observations.[7]

Other physiologic and psychological changes occur during the puerperium which are part of the process of regeneration undergone by the mother. There is a "taking-in" period which lasts for the first day or two, possibly three. During this restorative period the mother has a great need for sleep. Among other normal reactions associated with this taking-in phase is the mother's passive and dependent behavior. However, when the "taking-hold" phase follows, the mother is physically and psychologically ready to assume active care of her infant and seeks information and support to facilitate her mothering behaviors. Once her dependency needs have been met in the taking-in phase, she needs to move toward greater independence.[8] For further details of nursing care during the puerperium, refer to Chapters 28 and 29.

Effective patient teaching must take into account what is known about the processes occurring during labor and the puerperium, as well as individual variation and specific need. If the labor experience is as important as we suspect, health professionals have an obligation to assist parents in preparing for it and supporting them during this stressful time. When labor has started, a certain amount of teaching is possible, and sensitive care can be helpful, but this is not as effective as antenatal preparation. Although parents have long recognized the significance of being together with their new baby in the hours right after birth, until recently, health professionals have largely been oblivious to this in their concern for asepsis, technology, and immediate dangers to the newborn. Perhaps it is time to rethink delivery and recovery routines and educate both parents and professionals in the new data concerning mother–infant attachment.

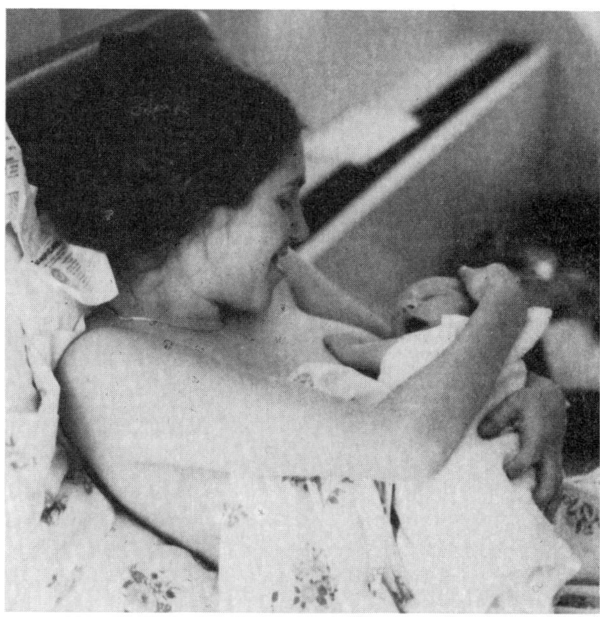

Figure 19-1.
En face position.

During the few days the postpartal woman spends in the hospital, her needs may conflict with the nursing staff's needs to maintain the routine or provide the teaching they believe necessary. Mothers will progress at different speeds in assuming the care-taking role, and will have individualized concerns. Finding a way to respond to individual needs yet conduct an efficient postpartal educational program is a major challenge to postpartal nurses. Parent teaching activities must also extend into the community to respond to the needs of families integrating a new member during the early years of childrearing.

Socioeconomic Factors

The learning process will vary according to culture and the socioeconomic situation. Mothering practices in lower income groups are influenced by economic circumstances that limit equipment, supplies, and mobility; by the organization of the family group and the authority structure; and by the accumulated folk knowledge which establishes specific practices for many common activities and problems of childrearing. Standard educational programs about breastfeeding or formula preparation, clothing and supplies for the baby, integration of the baby into the family, and the mother's nutritional and rest needs are often meaningless to low income mothers because of a lack of resources and a different value system. Family and friends are generally viewed as more reliable consultants for health concerns than professionals, whose assistance is sought only when community knowledge cannot solve the problem. Sometimes the use of language itself precludes useful exchange of information, as differences in terms used, accent, and speed of delivery vary substantially between middle-class nurses and low income mothers. In lower socioeconomic levels, the grandmother's word about baby care is often law, and she may be the major caretaker of the baby. Teaching given solely to the mother may thus be of little consequence to the actual care given to the baby. Different cultural groups also have their unique approaches to childrearing and patterns of assistance to new mothers. Values, language, style, and knowledge will exert influences within other cultural groups in a manner similar to that discussed previously.

The nurse must come to understand different cultural and low income lifestyles if effective antepartal and postpartal teaching is to occur. The approach to teaching used with these groups will probably need to shift from the giving of information to assessing present practices, supplementing these practices when necessary with information presented in a form that can be understood and accepted.[9]

Types of Education for Childbearing

Preparation for motherhood actually begins with the woman's own birth or earlier and is influenced by an accumulation of her experiences through infancy, childhood, adolescence, and maturity. The father's feelings and attitudes are influenced in a similar manner. There is an increasing tendency for schools to incorporate information about childbearing and parenthood into "health education" and "family life" courses. Classes about pregnancy, sexuality, and parenthood are becoming more common in college and university curricula, as well as more widely available in continuing education and private adult educational programs. Couples thus bring a wealth of previous learning to their experience of childbearing, some of it useful and positive and some frightening and inaccurate. With the advent of pregnancy, preparation for parenthood begins in earnest as the immediacy of the event escalates the need for information.

Types of Education for Childbearing

I. Individual teaching and counseling
II. Groups and classes
  A. Informational groups
  B. Discussion or counseling groups
  C. Prepared childbirth groups
    1. Dick-Read
    2. Lamaze or psychoprophylaxis
    3. Bradley
    4. Wright
    5. Kitzinger or psychosexual
  D. Other
    1. Yoga
    2. Hypnosis

Individual Teaching and Counseling

One-to-one teaching is widely used in all nursing settings, and is frequently effective in assisting patients to understand and adapt to a variety of health problems. In most nurse–patient contacts, some individual teaching occurs. Numerous opportunities are present during pregnancy for nurses to enhance the effectiveness of medical care through explanations of treatments and procedures, interpretations of what the physician tells parents, and specific instructions for carrying out the regimen of care. When the patient asks questions about symptoms or feelings or seeks general information, an on-the-spot response by the nurse meets that particular learning need.

Some clinics and offices have pamphlets or audiovisual material intended to provide individualized instruction to parents during the antepartal period. The amount of structure necessary to ensure that these materials are actually used varies widely. The effectiveness of written or media information without reinforcement through discussion is questionable.

Counseling, an interchange of opinions or giving of advice to help direct the judgment or conduct of others, is often hard to separate from teaching. While counseling is more personal and feeling-oriented, its use in combination with presentation of facts usually results in enhanced learning. Appropriate use of counseling takes into consideration the patient's viewpoint and works within an acceptable framework to bring about increased understanding, which leads to a change in behavior in the desired direction through the patient's internalization of the new goals.

Individualized nursing care in which the woman is assisted to recognize her feelings and fears, reassured that such feelings are normal, and given certain facts to dispel myths or anticipate and prepare for coming events is a common example of how teaching and counseling are combined in antepartal care.

Although individual teaching and counseling will continue to be a major mode of nursing intervention, concerns for more efficient use of the health professional's time have led to increased use of groups for antepartal education. Groups are also beneficial because the exchange of experiences among parents with common concerns provides support and encouragement, and expertise and knowledge of the group members combined often exceeds that of the professional alone.

Groups and Classes

Most institutions providing maternity care also offer some type of antepartal group instruction, but the goals and purposes of these groups vary widely. Many private organizations also offer programs in antepartal education, prenatal exercise and Yoga, and preparation for childbirth and parenthood. Classes may be affiliated with continuing education programs in colleges and universities, adult education programs in local communities and high schools, health professionals in private practice, or national health care organizations such as the Red Cross. The teachers in these groups or classes usually have some type of preparation or certification. They may represent one or, less commonly, several disciplines.

These educational programs can enhance, strengthen, and broaden the care and services provided by the physician and maternity nurse. Programs in parent education should be related segments in the total constellation of services provided to families. In order to make these sessions truly a preparation for parenthood and family-centered nursing, special attention has to be given to timing and availability of these courses. Sometimes hospitals and institutions arrange classes at times that are not feasible for the parents attending, especially for the father and often for the mother (*e.g.,* in the middle of a busy day). Therefore, attendance is sparse and limited and many valuable aims of the programs may be thwarted.

Informational Groups

The informational group is the most widely used type of program in this country. These groups are planned to serve everyone in the community and place emphasis on a general type of "education for childbirth." Courses usually include the physiology of childbearing, general hygiene, including nutrition during pregnancy and lactation, preparations for the baby, and the care of the mother and baby after delivery. In this type of program a multidisciplinary approach may be used in the teaching, or the nurse may be responsible for teaching all of the content.

In general, the material is usually covered in a lecture format with time allowed for questions and discussion. At times a semistructured approach may be used, with certain topics being suggested by the participants and additional relevant information introduced by the nurse–discussion leader as it seems appropriate. Audiovisual materials such as films and slides are often used, with a film depicting actual childbirth a standard component. Tours of the hospital labor unit, postpartum floor, and nursery are usually included.

Some of these classes are given for expectant mothers or fathers separately, in others the parents attend classes together. In the latter group the classes aid the parents in their mutual appreciation of the value of antepartal preparation and tend to promote the idea of sharing parenthood. The goals set for the parents in any of these classes are similar—namely, to gain increased knowledge about childbearing and increased understanding of ways to promote and to maintain optimum health through the practice of good health habits in daily living.

These classes are included as a part of the programs of private "public health" agencies such as the Visiting Nurse Association, official community health agencies such as the local and state departments of health, private organizations such as the Maternity Center Association in New York City, and many hospitals throughout the states.

Discussion or Counseling Groups

In this format no structured curriculum is set in advance. Group discussion is developed from the contributions of the group members. The leader is responsible for guiding the discussion and for opening essential areas not probed by the group members. The various areas described in informational programs (physiology of childbearing and general hygiene) are covered as the nurse–leader introduces these topics when they fit with the areas brought up by the participants.

The group situation demands that the nurse develop a new concept of self as a leader and acquire new skills. Knowledge and understanding of what material is relevant are essential so that it can be drawn upon as the group needs it. Hence, the nurse must be totally prepared each time that the group meets because the discussion may range from nutrition in the first trimester of pregnancy to the physiology of labor. In addition, she must be skilled in listening, probing, and reflecting so that she can help the group elaborate on germane comments and statements.

The nurse must recognize the importance and the implication of "iceberg questions," sometimes spoken of as "the question behind the question," knowing that such questions may indicate an underlying concern of the questioner. For example, an expectant mother in the last trimester of pregnancy asks, "How common is going crazy after having a baby?" In such instances the professional nurse should be able to explore and to sift alternatives until the real question can be asked and appropriate action may be taken. In this instance the patient really was not concerned with how often people became psychotic after childbirth but rather whether she is likely to experience this malady. Because of a history of mental illness in her family and her own extreme emotional lability during this pregnancy she was afraid that she might become psychotic after delivery.

Because training group leaders is a costly and time-consuming business (and it is essential that those who manage parents in this way be trained in the techniques), group education is not a commitment to be undertaken lightly by either the participating nurses or the sponsoring agencies. Unfortunately, many of these agencies rate the success of a program by the numbers attending; and in the group situation, by definition, only *small groups* can be served at any time.

Group discussion programs are usually well received by those who become involved on a continuing basis, with high levels of professional and patient satisfaction. Small groups are also quite effective in bringing about behavior change. Moreover, group education has the advantage of not limiting the discussion to certain topics usually discussed by particular class groups, and it can focus upon any of the aspects of pregnancy or childbearing which are of interest to the group.

Whatever the approach, the nurse who participates in parent classes is in a favorable position to help the patients and families develop a better understanding of their immediate situations, together with a balanced view of the sociology of pregnancy and parturition, growth and development, and the psychological and emotional aspects of family life.

Prepared Childbirth Groups

The interpretation of "labor" as "pain" has been held by women from time immemorial, with the result that many women approach childbirth in dread of a fearful ordeal. Orthodox Christian teaching considers pain the natural accompaniment of childbirth in partial reparation for Eve's enticing Adam into the original sin. As most body processes are free from discomfort, the question of labor pain as a social phenomenon is frequently raised. Whatever the basic causes and mechanisms of childbirth pain (see Chap. 24), concern developed gradually over finding a means to help relieve the suffering of women during labor.

The influence of the attitude of a woman toward her confinement upon the ease of labor was stressed for many years by the British obstetrician, the late Grantly Dick-Read. He emphasized certain psychological aspects of labor—that "fear is in some way the chief pain-producing agent in otherwise normal labor." The neuromuscular mechanism by which fear exerts a deleterious effect on labor is obscure, but the general validity of Dick-Read's contention is in keeping with common clinical knowledge. The woman builds up a state of tensions because she is frightened, and these tensions create an antagonistic effect on the muscular activity of normal labor and results in more pain. The pain causes more fear, which further increases the tensions, and so on, creating a vicious circle.

Dick-Read's approach included an educational component to help women comprehend the physiologic processes of labor, exercises to improve muscle tone, and techniques to assist in relaxation and prevent the fear-tension-pain mechanism. These three components are included in most childbirth preparation programs that developed after Dick-Read's work became well known.

The educational component during pregnancy is designed to eliminate fear. Facts which concern the anatomy and the physiology of childbearing and the appropriate care of the woman are taught. The woman not only learns how labor progresses but also is helped to gain an understanding of the sensations likely to accompany labor and methods of working cooperatively with them. The exercises that are included are designed for the muscles which will be used in labor, as well as those which will promote the general well-being of the body. The performance of any skill is more efficient if the muscles involved are in the best condition. The exercises are not strenuous and, for the most part, are ones that will contribute to improved posture, body balance, agility, and increased flexibility, strength, and endurance. The woman and her partner learn breathing techniques that will aid her ability to relax in the first stage of labor, and techniques that will help her to work effectively with muscles used in the delivery.

To enable the parents to better meet the needs of their baby after birth, information about growth and development is also included in these classes.

An important consideration throughout such programs is "to help the woman help herself," so that her pregnancy will be a healthy, happy experience and at the time of labor she will be better able to participate actively in having her baby. In former days when women often were given heavy sedation, they were unable to have this satisfying experience.

Currently most prepared childbirth programs include the father as an active participant in helping the woman cope with labor. In this way the father is made to feel involved and useful, and through learning the physiologic and emotional processes of pregnancy, he may gain an appreciation of the woman's experience. He is also able to explore his feelings and role as a parent and prepare psychologically for fatherhood.

Fathers also play another important role in labor. A study by Sosa, Kennel, and Klaus suggests that there may be major perinatal benefits of constant human support during labor.[10] The control group (no labor companion) showed a higher rate ($P<0.001$) of subsequent perinatal problems (*e.g.,* cesarean section and meconium staining). It was necessary to admit 103 mothers to the control group and 33 to the experimental group (supportive companions in labor) to obtain 20 in each group with uncomplicated deliveries. Also, in the final sample, the length of time from admission to delivery (primigravidas) was shorter in the experimental group (8.8 vs 19.3 hr $P<0.001$). Another study by Gaziano, Garvis, and Levine shows that the women in the study rated medication during labor of less importance than the presence of a labor companion.[11]

Prepared childbirth is variously called *natural childbirth, participant childbirth,* or by the particular program's founder as with Lamaze and Bradley. Early in the movement in the United States, prepared childbirth earned a bad name through publicity about its more overzealous advocates. "Painless childbirth" was held up as a goal by some extremist groups, and the woman who did experience pain and resorted to pain medication during labor was made to feel a failure. This can be extremely destructive to the woman's self-concept at a time when she needs positive reinforcement in her abilities to achieve and perform competently. Fortunately, current thinking recognizes the variability in individual responses to stress and the differing character of individual labors and teaches that pain medication used judiciously may enhance the woman's ability to use relaxation techniques, thus helping her to cope better with labor and to achieve a satisfying outcome.

For some years many obstetricians and labor room nurses resisted prepared childbirth. Couples who had been trained in a particular method often had to buck staff pressures in their attempt to use the relaxation techniques they had learned. Medication was at times forced upon the laboring woman because the physician felt it would be best for her, even when she protested that it was not necessary. Such practices as laboring in a semi-upright position instead of lying flat, having ice chips or sips of water, eliminating the perineal shave, holding and putting the baby to breast immediately after delivery, and constant presence of the father throughout labor and delivery caused much staff consternation and were often vetoed.

Although prepared childbirth advocates had long been reporting the increased satisfaction the couple experienced and the reduction of depressed babies when these methods were used, it took economic consumer pressure to bring about widespread acceptance of prepared childbirth. When childbearing couples began avoiding physicians and hospitals because they were not allowed to practice their method, the recalcitrants began to see the benefits of involvement and participation of the parents.

Because prepared childbirth classes differ, it is important that couples are aware of how to shop around for a teacher and class that suits their particular needs. (See Variables to Consider in Selecting a Childbirth Class.)

Lamaze or Psychoprophylactic Method. The *psychoprophylactic* method (PPM), or *Lamaze method*, is the most widely used prepared childbirth method in the United States today. It was first propounded by two Russian doctors, Nicolaiev and Velvovsky. The rationale of the program was based on Pavlov's concept of pain perception and his theory of conditioned reflexes (*i.e.,* the substitution of favorable conditioned reflexes for unfavorable ones).

The theory intrigued a Paris obstetrician, Ferdinand Lamaze, who studied Russian-trained mothers-to-be in a Leningrad clinic. Lamaze returned to France and began to prepare his patients in *psychoprophylaxis,* or *mental prevention* of pain in childbirth. He gradually introduced certain adaptations, the most important of which was the rapid shallow breathing which came to characterize the Lamaze method.

As the technique spread throughout Europe and Latin America the *Lamaze method* and psychoprophylaxis became synonymous. The late Marjorie Karmel was perhaps the most responsible for introducing this technique to America. There are now programs in psychoprophylaxis throughout this country. Many are under the auspices of the American Society for Psychoprophylaxis in Obstetrics, Inc.

Variables to Consider in Selecting a Childbirth Class

1. Professional credentials of instructor and type of training as a Childbirth Educator
2. Class size
   a. Eight couples or less—ideal for group interaction and supervised practice
   b. More than 12 couples—limited group interaction, limited supervised practice and decreased relaxation skills mastered by couple
3. Location of class
   a. Home—usually limits class size, informal, relaxed atmosphere
   b. Office, school, church, or hospital—class size may escalate and atmosphere may be less than ideal
4. Total hours of class time for the fee
5. Amount of supervised practice time per session
6. Fee payment by couple
   a. Directly to instructor—instructor accountable to consumer
   b. To group or sponsoring health facility—instructor accountable to agency

(ASPO), which was founded through joint efforts of Mrs. Karmel and a physical therapist, Elizabeth Bing, and others.

In general, the teaching in the program consists of combating the fears associated with pregnancy and childbirth by instructing the pregnant woman and her labor partner in the anatomy and the neuromuscular activity of the reproductive system and the mechanism of labor (Fig. 19-2). The underlying theory of these programs remains firmly based on the neurophysiology of cortical excitation and conditioned response. That is, the woman is taught to replace responses of restlessness and loss of control with more useful activity. Its usefulness lies in the fact that a high level of activity can excite the cerebral cortex sufficiently to inhibit other stimuli, in this case, the pain usually associated with labor. The responses also allow the woman to see herself as someone who is able to cope, which reinforces the probability of continued coping behavior (Fig. 19-3).

In some programs nutrition and general hygiene are included. Exercises which strengthen the abdominal muscles and relax the perineum are taught, and breathing techniques to help the process of labor are

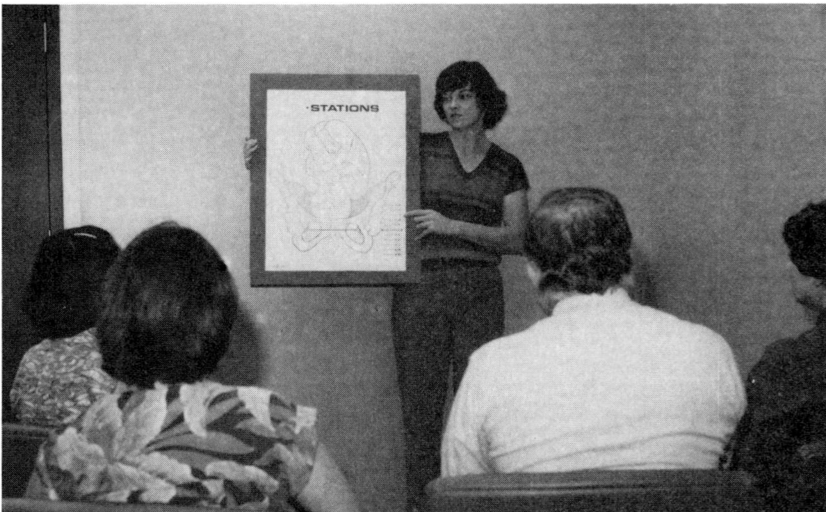

Figure 19-2.
Childbirth educator discussing labor process.

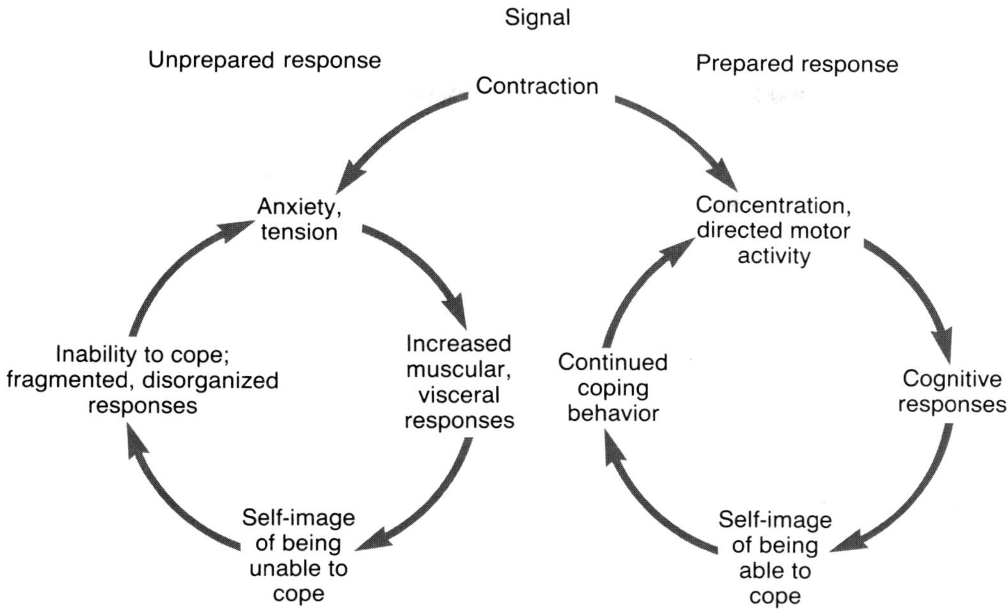

Figure 19-3.
The continuum of responses in the prepared and unprepared woman. (Redrawn from Hassid P: Textbook for Childbirth Educators. Hagerstown, MD, Harper & Row, 1978)

practiced (Fig. 19-4). Thus, the mother is conditioned to respond with respiratory activity and dissociation (or relaxation) of the uninvolved muscles. She then controls her perception of the stimuli associated with labor.

Several changes have occurred in the Lamaze method as a result of experiences gained over many years of use. Class content, flexible breathing techniques, theories of learning and motivation, and emphasis on the childbirth team constitute the major changes. Class content originally dealt mostly with exercises, relaxation, breathing techniques, and the normal labor and delivery experience. Childbirth educators have added information on such subjects as prenatal nutrition, infant feeding, cesarean birth, and other variations from usual labor, as well as discussions concerning sexuality, early parenting, and coping skills for the postpartum period.

The breathing technique has been modified to a moderate shallow breathing rather than rapid panting. Shallow effortless breathing, moderate in pace and high in the chest, is often taught in combination with the slower chest breathing to be used as labor intensifies when slow chest breathing is no longer effective by itself. Using this combined pattern, the woman begins her contraction with slow chest breathing, switches to shallow chest breathing for the peak of the contraction, and returns to slow chest breathing as the contraction declines. The shallow breathing itself has several variations. An acceleration-deceleration pattern or a pant-blow pattern may be used as transition nears. In the second stage of labor, the woman may assume any comfortable physiologic position (a 35° semisitting position, squatting, or side-lying, as in Fig. 19-4C). Pushing then may take one of two forms. The woman will take two deep breaths, hold her breath, relax the perineum (slightly bulge) and push out through the vagina. Grunting noises may accompany this effort and indicate the woman is responding to the physiological need to release air. Using the other method, the woman will take two deep breaths, relax the perineum and push out through the vagina while exhaling slowly through her mouth.[12]

This pushing effort is repeated throughout the contraction, timed, and coached by the partner. (For more specific techniques see Chap. 24, Table 24-2). Caldeyro–Barcia[13] found that when women *hold their breath* for pushing, bearing-down efforts which last more than 5 seconds resulted in late decelerations of the fetal heart rate and marked falls in the maternal systolic and diastolic blood pressures. He suggests that if the woman is not urged to bear down long and hard, which often occurs with the "cheering section" approach to pushing, her *spontaneous* efforts are usually within physiological limits—five seconds to six seconds long—and fetal acidosis is avoided.

Lamaze has progressed to a more individualized

approach of learning and motivation. The original psychoprophylactic training was rather rigid, with goals set by the teacher. Now, the couple sets its own goals for labor and delivery, and the teacher assists the couple in learning ways in which these goals can be realized. This approach removes any set criterion for the success of the labor experience, avoiding the disappointment of externally imposed goals which may be unrealistic for the particular couple.

Greater emphasis is also given to the childbirth team, in which the couple, obstetrician, nurse, and Lamaze teacher work together toward a satisfying labor experience. Rather than anticipating a thwarting of their goals, the couple is encouraged to discuss their goals with their physician so he or she can understand what they hope to do. They also gain appreciation of some of the physician's responsibilities and alternate plans, should labor not progress normally. Figure 19-5 can help couples plan their birth with their physician.

Labor room nurses tend to be better informed about methods of prepared childbirth and more committed to helping couples achieve their goals. Discussion of these goals with the nurses early in labor helps them understand and work more effectively with the couple.

Other Childbirth Methods. Several other approaches to prepared childbirth are used throughout the country, some of which are popular in specific geographic regions or even specific areas of a particular city. The *Bradley method,* also called husband-coached childbirth, emphasizes slow, deep breathing along with complete deep relaxation. The Academy of Husband-Coached Childbirth is the organization that trains teachers to conduct classes in the Bradley method.

The *Wright method* is based on psychoprophylaxis but uses less active breathing than is taught in the Lamaze method. The breathing "levels" become more complex as labor progresses. This method is also referred to as the *new childbirth.*

The *psychosexual method* of Shelia Kitzinger is not based on psychoprophylaxis but on a method using sensory memory as an aid to understanding and working with the body in preparation for birth. Included also is the Stanislavsky method of acting as a basis for teaching relaxation. Kitzinger advocates chest breathing but teaches release of the abdomen at the same time. Her method is called the psychosexual method because she saw sexuality as part of the larger whole encompassing family relationships, birth, cuddling, and feeding.[14]

Yoga, although not a method of prepared childbirth, has been used by numerous women in labor, sometimes in combination with other specific methods of childbirth preparation. Yoga teachings include relaxation, concentration, and a combination of abdominal and chest breathing called "complete breathing." It is not unusual to see childbirth educators teaching different techniques from several methods in an eclectic or "holistic" preparation for childbirth.

Although these programs may derive from different theories and vary in specific techniques, they have

A

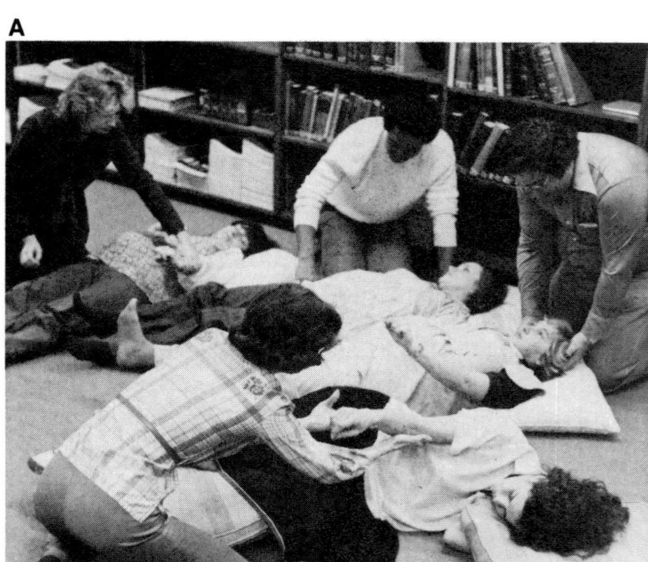

Figure 19-4.
(A) Couples practicing muscle relaxation for labor. *(B)* Couples practicing different positions and breathing for labor. *(C)* Couples practicing various positions for pushing—leg holding, squatting, relaxing legs, and lying on side.

many points in common including the following basic beliefs:

1. Fear enhances the perception of pain but may diminish or disappear when the parturient knows about the physiology of labor;
2. Psychic tension enhances the perception of pain, but the parturient may relax more easily if childbirth takes place in a calm and agreeable atmosphere and if good human contacts have been established between her and the personnel attending her;
3. Muscular relaxation and a specific type of breathing diminish the pain of labor.

Another reason for teaching correct breathing techniques is to avoid hyperventilation during labor. Nurses are often concerned about hyperventilation during labor when prepared childbirth breathing techniques are used. Undue fatigue, hyperventilation, and subsequent carpopedal spasm have been observed when breathing techniques are improperly used. Maternal respiratory alkalosis and a paradoxical acidosis in the fetus are also possibilities if hyperventilation is prolonged.

Hyperventilation can occur in any labor when the woman breathes improperly. Correct use of prepared childbirth breathing techniques can help prevent hyperventilation from occurring, which is another benefit of these programs.

Hypnosis

This technique is to induce a state of extreme suggestibility in which the patient is insensible to outside impressions, except the suggestion of her attendant. There is no particular "program" associated with the use of this technique; rather, training in achieving a hypnotic state or autohypnosis is usually given by an obstetrician who is especially trained in this area. Although there is no general regimen for learning this technique, the conditioning required is usually presented in several individual sessions at the time of the antepartal visits, usually in the latter half of pregnancy.

The modus operandi of hypnotically induced relaxation has been explained by suggesting that whenever all the voluntary muscles are completely relaxed during labor, the uterus has a monopoly on available energy and hence can work more efficiently. In addition, it is likely that when fears are abolished or diminished, efficient uterine action is promoted. The use of comfort measures, such as low back massage, has also been suggested as enhancing the hypnotic state. The major drawback to this technique lies in the difficulty of securing adequately prepared physicians.

Guide for Preparing Parents for Childbirth and the Puerperium

Whether or not the maternity nurse is involved in offering classes for parents or group preparation, it is important that education for childbirth and the puerperium be part of the professional repertoire. This information can be used for individual teaching or for

B

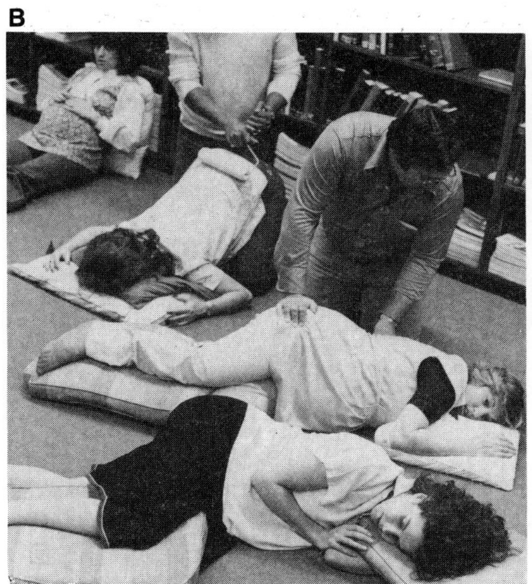

C

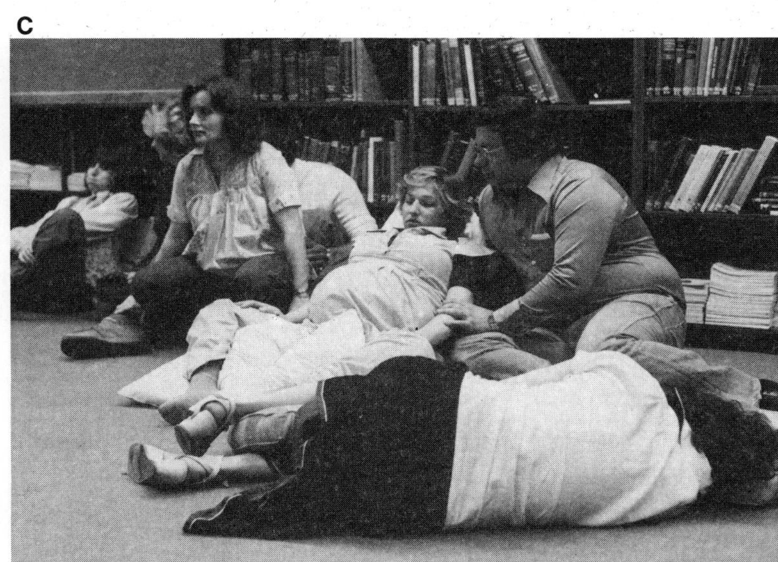

Choices in Childbirth

The two lists below do not represent an "Either-Or" situation. Most parents choose their options from both pathways. Very few doctors or midwives practice completely in accordance with either pathway. Consider and discuss each option and then decide which you prefer. Flexibility is necessary to ensure that the Birth Plan will apply in difficult or complicated labors as well as normal and typical labors.

(Which of these are routines and which are options in your hospital or birth center? Most parents choose some options from each list.)

	Medical Pathway	Physiologic Pathway
Labor	■ Mother in wheelchair upon arrival at hospital. ■ Shave, minishave, or clipping of long hairs on perineum. ■ Enema. ■ Partner is asked to leave during prep and exams. ■ Limit to one support person during labor and birth. ■ Confinement to bed and/or one position. ■ Induction of labor. Methods: Stripping membranes, amniotomy, oxytocin. ■ IV fluids for hydration and energy. ■ Frequent vaginal exams. ■ Electronic Fetal Heart Monitor. ■ Pain Relief through medication: analgesics or anesthetics.	■ Mother walks to labor & delivery. ■ No shave or clipping of hair. ■ Bowels emptied spontaneously, or enema self-administered at home. ■ Partner present throughout labor & delivery. ■ Presence of other friends, relatives, & siblings. ■ Freedom to walk and change positions as desired. ■ Spontaneous Labor. Alternatives: Making love, breast stimulation. ■ Drinking fluid or eating as desired. ■ Vaginal exams when requested by mother or for medical reasons. ■ Listening to fetal heart with fetal stethoscope. ■ Relaxation, emotional support, massage, breathing.
Birth	■ Lithotomy position or semi-sitting in labor bed for pushing. ■ Prolonged breathholding and bearing down for expulsion. ■ Limit of two hours on 2nd stage—then forceps or cesarean birth. ■ Delivery table for birth. ■ Lithotomy position with stirrups for birth. ■ Mother not allowed to touch sterile field. ■ Catheterization in second stage. ■ Episiotomy. ■ Forceps or vacuum extraction.	■ Choice of position and freedom to move. ■ Mother follows her urge to push. ■ Allow for longer 2nd stage and position variations to help progress. ■ Birth in labor bed, birth chair, or bean bag. ■ Sidelying, all fours, squatting, standing with leg up, semi-reclining with back support, no stirrups. ■ Mother allowed to touch baby's head as it crowns. ■ No catheterization and frequent voiding in first stage. ■ No episiotomy: massage, warm compresses, slower delivery, coaching to pant out baby, support to perineum. Late episiotomy with no anesthesic. ■ Spontaneous delivery.
After Birth	■ Intubation/Suctioning. ■ Immediate care of baby done out of sight of mother: e.g., identification, Apgar, heat lamp, replace hemostat with cord clamp. ■ Limit of 15-20 minutes on 3rd stage followed by manual extraction of the placenta. ■ Pitocin drip or injection for contraction of uterus after placenta is born.	■ Waiting to see if baby can handle own mucus. ■ Care done on mother's abdomen. Baby skin to skin with mother with heat lamp or blanket over them. Delay in non-essential routines. ■ Allow for longer time for placenta. Allow mother to move around, nurse baby. Let cord drain. ■ Evaluation of uterus before using uterine stimulant routinely. Breastfeeding.
Baby	■ Baby to isolette or nursery for 4-24 hours. Mother to recovery room for observation. ■ Eye drops–silver nitrate applied shortly after birth. ■ Baby's first feeding—glucose water by nurse. ■ Baby in Nursery except for scheduled 4 hour feedings. ■ Circumcision. ■ Home in 3 or more days after delivery.	■ Baby held by mother or father on delivery table and/or in recovery. ■ Omit eye drops or delay administration up to 2 hours. Use of other agent as alternative. ■ Colostrum by mother who plans to breastfeed or plain water given by mother. ■ Demand feeding, baby to mother when crying. Twenty-four hour rooming in. ■ No circumcision. Parents present to comfort baby after operation. ■ Early discharge from hospital.

■ The Unexpected ■

	Common Medical Procedures	Possible Options
Cesarean Birth	■ Scheduled surgery. ■ Mother without her support person in surgery. ■ General anesthesia. ■ Screen to prevent viewing surgery. ■ Mother not allowed to wear contacts or glasses. ■ Baby sent to Intensive Care Nursery.	■ Surgery after labor begins. ■ Father present to support mother. ■ Spinal or epidural. ■ Screen lowered at time of birth or baby held up for mother and father to see. ■ Mother to wear contacts or glasses. ■ Father to hold baby and mother to see baby, if baby is not in distress. Mother allowed to breastfeed in recovery if her and her baby's condition permits.
Premature/Sick Infant	■ Baby cared for by professionals. ■ Baby rushed to intensive care. ■ Baby sent to another hospital or another part of hospital. ■ Baby transported to hospital with intensive care unit. ■ Limited visits to baby from mother only. ■ IV and bottle feeding.	■ Parents involved in care of baby, diapering, touching, talking to baby in incubator, feeding baby. ■ Mother allowed to hold and see baby, if not distressed. ■ Baby close to mother in same part of hospital. ■ Father goes with the transport team, mother goes if she is able. ■ Father and/or extended family allowed to see baby. ■ Mother allowed to express her colostrum for the baby and encouraged and helped to get started at breastfeeding.

Figure 19-5.
Birth plan (Simpkin P, Reinke C: Planning your baby's birth. Seattle, The Pennypress, 1980)

reinforcing what has been learned from other sources. The guide for preparing parents presented here aims at helping the woman to manage her body well in activity and rest, to use her natural resources effectively during labor, and to achieve optimal postpartal restoration. Including the father in this instruction will assist him to understand his partner's needs during the childbearing process and offer support.*

There are great similarities between the Maternity Centers' breathing techniques and those used in other prepared childbirth methods; therefore, we present these breathing techniques as a general guide. The nurse must be aware, however, that this may vary somewhat in different parts of the country.

*The illustrative material and much of the information in the following section were provided through the courtesy of the Maternity Center Association, based upon their publication *Preparation for Childbearing,* ed. 4, New York, 1977.

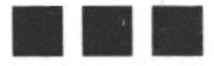

Comfort During Pregnancy

The majority of women can maintain their usual work and play activities during pregnancy. However, since changes do occur in weight and weight distribution, comfort in pregnancy can be significantly improved by good posture and body mechanics in everyday activities. It is often possible to reduce or overcome discomfort by correct positions, body movements, and exercises (Table 19-1). Since the major postural changes begin in the second trimester of pregnancy, this is the logical time for learning. Correct posture for standing, sitting, and stair climbing, and good body mechanics for carrying packages or lifting objects must be reinforced. The spinal muscles and joints should be protected from undue strain; thus the woman needs to know how her feet can be used efficiently for balance and for movement. (See chart, Principles for ADL During Pregnancy on page 340.)

(Text continued on page 340)

Table 19-1.
Relief of Common Discomforts that may Occur During Pregnancy

Discomfort	Exercise or Position
Swelling of feet, ankles	Leg elevating
Leaking urine when coughing, laughing	Pelvic floor contraction
Heaviness in pelvis	Knee–chest; pelvic floor contraction
Hemorrhoids and swelling around vagina	Knee–chest; pelvic floor contraction
Low back pain	Knee–chest
Cramps in thighs, buttocks	Knee–chest
Cramps in legs	Leg elevating; calf stretching
Tired legs	Leg elevating; calf stretching
Varicose veins in legs	Leg elevating; calf stretching
Shortness of breath	Good posture; good body mechanics; rib cage lifting; shoulder circling
Low backache	Pelvic rocking; good posture; pushing position; squatting
Middle backache	Pushing position
Upper backache	Shoulder circling; good posture
Numbness in arms and fingers	Shoulder circling; lying on side
Abdominal muscle spasm (stitch)	Pelvic rocking; deep abdominal breathing

PE Breathing Techniques

Complete Breath and Breath Control

A complete breath is one in which the chest wall expands and the diaphragm descends to its maximum extent. The breath is let out slowly under pressure so that a more complete exchange of oxygen and carbon dioxide can take place. It is used periodically during relaxation and should be followed by slow, quiet, easy respiration (Fig. 19-6).

1. Breathe in once as deeply as possible.
2. Hiss or blow the air out slowly, letting your whole body go limp.
3. Continue breathing quietly, easily, and rhythmically.
4. Let yourself go completely loose.
5. Soon your body will begin to feel very heavy and any exertion will be difficult.
   a. Gradually bend an elbow, bringing your hand toward your chin. Notice the effort.
   b. Slowly lower your arm to its resting position. Again you will find yourself actually working to prevent it from falling too quickly.

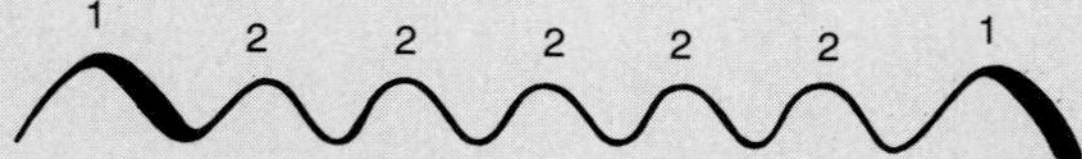

Figure 19-6.
Diagrammatic breath pattern. Complete breath and breath control. 1 = complete breath; 2 = slow rhythmic breathing.

The First Stage of Labor—Deep Breathing

1. Pretend that you are having a contraction that lasts 30 seconds to 45 seconds.
2. At the beginning of each contraction take a complete breath and hiss or blow it out.
3. Breathe deeply, slowly, and rhythmically throughout the remainder of the contraction.
4. When the contraction has ended, take another complete breath and hiss or blow it out slowly.
5. Breathe normally between contractions.
6. During labor, continue to use this pattern of breathing with contractions as long as it is helpful (Fig. 19-7).

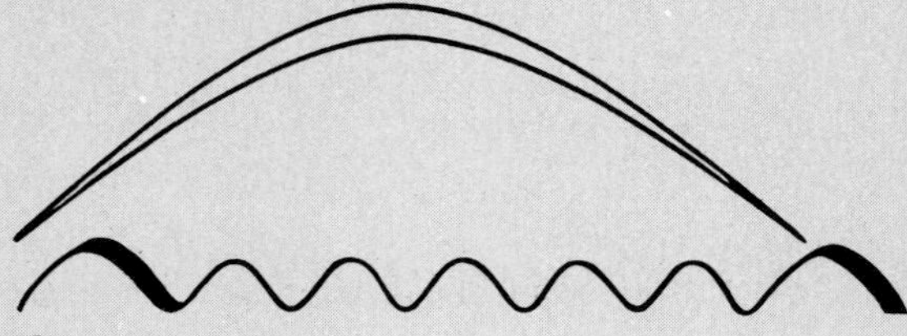

Figure 19-7.
Application of complete breathing to labor.

Modified Deep Breathing During Transition

As labor advances and contractions increase in strength, you often have a desire to keep the diaphragm as still as possible. Yet the uterus continues to need a good supply of oxygen. For this reason you should breathe deeply as the contraction begins and ends, and modify your breathing so that it is quiet and shallow at the peak of each contraction. To practice this do the following:

1. Pretend that you are having stronger contractions, lasting almost a minute.
2. Breathe in deeply as the contraction starts. Then slowly hiss or blow out, letting yourself go completely limp.
3. Make each of the next four or five breaths a little shallower than the previous one. You will notice that you are breathing very lightly.
4. Light breathing is quiet and effortless, almost like a throat breath. Experiment to find your own comfortable rate and continue for 15 seconds to 45 seconds. If you become dizzy or lightheaded, your breathing is too vigorous. If you have trouble getting enough air or difficulty maintaining the rhythm, try taking a quick, deep breath, and return to light breathing.
5. After the contraction has begun to subside, make each of the next four or five breaths a little deeper than the previous one.
6. End the breath pattern with one complete breath (Fig. 19-8).

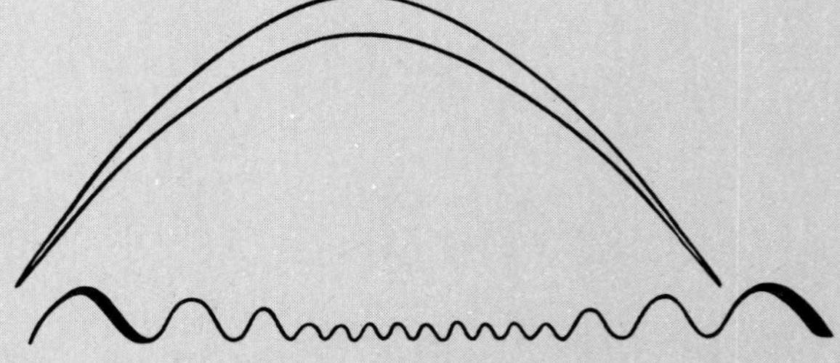

Figure 19-8. Modified complete breathing.

Further Adaptation for Transition

For the latter part of the first stage of labor (if you feel a tendency to hold your breath or to push during

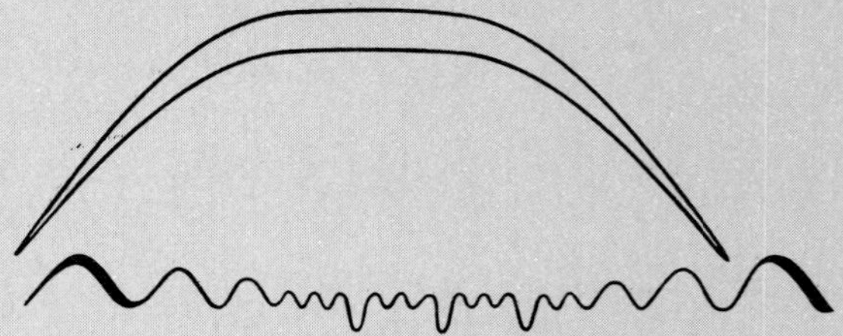

Figure 19-9. Modified complete breathing with adaptation for transition.

strong contractions) do the modified complete breath, but with the following important change:

1. During light breathing, puff out gently as you exhale on every third or fourth breath (Fig. 19-9).

The Second Stage—Pushing*

During the second stage of labor, you will find that pushing helps in the delivery of the baby. Contractions at this time last 60 seconds to 65 seconds and generally are accompanied by a strong urge to push. (However, if regional anesthesia is used, the pushing sensation diminishes.) To practice for this see Figure 19-10.

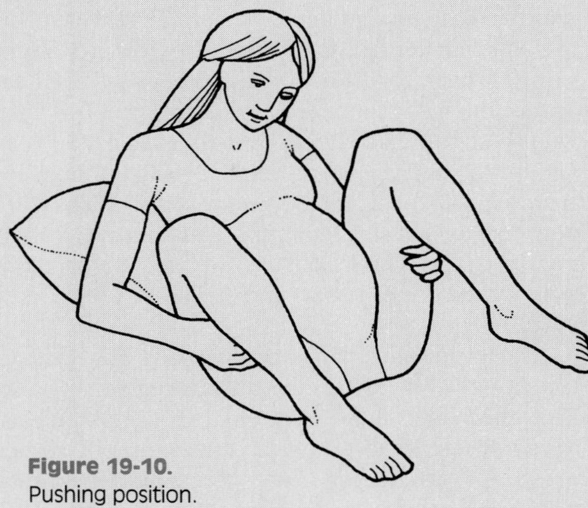

Figure 19-10.
Pushing position.

1. Lie on your back with head and shoulders elevated. Pillows may be used for practice at home. In the labor room the head of the bed should be elevated.
2. Bend your knees and separate your legs.
3. Take a deep breath and hiss or blow out.
4. Breathe in as quickly and deeply as you can; then hold your breath. (In labor, this "held" breath will help to fix your diaphragm so that your abdominal wall will make more effective downward pressure on the uterus and baby, aiding the baby's birth.)
5. Draw up your legs against your abdomen, in a squatting position, holding your thighs, ankles, or feet with your hands. If a delivery table is used, your feet and legs will be supported in stirrups so that you won't have to hold them, and there will be handles on which to pull. Raise head.
6. During practice, do *not* actually push. You will be able to do so in labor.
7. Take *catch breaths,* short breaths that may be taken whenever you can no longer hold your breath comfortably, as needed. Try to take no more than two or three catch breaths in each 60- to 65-second breath pattern (Fig. 19-11).
   a. Maintain the pushing position.
   b. Exhale, moving your head back.
   c. Take in a quick, deep breath.
   d. Tilt your head forward again and hold your breath.
8. When the contraction is over, relax completely, take a deep breath and sigh it out.

*For variations in positions and method see figure 19-4C and page 335.

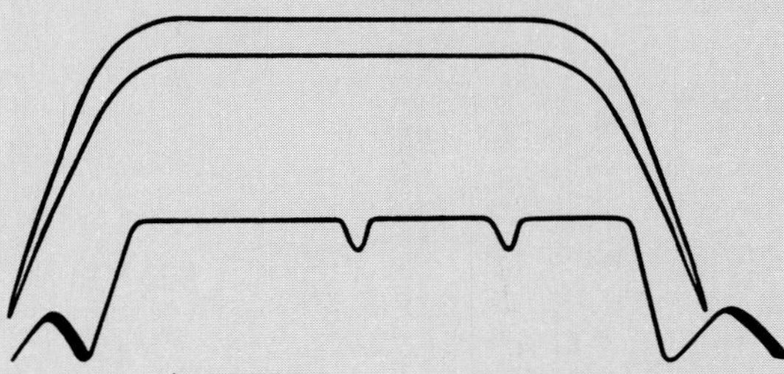

Figure 19-11.
Catch breath. (You may wish to practice breath holding and catch breaths without assuming the pushing position. You may do this while sitting in a chair by following the instructions relating to breathing described above.)

Panting

Your physician may tell you to pant or to stop pushing in the middle of a contraction. If so, begin panting immediately. This will make your diaphragm move up and down. Although this will not decrease the desire to push, it will physically prevent you from doing so. Forceful blowing will also accomplish the same purpose. To practice panting do the following:

1. Start doing the exercise described in the section on The Second Stage—Pushing.
2. All at once, raise your head and shoulders, allowing your arms and hands to relax.
3. Breathe in and out very quickly, keeping your mouth open like a panting dog.
4. Continue breathing this way until the contraction ends (Fig. 19-12).

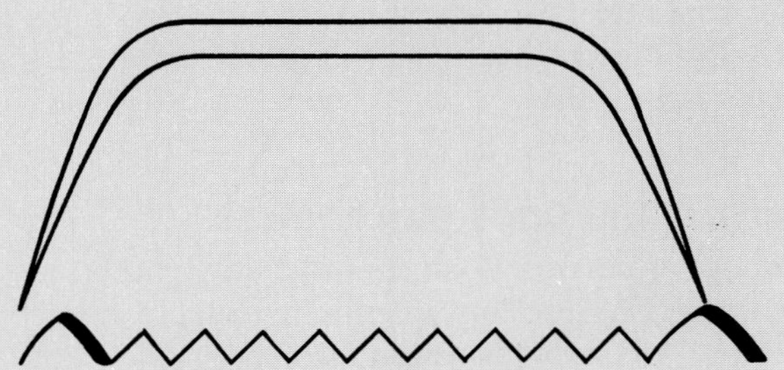

Figure 19-12.
Diagrammatic breath pattern for panting.

Principles for ADL During Pregnancy

1. Activities need to be varied (walking, standing, sitting).
2. Time period should be of short duration.
3. Walking back and forth is preferable to standing still.
4. Standing posture should be with one leg forward so that weight can be shifted easily and efficiently from foot to foot and the body turned comfortably.
5. Walking posture should be head erect, back upright, and chin up and pelvis tilted.
6. Use a footstool when sitting.
7. When climbing stairs, the entire foot should be placed on stair and leg muscles used to lift self up each step without leaning forward.
8. Stooping and lifting should be avoided; if stooping is necessary, it is best to squat down and reach and lift, with feet wide apart and back straight. The alternate squatting position, with one foot placed forward, may also be used. The body is lowered slowly to the other knee. The front foot, which should be flat on the floor, will be used for lifting. The rear foot, flexed at the toes, will serve for pushing and will act as a balance.
9. When carrying bulky packages (groceries) the load should be divided and carried in two hands. A cart that rolls easily should be used for heavy loads.

(Continued from page 337)

For rest and comfort during pregnancy, the woman can learn the position for lying on her side, on her back, in the side relaxation position, and equally important, how to get up and out of bed without strain.

Backache is one of the most common complaints, and the *pelvic tilt* performed daily will help to relieve abdominal pressure and low back pain during pregnancy and early labor. This exercise is also used to firm the abdominal muscles following the birth of the baby.

Other exercises to promote comfort and give relief from some of the common discomforts of pregnancy include *rib cage lifting, shoulder circling, leg elevating,* and *calf stretching.* (See pages 344–346.)

Posture and Body Mechanics

Maintaining correct posture and practicing good body mechanics are important in avoiding some of the more common discomforts of pregnancy. For example, a frequent cause of backache during pregnancy is poor posture. As pregnancy progresses, body proportion and weight distribution are altered. As the body's center of gravity is gradually shifted forward, the abdominal muscles often relax and the natural curvature of the spine becomes exaggerated, shortening the muscles of the lower back. The woman often compensates for this by leaning backward slightly at the waist, which shifts her weight to her heels when walking. This results in an awkward, waddling gait and frequently contributes to backaches, particularly of the lower back.

It is important to encourage the woman to be constantly mindful of her posture and to provide her with information on correcting her body alignment. (See Posture Checklist.) To help her get the feel of good body alignment it may be helpful to instruct her to stand with her feet about ten inches from a wall and to press her hips, spine, and the back of her head against the wall in an erect position (Fig. 19-13). The woman should take a deep breath, exhale, and relax and try to gain a sense of her body alignment as she stands in this position. Some exercises, such as the pelvic tilt, which strengthen the muscles of the abdomen and lower back, are also helpful in correcting poor posture and relieving backaches. (See Figure 19-18.)

The importance of practicing good body mechanics should also be taught to the pregnant woman. Body mechanics involve the efficient use of the body to evenly distribute weight and stress among several muscle groups rather than overtaxing a particular muscle group with undue strain. For example, pregnant women should be instructed to avoid stooping when lifting or reaching for low objects. Bending forward or stooping may put the woman off balance and will require the muscles of the back to assume the burden of returning the trunk (and any weight that is lifted) to an erect posture. A squatting posture is much preferred when reaching for low objects (Fig. 19-14). The woman should be instructed to squat with the back straight and the body properly aligned. Any weight to be lifted should be pulled close to the body and the muscles of the thighs and legs should be used to raise the body to an erect posture.

Good body mechanics relate directly to good posture. Throughout daily activities, such as household chores, walking, and climbing stairs, the woman should be encouraged to keep the back straight (but not rigid) and the body in proper alignment. Learning to maintain a correct posture and practicing good body mechanics often require a considerable amount of conscious thought and practice at first. It is not unusual for a person who has previously had a poor posture to feel strange or even uncomfortable when her body is in proper alignment. However, it should be emphasized that good posture and body mechanics are beneficial throughout life and, hopefully, the lessons learned during pregnancy will carry over to a more healthful future.

Comfort Positions

Pregnant women often comment that they find it difficult to relax because they are unable to find a comfortable position or that heartburn, backaches, or other common discomforts interfere with their ability to relax. A variety of positions have been found effective in providing comfort and in relieving some of the discomforts of pregnancy.

It should be noted that a position that works effectively for one woman may not necessarily work equally as well for another. For example, some women find the squatting position (see Fig. 19-14) relaxing and effective in relieving backaches while others find a pushing posture (see Fig. 19-10) or some other position or exercise more effective. Women should be encouraged to try a variety of positions until they find what works best for them.

Tailor Sitting

The tailor sitting position is helpful in stretching the muscles of the thighs, hips, and lower back. It is often helpful in relieving lower backache and many women find it relaxing. The woman should sit on the floor with her knees spread as far apart as comfortable, with one leg resting on the floor or chair in front of the other and the back straight (Fig. 19-15). Many women find it more comfortable to assume this position with the back against a wall or some other support. The beginner should remain in this position for about five minutes at a time, gradually increasing to intervals of 15 minutes to 30 minutes. Since this position significantly decreases circulation to the legs and feet, the woman should "shake out" her legs every few minutes and then return to the position. Many women find this a very comfortable position and assume it several times each day for relaxation. They may also find the tailor sitting exercise beneficial in strengthening thigh, hip, and lower back muscles and in providing additional relief from backache (see Fig. 19-15).

It should be noted that the tailor sitting position is not exactly the same as the "indian sitting" position that many people learn as children. In the indian

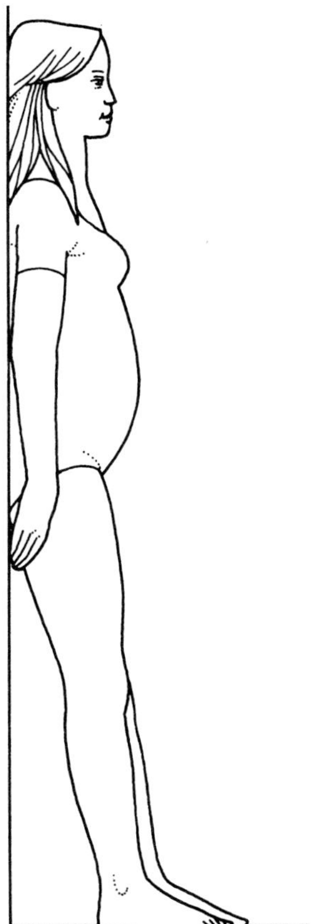

Figure 19-13.
Standing with the hips and back pressed against a wall can help the woman gain a sense of good body alignment.

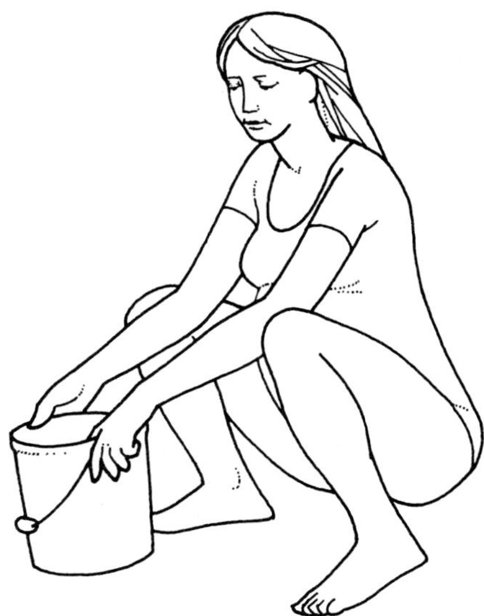

Figure 19-14.
The squatting posture is the preferred method of lifting or reaching for low objects during pregnancy.

Posture Checklist

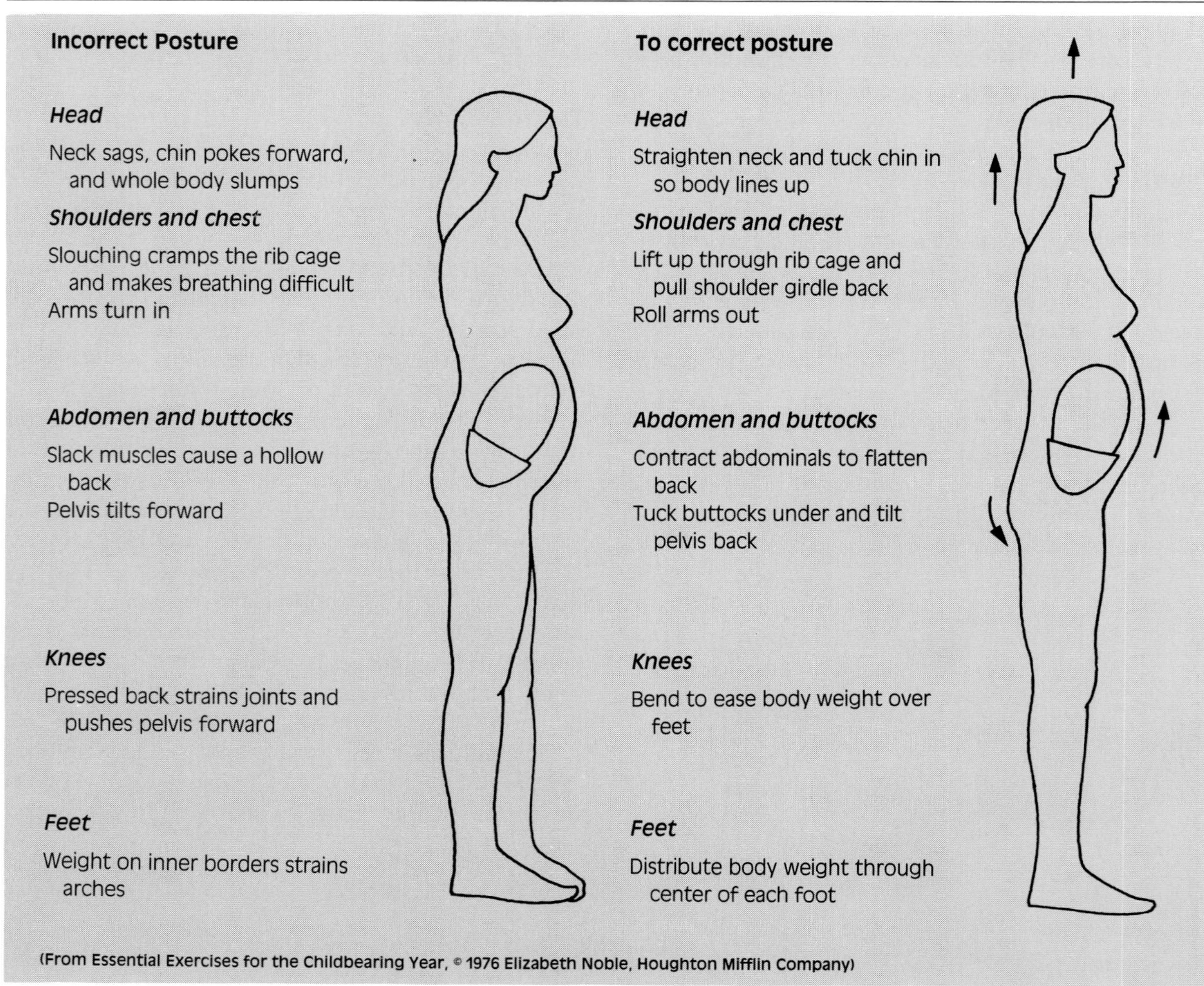

(From Essential Exercises for the Childbearing Year, © 1976 Elizabeth Noble, Houghton Mifflin Company)

sitting position the legs are often crossed with one leg resting on the other. Generally, the comfort positions in pregnancy place the body in good alignment, with no body part resting on any other body part to interfere with circulation.

Leg Elevation

Among the more common discomforts of pregnancy are fatigue, swelling, cramps, and varicosities of the legs. One method of relieving these discomforts and increasing circulation to the legs is to have the woman elevate her legs for two minutes to five minutes several times each day. It is often convenient to have the woman lie supine on her bed or on the floor with her heels resting against a wall (Fig. 19-16). Early in pregnancy, the body and legs can be nearly at a right angle with the buttocks either against the wall or very close to it. However, as pregnancy progresses, the right-angle position may become uncomfortable because of pressure on the diaphragm and the woman may find it more comfortable to move her body slightly away from the wall to reduce the angle. Eventually, she may find it more comfortable to lie with her legs supported by a footstool or chair. Women who experience swelling and varicosities of the vulva should be instructed to elevate both the legs and hips. When rising from the supine position, the woman should be instructed to relax for a few moments after lowering her legs and to rise slowly to avoid dizziness.

Sitting with the legs elevated will also provide some relief of discomfort.

Knee–Chest Position

Another position that has been found effective in relieving lower back pain is the knee–chest position. This position is also helpful in relieving the discom-

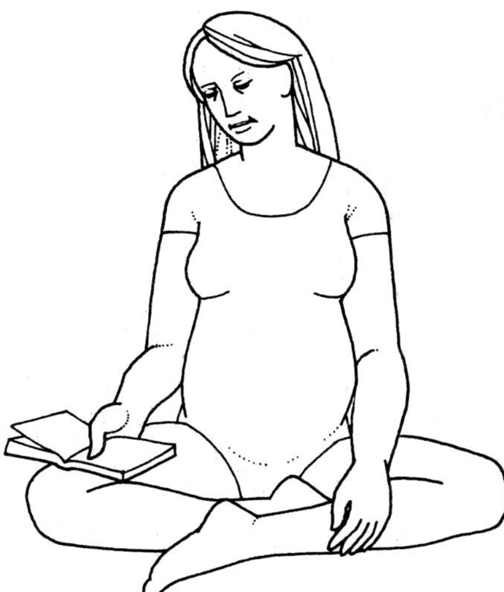

Figure 19-15.
The tailor sitting position is helpful in relieving lower backache.

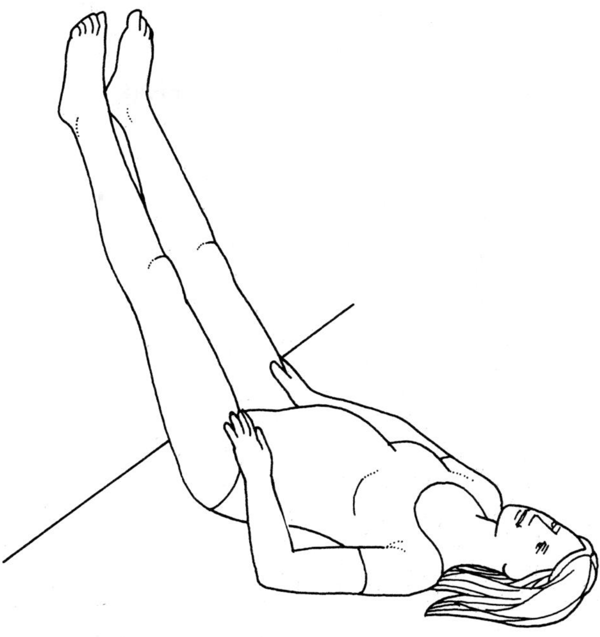

Figure 19-16.
Elevating the legs is helpful in relieving fatigue, swelling, cramps, and varicosities in the legs.

forts of hemorrhoids, swelling around the vagina, cramps in the thighs and buttocks, and heaviness in the pelvis. Instruct the woman to turn on her stomach and raise her body so that her knees and chest are close together (Fig. 19-17). Her chest should be against the floor and her knees should be about a foot apart. She should hold this position for about two minutes.

Exercises

Exercises done during pregnancy increase circulation, improve muscle tone, aid in prevention of fatigue, promote physical comfort, and encourage good posture. Exercises should be done smoothly, avoiding exaggerated or jerky movements. The woman should not do any exercise that causes pain or discomfort. Breathing should be coordinated with exercises, generally exhaling while doing the effort part of the exercise.

Many communities offer special exercise classes for pregnant and postpartum women. A group setting is often helpful because motivation is enhanced.

The following exercises are provided as a general guide for the pregnant woman.

Pelvic Floor Contractions. Pelvic floor exercises are useful in relieving the discomforts of heaviness in the pelvis and the leaking of urine during activity or when coughing or laughing. These exercises strengthen and increase the flexibility of the pelvic floor muscles. They also help the woman develop an awareness of tension and relaxation in the perineal area, which is important during childbirth. Pelvic floor contractions may also be helpful after childbirth to promote healing, provide comfort, and to help regain muscle tone after labor.

Pelvic floor contractions can be performed in a standing, sitting, squatting, or lying position. Instruct the woman to draw up the muscles of the pelvic floor as she would if she were attempting to avoid urinating. She should feel the squeeze as the muscles surrounding the vagina and urethra are tightened. She should hold this tightness for two or three seconds and then relax for a couple of minutes. Next, she should per-

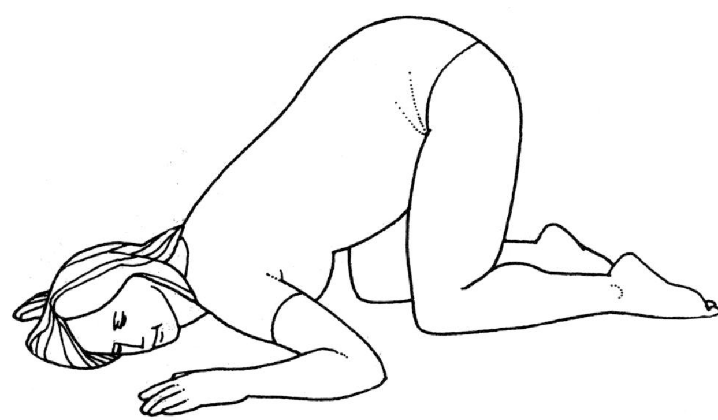

Figure 19-17.
The knee–chest position is helpful in relieving lower backache.

form the same exercise, tightening the muscles around the rectum and, eventually, tightening all of the muscles of the perineum at the same time. She should progress to doing 50 or more pelvic floor contractions each day in a series of five contractions, holding each contraction for five seconds.

Pelvic Tilt. The pelvic tilt is useful in strengthening the muscles of the abdomen and lower back and is also helpful in relieving backache. The pelvic tilt exercise may also be used during labor to relieve backache and to help in rotating the fetal head when the presentation is posterior.

To perform this exercise the woman should be on her hands and knees, with her hands directly under the shoulders and the knees under the hips. Her back should be in a neutral position with the small of the back flattened, *not hollowed*. Her head and neck should be aligned with a straight back and her elbows and knees should remain stationary throughout the exercise. Instruct the woman to pull in the abdominal muscles and buttocks and to press up with her lower back. She should hold this position for a few seconds and then relax to a neutral position (Fig. 19-18). Initially, many women will need assistance in assuming the neutral position and avoiding a sagging or hollow back posture. She should repeat the exercise about five times, maintaining a slow rhythmic motion. The pelvic tilt exercise may also be performed in a standing or supine position.

Calf Stretching. The calf stretching exercise is a particularly effective means of relieving leg cramps. If performed regularly, calf stretching is also helpful in preventing the cramps.

Instruct the woman to stand with her feet slightly apart and her hands on the back of a chair or some other object that will provide secure support. She should slide the heel of her right leg back as far as possible without letting her heel leave the floor. She should then bend the knee of her left leg, lowering herself slightly as she feels the stretching of the calf muscles in her right leg (Fig. 19-19). She should return to her original standing position, relax for a few minutes and repeat the exercise with the opposite leg. The exercise can be repeated several times, using the alternate leg each time. If the woman is performing the exercise to relieve a leg cramp, she may repeat the exercise several times with the affected leg until the cramp is relieved.

Rib Cage Lifting. Rib cage lifting is a useful exercise for increasing the flexibility of the intercostal muscles and for improving general muscle tone. This exercise may also be used to help relieve shortness of breath.

This exercise can be performed in either a standing, sitting, or tailor sitting position. The tailor sitting position is often recommended because performing the exercise in this position also helps to tone the muscles of the hips, thighs, and lower back. Instruct the woman to inhale while extending the right arm with the elbow slightly flexed above her head (Fig. 19-20). With the arm extended, she should then exhale, extending the arm further as she feels the muscles of her right side stretch. She should inhale again, return to the starting position, and repeat the exercise with the left arm. Initially, the exercise can be repeated five times with each arm and gradually increased to ten times.

Shoulder Circling. The shoulder circling exercise is useful in strengthening the muscles of the upper back and may be used to relieve upper backache and numbness in the arms and fingers.

This exercise can be performed in either a stand-

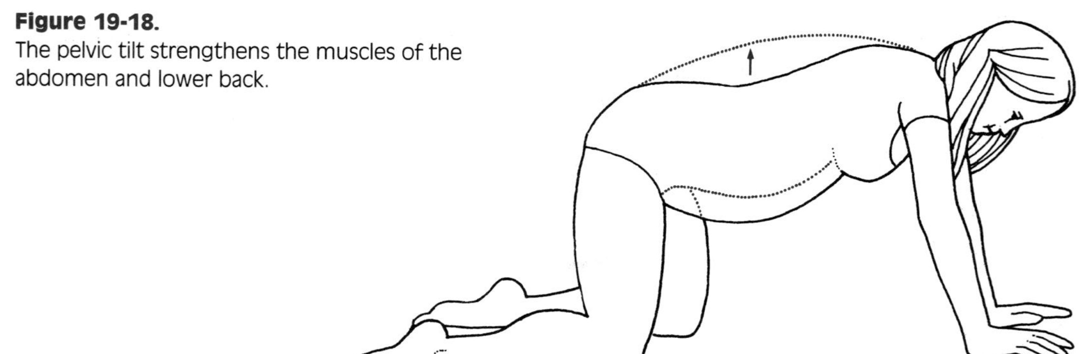

Figure 19-18.
The pelvic tilt strengthens the muscles of the abdomen and lower back.

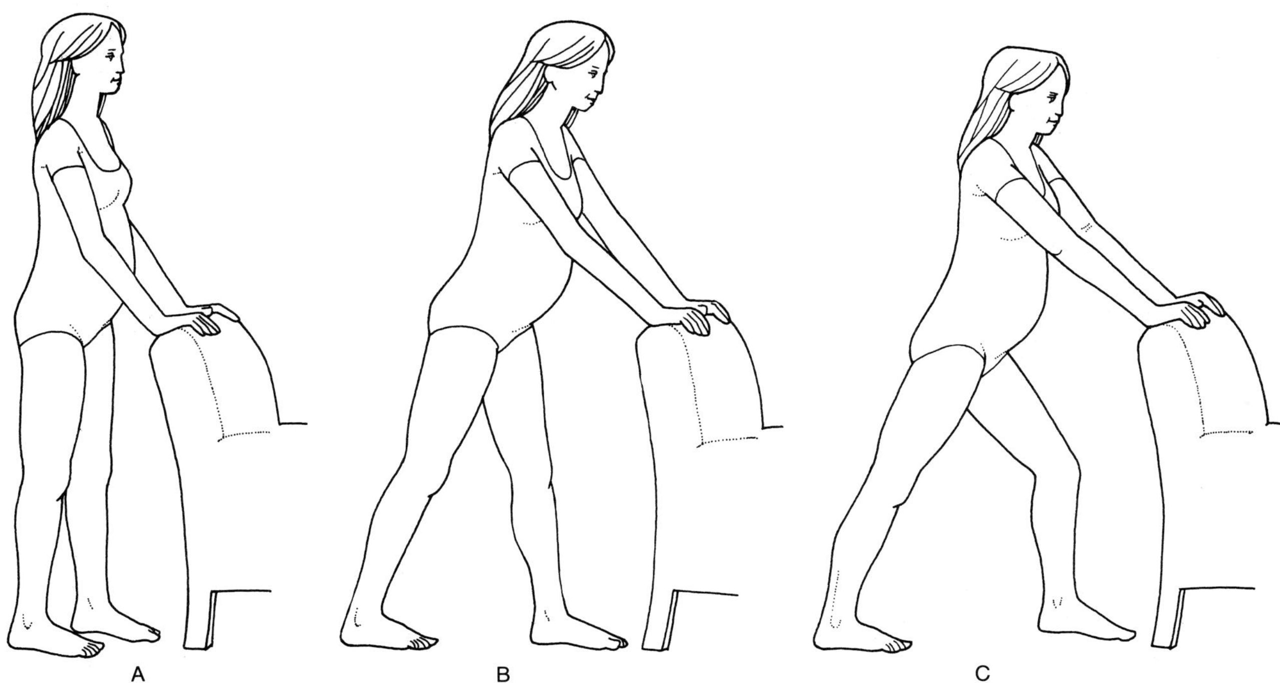

Figure 19-19.
Calf stretching is helpful in relieving lower leg cramps. Performed regularly, it can help to prevent the cramps. *(A)* Stand with your feet slightly apart and your hands on the back of a chair or some other object that offers secure support. *(B)* Slide the foot of the cramped leg as far back as possible, without letting the heel leave the floor. *(C)* Bend the knee of the other leg. Return to first position and relax. Perform several times.

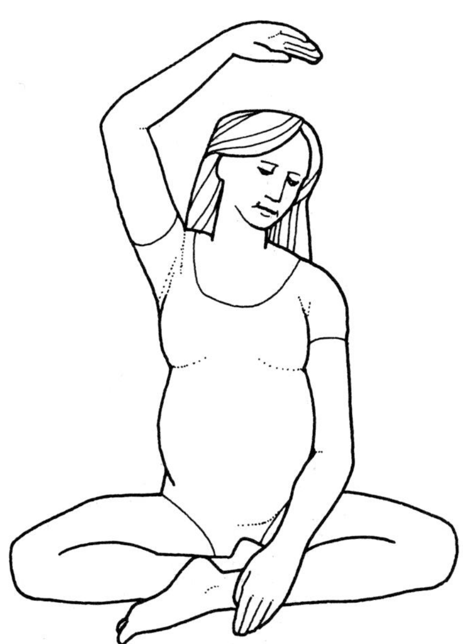

Figure 19-20.
Rib cage lifting can help to relieve shortness of breath.

ing or a sitting position. The woman should be instructed to keep her back, neck, and head straight throughout the exercise and to allow her arms to hang loosely at her sides. She should slowly rotate her shoulders up and back as far as they can comfortably go in a circular motion (Fig. 19-21). She should inhale as the shoulders are rotated and exhale as the circle is completed and the shoulders have returned to the starting position. The exercise can be repeated ten times, relaxing momentarily between each rotation.

Conscious Relaxation

It is also necessary to learn relaxation in pregnancy to prepare for labor and delivery. Controlled relaxation is the foundation of all the childbirth education techniques for labor. Humenick found that prenatal relaxation skill achievement was significantly related to medication used in childbirth.[15] She also found that larger childbirth class size correlated negatively with achievement of relaxation skill for expectant mothers.[16]

Tensing during labor is a natural response to the

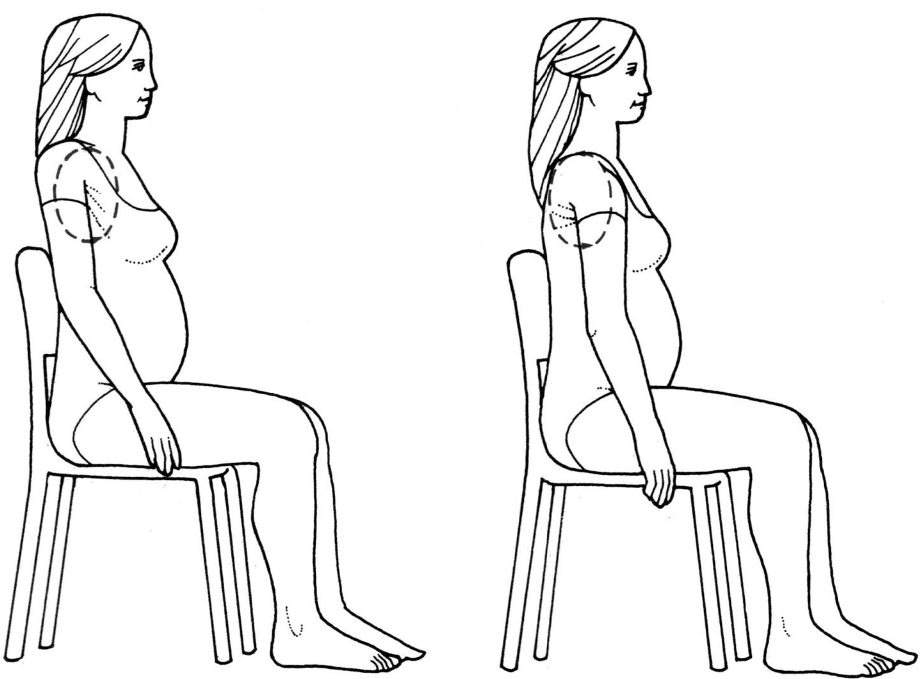

Figure 19-21.
Shoulder circling helps to strengthen the muscles of the upper back and can be used to relieve upper backache.

contracting uterus. Tension, however, causes exhaustion, oxygen depletion, lowers the pain threshold, and prolongs labor. Adrenaline, the hormone that accompanies the fear-tension-pain syndrome, inhibits the effects of oxytocin, which causes the uterus to contract. This interference with oxytocin actually makes the contractions of the uterus less effective and prolongs labor.[17]

The process of learning to relax is an active building of awareness of the state of the muscles, either tensed or relaxed, and a conscious control by the mind of that state. It is a learned activity, a process of isolating muscle groups, differentiating between tenseness and relaxation, and a conscious letting go of or total release of muscle groups. Relaxation is an active involvement of mind over body which requires awareness, concentration, and practice. A woman is taught and conditioned to respond in a given manner, that is, total body relaxation each time she experiences a contraction. Once the method is grasped, the response must be conditioned so that it will be automatically evoked during labor.

Constant practice or repetition of the technique is necessary to maintain a conditioned response of this nature. Continued practice establishes patterns that can be depended on if thought processes become cloudy in active labor. The response will be well ingrained and the body will respond as automatically as possible during labor and birth with this conditioning.

The woman and her labor partner should practice relaxation exercises during the last weeks of pregnancy. During labor, the exercise is not practiced as such but the skill the woman has learned by consciously relaxing her body while other body parts have been tensed will be used. During labor and birth all muscles that can be voluntarily controlled with the brain should be as relaxed as possible so the muscles of the uterus can work undisturbed, at maximum efficiency, and with the least amount of pain.

The skill of relaxation is not only helpful for birth but is a life-long skill that can be called upon during the daily stresses of life (See Preparatory Exercises for Controlled Relaxation and Practice Drill for Controlled Relaxation).

Postpartum Exercises

During the puerperium, the 6 weeks following childbirth, the body undergoes major changes. The organs that had adjusted during pregnancy to make room for the growing baby gradually return to their original positions in the woman's body. The uterus, cervix, and vagina slowly return to the nonpregnant state. Important hormonal changes also occur. In effect, a bodily

PE Preparatory Exercise for Controlled Relaxation*

Verbal cue	Action	Coaching role	Rationale
Take a deep breath and relax	Focus eyes on object, inhale, exhale and consciously release all tension		Begin with complete relaxation
Stretch down both heels	Extend legs, flex ankles, *keep rest of body relaxed*	Tap heels to signal contraction	Isolate tension, beginning with single body area
Relax	Relax both legs	Stroke to signal relaxation; look for relaxation	Associate word "relax" with stroking to signal release of tension
Tighten thighs	Tense both thighs	Tap thighs to signal tension	Isolate area to be tensed
Relax	Relax thighs	Stroke to signal relaxation	Associate verbal and tactile cues
Squeeze buttocks together	Tense gluteal muscles	Tap buttocks, or hips if woman is supine	Isolate area to be tensed
Relax	Relax buttocks	Stroke to signal relaxation	Associate verbal and tactile cues
Stretch arms down	Extend arms and hands fully	Tap hands	Isolate area to be tensed
Relax	Relax tension in hands and arms	Stroke arms	Associate verbal and tactile cue
Shrug your shoulders	Tense shoulders	Tap shoulders	Isolate area to be tensed
Relax	Relax shoulders	Stroke shoulders	Associate verbal and tactile cues
Make a face	Tense face; clench jaw	Tap cheek lightly	Isolate area to be tensed
Relax	Relax face	Stroke face; turn head gently side to side	Associate verbal and tactile cues; detect tension in neck
Take a deep breath and relax completely	Inhale, exhale, and completely relax	Observe for tension; where detected, stroke to signal release	Woman's awareness of feeling of complete relaxation; coach's awareness of the appearance of complete relaxation

*Exercises should be practiced in supine position with head and shoulders well supported by pillows with another pillow (or two) under the knees. (Hassid P: Textbook For Childbirth Educators. Hagerstown, Harper & Row, 1978)

PE Practice Drill for Controlled Relaxation*

Verbal cue	Action	Coaching role	Rationale
Contract right leg	Tense right thigh and calf; flex ankle Focus gaze on one spot to enhance concentration Think about the feeling of tension in the right leg and of relaxation in the rest of the body	Tap right leg; feel muscles for quality of muscle tension Look over rest of body for obvious signs of tension; lift left leg gently under knee to check relaxation; check both arms; turn head gently side to side to check relaxation of neck Where tension is detected, stroke and give cue, "Relax"	Isolate area to be tensed Detect tension and signal its release
Relax right leg	Relax completely	Stroke right leg; lift gently under right knee to detect tension	Detect hidden tension; signal its release; associate verbal and tactile cues
Contract left arm	Make a fist; tense entire arm and lift slightly off the floor Focus gaze on one spot to enhance concentration Think about the feeling of tension in the left arm and of relaxation in the rest of the body	Tap left arm; check for tension Check rest of body for signs of tension; lift right arm gently by hand, swing freely from shoulder; lift knees slightly; observe face; turn head gently side to side to detect neck tension; stroke to signal its release	Isolate area to be tensed Detect tension; signal its release
Relax left arm	Relax completely	Stroke left arm and shoulder Lift left arm gently by hand; swing from shoulder	Signal relaxation with tactile and verbal cues Detect hidden tension
Contract key areas	Tense jaw and perineum Focus gaze on one spot to enhance concentration Think about tension in jaw and perineum; feel relaxation in rest of body	Tap jaw lightly; note tension Check neck, arms and legs for tension; stroke to signal release as necessary	Isolate area to be tensed Awareness of impact of key areas on tension in shoulders, neck, legs, etc.
Relax key areas	Relax completely	Stroke jaw and other body areas to enhance and signal relaxation	With jaw relaxed, whole upper body can relax; with perineum relaxed, whole lower body can relax†

* The emphasis is always upon the relaxation, not on the tensing or on how quickly the woman can respond.

† Continue practice drill using arms, legs, and key areas in random pattern to enhance skills. Always begin and end with preparatory exercise (Table 19-2).

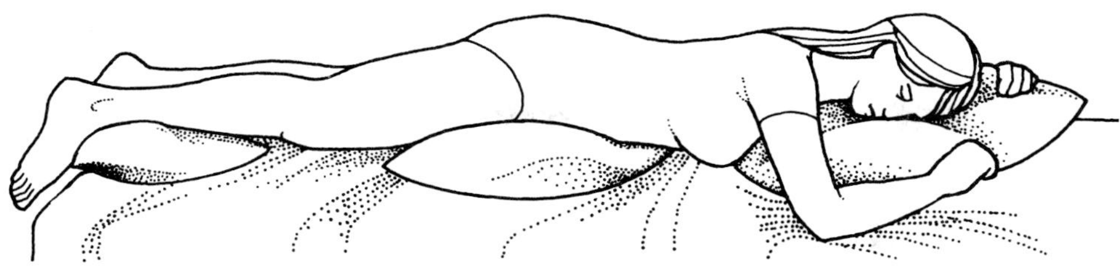

Figure 19-22.
Prone position for rest and relaxation postpartum.

transformation that took nine months to complete is being reversed in the course of a few weeks.

Good nutrition and adequate rest are essential during this period. A new mother needs at least one rest period each day. Lying on the abdomen may help the uterus to return to good position (Fig. 19-22). A pillow under the hips and ankles when she is lying in this position prevents back strain.

Postpartum exercises are important in restoring muscle tone and the woman's figure. Many of the exercises that are used during prepartum are also useful in the postpartal exercise program. In an uncomplicated delivery, simple exercises may be started during the first postpartum day. If the woman had an abnormal delivery or extensive perineal repair, exercises may need to be delayed.

A postpartal exercise program should progress in phases, beginning with simple exercises and progressing to more strenuous ones. When the mother is able to comfortably accomplish the repetitions of one phase, she is ready to progress to the next. Women progress at different rates and the same woman does not progress through all phases at the same rate. For example, the chart on Postpartal Exercises suggests two series of progressive exercises and it is not uncommon for a woman to easily progress through all of the phases of one series, but experience difficulty with one of the exercises in the other series. This should not be a matter of concern. The woman should progress through all exercises at her own pace. As with prepartal exercises, emphasis should be placed on avoiding fatigue and the mother should not do any exercise that causes pain. If the exercises are practiced properly, they should not be tiring. They should be done slowly and rhythmically, only a few times at first, and gradually increased.

The postural reflex needs to be reestablished postpartum so that the woman doesn't continue the stance she had during pregnancy. This means she must consciously contract the abdominal and pelvic floor muscles in order to balance the pelvis again after the sudden loss of its load. Because of the hormones of pregnancy the joints are still at risk for a few weeks and good body mechanics are essential to protect the joints and ligaments. The abdominal muscles are obviously in need of exercise. The goal is to achieve a flat abdomen and good posture, with the pelvis tilted back to realign correctly with the spine.[12] It is not uncommon for the longitudinal muscles (recti) of the abdomen to separate (diastasis) during pregnancy, labor, or delivery (see Fig. 19-23). The gaping can be slight or severe. If these muscles are not corrected,

(Text continues on page 353)

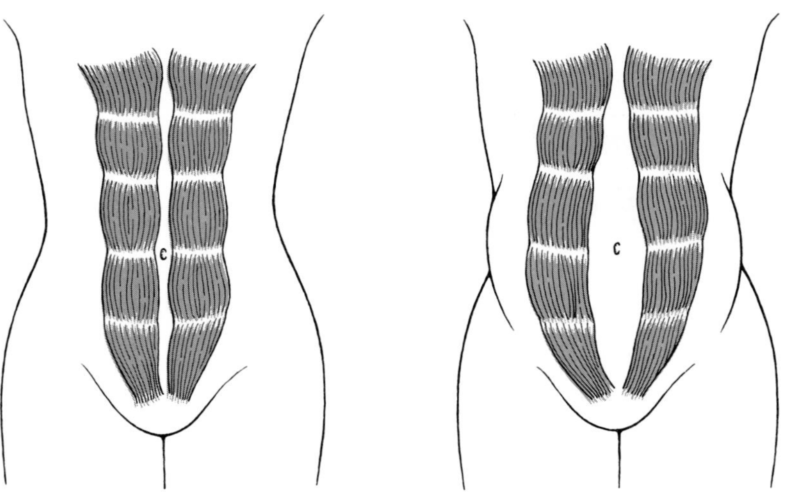

Figure 19-23.
Diastasis recti.

PE Postpartal Exercises

Postpartal exercises should be begun as soon as possible after birth. The exercise program can be presented in phases, beginning with simple exercises and progressing to ones that are more strenuous.

Firming the Abdomen

Phase I.
Abdominal Breathing

1. Lie on back with knees bent.
2. Inhale deeply through the nose, keeping ribs as stationary as possible and allowing the abdomen to expand up.
3. Exhale slowly but forcefully while contracting the abdominal muscles.
4. Hold for about 3 to 5 seconds while exhaling. Relax.
5. Begin with 2 repetitions, gradually progressing to 10.

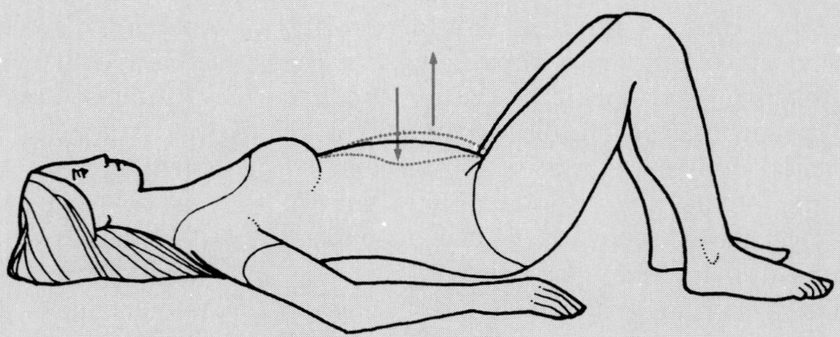

Phase II.
Combined Abdominal Breathing and Supine Pelvic Tilt

1. Lie on back with knees bent.
2. While inhaling deeply, roll pelvis back by flattening the lower back on the floor or bed.
3. While exhaling slowly but forcefully, contract the abdominal muscles and tighten the buttocks.
4. Hold for about 3 to 5 seconds while exhaling. Relax.
5. Begin with two repetitions, gradually progressing to 10.

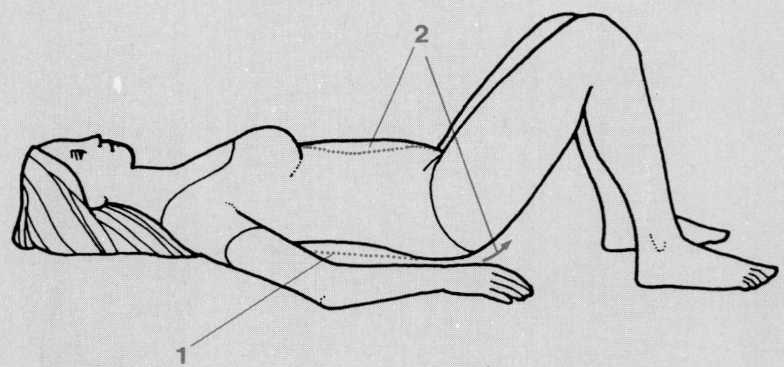

Phase III.
Reach for the Knees

1. Lie on back with knees bent.
2. While inhaling deeply, bring the chin onto the chest.
3. While exhaling, raise the head and shoulders slowly and smoothly, reaching for the knees with outstretched arms. The body should only rise as far as the back will naturally bend while the waist remains on the floor or bed (about 6 to 8 inches).
4. Slowly and smoothly lower head and shoulders to the starting position. Relax.
5. Begin with 2 repetitions, gradually progressing to 10.

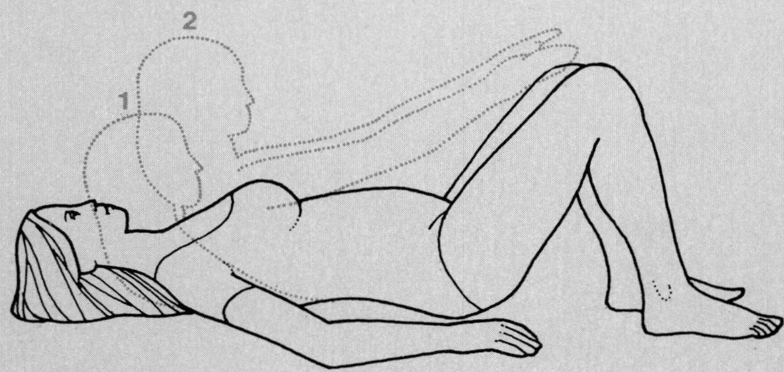

Firming the Waist

Phase I.
Double Knee Roll

1. Lie on back with knees bent.
2. Keeping shoulders flat and the feet stationary, slowly and smoothly roll the knees over to touch the right side of the bed.
3. Maintaining a smooth motion, roll the knees back over to touch the left side of the bed.
4. Return to starting position. Relax.
5. Begin with 2 repetitions, gradually progressing to 10.

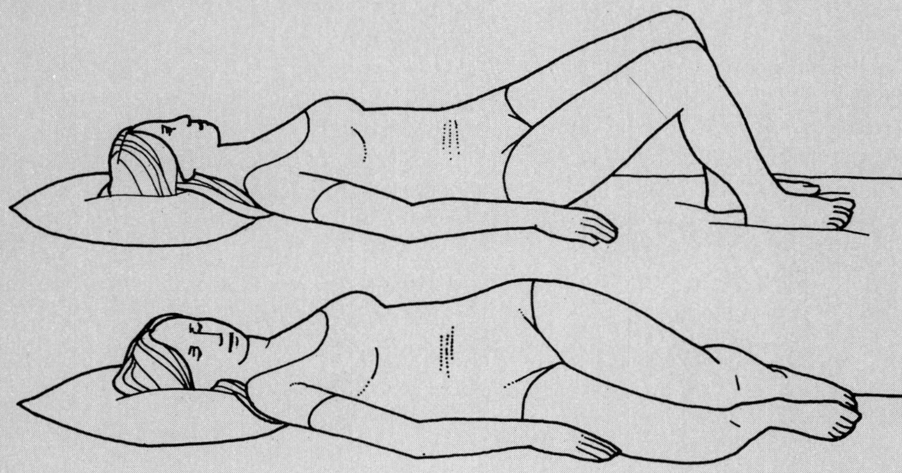

(Continued)

PE Postpartal Exercises (continued)

Phase II.
Single Knee Roll

1. Lie on back, right leg straight, left leg bent at the knee.
2. Keeping the shoulders flat, slowly and smoothly roll the left knee over to touch the right side of the bed and back to starting position.
3. Reverse position of legs, touch left side of the bed with the right knee and return to starting position. Relax.
4. Begin with 2 repetitions, gradually progressing to 10.

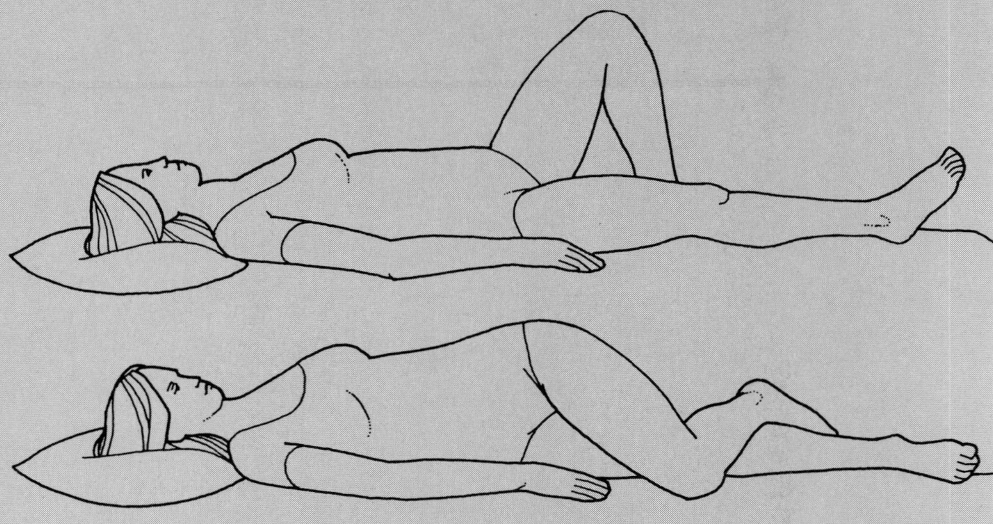

Phase III.
Leg Role

1. Lie on back with legs straight.
2. Keeping shoulders flat, slowly and smoothly lift the left leg and, keeping it straight, roll it over to touch the right side of the bed and return to starting position.
3. Repeat, using the right leg to touch the left side of the bed. Relax.
4. Begin with 2 repetitions, gradually progressing to 10.

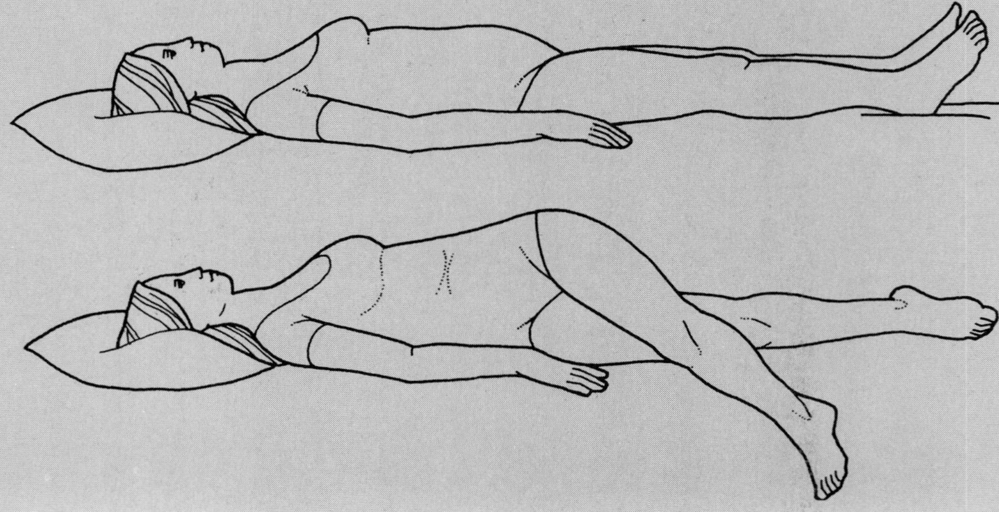

(Continued from page 349)
the abdominal wall will remain weakened and will not be supportive for a subsequent pregnancy. Because the recti muscles are important in controlling the tilt of the pelvis, their weakness can give rise to poor posture and pain in the lower back. A postpartum check of the recti muscles is done about the third day after delivery. Until this time the entire abdominal area feels so slack that the test is not reliable.

The following exercise may be done to see if diastasis has occurred. Lie on back with knees bent. Press the fingers of one hand firmly into the area around the navel. Slowly raise head and shoulders until neck is about 8 inches from the bed. The bands of muscles on each side will pull toward the midline, pushing the fingers out of the way. A slight gap, one or two fingers is just tissue slackness and will tighten by itself. A gap of three, four, or more fingers between the muscles requires a special exercise to restore the integrity of this area.

The following exercise is done to correct diastasis, if it has occurred. This exercise is done by lying on the back with knees bent. Cross hands over the abdominal area to pull the muscles toward the midline as head is raised. Take a deep breath. Raise the head (and later the shoulders to a 45° angle) off the bed while exhaling, and at the same time pull the muscles together. Return slowly to original position. Repeat exercise often and gradually work up to at least 50 times a day. Until the diastasis has closed, the woman should avoid exercises that rotate the trunk, twist the hips, or bend the trunk to one side.[12]

The purpose of the pelvic floor exercise after delivery is to enable the muscles to resume their role in supporting pelvic contents and to reestablish sphincter control. It is an excellent exercise to maintain life-long pelvic floor tone and to enhance sexual enjoyment. It is also widely used for women with sexual dysfunction to increase their capacity for orgasm, and it is helpful for minor degrees of cystocele.

Postpartum Teaching

Parenthood often constitutes a stress in the developmental processes of both mothers and fathers. The postpartum period is particularly stressful because of the numerous physical changes the mother undergoes, the incomplete integration of her pregnancy and labor experiences, the changing roles which must occur within the family complex, and the uncertainty of the nature of the early mother–child relationship. Fatigue, confusion, feelings of helplessness and inadequacy, and depression often complicate this period. Isolation from the extended family, lack of community resources, economic strains, and pressures upon the woman to resume her full previous role within the family as rapidly as possible create additional stresses. Table 19-2 outlines factors that may influence teaching and learning.

The nurse working on the postpartum unit has a unique opportunity to intervene early in the developing mother–child relationship and to assist the parents to anticipate and plan for the first few critical weeks at home. If the mother can attain a level of confidence in her ability to perform care-taking tasks and begin to recognize her baby's behavioral messages, a good foundation can be laid and later difficulties minimized. Sources for continuing care and counseling need to be available to parents during the baby's first few months at home, and the postpartum nurse can direct them to such sources in the particular community.

Individual Teaching

Part of the postpartum nurse's daily responsibility is to provide individual instruction and support to mothers who are under her care. This can range from information about infant sleep and activity patterns, growth and development, and how to dress the baby for different types of weather to sibling rivalry, contraception, and organizing the household to get the necessary tasks done. Mothers' concerns may be small and particular, such as getting the baby to stay awake and suck well, or they may be larger and more general, such as the changes in her own and the father's lifestyle after the advent of the baby. The nurse needs to be informed about a wide variety of topics including contraception, sexuality, and family dynamics, as well as infant care and involutional physiology.

Individual teaching allows the nurse to respond to the personal questions and concerns of mothers and to relate information to that particular situation. Reinforcement of mothering skills is particularly effective on an individual basis, as is counseling regarding family problems or emotions. However, the nurse may not have the time to give each mother the amount of individual teaching and counseling needed. Certain types of teaching can be effectively done in groups, and the use of postpartum groups has increased on hospital postpartum units. Baby-care classes seem well suited to group methods because

Table 19-2.
Factors Influencing Teaching and Learning

Factor	Implications
Infant's condition	Preparation of the parents of preterm infants or infant with significant neonatal problems differs considerably from parents of the healthy, full-term infant.
Parental age	Reflects development status. For example, the adolescent may need more concrete examples and be less able to assimilate written material.
Marital status	Marital status may influence paternal role. Whether married or not, there is need to determine desired paternal involvement. Father should be included in caretaking activities when interested. Marital instability usually increases the anxiety level and makes teaching more difficult.
Parity	When there are other siblings, the family usually needs more of a review of child care than actual teaching. Some teaching should be directed at interaction with the other children and meeting their needs as well as the infant's.
Socioeconomic status	Socioeconomic status influences parent's ability to provide material things for infant, and it usually influences child-rearing practices.
Educational level of parents	Appropriate vocabulary should be utilized for verbal instruction and written material.
Experimental readiness	Previous learning transfers to the new situation. Insight enables the learner to apply older learning to a new situation.
Health beliefs and behaviors of the family	When health beliefs deviate from the usual, teaching may be difficult and more time required to convince the family of the need to change.
Emotional state of the learner	Some anxiety may enhance the learning process, but high anxiety mitigates against learning. Efforts should be made to lower high anxiety levels before proceeding with instruction. Attempts should be made to help parents work through feelings about their child's illness before attempting to teach.
Physical state of the learner	Physical discomfort may preclude or reduce learning.
Parental questions	The type of questions asked indicates learning needs.
Parental motivation	Motivated parents are usually easier to teach. The nurse needs to find ways of stimulating the apparently unmotivated.
Interest in infant	Lack of interest in the infant makes teaching very difficult. When interest appears slight, there should be exploration of apparent disinterest.

(From Ochler JM: Family Centered Neonatal Nursing Care, Philadelphia, J.B. Lippincott Co, 1961.)

the more experienced mothers can add their wisdom and practices to the pooled knowledge available.

Postpartum Classes

The organization of classes for postpartum mothers, and sometimes for fathers as well, differs considerably from one institution to another. Each unit must work out the most convenient time for both staff and parents and a method of communicating to ensure maximum attendance. Sometimes a conference room on the unit is used, or a large patient room can be adapted and extra chairs brought in. The teachers may be postpartum nurses only, or they may be nursery nurses, physicians, social workers, nutritionists, and public health nurses. A variety of media aids can be used, ranging from films to flip charts, books, or other printed material. Closed-channel television which can be viewed by each mother in her room has also been explored as a method of postpartum group instruction.

The content of postpartum teaching varies, but generally it includes content about the mother and her needs and information about the care of a newborn. Content about the mother should include getting enough rest, postpartum blues, family adjustment to a new baby, involutional physiology, pericare, breast care, sexuality, contraception, nutrition, and postpartum exercises. Mothers should be instructed in bathing and dressing the baby, breast- or bottle-feeding, holding and handling, cord care and care of the circumcision, routine tests (*e.g.*, the PKU test), and the normal range of newborn behaviors, including sleeping and crying. Some classes may include time for the mother to practice what she has just been taught while the nurse is available for assistance.

Special Classes

Some postpartum units organize special classes for mothers with particular needs, for example, there may be breast-feeding classes. The mothers are instructed in techniques of nursing, and possible problems and their prevention are discussed. Mothers whose babies are in the intensive care nursery, but who plan to nurse, may also be invited to these classes. More experienced mothers can be encouraged to attend, as they are most helpful to new mothers who have never breast-fed before.

Common situations that breast-feeding mothers might encounter are discussed and group solutions are developed. Questions, such as what foods should be avoided, does breast-feeding ruin the breasts, and what to do when the mother plans to be away for several hours, are elicited from the mothers. Answers to these questions can be provided by the nurse or other mothers in the group. Having the telephone number of the nurse for consultation if problems arise after discharge is very helpful to mothers and promotes continued success with breast-feeding.

If the hospital is large enough to have a regular census of diabetic, adolescent, or low-income mothers, postpartum classes to address their particular needs and concerns are helpful. Perhaps women who had a cesarean birth could make up another group, as their physiologic problems often affect accomplishment of mothering tasks. If, however, the maternity service is relatively small and cannot support many different postpartum groups, the common concerns of baby care can be taught to a group of varied composition, with needs for particular information handled on an individual basis.

Outpatient Groups

Nurses and other health professionals are increasingly aware of the need to extend services to parents after discharge from the hospital. This care may be provided through the public health department, hospital-affiliated clinics, private physicians' offices, a community liaison nurse from the postpartum unit, or health professionals in private practice.

Parenting Groups

The importance of the first year of life in the child's development, both behaviorally and physically, has led to establishment of "parenting groups" in a variety of settings. Because most couples are unprepared for the realities of parenthood, there is a need to educate parents with respect to basic processes of parenting in order to foster more realistic expectations.

Such groups often meet prenatally and continue into the postpartum period. The goal is generally to promote healthy parent–child relationships by educating parents about the physical and psychological aspects of pregnancy, childbirth, infant care, parenting, and child development. The group also promotes independence and confidence in parents by teaching problem-solving techniques and by helping to establish and strengthen parents' support systems.[18] Parents' sense of self-esteem and worth, confidence in the parenting role, and realistic expectations regarding parenthood are key aspects in determining parenting behavior.[19] Such groups increase the confidence of mothers and fathers in their roles as parents as they develop a more relaxed feeling that makes them feel more in control of parenting situations, and have fewer behavioral problems with the children.[20]

Mothers' Groups

Mothers' groups provided by local facilities can also be helpful to new mothers. If mothers receive little or no instruction in the hospital before discharge, these groups can offer answers to many common concerns about care of the baby and support in mothering abilities. Cultural differences must be respected, and the structure must be informal and friendly if such groups are to be effective.

The content of each class varies, but information about infant nutritional needs and feeding methods is important and should be covered in detail, as inadequate nutrition and protein deprivation are common problems among this group, which may create serious implications for the baby. General care of the infant, particularly bathing, diaper care, and causes of simple skin rashes, is another standard topic.

Sharing among the mothers can also enhance learning. If the atmosphere is comfortable, these mothers can be encouraged to examine practices that might be contributing to the baby's health problems, and possibly to modify these practices.

The nurse has the opportunity to observe the infants for signs of illness and refer them to the pediatrician if needed. She is also able to identify serious emotional problems and make appropriate referrals.[21]

Cluster Visits

Cluster visits constitute one approach to pediatric care that uses the group method. A small number of mothers and their babies, usually four pairs, are scheduled for a joint visit with the pediatric nurse practitioner or pediatrician. Each baby is examined with the mother standing by, findings are explained, and instructions are given for minor illness or problems. Subjects of general interest are postponed until discussion time, which follows the examinations. While one mother and baby are involved in the examination, the others are getting acquainted and comparing notes.

During the discussion period, the nurse and mothers talk about childrearing, feelings related to motherhood and baby care, changes in the family structure, or other topics relevant to the baby's age or the mother's needs. The groups are formed to include mothers with babies of about the same age. The mothers generally take the lead in the discussion and often provide specific information and teaching for one another. During the last ten minutes, the next cluster visit is planned and immunizations are given to the babies as needed.

These cluster visits are usually alternated with individual visits. They permit more care to be provided to mothers and babies using less professional time. The mothers involved tend to respond very positively, as they enjoy the camaraderie, the sharing problems and anxieties, the chance to observe other babies, and the knowledge and support gained through the discussion. This group experience increases parental confidence and shows how babies are individuals whose weight and development vary. There appears to be no increased cross-contamination. Cluster visits are one way of providing improved health care at a lower cost to parents.[22]

Parent Effectiveness Training

Other outpatient groups for parents are those that train parents how to prevent behavior problems in their children. Parent Effectiveness Training (PET) was started in the early 1960s by Dr. Thomas Gordon, a clinical psychologist from Pasadena, California. Parents attend class one night a week for eight weeks and learn active listening and other communication skills, behavior modification, and methods of resolving parent–child conflicts. Content also includes dealing with infants and toddlers. PET classes are available in many communities in all 50 states and are sometimes sponsored by schools, social agencies, or organizations serving parents, as well as health professionals in private practice.[23]

References

1. Redman BK: The Process of Patient Teaching in Nursing. St Louis, CV Mosby, 1968
2. Gorman AH: Teachers and Learners in the Interactive Process of Education. Boston, Allyn and Bacon, 1969
3. Bibring GF, Huntington DS, Valenstein AF: A study of the psychological processes in pregnancy and of the earliest mother–child relationship. Psychoanal Study Child 16:9–71, 1961
4. Tanner LM: Developmental tasks of pregnancy. In Bergersen BS (ed): Current Concepts in Clinical Nursing, Vol. II, pp 292–297. St Louis, CV Mosby, 1969
5. Klaus M, Kennell J: Care of the mother. In Klaus M, Fanaroff A (eds): Care of the High-Risk Neonate, pp 98–118. Philadelphia, WB Saunders, 1973
6. Kennell J, Klaus M: Care of the mother of the high-risk infant. Clin Obstet Gynecol 14:926, 1971
7. Rubin R: Maternal touch. Nurs Outlook 11:829–831, November 1963
8. Editorial: Puerperal change. Nurs Outlook 9:753–755, 1961
9. Spaulding MR: Adapting postpartum teaching to mothers' low-income lifestyles. In Bergersen BS (ed): Current Concepts in Clinical Nursing, Vol. II, pp 280–291. St Louis, CV Mosby, 1969
10. Sosa R, Kennell J, Klaus M: The effect of a supportive companion on perinatal problems, length of labor, and mother infant interaction. New Engl J Med 303:597–600, 1980
11. Gaziano E, Garvis M, Levine E: An evaluation of childbirth education for the clinic patient. Birth and the Family Journal 6:89, Summer 1979
12. Noble E: Essential Exercises for the Childbearing Year. Boston, Houghton-Mifflin, 1982
13. Caldeyro–Barcia, R: The influence of maternal bearing-down efforts during second stage on fetal well-being. Birth and the Family Journal 6:17, Spring 1979
14. Bean CA: Methods of Childbirth. New York, Doubleday, 1972
15. Humenick S: Assessing the quality of childbirth education: Can teachers change? Birth and the Family Journal 7:82–90, Summer 1980
16. Humenick S, Marchbanks P: Validation of a scale to measure relaxation in childbirth education classes. Birth and the Family Journal 8:141, Fall 1981
17. Ewy D, Ewy R: Preparation for Childbirth. New York, New American Library, 1976
18. Smith D, Smith H: Toward improvements in parenting: A description of prenatal and postpartum classes with teaching guide. Journal Obstetrics, Gynecology and Neonatal Nursing 7:22–27, November/December 1978
19. Wuerger M: Stepping into parenthood. Am J Nurs 76:1283–1285, August 1976
20. Shaw NR: Teaching young mothers their role. Nurs Outlook 22:695–698, November 1974
21. Cooper I: Group sessions for new mothers. Nurs Outlook 22:251, April 1974
22. Feldman M: Cluster visit. Am J Nurs 74:1485–1488, August 1974
23. Gordon T: Parent Effectiveness Training. New York, New American Library, 1975

Suggested Reading*

Bing E: Six Practical Lessons for an Easier Childbirth. New York, Bantam Books, 1977

Dick-Read G: Childbirth Without Fear. New York, Harper & Row, 1972

*If not available locally write to International Childbirth Education Association Book Center, PO Box 20048, Minneapolis, MN 55420 USA

Karmel M: Thank You, Dr. Lamaze. Philadelphia, JB Lippincott, 1959

Noble E: Essential Exercises for the Childbearing Year. Boston, Houghton-Mifflin, 1982

Rozdilsky ML, Banet B: What Now? A Handbook for New Parents. New York, Charles Scribner's Sons, 1975

Salk L: Preparing for Parenthood. New York, Bantam Books, 1975

CHAPTER

20

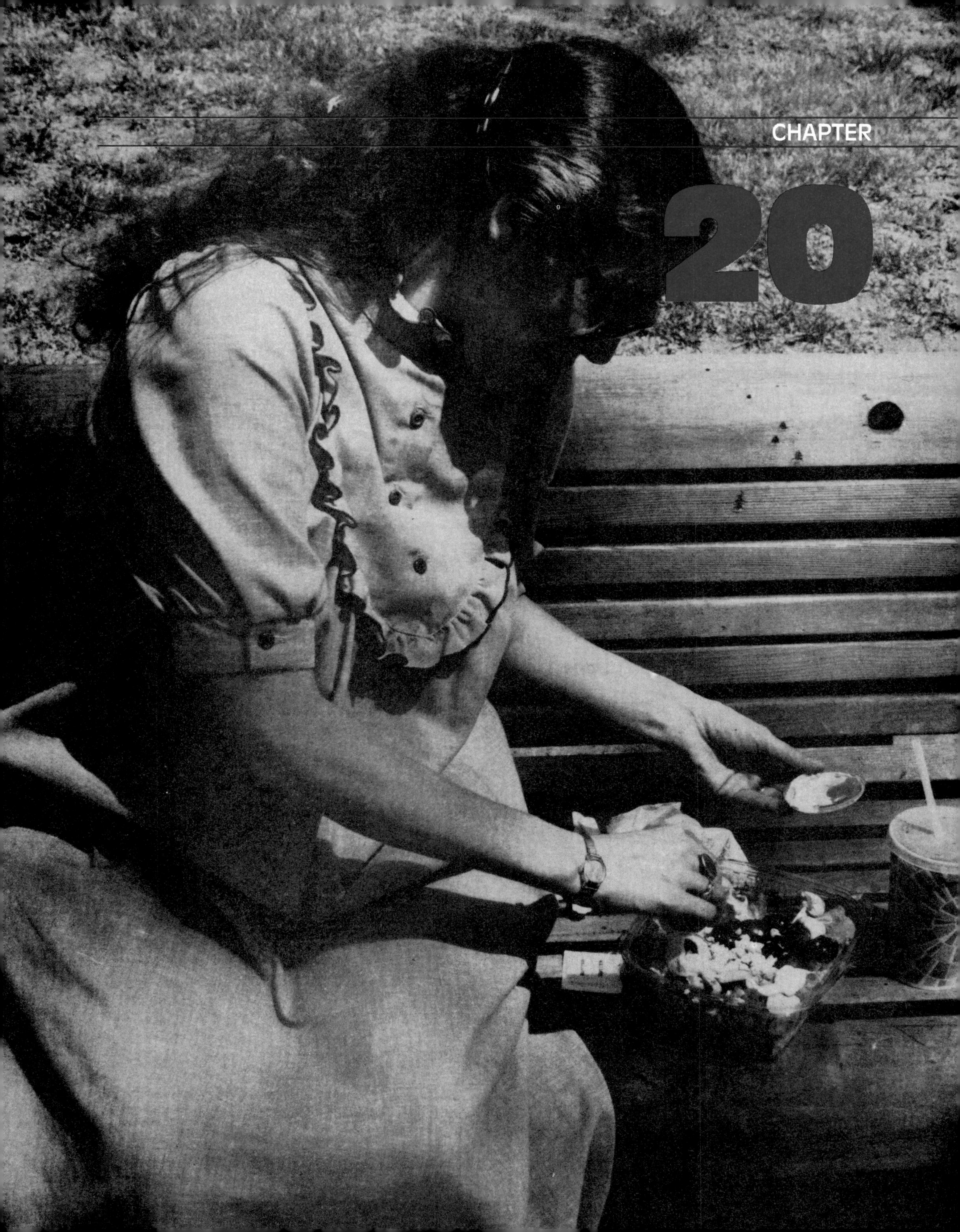

CHAPTER 20

Nutrition in Pregnancy

Nutrition plays a key role in the outcome of pregnancy. A woman's nutritional status at conception, and the quality of the diet she consumes during the following months, help to determine her health and well-being and that of her child. Ensuring optimum nutrition for all childbearing women might not eliminate all the problems of pregnancy, but it is a giant step in the right direction.

Importance of Nutrition During Pregnancy

In 1970, the National Academy of Sciences issued a report, *Maternal Nutrition and the Course of Pregnancy.*[1] This report reviewed studies of reproductive experiences and concluded that adequate prenatal nutrition is one of the most important environmental factors affecting the health of pregnant women and their babies.

The importance of maternal nutrition during pregnancy has long been recognized. In the Old Testament, Samson's mother was advised to eat well while she was pregnant. Over the years a wide variety of dietary advice has been given to the pregnant woman. This includes instructions that ranged from severe restriction of intake to admonitions to eat large quantities, and from limitation of protein to high protein diets.[2] The final words on the effects of nutrition during pregnancy have not been written, but at present, stress is being placed on the importance of adequate nutrition before, during, and after pregnancy.

Effects of Poor Nutrition

Controlled studies on animals have shown a direct relationship between maternal diet and pregnancy outcome. Although it is not possible to show a direct cause and effect relationship between specific nutrients and specific problems in human studies, general correlations have been found. Chronic malnutrition in developing countries and in low-income populations of developed countries has been shown to be related to reproductive problems, including difficulties during pregnancy, labor, and delivery; increased perinatal mortality; low birth weight, and other problems of the newborn.

Some historical occurrences have provided study populations that demonstrate the effects of nutritional deprivation under conditions that would not have been purposely set up. During World War II, a seven-month food embargo of western Holland decreased the population's average daily food ration to fewer than 750 calories. In a retrospective study, women who were pregnant or who conceived during the famine were shown to have a higher incidence of stillbirth and neonatal mortality, and decreased infant birth weight.[3] Similar effects on pregnancy were found during the siege of Leningrad in 1941 and 1942.

Effects of Supplementation

There have been a number of studies in the last few decades that are designed to demonstrate the effects of improved nutrition on the pregnancies of women with deficient nutrition. In some of these studies supplementation is by means of additional food and in others it is by provision of a prepared supplement of either protein and calories or just calories. One of the supplemental food programs was carried out at the Montreal Diet Dispensary.[4] The study showed a lower incidence of preeclampsia and other diseases of pregnancy, easier deliveries with fewer Cesarean sections, and a greater mean birth weight with considerably lower neonatal morbidity and mortality.

Effects on Mental Development

When discussing the effects of nutrition on mental development, it is difficult to differentiate between the prenatal and postnatal nutritional effects. The critical period for brain cell development begins during pregnancy and continues during the first year of life. The nutritionally deprived fetus may have decreased development of brain cells, but if optimum nutrition is provided after birth, the effects may be reversible.[5]

Inductees into the Dutch armed forces whose conception, gestation, or birth occurred during the 1944-1945 famine were compared with other Dutch inductees who were born in the same time period, but not living in the famine area. Although birth weights in the famine area were significantly lower than in other areas, intelligence tests failed to show significant differences between famine and non-famine subjects.[5] A possible explanation for the good mental outcomes of the survivors of the famine in spite of their prenatal nutritional deprivation is that

Possible Adverse Effects of Poor Nutrition on the Reproductive Cycle*

- Infertility
- Reproductive casualty
  - Abortion
  - Stillbirth
  - Neonatal death
- Pregnancy problems
  - Preeclampsia and eclampsia
  - Placental abnormalities
  - Gestational diabetes
- Difficult labors and deliveries
- Low-birth-weight infants
- Slow postpartum recovery of mother
- Difficulties with lactation
- Delayed mental and physical development of infant.

*Obviously there are many other factors which influence the occurrence of these problems, but prepregnant nutritional status and nutrient intake during pregnancy play a significant role.

the Dutch were generally well nourished before and after the famine, in contrast to many other study populations who suffer from chronic malnutrition and other deprivations.[6]

On the other hand, when malnutrition during and following pregnancy is associated with other forms of environmental deprivation, mental retardation and severe, long-lasting behavioral effects, such as learning disabilities, are more frequent. The Montreal Diet Dispensary study indicates that improved nutrition during pregnancy and lactation improved the mental development of the children in the study, compared to siblings who were born before the mother received supplements.[7]

Nutritional Assessment

Each woman who becomes pregnant has a unique nutritional background. Many factors influence her nutritional status and her daily food intake. To be able to help these women choose the best possible diets during their pregnancy, the nurse needs to be aware of the factors, their effect on each individual, and ways of obtaining information about them.

Assessing Dietary Intake

To gather information about the patient's food habits and actual food intake, an atmosphere and opportunity must be provided for the woman to discuss her concerns about food and diet and to give information about her current dietary patterns. Nutritional evaluation requires information on what is eaten, as well as the quantities and the method of preparation. Information regarding purchasing practices is also needed, as certain foods may not be purchased because of cost and more economical substitutions may be needed.

The *Nutrition Questionnaire* which was developed by the California Department of Health Services is a useful tool in assessing the patient's food habits. It should be completed by the patient on her first prenatal visit and used as a basis for a nutritional counseling interview. Some questions may not be applicable to all client populations and other questions may need to be added in some areas.

To provide appropriate guidance for the woman and to better assess her level of understanding and knowledge about her diet, a *diet history* can be taken to determine actual eating patterns. The nurse may ask the woman to describe or write down her food intake for the past 24 hours or for a typical day. This should include the time, place, type of food and amount. There are a variety of forms available that may be useful in obtaining a diet history (see Diet History and Evaluation Form).

Another method of obtaining the information is to have the woman keep a *diary* of everything she eats for two or three days. She should be advised to avoid holidays or days with atypical diet patterns, to record everything as soon after eating as possible, to write down amounts of each food as accurately as she can, and to describe sauces and condiments, such as cheese sauce or soy sauce. Some women have difficulty remembering to write things down, but even if the diary is incomplete, it can still provide useful information.

The *Guide to Food Frequency* can provide useful information for identifying food preferences and dislikes that might lead to diet inadequacies. However, it should be used only with a diet history or food intake diary because it does not show daily food patterns and amounts.

Assessing Nutritional Status

Gathering information about a variety of maternal characteristics can help in assessing a woman's nutritional status.

Anthropometric evaluation includes various measurements of the body. Height and weight are the most common measurements taken. Comparing height to pregravid weight gives an estimate of body build, which is useful in determining standard weight and identifying the underweight person. Recording weight at intervals throughout the pregnancy also

(Text continues on page 370)

AT Nutrition Questionnaire

A nutritional questionnaire such as this one developed by the California Department of Health Services can be an invaluable tool in helping to assess a client's nutritional intake.

Name: ______________________________ Date: ____________

Please answer the following by checking the appropriate box or filling in the blank. Answer only those questions which apply to you. All information is confidential.

I. a) Before this pregnancy, what was your usual weight?
   ________ lbs. ( ) Don't Know

b) During your last pregnancy, how much weight did you gain?
   ________ lbs. ( ) Don't Know

c) How much weight do you expect to gain during this pregnancy?
   ________ lbs. ( ) Don't Know

d) Have you ever had any problems with your weight?
   ( ) Yes ( ) No
   If yes, what? ( ) Underweight
   ( ) Overweight
   ( ) Other ________

II. a) How would you describe your appetite?
   ( ) Hearty ( ) Moderate ( ) Poor

b) With this pregnancy, have you experienced either of the following?
   ( ) Nausea ( ) Vomiting

III. a) How would you describe your eating habits?
   ( ) Regular ( ) Irregular

IV. a) Indicate the person who does the following in your household:
   Plans the meals ________
   Buys the food ________
   Prepares the food ________

b) How much is spent on food each week for your household:
   $ ________ ( ) Don't Know
   How many people does this feed? ________

c) Indicate the types of kitchen equipment you have in your home:
   ( ) Refrigerator ( ) Stove
   ( ) Hot plate

V. a) Are you *now* taking any vitamin or mineral supplement?
   ( ) Yes ( ) No

b) Do you take any pills to control your weight?
   ( ) Yes ( ) No

c) Do you take diuretic (water) pills?
   ( ) Yes ( ) No

VI. a) Are you now on a diet to lose weight?
   ( ) Yes ( ) No

b) Are you *now* on a special diet (low salt, diabetic, gallbladder)?
   ( ) Yes ( ) No
   If yes, what kind of diet? ________

c) If you have been on a special diet in the past, indicate what kind and when.
   ____
   ____

VII. a) Is there any food you *can't* eat?
   ( ) Yes ( ) No
   If yes, what foods? ________
   ____
   What happens when you eat this food?
   ____

b) Do you have any cravings for things such as the following:
   ( ) cornstarch
   ( ) plaster
   ( ) dirt or clay
   ( ) other ________

VIII. Do you have any of the following problems?
   ( ) constipation
   ( ) diarrhea

IX. a) Do you smoke? ( ) Yes ( ) No

b) Do you drink any alcoholic beverages (liquor, wine, beer)? ( ) Yes ( ) No

X. Are you receiving either of the following?
   ( ) food stamps
   ( ) WIC vouchers

XI. How do you want to feed your baby?
   ( ) breast feed
   ( ) evaporated milk formula
   ( ) commercial formula
   ( ) undecided

Nutrition During Pregnancy and Lactation. Maternal and Child Health Unit, California Department of Health, 1975

AT A Diet History

A "diet history" or "food diary" could use a simple form such as the one below.

Daily Food Intake

Patient's name: ______________________________

Date: ______________ Food intake recorded by: ______________________________

Instructions

1. Include everything eaten from the time she gets up until she goes to bed.
2. Food should be described in terms of how it was prepared and served (*e.g.*, Mashed potatoes and gravy; salad of raw carrots with raisins and mayonnaise).
3. Approximate amounts should be listed for each individual food (*e.g.*, 1 small carrot; ¼ cup raisins; 1 tablespoon mayonnaise).

Time	Place	Food Eaten (description)	Amount

Nutrition During Pregnancy and Lactation. Maternal and Child Health Unit, California Department of Health, 1975

AT Diet History and Evaluation Form

It is desirable to obtain a dietary history as early as possible in pregnancy and before recommending a specific diet for an individual mother. This history should include information concerning the expectant mother's usual food practices, meals often omitted, typical menu patterns, food likes and dislikes, cultural factors, methods of food preparation, financial situation, and so on. Nutritional gaps will be obvious from an evaluation of this information. During the process of taking a diet history, useful information is obtained concerning the patient's level of nutrition knowledge and clues to methods of counseling. Explaining any recommended changes will help the expectant mother understand her present needs. If history is kept in patient's chart and information is recorded elsewhere, interviewer may prefer to omit some questions. Sample form may be changed to fit situation.

Name ______________________ Date ______________________

______________________ Due Date ______________________

Patient's childhood home ______________________ Height ______________________

(State or country) ______________________ Present weight ______________________

Patient's occupation ______________________ Pregravid weight ______________________

Last year school completed ______________________

Husband's occupation ______________________ Birth date ______________________

Money available for food weekly ______________________ Number in household ______________________

Food currently bought by ______________________

Meals currently prepared by ______________________

Foods liked especially, including cravings ______________________

Foods never eaten and why (storage problems, equipment, and so on) ______________________

Nutritional supplements currently used during pregnancy (kind and amount used) ______________________

Diet modified previously or currently (type of diet and date) ______________________

Meals and snacks often eaten at the following times:

Morning: ______________________

Midmorning: ______________________

Midday: ______________________

(Continued)

AT Diet History and Evaluation Form (continued)

Afternoon: ______

______

Evening: ______

______

______

______

Before bedtime: ______

______

Prenatal diet prescribed and date ______

Instruction received on prenatal diet including materials given ______

______

______

Additional information ______

______

Follow-up remarks ______

______

Prenatal dietary history recorded by: ______

______

______

______

______

(Cross AT, Walsh HE: Prenatal Diet Counseling. Journal of Reproductive Medicine, 7:269–270, 1971. From Nutrition—During Pregnancy and Lactation, Berkeley, CA, California State Dept. of Public Health, 1971)

AT Guide to Food Frequency

This guide to food frequency can be a helpful tool in a nutritional assessment. However, it should only be used with a diet history or food intake diary.

Name: ______ Date: ______

Instructions

Indicate whether or not you eat the following foods by checking the columns **"Don't eat"** or **"Do eat"** for each item. For each food you have checked **"Do eat"** write the approximate number of times you eat it in a week. If you eat any particular food less than once a week, do not write anything in the column **"Times eaten per week."**

In some cases more than one food has been listed on a line. If you do not eat all of these foods, underline the specific foods you eat. A space has been provided at the end for you to write in foods not listed which you regularly eat.

Food	Don't Eat	Do Eat	Times Eaten Per Week	For Office Use Only
I. Chicken				
Beef, hamburger, veal				
Liver, kidney, tongue				
Lamb				

AT Guide to Food Frequency (continued)

Food	Don't Eat	Do Eat	Times Eaten Per Week	For Office Use Only
Cold cuts, hot dogs				
Pork, ham, sausage				
Bacon				
Fish				
Kidney beans, pinto beans, lentils (all legumes)				
Soybeans				
Eggs				
Nuts or seeds				
Peanut butter				
Tofu				
II. Milk (fluid, dry, evaporated)				
Cottage cheese				
Cheese (all kinds other than cottage)				
Condensed milk				
Ice cream				
Yogurt				
Pudding and custard				
Milkshake				
Sherbert				
Ice milk				
III. Whole grain bread				
White bread				
Rolls, biscuits, muffins				
Bagel				
Crackers, pretzels				
Pancakes, waffles				
Cereals				
White rice				
Brown rice				
Noodles, macaroni, grits				
Tortillas (flour)				
Tortillas (corn)				
IV. Tomato, tomato sauce, or tomato juice				
Orange or orange juice				
Tangerine				
Grapefruit or grapefruit juice				
Papaya, mango				
Lemonade				
White potato				
Turnip				
Peppers (green, red, chili)				
Strawberries, cantaloupe				

(Continued)

AT Guide to Food Frequency (continued)

	Food	Don't Eat	Do Eat	Times Eaten Per Week	For Office Use Only
V.	Dark green or red lettuce				
	Asparagus				
	Swiss chard				
	Bok choy				
	Cabbage				
	Broccoli				
	Brussels sprouts				
	Scallions				
	Spinach				
	Greens (beet, collard, kale, turnip, mustard)				
VI	Carrots				
	Artichoke				
	Corn				
	Sweet potato or yam				
	Zucchini				
	Summer squash				
	Winter squash				
	Green peas				
	Green and yellow beans				
	Hominy				
	Beets				
	Cucumbers or celery				
	Peach				
	Apricot				
	Apple				
	Banana				
	Pineapple				
	Cherries				
VII.	Cakes, pies, cookies				
	Sweet roll, doughnuts				
	Candy				
	Sugar or honey				
	Carbonated beverages (sodas)				
	Coffee or tea				
	Cocoa				
	Wine, beer, cocktails				
	Fruit drink				
VIII.	Other foods not listed which you regularly eat				

Nutrition During Pregnancy and Lactation. Maternal and Child Health Unit, California Department of Health, 1975

AT Prenatal Weight Gain Grid

Guide to prenatal weight gain grid.

Recommended weight gain during pregnancy is 2 to 4 pounds (1–2 kg) during first trimester and 0.9 pound (0.5 kg) per week for second and third trimesters. For optimum care, the prenatal weight gain grid should be used with all pregnant women. This tool provides a visual representation of the patient's weight gain during pregnancy by plotting the patient's weight gain at every visit.

Patient's Name: ______________________________

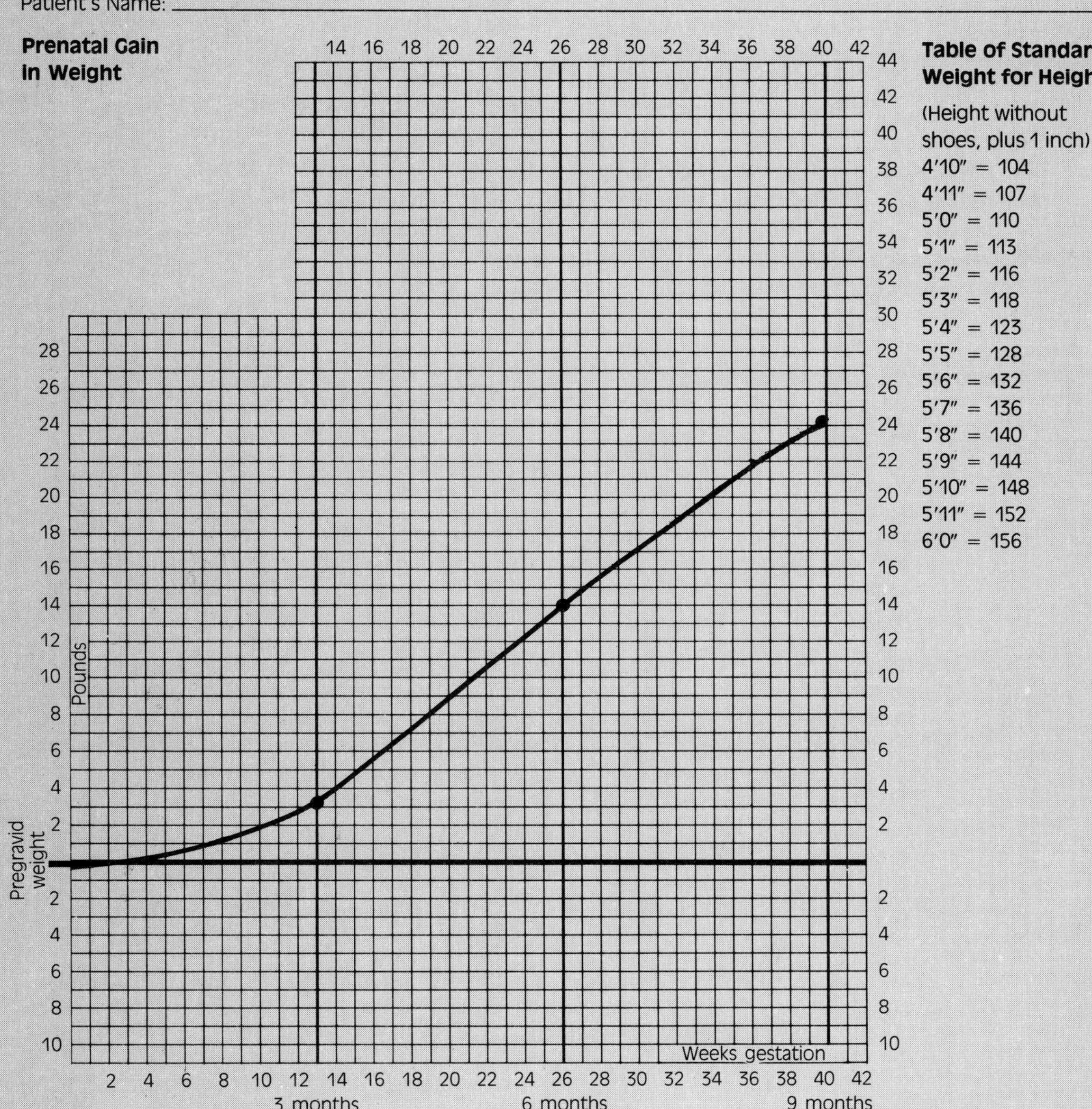

Table of Standard Weight for Height*

(Height without shoes, plus 1 inch)

4′10″ = 104
4′11″ = 107
5′0″ = 110
5′1″ = 113
5′2″ = 116
5′3″ = 118
5′4″ = 123
5′5″ = 128
5′6″ = 132
5′7″ = 136
5′8″ = 140
5′9″ = 144
5′10″ = 148
5′11″ = 152
6′0″ = 156

*The above weights were taken from Metropolitan Life Insurance Company, Actuarial Tables, 1959 and adjusted to comply with instructions appearing on the Prenatal Weight Gain Grid, namely, height in inches without shoes plus 1 inch to establish a standard for heels. Pacients should be weighed with shoes as normally worn. The table above is for medium body build and, except for extreme body build deviations, these figures should be used.

For example, a patient whose height, measured without shoes, is 5 feet 4 inches would have one inch added; therefore, her standard weight for height would be 128 pounds.

Ranges are not acceptable in estimating standard weight since this is an objective observation and represents the mid-point. This mid-point must be used for recording purposes.

For patients under age 25 one pound should be deducted for each year.

Nutrition During Pregnancy and Lactation. Maternal and Child Health Unit, California Department of Health, 1975

(Continued from page 362)
allows comparisons of the individual's weight gain pattern with the recommended pattern (see Prenatal Weight Gain Grid). Measurement can also include the use of tape measures and calipers for skin fold width, but these are not usually done and are not necessary for most women.

Laboratory tests are used to determine the presence of adequate amounts of certain nutrients. Hemoglobin and hematocrit are done routinely to evaluate the woman's iron status and need for supplements. The serum folacin level may be used as an indicator of nutritional intake.[8] Determination might also be made of serum albumin, total serum protein, and serum vitamin B_{12}. Additional hematologic values may be obtained in assessing specific nutrient-related problems.[9]

General physical assessment of the pregnant woman can provide useful information in assessing nutritional status. Alone, the signs may not be reliable indicators, but considered together, and with laboratory tests and dietary history, they can provide useful clues for further investigation (see Table 20-1).

Factors in Planning the Diet

Individual Factors Involved in Food Choices

The psychological aspects of nutrition are important determinants of food choice, but do not lend themselves to clear-cut analysis. Food is a basic need for survival, and hunger is one of the most fundamental of all sensations.

Table 20-1.
Physical Indicators of Nutritional Status

Body Area	Normal Appearance	Signs Associated with Malnutrition
Hair	Shiny, firm, not easily plucked	Lack of natural shine; hair dull and dry; thin and sparse; hair fine, silky and straight; color changes (flag sign); can be easily plucked
Face	Skin color uniform; smooth, pink, healthy appearance; not swollen	Skin color loss (depigmentation): skin dark over cheeks and under eyes (malar and supraorbital pigmentation); lumpiness or flakiness of skin of nose and mouth; swollen face; enlarged parotid glands; scaling of skin around nostrils (nasolabial seborrhea)
Eyes	Bright, clear, shiny; no sores at corners of eyelids; membranes a healthy pink and are moist; no prominent blood vessels or mound of tissue on sclera	Eye membranes are pale (pale conjunctivae); redness of membranes (conjunctival injection); Bitot's spots; redness and fissuring of eyelid corners (angular palpebritis); dryness of eye membranes (conjunctival xerosis); cornea has dull appearance (corneal xerosis); cornea is soft (keratomalacia); scar on cornea; ring of fine blood vessels around corner (circumcorneal injection)
Lips	Smooth, not chapped or swollen	Redness and swelling of mouth or lips (cheilosis); especially at corners of mouth (angular fissures and scars)
Tongue	Deep red in appearance; not swollen or smooth	Swelling; scarlet and raw tongue; magenta (purplish color) of tongue; smooth tongue; swollen sores; hyperemic and hypertrophic, and atrophic papillae
Teeth	No cavities; no pain; bright	May be missing or erupting abnormally; gray or black spots (fluorosis); cavities (caries)
Gums	Healthy; red; do not bleed; not swollen	"Spongy" and bleed easily; recession of gums
Glands	Face not swollen	Thyroid enlargement (front of neck); parotid enlargement (cheeks become swollen)

(Continued)

Related to hunger, but of a very different origin, is appetite. Appetite is Nature's primary defense for the prevention of hunger. Based on the anticipation of eating, the impulse is determined by the person's previous experience. Only by coincidence and training does appetite become associated with health-giving foods. Factors affecting food-seeking behavior are the main determinants of eating (*i.e.,* hunger, appetite, and custom). The great deterrents to normal appetite are worry, fear, and preoccupation with troublesome or difficult problems. These may be reflected in either an increase or a decrease of appetite. Some of the positive emotional stimulants include situations that encourage feelings of calm contentedness, mild elation, or ego-stimulation.

Present-day cuisine is a potpourri of heritage, superstition, custom, knowledge, and opportunity. Subtle cravings are passed along from one generation to the next by the process of training and imitation. Unique methods of food preparation as well as food selection, combinations, and prejudices are embodied in this training. Congeniality and hospitality are enhanced by the serving of good food; and it has become the custom to serve food at practically all functions, business as well as social.

From infancy onward, food and closeness are associated with love and security. Food and eating are looked upon as symbolizing interpersonal acceptance, warmth, and sociability. Throughout all societies this symbolic undertone is unmistakable, from the "breaking of bread" in antiquity to the modern banquet the serving of food is a vehicle for expressing honor, joy, or mutual bonds. It is easy to see why food has become associated with the symbolism of motherliness. Feeding is not only kindly and warm in its emotional meaning to those who receive food, but it is also essential to growth and well-being; hence, it has become bound up with the idea of the

Body Area	Normal Appearance	Signs Associated with Malnutrition
Skin	No signs of rashes, swellings, dark or light spots	Dryness of skin (xerosis); sandpaper feel of skin (follicular hyperkeratosis); flakiness of skin; skin swollen and dark; red, swollen pigmentation of exposed areas (pellagrous dermatosis); excessive lightness or darkness of skin (dyspigmentation); black and blue marks due to skin bleeding (petechiae); lack of fat under skin
Nails	Firm, pink	Nails are spoon shaped (koilonychia); brittle, ridged nails
Muscular and skeletal systems	Good muscle tone; some fat under skin; can walk or run without pain	Muscles have "wasted" appearance; baby's skull bones are thin and soft (craniotabes); round swelling of front and side of head (frontal and parietal bossing); swelling of ends of bones (epiphyseal enlargement); small bumps on both sides of chest wall (on ribs)—beading of ribs; baby's soft spot on head does not harden at proper time (persistently open anterior fontanelle); knock knees or bow legs; bleeding into muscle (musculoskeletal hemorrhages): person cannot get up or walk properly
Internal systems		
Cardiovascular	Normal heart rate and rhythm; no murmurs or abnormal rhythms; normal blood pressure for age	Rapid heart rate (above 100 tachycardia); enlarged heart; abnormal rhythm; elevated blood pressure
Gastrointestinal	No palpable organs or masses (in children, liver edge may be palpable)	Liver enlargement; enlargement of spleen (usually indicates other associated diseases)
Nervous	Psychological stability; normal reflexes	Mental irritability and confusion; burning and tingling of hands and feet (paresthesia); loss of position and vibratory sense; weakness and tenderness of muscles (may result in inability to walk); decrease and loss of ankle and knee reflexes

(Reprinted with permission from Nutritional Assessment in Health Programs, American Journal of Public Health, 63: November, 1973 Supplement.)

mother, the one who originally nurtured, loved, and supported.

The pregnant woman makes a close identification with the concept of the mother, and selections and choices may be influenced profoundly by these symbolic meanings of food. She may crave certain foods and reject others, and not because of physiologic factors. For instance, she may feel that certain foods will "mark" her baby or will give him strength. It is crucial that the meaning which food has for the patient be explored and that her feelings and attitudes be respected.

The *stage of growth and development* of the patient may also influence her food choices. For instance, foods enjoyed by adolescents are often different from those enjoyed by older people.

When people marry younger and become parents at an earlier age, they carry these eating patterns into marriage with them. In addition, adolescence is a time for developing independence, and this is healthy. However, many foods may be rejected (*e.g.,* milk, vegetables, cereal, and the like), because they are associated with "home" and a dependency period. The desire to be free and to select the "forbidden" foods is very strong.

The *religious, racial,* and *ethnic background* of the patient and her family is also an important consideration. Certain foods may be highly valued and oth-

Table 20-2.
Ethnic Dietary Characteristics

Ethnic Group	Protein Foods	Milk and Milk Products	Grain Products	Vegetables and Fruits	Counseling Suggestions
Mexican–American	Variety of meats, poultry and legumes, eggs	Not usual part of adult diet as beverage; small quantities of cheese in cooking	Tortillas and rice are staples	Tomatoes, chili peppers, fried potatoes, other raw or boiled vegetables, oranges, apples, bananas	Increase cheese and milk in cooking, and milk as beverage. Encourage variety of vegetables eaten raw or cooked for short time in small amount of water. Decrease consumption of carbonated beverages and other empty calorie foods Encourage use of enriched flour for tortillas
Black/Southern	Beef, pork, chicken; legumes as accompaniment	Some milk, buttermilk, cheese, ice cream	Rice, biscuits, white and corn bread	Greens, sweet potatoes, okra, cabbage, corn, green beans, usually boiled; seasonal fruits, limited citrus	Increase milk and decrease carbonated beverages Encourage whole grain cereals and bread. Decrease water and time for cooking greens and other vegetables Eat some raw vegetables Increase vitamin C sources

(Continued)

ers excluded from the diet. Methods of preparation may also be different. Many families are fond of their regional or national diet and prefer it to the American "meat and potatoes" regimen.

Knowing the patient's ethnic background can be helpful in understanding her dietary habits, but there is much variation within ethnic groups. These differences may be related to climate, growing conditions, geographic relocation, intermarriage, and individual differences. Therefore, assumptions should not be made about a patient's food habits based on surname or language spoken (see Table 20-2).

Food allergies or *intolerances* can develop to a number of different foods. Adjustments in the diet may be required to avoid these foods and still obtain adequate amounts of the essential nutrients. Intolerance to the milk sugar, lactose, is a particular problem during pregnancy because it is difficult to meet the pregnant woman's need for calcium, protein, and certain vitamins and minerals without using milk.

Nutritional Risk Factors

There are certain factors that place women "at risk" for nutritional problems related to pregnancy and require special attention to nutritional needs. These factors can be grouped into categories (Table 20-3).

Ethnic Group	Protein Foods	Milk and Milk Products	Grain Products	Vegetables and Fruits	Counseling Suggestions
Chinese	Fish, chicken, pork, legumes, eggs, nuts	Ice cream, flavored milk, some milk in cooking	Rice, millet, noodles	Variety of vegetables, often stir-fried with minimal nutrient loss; many fruits, usually fresh	Increase serving sizes of protein foods, or use as snacks Increase calories Encourage dairy products in cooking and use of tofu (soy bean curd) Discourage washing rice because of nutrient loss
Japanese	Variety of meat and fish, eggs, nuts, legumes, tofu (soy bean curd)	Milk and milk products limited	Polished rice, some wheat products	Variety of fruits and vegetables	Encourage use of dairy products to overcome major dietary problem Use calcium and vitamin D supplements if necessary Avoid par-cooking of vegetables and washing of rice to avoid nutrient loss
Puerto Rican	Chicken, pork, beef, eggs, beans; ham butts and sausage used for flavoring, not as a protein source	Limited use—"cafe con leche" may contain 2 oz to 5 oz milk	French bread, rolls, crackers, rice; increasing use of cereals	Pumpkins, carrots, green pepper, tomatoes, sweet potatoes, canned fruits and nectars	Encourage milk and cheese Suggest meat source with bean meal Urge more leafy green vegetables Increase use of citrus and other fresh fruits, and use of whole grain or enriched breads, cereal and rice

Table 20-3.
Nutritional Risk Factors

Category	Factor	Significance
Age	Adolescence	Increased nutritional needs; possible poor food habits
	Older gravidas	Possible increased incidence of other risk factors
Obstetrical history	High parity or frequent conceptions	Depletion of maternal nutrient stores
	Previous obstetrical complications	Possible nutritional relationship may recur
Medical history	Preexisting medical problems	May affect ingestion, utilization, or absorption of nutrients
Complications of current pregnancy	Development of complications, such as anemia, preeclampsia, or gestational diabetes	Development of nutritional deficiencies due to increased nutritional needs
Maternal weight	Low prepregnancy weight	Increased incidence of pregnancy and neonatal complications
	Insufficient weight gain	Indication of poor maternal and fetal nutrition; increased number of low-birth-weight infants
	Obesity	Possible poor nutritional habits; increased incidence of pregnancy complications
	Excessive weight gain	If sudden, may indicate preeclampsia; lack of agreement on other possible risks
Dysfunctional dietary patterns	Dietary faddism	Diets often inadequate to meet fetal or maternal nutritional needs
	Pica	Displacement of nutritious foods, often related to iron deficiency anemia
	Excessive use of alcohol, drugs, or tobacco	Interference with appetite and with utilization of some nutrients
Socioeconomic status	Low income	Limited ability to buy sufficient food; possible chronic malnutrition
Cultural or ethnic group	Ethnic or language differences	Interference with ability to find usual foods; misinterpretation of dietary instructions
Psychological conditions	Depression, anorexia nervosa	Possible reduced caloric and nutrient intake

Age

A woman's age can affect her nutritional needs during pregnancy as well as her dietary habits. *Women under the age of 17,* who become pregnant, have their own growth needs to satisfy in addition to their pregnancy needs and those of the fetus. This increases their nutritional requirements at a time when they may be reluctant to follow dietary instructions or to gain weight. Adolescent pregnancies have been associated with low birth weight, prematurity, and increased perinatal mortality. *Older gravidas* may also be at increased nutritional risk, mostly because they have a greater chance of being in one of the other risk categories.

Obstetrical History

High parity or frequent conceptions can cause depletion of maternal nutrient stores, leading to pregnancy complications, unless the diet is of very high quality.

Previous obstetrical complications, such as inadequate weight gain, preeclampsia/eclampsia, anemia, gestational diabetes, antepartum hemorrhage, premature or small for gestational age infants, and fetal or neonatal death have nutritionally related factors and may recur in the present pregnancy. These women need very good nutritional guidance.

Pregnancy Complications

Complications that develop during the current pregnancy, such as anemia, gestational diabetes, or preeclampsia, may indicate the development of nutritional deficiencies due to increased nutritional needs. Continuing emphasis on a well-balanced diet is important, as well as specific help, possibly from a dietitian, to meet the individual needs related to the condition.

Medical History

Preexisting medical problems, including anemia, cardiac disease, diabetes, hypertension, and infections, may affect the ingestion, absorption, or utilization of nutrients. These patients will need nutritional guidance to meet their pregnancy needs and to incorporate any diet therapy for the particular condition.

Maternal Weight

Low prepregnancy weight is defined as 10% or more under the standard weight for height. Underweight women have been shown to have more pregnancy complications, and their infants a higher incidence of prematurity and low birth weight, lower Apgar scores, and increased neonatal morbidity. Improved nutrition with adequate weight gain during the pregnancy has been shown to improve the outcome.

Insufficient weight gain during pregnancy has been shown to be correlated with low birth weight infants and may indicate poor maternal and fetal nutrition. Pitkin defines it as a gain of 1 kg or less per month during the second or third trimester.[10]

Obesity is defined as a weight 20% above the standard weight for height (see the "Prenatal Weight Gain Grid" on p. 369 for standards). The obese maternity patient is at risk for developing such problems as hypertension, gestational diabetes, and thrombophlebitis. The obesity also indicates, in most cases, that her nutritional habits are not optimal. It is sometimes tempting for the obese patient to try to lose weight during pregnancy, but this can be dangerous to the fetus. When caloric intake is low enough to cause weight loss, maternal fat stores are catabolized for energy, resulting in ketonemia. Evidence suggests that ketosis is poorly tolerated by the fetus and maternal acetonuria during pregnancy has been associated with significant lowering of the IQ scores of the offspring.[11]

Kitay advised that "education in the proper foods to eat, rather than weight reduction, should be paramount during pregnancy" for the obese patient.[8] Improved dietary habits learned during pregnancy may lead to easier weight reduction after pregnancy.

Excessive weight gain during pregnancy has not been well defined, nor is there agreement on whether or not it should be considered a risk factor.

Pitkin defines excess weight gain as a gain of three kg or more per month.[11] Some studies have shown that pregnancy outcome continues to improve as maternal weight gain increases, but others indicate that there can be problems above a certain optimal gain.[12] Those favoring unrestricted weight gain cite concern that any limitation will possibly limit needed nutrients.

Dysfunctional Dietary Patterns

Dietary faddism refers to diets which are very restrictive or food habits which concentrate on certain foods or food groups to the exclusion of others. Food regimens such as the macrobiotic diet, the Atkins diet, or the Stillman diet, are insufficient for even a nonpregnant woman if pursued for a prolonged period of time. For the pregnant woman, with her increased nutritional needs, they should not be used at all. Besides endangering the fetus, they sometimes induce harmful metabolic changes in the mother.

Pica is usually defined as the craving for and ingestion of nonnutritive substances such as clay, laundry starch, raw flour, or ice. In some cases there are regional preferences for certain substances. The cause is unknown, but in many instances it appears to be related to iron deficiency anemia as either a cause or an effect. Some studies indicate that the ingested substances could lead to anemia by displacing iron-containing foods, but others have demonstrated that iron therapy can stop the cravings.[13] When large quantities are ingested there is usually some displacement of nutritious foods to the detriment of the woman's nutritional status.

Excessive use of alcohol, drugs, or *tobacco* can interfere with appetite and with the utilization of some nutrients, sometimes resulting in congenital anomalies, low birth weight, and in the case of alcohol and drugs, withdrawal symptoms in the infant after delivery. See Chapter 6 for further discussion.

Socioeconomic Status

Low income limits the amount of money available for food and may be related to an inadequate nutrient intake. Low maternal nutrient stores may also be a problem due to chronic malnutrition. There is an increased likelihood of low-birth-weight babies and other reproductive problems in low socioeconomic groups.

Ethnic or Language Differences

Ethnic or language differences may contribute to nutritional problems in the pregnant woman. She may not be able to find the foods she is used to cooking and substitutions may not furnish the same nutrients. Also, if English is not spoken, she may misunderstand or misinterpret dietary instructions or recipes.

Psychological Conditions

Depression, anorexia nervosa, and other mental problems may lead to a reduced caloric and nutrient intake. The result may be poor maternal weight gain with the possibility of low-birth-weight infants and perinatal mortality.

Dietary Counseling

Dietary evaluation and counseling may be done by one person, or it may be a shared responsibility between the doctor, nurse, nutritionist, and other members of the health-care team, depending on who is available. In any case, the nurse plays an important role because she usually sees the patient at each visit and often is the one available to answer questions. If more than one person is involved in the counseling, it is important that there be consistency in the nutritional information taught and the advice given.

Ideally, counseling about nutrition begins at the first prenatal visit, starting with the assessment of dietary intake.

As the nurse and the woman plan together, the patient's likes and dislikes are recognized, and those foods that provide the essential nutrients are encouraged. Suggestions may be given for the addition of certain foods or the modification of existing methods of selecting or preparing it. Incorporating the woman into the planning and allowing her choices whenever possible, helping her to increase her knowledge of nutrients, encouraging and reinforcing correct choices or willing adaptations, and giving firm guidance when indicated, all help the patient and the nurse to achieve their respective goals.

Many women are already eating an adequate diet. They may only need reinforcement of their dietary habits and encouragement to continue what they are doing. For those women whose dietary intake is not adequate or whose history indicates one or more risk factors, consistent counseling toward optimum nutritional intake is vitally important.

The nurse must have a tolerant and nonjudgmental attitude and should respect the patient's right to reject dietary information if she chooses. This attitude may be difficult for the nurse to achieve as health care providers traditionally expect their advice to be followed. However, more may be gained in the long run by accepting the "patient's right to choose." A patient is more likely to seek care from those she feels respect her views, even when these views differ from those of the provider.

Dietary counseling should be an ongoing aspect of prenatal care. It is not enough to talk about it at the first visit and hand out a suggested diet plan or food guide. There should be some discussion of nutrition at each follow-up visit with reinforcement or additional suggestions as needed. Periodic use of diet recall or a food diary can be helpful in assessing the extent to which the suggestions are being followed. The following sections include information on specific areas that may be helpful in counseling.

Calorie Intake and Weight Gain

Calories provide the energy requirements for the body and are needed to maintain bodily processes, thermal balance, and physical activity. Caloric allowances are established to provide for adequate energy requirements and to support growth and body weight levels for the fetus and mother which are commensurate with health and well-being.

In the past, it was generally recommended that weight gain be limited by caloric restriction, with the purpose of preventing and controlling preeclampsia and eclampsia. This idea goes back to some observations that were made after World War I. It was noted that pregnant women in Germany and Austria–Hungary gained less because of protein and fat scarcity and seemed to have a lower incidence of preeclampsia. Subsequent studies were not done and from these unsystematic observations came the notion that caloric restriction to limit weight gain protected women from preeclampsia and other pregnancy complications.

In recent years, controlled studies have been undertaken and the evidence does not support the contention that caloric intake as reflected by weight gain causes preeclampsia. To the contrary, there is evidence that limiting weight gain decreases essential nutrient intake, which is thought to be one of the contributing factors in the development of preeclampsia.

In pregnancy there is an increased need for calories to meet the energy requirements for building fetal and placental tissue and for maintaining the woman's tissue requirements. The recommended dietary allowance (RDA) is 300 Kcal/day above the woman's usual RDA. For the individual woman actual needs could vary according to many factors, including her size and activity. Vermeersch suggests calculating individual needs by allowing approximately 40 Kcal/kg of pregnant body weight or about 18 Kcal/lb.[14] In a study group at the Montreal Diet Dispensary, additional calories are recommended for specific conditions such as protein deficiency, underweight, and special conditions of stress.[7]

One of the main risks to the newborn is low birth weight and the problems that accompany it. The outcome for the infant has been shown to improve as the birth weight increases. Many studies have shown the relationship between maternal weight gain and birth weight. It is these findings, coupled with concern over the relatively high United States perinatal mortality rate, that have led to the recommendation of more liberal weight gain for the mother during pregnancy. The weight gain recommended varies from one source to another. Some suggest that unlimited weight gain might be best to ensure an adequate intake of nutrients. Others advocate a minimum gain of 24 lb or 25 lb, with a range of 24 lb to 30 lb.

In a study conducted by Naeye, optimum pregnancy weight gain was shown to be related to prepregnancy weight.[12] According to his findings mothers who began pregnancy very overweight had the lowest perinatal mortality rates when they gained 15 lb to 16 lb. For the very thin mothers, the most favorable gain was about 30 lb, and for the average weight mothers, about 20 lb. Ademowore and colleagues demonstrated that maternal weight gain alone is less important as an indicator of birth weight than the quality of nutrition.[15]

For some time, it was taught that maternal weight gain was adequate if it consisted only of the amount necessary for the products of conception, and that anything over that would just be stored by the mother as "unwanted fat." Although the exact components of weight gain and the proportions of each are not known, and probably vary from one pregnancy to another, Pitkin has diagrammed a possible distribution of average weight gain (Fig. 20-1). The following figures illustrate the approximate distribution of the chart:

	kg	lb
Fetal components		
Fetus	3.4	7½
Placenta	0.6	1½
Amniotic fluid	1.0	2¼
Maternal components		
Uterus and breasts	1.6	3½
Blood	2.0	4½
Extracellular fluid	1.6	3½
Other tissue (fat)	0.8	1¾

Please bear in mind that these figures are just rough estimates, and that if actual weights could be measured, they might differ considerably. The fat compo-

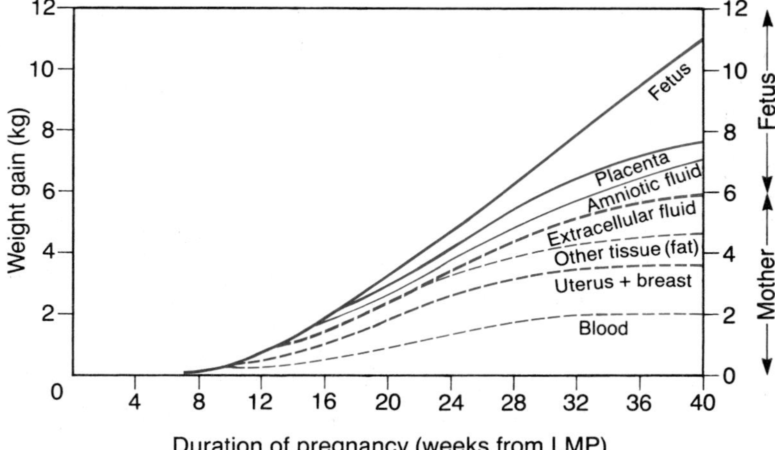

Figure 20-1. Pattern and components of cumulative gain in weight during pregnancy, assuming total gain of 11 kg. (Pitkin RM: Nutritional support in obstetrics and gynecology. Clin Obstet Gynecol 19, 3:491, September 1976)

nent is sometimes quoted as being closer to 2 kg, and in some analyses, part of the maternal gain is credited to lean muscle mass.

It is apparent from Figure 20-1 that most of the gain during the second trimester is related to maternal tissues, while the fetus gains the most during the third trimester. The pattern of total weight gain is also illustrated in this figure. This pattern is believed to be much more important than the actual amount of weight gained. The usual pattern consists of a 1 kg to 2 kg (2 lb–4 lb) weight gain during the first trimester, followed by an average, fairly steady, gain of about .4 kg (.9 lb) per week during the last two trimesters.[10]

The "Prenatal Weight Gain Grid" on page 369 shows the recommended pattern. It can be used to plot the pattern of each individual's weight gain and to detect any deviation. For example, a sudden, sharp increase in weight after the 20th week may indicate excessive water retention and the onset of pre-eclampsia. Inadequate weight gain or weight loss can also be noted.

Promoting Adequate Weight Gain

Counseling in regard to weight gain varies from one patient to another. Some women have been counseled to restrict weight with previous pregnancies or have heard about this practice from friends and believe it is the best way. They may need reassurance that gaining over 20 lb is beneficial for both themselves and the baby. Other women may think that they can limit the size of the baby and have an easier delivery if they eat less. They can be helped to understand that if the mother's nutritional status is poor, the labor and delivery might be difficult regardless of the size of the baby.

Some women are very weight conscious and may resist gaining adequate weight because of fears that they will not be able to lose it after the baby is born. Careful explanation of the distribution of the additional weight and the importance of good nutrition to the outcome of pregnancy may help them accept the weight gain. Holey states, "Knowing from her first prenatal visit that her 'temporary pounds' will influence her unborn child and prepare her for the work of motherhood is not only fascinating to the mother, but makes sense of the puzzle—'Why should I gain so much weight?'"[16]

Women who gain weight rapidly during the first two trimesters may reach what they consider to be maximum gain by the 7th month. They then attempt to cut down on what they eat to try to avoid gaining any more weight. This deprives them of adequate nutrients at the time when fetal brain cells are growing the fastest, and when the fetus is depositing a protective layer of fat.[17]

Making Calories Count

"Making calories count" is not the same as saying that pregnant women should count their calories; it is to emphasize the importance of eating only foods that contribute necessary nutrients to the diet. "Empty calories" are to be avoided, especially if the woman's appetite is poor or her food dollar is limited. The obese woman also benefits from this kind of instruction, not only during pregnancy, but also in planning a weight reduction program after pregnancy. "Eat to appetite" may be a good slogan to promote adequate weight gain during pregnancy, but it is only valid when the woman is taught which foods to eat in order to obtain the most nutrients.

The woman whose diet consists mainly of foods such as donuts, candy bars, and soda pop may satisfy her appetite, but her nutritional status suffers and she gets a very poor return for her food dollar. This does not mean that desserts must be eliminated from the diet. Custard, made from eggs and milk, is an example of a nutritious dessert. The nutritive value of other desserts such as baked goods can be improved by the use of whole grain flour and the addition of wheat germ or extra eggs and milk.

Nutrient Needs

A brief review of basic nutrition may be helpful to the nurse in teaching her clients about good nutrition during pregnancy. All foods are made up of a combination of classes of nutrients—carbohydrates, proteins, fats, vitamins, minerals, and water. Carbohydrates, proteins, and fats constitute the group referred to as "energy nutrients" because they contribute energy or "calories" to the diet. Vitamins, minerals, and water do not contribute to the caloric content of food.

Recommended Dietary Allowances (RDA)

The Food and Nutrition Board of the National Research Council sets standards for the daily intake of calories and nutrients by people in the United States (Table 20-4). The RDA is set for 18 of the 40 or so nutrients known to be needed to promote growth and maintain health. The allowances are based on available scientific data and are updated periodically. Those for the adult woman are based on the needs of a well-nourished, semisedentary reference woman between 23 years of age and 50 years of age, who weighs 120 pounds and is 64 inches tall. Allowances vary for the older or younger woman, and are increased for pregnant or lactating women. They are meant to be used as a basic reference and changed according to individual needs.

Carbohydrate

The main function of a carbohydrate is to produce energy. It is necessary in adequate amounts to spare protein for growth needs. The main sources of carbohydrate in the diet are fruits, vegetables, and grain products. The unrefined sources contribute valuable fiber. Sugars and sweets are also sources of carbohydrates, but are often called "empty calories" because they do not contribute many nutrients to the diet.

Fat

Fat is a concentrated source of energy, yielding over twice as many calories as carbohydrates. Besides supplying energy, fat in the diet provides essential fatty acids and supplies and carries the fat soluble vitamins, A, D, E, and K. Also, fats, such as butter, margarine and salad oil, add to the palatability of food.

Protein

The main function of protein is to build and repair all body cells. An increased amount is needed during pregnancy for growth and maintenance of maternal and fetal tissues. Proteins are made up of different combinations of the more than 20 amino acids. Eight of these cannot be synthesized by the body and are referred to as *essential amino acids,* which must be supplied by the diet. All eight must be present in the correct proportion at the same meal in order to be used by the body.

Proteins that contain adequate amounts of all eight essential amino acids are called *complete proteins.* Most animal sources fall into this category. Most vegetable protein sources are deficient in one or more of the essential amino acids. Those amino acids that are in short supply in any given protein are called *limiting amino acids.* The body can only use the protein to the level of the limiting amino acid, and what is left over is used for energy. Two or more "incomplete" protein sources with different limiting amino acids can be combined in the same meal and are then used as a complete protein.[18]

Vitamins

Vitamins are organic substances that are essential to life and must be supplied by the diet in minute amounts daily. They are directly involved in regulating the metabolism of carbohydrate, protein, and fat, and they assist in regulating reactions by which body tissues are maintained. Many reactions in the body require more than one vitamin, and the lack of any one can interfere with the function of another. Most vitamins cannot be synthesized by the body.

Fat-soluble vitamins are stored by the body, so large doses, especially of vitamins A and D, can be toxic. Excesses usually come from excessive supplementation, not from food sources.

Vitamin A assists in maintaining the integrity of the mucous membrane, which increases the body's resistance to infection. It is also essential for normal skeletal and tooth development and plays a role in night vision. Carotene, which is synthesized by plants and is the usual form of the vitamin in foods, is the precursor of vitamin A. Dark green and deep yellow vegetables and fruits are the best sources of vitamin A. Some foods such as milk, are fortified with vitamin A.

Vitamin D is important for its role in the absorption and utilization of calcium and phosphorus in skeletal and tooth bud formation. Egg yolk, liver, and some fish contain small amounts of vitamin D. Cod liver oil was used as a supplement for years to prevent rickets in children. Currently, most milk is fortified with 400 I.U. of vitamin D per quart. Although some vitamin D can be produced by the body from sunlight on the skin, this is not a reliable source because of the variability of exposure to the sun and interferences with the rays, such as smog or dust.

Vitamin E is primarily an antioxidant. It reduces oxidation of the polyunsaturated fatty acids, helping to maintain the integrity of the cell membranes. It is also involved in certain enzymatic and metabolic reactions. The main sources of vitamin E in the diet are vegetable fats and oils, leafy green vegetables, grains, nuts, and egg yolks.

Vitamin K is an essential factor in the formation of prothrombin, and is therefore necessary for normal blood clotting. Leafy green vegetables and pork liver are excellent dietary sources of this vitamin. Vitamin K is also synthesized by bacteria of the lower intestinal tract. Dietary deficiency is not usually a problem.

Water-soluble vitamins are not stored in any significant amount, so it is easier for deficiencies to develop than with the fat-soluble vitamins. *The B complex* actually consists of a number of different vitamins that are essential to good nutrition. The Food and Nutrition Board lists allowances for thiamin (vitamin B_1), riboflavin (vitamin B_2), niacin (vitamin B_6), folacin (folic acid), and vitamin B_{12}. They serve as components of enzymes and coenzymes in many reactions in the body, such as cell respiration, glucose oxidation, and energy metabolism. Requirements are increased to meet the increased metabolic and growth needs of pregnancy. The B vitamins are not all found together in the same foods; however, if the diet includes milk, organ and other meats, eggs, whole grain or enriched cereals and breads, legumes and dark green vegetables, most of them will probably be present. Vitamin B_{12} is only found in foods of animal origin.

Folic acid is one of the B vitamins that has received increasing attention in recent years. It is involved in

Table 20-4.
Recommended Daily Dietary Allowances for Pregnancy

	Age				Differences for Lactation
	11–14	15–18	19–22	23–50	
Body size					
Weight					
kg	46	55	55	55	
lb	101	120	120	120	
Height					
cm	157	163	163	163	
in	62	64	64	64	
Nutrients					
Energy, Kcal	2500	2400	2400	2300	+200
Protein, g	76	76	74	74	− 10
Vitamin A, RE*	1000	1000	1000	1000	+200
IU*	5000	5000	5000	5000	+1000
Vitamin D,† μg	15	15	12.5	10	same
Vitamin E,‡ Q-TE	10	10	10	10	+ 1
Ascorbic Acid, mg	70	80	80	80	+ 20
Niacin, mg NE§	17	16	16	15	+ 3
Riboflavin, mg	1.6	1.6	1.6	1.5	+ 0.2
Thiamin, mg	1.5	1.5	1.5	1.4	+ 0.1
Vitamin B_6, mg	2.4	2.6	2.6	2.6	− 0.1
Folacin, μg[11]	800	800	800	800	−300
Vitamin B_{12}, μg	4.0	4.0	4.0	4.0	same
Calcium, mg	1600	1600	1200	1200	same
Phosphorus, mg	1600	1600	1200	1200	same
Iodine, μg	175	175	175	175	+ 25
Iron, mg**	18+	18+	18+	18+	**
Magnesium, mg	450	450	450	450	same
Zinc, mg	20	20	20	20	+ 5

(After Food and Nutrition Board, National Research Council, National Academy of Sciences, Recommended Dietary Allowances, 9th ed, Washington, D.C., 1980)
The allowances are intended to provide for individual variations among most normal persons as they live in the United States under usual environmental stresses. Diets should be based on a variety of common foods in order to provide other nutrients for which human requirements have been less well defined.
*RE = Retinal Equivalent; 1 retinol equivalent = 1 μg retinol or 6 μg β carotene. 1 RE = 10 International Units.
†As cholecalciferol. 10 μg cholecalciferol = 400 IU of vitamin D.
‡α-tocopherol equivalents. 1 mg d-α tocopherol = 1 α-TE.
§1 NE (niacin equivalent) is equal to 1 mg of niacin or 60 mg of dietary trypotophan.
[11]The folacin allowances refer to dietary sources as determined by *Lactobacillus casei* assay after treatment with enzymes (conjugases) to make polyglutamyl forms of the vitamin available to the test organism.
**The increased requirement during pregnancy cannot be met by the iron content of habitual American diets nor by the existing iron stores of many women; therefore, the use of 30 mg–60 mg of supplemental iron is recommended. Iron needs during lactation are not substantially different from those of nonpregnant women, but continued supplementation of the mother for 2 months to 3 months after parturition is advisable in order to replenish stores depleted by pregnancy.

deoxyribonucleic acid (DNA) and ribonucleic acid (RNA) synthesis. If there is a lack of folic acid, cell division cannot proceed normally. Needs are increased during pregnancy for growth of the fetus and in expansion of maternal blood volume. Maternal serum folate levels are often low during pregnancy, but megaloblastic anemia, a sign of folic acid deficiency, is seldom seen. Leafy green vegetables, other green vegetables, liver, yeast, legumes, nuts, and whole grains are sources of folic acid, but as much as 80% of the vitamin may be destroyed in cooking or storage, so supplementation is often advised.[14]

Vitamin C (ascorbic acid) is essential for the formation of *collagen,* which is sometimes called the "cement" that holds the body's cells and tissues together. This helps explain the importance of vitamin C in building strong bones and teeth, healing wounds and aiding the ability of the body to withstand the stresses of injury and infection. Vitamin C is found in fresh vegetables and fruits, especially citrus fruits. Fresh strawberries, cantaloupe, pineapple, guavas, tomatoes, and the green vegetables are also good sources. Other fruits and vegetables can be important dietary sources if eaten in sufficient quantity. Vitamin C is easily destroyed by exposure to air, overcooking, or cooking in too much water. The exact amount of vitamin C needed in the diet to promote optimum health is not known, but it probably varies from person to person. Infections and stress may increase requirements. The current RDA is 60 mg for adults, with an additional 20 mg for pregnant women.

Minerals

There are 14 or more mineral elements that are essential for good nutrition. Some of these are found in fairly large amounts in the body, and others, called *trace elements* or *micronutrients,* are found in minute amounts. The minerals are constituents of vital body materials and some act as regulators and activators of body functions.

Calcium is an important constituent of bone and teeth. It is also used by the body for other functions, such as normal blood clotting, promoting muscle tone, and regulating the heart beat.

Although two thirds of the calcium in the fetus is deposited during the last month of pregnancy, the mother's daily requirement of calcium is increased during the entire course of pregnancy to prepare adequate storage for this demand. The principal foods from which calcium is obtained are cheese, eggs, oatmeal, vegetables, and milk. A quart of milk alone supplies 1.2 g of calcium.

Phosphorus is an essential constituent of all the cells and the tissues of the body. Milk provides an abundant source of phosphorus. Actually, because phosphorus is an almost invariable constituent of protein, a diet which includes sufficient protein-rich foods, such as eggs, meat, cheese, oatmeal, and green vegetables, will provide also an adequate amount of phosphorus.

Iron is one of the chief components of hemoglobin, the substance in the blood responsible for carrying oxygen to the cells. During pregnancy iron is needed to manufacture hemoglobin for fetal red blood cells as well as maternal red blood cells. During the first two trimesters of pregnancy, iron is transferred to the fetus in moderate amounts, but during the last trimester, when the fetus builds up its reserve, the amount transferred is accelerated about ten times. The diet should be rich in iron-containing foods, for example, liver, wheat germ, and egg yolks, but dietary sources of iron and limited maternal stores often cannot supply the amounts needed for pregnancy. Therefore, supplementation of 30 mg to 60 mg of elemental iron daily is recommended. A glass of citrus juice taken with the iron can enhance absorption.[19]

Iodine is only needed in very small amounts for the health of the woman and the fetus. This mineral is obtained very readily from seafoods and cod liver oil. In certain localities around the Great Lakes and in parts of the Northwest the water supply and the vegetables grown are poor in iodine. Hence, daily use of iodized salt ensures an adequate intake of iodine and prevents deficiency.

Zinc has recently been shown to be important during pregnancy. Deficiency has been linked to congenital malformations and labor and delivery complications, including prolonged labor. Meats, fish, egg yolks, and most other protein foods, have a relatively high zinc content, so a diet meeting the RDA for protein should also furnish sufficient amounts of zinc.[20]

Sodium is present in foods of animal origin, and in some vegetables, but the major dietary source is salt. There is increasing recognition of the importance of adequate sodium intake during pregnancy. In the past, like calorie restriction, restriction of salt was thought to be an important factor in the prevention of toxemia. Clinical and laboratory data now indicate that sodium requirement is increased during pregnancy. Restriction, therefore, can be harmful when imposed indiscriminately. Flowers has noted that there is a mechanism present in pregnancy that increases sodium reabsorption and retention when there is a reduction in sodium intake.[21] An adequate renal and placental blood flow demands an adequate circulating blood volume. When there is a stringent reduction in sodium intake, there is a reduction in circulating blood volume which is intolerable during pregnancy and causes damage to both the mother and fetus. Thus, the routine restriction of salt is no longer practiced. The use of diuretics for reduction of edema that was previously thought to be associated with sodium retention caused by excessive salt in the diet has also been discontinued.

Many physicians now advise patients early in the pregnancy to simply "salt their food to taste." However, this does not mean that salt intake needs to be increased, because the usual diet of most women in the United States easily meets even the increased pregnancy needs.[22]

Water and Other Fluids

Water is often omitted when nutrients are listed, but it is, in fact, a very essential nutrient. It is an important solvent that is necessary for digestion, nutrient transport to the cells, and removal of body wastes. It is also a lubricant and helps regulate body temperature.

Fluids should be taken freely, averaging six to eight glasses daily. Water and juices are good choices. Some other beverages contain ingredients that should be used sparingly in the prenatal diet. For example, regular soft drinks contain many empty calories, dietetic soft drinks contain artificial sweeteners, and cola, tea, and coffee contain caffeine (see Food Additives, p 389). Women who drink large quantities of any of these beverages should be counseled to decrease their intake. There is no definite evidence at present that tea and coffee should be eliminated from the prenatal diet. Using decaffeinated coffee and removing the teabag promptly when brewing tea helps to decrease the amount of caffeine per cup.

Vitamin and Mineral Supplements

The use of vitamin and mineral supplements during pregnancy is not universally agreed upon. Ideally, the diet should supply all the nutrients so that supplements are not necessary. Some doctors prescribe a multivitamin and mineral preparation to be "on the safe side." Others prescribe just iron and folacin because these two nutrients are difficult to obtain adequately by diet alone. Other supplements might be needed in specific circumstances, such as calcium for the woman who drinks little or no milk and vitamin B_{12} for the *vegan* vegetarian. If any vitamin or mineral supplements are used, it is important for the woman to understand that they are in addition to, not instead of, her recommended dietary intake.

Planning the Diet

The following discussion and tables provide guidelines to assist the nurse in helping the pregnant woman plan her diet. Planning a menu to include all the essential nutrients would seem impossible if each nutrient had to be considered individually. Fortunately, they are found in foods in certain combinations, so division of foods into groups according to the nutrients they supply can simplify the planning. The four basic food groups are protein foods, milk and milk products, breads and cereal, and fruits and vegetables. The Daily Food Guide further differentiates between Vitamin C-rich fruits and vegetables, dark green vegetables, and other fruits and vegetables (Table 20-5).

The Daily Food Guide is meant to be used to plan nutritionally adequate diets with patients. The woman should eat the number of servings recommended from each food group every day. The "Nutritional Teaching Guides" are helpful in selecting the foods. The "Sample Meal Plan" illustrates how the guide can be used. Note that the guide serves as a framework for the menu, but does not limit the foods that can be included. Intake varies depending on the foods selected, but using the guide leads to an average intake of adequate amounts of most of the essential nutrients. The woman should be counseled to include additional nutritious food to meet her caloric needs.

Protein Foods

Four or more servings of beef, pork, lamb, veal, or organ meats are recommended daily. Legumes (*e.g.,* dried beans, peas, and lentils) or nuts may be used as alternates. In addition to their main value of providing amino acids, these foods are also good sources of many vitamins and minerals.

Often the family's budget restricts the quantity and the variety of these proteins, especially meat. The substitution of cheese, peanut butter, poultry, fish, or legumes may then be suggested. The mother may also need advice regarding the preparation and the use of

Table 20-5.
Daily Food Guide*

Food Group	Daily Servings		
	Nonpregnant	Pregnant	Breast-Feeding
Protein foods	4	4	4
Milk and milk products	2	4	5
Breads and cereals	4	4	4
Vitamin C-rich fruits and vegetables	1	1	1
Dark green vegetables	1	1	1
Other fruits and vegetables	1	1	1

*Additions—(a) 2 tablespoons (30 ml) fats and oils each day (*e.g.,* vegetable oil, margarine, mayonnaise, salad dressing); fats and oils provide essential nutrients such as fatty acids and vitamin E; (b) Plenty of liquids—at least six 8-ounce (240 ml) glasses each day during pregnancy; plus eight 8-ounce glasses a day during breast-feeding (*e.g.,* water, milk, cocoa, fruit juice, soups, coffee, tea).

Eating Right for Your Baby. Sacramento, CA, California Department of Health Services, 1978

Sample Meal Plan

	Pregnant Woman		Lactating Woman	
Breakfast	1 svg Vitamin C-rich fruits and vegetables 1 svg grain products 1 svg milk and milk products	4 oz orange juice ½ c oatmeal with brown sugar* 8 oz milk coffee or tea*	1 svg vitamin C-rich fruits and vegetables 1 svg grain products 1 svg milk and milk products	4 oz orange juice ½ c oatmeal with brown sugar* 8 oz milk coffee or tea*
Morning Snack	Optional	*	Optional	*
Lunch	2 svgs grain products 1 svg protein foods 1 svg other fruits and vegetables 1 svg milk and milk products	1 tuna fish sandwich made with 2 slices whole wheat bread, ½ c tuna fish, diced celery and onion to taste*, mayonnaise*, lettuce* 1 small banana 8 oz milk	2 svgs grain products 1 svg protein foods 1 svg other fruits and vegetables 1 svg milk and milk products	1 tuna fish sandwich made with 2 slices whole wheat bread, ½ c tuna fish, diced celery and onion to taste*, mayonnaise*, lettuce* 1 small banana 8 oz milk
Afternoon Snack	1 svg protein foods ½ svg milk and milk products	½ c salted peanuts 4 oz milk	1 svg protein foods 1 svg milk and milk products	½ c salted peanuts 8 oz milk
Dinner	2 svgs protein foods 2 svgs leafy green vegetables 1 svg milk and milk products	6 oz roast beef ½ c egg noodles* with sauteed poppy seeds* ¾ c cut asparagus salad made with 1 c torn spinach, sliced mushrooms, and radishes to taste*, and oil and vinegar* 8 oz milk coffee or tea*	2 svgs protein foods 2 svgs leafy green vegetables 1 svg milk and milk products	6 oz roast beef ½ c egg noodles* with sauteed poppy seeds* ¾ c cut asparagus salad made with 1 c torn spinach, sliced mushrooms and radishes to taste*, oil and vinegar 8 oz milk coffee or tea*
Evening Snack	½ svg milk and milk products	2 oatmeal raisin cookies* 4 oz milk	1 svg milk and milk products	2 oatmeal raisin cookies* 8 oz milk

*This food is optional and is added to the basic diet.
(After Nutrition During Pregnancy, Sacramento, CA, California Department of Health Services pp 35–36)

the organ meats that are so rich in protein, vitamins, and minerals. Because some of these are relatively inexpensive, many women do not realize their nutritional worth and further avoid them because of the aesthetics that may be involved in the preparation—skinning, soaking, and so on. Taste also is sometimes a factor.

Nevertheless, with a little ingenuity and suggestions from a good nutrition book or cookbook, the nurse can do much to help the family use this valuable and inexpensive source of protein. Liver, for instance, can be lightly broiled, ground, and incorporated into a meatloaf or ground meat patties. The taste and looks are disguised, the nutritional value is retained, and the meat goes further.

Vegetarianism has become the dietary choice of an increasing number of people in recent years. Some abstain from eating meat for religious or health reasons, while others choose the vegetarian way to make more efficient use of the world's resources or to economize on their food bills.

Vegetarian diets vary in the extent to which they

(Text continues on page 386)

PE **Nutritional Teaching Guides**

Protein Foods

Protein builds muscle and tissue for the mother and the fetus. Besides protein, protein foods provide B vitamins and iron. B vitamins help you obtain energy from food. Iron is needed to form red blood cells.

Protein comes from both animal and vegetable sources. Each day eat a total of four servings. Try to include two servings from animal protein foods and two servings from vegetable protein foods.

Animal Protein

A serving is two oz. (60 g) unless otherwise noted.

Beef (ground, cube, roast, or chop)	
Clams	4 large or 9 small
Eggs	2 medium
Fish (fillet or steak)	
Fish sticks	3 sticks
Frankfurters	2
Lamb (ground, cube, roast, or chop)	
Luncheon meat	3 slices
Organ meats: heart, kidney, liver, tongue	
Oysters	8–12 medium
Pork, ham (ground, roast, or chop)	
Poultry (chicken, duck, turkey)	
Rabbit	
Sausage links	4 links
Shellfish (crab, lobster, scallops, shrimp)	
Spareribs	6 medium ribs
Tuna fish	
Veal (ground, cube, roast or chop)	

Vegetable Protein

Beans are the best choice from vegetable protein foods. A serving of beans contains more vitamins and minerals than a serving of nuts or seeds. A serving is any of the following:

Canned beans (garbanzo, kidney, lima, pork and beans)	1 cup (240 ml)
Dried beans and peas	1 cup (240 ml)
Nut butters (cashew butter, peanut butter, *etc*)	¼ cup (60 ml)
Nuts	½ cup (120 ml)
Sunflower seeds	½ cup (120 ml)
Tofu (soybean curd)	1 cup (240 ml)

One can get the protein needed by eating only vegetable protein foods. However, these foods should be combined with eggs and milk. Ask the physician, dietitian, or nutritionist for further information.

Milk and Milk Products

Milk and milk products are the best food sources of calcium. Calcium builds strong bones and teeth in your baby. It also keeps nerves and muscles healthy.

Milk and milk products also contain protein, several B vitamins, and vitamins A and D. Vitamin D helps the body use calcium. Vitamin A is needed for growth and vision. It also protects you from infection.

Choose four servings of milk and milk products each day if you are pregnant. Choose five servings if you are breast-feeding. A serving is 1 cup (8 oz or 240 ml) unless otherwise noted.

Cheese (except camembert and cream)	1 slice (1½ oz or 45 g)
Cheese spread	4 tablespoons (60 ml)
Cocoa made with milk	1¼ cups (10 oz or 300 ml)
Cottage cheese	1⅓ cups (320 ml)
Custard (flan)	
Ice cream	1½ cups (360 ml)
Ice milk	
Milk	
buttermilk	
chocolate (not drink)	1¼ cups (10 oz or 300 ml)
evaporated	½ cup (4 oz or 120 ml)
goat	
lowfat	
nonfat	
nonfat (made from dry milk powder)	
nonfat dry milk powder	⅓ cup (80 ml)
whole	
Milkshake	
Pudding	
Soups made with milk	1½ cups (12 oz or 360 ml)
Yogurt (plain)	

Not all milk and milk products contain vitamins A and D. Check the label.

Breads and Cereals

Breads and cereals have several nutrients important for you and your baby including B vitamins and iron. These foods may be either whole grain or enriched. It's best to eat whole grains because they contain more vitamins and minerals. Whole grains also provide fiber that helps prevent constipation.

Choose four servings of breads and cereals each day. A serving is any of the following:

Whole Grain Items

Bread (cracked, whole wheat, or rye)	1 slice
Cereal, hot (oatmeal, rolled oats, rolled wheat, cracked wheat, wheat and malted barley)	½ cup cooked (120 ml)
Cereal, ready-to-eat (puffed oats, shredded wheat, wheat flakes, granola)	¾ cup (180 ml)
Rice (brown)	½ cooked (120 ml)
Wheat germ	1 tablespoon (15 ml)

In some communities you can also buy whole wheat macaroni, noodles, and spaghetti.

Enriched Items

Bagel	1 small
Bread (all except those listed above)	1 slice
Cereal, hot (cream of wheat, cream of rice, farina, cornmeal, grits)	½ cup cooked (120 ml)
Cereal, ready-to-eat (all except those listed above)	¾ cup (180 ml)
Crackers	4
Macaroni, noodles, spaghetti	½ cup cooked (120 ml)
Pancake, waffle	1 medium (5-in or 13-cm diameter)
Rice (white)	½ cup cooked
Roll, biscuit, muffin, dumpling	1
Tortilla	1 (6-in or 15-cm diameter)

Doughnuts, cakes, pies, and cookies are not included in the breads and cereals group. These foods contain mostly calories and very few nutrients.

Vitamin C-rich Fruits and Vegetables

Vitamin C-rich fruits and vegetables contain ascorbic acid (vitamin C). This vitamin is needed to hold body cells together and to strengthen blood vessel walls. Ascorbic acid also aids in healing wounds.

Choose one serving of Vitamin C-rich fruits and vegetables each day. A serving is ¾ cup (180 ml) unless otherwise noted.

Vegetables

Bok choy	
Broccoli	1 stalk
Brussels sprouts	3–4
Cabbage	
Cauliflower	
Chili peppers (green or red)	¼ cup
Greens (collard, kale, mustard, turnip)	
Peppers (green or red)	½ medium
Tomatoes	2 medium
Watercress	

Fruits

Cantaloupe	½ medium
Grapefruit	½ large
Guava	½ small
Mango	1 medium
Orange	1 medium
Papaya	½ small
Strawberries	
Tangerine	2 large

Juices

Fruit juices and drinks with vitamin C added

Grapefruit	½ cup (4 oz or 120 ml)
Orange	½ cup (4 oz or 120 ml)
Pineapple	1½ cups (12 oz or 360 ml)
Tomato	1½ cups (12 oz or 360 ml)

Dark Green Vegetables

Dark green vegetables are an excellent source of vitamin A and folacin. A fetus needs vitamin A for bone growth and tooth formation. Vitamin A is also important for vision and resisting infections.

Folacin, a B vitamin, is needed to form red blood cells and other body cells. Cooking temperatures destroy folacin, so eat dark green vegetables raw whenever possible.

Choose one serving of dark green vegetables each day. A serving is 1 cup (240 ml) raw or ¾ cup (180 ml) cooked.

Asparagus
Bok choy
Broccoli
Brussels sprouts
Cabbage
Chicory
Endive
Escarole
Greens (beet, collard, kale, mustard, turnip)
Lettuce (dark leafy, red leaf, romaine)
Scallions
Spinach
Swiss chard
Watercress

(Continued)

PE Nutritional Teaching Guides (continued)

Other Fruits and Vegetables

Other fruits and vegetables add vitamins and minerals to your diet. Those dark yellow in color contain vitamin A. Fruits and vegetables also provide fiber which is important for normal bowel movements.

Choose one serving of other fruits and vegetables each day. A serving is ½ cup (120 ml) unless otherwise noted.

Vegetables

Artichoke	1 medium
Bamboo shoots	
Beans (green, wax)	
Bean sprouts	
Beet	
Burdock root	
Carrot	
Cauliflower	
Celery	
Corn	
Cucumber	
Eggplant	
Hominy	
Lettuce (head, boston, bibb)	
Mushrooms	
Nori seaweed	
Onion	
Parsnip	
Peas	
Pea pods	
Potato	1 medium
Radishes	
Summer squash	
Sweet potato	1 medium
Winter squash	
Yam	1 medium
Zucchini	

Fruits

Apple	1 medium
Apricot	2 medium
Banana	1 small
Berries	
Cherries	
Dates	5
Figs	2 large
Fruit cocktail	
Grapes	
Kumquats	3
Nectarine	2 medium
Peach	1 medium
Pear	1 medium
Persimmon	1 small
Pineapple	
Plums	2 medium
Prunes	4 medium
Pumpkin	¼ cup (60 ml)
Raisins	
Watermelon	

Dark yellow fruits and vegetables, such as carrots, sweet potatoes, yams, winter squash, apricots, and persimmons, are an excellent source of vitamin A.

(After Eating Right for your Baby. Sacramento, CA, California Department of Health Services, 1978)

(Continued from page 383)
exclude animal sources of protein. Lacto-ovovegetarians exclude meat, but include eggs and dairy products, and sometimes fish, poultry, and liver. Lactovegetarians exclude all animal protein sources, except dairy products, and the "pure" vegetarians or *vegan* vegetarians, exclude *all* animal sources of protein. The vegan vegetarians run the risk of developing a vitamin B_{12} deficiency because this vitamin is found only in foods of animal origin.

Vegetarian diets can be adequate if the individual is knowledgeable about the complementarity of protein and includes an appropriate selection of protein foods with different limiting amino acids to assure the presence of complete proteins (see Table 20-6). However, some of the people who subscribe to these diets do not have the requisite knowledge and resources to procure the appropriate foods. They need assistance in finding sources of information and in planning menus.

Milk and Milk Products

The expectant mother needs a quart of milk or its equivalent daily. Milk is nature's most nearly perfect food and is invaluable as a nutrient. It contains all the different kinds of mineral elements that are needed for fetal development. The high content of calcium and phosphorus in milk makes it almost indispensable for good growth of bone and teeth; it provides these minerals in the correct proportions and in a digestible form which permits optimum utilization by both mother and fetus. It is not only an excellent source of protein, but it is also the most readily digested and easily absorbed of all food proteins.

Finally, milk contains some of the most important vitamins, particularly vitamin A, which increases resistance to infection and safeguards the development of the fetus.

When a woman indicates that she does not drink milk or drinks very little, it is important to pursue the

Table 20-6.
Complementary Plant Protein Sources

Food	Amino Acids Deficient	Complementary Protein
Grains	Isoleucine	Rice + legumes
	Lysine	Corn + legumes
		Wheat + legumes
		Wheat + peanut + milk
		Wheat + sesame + soybean
		Rice + sesame
		Rice + brewer's yeast
Legumes	Tryptophan	Legumes + rice
	Methionine	Beans + wheat
		Beans + corn
		Soybeans + rice + wheat
		Soybeans + corn + milk
		Soybeans + wheat + sesame
		Soybeans + peanuts + sesame
		Soybeans + peanuts + wheat + rice
		Soybeans + sesame + wheat
Nuts and seeds	Isoleucine	Peanuts + sesame + soybeans
	Lysine	Sesame + beans
		Sesame + soybeans + wheat
		Peanuts + sunflower seeds
Vegetables	Isoleucine	Lima beans, Green peas, Brussels sprouts, Cauliflower, Broccoli } + sesame seeds or Brazil nuts or mushrooms
	Methionine	Greens + millet or converted rice

(After Lappé FM: Diet For a Small Planet. Ballantine, NY, 1975) by Frances Moore Lappé, Friends of the Earth/Ballantine, New York, 1975.

subject and find out the basis for the avoidance. She may not like milk, or be able to tolerate it well. After the cause is established, a plan can be developed with her to make milk more palatable or to include adequate substitutes.

The instant nonfat and whole dry milks may be used in a quantity that provides an adequate intake. Approximately five tablespoons of dried skim milk equals one pint of fluid milk. The milk may be used dry and worked into meatloaf, mashed potatoes, cereals, sandwich spreads, baked articles, and so on. Reconstituted with less than the usual amount of water, it has a richer taste than the regular liquid skim milk. Certain condiments and flavorings (*e.g.,* vanilla, nutmeg, cinnamon) enhance the flavor of milk. Some patients may prefer evaporated milk, buttermilk, nonfat, or lowfat milk instead of whole milk. Milk can also be taken in some other form, such as soups or custards.

Other dairy products, such as cottage cheese, ricotta cheese, farmer's cheese, hoop cheese, yogurt, and the hard cheeses are also adequate substitutions. One ounce of cheese contains approximately the same amount of minerals and vitamins as a large glass of whole milk. However, the total protein and fat content varies and must be considered when making substitutions. Cream cheese has a high percentage of fat and a low calcium content so it is not a good substitute for the other cheeses. Also, products such as "cheese foods" and "cheese spreads" are diluted and therefore contain fewer nutrients per serving.

Lactose intolerance has received increasing attention in recent years. Many adults, especially those from certain geographical areas, have difficulty digesting milk because of an insufficient amount of the enzyme lactase in the small intestine. Lactase is responsible for breaking down lactose (milk sugar) into glucose and galactose. If the available lactase is not sufficient to hydrolyze the amount of lactose ingested, fermentation occurs in the large intestine and causes abdominal cramps, diarrhea, bloating, and flatulence.

Groups of people most likely to be lactose intolerant include those whose traditional cultural food habits did not include much milk in the adult diet. These include Eskimos, aborigines of Australia, natives of New Guinea, Chinese, Thais, Filipinos, and most African Blacks.[23] Lactose intolerance is not, of course, limited to these groups. On the other hand, not every woman who says "I don't like milk" or "Milk doesn't agree with me," is lactose intolerant.

In counseling these women, special attention should be directed to meeting calcium, protein, vitamin, and mineral requirements. Some dairy products are lower in lactose than others, (see Table 20-7) and can be used in place of milk. Encouraging the lactose intolerant individual to "drink more milk" can be counter productive if it causes symptoms. Besides the discomfort from the symptoms, the increased stool frequency and mass can lead to the increased loss of nutrients, including calcium, in the feces. This, in turn, can cause a negative calcium balance.

Bread and Cereal

Four or more servings should be included from this group daily. Women should be encouraged to substitute whole grain products for white bread and cereals. Whole grains contain vitamins and minerals not

Table 20-7.
Composition and Comparison of Dairy Products

Products and Amount	Calories	Protein (g)	Lactose (g)	Lactose Ratio to Milk	Calcium (mg)	Calcium Ratio to Milk
Sandwich cheese (2 oz)						
American	210	12.6	0.96	0.09:1	364	1.4:1
Cheddar	230	14.2	1.18	0.11:1	386	1.5:1
Cream cheese	196	4.8	1.14	0.11:1	40	0.15:1
Swiss	210	15.6	0.96	0.09:1	522	2.0:1
Cottage Cheese (4 oz)						
Plain, creamed	108	14.0	2.4	0.23:1	68	0.3:1
Lowfat (2%)	96	15.6	3.7	0.36:1	100	0.4:1
Uncreamed	92	21.2	0.8	0.08:1	28	0.1:1
Ice Cream (4 oz)						
Vanilla (12% fat)	254	4.4	8.0	0.77:1	164	0.6:1
Ice Milk (4 oz)						
Vanilla	166	4.4	8.4	0.8:1	156	0.6:1
Milk (8 oz)						
Whole milk (3.5% fat)	141	7.3	10.4	1:1	260	1:1
Chocolate drink	136	7.3	9.6	0.9:1	247	0.95:1
Egg nog (6% fat)	304	10.4	12.8	1.2:1	343	1.3:1
Skimmed	73	7.3	10.4	1:1	266	1:1
Yogurt (8 oz)						
Blueberry	257	9.6	10.4	1:1	282	1:1
Plain	134	12.0	13.6	1.3:1	362	1.4:1
Strawberry	232	10.4	12.0	1.2:1	314	1.2:1
Vanilla	195	11.2	12.8	1.2:1	336	1.3:1
Milk (reconstituted; 8 oz)						
Nonfat dry	80	8.0	12.4	1.2:1	300	1.2:1
Evaporated whole	174	8.8	12.5	1.2:1	325	1.3:1
Evaporated skim	96	9.6	13.9	1.3:1	350	1.4:1
Liquid breakfast mix (1-serving envelope)						
Vanilla	130	7.0	12.2	1.2:1	50	0.2:1

Figures are calculated from nutritional analysis information provided by the Kraftco Corporation and the Carnation Company on their own products. (Luke B: Lactose intolerance during pregnancy: Significance and solutions. MCN Vol 2, No 2:95, March/April 1977)

found in refined flour and not replaced by the enriching process. When cereals are supplemented by milk, they become adequate for growth, as well as for maintaining life. The *germ* of the grain, removed in the refining process, also contains protein of value comparable to that from animal sources. Wheat germ can be purchased separately and eaten as a cereal or added to foods, such as baked goods or meatloaf to increase the nutritional value.

Cereal products are a primary source of energy in the diet, and they make an important contribution to every nutrient need except calcium, ascorbic acid, and vitamin A. When bread is buttered, it even contributes to the vitamin A intake. Whole grain cereal and breads also add fiber to the diet to help counteract constipation.

Vegetables and Fruits

Three or more servings should be included from this group. At least one serving of dark green vegetables and one serving of citrus fruits or tomatoes should be included. Some fruits and vegetables each day should be served raw.

Vegetables

Vegetables are particularly rich sources of iron, calcium, and several vitamins. The dark green vegetables are good sources of vitamin A, folacin, and iron. The deep yellow fruits and vegetables are also good sources of vitamin A. Fresh or frozen vegetables can be used interchangeably. Canned vegetables may be used if necessary, but some nutrients are lost in the cooking and canning process.

Careful preparation and cooking of vegetables helps to retain the maximum vitamin and mineral content. Presoaking should be avoided. Steaming and stir-frying are preferred methods of cooking. Steamer baskets to fit standard size pans are widely available. Some vegetables contain several incomplete proteins that add to the total protein intake.

In addition to their value as nutrient agents, these vegetables deserve an important place in the diet as laxative agents because their fibrous framework increases the bulk of the intestinal content and thereby stimulates elimination.

Fruits

Citrus fruits such as oranges, lemons, and grapefruit are the best sources of vitamin C. Most of these fruits also supply vitamins A and B. Tomatoes are also an excellent source of vitamin C, the amount, however, must be twice that of the citrus fruits to supply the same amount of vitamin. Other fruits, raw and cooked, such as prunes, raisins, apricots, contain important minerals (*e.g.,* iron and copper) as well as vitamins. Fruits may stimulate a lagging appetite and counteract constipation. They may be used as juices, combined in salads, as additions to cereals, or plain yogurt, as in between meal refreshments and in desserts, such as gelatins and puddings. Fruits contain some incomplete proteins but only supplement the other proteins.

Food Quality

Women may need to be reminded to select foods that are fresh and of good quality, as they are more appealing and safer as well. Foods that have been on the shelf a long time are more likely to begin to deteriorate or become rancid, interfering with their nutritive value. Aflatoxins and other mycotoxins are produced by fungal growths on a wide variety of foodstuffs. They can be toxic to humans and are suspected of being teratogenic and carcinogenic. Therefore, pregnant women should be warned against eating any foods that are fermented, moldy, rotten, discolored, or malodorous because they are potentially contaminated.[24]

Food Additives

Food additives are substances, added either directly or indirectly to a food, that become a component of the food or affect its functional characteristics.[25] Some additives are necessary to our food supply to prevent spoilage and ensure that certain products are safe to eat. Other additives are used to improve the flavor, odor, texture, color, or the nutritional quality of foods.

The FDA monitors additives and bans those that cause cancer or other problems in animals. There is often controversy over the safety of additives. Nitrates and nitrites, for example, can be converted by the body to nitrosamines, which have been shown to be teratogenic and carcinogenic in rats, but they are still used to preserve processed meats and other foods until adequate substitutes can be found. Recently, one of the artificial sweeteners, saccharin, has received publicity because of the possibility that it causes bladder cancer. The FDA is considering a ban on its use. BHA and BHT, which are used in many foods including cereals, oils, and snack foods, are other additives whose safety has been questioned.

Although caffeine is not really an additive, it is a substance of potential concern to the pregnant woman. There have been conflicting results, but it has been shown to be teratogenic and mutagenic in some experiments on rats and mice. There is insufficient evidence to label it as a teratogen in humans, but it should be used with caution.

Streitfeld points out that teratogenicity is usually considered to be dose related, so that, although it may

NC Nursing Care: Nutrition During Pregnancy

Assessment	Intervention	Evaluation
Nutritional status Physical Current food intake Individual factors in food selection Risk factors Patient understanding of nutrition Why good nutrition is important during pregnancy What are important nutrients Why weight gain is important	Dietary counseling Involve mother in planning Consider individual needs, preferences, and attitudes, family needs, cultural or ethnic background Provide information about nutrient needs Encourage and reinforce appropriate food choices and preparation Plan menus with patient, including foods she likes, can afford, and is able to prepare Give careful, thorough explanation of rationale for any suggested changes Teach importance of weight gain; use and discuss weight gain grid at each visit Refer to dietitian when appropriate.	Weight gain is adequate and follows recommended pattern Repeat dietary recall or food diary indicates use of Daily Food Guide and suggested changes Absence of nutritionally related problems such as preeclampsia and anemia

be impossible to eliminate additives from the diet, reducing the amount during pregnancy would lower the risks.[25] Until more is known, it is wise for the pregnant woman to read labels carefully and choose products with as few additives as possible.

Additional Resources

When consultation with a nutritionist is advisable and one is not available on the clinic or hospital staff, one may be found in the area through the local community health department or a home economist's office. Publications, visual aids, charts, and so on may be secured from city, county, and state health departments. The March of Dimes Birth Defects Foundation also provides many teaching aids and reminders about nutrition during pregnancy.

The United States Government Printing Office is another invaluable source of publications. The Food and Nutrition Board, National Research Council, Council on Foods and Nutrition, American Medical Association, American Home Economics Association, American Public Health Association are all professional organizations that offer additional resources. The above associations are only a few of the resources that the nurse and the physician have to assist their patients in planning for adequate nutrition.

If counseling is to be effective and the results lasting, the nurse should strive to elicit wholehearted cooperation from the patient. This may be facilitated by involving her in the planning; considering her needs, background, preferences, and attitudes, and those of her family; providing information; encouraging and reinforcing appropriate choices and preparation; providing gentle but firm limit setting when indicated; and giving careful, thorough explanation regarding the rationale behind the advice.

If the pregnant woman is helped to understand the importance of good nutrition for herself and her

Basic Guidelines for Good Nutrition During Pregnancy

1. Use the "Daily Food Guide" to plan each day's meals.
2. Include a wide variety of foods.
3. Gain weight gradually and steadily.
4. Salt food to taste with iodized salt.
5. Do not diet to lose weight.
6. Use supplements as prescribed.

fetus, she may be more motivated than at other times in her life to improve her dietary habits. She should be encouraged to continue her new interest in nutrition after the baby arrives. These improvements can have long-lasting effects on her family. Not only does improved nutrition promote better health for the present family, but it can have a positive effect on future pregnancies of the mother and her children.

References

1. Committee on Maternal Nutrition, Food and Nutrition Board, National Research Council: Maternal Nutrition and the Course of Pregnancy. Washington, DC, National Academy of Sciences, 1970

2. Luke B: Maternal Nutrition. Boston, Little, Brown & Co, 1979

3. Rosso P, Cramoy C: Nutrition and Pregnancy. In Winick M (ed): Nutrition—Pre and Postnatal Development, p. 176. New York, Plenum Press, 1979

4. Primrose T, Higgins A: A study in human antepartum nutrition. J Reprod Med 7, 6:257–264, December 1971

5. Winick M: Malnutrition and mental development. In Winick M (ed): Nutrition—Pre and Postnatal Development, p 52. New York, Plenum Press, 1979

6. Stein Z (ed): Famine and Human Development: The Dutch Hunger Winter of 1944–1945. New York, Oxford University Press, 1975

7. Higgins A: Montreal diet dispensary study. In Nutritional Supplementation and the Outcome of Pregnancy, p 93–110. Washington, DC, National Academy of Sciences, 1973

8. Kitay DZ: Dysfunctional antepartum nutrition. J Reprod Med Vol 7, No. 6: 251–256, December 1971

9. Nutrition During Pregnancy and Lactation. Maternal and Child Health Unit, California Department of Health, 1975

10. Pitkin RM: Nutritional support in obstetrics and gynecology. Clin Obstet Gynecol 19, 3:489–513, September 1976

11. Pitkin RM: Nutritional influences during pregnancy. Med Clin North Am 61, 1:3–14, January 1977

12. Naeye RL: Weight gain and the outcome of pregnancy. Am J Obstet Gynecol 135, 1:3–9, September 1979

13. Luke B: Understanding pica in pregnant women, MCN 2, 2:97–100, March/April 1977

14. Vermeersch J: Physiological basis of nutritional needs. In Worthington B (ed): Nutrition in Pregnancy and Lactation, 2nd ed, St Louis, CV Mosby, 1981

15. Ademowore AS, Courey NG, Kime JS: Relationships of maternal weight gain to newborn birthweight. Obstet Gynecol 39:460, 1972

16. Holey ES: Promoting adequate weight gain in pregnant women. MCN 2, 2:86–89, March/April 1977

17. Shearer M: Malnutrition in middle-class pregnant women, Birth and the Family Journal 7, 1:27–35, Spring 1980

18. Lappe FM: Diet for a Small Planet. New York, Ballantine Books, 1975

19. Robinson CH: Basic Nutrition and Diet Therapy, 4th ed. New York, Macmillan, 1980

20. Lemasters GK: Zinc insufficiency during pregnancy. JOGN Nurs 10, 2:124–125, March/April 1981

21. Flowers CE: Editorial: Nutrition in pregnancy. J Reprod Med 7:264–274, November 1971

22. Food and Nutrition Board: Recommended Dietary Allowances, 9th rev ed. Washington DC, National Research Council, Committee on Dietary Allowances, 1980

23. Luke B: Lactose intolerance during pregnancy: Significance and solutions. MCN 2, 2:92–96, March/April 1977

24. Streitfeld PP: Congenital malformation: Teratogenic foods and additives. Birth and the Family Journal 5:1, Spring 1978

25. Green ML, Harry J: Nutrition in Contemporary Nursing Practice, p 228. New York, John Wiley & Sons, 1981

Suggested Reading

California Department of Health Services: Eating Right for Your Baby, Using Vitamin/Mineral Pills and Salt, Your Weight and Weight Gain, Relief from Common Problems: Nausea, Constipation, Heartburn. In Nutrition for Pregnancy and Breastfeeding Series. Sacramento, California, 1978*

Lappe, FM: Diet for a Small Planet. New York, Ballantine, 1971

Luke B: Maternal Nutrition, Boston, Little Brown & Co. 1979

Nutrition During Pregnancy and Lactation. Sacramento, California, Maternal and Child Health Unit, California Department of Health, 1975*

Rang ML: Bibliography for nutrition in pregnancy, JOGN Nurs 9, 1:55–58, January/February 1980

Rush D, Stein Z, Susser M et al: Diet in Pregnancy: A Randomized Controlled Trial of Nutritional Supplements, New York, AR Liss, 1980

Williams ER: Vegetarian diets in pregnancy. Birth and the Family Journal 3:2, Summer 1976

Williams P: Nourishing Your Unborn Child. New York, Avon Books, 1974

Worthington–Roberts BS, Vermeersch J, Williams SR et al: Nutrition in Pregnancy and Lactation, 2nd ed. St Louis, CV Mosby, 1980

*Available without charge by writing to Department of Health, 714 P. Street, Sacramento, California 95814.

CHAPTER

21

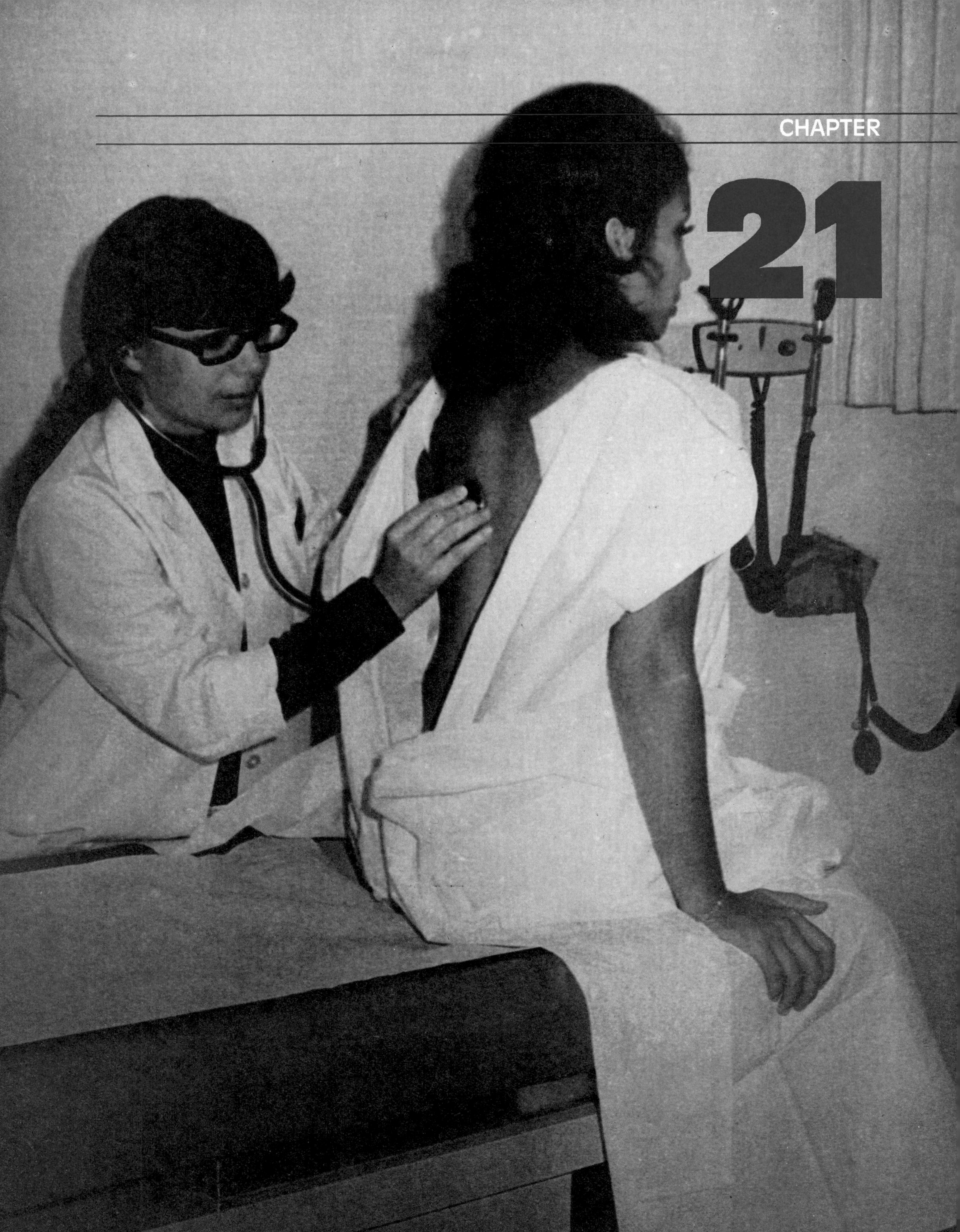

Antepartal Care

Pregnancy is a normal physiological process which only occasionally is complicated by pathological conditions dangerous to the health or life of the mother, fetus, or both. The vast majority of all births do not require active management by health professionals, as the natural reproductive process unfolds according to biological patterns adaptive for the species. Normal pregnancy does, however, significantly alter the woman's physiological systems and there is always the potential for reduction of general health status and the development of hazards for mother and fetus. The concept that pregnant women need special attention is ancient and interwoven into the social fabric of the culture.

Modern prenatal care is a relatively recent development, in which the organized health-care system assumes primary responsibility for the supervision of pregnancy and the conduct of labor and delivery. This nursing practice originated around the turn of the century in the United States when the Instructive Nursing Association in Boston began making house calls on mothers registered at the Boston Lying-In Hospital for delivery. The goal was to contribute to the health of pregnant women, who then visited the physician only for confirmation of pregnancy and were not seen again until they appeared at the hospital in labor.

Antepartal care refers to the medical and nursing supervision and care given to the pregnant woman during the period between conception and the onset of labor. Opinions vary, but generally in current practice, adequate antepartal care is that care which considers the physical, emotional, and social needs of the woman and her unborn baby, her mate, and their other children. It attempts to provide the best of medical and nursing science to protect the life and health of the mother and fetus. In addition, it takes into consideration the social conditions under which the family lives (*i.e.,* its economic status, educational level, housing, nutrition, and so on; see Chap. 5) so that the mother and fetus may pass through pregnancy, labor, and the puerperium with a maximum of mental and physical fitness. Innovative styles in delivery of care, together with the use of personnel who have a better understanding of the lifestyles of the patients they serve, are gradually and surely improving the use of health services. The goals of antepartal care are accomplished through the combined efforts of the expectant parents, the physician, the nurse, and the various other members of the health team. These goals include increasing the knowledge of the mother-to-be and her family, so that all members may experience pregnancy in a positive way, the health of mother and infant are promoted, and the family transition to include its new member proceeds smoothly.

Antepartal care may be considered the foundation for the normal development, adequate growth, and good health of the baby. During this formative period, the teeth, bones, and various systems of the body have their beginnings, and the foundations for the infant's future health are laid. Adequate antepartal care also aids in stabilizing the daily health of the mother. As pregnancy advances, the demands of the fetus increase. Since individuals react differently to pregnancy, the careful monitoring of regular care is of the utmost importance in detecting these reactions; this not only helps to relieve discomforts and to prevent accidents and complications, but it also aids in ensuring a more rapid convalescence and continued good health.

Concepts of Prevention and Early Detection

Antepartal care is often thought of as preventive care, and the relationship between early and continued medical supervision during pregnancy and positive outcome for mother and fetus are well established. Although studies that associate prenatal care with improved pregnancy outcome have been criticized on the basis that the type of woman seeking early care, rather than the care itself, is the important factor, a strong relationship is still found between prenatal care and pregnancy outcome when sociodemographic factors are taken into account.[1]

It is not clearly established which factors are really important within this complex interaction between the individual-family reproductive unit and the multiple-dimension prenatal component of the health-care delivery system. To consider but a few aspects, there is patient self-selection for timing of entry into the system, degree of compatibility between personal values and goals and norms of professionals, physical and economical access considerations, the impact of patient education and monitoring on health-promoting behaviors, and the effects of early detection of potential problems on the incidence of complications. This last factor is probably responsible for most statistical correlates between antepartal care and infant and maternal morbidity and mortality. Early detection of such problems as anemia, urinary tract infections, and preeclampsia can contribute greatly to preventing the serious consequences of these conditions which can occur if they are not treated in time.

The actual prevention of disease, and thus, promotion of better health status, precedes the development of specific illnesses. Prevention involves macroecological issues that must be addressed on the societal level. Such factors as lifestyle and associated habits related to substance abuse; exercise and diet; poverty and its relations to education, housing, living conditions, nutritional status, and vital reserve; and environmental hazards such as air pollution, chemical toxins, noise, and crowding have much more to do with health status of the population than the interventions of the medical-care system. Real prevention means alleviation of the conditions leading to poor health and establishment of conditions which encourage health-promoting behaviors. The lack of a coordinated national health policy in the United States continues to fragment and render less effective our efforts to deal with these macroecological problems.

Quality and Equity Concerns

To a large degree, the structure in which antepartal care is delivered reflects values and assumptions of the middle class. For this group, it is quite effective in assuring healthy outcomes. However, there is a disparity in pregnancy outcomes of middle-income groups and low-income groups, which is usually taken to indicate that the prevalent model of antepartal care is not effective for certain segments of the population. Many factors are involved in this disparity, including quality of medical services, use and compatibility with cultural norms and values, ability to comply with remedies and treatments prescribed, and baseline health status that often span several generations.

The lower socioeconomic groups, generally those in greatest need of good maternity care, with the highest death and sickness rates, often lack confidence in the community facilities for their care. They believe that adequate health care is a right of citizenship; however, when they seek it, they often find that two kinds of care exist—one for those who can pay and another for those who cannot. Since so many people now feel that proper health care is a right of citizenship, the provision of adequate health services for all requires a restructuring of present national priorities and an escalation of the public's social consciousness. Most health professionals agree that any worthwhile program should provide financial support and maintain the mother's dignity as well. The concept of comprehensive health planning by states and localities, including area health-education centers, community clinics, and innovative programs in hospital clinics have been an attempt to provide a higher caliber of care for all segments of society.

Within the last ten years, the focus of service in many outpatient departments and clinics of hospitals has changed from dispensing first aid to giving ambulatory care. As a result, the ambulatory care department is now one of the most dynamic, change-oriented departments in many hospitals.

As part of this change, nursing service in these ambulatory care settings has replaced the managerial role with a care-centered, more independent role in which nurses are expanding their functions of educating patients, providing supportive guidance, and making observations. In this role, the professional nurse becomes the health professional who is primarily responsible for maintaining continuity of health care for a specific patient population.

Increasingly, expanded nursing roles such as the nurse practitioner and clinical specialist are used to provide routine prenatal care in outpatient, ambulatory settings.

Distribution and Manpower Concerns

The maldistribution of health personnel, which is characteristic of our urban specialty orientation in health care, contributes to the disparity in outcomes noted among various population groups. Rural and geographically isolated communities have traditionally experienced difficulties obtaining adequate health and medical care because professional socialization and economic considerations promote practice in highly populated metropolitan areas. Inner-city areas also suffer a lack of health-care resources, largely due to economic factors and cultural differences between providers and patients.

It is becoming more and more accepted that quality maternity care in the future will be provided by a closely integrated team of physicians, professional nurses, nurse–midwives or nurse practitioners, laboratory technicians, social workers, nutritionists, health educators, and homemakers. None of these are available in sufficient numbers at the present. However, the development of expanded roles for nurses, together with training programs for the education of paraprofessionals, are proving to be viable efforts to ease this aspect of the present crisis. Research has indicated that when nurses use expanded roles and are integral members of the health-care team, there are considerably fewer broken antepartal appointments, better postpartal clinic attendance, better use of family planning services and techniques, and reduction of infant mortality.[2,3]

Government programs have been developed to encourage health professionals to enter practice in medically underserved rural or inner-city urban areas. Efforts such as the National Health Service Corps, which supports team practices between physicians and nurse practitioners in rural communities; Medicare reimbursement of nurse practitioners and physician's assistants in rural clinics; scholarships and educational subsidies for primary-care providers; and program grants for primary care to schools of nursing and medicine are steps toward ensuring greater availability and appropriate distribution of health personnel.

One of the most effective methods of providing care to underserved populations, whether they are geographically isolated or culturally unique, has been training of indigenous community members through decentralized educational programs. This often improves the quality of care. Their familiarity with the lifestyles of childbearing families, their knowledge of the socioeconomic factors to be considered, and their willingness to provide whatever service is needed, be it transportation or referral for counseling, are salient factors in the improvement of reproductive outcomes. There is a very important message in the majority of the current research on the delivery of antepartal services to the various segments of society. Programs that are planned by outsiders and that do not consider the involvement of those whom they serve are doomed to failure and in no way deliver the quality of care that they ostensibly were designed to give.

Lack of coordination and overlap in agencies presents another dimension of maldistribution of health services. For example, there may be several community-health nursing services in one area, such as the health department, a voluntary nursing agency, and school nursing services. Many times they all serve one family, but they seldom communicate with one another regarding the total needs of the family. Similarly, some hospitals may be overcrowded, while others have empty beds. Nothing is done to relieve the shortage because the first hospital may be governed by economic considerations to the exclusion of the comfort and safety of its patients.

Public Law 93-641, the National Health Planning and Resources Development Act of 1974, was intended to affect the distribution and quality of maternity services as well as other health-care services. This act established Health Systems Agencies, which are regional organizations within states that have primary responsibility for health planning and development of health services, manpower, and facilities to meet the needs of their service areas. The Health Systems Agencies are charged with the following:

1. improving the health of residents of a health-service area,
2. increasing the accessibility (including overcoming geographic, architectural, and transportation barriers), acceptability, continuity, and quality of the health services provided them,
3. restraining increases in the cost of providing them health services,
4. preventing unnecessary duplication of health resources.[4]

Guidelines for implementation of this law have been issued by the Secretary of the Department of Health, Education, and Welfare. The general thrust is to set a minimum number of deliveries per year for a hospital to maintain an obstetrical service, therefore promoting concentration of deliveries in larger regional centers to increase efficiency and cost effectiveness. There are exception clauses for small, rural communities, isolated geographic areas, and transportation distances. The continued influence of Public Law 93-641 will depend upon the levels of support provided by Congress and the administration for operation of the Health Systems Agencies.

The development of innovations such as community clinics and alternative birth centers are attempts by the health system to respond to consumer needs. Community clinics are initiated and organized by the indigenous population and are staffed largely by local people. Health professionals who share the ethnic and cultural background of the community are usually recruited. Supported largely by federal funds, community clinics can be very effective in responding to specific health-care needs of the population, served in a setting compatible with the values and style of the culture.

Alternative birth centers are special units associated with an acute hospital, which offer a more homelike atmosphere for labor and delivery. Low-risk mothers undergo labor in a comfortable room without the usual equipment and requirements of standard labor rooms and deliver in a natural position in the same bed (Fig. 21-1). Companions may be present in varying mix, and there is little intervention by the health provider beyond basic safety monitoring (see Chap. 45, Alternatives in Maternity Care).

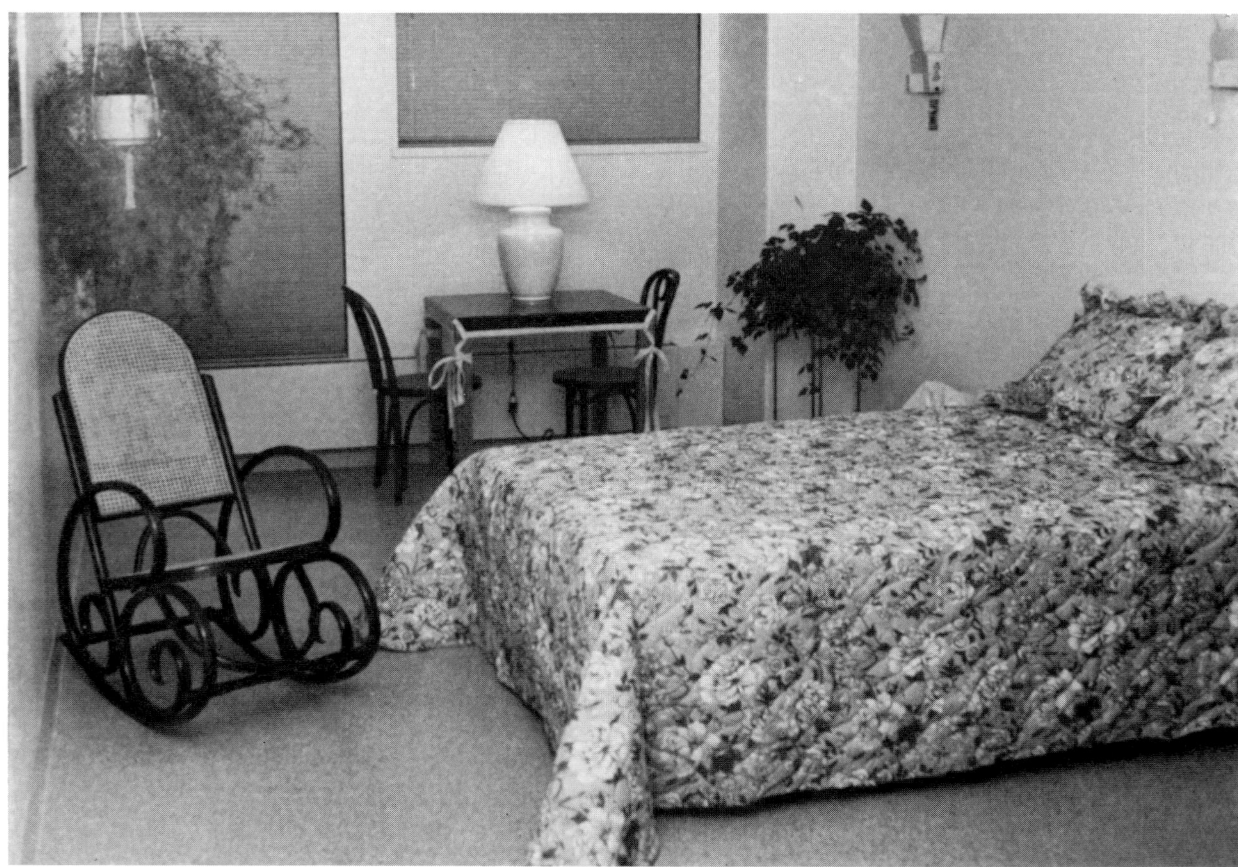

Figure 21-1.
Alternative birthing center. (Photo by Don Lorenzo, Mt. Zion Hospital and Medical Center, San Francisco. All rights reserved.)

Concerns Related to Economics of Health Care

Although the stated goals for health care on the national level include assuring quality, access, and control of costs, methods of financing services continue to support disparities among population groups. The chief protection for the medical needs of most of America's young parents is voluntary and commercial prepayment insurance. Unfortunately, the maternity benefits traditionally have been distressingly low. Young people with low incomes are frequently saddled with a large medical and hospital bill at a time when they can least afford to pay. Many professionals feel that maternity care should be entirely covered, but the actuarials believe that the rates for this kind of coverage would be prohibitive. However, it might be noted that insurance companies have had this opinion about other forms of coverage and under public pressure have increased benefits. Many community health leaders feel that the resources of this country are so vast that full coverage is feasible if there is a public mandate to provide it.

Various bills for national health insurance have been introduced in the United States Congress, but conflicting goals and assumptions continue to make it very difficult for legislators to develop a comprehensive, widely acceptable plan. Many question the commitment of the majority to the concept that equitable health care is a right of all people. Certainly our values supporting individual rights and minimum government interference and our pluralistic governmental structure provide significant obstacles to a sense of national-social purpose. The involvement of concerned health professionals in the governmental processes can help promote an equitable health-care system which is responsive to promotion of health and prevention of illness (Fig. 21-2).

Antepartal Management

Maternity care is provided by a mixture of health professionals, including physicians, nurses, nurse practitioners or clinicians, nurse specialists, social

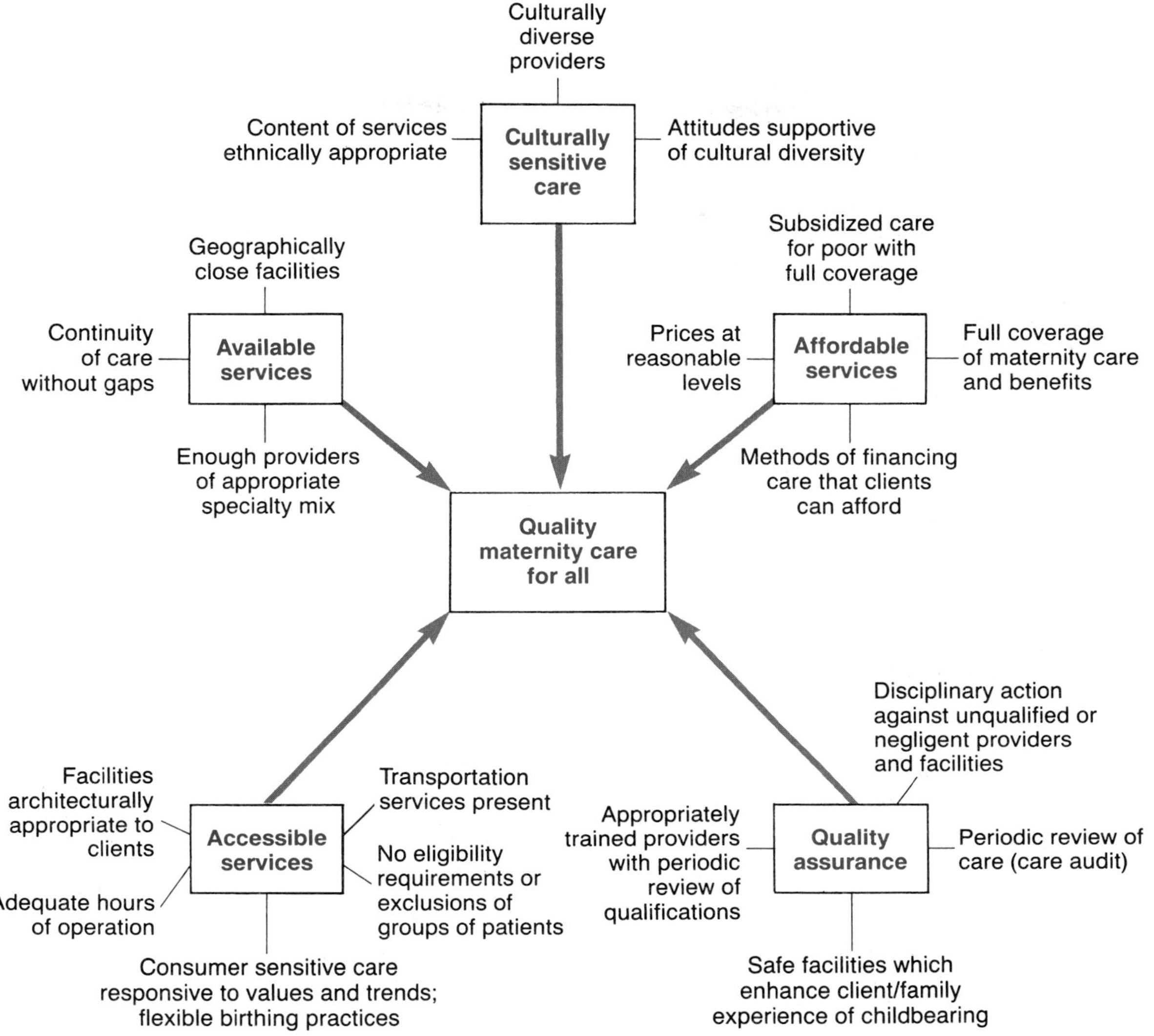

Figure 21-2.
Health-care system requirements for providing quality maternity care for all.

workers, dietitians, and other specialized personnel. Although often thought of as a team, the actual interrelations vary from an integrated, collaborative arrangement to a loosely structured, referral-type situation.

In general, physicians are diagnosticians of normal and abnormal conditions associated with the childbearing cycle. They are also technical specialists in the sense that they carry through the technical medical procedures associated with the childbearing cycle, including, of course, delivery of the infant. The nurse–midwife also shares some of these activities. However, she works under the supervision of the physician and is not responsible for the complicated or abnormal patients. She can also be teacher, counselor, and coordinator for the patient. The role of the nurse as clinician or practitioner is somewhat newer in the health-care spectrum. This nurse can be responsible for physical assessment of the patient as well as the teaching, counseling, and coordination aspects of care.

In some settings family, obstetric-gynecological, or maternity nurse practitioners assume primary responsibility for the management of uncomplicated pregnancies. Working in collaboration with a physician, who may be remote from the site, these nurse practitioners do the initial obstetrical workup, supervise the pregnancy and manage minor difficulties, coordinate other needed services, and may be involved in intrapartal care, although delivery is more commonly done by the physician or midwife. Infant care and postpartal follow-up are also assumed by the nurse practitioner.

The nurse is primarily the teacher, counselor, developer, and implementer of teaching programs and coordinator for assuring continuity of care in the total patient experience. It is apparent that all of these health professionals have some similar skills, but may differ in their orientations and their primary responsibilities.

Several variables interact to determine who provides which services to the family. The number and availability of health professionals, for instance, are crucial factors. In some rural areas, both physicians and allied health personnel are in short supply; hence, the nurse–midwives and nurses must truly fulfill every aspect of their roles. Usually a minimum of time is available and patients with the greatest need are seen in triage. This emphasizes the necessity for accurate and thorough patient assessments so that appropriate referrals can be made to other professional services. In some of the larger metropolitan clinics, there may be a surfeit of various personnel but a large patient population, and the nurse finds that coordinating and providing continuity of care must be emphasized.

Another variable influencing who provides what services is the orientation of the nurse. A nurse who is technically oriented concentrates on the technical aspects of the care. A nurse who is interested and skilled in the interpersonal and teaching aspect spends time in supportive, interpretive, and counseling activities. The nurse's strong preparation in interpersonal communication and supportive techniques as well as formal and informal teaching techniques provides an ideal background for working with total families as they move through the reproductive cycle.

Initial Prenatal Visit

When the woman thinks she may be pregnant, she makes an appointment with the physician or clinic. The visit for confirmation of pregnancy may be combined with the prenatal workup or two visits may be required, depending upon office or clinic routines. The prenatal workup consists of a thorough history, a physical examination, and laboratory tests. Prenatal forms are used by most facilities to summarize data and to serve as a flow sheet for continuing visits throughout pregnancy. Frequently the nurse is responsible for obtaining the history, collecting specimens, participating in the physical examination, and providing initial patient education and orientation to the services which are offered.

The *initial contact* with the patient is particularly important. By greeting the patient in a pleasant and professional manner the nurse can initiate a productive relationship that conveys interest and concern for the patient. In making a patient comfortable while the woman waits for her appointment with the physician, the nurse can use the opportunity to find out any questions, symptoms, or problems that the mother may have and deal with them or report them to the proper person. This is an example of one way that the nurse can use limited contacts with the patient constructively.

The History

The name and address of the patient, her age and parity, and the date of the latest menstrual period are recorded, and the date of delivery is estimated. Inquiries are made into the family history, with special reference to any condition likely to affect childbearing, such as hereditary diseases, tuberculosis, or multiple pregnancy. Then the personal history of the patient is reviewed, not only with regard to previous diseases and operations, but particularly in relation to any difficulties experienced in previous pregnancies and labors, such as miscarriages, prolonged labor, death of infant, hemorrhage, and other complications.

Inquiry is made into the history of the present pregnancy, especially in relation to nausea, edema of the feet or the face, headache, visual disturbance, vaginal bleeding, constipation, breathlessness, sleeplessness, cramps, heartburn, lower abdominal pain, vaginal discharge, and varicose veins.

As time permits, the nurse can use the initial visit to expand upon historic information for assessment purposes, both nursing and medical. The following areas are generally included:

1. Social and personal characteristics of the patient—age, marital status, occupation, ethnicity, religion, height, weight, number of children in the home;
2. Information summary of spouse (father of baby)—name, address, age, height, weight, ethnicity.
3. Characteristics influencing the course of pregnancy—estimated date of confinement (EDC), last menstrual period (LMP), blood type and Rh, pertinent medical conditions or hospitalizations, current medications and medication habits, usual bowel patterns, usual sleep patterns, resumé of dietary habits;
4. Attitudes toward the pregnancy—
   Was this child planned?
   What are the patient's goals and values regarding this pregnancy and other relevant areas?
   Does she view this pregnancy positively or as an interference in her life?

What is her knowledge about health in general and pregnancy and childrearing in particular?
Does she have any previous experience with pregnancy or childrearing?
What are her expectations and concerns about this pregnancy, birth, and care of the infant?
What is her apparent willingness or disinclination to prepare herself in the areas that need attention?

5. Resources—
   What appears to be her general level of intelligence or education?
   What is the level of economic stability?
   Is the family intact?
   Is there extended family available to her?
   Does she have sufficient friends from whom she can get tangible help and emotional support if necessary?
6. Resumé of antenatal classes and instruction—antenatal classes and films attended, individual and group instruction and counseling.

Physical Examination

A thorough physical examination is usually performed to establish a baseline for the woman's general state of health and to evaluate the pregnancy. Vital signs including temperature, blood pressure, pulse, respiration, height, and weight are taken by the nurse or attendant. The physician or nurse practitioner then performs the physical examination, paying particular attention to the teeth and throat, thyroid gland and lymph nodes, lungs, heart, breasts, skin, extremities, and abdomen (Fig. 21-3). Characteristic changes of pregnancy are noted (see Chap. 17), and signs of infection or systemic disease identified if present.

Physical indicators of high-risk pregnancy can often be determined in initial examination, such as obesity, hypertension, severe varicosities, preeclampsia, or inappropriate uterine size for dates.

Pelvic examination provides data relevant to confirming the pregnancy and determining the length of gestation, pelvic characteristics, and any abnor-

(Text continues on page 404)

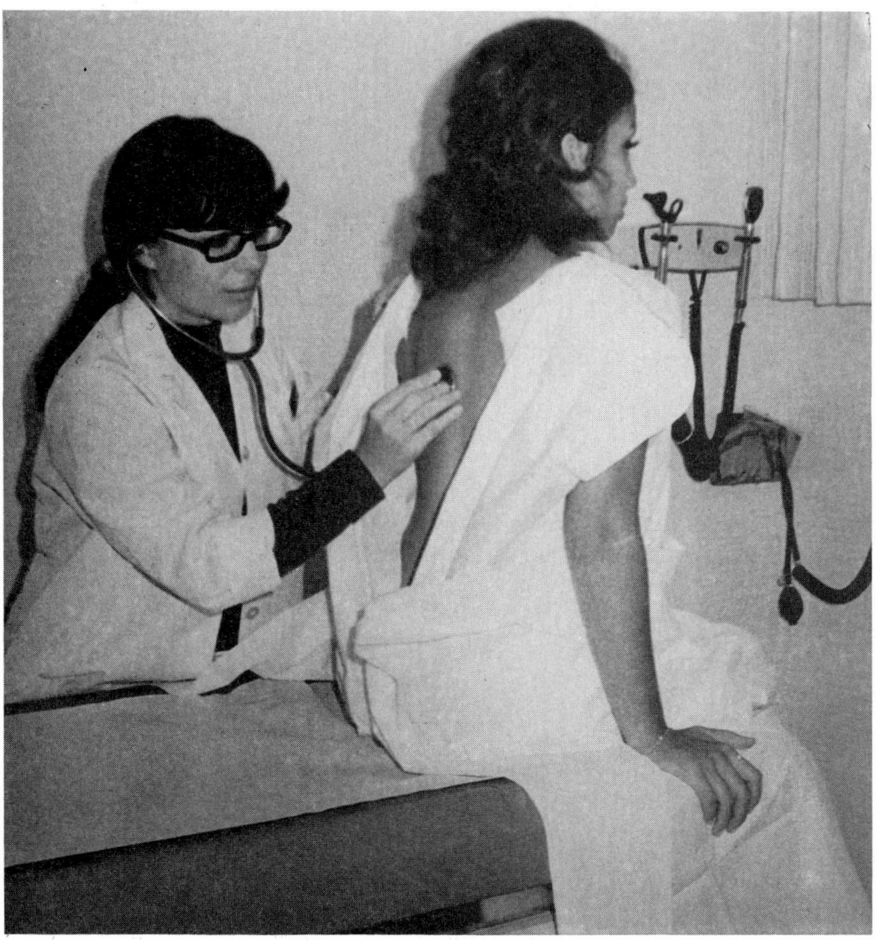

Figure 21-3.
An important part of antepartal care is the initial physical examination.

AT Prenatal Physical Examination

B.P.: ____ Height: ____ Weight: ____ Usual Weight: ____

General Appearance: ____

General Examination: ____

Head: ____ Eyes: ____ Pharynx: ____ Teeth: ____

Thyroid: ____ Skin: ____ Adenopathy: ____ Breasts: ____

Lungs: ____ Heart: ____

Extremities: Varicosities: ____ Edema: ____

Other: ____

Obstetrical Examination:

Abdominal Scars: ____ Masses: ____ Herniae: ____

Uterus: McDonald's measurement: ____ cm. F.H.: ____

Presentation: ____ Duration of gestation (estimated). ____ wks.

Abnormalities noted: ____

Pelvic examination: Introitus: ____ Vagina: ____

Cervix: ____ Corpus; Contour: ____ Size: ____

Adnexa: ____

Clinical Pelvimetry:

Examiner	Consultant
Subpubic angle: ____	Subpubic angle: ____
Bi-ischial: ____	Bi-ischial: ____
Diagonal conjugate: ____	Diagonal conjugate: ____
Sacrum: ____	Sacrum: ____
Ischial spines: ____	Ischial spines: ____
S.S. notch: ____	S.S. notch: ____
Clinical Classification: ____	Clinical Classification: ____
____ Examiner	____ Consultant M.D.

Laboratory Examination:

V.D.R.L. ____ G - C Culture ____

Chest X-Ray: ____ Tine Test - Date ____ Results ____

Hgb: ____ Hct: ____ Blood Group: ____ Rh Type: ____

Rubella titer: ____ Antibody screen: ____ Husband's Rh Type: ____

Urinalysis: Protein: ____ Glucose ____ Culture ____

Pap Smear ____

Other ____

Additional Comments: ____

____

____

____ M.D.

Name: ____ P.F.# ____

History of Previous Pregnancies (Include abortions)

No.	Year	Labor				Delivery			Child at Birth			Duration of nursing	Present health of child	Complications of pregnancy, labor, delivery, puerperium
		Spont.	Induc.	wks a EDC wks p	Hours	Method	Perineum	Place	Weight	Condition	Sex			

Family History: (Underline positive items and elaborate below): 1) Congenital anomalies 2) Diabetes 3) Heart disease 4) Hypertension 5) Renal disease 6) Tuberculosis 7) Convulsions 8) Multiple pregnancies 9) Psychiatric 10) Other ______

Past History: Operations and Injuries ______

(Underline positive items and elaborate below): 1) Transfusions 2) Drug sensitivities 3) Asthma, Hay fever 4) Allergies 5) Diabetes 6) Rheumatic fever 7) Heart disease 8) Hypertension 9) Tuberculosis 10) Urinary tract disease 11) Vascular disease 12) Venereal disease 13) Psychiatric disease 14) Other ______

Menstruation: Age of Menarche ______ Duration of Cycle ______ Amount Flow ______ Pain ______ IMB ______

History of Present Pregnancy

Vomiting Nausea ______ Urinary Symptoms ______ Date of Quickening ______ LMP ______ { Normal Abnormal

Headache ______ Abdominal Pain ______ Bleeding ______ PMP ______

Pruritus Leucorrhoea ______ Edema ______ Constipation ______ EDC ______

Medications ______ Other ______

Age ______ yrs. M S W D Sep Race: BL ______ Wh ______ Y ______ Br ______ Religion ______

Husband: Age: ______ yrs. Ht ______ Wt ______ Significant medical history ______ Husband's Occupation ______

Parity: Prior pregnancies ______ Full term ______ Premature ______ Abortions ______ Living children ______

Interviewed by ______ Physician ______ M.D.

Date	Wt.	Urine		BP	Weeks	MCD	Position	FHT	Quickening	Return

(Continued from page 401)
malities which might produce complications of pregnancy. At the same time, specimens are obtained to screen for potential problems. The pelvic examination includes both speculum and bimanual examinations. On speculum exam, the characteristics of the vaginal and cervical mucosa are examined, and vaginal discharge is evaluated. Unusual lesions are identified and biopsies are taken, as well as smears for vaginitis and cultures for gonorrhea. Papanicolaou smears to screen for cervical cancer are done routinely.

The bimanual examination provides information about the consistency of the cervix; the size, shape, and consistency of the uterus; the condition of the fallopian tubes and ovaries; and the configuration of the bony pelvis. Uterine size is useful in determining length of gestation, and pelvic measurements enable a clinical appraisal of potential pelvic contractions which might lead to cephalopelvic disproportion in labor. Other abnormalities of the birth canal, such as soft tissue masses, can also be identified.

Abdominal examination is useful in providing information about the position of the fetus after the 13th week of gestation. Leopold's maneuvers help determine position and presentation of the fetus, and auscultation of the fetal heart tones can provide an indication of fetal conditions. Fetal activity can be assessed, and the height of the fundus can be used to approximate the length of gestation by means of McDonald's technique. A flexible tape measure is used to measure the distance from the upper border of the symphysis pubis to the top of the fundus. Frequently the tape measure is curved over the mother's abdomen (Fig. 21-4) although some providers hold it straight between the fingers with the hand at a right angle to the top of the fundus. The distance measured in centimeters, multiplied by two and divided by seven gives the duration of pregnancy in lunar months. Generally, up until about 32 weeks, this distance in centimeters corresponds to the length of gestation.

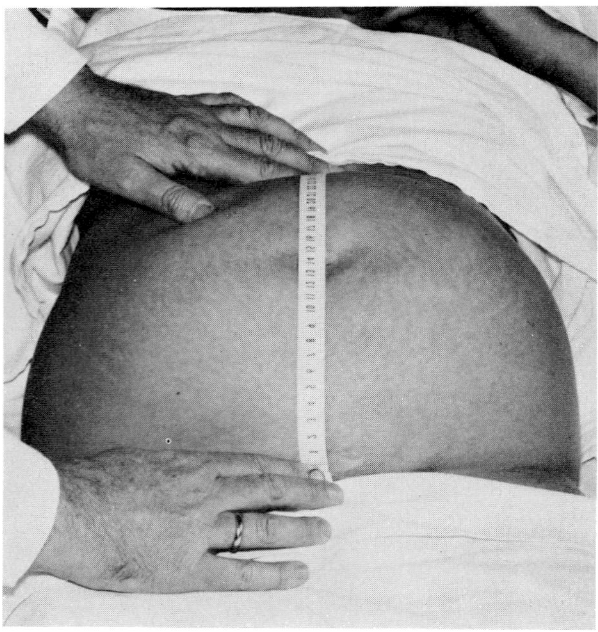

Figure 21-4.
Measuring fundus-to-symphysis distance by McDonald's method. (Danforth DN (ed): Obstetrics and Gynecology, 4th ed. Philadelphia, Harper & Row, 1982)

Role of the Nurse

While assisting the physician with the physical examination, the nurse has an opportunity to learn more about the patient's condition. Being alert to the cues and the events that transpire during this time helps the nurse interpret the physician's instructions or answer questions which the patient may ask afterward. Often a patient hesitates to discuss some matter with the physician because she considers it too trivial, but she may feel comfortable talking about it with the nurse. In turn, the nurse may consider this a problem of some importance, and on reporting it to the physician may find that it has a bearing on the course of treatment that is prescribed.

Another of the nurse's responsibilities is to prepare the patient for the physical examination. Since the initial examination is thorough, it is desirable that the patient disrobe completely and wear a gown that opens easily. In addition, the expectant mother should be covered with a small sheet to prevent unnecessary exposure and chilling. The nurse should instruct the patient to empty her bladder because a full bladder is uncomfortable and may interfere with the manipulations carried out during the examination. A good footstool is imperative if the patient is to mount the table in safety and comfort. Many patients move somewhat awkwardly, especially as they near term, and the nurse can contribute a great deal to their safety and also help alleviate embarrassment by assisting the mother to move slowly but steadily when she changes position.

The vaginal or pelvic examination deserves special consideration because often it is the most stressful part of the experience for the patient. This examination is carried out with the patient in the dorsal recumbent position. In this position the patient lies on her back with the lower extremities flexed and rotated outward. Her heels are supported in stirrups, which are level with the table, perhaps a foot in front of her buttocks. In this position the anxious patient, already under stress during the physical examination, is likely to tense her abdominal, pelvic, and thigh muscles, attempting to adduct her thighs. Moreover, if the patient arches her back as her tension increases, her pelvis will be tilted downward, a position that makes the pelvic examination almost impossible to achieve.

The nurse can be most effective in assisting the patient to relax if she encourages her to keep breathing naturally, reminds her to breathe if she holds her breath, and helps her to let the small of her back press down on the table. Merely telling the anxious patient to relax is of no avail; thus, the nurse needs to give the patient direct guidance, often step by step. For example, if the patient is clenching her fists, the nurse may say, "See, your wrists and hands are tense. Try to let them go limp—very limp—like a rag doll's. That's it—very limp." And a moment later, "Keep breathing naturally." Such short, explicit requests and instruction give the mother a simple task that she can do with guidance. This diverts her attention from the anticipated discomfort and promotes relaxation.

Steps in the Pelvic Examination

To see the cervix clearly, the examiner sits on a stool and focuses a good light into the vagina. Any equipment that is needed, such as vaginal speculum, swabs, cotton balls, slides, and lubricating jelly, should be within reach.

The pelvic examination begins with an examination of the external genitalia, including the urethra and Skene's and Bartholin's glands. If any unusual discharge is present, a specimen may be obtained for culture or microscopic examination.

Usually, the next step is to insert a speculum into the vagina to distend the folds so as to provide a clearer view of the cervix (Fig. 21-5). If a Papanicolaou smear is to be taken, no lubricating jelly is used; instead, the speculum may be rinsed under *tepid* running water to facilitate the ease of insertion. Occasionally, the dilatation of the vagina by the speculum may cause an unpleasant sensation of stretching (Fig. 21-6).

As the examination proceeds, the cervix is visualized, and the examiner notes its color and character. Normally, the cervix of the primigravida is pink or bluish and smooth, with a dimple for the os. The

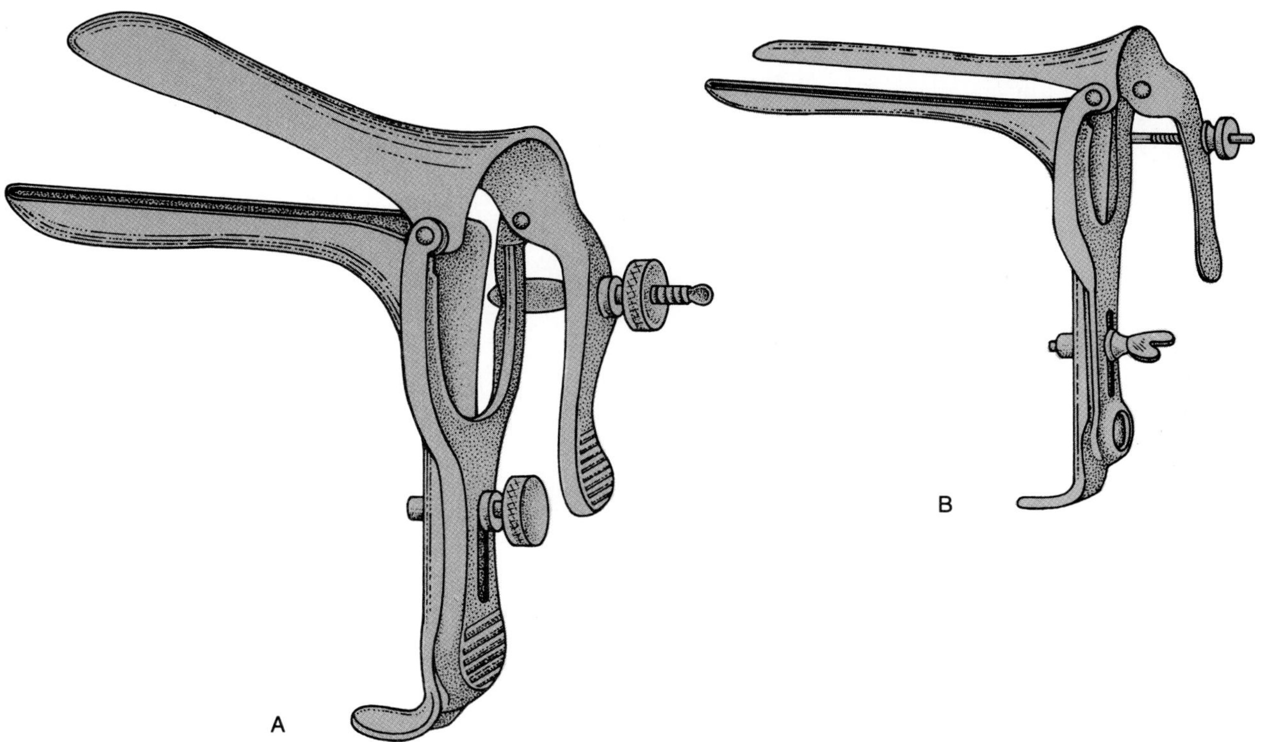

Figure 21-5.
Instruments of the gynecological examination. *(A)* Graves speculum, *(B)* Pederson speculum.

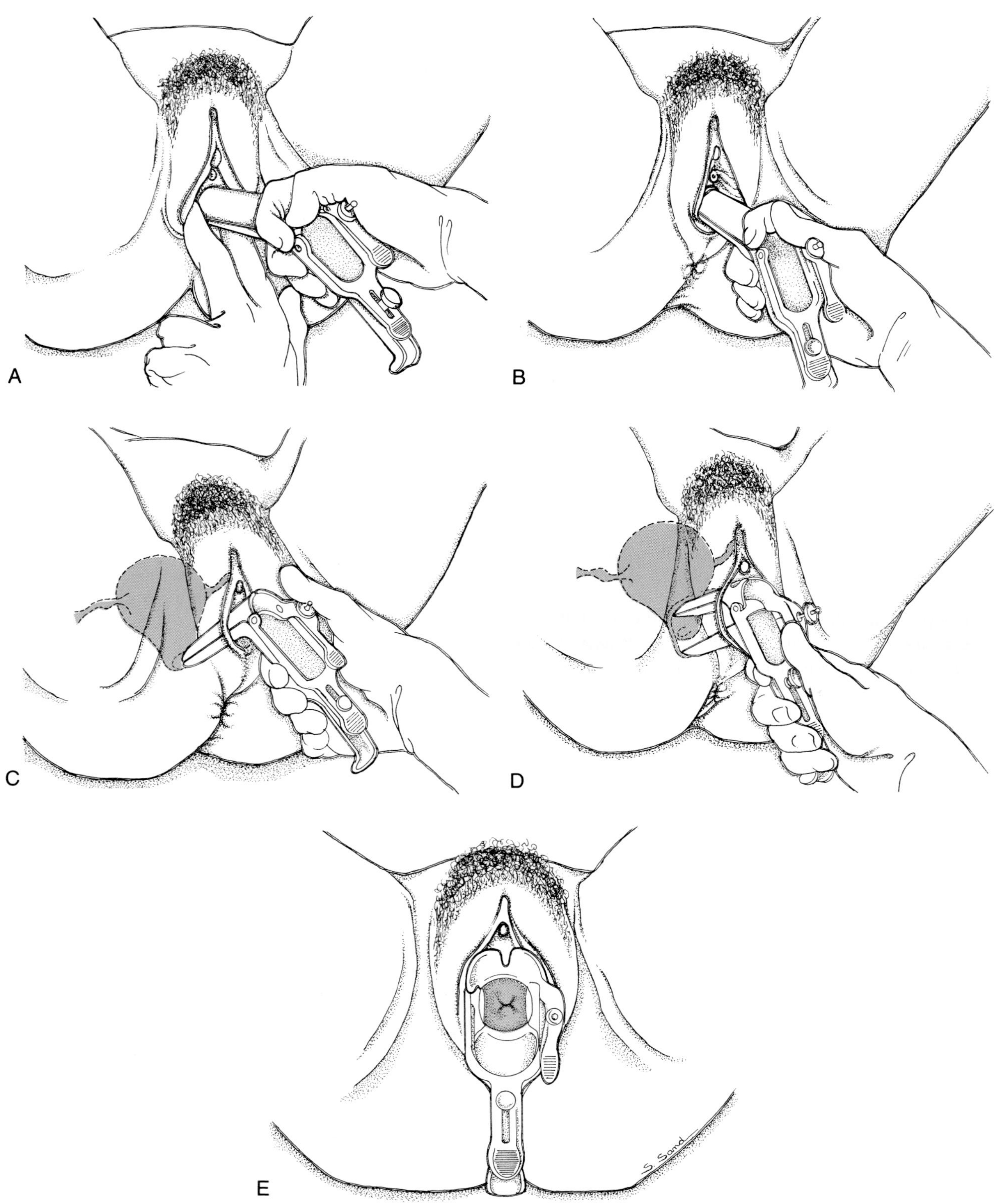

Figure 21-6.
Insertion of the speculum. *(A)* opening the introitus, *(B)* oblique insertion of speculum, *(C)* final insertion of speculum, *(D)* opening the blades of the speculum, *(E)* view of cervix through the speculum.

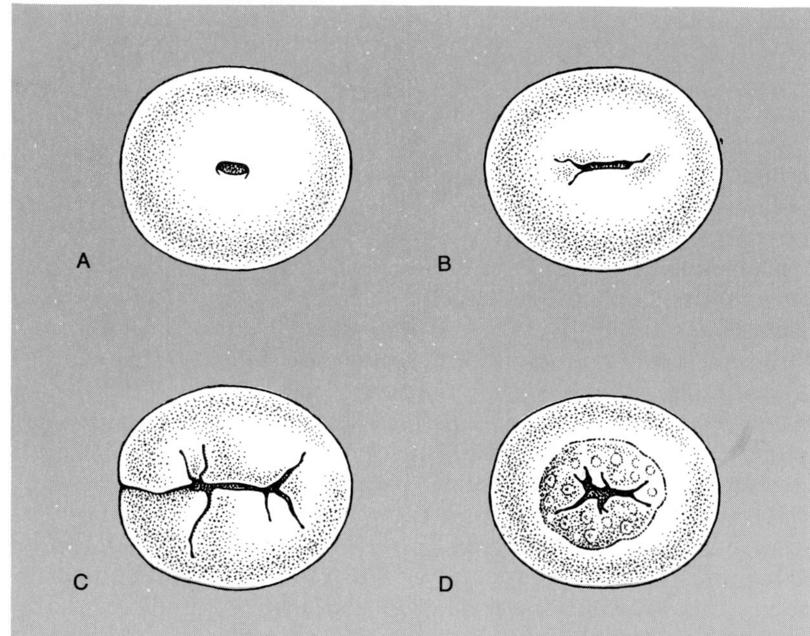

Figure 21-7.
Common appearance of the cervix. *(A)* The nulliparous cervical os is small and either round or oval. *(B)* After childbirth the os presents a slitlike appearance. *(C)* Difficult deliveries may tear the cervix, producing permanent lacerations. *(D)* Ectopion, often present in multigravidas, is a pinkish-red, bumpy tissue composed of columnar epithelium. (Redrawn from Bates B: A Guide to Physical Examination, 2nd ed. Philadelphia, JB Lippincott, 1979)

cervix of a multigravida may have an irregular os due to lacerations from previous deliveries (Fig. 21-7). Ectropion is often present around the os in multigravidas; this is a darker pinkish-red, bumpy tissue composed of columnar epithelium, which lines the endocervical canal. Unless infection is present, this tissue is considered a normal variant during the years of active estrogen secretion. Any discharge that is purulent, greenish, or frothy is considered to be abnormal, and a specimen may be secured for microscopic examination or culture.

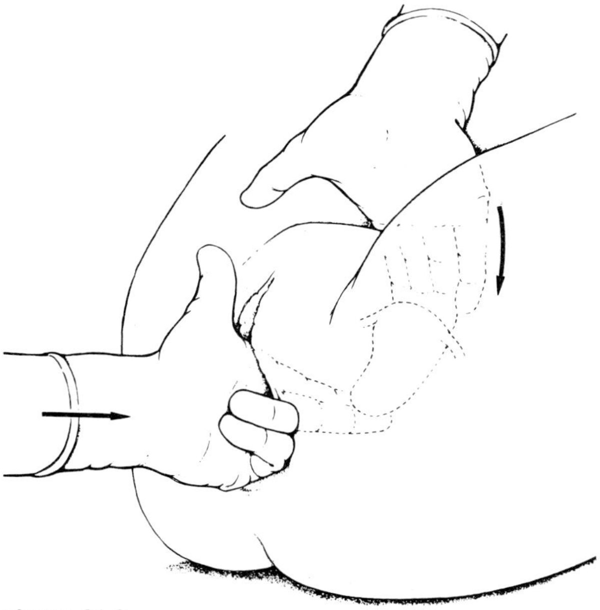

Figure 21-8.
Bimanual palpation of the uterus.

After the cervix has been examined, the examiner withdraws the speculum and proceeds with the bimanual examination to evaluate the uterus and the adnexa (Fig. 21-8). The size, consistency, and contour of these organs, as well as the relationship of the uterus to the pelvis, are determined. Pelvic measurements are taken at the same time. The examination is usually completed with an examination of the rectum to ascertain the presence of hemorrhoids, polyps, or other abnormalities.

When the examination is completed, disposable tissues should be offered the patient to wipe the perineum adequately. Optimally, further activity and demands should be kept at a minimum, so that the mother may recoup the energy which has been dissipated through trying to absorb all the new experiences and information. It is better to postpone further specific health teaching and counseling until a subsequent visit, when the patient is not so overloaded with new stimuli and fatigue.

Pap Smear. The Pap smear is obtained during speculum examination. The cervix is cleansed with a dry cotton ball to remove excess mucus, and a saline-moistened cotton-tipped applicator is introduced into the endocervical canal. It is rotated several times, withdrawn, and rolled on a glass slide. The smear is fixed immediately with commercial fixatives or immersed in 95% ethyl alcohol to prevent the specimen from drying, which distorts the cells. Next, a wooden or plastic spatula is used to obtain the ectocervical sample. The shaped end is introduced slightly into the cervical os and turned firmly several times to scrape the tissue of the squamocolumnar junction (where the endocervical epithelium meets that of the ectocervix) (Fig. 21-9). This is the area where most malignancies arise and can be seen as a color change of cervical epithelium. This specimen is smeared on a glass slide and fixed as above. Some providers place both endo- and ectocervical specimens on one slide. A vaginal pool sample may also be taken by introducing the rounded end of the spatula into the posterior vaginal fornix, or by aspirating fluid with a vaginal pipette. The smears should be accompanied with data about the woman's age, LMP, pregnancy, or postpartum, gynecological surgery, and use of hormones. Components of the Prenatal Physical Examination summarizes the techniques for examination and normal and abnormal findings, which are generally included in the prenatal physical examination.

Laboratory Tests

The laboratory tests carried out in antepartal care are the urine examination, the blood test for syphilis, complete blood count or hemoglobin, tests for the Rh factor and blood type, and often rubella titer (tests for the mother's status to rubella immunity), gonorrhea culture and antibody screening (see chart on Laboratory Tests During Pregnancy).

Urine Test

At the first and subsequent examinations, the urine is tested for albumin and sugar. The patient is instructed to collect part of the first urine voided in the morning before breakfast. The reason for this is that glucose may spill into the urine of a normal pregnant woman due to a decreased kidney threshold for glucose. Hence, it is more likely to appear in the urine after a meal. The test for sugar is the same as that used to test a diabetic's urine; several simple tests are available today and may be completed quickly and accurately in a matter of minutes.

Any positive reaction to sugar is reported so that the possibility of diabetes or a prediabetic condition can be ruled out.

The test for albumin is simple also. The principle involved here is the application of heat in chemical form, which solidifies any albumin present and causes a whitish precipitate. *The presence of albumin in the urine is another symptom of possible preeclampsia and should be reported immediately.*

Dipsticks with reagents for sugar, albumin, acetone and other urine constituents are widely used for their simplicity and convenience.

Figure 21-9.
The Pap smear. *(A)* Obtaining the endocervical sample, *(B)* obtaining the ectocervical sample.

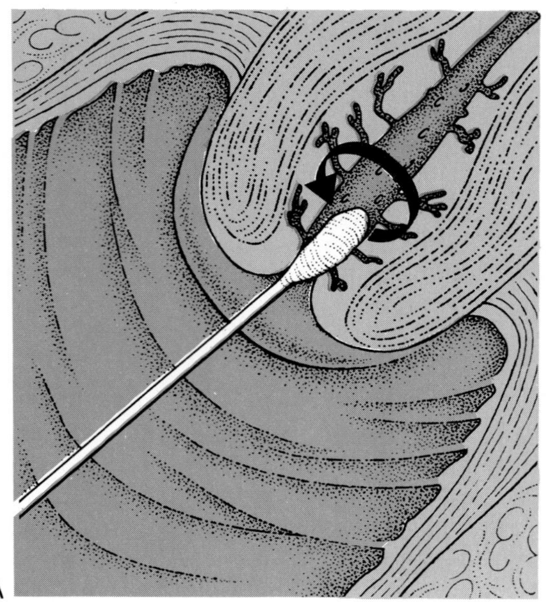

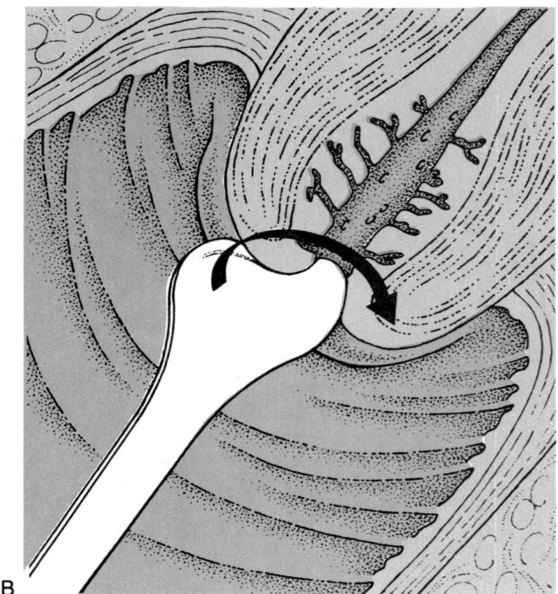

NC Nursing Care: Components of the Prenatal Physical Examination

Part Examined Examination Technique	Normal Findings	Abnormal Findings
Head and neck		
Palpation, inspection with oto-opthalmoscope, and visual inspection of mouth	Hyperemia of nasal and buccal mucous membranes, slight diffuse enlargement of thyroid	Enlarged lymph nodes, thyroid nodules or irregular enlargement, lesions of eyes or mouth, caries and abscesses of teeth, ear infections
Chest and heart		
Auscultation with stethoscope, percussion and visual inspection	Lungs clear, heart in regular rhythm (occasionally a soft, short functional murmur due to hemodynamic changes of pregnancy)	Adventitious lung sounds (rales, wheezes, ronchi), irregular cardiac rhythm, nonphysiological murmurs
Breasts		
Palpation and visual inspection	Enlargement of breasts with increased vascular patterns, darkened areola with prominant tubercles, clear fluid from nipples in later pregnancy	Masses or nodules, bloody or serosanguinous nipple discharge, nipple lesions, erythema
Skin		
Visual inspection	Pigmentation changes (linea negra, mask of pregnancy), enlargement of nevi, appearance of spider angiomas, mottled erythema of hands	Pallor, jaundice, rash, skin lesions
Extremities		
Visual inspection and palpation Percussion with reflex hammer	Mild pretibial and ankle edema in third trimester, slight edema of hands in hot weather	Limitations of motion, varicosities, more than slight pretibial, hand, or ankle edema, edema of face or sacrum, hyperreflexia and clonus
Abdomen		
Palpation, visual inspection, auscultation, percussion	Enlarged uterus, palpation of fetal outline in later pregnancy, fetal heart sounds, contractions in last trimester	Uterus too large or too small for dates, absence of fetal heart sounds beyond 10 weeks (using doppler), transverse lie of fetus, fetal head in fundus, tonic uterine contractions, enlarged liver or spleen

(Continued)

Nursing Care: Components of the Prenatal Physical Examination (Continued)

Part Examined Examination Technique	Normal Findings	Abnormal Findings
Pelvis		
Speculum exam, bimanual exam with inspection and palpation, collection of specimens	Speculum exam Bluish discoloration of mucosa of vagina and cervix, congested cervix, ectropion in multigravidas, increased leukorrhea	Speculum exam Yellow, purulent, frothy, cheesy white or homogeneous grey, foul-smelling discharge; friable, bleeding lesions of cervix; vaginal lesions; bleeding from cervical os, amniotic fluid
	Bimanual exam Cervix soft, admits a finger or two (depending upon gravida and length of pregnancy), uterus soft and enlarged, fetal head or parts may be felt in lower uterine segment, gynecoid pelvic configuration	Bimanual exam Cervix dilated and effaced (unless labor has begun); cervical or vaginal masses; excessive amniotic fluid (uterus unusually enlarged); adnexal masses or fullness; rectal masses; hemorrhoids; contractions of the pelvic inlet, midpelvis, or outlet
	Pap smear Squamous metaplasia, negative or normal, adequate or increased estrogen, endocervical cells present, hyperplasia is considered borderline	Pap Smear Inflammation, presence of *trichomonas* or fungi, diminished or absent estrogen, atypical or suspicious cells, atypical hyperplasia, dysplasia, neoplasia, or carcinoma

Blood Tests

Blood for the Venereal Disease Research Laboratories (VDRL) or other serologic tests for syphilis is usually obtained by venipuncture. A sufficient quantity of blood is drawn at this time so that a portion may be used for the Rh factor and complete blood count (CBC) or hemoglobin estimation. Since many pregnant women develop anemia, the latter examination is highly important.

If the test for the *Rh factor* shows that the patient is Rh negative, it may be necessary to check the father and do serial antibody titers throughout pregnancy. It is also a wise precaution to obtain the father's blood type (see Chap. 39).

In some states, a blood test for presence of rubella antibodies is required. Since maternal rubella during the first trimester has such devastating effects upon the fetus, it is important to know the mother's immune status so she may be counseled about possible rubella exposure during pregnancy. If the mother's titer is negative, she has no immunity and is strongly advised to stay away from small children, particularly with any symptoms of upper respiratory infections (rubella prodromal symptoms). Immunization is not done during pregnancy but should be done in nonimmune women after delivery.

Gonorrhea Culture

It is often routine to perform gonorrhea cultures as part of the prenatal workup, without ascertaining a history of exposure. This is done because gonorrhea is frequently asymptomatic in women, and is a widespread infectious disease. If the culture is positive, treatment during pregnancy can prevent possible maternal and fetal complications. Any regular sexual partner and known contacts must also be treated. (See Laboratory Tests During Pregnancy.)

Return Visits

Regular return visits are scheduled throughout pregnancy to provide continuing monitoring of maternal and fetal status, to institute treatment and further diagnostic tests as necessary, and to offer ongoing opportunity for support and education. The usual schedule

Laboratory Tests During Pregnancy

Test	Source of Specimen	Purpose
Urinalysis Sugar Albumin	Clean voided urine	Sugar (glycosuria)—screen for diabetes Albumin (proteinuria)—screen for preeclampsia, kidney stress, or renal problems
CBC Hematocrit and hemoglobin White blood count and differential Platelets	Venous blood	Hematocrit and hemoglobin—screen for anemia White blood count and differential—identify infectious processes, screen for blood dyscrasias, folic acid deficiency Platelets—assess blood clotting mechanisms
Urine culture	Clean voided urine	Diagnose urinary tract infections; often done routinely on all pregnant women; done when urinary symptoms are present to identify organism
Serological test for syphilis	Serum	Screen for syphilis (if positive must confirm with FTA-ABS)
Rh factor and blood type	Venous blood	Determine the blood type and Rh factor (positive or negative), blood type is important in case of hemorrhage; Rh factor alerts providers to possible incompatibility disease in fetus
Rh titers	Venous blood	Done when mother is Rh negative and father is Rh positive to assay danger to fetus (signified by rising titer)
Rubella antibodies	Venous blood	Determine if mother has been exposed previously to rubella and has built up antibodies (*i.e.*, is immune or not)
Gonorrhea culture	Cervical discharge	Diagnose gonorrhea; often done routinely as gonorrhea is frequently asymptomatic in women

of visits is once a month until the seventh month, every 2 weeks during the seventh and eighth months, and weekly during the ninth month until delivery. Visits are scheduled more frequently if problems arise. Routine return visits consist of follow-up history, physical examination, and patient education (See Schedule of Return Prenatal Visits and Prenatal Education Checklist).

General inquiry is made about how the patient and family are feeling and the presence of any concerns or symptoms. New signs or physical findings, such as excessive weight gain or glycosuria, are explored through a series of questions. The woman is queried about any untoward signs and symptoms, including edema of the fingers or face, bleeding, constipation, and headaches. During these visits the woman is encouraged and given ample opportunity to ask any questions of concern to her.

Weight, blood pressure, fundal height, and fetal heart tones are taken during each return visit. Weight is plotted on a graph or flow sheet and deviations from expected progression are noted and explored. The abdomen is examined for fetal position and measured according to McDonald's technique as described earlier. Legs and feet are examined for edema and development of varicosities. Other aspects of the physical examination are performed if indicated by signs or symptoms.

Vaginal examinations are usually not done on return visits until the patient nears term. Frequently vaginal exams begin about 2 weeks or 3 weeks from EDC to assess the status of the cervix, fetal presentation, and the degree of engagement. The urine is tested on each return visit for sugar and protein (albumin), and hematocrit is repeated at 32 weeks to 34 weeks as a precaution against anemia.

Schedule of Return Prenatal Visits

First through sixth month—visits once per month
Seventh and eighth months—visits every two weeks
Ninth month until delivery—visits once per week

Included in Visit	When Done
Weight	Each visit
Blood pressure	Each visit
Fundal height (McDonald's)	Each visit
Fetal heart rate	Each visit
Check for edema	Each visit
Pelvic examination	Middle of ninth month, then weekly as indicated
Other examination	As indicated by symptoms
Inquiry about symptoms, signs, or problems	Each visit
Prenatal education*	Each visit
Nutrition and appetite	Each visit
Family and personal adjustment	Each visit
Urinalysis for glucose and albumin	Each visit
Hematocrit and hemoglobin	At 32 to 34 weeks (more often if anemic)
Urine culture	As indicated by symptoms or signs
Rh titers	If initially negative, twice more during pregnancy; if positive, more often as indicated by titer levels
Other tests	As indicated by symptoms or signs

*See Prenatal Education Checklist.

AT Prenatal Education Checklist

Pregnancy and Health Status

Date	Initials	
________	________	Prenatal history and physical examination results discussed
________	________	Prenatal laboratory panel results discussed
________	________	Medications and teratology discussed
________	________	Nutritional counseling
________	________	Preferred weight gain ______________________________
________	________	Emotions of pregnancy
		The following minor problems discussed:
________	________	Constipation or hemorrhoids
________	________	Backache
________	________	Leg cramps
________	________	Stretch marks
________	________	Difficulty sleeping
________	________	Ankle edema
________	________	Nausea and vomiting
________	________	Heartburn
________	________	Varicosities
________	________	Headache
________	________	Stuffy nose and allergies

AT Prenatal Education Checklist (continued)

Pregnancy and Health Status

Date Initials

The following danger signs discussed:

- ______ ______ Vaginal bleeding
- ______ ______ Swelling of face and fingers
- ______ ______ Severe continuous headaches
- ______ ______ Dimness or blurring of vision
- ______ ______ Flashes of light before eyes
- ______ ______ Severe abdominal pain
- ______ ______ Persistent vomiting
- ______ ______ Chills and fever
- ______ ______ Sudden escape of fluid from vagina

Preventive Health Care

- ______ ______ Smoking discussed
- ______ ______ Activity, exercise, travel, working discussed
- ______ ______ Sexual activity discussed
- ______ ______ Accident prevention
- ______ ______ Dental care
- ______ ______ Alcohol discussed
- ______ ______ Community health resources
- ______ ______ Contraception discussed. Plans: ______ birth control pills, ______ IUD, ______ diaphragm, ______ foam and condom, ______ tubal ligation, ______ vasectomy, ______ rhythm or ovulation, ______ none

Preparation for Labor, Delivery, and Parenthood

- ______ ______ Prenatal classes discussed
- ______ ______ Enrolled in class: date ______ type ______
- ______ ______ Hospital arrangements discussed (visit and register)
- ______ ______ Breast-feeding versus bottle feeding discussed

  Type selected ______. Breast care taught ______.
- ______ ______ Management of labor and delivery discussed

  Anesthesia/analgesia ______

  Prepared childbirth ______
- ______ ______ Partner in delivery room discussed. Yes ______ No ______
- ______ ______ Signs of labor discussed (when to go to hospital)

Instructed on what to do about the following:

- ______ ______ Ruptured membranes
- ______ ______ Bleeding
- ______ ______ Fever
- ______ ______ Fetal monitoring equipment discussed
- ______ ______ Circumcision discussed
- ______ ______ Special requests related to birth ______.
- ______ ______ Infant care
- ______ ______ Rooming-In
- ______ ______ Pediatrician
- ______ ______ Layette

Instructions to Patients

After the routine examination the patient may be instructed regarding diet, rest and sleep, daily intestinal elimination, proper exercise, fresh air and sunshine, bathing, clothing, recreation, and dental care.

It is usually possible and always desirable to assure the woman that the findings on examination were normal and that, barring complications, she may anticipate an uneventful pregnancy followed by an uncomplicated delivery. However, at the same time, she is tactfully instructed about certain danger signals which she must report immediately. These symptoms are as follows:

Vaginal bleeding, no matter how slight
Swelling of the face or the fingers
Severe continuous headache
Dimness or blurring of vision
Flashes of light or dots before the eyes
Pain in the abdomen
Persistent vomiting
Chills and fever
Sudden escape of fluid from the vagina

In addition, the patient needs an explanation of the changes that are taking place within her body. This point cannot be stressed enough. Intelligent exploration with the patient regarding her concerns about these changes and appropriate instruction gives her greater reassurance and self-confidence. An understanding and empathic attitude does much to buoy the patient's morale and to diminish unnecessary anxiety.

As the patient approaches full term, she can also be instructed about the signs and symptoms of oncoming labor, so that she may know when the process is beginning and when to notify the physician. At this time she needs to report the frequency of contractions and any other pertinent symptoms.

Most hospitals conduct routine tours of the maternity division for the expectant parents. It is advisable to encourage them to take advantage of this opportunity sometime during the pregnancy. Becoming familiar ahead of time with the surroundings where the mother-to-be will deliver the baby reduces the anxiety that may be experienced in going to a strange hospital for the first time after labor begins. The details of the hospital admission routine are explained, so that the mother is familiar with this procedure before being admitted for delivery.

Weight

The routine estimation of weight at regular intervals during pregnancy is an important detail of antepartal care. A *marked gain* or *loss* in weight is discussed by the obstetrician. At first the average gain in weight of the fetus is 1 g daily; nine tenths of the weight is gained after the fifth month, and one half of the weight of the fetus is acquired during the last eight weeks. Most specialists agree that a weight gain of about 25 pounds to 30 pounds is desirable for a woman who is average or "normal" in her prepregnant weight. However, there is increasing evidence among investigators that the weight gain for pregnancy needs to be individualized for every patient, particularly those of under and over average prepregnant weights. In the former case, a gain of 30 pounds or more has had no deleterious effects on the mother and has resulted in a healthy normal weight infant. For all patients the emphasis is becoming less on gain per se than on a balanced nutritional status related to the patient's general physical condition.

Certainly no woman should try to lose weight during pregnancy, and even those who begin pregnancy significantly overweight must expect to gain additional weight. Explaining to the patient how pregnancy weight is distributed (see Chap. 20) helps her understand why it is necessary for normal progression of fetal development.[5]

Visual Aids and Teaching Groups

In hospitals and offices where the appointment system is used, the waiting time for the patient is minimized. In others the patient may have to wait longer periods. Waiting time in any setting may be used advantageously by providing reading material that contributes to the patient's knowledge of her condition. Visual aids such as posters and charts may be both instructive and diverting. Flannelboard posters are excellent in this respect, because they can be changed frequently. These visual aids also provide an outlet for the creative ideas of the staff.

Some offices and more and more clinics are using a group approach for discussion, teaching, and guidance. These groups are usually under the leadership of the nurse and provide a maximum amount of instruction for a large number of patients in a short period of time. In addition, in the large, busy clinic, this group discussion technique provides patients with a feeling of continuity of care since the nurse leader remains a stable figure.

Referrals

The problems that come to light are not always of a physical nature; emotional and social problems also may interfere with the patient's ability to derive full benefit from health services. It is the responsibility of the nurse to find out in what ways the patient needs help and to make appropriate referrals when they are indicated (*e.g.,* to the nurse in the community, to community services, or to other members of the extended health team). Through the use of such referrals, lines of communication can be kept open between the particular health agency, the community, and the members of the health team. This is one of the nurse's most important functions. Thus, comprehensive care for the patient is assured.

Anticipatory Guidance

The nurse in the office or the clinic can devote much nursing care to health teaching and anticipatory guidance (*i.e.,* informing mothers about what to expect regarding their pregnancy, delivery, postpartal, and childbearing periods before they begin to worry or to make mistakes). Therefore, it is necessary to have broad knowledge and understanding about the physiology of pregnancy and childbearing, general hygiene, nutrition, the emotional, psychological, and socioeconomic aspects of family living, and the part played by a family in the larger community. Teaching sessions are individualized for each patient, and should include instruction in ways of maintaining good health habits in daily living, interpretation of the reasons that these practices are important, and suggestions of ways in which undesirable habits may be changed or modified.

The first step toward this goal is to identify the level of knowledge and understanding of the patient through exploration of what the patient knows and feels about the topic in question. Second, any misinformation or misconceptions must be clarified. The final step is to add to the base of knowledge and understanding through reinterpretation, clarification, reemphasis, and reinforcement.

General Health Maintenance in Pregnancy

Pregnancy ought to be a normal, happy, healthy experience for a woman. If a woman has a good general state of health, there is no reason why pregnancy should produce physical or emotional symptoms that would significantly interfere with her ability to function and participate in her usual activities. Women are encouraged to continue their usual habits with very little change, unless they have previously been living in ways not conducive to health and well-being. Although pregnancy creates numerous physiological and psychoemotional changes, women with basically positive attitudes and good health are able to adapt without undue stress. Many find these changes intriguing and enjoyable—part of the mystery of the phenomenon of childbearing. During the months of antepartal care, the nurse has many opportunities to assist patients to attain healthier patterns of living and to reinforce health-promoting behaviors.

Rest, Relaxation, and Sleep

Because rest and sleep are so essential to health, it is important to emphasize this detail in the parent-teaching aspect of the antepartal period. Pregnant women become tired more readily; therefore, the prevention of fatigue must be stressed. The body is made up of various types of cells, each of which has a specific function. Depletion of nerve-cell energy results in fatigue, and fatigue causes certain reactions in the body that are injurious. For all body processes, such as digestion, metabolism, working, playing, and studying, nerve-cell energy is used. Nature has made provision for some reduction in normal energy without injury to health. Beyond this limit the symptoms of fatigue are evidenced in irritability, apprehension, a tendency to worry, and restlessness. These symptoms are sometimes very subtle and misleading, but in contrast, human beings are very conscious of tired muscles. It is better to avoid fatigue than to have to recover from overfatigue. The pregnant woman should rest to prevent this fatigue. Rest and sleep replenish the cell energy.

If patients cannot sleep, they can attempt to rest. Rest is the ability to relax. Patients often need to learn how to relax. There is no code so variable, so necessarily adapted to the individual, as that of rest and sleep. The final test is whether the day's work is done with zest and energy to spare.

The expectant mother ought to get as much sleep as she feels she needs. Some people need more than others. In addition to a good night's sleep, it is advisable that the mother take a nap or at least rest for a half hour every morning and afternoon. If this is not possible, shorter rest periods, preferably taken lying down (several times a day) are beneficial.

Not all mothers are able to follow the recommended rest periods. Both the woman who works throughout her pregnancy, and the mother of preschool children need special attention in planning for adequate rest. Rigid recommendations are to be avoided, and the nurse can search with the mother for minutes in her busy day that can be used for rest; again, counseling the family may be necessary to maximize the mother's free moments. Although the nurse strives for flexibility, she also needs to emphasize the necessity of this aspect of general hygiene. It can be explained that rest means not only to lie down and perhaps to sleep, but also to lie down or to sit comfortably—to rest the body, mind, abdominal muscles, legs and back, and to stretch out whenever possible, and so make it easier for the heart to pump the blood to the extremities.

During the last months of pregnancy, a small pillow used for support of the abdomen while the patient lies on her side does much to relieve the discomfort common during this period and adds materially to the degree of rest that the patient gets in a given time.

It should be suggested that the patient sit whenever possible, even while doing her housework. Sitting to rest for other brief periods during the course of the day can be beneficial if the feet and legs are elevated.

Often certain minor discomforts of pregnancy can be overcome by rest. Rest and the right-angle position (see Fig. 19-16) are advised for swelling, edema, and varicosities of the lower extremities. Rest and Sims's position (see Fig. 21-11) are advised for varicosities of the vulva and the rectum. Even for the more serious abnormalities, the simple aids included in "diet and rest" may help measurably until more specific orders from the obstetrician can be obtained. In such instances, the nurse must be aware of the mother's interpretation of "rest," and, if indicated, she can provide the necessary guidance to help the mother to understand and to plan for it.

Exercise

Outdoor exercise during pregnancy is usually very beneficial because it affords diversion in the sunshine and fresh air. However, the degree of exercise recommended depends on the individual woman, her general condition, and the stage of pregnancy.

There are differences in the amount of exercise for the early and late periods of pregnancy. When pregnancy is advanced, exercise may be limited in comparison with the amount advised previously. Exercise provides a welcome diversion, reduces anxiety and tension, quiets the mind, promotes sleep, and stimulates the appetite, all of which are valuable aids to the pregnant mother.

Walking in the fresh air is generally a preferred form of exercise during pregnancy because it stimulates the muscular activity of the entire body, strengthens some of the muscles used during labor, and is available to all women. Exercise of any kind should not be fatiguing; to secure the most beneficial results, it should be combined with fresh air and sunlight, as well as periods of rest.

Interest in active exercise has been increasing among pregnant women, as in the general population. More women are exercising strenuously during pregnancy than in previous years. It is not unusual to see pregnant women regularly engaged in physically demanding work or sports and doing aerobic exercises such as running, bicycling, climbing stairs, and swimming. The research to date indicates that most fetuses can tolerate strenuous maternal exercise when women are accustomed to this level of activity and continue exercise programs into their pregnancies. New strenuous exercise should not begin during pregnancy, and women need their physician's approval before undertaking any strenuous exercise program. In physically fit women, the ventilatory reserve and cardiovascular changes of pregnancy contribute to increased fetal tolerance of the circulatory and respiratory challenges of strenuous maternal exercise.[6]

Prenatal exercises are a standard component of childbirth education, but approaches vary widely according to the type of childbirth preparation. Most programs include exercises that strengthen abdominal muscles, relax muscles of the pelvic floor, teach the pelvic tilt, stretch and adduct the thighs, limbering exercises such as arm swinging and squatting, and bridging exercises such as tailor sitting, back arching, and ankle circling (see Chap. 19). For women who are not accustomed to exercising regularly, data indicate that even well-motivated patients do not remember to practice more than three exercises daily.[7] Exercises must therefore be adapted to each individual, and concentrate on those areas most in need of attention. Women with poor posture, (*e.g.,* lordosis, protruding abdomen, and locked knees) need to learn the pelvic tilt which flattens the low back, rotates the pelvis upward in front, pulls the abdomen in, and unlocks the knees. Maintaining this posture for increasing amounts of time, while remembering to breathe regularly, is a great aid to prevention of backache and fatigue. Other women may need abdominal strengthening exercises such as sit-ups or leg lifts, or thigh stretching exercises such as tailor sitting (See Common Prenatal Exercises).

Most pregnant women benefit from a combination of moderate aerobic exercises and specific prenatal exercises. Standing or sitting for long periods of time should be avoided. Adequate exercise not only promotes a general sense of well-being, but can also aid in preventing several minor discomforts of pregnancy. Lifting heavy objects, moving furniture, reaching to hang curtains, any activity which might involve sudden jolts, sudden changes in balance which might result in a fall or the likelihood of physical trauma should be avoided.

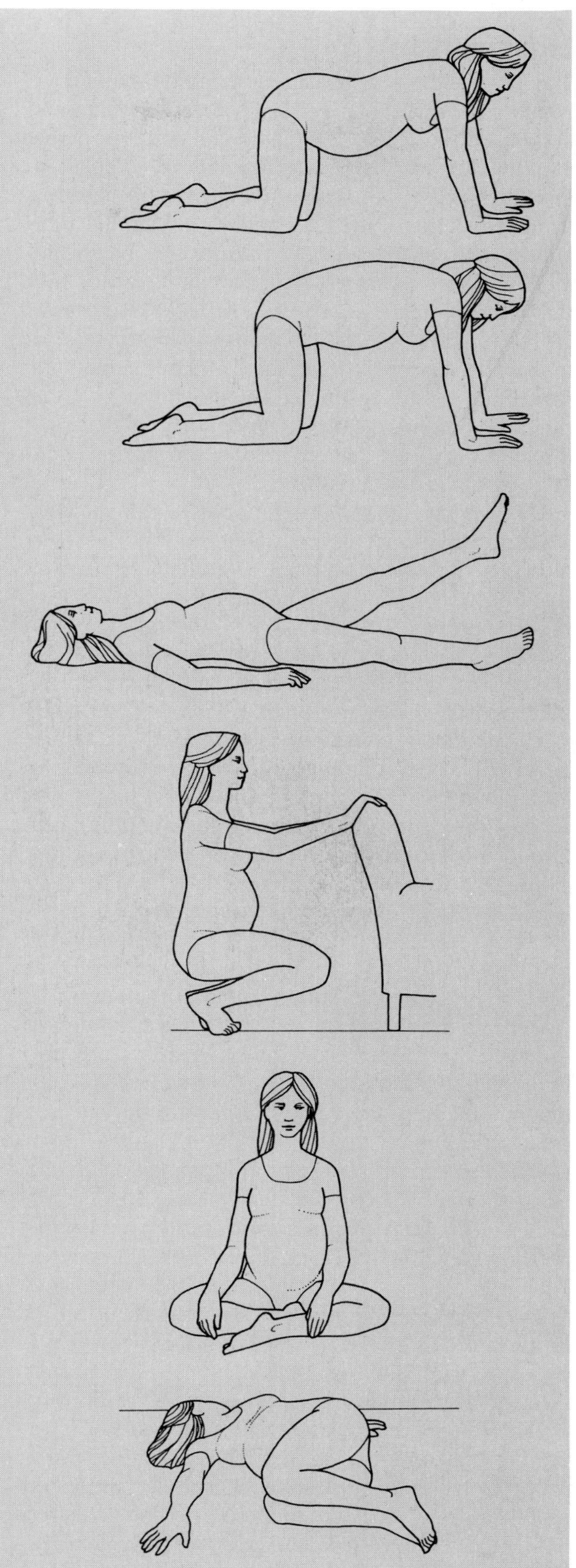

Pelvic Tilt

Buttocks are tucked under to flatten out the hollow of the lower back. Hold for 3 seconds. Then relax, allowing hips to move back to former position. Repeat several times. This exercise may be done sitting, standing, on the hands and knees, or lying on the floor. This exercise strengthens back and abdominal muscles and relieves backache.

Leg Raising

Alternate raising of the legs while lying on the floor strengthens abdominal muscles and improves their tone.

Knee Bends

Deep knee bends using a chair for stabilization will strengthen back muscles, and will keep leg and hip joints supple.

Tailor Sitting

Sitting on the floor with one foot in front of the other, tucked inward toward the perineum, and with the knees pressed downward toward the floor, is tailor sitting. This aids in relaxing muscles of the pelvic floor, helps relieve backache, and stretches thigh muscles.

Knee–Chest Twist

Lying on the back, the knees are pulled to the chest and arms stretched straight to the sides. The knees are rolled to one side, while the head is turned to the opposite side. Sides are switched and repeated. This stretches the spine and relieves backache.

Employment

The same attitude of moderation can be maintained whether for work or play. Ideally, any activity should not be continued to the extent of even moderate fatigue; however, it is not realistic to expect the mother to willingly discontinue her job because it is tiring, especially if it is essential to the family sustenance. If her employment is influencing her health adversely, the matter needs conscientious exploration by the health team to see what realistic adjustments can be made. A referral to a social worker may be indicated to better ascertain the economic situation of the family or the resources in the community that might be helpful. Different job opportunities can be discussed, and the patient's skills, satisfactions, and preparation can be considered.

In general, jobs requiring moderate manual labor should be avoided if they must be continued over long hours, or if they require delicate balance, constant standing, or constant working on night shifts. Actually, the woman who has a "desk job" in an office often does less strenuous work than the average homemaker who does not go out to work. Nevertheless, positions which require the worker to sit constantly can be extremely tiring. Adequate rest periods should be provided for all pregnant women employed in such positions.

In some countries the time of discontinuing routine jobs has been regulated by law, and the limits, although arbitrary, are generally from six to eight weeks prior to the expected date of confinement.

Many women are employed in industry, and the problem of pregnancy for the working mother in this type of employment is a most important one. To safeguard the interests of expectant mothers so engaged, the Standards for Maternity Care and Employment of Mothers in Industry have been recommended by the United States Children's Bureau (see chart on page 42).

The environmental risks to pregnant women and occupational hazards to those employed in certain industries have received considerable attention in recent years. Ten percent of all birth defects are known to be caused by environmental agents, and another sixty-five percent to seventy percent are of unknown origin. Environmental and workplace exposure to toxins may be responsible for most of these developmental defects. With women composing nearly half of the work force, the problem of intrauterine exposure to toxic substances is one of major proportions. Many industrial chemicals have been found hazardous to reproduction. Vinyl chloride used in the plastic industry, the agricultural pesticide dibromochloropropane, chloroprene, which is used in rubber industries, and hydrocarbons which are used in numerous industries, are capable of causing reproductive failure in both men and women. Among wives of male operating room personnel exposed to anesthetic gases, a 25% increase over expected incidence of birth defects was found. Hexachlorophene and radiation exposures among health workers are associated with congenital malformations and diseases. Hair dyes used by beauticians are capable of causing mutations in lab experiments. Textile workers exposed to cotton dust are at risk for byssinosis (brown lung), which reduces fetal oxygenation as a result of maternal bronchial disorders. Benzene, used in textile industries, can cause chromosomal aberrations. Exposures to lead, mercury, lithium, and the solvents toluene and xylene occur among workers in the arts and crafts industry. Chronic poisoning by such compounds has implications for fetal development and well-being.[8]

Environmental contamination poses a risk to any pregnant woman exposed to toxic substances. The use of pesticides in agriculture, forestry, and lawn care is of growing concern. Dioxin, a degradation product of the pesticide 2,4,5T (Agent Orange, used as a defoliant in Vietnam) is known to cause mutations and birth defects and miscarriages in laboratory animals. When this agent was sprayed in Alsea, Oregon in 1979, the incidence of miscarriage among women living in the area increased significantly. Two other widely used pesticides, heptachlor and chlordane, are carcinogenic in animals, and possibly linked to causing neuroblastomas and leukemia in prenatally and postnatally exposed children.[8] Pregnant women are advised to avoid using such agents at home (on lawn and gardens) and prevent exposure at work (*i.e.*, nurseries).

The prenatal history should include assessment of possible work, home, or environmental exposure to toxins. Appropriate teaching and counseling by the nurse helps the patient to make a more informed decision about the risks and benefits of working in a potentially hazardous environment. Steps to avoid or minimize exposure can be identified. Table 21-1 summarizes occupations commonly held by women, potential occupational hazards, and known or suspected effects on reproduction.

Recreation

Recreation is as necessary during pregnancy as it is at any other time in life. The patient is preparing for one of the most important role changes that she will undergo during her lifetime, and concomitant with any such change is the production of anxiety. It is to be

Table 21-1.
Occupations Commonly Held by Women and Potential Occupational Hazards

Occupation	Potential Hazard	Known or Suspected Effects on Reproduction
Hospital workers Nurses Anesthetists Lab technicians Physicians Dentists Dental assistants	Radiation	Chromosomal aberrations, sterility, birth defects, leukemia, miscarriages, retarded fetal development, carcinogen
	Benzene	Chromosomal aberrations, aplastic anemia and leukemia, prolonged menstrual periods
	BIS (Chloromethyl ether)	Known human carcinogen, possible fetal effects (BIS ether formed by combination of formaldehyde and HCl in warm, moist air)
	Toluene	Chromosomal aberrations (derivative of benzene, less toxic)
	Anesthetic gases	Birth defects, miscarriages, infertility, low-birth weight infants
	Hexachlorophene	Congenital malformations
	Mercury	CNS damage in humans, cerebral palsy symptoms in exposed infants, behavioral alterations in animal offspring
	Estrogens	Birth defects (teratogenic), carcinogenic in offspring (DES), heavier and more frequent menses, enlarged breasts and impotence in male workers
Clerical workers	Asbestos	Chronic lung disease (asbestosis) with reduced fetal oxygenation
	Trichloroethylene	Liver and kidney damage, suspected carcinogen
	Benzene	See above
	Toluene	See above
Laundering and dry cleaning	Perchlorethylene	Liver damage, suspected carcinogen, CNS effects (dizziness, nausea), extended exposure can cause death, fetal studies not complete
	Carbon tetrachloride	Specific toxicity to liver and kidneys, suspected carcinogen, passes placental barrier to cause fetal liver damage in animals
	Petroleum solvents	Reproductive failure in both men and women
	Trichloroethylene	See above
	Benzene	See above
Textile and apparel	Carbon disulfide	Menstrual irregularities, decreased fertility, miscarriage, decreased sex drive and sperm abnormalities in men
	Dyes, aniline	Carcinogenic
	Chloroprene	Functional disruption of spermatogenesis in men, miscarriage rate increased three times in their wives, chemically related to vinyl chloride
	Cotton dust	Chronic lung disease (byssinosis, brown lung) with reduced fetal oxygenation
	Benzene	See above
	Toluene	See above
	Asbestos	See above
	Trichloroethylene	See above
	Perchlorethylene	See above
Electronic workers, rubber workers	Nitrosamides	100% incidence of nervous system tumors in animal studies in offspring
	Lead	Sterility, birth defects, prematurity, mental retardation, chromosomal aberrations, menstrual disorders
	Polychlorinated biphenyls (PCB)	"Cola-colored babies" with high frequency of growth retardation, gingival hyperplasia, spotted skull calcification, stillbirths, liver cancer, and reduced fertility in animals
	Arsenic	Carcinogenic; can cause death
	Mercury	See above
	Trichloroethylene	See above

(Continued)

Table 21-1.
Occupations Commonly Held by Women and Potential Occupational Hazards (Continued)

Occupation	Potential Hazard	Known or Suspected Effects on Reproduction
Agricultural workers	Pesticides (chlorinated hydrocarbons)	Carcinogenic, abnormalities in offspring and infertility in animals, kepone causes decreased sex drives and sterility in human males
	Dioxin (2,4,5T)	Miscarriages in humans, mutations, birth defects and miscarriages in animals.
	Heptachlor and Chlordane	Carcinogenic in animals; possibly cause neuroblastomas and leukemia in prenatally or postnatally exposed children
	Chloroprene	See above
Outdoor work Toll booth workers Traffic controllers Airline stewardesses	Carbon monoxide	Acute exposure has caused fetal and fetal-maternal deaths; chronic exposure causes decreased birth weight and increased neonatal mortality in animals
Hairdressers and Cosmetologists	Hair dyes	Mutations in bacterial lab cultures, possibly carcinogenic, chromosomal damage in women using hair dyes
	Vinyl chloride (aerosol sprays)	Documented carcinogen, linked to angiosarcoma of the liver, possible chromosomal aberrations of sperm, increased miscarriage rate and birth defects in humans
	Asbestos (hair dryers)	See above
	Benzene, toluene	See above
Arts and crafts	Benzene, toluene	See above
Painters	Lead	See above
Printers	Mercury	See above
Potters	Lithium, barium	Heavy metal poisoning
Silkscreen, wood-work, stained glass	Chromium	Suspected carcinogen
	Benzidine dyes	Suspected carcinogen
Various	Cadmium	Implicated in bronchogenic and prostatic cancer, testicular damage, sterility, teratogenic effects, low-birth weight in animals, cigarette smoke high in cadmium and heavy smoking increases risk
	Manganese	Impotence and decreased sex drive in exposed males

(After Greenberg, J: Implications for primary care providers of occupational health hazards on pregnant women and their infants. Journal of Nurse–Midwifery 25, 4:21–30, July/August 1980)

expected that a certain amount of concern about the impending labor will be present; the additional responsibility of having a helpless new baby in the household, plus caring for and integrating him into the family unit is also anxiety provoking. The parents will have occasion to wonder whether they are equal to the enormous responsibility of rearing children, and whether or not they will be "good" parents. Therefore, activities which are diverting, healthful, and relaxing help the patient and the family to keep things in proper perspective. The nurse can discuss with the mother some types of recreation that are most relaxing and pleasing for her and her family. Family group activities can still be enjoyed, even though the mother's energy and dexterity may be somewhat curtailed.

Consideration and understanding on the part of the father, the family, the physician, and the nurse can do much to relieve any uncertainties or concerns that the mother may have. When the father, in particular, understands more about the processes involved in the pregnancy (see Suggested Reading), his helpful-

Standards for Maternity Care and Employment (United States Children's Bureau)

1. Facilities for adequate prenatal medical care should be readily available for all employed pregnant women, and arrangements should be made by those responsible for providing prenatal care, so that every woman has access to such care. Local health departments should make the services of prenatal clinics available to industrial plants, and the personnel management or physicians and nurses within the plant should make information about the importance of such services and where they can be obtained available to employees.
2. Pregnant women should not be employed on a shift including the hours between 12 midnight and 6 A.M. Pregnant women should not be employed more than 8 hours a day nor more than 48 hours per week, and it is desirable that their hours of work be limited to not more than 40 hours per week.
3. Every woman, especially a pregnant woman, should have at least two 10-minute rest periods during her work shift, for which adequate facilities for resting and an opportunity for securing nourishing food should be provided.
4. It is not considered desirable for pregnant women to be employed in the following types of occupations, and they should, if possible, be transferred to lighter and more sedentary work:
   a. Occupations that involve heavy lifting or other heavy work,
   b. Occupations that involve continuous standing and moving about.
5. Pregnant women should not be employed in the following types of work during any period of pregnancy:
   a. Occupations that require a good sense of bodily balance, such as work performed on scaffolds or stepladders and occupations in which the accident risk is characterized by accidents causing severe injury, such as operation of punch presses, power-driven woodworking machines, or other machines having a point-of-operation hazard,
   b. Occupations involving exposure to toxic substances considered to be extrahazardous during pregnancy, including the following:
      Aniline
      Benzene and toluene
      Carbon disulfide
      Carbon monoxide
      Chlorinated hydrocarbons
      Lead and its compounds
      Mercury and its compounds
      Nitrobenzol and other nitro compounds of benzol and its homologs
      Phosphorus
      Radioactive substances and x-rays
      Turpentine
      Other toxic substances that exert an injurious effect upon the blood-forming organs, the liver, or the kidneys.

   Because these substances may exert a harmful influence upon the course of pregnancy, may lead to premature termination, or may injure the fetus, the maintenance of air concentrations within the so-called maximum permissible limits of state codes, is not, in itself, sufficient assurance of a safe working condition for the pregnant woman. Pregnant women should be transferred from workrooms in which any of these substances are used or produced in any significant quantity.
6. A minimum of six weeks' leave *before* delivery should be granted with the presentation of a medical certificate of the expected date of confinement.
7. At any time during pregnancy, a woman should be granted a reasonable amount of additional leave with the presentation of a certificate from the attending physician to the effect that complications of pregnancy have made continuing employment prejudicial to her health or to the health of the child.

   To safeguard the mother's health she should be granted sufficient time off after delivery to return to normal and to regain her strength. The infant needs her care, especially during the first year of life. If it is essential that she return to work, the following recommendations are made:
   a. All women should be granted an extension of at least two months leave of absence after delivery.
   b. Should complications of delivery or of the postpartum period develop, a woman should be granted a reasonable amount of additional leave beyond two months following delivery with presentation of a certificate to this effect from the attending physician.

ness can be increased. If a "blue" day comes, the father can make it his particular responsibility to provide a means of counteracting it. During a home visit the nurse might discuss with the family ways in which they might help to diminish the strain in this period. This may necessitate changes in attitudes, understanding, and habits. Certainly, it means increased tolerance and forbearance on the part of those involved; yet, this is one of the ways that others can make their contribution to a successful pregnancy. The father's gentleness and tenderness are especially appreciated and therapeutic at this time; the mother can help him maintain his supportive attitude and behavior by letting him know when his actions are helpful and gratifying. This type of "feedback" conveys her appreciation to the father and leads to reinforcement of his positive behavior. He is perhaps the key person in helping the mother to secure the kind of social relaxation that she enjoys most.

Books, radio, music, movies, sporting events, television, sewing clubs, church functions, visiting, drives, walks, and entertaining friends are some of the means of providing relaxation and diversion. However, the mother should avoid situations that are likely to cause discomfort. Amusements, exercise, rest, and recreation at proper intervals help to keep the pregnant mother well and happy in an environment conducive to her well-being and happy anticipation of the baby.

Traveling

This is perhaps a detail of antepartal care which most patients think very little about, unless they have a tendency to become nauseated or have had a previous miscarriage which precludes any extensive strain.

Even though there is little restriction on travel from a medical point of view, it should be discussed with the mother, so that any of her concerns or misinformation may come to light. The general information that is usually given to a pregnant woman is to avoid any trip which will cause undue fatigue, since she is prone to tiring easily. For traveling long distances, the railway or airplane is safest and provides greatest comfort. If travel is by private automobile, rest periods of 10 minutes to 15 minutes ought to be planned at least every two hours. This not only helps to avoid fatigue, but also benefits the general circulation by providing the chance to stretch and walk.

The pregnant woman should be advised to use seatbelts because they have been found to decrease maternal mortality in severe car accidents. They should be worn low and comfortably under the abdomen and in conjunction with the shoulder strap if one is available. Both belts can be adjusted so that they are not too tight or pressing tightly against the neck and abdomen.

Thus, while traveling in general is not usually contraindicated during pregnancy, each expectant mother should seek individual consultation concerning the advisability of extensive travel at any time during the period of pregnancy.

Immunizations and Vaccinations

Another important topic which is interrelated with travel is that of immunization and vaccination protection for the pregnant woman. The diseases that she will be exposed to during her travels, as well as in the course of her daily life, must be considered. In *The Medical Letter on Drugs and Therapeutics,* the Advisory Committee on Immunization of Infectious Diseases of the American Academy of Pediatrics reviewed the following vaccinations and made these recommendations.[9]

Cholera. This is a killed bacterial vaccine and should be given only if there is danger of infection. As yet there is no definitive evidence of abortigenic effect.

Mumps and measles (rubeola). These are live viruses and should never be given to pregnant patients.

Poliomyelitis. Immunization during pregnancy is rarely indicated because this disease has been almost eradicated in *the United States.*

Rubella. Pregnancy is a contraindication for administration of the live rubella vaccine. This virus has been shown on occasion to infect both the placenta and the fetus and for this reason is avoided.

Smallpox. Vaccinia virus administered during pregnancy occasionally infects the fetus. This fetal vaccinia has almost always been associated with primary vaccination. Hence, primary vaccination should only be given to pregnant women who have been exposed to an endemic area.

Yellow fever. Since this is a live virus, it should be given to pregnant women only if there has been an exposure or if there is a great risk of exposure.

Other vaccines and immunizations. There were no recommendations made by the Committee regarding vaccination against influenza, epidemic typhus, and typhoid. Tetanus and diphtheria toxoids are considered safe and the tuberculin and histoplasmin test are also permitted.

As there is at least somewhat of a risk with many of these vaccinations, it is important to counsel patients regarding the spacing of conception well after receiving these injections. The patient can be counseled also to plan vacations and travels during pregnancy to minimize the opportunity for disease exposure and the consequent need for post hoc vaccination. In addition, all patients should be advised to report any illness, no matter how trivial, to their physician so that appropriate follow-up can be done.

Skin Care

The glands of the skin may be more active during pregnancy, and there may be increased or decreased perspiration, resulting in irritation or dryness. Since the skin is one of the organs of elimination, bathing is obviously important. A bath or a shower should be taken daily because it is stimulating, refreshing, and relaxing. They not only act as a tonic and a general invigorator but also favor elimination through the skin as well. Elimination through the skin is thought to lessen the strain of elimination by the kidneys. The old idea that tub baths should be avoided because the wash water enters the vagina and thereby carries infection to the uterus now is believed to have little validity. However, tub baths should not be taken after rupture of the membranes. The only objection to tub baths during the last trimester of pregnancy is that at this period the heavy weight of the large abdomen may put pregnant women off balance and make climbing in and out of the tub awkward. Therefore, the likelihood of slipping or falling in the bathtub is increased.

Chilling the body should be avoided; thus, cold baths, sponges, or showers should be avoided if they produce this sensation.

Breast Care

Special care of the breasts during pregnancy is an important preparation for breast-feeding. During the antepartal period the breasts often have a feeling of fullness and, in fact, do become larger, heavier, and more pendulous. A well-fitted supporting brassière that holds the breasts up and in may relieve these discomforts. It may also help to prevent the subsequent tissue sagging so often noticeable after delivery due to the increased weight of the breasts during pregnancy and lactation.

There may be sufficient secretion of colostrum from the nipples to necessitate wearing a pad to protect clothing. The daily care of the nipples and the reason for it, as well as the actual procedure, should be explained to the patient as follows.

Early in pregnancy the breasts begin to secrete colostrum. This secretion often oozes out on the surface of the nipple, and as it dries, it forms fine imperceptible crusts. If these crusts are allowed to remain, the skin underneath becomes tender; if left until the baby arrives and begins nursing, this tender skin area is likely to crack. This condition may cause infection. Nipples that are kept clean and dry do not have a tendency to become sore or cracked.

The breasts are to be bathed daily; this may be done at the beginning of the shower bath. The patient should use a clean washcloth and warm water. Some studies have demonstrated that the use of soap, alcohol, and other such materials during the antepartal period and puerperium tends to be detrimental to the integrity of the nipple tissue because they remove the protective skin oils and leave the nipple more prone to damage (see Suggested Reading). Therefore, the possible disadvantages of using these substances should be discussed with the woman in the early stages of antepartal care.

The woman should be taught to bathe her breasts as follows. She begins cleansing each breast by washing the nipple thoroughly with a circular motion, making sure that any dried material has been removed. She gradually continues working away from the nipple in this fashion until the entire breast is washed. The breast is then rinsed in this manner and dried with a clean towel. Rubbing the nipples with a rough towel during the last trimester of pregnancy may be helpful in attempting to toughen them.

Some specialists advise the use of nipple cream, a hydrous lanolin preparation, to prepare the nipples for nursing. This can be applied after the breasts are bathed. First, a small quantity of cream is placed on the thumb and the first finger; then the nipple is grasped gently between the thumb and this finger. With a rolling motion, the cream is worked into the tiny creases found on the surface of the nipple. The position of the thumb and finger should be gradually shifted around the circumference of the nipple until a complete circuit has been made. This procedure is limited to about 30 seconds on each breast.

A nipple that is flat or even slightly inverted in early pregnancy very probably will become protractile by delivery. If the nipples are inverted, special care can be started by the woman in the fifth or sixth month of pregnancy or earlier. In one such treatment, the thumbs are placed close to the inverted nipple, the breast tissue is pressed firmly while the thumbs are gradually pushed away from the areola. The strokes should follow an imaginary cross drawn on the breast and be done four or five times in succession on awakening each morning. The nipple will assume an erect, projected position and then can be grasped as a unit and gently teased out a bit further. This is done daily, so that the nipples may be made more prominent for the baby to grasp (Fig. 21-10).

Clothing

During pregnancy the clothes should be given the same or perhaps even a little more attention than at other times. The mother who feels that she is dressed attractively and is well groomed reflects this in her

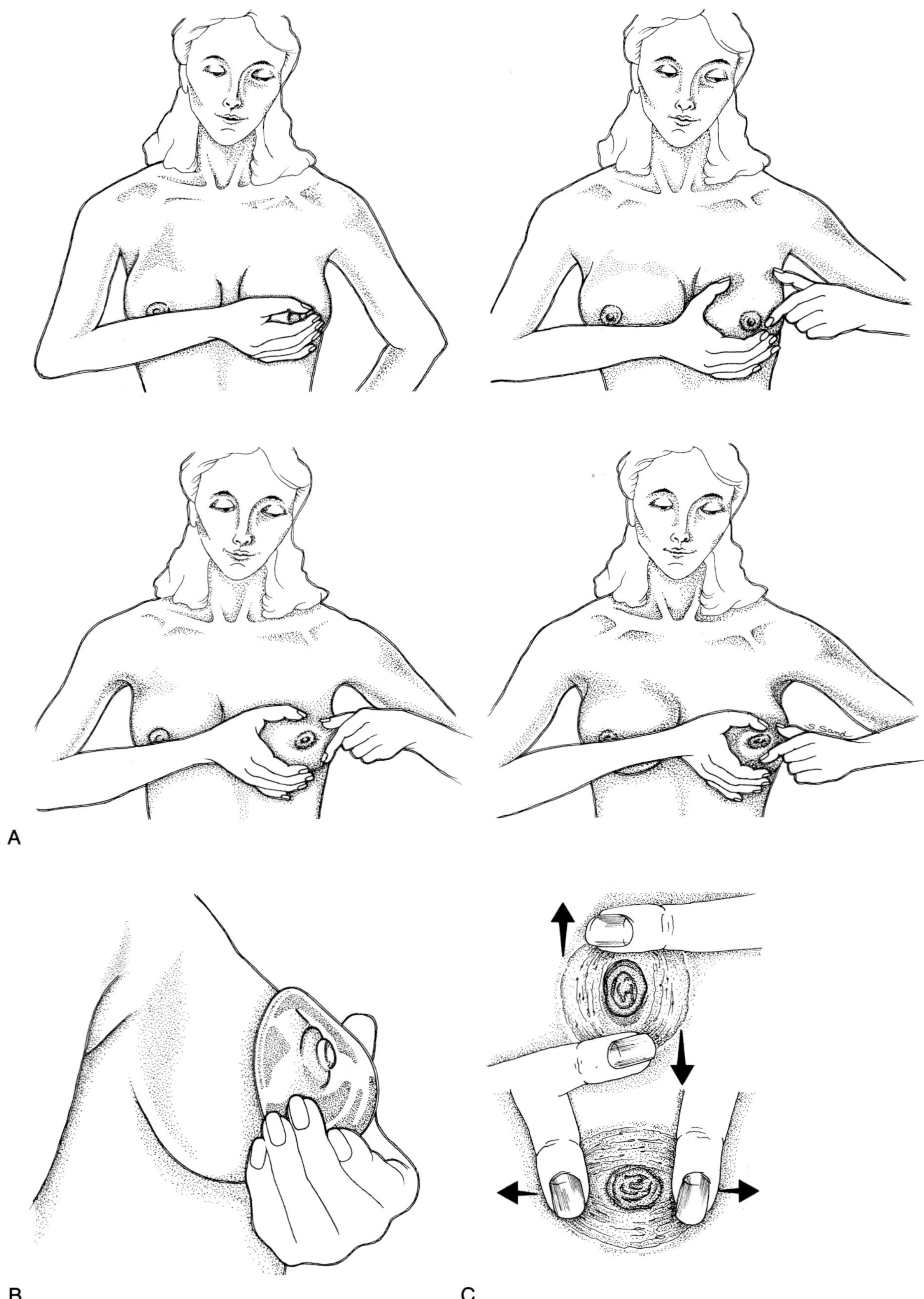
A
B
C

manner. Her clothing should be practical, attractive, and nonconstricting. Most women are able to dress in their usual manner until the enlargement of the abdomen becomes apparent. Maternity specialty shops and department stores have made maternity fashions widely available.

Today designers and stylists are giving consideration to the pregnant mother's clothing, so that she may dress attractively and feel self-confident about her appearance. The clothes are designed to be comfortable and "hang from the shoulders," thus avoiding any constriction; they are made in a variety of materials. The expectant mother can dress according to the climate and the temperature for her comfort.

Abdominal Support

Women who have been unaccustomed to wearing a girdle scarcely feel the need of abdominal support, especially during the early months of pregnancy. Later, however, a properly fitted maternity girdle often gives the support needed to avoid fatigue. The natural softening of the pelvic joints which accompanies pregnancy and the increasing weight of the abdomen may cause a change in posture and result in a severe backache.

If the mother's abdomen is large or if previous pregnancies have caused her abdomen to become lax or pendulous, a properly made and well-fitting maternity girdle gives support and comfort. The purpose of the garment is support, not constriction of the abdomen.

Breast Support

It is advisable that every pregnant woman wear a well-fitted brassière to support the breasts in a normal uplifted position. Proper support of the breasts is conducive to good posture and thus helps to prevent backache.

Figure 21-10.
Care of the breasts. The nipple and areola should be kept clean with mild soap and water to avoid the formation of crusts of colostrum. Such crusts may cause skin irritation. *(A)* The nipple and areola should be soft and protractable. During the last two months of pregnancy, the breasts should be massaged to milk the colostrum and prevent it from blocking the ducts. *(B)* Inverted nipples can sometimes be encouraged to become mobile by the use of Waller's shields. The shield is pressed close to the breast by a brassiere and the nipple is pushed forward through the hole in the base of the shield. *(C)* Inverted nipples can also be treated by placing the thumbs close to the inverted nipple, pressing firmly into the breast tissue, then gradually pushing away from the areola. The strokes should be directed vertically *(top)* and horizontally *(bottom)* and done four or five times in succession.

The selection of a brassière is determined by individual fitting and is influenced by the size of the breasts and the need for support. It is important to see that the cup is large enough and that the underarm is built high enough to cover all the breast tissue. Wide shoulder straps afford more comfort for the woman who has large and pendulous breasts. Again, the size of the brassière is determined by the size of the individual, but in most instances the brassière is approximately two sizes larger than that usually worn. The mother who is planning to breast-feed finds it practical to purchase nursing brassières which can be worn during the latter months of pregnancy, as well as during the postpartal period for as long as she is nursing her baby.

Garters

Round garters or any tight bands (*e.g.,* rolled stockings or elastic tops on knee-high stockings) that encircle the leg tend to aggravate varicose veins and edema of the lower extremities and should be discarded in favor of suspender garters or some form of stocking supporters attached to an abdominal support. If pantyhose do not aggravate any discharge that the mother may have, she may use these.

Shoes

A comfortable, well-fitting shoe is essential for the expectant mother. The postural changes which occur as the mother's abdomen enlarges may be aggravated by wearing high-heeled shoes and create backache and fatigue. It is advisable that low-heeled shoes be worn during working hours and for busy daytime activities. For evening or more fashionable afternoon attire, a 2-inch heel is acceptable if the patient does not develop backache from the increased lordosis induced by the heels, and if she can maintain adequate balance. Platform shoes contribute to precarious balance and are not advised.

The height of the heel is but one consideration; the support which the shoe gives the foot adds materially to the mother's comfort. Many flat-heeled shoes give little or no support to the feet and thus may cause fatigue and aching legs and back. A simple method to check the support of a shoe is to place the shoe flat on the floor, and press the thumb down on the inner sole against the shank (the part that would come under the arch of the foot). If the shoe gives under pressure, it will give weak support to the foot.

Care of the Teeth

Good dental care is necessary because the teeth are important for adequate mastication of food. The teeth should be brushed carefully on arising, after each meal, and before retiring at night. An alkaline mouthwash may be used if desired. It is advisable for the expectant mother to visit her dentist at the very beginning of pregnancy and follow any recommendations made. Any extensive elective work is better postponed until after the pregnancy. The most favorable period for routine, minor procedures is from the fourth to the seventh month. The mother is usually less nauseated and, in general, feeling well.

Diagnostic dental roentgenograms should be postponed until the latter half of pregnancy. A lead apron over the abdomen gives sufficient protection.

The old saying, "For every child a tooth," based on a belief that the fetus takes calcium from the mother's teeth, has no real scientific basis. It should be carefully explained to the mother that an adequate diet during pregnancy supplies the baby with lime salts and other necessities in sufficient amounts to build his bones and teeth. Therefore, this old adage need not be true if proper attention is given to the care of the teeth and nutrition during pregnancy.

Bowel Habits

The pregnant woman with regular elimination habits usually experiences little or no change in the daily routine. Those who have a tendency toward constipation become noticeably more irregular during pregnancy because of decreased physical exertion, relaxation of the bowel in association with the relaxation of smooth-muscle systems all over the body, and pressure of the enlarging uterus. The presenting part of the fetus exerts pressure on the lower bowel, especially during the latter part of pregnancy. Iron supplementation during pregnancy is an additional contributing factor to constipation.

Constipation may be prevented or alleviated by maintaining regular bowel elimination, drinking a large amount of fluids daily, and maintaining a diet that contains several daily servings of fresh fruit and raw vegetables, whole grain breads and cereals, and particularly products with whole bran. If these measures are not effective, a stool softener such as dioctyl sodium sulfosuccinate or a mild laxative such as milk of magnesia may be recommended. Harsh laxatives and purgatives are contraindicated. Mineral oil should not be used because it prevents absorption of fat-soluble vitamins from the gastrointestinal tract. Lack of vitamin K can lead to hemorrhagic disease of the newborn.

Hemorrhoids

Pregnancy often precipitates the occurrence of hemorrhoids (anal varicosities), partially as a result of constipation. Maintaining regular bowel habits, keeping the stool soft, and avoiding straining at stool can help prevent or minimize hemorrhoids. Standing for long periods of time and wearing constricting clothing are aggravating factors. Passage of hard fecal material can injure the rectal mucosa and cause bleeding from fissures or hemorrhoids. Hemorrhoids may become thrombosed or protrude through the anus. The little bumps and nodules seen in a mass of hemorrhoids are the distended portions of the affected vessels. Like varicosities in other areas, they are caused by pressure interfering with return venous circulation and are aggravated by constipation. They often cause great discomfort to the pregnant patient and, due to pressure at the time of delivery, may cause great distress during the postpartal period.

The first step is the prevention and the treatment of constipation. The guidance that the nurse gives the mother in this respect cannot be stressed enough. In

Kegel's Exercises

Tightening and relaxing the pubococcygeal muscle keeps the vagina toned, increases the strength of the perineum, and helps prevent or control hemorrhoids. This contributes to the strength of the pelvic sling in supporting the fetus, increases sexual pleasure, and enhances urinary control.

The muscle that is used to stop the flow of urine is the pubococcygeal muscle. Practice stopping urine by squeezing this muscle several times to become familiar with it. When lying down, insert one finger into the vagina and contract the pubococcygeal muscle; note the feeling of the contraction around your finger.

Exercises:

1. Squeeze the pubococcygeal muscle for 3 seconds, relax for 3 seconds, and squeeze again. Begin with 10 three-second squeezes per day, and increase gradually until you are doing 100 twice daily.
2. Squeeze and release, then squeeze and release alternately as rapidly as you can. This is called the "flutter" exercise.
3. Bear down as during a bowel movement, but concentrate on the vagina instead of the rectum. Hold for 3 seconds.

Kegel's exercises can be done anywhere and anytime. The increased control gained over the pubococcygeal muscle is useful throughout pregnancy, during labor, during intercourse, and to prevent loss of vaginal tone with aging. This exercise, done regularly, is useful for the rest of your life.

addition, when internal hemorrhoids protrude through the rectum, the mother can be instructed to replace them carefully by pushing them gently back into the rectum. Usually the patient can manage this quite well, after a thorough explanation or demonstration. She lubricates her finger with petrolatum or mineral oil to aid ease of insertion and to avoid trauma to the veins. If the patient wishes, a finger cot can be used to cover her finger. Also, taking either the knee–chest position or elevating her buttocks on a pillow facilitates replacement through gravity (see Fig. 21-11).

The application of an icebag or cold compresses wet with witch hazel or Epsom salts solution, gives great relief. The physician may order tannic acid in suppositories, or compresses of witch hazel and glycerin. If the hemorrhoids are aggravated the first few days after labor, the same medications usually give relief. Surgery is seldom resorted to during pregnancy. Doing Kegel's exercises regularly helps prevent and control hemorrhoids. (See page 426.)

Douches and Vaginal Hygiene

Vaginal douching, long considered a requisite of feminine hygiene by some women, should be kept at a reasonable minimum during pregnancy. If excessive vaginal secretion or infection exist, then the kind of douche and the frequency with which it is to be taken will be prescribed. In the absence of excessive secretions or infection, the nurse might reassure the patient that a washcloth and soap and water are quite adequate for general cleanliness, emphasizing washing anteriorly first, and the rectal area last. The use of moist towelettes that are sold in foil packages is not contraindicated.

Deodorant "feminine hygiene" sprays are contraindicated as they have been found to cause severe perineal irritation in many women, as well as urethritis and cystitis. During pregnancy, the sebaceous glands in the genital area are quite active and there may be a characteristic odor that some women find quite unpleasant. Plain soap and water are very effective agents to keep this odor under control. Any suggestions that the nurse might give for general cleanliness is usually appreciated. Women may find that the genital area is a little more sensitive to heat and cold and pressure during pregnancy, but they should be reassured that regular cleansing procedures do not cause any harm.

Specific instructions about douching are to be given if the woman so desires. Having copies of the instructions for douching that agree with the philosophy of the office or clinic is an effective method of conveying this information. The instructions should be clear enough for the patient who has never douched and knows nothing about it (see list below).

Sexual Relations

From the standpoint of all parties involved—patient, nurse, and physician—the area of sexual relations, because of its intimate nature, often becomes one of the most difficult in which to give appropriate guidance. Many patients are reluctant to discuss sex, especially when the patient–physician–nurse rela-

PE Douching During Pregnancy

The following points can be included in the instructions and stated in language and vocabulary that is understandable to the patient.

It is a four-minute procedure (after the initial few times.)

It can be done while sitting on the toilet.

A gravity bag must be used (never a hand bulb syringe).

The douche tip should not be inserted more than 3 inches.

The frequency and the solution are prescribed according to the needs of the patient.

The douche bag may be placed (hung or held) no higher than 2 feet above the level of the vagina.

The douche tip should be held at about the 3-inch length and inserted in the vagina, and the labial tissue in that area should be held around the douche tip with the same hand.

The solution is allowed to run in until there is a slight feeling of fullness, then it is expelled (the douche bag holds enough solution to do this four or five times).

The bag and the tube should be rinsed and hung to dry with a towel underneath.

For comfort, the solution should only be barely warm to the hand. Holding the labial tissue around the douche tip allows the water to flow in without flowing out immediately, and this, along with rapid expelling, enables the solution to get into the folds of the wall of the vagina. In the nonpregnant woman there is no contraindication to inserting the entire douche tip or as much of it as the vagina can accommodate.

tionship is new; yet, they are disturbed because of the changes which may be taking place in their bodies and emotions, with consequent influences on their sexual relationship.

Because of this reluctance, nurses and physicians often avoid exploring the possibility of an existing problem with the patient. The counseling then consists mostly of prohibitions regarding the time and frequency of intercourse. However, when there is a need, most patients discuss the subject, with a little help, especially when the physician or the nurse conveys the idea that these are "expected" changes and that there is nothing "shameful" or unique about them. Thus, the nurse should be prepared to fulfill this counseling activity and act as a resource person when called upon.

It is important to understand the anatomical, physiological, and psychological aspects of sexual response and sexuality during pregnancy (see Chaps. 9 and 12). The approach here is extremely important and requires adroit use of communication skills, especially those of listening, reflecting, and gentle probing. Finally, one's own feelings and attitudes about sexuality, pregnancy, and motherhood need to be examined in order to understand and better empathize with the patient's situation.

While sexuality has become a more open topic in today's society, there is a wide variety of views among people of different cultural backgrounds. Nonetheless, there is a growing expectation on the part of patients that health professionals will offer counseling related to sexuality as an integral part of health care. Particularly in maternity nursing, sexual concerns are close to the surface, providing a ready situation for intervention and satisfying sexual adjustments. Being willing to explore and respond to patient's sexual concerns and having knowledge of appropriate sources of referral for sexual counseling are part of the function of the maternity nurse (see Chap. 12 for a full discussion of this area).

Smoking

The Surgeon General's report, as well as other recent studies, has indicated that cigarette smoking is a health hazard of sufficient importance in this country to warrant remedial action. Lung cancer, vascular thrombotic problems, and heart disease have been linked significantly with cigarette smoking. With respect to pregnancy, several studies have found a relationship between smoking and lower birthrates, higher rates of prematurity, and higher neonatal mortality.

Adverse effects of maternal smoking have been confirmed in recent studies. Smoking during pregnancy is related to increased spontaneous abortions, stillbirths, premature infants, placental abruptions, placenta previa, early and late bleeding in pregnancy, and premature and prolonged rupture of the membranes. Increased incidence of Rh disease and anomalies of the heart and other organs have also been found. Women who smoke deliver small-for-gestational-age infants almost twice as often as women who do not smoke. These newborns (weighing less than 2500 g) are at increased risk for hypoglycemia, which can result in permanent brain damage. Small-for-date infants have more learning disorders, lower IQ, mental retardation, and are more prone to neurologic deficits such as cerebral palsy and epilepsy.[10]

Smoking prevents efficient assimilation of essential vitamins and minerals in the mother. The fetus can be adversely affected by inadequate maternal nurition. Smoking causes rapid calcium mobilization, which can reduce calcium stores, reduces vitamin B_{12} levels, causes significantly lower vitamin C levels (one cigarette depletes vitamin C levels by 25 mg, the amount from an average orange), and may cause deficiencies of vitamins B_6, B_1, and A. There is also evidence that components of tobacco smoke interfere with placental processes involved in metabolization of hormones and transport of amino acids, vitamins, and other nutrients.

Data from the United States Collaborative Perinatal Project indicate that the negative effects of smoking continue even if the woman quits before becoming pregnant. Placenta previa and the presence of abnormally large areas of dead tissue on the placenta are common for smoking mothers, and could be related to past smoking (measured as cigarettes per year over a period of time). It is unclear how long these effects of smoking continue. This study also found a direct link between smoking and sudden infant death syndrome. Although prematurity and respiratory and prenatal infections are the greatest risk factors in crib death, smoking alone increases the risk by 52%.[11]

The mechanism by which smoking affects fetal well-being is somewhat obscure, but it is thought that the nicotine in the cigarettes causes peripheral vasoconstriction, with subsequent changes in the heart rate, blood pressure, and cardiac output that appear to have a detrimental effect on the development and the health of the fetus. Carbon monoxide also is found in higher concentrations in smokers, with a consequent decrease of oxygen, which also affects the fetus. The lack of key nutrients is believed important, and even mild maternal under-nutrition in the last few weeks of gestation may compromise the intricate process of brain cell division.

Data from a large perinatal mortality study revealed that birth weight distributions shifted downward as maternal smoking level increased. However, maternal weight gain distributions were the same for smokers and nonsmokers, indicating that smoking does not reduce maternal weight gain. Within each level of maternal weight gain, from below 5 pounds to over 40 pounds, the more the mothers smoked, the greater percentage of neonates weighing less than 2500 g. Evidence supports a direct effect of maternal smoking on infant birth weight, possibly due to hypoxic effects of carbon monoxide, rather than an effect mediated through eating. Thus, efforts to prevent smoking should have greater benefits than efforts to increase maternal food intake.

Some disturbing observations from long-term studies indicate that low-birth weight babies of smokers are small for dates at birth and continue to grow at low percentiles for height and weight after birth.[12]

On the first prenatal visit, assessment of whether and how much the woman smokes is important. Previous obstetrical history and presence of other risk factors are taken into consideration to inform the woman of problems which might occur as a result of smoking. It is strongly advised that smoking be stopped, ideally as early before conception as possible. The nurse can discuss whether the woman has ever quit smoking before and if she thinks she could quit now. Pregnancy can be a motivation to stop smoking based on concern about harming the baby. Information about quitting smoking is available from several sources, and smoking clinics or support groups are common. On follow-up visits, if the mother has not been successful in quitting smoking, she can be encouraged further or provided more direct guidance. As a minimum, she can be advised to reduce the number of cigarettes smoked daily and to smoke low tar and low nicotine brands. Women who continue smoking during pregnancy need careful nutritional teaching to ensure adequate intake of nutrients. Their pregnancy is then considered high risk and is followed accordingly (see chart on Smoking and Alcohol Risks).

Alcohol

Alcohol consumption during pregnancy is now recognized as a major health problem. In 1973 the fetal alcohol syndrome (FAS) was first identified as a distinct clinical entity caused by maternal alcohol consumption. Infants born with this syndrome have altered patterns of growth and morphogenesis, having characteristic facies, growth deficiencies, and mental retardation (see Chap. 43). The severity of FAS depends on the amount of alcohol consumed and the time during pregnancy it is consumed. About 40% of women who drink heavily during pregnancy give birth to infants with FAS. Maternal alcohol consumption may be related to a number of other neurologic, behavioral, and psychosocial disorders, and may possibly cause abortion and stillbirth. Intrauterine alcohol damage may be the most common fetal teratogen and the leading cause of mental retardation in this country.[13]

No minimum safe level of alcohol consumption during pregnancy has been established. Therefore, it is recommended that the mother abstain from alcohol while pregnant. It is important for the nurse to assess alcohol usage early in pregnancy. A decrease in consumption at any time, however, even in the third trimester, may limit fetal damage. Counseling and education about the FAS are important in assisting women to understand the risk involved and to help her make informed choices.

Alcoholism is often a difficult problem to identify and remedy. The nurse may need to be alert to indirect cues, such as missed clinic appointments, women with isolated lifestyles, or women in lower status jobs than their educational level indicates. Problems brought up by the patient about behavior problems with children, sexuality, and family conflicts may be symptoms of alcoholism. The history may be suggestive, especially if there has been a previous failure-to-thrive infant or an unexplained neonatal death. Women with a family history of either alcoholism or teetotalism seem more prone to have alcohol problems. Avoidance of discussion of drinking may be a cue to alcoholism, as people who drink socially are usually not defensive or elusive when discussing drinking habits.

Mothers with mild to moderate drinking problems may respond to education and encouragement to stop or limit intake. Specific suggestions for avoiding drinking, or limiting the amount of alcohol in drinks or times of consumption can be helpful. Depending on the patient's response, and when alcoholism is severe, referral to an alcohol counselor or program may be necessary. Detoxification procedures must be carefully selected because of potential effects on the fetus. Disulfiram (Antabuse) is contraindicated during pregnancy because of its inhibitory action on several enzymes.

Smoking and Alcohol Risks

	Fetal Risks	Maternal Risks
Smoking	Abortion, stillbirth, prematurity Placenta abruptio and previa Premature rupture of membranes Low-birth weight (brain damage, mental retardation, learning disorders, neurologic deficits, lower IQ) Deficiency in key nutrients Sudden infant death syndrome	Hemorrhage (from placenta abruptio and previa) Sepsis (from ruptured membranes) Vitamin and mineral deficiencies Bronchitis, emphysema, bronchiectasis Lung cancer Hypertension and cardiovascular disease, heart attacks
Alcohol	Fetal alcohol syndrome (developmental defects, mental retardation) Withdrawal after birth Neurologic, behavioral, and psychosocial disorders Abortion, stillbirth (results tentative)	Cirrhosis Malnutrition, vitamin and mineral deficiencies Withdrawal (delirium tremans) Chronic brain syndrome Family and social disruption Sexual problems

Minor Discomforts

The minor discomforts of pregnancy are the common complaints experienced by most expectant mothers, to some degree, in the course of a normal pregnancy. However, all mothers do not experience all of these discomforts, and, indeed, some mothers pass through the entire antepartal period without any complaints of this type. Although the discomforts are not serious in themselves, their presence detracts from the mother's feeling of comfort and well-being. In many instances they can be avoided by preventive measures, or entirely overcome by common sense in daily living once they do occur.

Frequent Urination

One of the first signs the woman may notice to make her suspect she might be pregnant is the frequent desire to empty her bladder. This is caused by the pressure of the growing uterus against the bladder and subsides about the second or the third month, when the uterus expands upward into the abdominal cavity. Later, during the last weeks of pregnancy the symptoms recur.

Nausea

Nausea and vomiting to mild degree, the so-called morning sickness, constitute the most common disorder of the first trimester of pregnancy. Symptoms usually appear about the end of the fourth or sixth week and last until about the twelfth week. Nausea occurs in about 50% of all pregnancies; of these, about one third experience some vomiting. Usually, it occurs in the morning only, but a small percentage of patients may have nausea and vomiting throughout the entire day.

Altered hormonal status, with high levels of HCG and progesterone, are involved in producing these symptoms through their effects upon gastrointestinal smooth musculature. Changes in carbohydrate metabolism and other metabolic processes may also contribute.

For many years it has been thought that this condition has an emotional basis. In all life's encounters, there are probably few experiences that are as anxiety provoking as the realization of being pregnant. At first there is the anxious uncertainty before she can be sure of the diagnosis. Then, there are numerous adjustments that have to be made and responsibilities that may seem to be overwhelming. Emotionally, the implications of pregnancy extend far back into her childhood. It is understandable that women who cannot adjust to all these new circumstances could have problems. Moreover, whether causative or not, the stress of pregnancy and all its ramifications can contribute to the symptoms caused by the metabolic changes associated with pregnancy.

Manifestations

The typical sign of morning sickness starts with a feeling of nausea when the woman is getting out of bed in the morning. She is unable to retain her breakfast but by noon she has completely recovered and has no further episodes until the next morning. The nausea does not always occur in the morning but may happen in the afternoon or in the evening. In a small percentage of women the nausea and vomiting may persist throughout the day and even be worse in the afternoon. With the majority of women this problem lasts from one month to three months and then suddenly ceases. There may be a slight loss of body weight but no other signs or symptoms.

Management

Often this condition can be controlled or at least relieved. Various before-breakfast remedies are used often. Taking a dry piece of toast or a cracker a half hour before getting out of bed may produce relief. In some instances sips of hot water (plain or with lemon juice), hot tea, clear coffee, or hot milk have been tried and found successful. However, the dry carbohydrate foods seem to be more effective. After remaining in bed for about a half hour after taking these remedies, the woman gets up and dresses slowly (meanwhile sitting as much of the time as possible). After this she is usually ready for her breakfast.

Greasy foods and those known to cause disagreeable after effects should be avoided in the diet. Other suggested remedies include eating an increased amount of carbohydrate foods during this period of disturbance or eating simple and light food five or six times a day instead of three regular full meals. Unsweetened popcorn during the morning is sometimes advised. Another helpful remedy is sweet lemonade, about half a lemon to a pint of water sweetened with milk sugar. Such a drink is usually welcome following a bout of vomiting. Small amounts of ginger ale or cola drink, spearmint, raspberry, or peppermint tea also may be helpful.

Once nausea and vomiting are established, they are difficult to overcome; therefore, it is especially desirable to prevent the first attack, or at least to control this condition as soon as possible after it develops. Vomiting can deplete the system of necessary nutrients at a time when daily health should be maintained. Eating high-protein meals (*e.g.*, eggs, cheese, meat), fruit, and fruit juices may help prevent morning sickness by avoiding hypoglycemia, which is a cause of nausea. Taking 10 mg of vitamin B_6 at bedtime may be helpful also.

Pregnancies differ, and what may help one person may not benefit another. The trial-and-error method often is necessary to obtain results. If persistent vomiting develops, as it does with a small number of women, the condition is no longer considered to be a minor discomfort but a serious complication (see Chap. 34).

Heartburn

This is a neuromuscular phenomenon which may occur any time throughout gestation. As a result of the diminished gastric motility which normally accompanies pregnancy, reverse peristaltic waves cause regurgitation of the stomach contents into the esophagus. It is this irritation of the esophageal mucosa which causes heartburn. It may be described as a burning discomfort diffusely localized behind the lower part of the sternum, often radiating upward along the course of the esophagus. Although it is referred to as heartburn, it really has nothing to do with the heart. Often it is associated with other gastrointestinal symptoms, of which acid regurgitation, belching, nausea, and epigastric pressure are most troublesome. Nervous tension and emotional disturbances may be a precipitating cause. Worry, fatigue, and improper diet may contribute to its intensity.

Very little fat should be included in the diet. Although fatty foods are especially aggravating in this disturbance, strangely enough, the taking of some form of fat, such as a pat of butter or a tablespoon of cream, a short time before meals acts as a preventive because fat inhibits the secretion of acid in the stomach. However, this does not help if the heartburn is already present. Coffee and cigarettes tend to make heartburn worse because they stimulate acid secretion in the stomach and irritate the mucosa.

Eating several small meals daily instead of three large ones may help prevent heartburn. Wearing clothes that are loose around the waist may also be helpful. When heartburn occurs, it may be relieved with small sips of water, milk, or a carbonated drink. Lying down makes regurgitation worse, so it is best to sit upright. Relaxing and breathing deeply for several minutes may help. The "flying exercise" is also suggested—sitting tailor fashion, the arms are raised and lowered quickly, bringing the hands together over the head, and repeated several times.

When antacids are used, those with an aluminum or magnesium base should be taken. Many over-the-counter remedies contain sodium, which promotes water retention and could lead to serious problems. Women are advised to avoid Alka-Seltzer, Fizrin, and baking soda (sodium bicarbonate), which are high in sodium ions. Equally effective medications are aluminum compounds, such as aluminum hydroxide gel, or this medication in tablet form with magnesium trisilicate.

Flatulence

This is a somewhat common and often disagreeable discomfort. Usually it is due to undesirable bacterial action in the intestines, which results in the formation of gas. Eating only small amounts of food which are well masticated may prevent this feeling of distress after eating. Regular daily elimination is of prime importance, as is the avoidance of foods that form gas (*e.g.,* beans, parsnips, corn, sweet desserts, fried foods, cake, and candy). If these measures fail to relieve the condition, the physician should be consulted.

Backache

Most pregnant women experience some degree of backache. As pregnancy advances, the woman's posture changes to compensate for the weight of the growing uterus. The shoulders are thrown back as the enlarging abdomen protrudes, and, in order for body balance to be maintained, the inward curve of the spine is exaggerated. The relaxation of the sacroiliac joints, in addition to the postural change, causes varying degress of backache following excessive strain, fatigue, bending, or lifting.

The woman can be advised early in pregnancy how to prevent such strain through measures such as good posture and body mechanics in everyday living and avoidance of fatigue. Appropriate shoes worn during periods of activity and a supporting girdle may be helpful (see Clothing).

The key to good posture is to sit, stand, walk and lie in a way that minimizes the hollow or curvature of the lower back. To do this, the abdominal and gluteal muscles are contracted and those of the lower back are relaxed, while the pelvis is tilted slightly upward and forward. The pelvic tilt exercise brings the pelvis into this alignment (See also Chap. 19, Table 19-4). Sitting posture can be improved by using armrests, foot supports, and a pillow for the back. The tailor position or lotus position used for yoga are useful for relief of back pain. The mother should always bend from the knees rather than the back when lifting, keeping the spine straight. Avoiding forward leaning while doing chores helps prevent strain on the back and is facilitated by adjusting the height of the work surface or the mother's position to maintain proper posture when standing or sitting.[14]

Daily exercises such as walking, swimming, and stretching are effective ways of preventing backache. Prenatal exercises or yoga are also helpful. The knee–chest twist is a particularly beneficial exercise. When backache occurs, it may be relieved by applying a heating pad or hot water bottle to the lower back, by having a backrub, or by sitting in a jacuzzi that is not too hot.

Dyspnea

Difficult breathing or shortness of breath occasionally results from pressure on the diaphragm by the enlarged uterus and may interfere considerably with the patient's sleep and general comfort during the last weeks of pregnancy. Usually it is not a serious condition, but unfortunately it cannot be wholly relieved until after "lightening" (the settling of the fetus into the pelvic cavity with relief of the upper abdominal pressure) or after the birth of the baby, when it will disappear spontaneously. It is most troublesome when the patient attempts to lie down, so that her comfort may be greatly enhanced by propping her up in bed with pillows. In this semisitting posture she can sleep better and longer than with her head low. It is well for the nurse to demonstrate how these pillows may be arranged comfortably so that the patient's back is adequately supported.

In patients with known heart disease, shortness of breath, especially of rather sudden onset, may be a sign of oncoming heart failure and should be reported at once to the physician.

Varicose Veins

Varicose veins or varices may occur in the lower extremities and, at times, extend up as high as the external genitalia or even into the pelvis itself. A varicosity is an enlargement in the diameter of a vein due to a thinning and stretching of its walls. Such distended areas may occur at short intervals along the course of the blood vessel; they give it a knotted appearance. Varicosities generally are associated with hereditary tendencies and are enhanced by advancing age, multiple pregnancy, and activities which require prolonged standing.

During pregnancy the pressure in the pelvis due to the enlarged uterus, which presses on the great abdominal veins, interferes with the return of the blood from the lower extremities. Added to this, any debilitating condition favors the formation of varicosities in the veins because of the general flabbiness and lack of tone in the tissues.

Naturally, the greater the pressure in the abdomen, the greater the chance of varicose veins of the lower extremities and the vulva. Therefore, any occupation which keeps a patient constantly on her feet, particularly in the latter part of pregnancy, causes an increase in abdominal pressure and so acts as an exacerbating factor.

Symptoms

The first symptom of the development of varicose veins is a dull aching pain in the legs due to distention of the deep vessels. Inspection may show a fine purple network of superficial veins that cover the skin in a lacelike pattern, although this does not always appear. Later, the true varicosities appear, usually first under the bend of the knee, in a tangled mass of bluish or purplish veins, often as large as a lead pencil. As the condition advances, the varicosities extend up and down the leg along the course of the vessels, and in severe cases they may affect the veins of the labia majora, the vagina, and the uterus.

Management

Treatment for varicose veins begins by promptly abandoning any constricting garters, stockings, or other clothing that causes pressure, particularly on the legs or thighs. If varicosities persist in spite of this precaution, the patient can be taught to take the right-angle position, that is, to lie on the bed with her legs extended straight into the air at right angles to her body, with her buttocks and heels resting against the wall (see Fig. 19-16). At first, this position is taken for two to five minutes several times a day. For some patients this position is very uncomfortable at first, but if it is explained, and the discomfort is therefore anticipated, the patient is less likely to discontinue the exercise. Late in pregnancy this position may be too difficult to assume because of pressure against the diaphragm.

To give support to the weak-walled veins, either an elastic stocking or elastic bandage often is recommended. The initial cost of elastic stockings is somewhat more than that of bandages, but they are easier to put on, more effective, have a neater appearance and a longer usefulness than bandages. A regular nylon stocking put on over the elastic hose further improves the appearance. Many hosiery companies are manufacturing "support" hose which do not have the strength of the elastic stockings but are very effective in giving a moderate amount of support. This type of stocking is useful in cases in which the varicosities are very mild or may not even be apparent peripherally but are suspected because of the ache they produce. Many women who must be on their feet a great deal and do not have the opportunity to rest frequently wear these stockings during working hours as a "prophylactic" measure. The nurse can be very helpful in apprising mothers of the varieties of hose now available which meet the needs of individual patients.

The patient also must be told that the stocking or the bandage should be removed at night for greater comfort and reapplied in the morning after the legs have been elevated so that the vessels will be less dilated. The longer stockings or bandage is more satisfactory when the varicosities are above the knee. Both the elastic stocking and bandage are washable, which helps to maintain their original elasticity. However, mild soap rather than detergent should be used.

Varicosities of the vulva may be relieved by placing a pillow under the buttocks and elevating the hips for frequent rest periods or by taking the elevated Sim's position for a few moments several times a day (See Fig. 21-11). Patients suffering from this condition

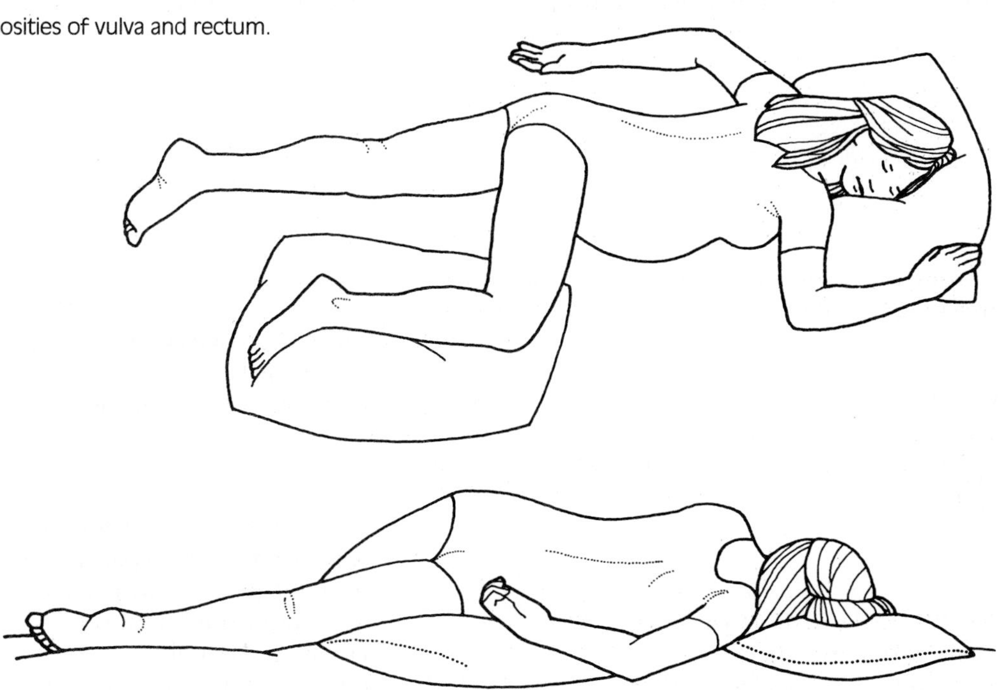

Figure 21-11.
Sims's position for varicosities of vulva and rectum.

should not stand when they can sit, and they should not sit when they can lie down.

More important than the treatment of this condition is its prevention. Every pregnant woman should be advised to sit with her legs elevated whenever possible. And when the legs are elevated, care should be taken to see that there are no pressure points against the legs to interfere with the circulation, particularly in the popliteal space. Tight constricting garments, round garters, constipation, standing for long periods of time and an improper amount of rest all tend to aggravate this condition.

A *varicose vein in the vagina* may rupture during the antepartal or intrapartal period, but this is rare. The hemorrhage is venous and can be controlled readily by pressure. The foot of the bed can be markedly elevated.

Cramps

Cramps are painful spasmodic muscular contractions in the legs. They may occur at any time during the pregnancy but more generally during the later months due to pressure of the enlarged uterus on the nerves affecting the lower extremities. Other causes have been attributed to fatigue, chilling, tense body posture and insufficient or excessive calcium in the diet. They are commonly noted after the use of diuretics.

A quart of milk in the daily diet has been generally recommended to meet the calcium needs during pregnancy. However, studies show that large quantities of milk or dicalcium phosphate predispose to muscular tetany and leg cramps as a result of the excessive amount of phosphorus absorbed from these products. Some authorities suggest that small quantities of aluminum hydroxide gel be taken with the quart of milk because it removes some of the dietary phosphorus from the intestinal tract. Immediate relief may be obtained by forcing the toes upward and by putting pressure on the knee to straighten the leg. Elevating the feet and keeping the extremities warm are preventives.

Cramps, while not a serious condition, are excruciatingly painful for the duration of the seizure. Regular exercise to keep circulation good in the legs

Figure 21-12.
Elevate legs to relieve edema. Swelling and discomfort are reduced if the legs can be elevated as much as possible, even at work.

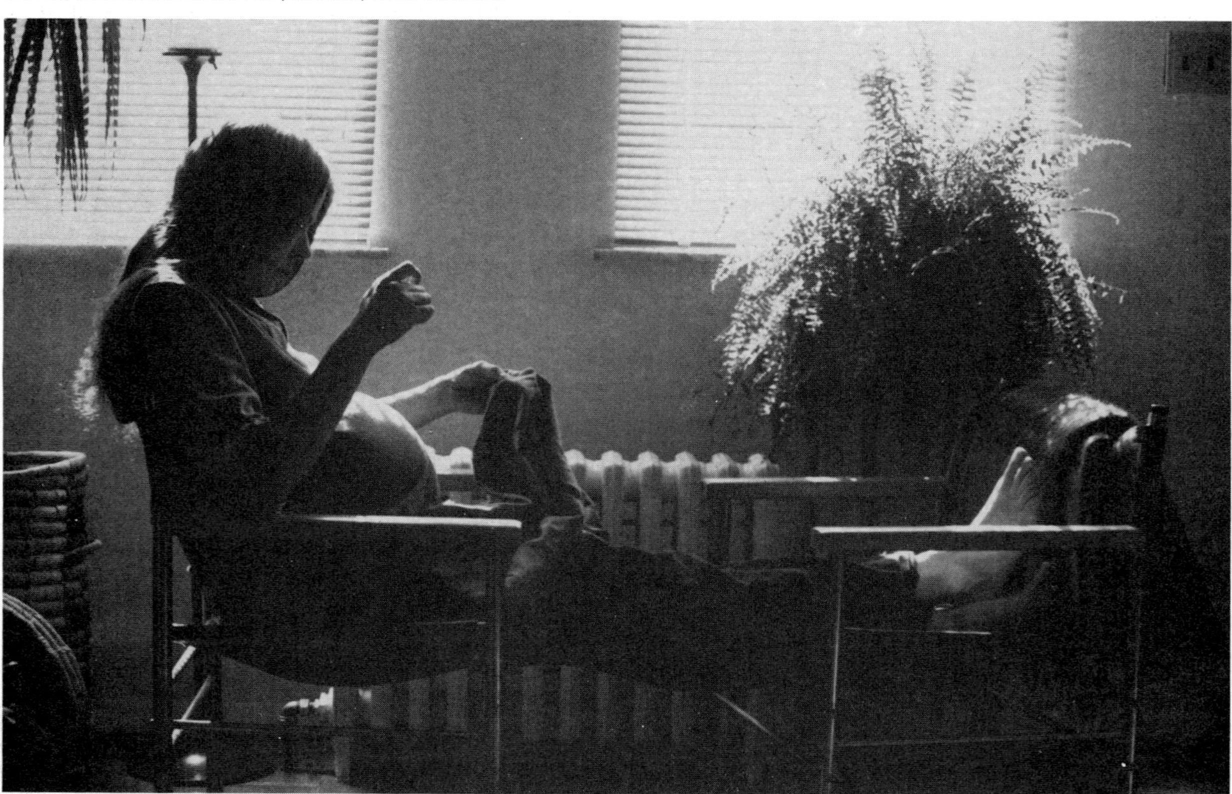

helps prevent cramps. Taking a warm bath before bedtime can improve circulation at night. Cramps are often brought on by pointing the toes when stretching; the woman needs to be reminded to avoid this. Massaging the cramped muscle, soaking it in warm water, using a heating pad, and standing and walking when able relieve cramps.

Edema

Swelling of the lower extremities is very common during pregnancy and is sometimes very uncomfortable. It is especially likely to occur in hot weather. Often it may be relieved by a proper abdominal support or by resting frequently during the day. Elevating the feet or taking the right-angle position often gives relief.

Edema may be prevented by avoiding highly salted foods, eating high-protein foods, and avoiding tight clothing. Women who work or must remain standing or sitting for long periods need to rest two to three times daily with legs raised for about 20 minutes. When edema occurs, elevating the legs as much as possible reduces swelling and discomfort (Fig. 21-12).

Although edema of the ankles, feet, and even hands are common, particularly in late pregnancy, the nurse must always be alert for possible complications. *Edema is one of the signs of preeclampsia and must not be overlooked.* Sudden weight gain of more than 2 lb per week needs careful evaluation. The nurse should look for distribution of edema on the face and sacrum as additional indices of preeclampsia. This must be brought to the physician's attention. Natural Remedies for Minor Discomforts of Pregnancy, describes the prevention of various minor discomforts of pregnancy, medications to avoid, and safe natural remedies.

Natural Remedies for Minor Discomforts of Pregnancy

Prevention	Natural Remedies	Medicines Not to Be Used*
Nausea and vomiting		
High-protein meals, fruit and fruit juices to avoid hypoglycemia Several small meals daily Avoid fried foods Drink liquids between meals rather than with meals Get out of bed slowly, avoid sudden movements Eat dry bread or crackers before rising (keep by bed) Eat yogurt or milk at night or before arising	Eat dry bread or crackers Sip soda water Take a walk in fresh air Drink spearmint, raspberry leaf, or peppermint tea	Antihistamines (contained in most antinausea medicines)
Headache		
Get enough sleep at night and enough rest during the day Do not go for long periods without eating Drink plenty of fluids Avoid things which contribute to headaches (*e.g.*, eye strain, stuffy rooms, cigarette smoke, rushing around)	Apply a cool, wet washcloth to forehead and back of neck (some prefer warm cloth) Massage neck, shoulders, face, scalp, forehead Take a walk in fresh air Take a warm bath Find a quiet place and relax Meditate or do yoga	Narcotic analgesics Aspirin, Excedrin, Percogesic, Cope

(Continued)

Natural Remedies for Minor Discomforts of Pregnancy (Continued)

Prevention	Natural Remedies	Medicines Not to Be Used*
Heartburn		
Avoid foods known to cause gastric upset Avoid greasy, fried foods Avoid highly seasoned foods Eat several small meals daily Avoid coffee and cigarettes Wear loose clothes at waist Drink 6–8 glasses water daily	Take small sips of water Sip carbonated beverage Sit upright Relax and breathe deeply for several minutes Do the flying exercise Use aluminum base antacids	Sodium base antacids (*e.g.,* Alka-Seltzer, Fizrin, Soda Mint, baking soda)
Fatigue		
Get enough sleep and rest Take naps during the day Pace daily life to provide for extra rest Eat well-balanced meals Exercise regularly	Take the time to rest when the body demands it Sit with feet up whenever possible Use suggestions under Prevention	Caffeine (*e.g.,* coffee, tea, cola drinks, stay-awake pills) Amphetamines
Leg Cramps		
Get enough calcium (milk, dark green leafy vegetables, supplements) Exercise regularly Keep the legs warm Take a warm bath at bedtime Do not point the toes when stretching	Sit down, straighten the leg, point or pull toes upward toward the knees Massage the cramped muscle Walk around when able Soak cramped muscle in warm water or use heating pad	Quinine Muscle relaxants
Constipation		
Drink plenty of fluids (6–8 glasses of water daily) Exercise regularly Eat raw vegetables, cooked fruit (*e.g.,* prune juice, 3 tbsp bran daily, whole grain bread and cereal, oatmeal, brown rice *Caution*—raw apples and coffee increase constipation Chew food thoroughly Have good bowel habits (do not force bowel movements, go when having the urge, take time for bowel movements, raise feet on stool to reduce strain)	Drink either hot or very cold liquid on an empty stomach Follow suggestions under prevention Bulk-producing laxatives (*e.g.,* Metamucil, Effersyllium)	Laxatives which are other than bulk producing (best to avoid all laxatives; at least use only twice per week; taking too many laxatives causes more constipation)

Natural Remedies for Minor Discomforts of Pregnancy (Continued)

Prevention	Natural Remedies	Medicines Not to Be Used*
Varicose veins		
Regular exercise Avoid tight or binding clothes (especially garters, knee-length stockings) Wear full-length support hose when standing or walking for a long time Avoid sitting or standing for a long time Wear shoes with well-padded soles to absorb shock	Lie with feet raised several times daily Lie with feet against wall Wear elastic support hose (put on before arising)	No medications
Hemorrhoids		
Prevent constipation and straining during bowel movements Follow good bowel habits Do not sit for a long time on the toilet Regular Kegel's exercises	Sit in warm tub for 15 min–20 min 3–4 times daily Apply dilute lemon juice or vinegar compresses, use Tucks or witch hazel compresses Use bulk-producing laxatives to keep stool soft	Local anesthetic creams (Preparation H, Americaine, Anusol)
Backache		
Good posture Bend from knees when lifting Wear supportive shoes with low heels Exercise regularly Prenatal exercises or yoga Maintain normal weight gain	Prenatal exercises (especially the pelvic tilt and knee–chest twist) Apply heat to the lower back Have a backrub or back massage Rest the back	Analgesics Aspirin, Tylenol
Edema		
High-protein foods Avoid highly salted foods Avoid standing for long periods Avoid tight clothing and constrictions of legs Rest and elevate legs 2–3 times daily for 20 min	Sit with legs raised as much as possible Follow suggestions under prevention	Diuretics (prescriptions and over-the-counter water pills)

(Continued)

Natural Remedies for Minor Discomforts of Pregnancy (Continued)

Prevention	Natural Remedies	Medicines Not to Be Used*
Difficulty sleeping		
Exercise daily Take a warm bath at bedtime Drink hot water with lemon, or warm milk, at bedtime Do not eat a large meal within 2–3 hr of bedtime Decrease noise and lights Do relaxation exercises Use pillows under knees, back, or abdomen Avoid caffeine	Relax and do not worry about not sleeping; even lying in bed is restful to the body Read for a while Follow suggestions under prevention	Sleeping aids (Sleep-Ez, Nytol, Sominex, Compoz, etc) Sedatives Tranquilizers
Stuffy nose and allergies		
Avoid allergens Do not smoke cigarettes, avoid smoke-filled rooms	Breathe steam from hot shower, pot of boiling water, or vaporizer/humidifier Drink plenty of liquids Salt-water nose drops (¼ tsp salt in 1 cup warm water) Warm, moist towel on sinuses; massage sinuses	Antihistamines (in most cold remedies—Contac, Coricidin, Allerest, Dristan, etc)

*In severe cases, the physician may prescribe a medication after weighing the benefits to the mother and risks to the fetus.

Vaginal Discharge

In pregnancy there is increased vaginal secretion so that a heavier discharge at this time usually has no particular significance. However, it is wise to instruct the patient to call any copious or yellow or greenish foul-smelling or irritating discharge to the attention of the physician. For instance, a profuse yellow discharge may be regarded as a possible evidence of gonorrhea or Trichomonas (see Chap. 35), especially when it is accompanied by such symptoms as vaginal itching or burning, or by such urinary manifestations as burning on urination and frequency. The microscopic result of a smear or culture indicates whether or not definite treatment is necessary.

If any discharge becomes irritating, the patient may be advised to bathe the vulva with a solution of sodium bicarbonate or boric acid. The application of KY jelly after bathing often relieves the condition entirely. Instructing a patient to wear a perineal pad is sometimes all the advice that is needed. A douche should never be taken unless prescribed by the physician.

Trichomonas

A particularly stubborn form of leukorrhea in pregnancy is caused by the parasitic protozoan known as the *Trichomonas vaginalis.* It is characterized not only by a profuse frothy discharge (yellow–green in color), but also by irritation and itching of the vulva and the vagina. The diagnosis is easily made by taking a small quantity of the fresh vaginal discharge and examining it under the microscope in a hanging-drop or wet prep. Here the spindle-shaped organisms, somewhat larger than leukocytes, with whiplike processes attached, can be seen in active motion.

Trichomonas vaginitis is treated with sulfanilamide, aminacrine hydrochloride, and allantoin (AVC cream), aminoacridine hydrochloride, polyox-

Vaginal Discharge Caused by Infections

Type	Causative Organism	Signs and Symptoms	Treatment
Candidiasis	*Candida albicans,* yeast	Thick, white, cottage-cheese or curdy discharge on cervix and vagina Pruritis (itching) of perineum, labia, thighs Erythema of labia, perineum Edema of genitalia if severe	Fungicidal creams or suppositories (Nystatin, Mycostatin, Nilstat)
Trichomonas	*Trichomonas vaginalis,* protozoan	Copious yellow–green, frothy discharge Pruritis (itching) of perineum, labia, thighs Erythema of labia, perineum Petechiae of cervix and vagina	AVC cream, trichofuron cream or suppositories, Vagisec suppositories Note. *Flagyl (metronidazole), although highly effective, is contraindicated during pregnancy due to its teratogenic effects*

yethylene nonyl phenol, sodium edetate, sodium dioctyl sulfosuccinate (Vagisec suppositories) or trichofuron cream. Although oral metronidazole (Flagyl) is highly effective, it is contraindicated during pregnancy because of its potential for fetal abnormalities.[15] Simultaneous treatment of the sexual partner is recommended, usually with oral Flagyl, as the infection is transmitted through sexual contact, although males are generally asymptomatic.

Candidiasis

Candidiasis, a yeast infection caused by the *Candida albicans,* is another common cause of profuse vaginal discharge. The organism is frequently present in the vaginal canal without producing symptoms, but during pregnancy the physical changes in the vagina produce conditions that foster development of infection. It is characterized by white patches on the vaginal mucosa and a thick cottage-cheeselike discharge which is extremely irritating, so that burning or pruritus is present. Even the external genitalia often become inflamed, and occasionally extensive edema is observed. Bleeding may accompany the other symptoms if the patches on the mucosa are removed.

It is not necessary to treat patients in whom *Candida* are found if signs and symptoms are not present. Specific fungicidal suppositories, such as Mycostatin, are used to treat this condition. Although this treatment is effective, the infection is stubborn and likely to recur and require repeated treatment during the pregnancy. The *pruritis,* or itching of the skin, may be relieved to a marked degree if proper hygienic measures are employed to keep the area free of the irritating discharge being deposited on the skin surface.

The woman who has this infection may transmit it to her infant during the process of delivery. *Thrush* develops when the organisms colonize the mucous membrane of the infant's mouth.

Drugs During Pregnancy

The use of all medication is to be minimized during pregnancy. Evidence regarding the adverse effects of many chemical substances when taken by a pregnant woman continues to accumulate. Because of the rapid formation of fetal organ systems and development of cellular functions, the first trimester is a particularly susceptible time. However, ingestion of drugs at any time during pregnancy holds potential for fetal damage. The impact of a drug on the developing fetus may range from no measurable effect to such marked toxicity that the embryo is killed (aborted). Sublethal doses of drugs may result in gross anatomical defects or a permanent subtle metabolic or functional deficit.

The effects of drugs and other substances, such as toxic chemicals used in industry or agriculture, upon the embryo or fetus can be grouped into three classes—(1) *Mutagens* are chemicals or substances that cause a change in gene structure; they alter genetic information. When sperm or ova are affected, such mutations can cause miscarriage, congenital defects, mental retardation and other mental and physical abnormalities in the infant. Radiation is one classic cause of mutations, but many other substances are known or suspected causes of mutagenic action. (2) *Carcinogens* are chemicals or substances which can induce or promote cancer. Transplacental carcinogens are often difficult to identify because of the long latency period in development of tumors. In prenatally exposed females, vaginal adenomas caused by administration of diethylstilbestrol to their mothers do not appear in the daughters for some 18 to 20 years. Many agents have been identified as carcinogenic in either humans or animals. It is suggested that the recently discovered rise of cancer in children may be due to chemical exposures during pregnancy. (3) *Teratogens* are chemicals or substances that interfere with fetal development after conception. This is an acute toxicologic event which requires only short or instantaneous exposure. The pathological results

Recommendations for Drug Use During Pregnancy

Drugs Contraindicated Throughout Pregnancy

- Antineoplastic agents
- Diethylstilbestrol
- Oral hypoglycemics
- Radioactive iodine
- Tetracycline
- Metronidazole (Flagyl)
- Oral contraceptives
- Quinine
- Corticosteroids
- Thalidomide
- Sedatives and tranquilizers (*i.e.,* Librium, Valium, Meprobamate, Tofranil)
- Diphenylhydantoin (Dilantin)
- Trimethadione (Tridione)
- Lasix
- Propylthiouracil
- Indomethacin (Indocin)
- Streptomycin
- Chloramphenicol (Chloromycetin)
- Chloroquine (Aralen)
- Dextroamphetamines
- Vitamins A, C, D, or K in excess

Drugs Used with Caution During Pregnancy

- Diuretics
- Antihypertensives
- Anticonvulsants
- Oral anticoagulants
- Phenothiazines
- Antithyroid drugs (except those contraindicated above)
- Antibiotics (except those contraindicated above)
- Antihistamines
- Theophylline
- Caffeine (anomalies, abortion with more than 600 mg/day)
- Salicylates
- Laxatives (other than bulk-producing)
- Local anesthetics
- Nicotine

Drugs to Avoid Near Term or During Delivery

- CNS depressants
- Narcotic analgesics
- Nitrofurantoin
- Oral anticoagulants
- Salicylates
- Sedatives
- Sulfonamides
- Vitamin K
- Lithium

are seen within a relatively short time. Many drugs are known to have teratogenic effects on the fetus if taken during pregnancy, causing such anomalies as bone and limb deformities, deafness, cardiac defects, growth retardation, prematurity, and metabolic abnormalities.

A drug's potential for teratogenesis or other adverse effects depends upon the degree to which it enters fetal circulation, the dosage, duration of administration, stage of pregnancy, and physical condition of mother and maturity of infant at birth. Most drugs cross the placenta by simple diffusion. Diffusion of a substance depends on its concentration, degree of ionization, lipid solubility and molecular weight. Nonionized and highly lipid-soluble compounds diffuse more readily across the placenta; substances with molecular weights greater than 1000 do not pass by diffusion. The fetus and infant are particularly susceptible to drugs as they have a limited ability to metabolize and excrete drugs, and there may be inefficiency in the blood–brain barrier, and increased affinity of various receptor sites.[16]

Prenatal counseling stresses the importance of avoiding use of self medication and prescription medication. The vast majority of drugs has not received adequate clinical testing to establish their safety during pregnancy. Those drugs with known or suspected toxicity should be avoided. All other drugs must be given very cautiously to pregnant women, with the benefits of administering the drug weighed against the potential risk to the fetus. The nurse assesses medication and street-drug use during the prenatal history, and discusses the risks involved if the mother is taking drugs. When the physician does prescribe a drug for a necessary treatment, the smallest dosage for the shortest period of time is given (see chart on Recommendations for Drug Use During Pregnancy).

When assisting the pregnant women find relief from the minor discomforts of pregnancy, the nurse can suggest natural remedies which do not rely upon medications. The safest course for the baby is to avoid taking any drugs at all (see Natural Remedies for Minor Discomforts of Pregnancy).

Preparations for the Baby

Layette

The baby's layette and equipment are of real interest to all parents, in fact, they are interesting to almost everyone. The cost of the layette should be in keeping with the individual economic circumstances.

Baby clothing should have the following characteristics. It should be comfortable, lightweight, and easy to put on and launder. Any clothing which comes in contact with the infant's skin should be made of soft cotton material. Wool should be avoided because it can irritate an infant's skin. Knitted materials are preferred because they are easy to launder and can stretch sufficiently to allow more freedom in dressing the baby. Caution should be taken that the materials are fire resistant. Garments that open down the full length and fasten with ties or grippers are easier to put on. Ties or grippers are also safer than buttons.

The geographic location and climate greatly influence the selection of the infant's clothing. Size 1 shirts and gowns are recommended, since the infant grows rapidly in the first 6 months and quickly outgrows garments. It is important to remember that clothing should not inhibit the baby's normal activities. The complete outfit of clothes that the baby wears need not weigh more than 12 oz to 16 oz.

The mother can be advised to prepare a very simple layette. As she sees how fast her baby grows, and what is needed, the additional items can be secured. The complete layettes which can be purchased often contain unnecessary items and are costly. Also, many articles may be received as baby gifts. Therefore, it is wise to choose only those things which are necessary for immediate use.

Some further suggestions in relation to the selection of specific items are as follows.

Shirts, Gowns, and the Like

The sleeves should have roomy armholes, such as the raglan-type sleeve. If a pullover-type garment is used, the neck opening should be so constructed that it is large enough to be put on easily over the feet or the head.

Diapers

The selection of diapers should be considered from the standpoint of their comfort (soft and light in weight), absorbency, cost and washing and drying qualities. The mother who plans to use a commercial diaper service may either use the company's diapers or her own. Disposable diapers are frequently used but they may be more expensive in the long run than cloth diapers or a diaper service.

Receiving Blankets

Receiving blankets should be made of cotton flannelette, 1 yard square. This square is used to fold loosely about the baby. If the blanket is properly secured, the baby may lie and kick and at the same time keep covered and warm. In the early weeks these squares take the brunt of the service and in this way save the finer covers from becoming soiled so quickly.

Afghans or Blankets
These can be of very light-weight cotton or polyester material. The temperature and the weather will determine the amount of covering needed.

Sheets
Crib sheets are usually 45 inches by 72 inches and are available in muslin, percale, and knitted cotton materials. The knit sheets are practical for bottom sheets and do not need to be ironed. Pillowcases are very usable for the carriage or the basket mattress. Receiving blankets may be used for top sheets.

Waterproof Sheeting
Various waterproof materials are suitable to protect the mattress and to be used under the pads. Even though the mattress may have a protective covering, it is necessary to have a waterproof cover large enough to cover the mattress completely–something that can be removed and washed.

Waterproof Pants
These offer protection for special occasions. If the plastic variety is used, they should not be tight at the leg or the waist. For general use, a square of protective material such as Sanisheeting or a cotton quilted pad can be used under the baby next to the diaper.

Bath Apron
This is a protection for both mother and baby and may be made of plastic material covered with terry cloth.

Nursery Equipment
In choosing the equipment, again the individual circumstances should be considered. Expense, space, and future plans all influence the selection. Most nurseries are planned for the satisfaction of the parents. Eventually the baby's room becomes the child's room; and if economy must be considered, furniture should be selected that will appeal to the child as he grows and develops.

Bed
A basket, bassinet, or crib may be used as the baby's bed. The trimming on the basket or the bassinet should be such that it can be removed easily and laundered. A bed may be improvised from a box or a bureau drawer, placed securely on a sturdy table or on chairs which are held together with rope. Many parents may have a carriage that may be used as a bed. However, after about the first 2 months, the baby needs a crib. The crib should be constructed so that the bars are close enough together to prevent the

Layette

Layette Necessities

Five or six shirts

Three to four dozen diapers (if diaper service is not used)

Four to six receiving blankets (These are very versatile items and can be used in various ways. For instance, they can be rolled firmly and used to support the back when the infant is on his side; in emergencies, they can be used as bathtowels, diaper pads, and sheets.)

Three to six nightgowns, kimonos, or sacques

Six cotton covered waterproof diaper pads (11″ x 16″)

Two waterproof protectors for under diaper pads

Two afghans or blankets } (if climate is cold)
One bunting }

Two to four soft towels (40″ x 40″)

Two to four soft washcloths

Nursery Equipment

Basket, bassinet, or crib

Mattress (firm, flat and smooth)

Mattress protector (waterproof)

Sheets or pillowcases for mattress

Chest or separate drawer

Cotton crib blankets

Bathtub

Diaper pail

Equipped toilet tray

Absorbent cotton or cotton balls

Baby soap (bland, white, unscented)

Rustproof safety pins

Soapdish

Bath apron (for mother)

Table for bathing or dressing

Chair (for mother)

Additional Suggestions for Layette and Equipment

Sweaters	Footstool
Crib spreads	Diaper bag (for traveling)
Bibs	Disposable diapers
Clothes drier	Nursery light
Chest of drawers	Carriage or stroller
Nursery stand	Car seat

baby's head from being caught between them. If it is painted, a nonleaded paint that is "safe for babies" should be used.

Mattress

The mattress is to be firm (not hard) and flat. All mattresses, including the waterproof-covered type, can be protected by a waterproof sheeting to prevent the mattress from becoming stained and from absorbing odors. The waterproof sheet is easily washed and dries quickly.

Bathtub

The plastic tub is safe and easy to keep clean. Some mothers adapt the kitchen or bathroom sink for the baby's bath.

Diaper Pail

This should be large enough for at least the day's supply of soiled diapers. It may be used also for boiling the diapers.

Use of Community Resources

The nurse in the office or the clinic who is alert to actual or potential health problems that affect both the woman and her family recognizes that a home visit by a community-health nurse often is very helpful. If such a situation arises, the woman can be informed about available community-health services, and what the community-health nurse (CHN) might do while making a home visit and how such a visit can be beneficial. With the physician's knowledge and the woman's permission, a referral can be made through the proper channels. Each institution or agency has its own procedure.

Real value may be derived from a visit in which the nurse is able to see the woman in her usual surroundings. For instance, if the woman has the problem of excessive weight gain and is not responding to clinic therapy, the CHN can visit the home and gain some insight into the basis of the problem. In her report to the clinic or the office staff, she relates information that contributes to both the medical and the nursing management of this pregnancy.

In situations in which the clinic program is limited in educational opportunities, such as parents' classes or individual guidance, the community-health nurse's visit to the home may be necessary to supplement the health-care teaching and anticipatory guidance done in the clinic.

Role of the Community-Health Nurse

The nurse in the community is "home based" in either an official or a voluntary agency. The official health agency may have an antepartal clinic offering complete antepartal services for those families who are having financial crises that may or may not be a result of the pregnancy.

If the woman or her family has a problem that the clinic nurse thinks needs to be followed up in the home (between clinic visits), she contacts the CHN and communicates the necessary information. In turn, the CHN informs the clinic personnel of any pertinent findings. If complete comprehensive care is to be given to patients, open lines of communication and an expeditious interagency referral system are basic to the best service of all members of the health team, whatever their level of responsibility.

Home Visits

The district CHN does not follow a stereotyped routine when she makes her home visits, since each visit involves an individual patient in her own home setting. She does not have the "captive audience" that the hospital nurse does; rather she is a guest in the woman's home, and this involves a somewhat different approach and orientation. In such a situation, it is especially important to orient the visit to what the woman wants and needs to know. Repeated visits based on the *nurse's* needs (to impart certain information, instruction, and so on) may very well result in a firmly closed door and a consequent severing of the nurse–patient relationship.

Astute assessment of the situation at each visit includes, first of all, finding out what the woman needs to know. Communication and observation skills (previously mentioned) are, of course, of paramount importance here. It is the wise nurse who takes her cues from the mother and handles each need as it arises without feeling compelled to "teach" a certain amount of material each visit. If the visits are managed in this way, topics may include basic information about pregnancy, hygiene, and nutrition, specific preparations for the baby, how to handle sibling rivalry, and so on. These subjects may come up naturally in the course of the visits, or the nurse can guide conversation around to them as she explores with the mother certain areas of need. By the end of the antepartal supervision period, all necessary counseling usually can be accomplished.

Opportunities for Family-Health Supervision

During the course of antepartal care, the nurse has many opportunities for family-health supervision. In her observation of other children in the home, she

NC Nursing Care: Antepartal Nursing Care

Assessment	Intervention	Evaluation
Physiological status of pregnancy	Take general health history and obstetrical history, physical examination and laboratory tests as part of antepartal workup; continue surveillance at return visits	Identification of EDC, minor health problems (*i.e.*, anemia, urinary tract infection), complications of pregnancy, concurrent disease, high risk factors
Psychosocial status of pregnancy	Provide patient profile, identifying data, family composition, attitudes toward pregnancy, knowledge levels, expectations related to pregnancy, family and personal resources, coping mechanisms, and economic situation	Identification of actual and potential problems, sources of strength, resource networks, and information gaps
Health maintenance needs	Provide information about ways to promote health and well-being during pregnancy (*i.e.*, rest, exercise, work, recreation, travel, medications and immunizations, skin care, breast care, clothes, teeth, bowel habits, douching, smoking, sexual relations, drug and alcohol use)	Identification of areas needing improvement; inquire into changes in behaviors; determine if sense of well-being is improved following changes; note areas that continue to be problems
	Refer to appropriate health professional or agency when significant problems are identified	Follow-through of referral, recommendations, and treatment plans
Minor discomforts	Provide information and instruction about occurrence and alleviation of such discomforts as urinary frequency, nausea and vomiting, heartburn, constipation, flatulence, hemorrhoids, backache, dyspnea, varicosities, leg cramps, and vaginal discharge	Identify present discomforts and determine whether remedies advised improved symptoms, or if understanding alleviated concern

may be the first person to notice a neglected orthopedic condition, to suspect a need for a chest roentgenogram, or to observe a possible vision or hearing difficulty. In addition, observation of the mother's interaction with her children may give valuable clues to the woman's mothering patterns. This aids the nurse in planning more effective anticipatory guidance and health teaching.

The Medical Social Worker

The medical social worker, a member of the extended health team, works closely with the nurse in the care of the pregnant woman. Most hospitals and community-health agencies have a substantial Social Service Department.

The function of social-service workers is to help people meet and cope with problems that interfere with social functioning. These problems may include unmarried parenthood, divorce, desertion, placing older children during the mother's hospital stay, arranging for a working housekeeper, planning convalescent care for the mother, or arranging financial or material assistance.

In their professional role, social workers are called on to evaluate these problems. Then, with the patient's cooperation, they help her to mobilize her resources and assist her, when necessary, through referral and

Assessment	Intervention	Evaluation
Minor discomforts (continued)	Refer to physician or other health professional if difficulties persist or if there is present significant interference with daily activities	Follow-through of referral, recommendations, and treatment plans
Prenatal educational needs	Provide specific information and instruction related to growth and development of the fetus, progression of pregnancy, physical and emotional changes, prenatal management routines, preparation for childbirth, or refer to sources providing these educational services (*i.e,* childbirth classes, nutritionist)	Patient affirms understanding, has no further questions, has become involved in classes, has made preparations for labor and delivery and for infant care at home
Indicators of complications of pregnancy (*i.e.,* rising blood pressure, facial edema, bleeding, excessive weight gain, inappropriate fundal measurements for dates)	Notify physician, obtain additional physical data and laboratory tests as indicated, explain to patient the meaning of symptoms and signs and the plan of care	Control or alleviation of signs and symptoms of complications; patient affirms understanding and cooperates with treatment plans
Indicators of stress and psychosocial problems (*i.e.,* missed appointments, noncompliance, affect, direct expression of concerns, acting out behavior of children, complaints)	Determine sources of problems, whether economic, interpersonal, due to emotional illness, cultural discrepancies, or conflicts with the system of health care; provide counseling according to level of skills, refer as needed for more intensive therapy; use community resources for socioeconomic, cultural disparity problems; work with agency and health team to improve patient relations if this is a problem	Patient affirms improvement of the problem, follows through on referrals, implements suggestions and recommendations, and reports that these have been helpful; some concrete indicators could be initiation of family therapy, application for social relief or medical care assistance, keeping appointments, and complying with treatment

counseling to alleviate the condition. They may make home visits and interview the patient, and perhaps other family members, to aid them in diagnosing the extent of the problems.

Social problems may seem overwhelming if the patient's physical condition is affected, and these concerns, in turn, may interfere with the benefit that the patient may derive from medical services. The social worker may act as an understanding counselor between the family and the patient during her hospital stay. In many hospitals the need for a social service referral is apparent when the patient is registered early in pregnancy. In that event, the patient is interviewed after the initial medical examination, and from both the physical and the social findings plans are made with the patient to mobilize her resources.

By observation, counseling, and liaison work, the social worker combines efforts with the other members of the health team to see the patient not only as an individual maternity patient, but also as an important member of the family, and the family as an integral part of the community.

Summary

Comprehensive antepartal care is a quality of patient care that is goal directed toward the total health and the well-being of the pregnant woman and her family.

With this as the central objective, the combined efforts of several disciplines in addition to those of medicine and nursing, may be required in the cooperative plan to achieve the ultimate goals. The practitioner–patient relationship is reciprocal, involving giving and receiving by both parties, and, to be meaningful, it must be a positive interaction. This type of interaction can be achieved only if the patient and her problems are understood and viewed with respect. The patient, in turn, must be helped to understand the goals of the health practitioners.

A positive effort on the part of the health team becomes possible if each member has a clear understanding of his or her own role, appreciates and understands the contribution of the other professions represented on the team, knows something of the processes involved in the differing approaches, recognizes commonality of interest and skill, and has the intellectual and the emotional capacity to enter into a team relationship.

References

1. Quick JD, Greenlick MR, Roghmann KJ: Prenatal care and pregnancy outcome in an HMO and general population: A multivariate cohort analysis. American Journal of Public Health 71, 4:381–390, April 1981

2. Grimm LM: Changed patterns of obstetric care: Maternity continuity clinic. Am J Nurs 73:1723–1725, October 1973

3. Thompson HE, McFee JG, Haverkamp AD, Longwell FH: Factors contributing to improved maternal care and fetal outcome in a medium-sized city-county hospital. Am J Obstet Gynecol 116, 229–238, May 15, 1973

4. Public Law 93–641, 88 Stat. 2236, 93rd Congress, S. 2994, 4 January, 1975, pp 6–7

5. Holey ES: Promoting adequate weight gain in pregnant women. MCN 2, 2:86–89, March/April 1977

6. Woodward SL: How does strenuous maternal exercise affect the fetus? A review. Birth and the Family Journal, 8, 1:17–24, Spring 1981

7. Shearer MH: Teaching prenatal exercise: Part 1—Posture. Birth and the Family Journal, 8, 2:105–108, Summer 1981

8. Greenberg J: Implications for primary care providers of occupational health hazards on pregnant women and their infants. Journal of Nurse–Midwifery, 25, 4:21–30, July/August 1980

9. Drugs and therapeutic information. In Safety of Immunizing Agents in Pregnancy. Med Lett Drugs Ther 18, 291:5, March 6, 1970

10. Deibel P: Effects of cigarette smoking on maternal nutrition and the fetus. JOGN Nurs 9, 6:333–336, November/December 1980

11. New smoking risk found: Quitting before pregnancy no safeguard. Journal of Nurse–Midwifery 24, 2:24, March/April 1979

12. Meyer MB: How does maternal smoking affect birth weight and maternal weight gain? Am J Obstet Gynecol 131:888–893, August 15, 1978

13. Stephens CJ: The fetal alcohol syndrome: Cause for concern. MCN 6:251–256, July/August 1981

14. Cooper SB: Preventing back abuse in young mothers. MCN 2, 4:260–263, July/August 1977

15. Is Flagyl dangerous? Med Lett Drugs Ther 17:53–54 1975

16. Gullekson DJ, Temple AR: Maternal drug use during the perinatal period. Family and Community Health, 1, 3:31–41, November 1978

Suggested Reading

Anderson SF: Childbirth as a pathological process: An American perspective. MCN 2, 4:240–244, July/August 1977

Bancroft AV: Pregnancy and the counter-culture. Nurs Clin North Am 8:67–76, March 1973

Block D: Some crucial terms in nursing: What do they really mean? Nurs Outlook 22, 11:689–694, November 1974

Erikson MP: Trends in assessing the newborn and his parents. MCN 3, 2:99–103, March/April 1978

Jordan AD: Evaluation of a family-centered maternity care hospital program. JOGN Nurs 2, 1:13–35, January/February 1973

Kowalski KE: Changed patterns of obstetric care on call staffing. Am J Nurs 73, 10:1725–1727, October 1973

LaFage WL: A reversal of roles for the maternity nurse—New insights. MCN 2, 5:313–314, September/October 1977

Martin LM: Health Care of Women. Philadelphia, JB Lippincott, 1978

Otte MJ: Correcting inverted nipples. Am J Nurs 75:454–456, March 1975

Over-the-Counter-Drug Committee of the Coalition for the Medical Rights of Women: Safe natural remedies for discomforts of pregnancy. 1638B Haight Street, San Francisco, CA 94117

Study Aids for Unit IV: Antepartal Assessment and Management

Conference Material

1. A mother in her first trimester is undergoing a difficult divorce. She appears very anxious and upset and tells you that she sometimes feels like she is losing her mind. What do you know about the psychological and physiological effects of anxiety during pregnancy. What specific interventions would you plan to help this mother?

2. A couple comes to childbirth education classes and the husband complains that he had symptoms of morning sickness during the first trimester and is now experiencing low back pain and aching legs. What might your counseling be for this couple?

3. A young husband complains to you that his wife's sexual desire has changed since she has become pregnant. When he tells you, you note that his wife becomes flushed and tense. What would you tell this couple to reassure them about their apparent problem?

4. What childbirth education classes are available in your community? How do they compare to the "variables to consider in selecting a childbirth class?" (See Table 19-3)

5. What community resources are available for prenatal and postpartum exercise classes and parenting classes?

6. A 34-year-old woman delivered her first baby a few hours ago. She and her husband attended childbirth classes. The woman requested and received 50 mg demerol during her labor. She tells you how guilty she feels because she needed medication for pain, as she and her husband had hoped to have a "natural birth." How would you respond to this patient?

7. Examine several women on their third postpartum day for diastasis recti. Depending on the results of your findings teach each woman an appropriate exercise to strengthen her abdominal muscles.

8. A 15-year-old mother from a low-income family will be going home with her baby in 2 days. She will be living with her mother and father. What specific teaching measures would you include in discharge planning for this patient?

9. Dorothea W. is a 28-year-old married mother of two, presently in the seventh month of her third pregnancy. Her husband Sam works as a printer; the children are both boys, ages seven and four. Dorothea quit her secretarial job last month, and plans not to work until the new baby is about 2 years of age. Her pregnancy has been progressing normally; she has experienced recent discomfort with hemorrhoids and heartburn. At her prenatal visit, you notice that she has gained 8 lb since the last visit 1 month ago, and she has moderate edema of the ankles and hands. The couple will begin childbirth classes in 2 weeks; both previous deliveries have been conscious and participative, without complications. In conducting Dorothea's prenatal visit, discuss how you would approach and manage the following areas:

Conference Material (continued)

A. Assessment of potential occupational hazards to the fetus
B. Counseling her about prevention and control of hemorrhoids and heartburn
C. Evaluation of her weight gain and edema
D. Assessing the family's economic situation
E. Determining her educational and informational needs at this stage of pregnancy

10. Sally S. has come to the clinic for her first antepartal visit. She is 20 years old, unmarried, and is 16 weeks pregnant. She is presently unemployed and is receiving welfare assistance; she lives at home with her divorced mother and two siblings. Sally is in good general health, but is 30% overweight and smokes one and one half packs of cigarettes per day. She wants to keep the baby, and relates that her mother will help her care for it. In your antepartal assessment, what areas will receive particular attention, both psychosocial and physical? What types of problems and complications are potentially present in Sally's situation? Based upon the information given, what risks can you identify for Sally, and what risks for the baby? How will you counsel Sally about weight gain during pregnancy? How will you counsel her about cigarette smoking? What types of community agency or specialist referrals might be appropriate for Sally?

11. One of the patients you have been following in the prenatal clinic, Mrs. Scott, has missed several appointments. She is a 43-year-old multipara with several moderately severe physical problems, including vulvar varicosities and gestational diabetes. Because of her missed appointments, a thorough antepartal assessment has not been done. However, the history does reveal that her last pregnancy, 3 years ago, ended in an unexplained stillbirth. Today Mrs. Scott has kept her appointment. When discussing the missed appointments, she mentions that she has been preoccupied with family troubles and difficulties with the children. She appears distracted and has a hard time keeping focused in the discussion. What specific problems will you consider as potential causes of Mrs. Scott's behavior? How will you further assess these problems? What risks are present for the fetus with each problem? What nursing intervention is appropriate, and what types of referrals might be indicated?

Multiple Choice

Read through the entire question and place your answer on the line to the right.

1. Below are some signs, symptoms, and conditions commonly associated with pregnancy. Those which the patient might notice and describe in the first trimester of pregnancy are:
A. Amenorrhea
B. Enlargement and tenderness of breasts
C. Enlargement of uterus
D. Frequent micturition
E. Goodell's sign

Select the number corresponding to the correct letters.
1. A and C
2. A, B and D
3. B, D and E
4. All of them _____

2. In pregnancy, morning sickness is most common during which of the following periods?
   A. First month
   B. First 6 weeks
   C. Sixth week to twelfth week
   D. First 4 months
   E. Eighth week to sixteenth week _____

3. A pregnant woman seen for the first time in the antepartal clinic has a hemoglobin of 10 g. The nurse should understand that this condition is:
   A. A true anemia
   B. Caused by increased blood volume
   C. Dangerous to baby's development
   D. Predisposing to postpartal hemorrhage _____

4. Active fetal movements are usually first perceived by motion
   A. In the third month of gestation
   B. Towards the end of the fifth month
   C. Between the sixth and seventh months _____

5. Which of the following placental hormones are the commonly employed tests for pregnancy designed to detect?
   A. Estrogens
   B. Progesterone
   C. Human placental lactogen (HPL)
   D. Human chorionic gonadotropin (HCG) _____

6. During her first visit to the clinic the mother confides to the nurse that she is afraid to have a baby. The most appropriate response of the nurse might be:
   A. "Modern obstetrics makes having a baby so safe that you have absolutely nothing to fear."
   B. "Perhaps if you discussed this with a psychiatrist he would help you to overcome this feeling."
   C. "Many women feel this way, so I wouldn't be concerned about it if I were you."
   D. "I can understand that you might feel this way. What is it in particular that you are worried about?" _____

7. Pregnancy has been referred to as a critical event in the lives of parents. Which of the following descriptions best describes pregnancy?
   A. Pregnancy is always a crisis
   B. Pregnancy is a role transition
   C. Pregnancy is just a normal developmental stage people go through _____

(continued)

8. Current research on pregnancy demonstrates that:

A. Men as well as women experience changes in body image during pregnancy
B. Men often have the physiological symptoms of pregnancy that their mates experience
C. Men do not identify with their mates very well during pregnancy

Select the number corresponding to the correct letters:

1. All of the above
2. A and B
3. A and C
4. B and C
5. C only ____

9. Several psychological tasks have to be accomplished by the mother during pregnancy. Which of the following is *not* a usual task?

A. Preparation for physical separation from the infant
B. Belief that she is pregnant and incorporation of the fetus into her body image
C. Working through the anger that usually accompanies pregnancy
D. Resolution of the identity confusions that accompany role transition ____

10. Certain specific psychological tasks of pregnancy seem to occur at specific times during gestation. Which one is not evident during later stages of pregnancy?

A. Perception of the fetus as a separate object
B. Readiness to assume the care-taking relationship with the baby
C. Incorporation and integration of the fetus
D. Preparation for labor ____

11. Expectant parents should consider which of the following variables when selecting a childbirth class?

A. Class size
B. Instructor's age
C. Whether or not the instructor has given birth
D. Professional credentials of instructor and type of training as a Childbirth Educator
E. Amount of class hours for the fee

Select the number corresponding to the correct letters.

1. A, C, D, and E
2. D and E
3. A, D, and E
4. A, B, D, and E
5. All of them ____

12. The purpose of breathing techniques for labor is to:

A. Increase pain perception
B. Provide oxygenation

C. Aid in relaxation
D. Obviate the need for analgesics

Select all that are correct. _____

13. Which exercise can help relieve low backache in pregnancy?
A. Shoulder circling
B. Back massage
C. Calf stretching
D. Pelvic rocking or pelvic tilt _____

14. Both prenatal and postpartum exercises are concerned with the following:
A. Improving circulation
B. Strengthening abdominal muscles
C. Improving tone of pelvic floor muscles
D. Strengthening leg muscles
E. Improving posture
F. Developing an awareness of relaxation of pelvic floor muscles

Select all that are correct. _____

15. Relaxation is:
A. A learned activity
B. A passive process
C. An active process
D. Requires awareness and concentration
E. A natural reaction

Select the number corresponding to the correct letters.
1. A, B, D, and E
2. A, C, D, and E
3. A, D, and E
4. A, C, and D
5. A, B, and D _____

16. Which of the following statements is true regarding weight gain during pregnancy?
A. Excessive weight gain is a cause of preeclampsia.
B. The obese client should be advised to limit her weight gain to 10 lb or less.
C. Inadequate weight gain during pregnancy is related to an increased incidence of low-birth-weight infants.
D. A weight gain of 20 lb is sufficient for most women during pregnancy. _____

17. Protein needs:
A. are decreased during pregnancy
B. can be met by a combination of foods from plant and animal sources
C. require inclusion in the diet of 20 essential amino acids
D. are more important than the need for other nutrients _____

(continued)

18. Which of the following questions would be helpful in the dietary assessment of a pregnant woman?
   A. Where are you from?
   B. Who purchases the food for your household?
   C. Are there any foods you cannot eat?
   D. All of the above. ____

Discussion

19. Name four components of quality maternity care that is available to all women in the population.

20. Name two procedures done in antepartal physical examinations to assess the condition of the fetus, and describe the information each provides.

21. What physical examination procedures and questions of the mother are included in each return visit during pregnancy?

22. Name six danger signals that a pregnant woman should report immediately to the physician.

23. What is considered an acceptable weight gain during pregnancy? What principles are followed in counseling the mother about weight gain?

24. Why is regular exercise so important during pregnancy? What are some exercises the nurse could advise the mother to do?

25. Name three occupational hazards to which women are frequently exposed, and describe the dangers to the fetus or mother from these.

26. What types of immunizations are contraindicated during pregnancy?

27. Describe preventive measures in breast care during pregnancy that help mothers avoid nipple cracking and infection later while nursing.

28. Why is constipation such a frequent problem among pregnant women?

29. How may hemorrhoids be prevented and controlled during pregnancy?

30. Name four risks to the fetus from maternal smoking.

31. What advice should be given pregnant women regarding alcohol consumption?

32. Describe natural remedies to prevent and control nausea and vomiting.

33. How may backache during pregnancy be avoided and relieved?

34. What is the management of varicose veins during pregnancy?

35. What measures provide immediate relief of leg cramps?

36. In evaluating edema in later pregnancy, what signs would raise your suspicion of preeclampsia?

37. Name the two common vaginal infections which frequently occur during pregnancy.

38. What general advice is given to pregnant women about use of drugs?

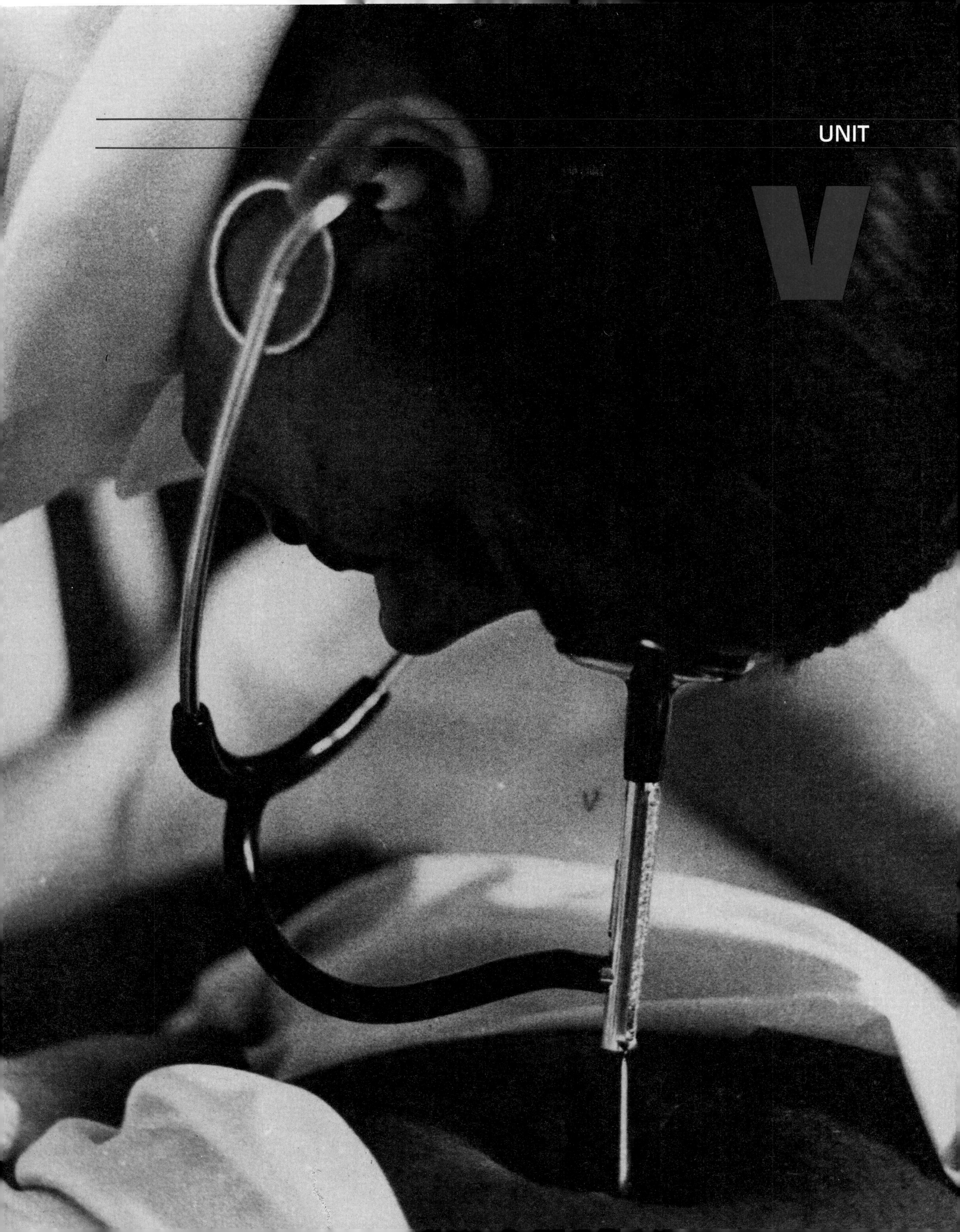

UNIT

V

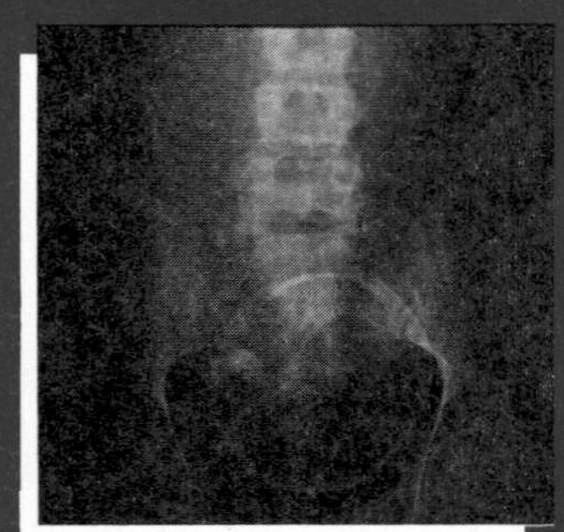

22 Presentations and Positions

Fetal Habitus

Fetal Head

Presentation

Positions

Fetal Skull Measurement

Diagnosis of Fetal Position

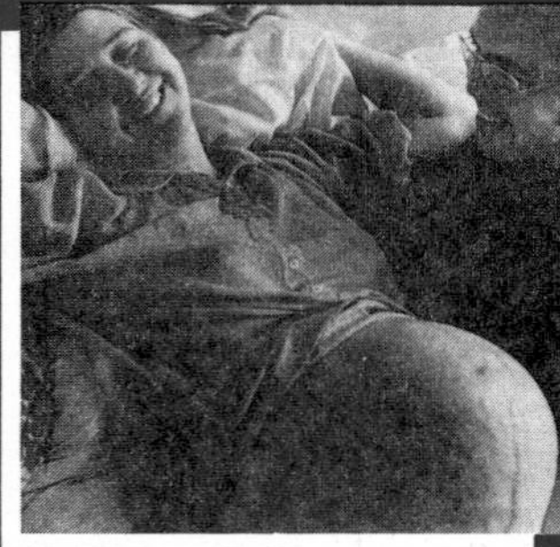

23 Phenomena of Labor

Premonitory Signs of Labor

Cause of Onset of Labor

Uterine Contractions

Duration of Labor

The Three Stages of Labor

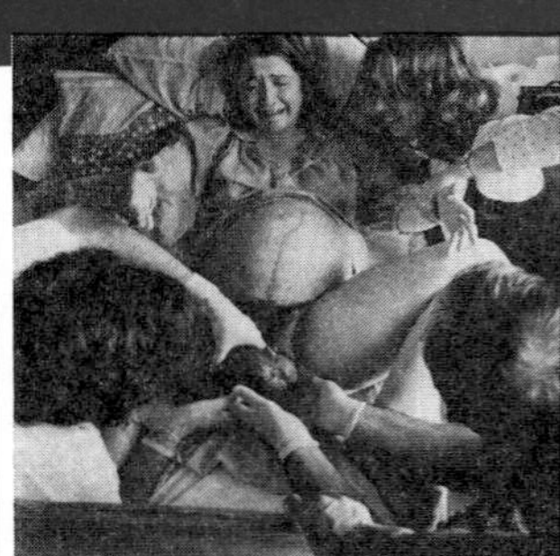

24 The Conduct of Normal Labor

Dimensions of Effective Nursing Care

Prelude to Labor

The Onset of Labor

Examinations in Labor

Conduct of the First Stage

Conduct of the Second Stage

Conduct of the Third Stage

Lacerations of the Birth Canal

Episiotomy and Repair

Conduct of the Fourth Stage

UNIT V

Intrapartal Assessment and Management

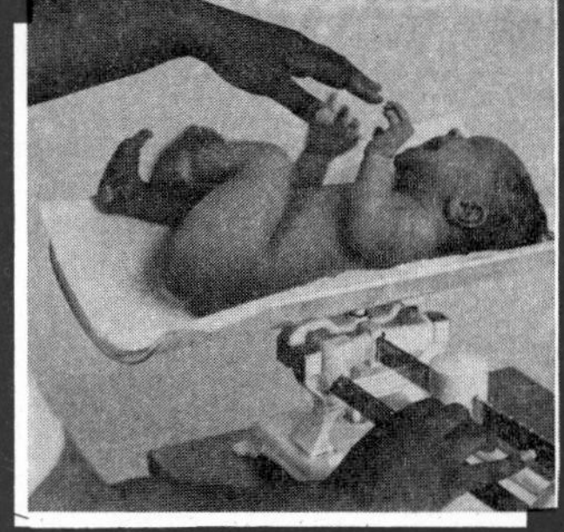

25 Immediate Care of the Newborn

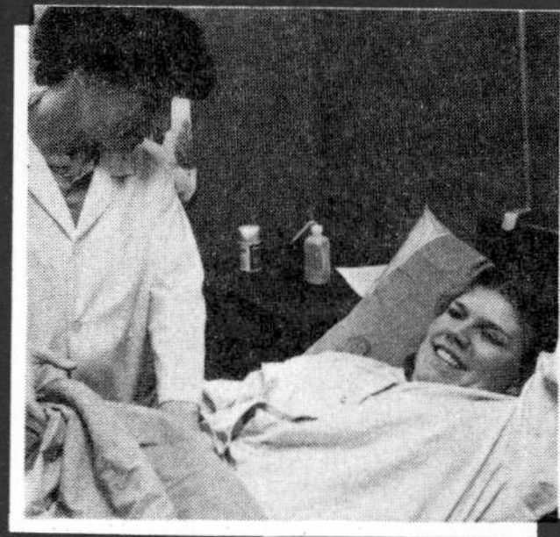

26 The Nurse's Contribution to Pain Relief During Labor

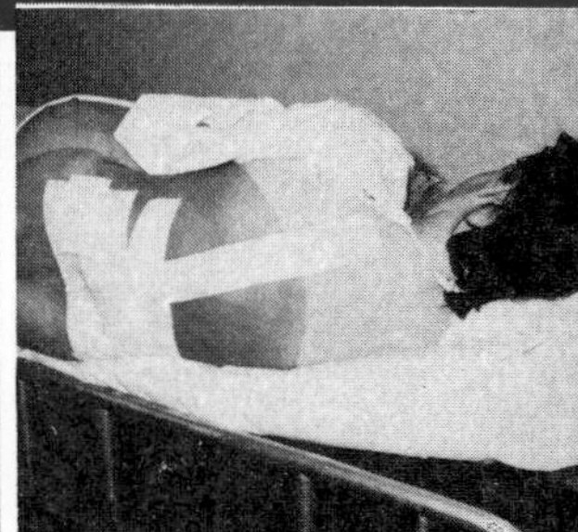

27 Analgesia and Anesthesia for Childbirth

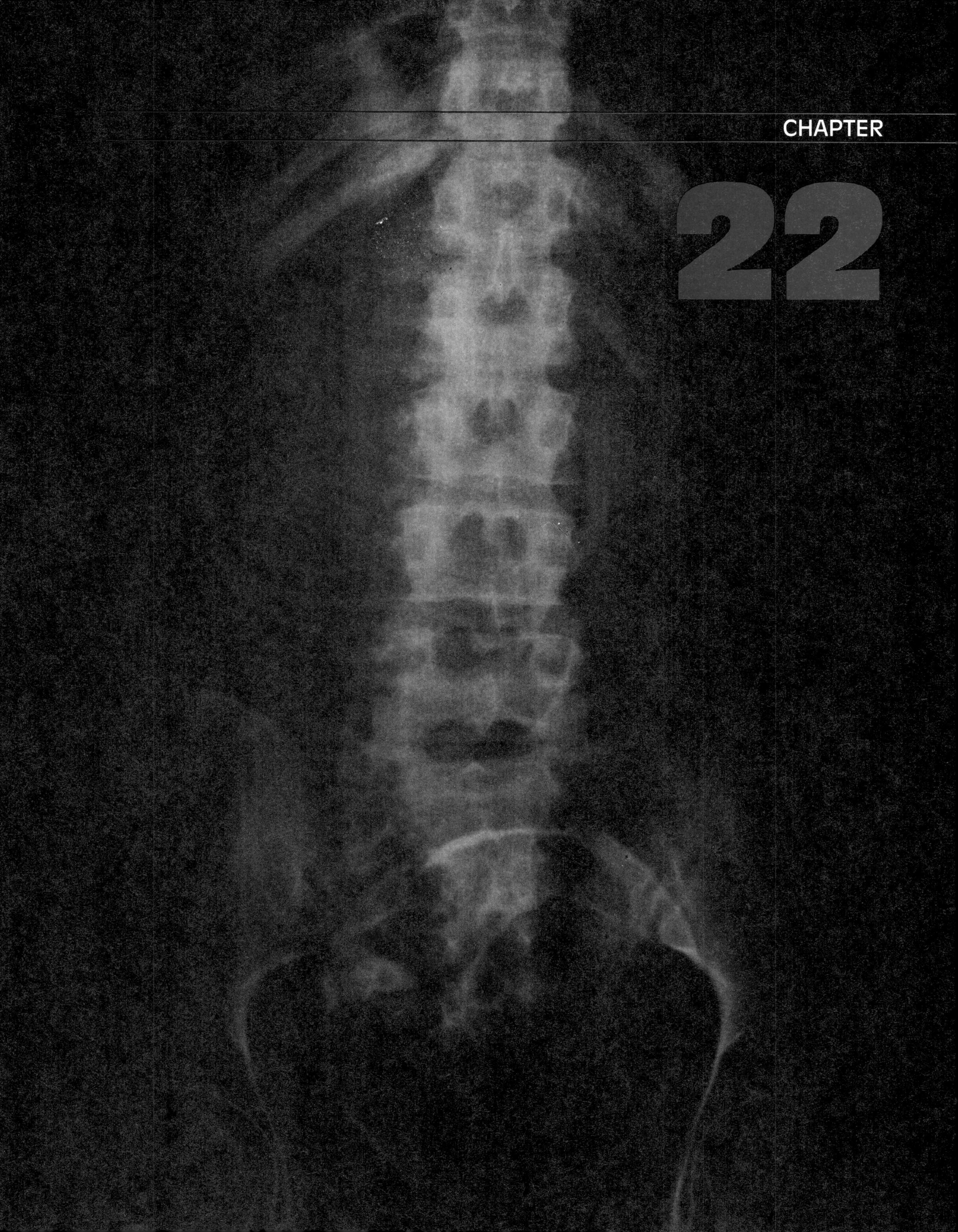

CHAPTER

22

CHAPTER 22

Presentations and Positions

Fetal Habitus

Habitus, or attitude, of the fetus means the relation of the fetal parts to one another. The most striking characteristic of the fetal habitus is flexion. The spinal column is bowed forward, the head is flexed with the chin against the sternum, and the arms are flexed and folded against the chest. The lower extremities also are flexed, the thighs are on the abdomen and the calves of the lower legs are against the posterior aspect of the thighs. In this state of flexion the fetus assumes a roughly ovoid shape, occupies the smallest possible space, and conforms to the shape of the uterus. In this attitude it is about half as long as if it were completely stretched out. However, there are times when the fetus assumes a different position.

Fetal Head

From an obstetrical viewpoint the head of the fetus is the most important part. If it can pass through the pelvic canal safely, there is usually no difficulty in delivering the rest of the body, although occasionally the shoulders may cause trouble.

The cranium, or skull, is made up of eight bones. Four of the bones—the sphenoid, the ethmoid, and the two temporal bones—lie at the base of the cranium, are closely united, and are of little obstetrical interest. On the other hand, the four bones forming the upper part of the cranium—the frontal, the occipital, and the two parietal bones—are of great importance. These bones are not knit closely together at the time of birth but are separated by membranous interspaces called *sutures.* The intersections of these sutures are known as *fontanels* (Fig. 22-1).

By means of this formation of the fetal skull, the bones can overlap each other somewhat during labor and so diminish materially the size of the head during its passage through the pelvis. This process of overlapping is called "molding," and after a long labor with a large baby and a snug pelvis, the head often is so definitely molded that several days may elapse before it returns to its normal shape.

The most important sutures are the sagittal, between the two parietal bones; the frontal, between the two frontal bones; the coronal, between the frontal and the parietal bones; and the lambdoid, between the posterior margins of the parietal bones and the upper margin of the occipital bone. The temporal sutures, which separate the parietal and the temporal bones on either side, are unimportant in obstetrics because they are covered by fat parts and cannot be felt on the living baby.

The important fontanels are the anterior and the posterior. The anterior fontanel is large and diamond shaped, and is located at the intersection of the sagittal and the coronal sutures, while the small triangular posterior fontanel lies at the junction of the sagittal and the lambdoid suture. The sutures and the posterior fontanel ossify shortly after birth, but the anterior fontanel remains open until the child is over a

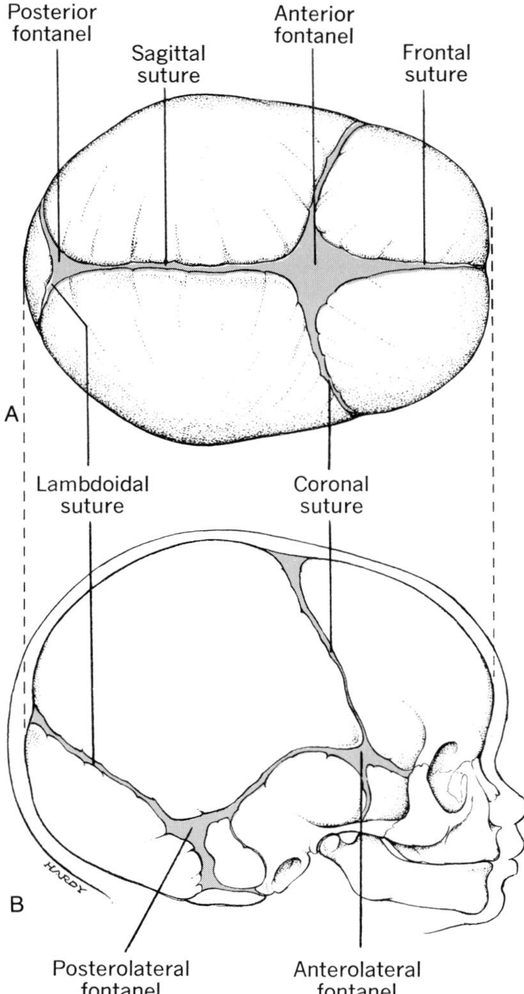

Figure 22-1.
Fetal skull showing fontanels and sutures: *(A)* superior aspect; *(B)* lateral aspect.

year old, constituting the familiar "soft spot" just above the forehead of an infant.

By feeling or identifying one or another of the sutures or fontanels and considering its relative position in the pelvis, one is able to accurately determine the position of the head in relation to the pelvis.

Presentation

The term *presentation* or *presenting part* is used to designate that portion of the infant's body which lies nearest the internal os, or, in other words, that portion which is felt by the examining fingers when they are introduced into the cervix. When the presenting part is known, by abdominal palpation, it is possible to determine the relation between the long axis of the baby's body and that of the mother.

Head or *cephalic presentations* are the most common, being present in about 97% of all cases at term. Cephalic presentations are divided into groups, according to the relation of the infant's head to its body (Fig. 22-2). The most common is the *vertex presentation,* in which the head is sharply flexed so that the chin is in contact with the thorax, thus the vertex is the presenting part. The *face presentation,* in which the neck is sharply extended so that the occiput and the back come in contact, is more rarely observed.

Breech presentation is the next most common, being present in about 3% of cases. In breech presentations the thighs may be flexed and the legs extended over the anterior surface of the body *(frank breech presentation),* or the thighs may be flexed on the abdomen and the legs on the thighs *(full breech presentation),* or one or both feet may be the lowest part *(foot or footling presentation).*

When the fetus lies crosswise in the uterus, it is in a "transverse lie" and the shoulder is the presenting part—*shoulder presentation.* The common causes of a transverse lie are abnormal relaxation of the abdominal walls due to great multiparity, pelvic contraction, and placenta previa. Shoulder presentations are relatively uncommon, and, with very rare exceptions, the spontaneous birth of a fully developed child is impossible in a "persistent transverse lie."

Positions

In addition to knowing the presenting part of the baby, it is important to know the exact position of the presenting part in relation to the pelvis. This relationship is determined by finding the position of certain

Figure 22-2.
Fetal presentations. (Redrawn from Benson, RC: Handbook of Obstetrics and Gynecology, 7th ed. Los Altos, California, Lange Medical Publications, 1980)

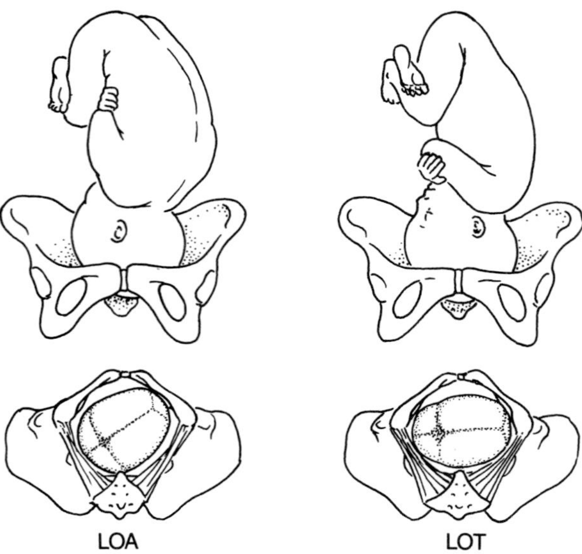

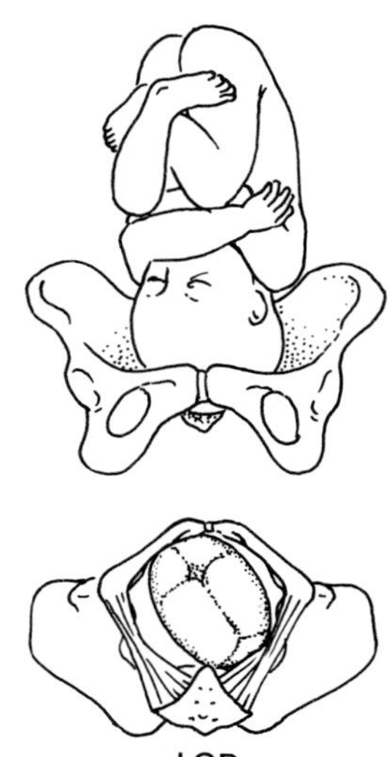

Vertex Presentations

points on the presenting surface and relating these to the four imaginary divisions or regions of the pelvis. For this purpose the pelvis is considered to be divided into quadrants—left anterior, left posterior, right anterior, and right posterior. These divisions aid in indicating whether the presenting part is directed toward the right side or the left side and toward the front or the back of the pelvis.

Certain points on the presenting surface of the baby have been arbitrarily chosen as points of direction in determining the exact relation to the presenting part of the quadrants of the pelvis. In vertex presentations the occiput is the guiding point; in face presentations, the chin (mentum); in breech presentations, the sacrum; and in shoulder presentations, the scapula (acromion process).

Position, then, has to do with the relation of some arbitrarily chosen portion of the fetus to the right or the left side of the mother's pelvis. Thus, in a vertex presentation, the back of the head (occiput) may point

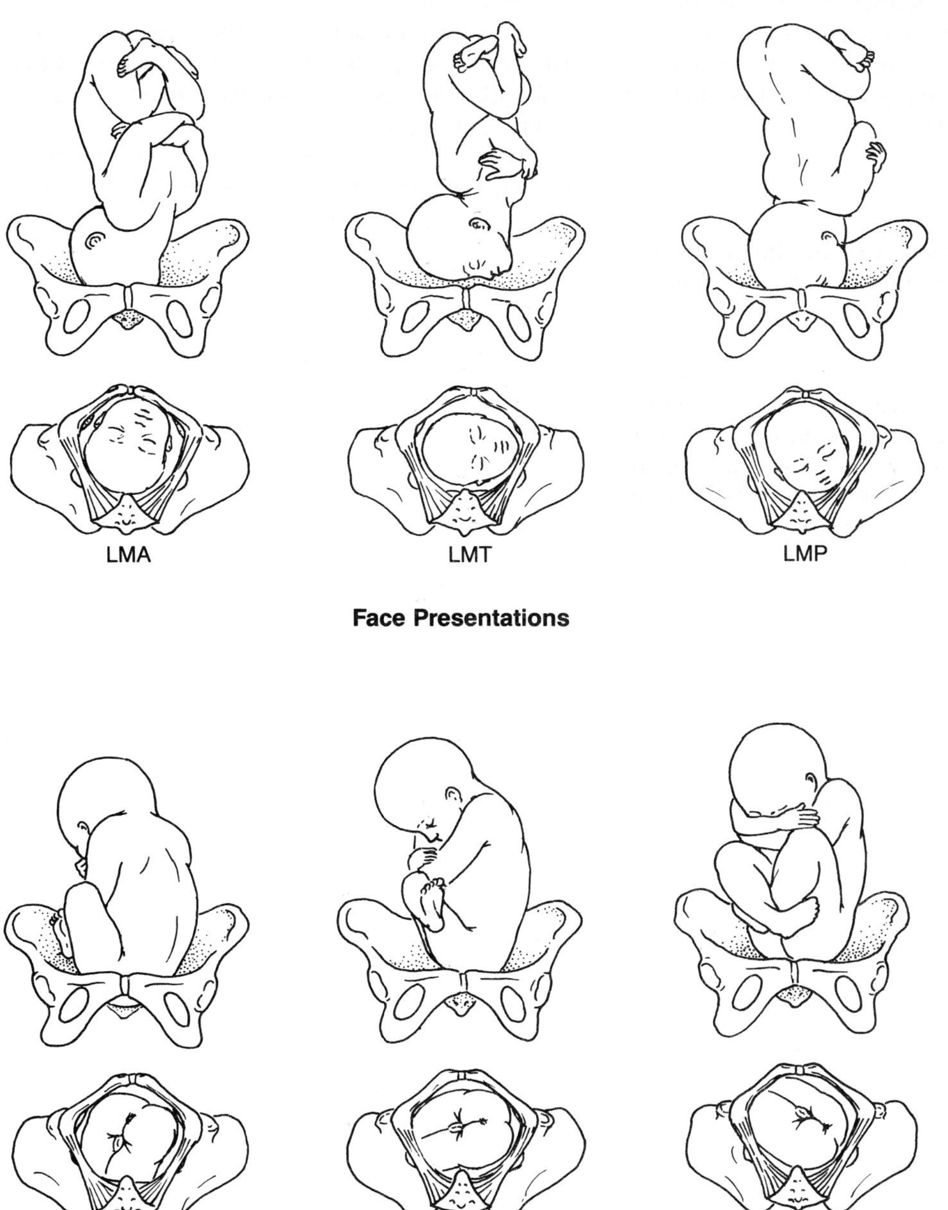

Abbreviations for Fetal Presentations

Positions—Vertex Presentation

L.O.A.—Left occipitoanterior
L.O.T.—Left occipitotransverse
L.O.P.—Left occipitoposterior
R.O.A.—Right occipitoanterior
R.O.T.—Right occipitotransverse
R.O.P.—Right occipitoposterior

Positions—Breech Presentation

L.S.A.—Left sacroanterior
L.S.T.—Left sacrotransverse
L.S.P.—Left sacroposterior
R.S.A.—Right sacroanterior
R.S.T.—Right sacrotransverse
R.S.P.—Right sacroposterior

Positions—Face Presentation

L.M.A.—Left mentoanterior
L.M.T.—Left mentotransverse
L.M.P.—Left mentoposterior
R.M.A.—Right mentoanterior
R.M.T.—Right mentotransverse
R.M.P.—Right mentoposterior

Positions—Shoulder Presentation

L.A.D.A.—Left acromiodorso-anterior
L.A.D.P.—Left acromiodorso-posterior
R.A.D.A.—Right acromiodorso-anterior
R.A.D.P.—Right acromiodorso-posterior

to the front or to the back of the pelvis. The occiput rarely points directly forward or backward in the median line until the second stage of labor, but usually it is directed to one side or the other.

The various positions are usually expressed by abbreviations made up of the first letter of each word which describes the position (see Abbreviations for Fetal Presentations). Thus, left occipitoanterior is abbreviated L.O.A. This means that the head is presenting with the occiput directed toward the left side of the mother and toward the front part of the pelvis. If the occiput is directed straight to the left with no deviation toward front or back of the pelvis, it is termed left occipitotransverse, or L.O.T. The occiput might also be directed toward the back or posterior quadrant of the pelvis, in which case the position is left occipitoposterior, or L.O.P. There are also three corresponding positions on the right side—R.O.A., R.O.T., and R.O.P.

The occipital anterior positions are considered the most favorable for both mother and baby, and of these, the L.O.A. position is most common.

The same system of terminology is used for face, breech, and shoulder presentations, as indicated in the Abbreviations for Fetal Presentations.

Although it is customary to speak of all "transverse lies" of the fetus simply as shoulder presentations, the examples of terminology sometimes used to express position in the shoulder presentation are listed. Left acromiodorso-anterior (L.A.D.A.) means that the acromion is to the mother's left and the back is anterior.

Fetal Skull Measurement

Figure 22-3 shows the principal measurements of the fetal skull. The most important transverse diameter is the biparietal; it is the distance between the biparietal protuberances and represents the greatest width of the head. It measures, on an average, 9.25 cm.

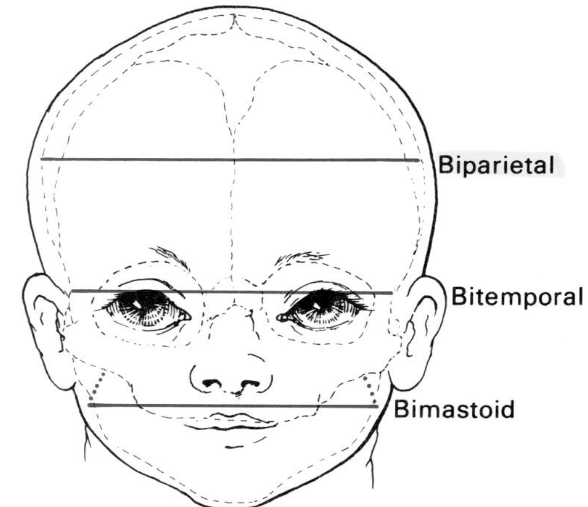

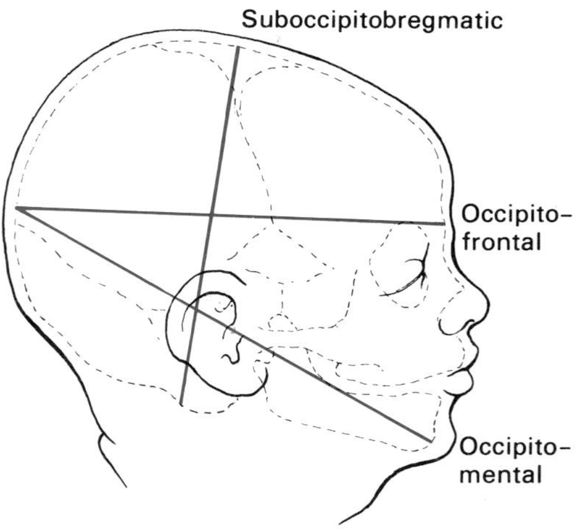

Figure 22-3.
Fetal skull showing various diameters.

There are three important anteroposterior diameters—the suboccipitobregmatic, which extends from the undersurface of the occiput to the center of the anterior fontanel and measures about 9.5 cm; the occipitofrontal, which extends from the root of the nose to the occipital prominence and measures about 12 cm; and the occipitomental, which extends from the chin to the posterior fontanel and averages about 13.5 cm.

In considering these three anteroposterior diameters of the fetal skull, it is important to note that with the head in complete flexion and the chin resting on the thorax, the smallest of these, the suboccipitobregmatic, enters the pelvis, whereas if the head is extended or bent back (with no flexion whatsoever), the greatest anteroposterior diameter presents itself to the pelvic inlet. Herein lies the great importance of flexion; the more the head is flexed, the smaller is the anteroposterior diameter which enters the pelvis. Figure 22-4 shows this basic principle in diagrammatic form.

Diagnosis of Fetal Position

Diagnosis of fetal position is made in five ways—abdominal palpation; vaginal examination; combined auscultation and examination; ultrasound; and in certain doubtful cases, the roentgenogram.

Palpation

It is extremely helpful to palpate the abdomen before listening to the fetal heart tones. The region of the abdomen in which the fetal heart is heard varies according to the presentation and the extent to which the presenting part has descended. The location of the fetal heart sounds by itself does not give very important information as to the presentation and the position of the child, but it sometimes reinforces the results obtained by palpation. To obtain satisfactory information by abdominal palpation for the determination of fetal position, the examination should be

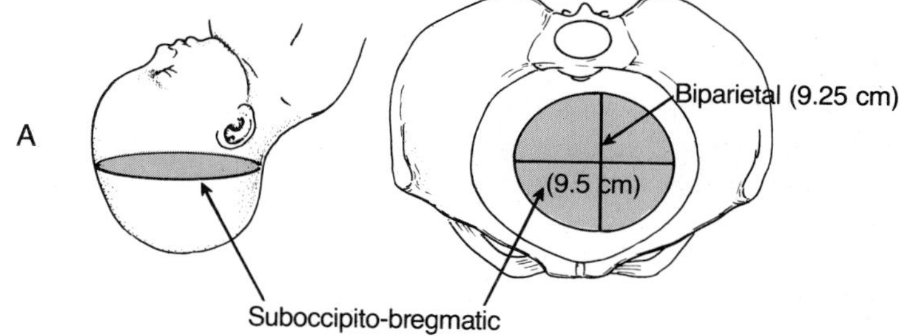

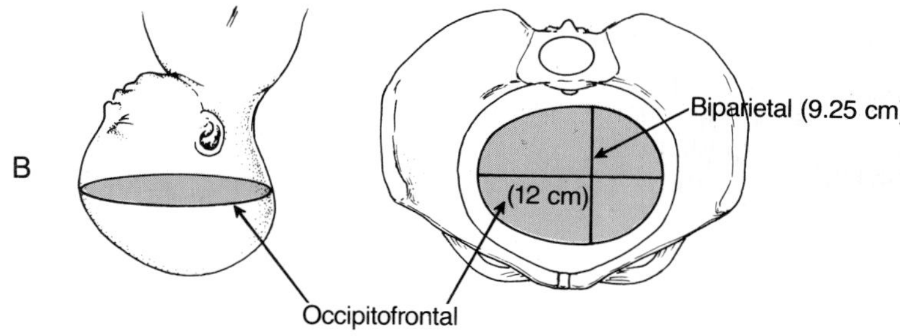

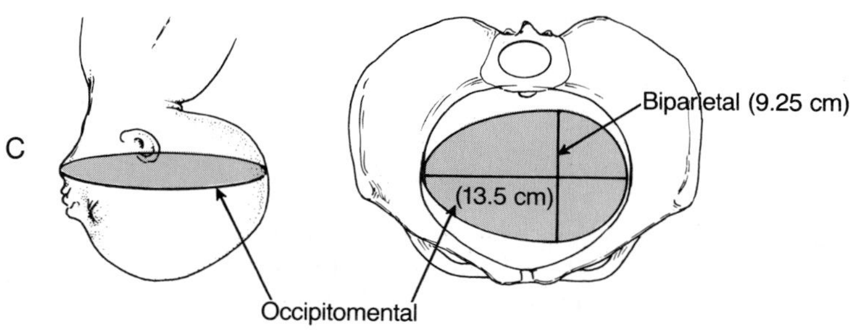

Figure 22-4.
(A) Complete flexion allows smallest diameter of head to enter pelvis. *(B)* Moderate extension causes larger diameter to enter pelvis. *(C)* Marked extension forces largest diameter against pelvic brim, but head is too large to enter pelvis.

The Four Maneuvers of Leopold

1. Palpate upper abdomen to determine contents of fundus.
2. Locate fetal back in relation to right and left sides.
3. Locate presenting part at inlet and check for engagement by evaluating mobility.
4. Palpate just above the inguinal ligament on either side to determine the relationship of the presenting part to the pelvis.

made systematically by following the four *Leopold maneuvers* (Fig. 22-5).

The patient should empty her bladder before the procedure begins. This not only contributes to the patient's comfort but also aids in gaining more accurate results in the latter part of the examination. The first three maneuvers are conducted at the side of the bed, facing the patient; during the last one the examiner stands to the side, facing the patient's feet.

Although a diagnosis should not be made on the basis of inspection, actual observation of the patient's abdomen should precede palpation. For the examination the patient should lie flat on her back, with her knees flexed to relax the abdominal muscles. The examiner should lay both hands gently and, at first, flat upon the abdomen. If done in any other manner than this, or if the hands are not warm, the stimulation of the fingers will cause the abdominal muscles to contract. One should become accustom to palpating the uterus in a definite, methodical way.

First Maneuver

The examiner should ascertain what is lying at the fundus of the uterus by feeling the upper abdomen with both hands (Fig. 22-5A). Generally, one will find that there is a mass, which is either the head or the buttocks (breech) of the fetus. The pole of the fetus can be ascertained by observing the following three points:

1. Its relative consistency—the head is harder than the breech.
2. Its shape—the head is round and hard, and the transverse groove of the neck may be felt; the breech has no groove and usually feels more angular.
3. Mobility—the head moves independently of the trunk, but the breech moves only with the trunk; the ability of the head to be moved back and forth against the examining fingers is spoken of as ballottement.

Second Maneuver

Having determined whether the head or the breech is in the fundus, the next step is to locate the back of the fetus in relation to the right and the left sides of the mother. Still facing the patient, the examiner places

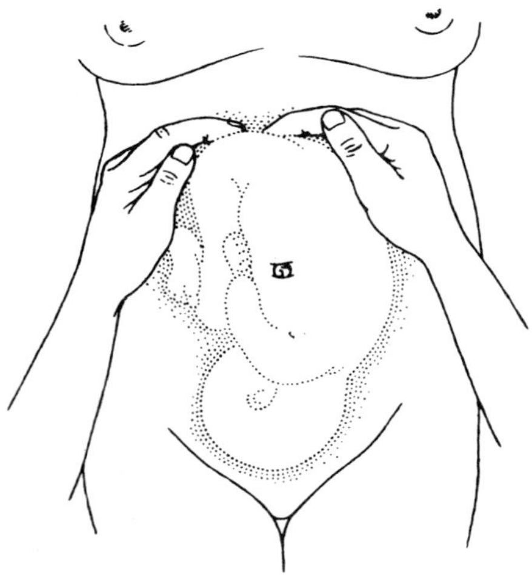

A

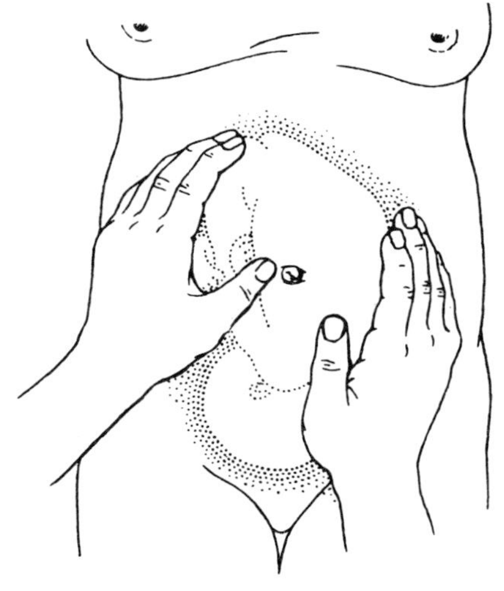

B

Figure 22-5.
Leopold maneuvers, or palpation of fetal position. *(A)* First maneuver; *(B)* Second maneuver; *(C)* Third maneuver; *(D)* Fourth maneuver.

the palmar surfaces of both hands on either side of the abdomen and applies gentle but deep pressure (Fig. 22-5B). If the hand on one side of the abdomen remains still to steady the uterus, a slightly circular motion with the flat surface of the fingers on the other hand can gradually palpate the opposite side from the top to the lower segment of the uterus to feel the fetal outline. Then, to palpate the other side, the functions of the hands are reversed (*i.e.,* the hand which was used to palpate now remains steady), and the other hand palpates the opposite side of the uterus.

A smooth, hard, resistant plane—the back—is felt on one side, while on the other, numerous angular nodulations are palpated—the knees and the elbows of the fetus.

Third Maneuver

This maneuver is an effort to find the head at the pelvic inlet and to determine its mobility. It should be conducted by gently grasping the lower portion of the abdomen, just above the symphysis pubis, between the thumb and the fingers of one hand and then pressing together (Fig. 22-5C). If the presenting part is not engaged, a movable body is felt, which is usually the head.

Fourth Maneuver

This maneuver is conducted while facing the patient's feet. The tips of the first three fingers are placed on both sides of the midline about 2 inches above Poupart's ligament. Pressure is now made downward and in the direction of the birth canal, the movable skin of the abdomen being carried downward along with the fingers (Fig. 22-5D). The fingers of one hand meet no obstruction and can be carried downward well under Poupart's ligament; these fingers glide over the nape of the baby's neck. The other hand, however, usually meets an obstruction an inch or so above Poupart's ligament; this is the brow of the baby and is usually spoken of as the "cephalic prominence." This maneuver gives several kinds of information, such as the following:

1. If the findings are as described above, it means that the baby's head is well flexed.
2. Confirmatory information is obtained about the location of the back, as naturally the back is on the opposite side from the brow of the baby, except in the uncommon cases of face presentation, in which the cephalic prominence and the back are on the same side.
3. If the cephalic prominence is very easily palpated, as if it were just under the skin, a posterior position of the occiput is suggested.
4. The location of the cephalic prominence tells how far the head has descended into the pelvis. This maneuver is of most value if the head has engaged, but may yield no information with a floating, poorly flexed head.

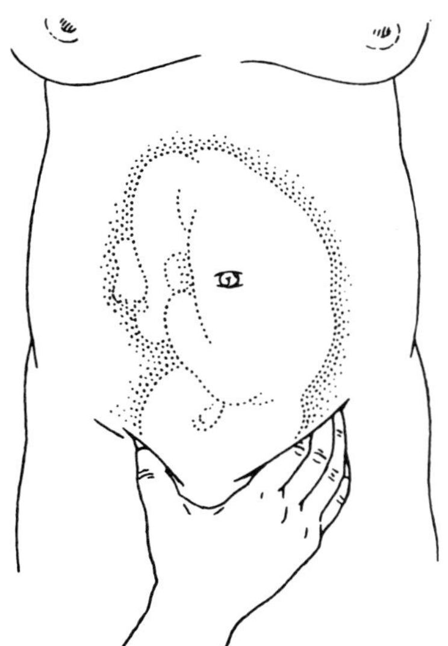

C

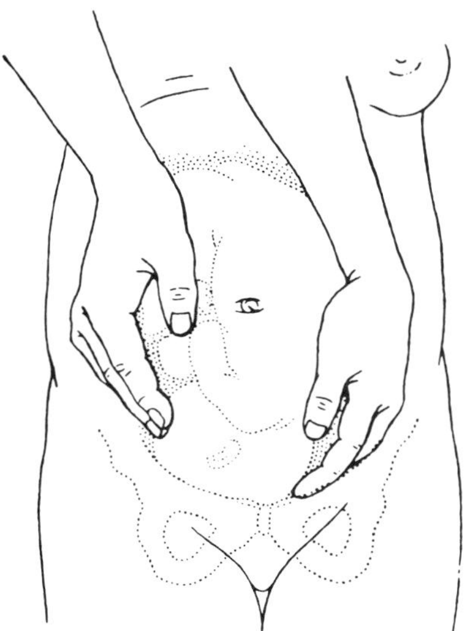

D

Vaginal Examination

During a vaginal examination, the fontanels and the suture lines of the fetal skull are identified. Prior to the onset of labor, the vaginal examination gives limited information concerning the position of the fetus because the cervix is closed. However, during labor, after dilatation of the cervix, important information about the position of the fetus and the degree of flexion of its head can be obtained, by palpating and identifying the fontanels. When the head is well flexed, the posterior fontanel is easily identified by palpating the junction point of the sagittal suture and the two lambdoid sutures (Fig. 22-6). When the fetal head is well flexed, the anterior fontanel is located well within the birth canal. It is diamond shaped and has four sutures which lead to it—the sagittal posteriorly, two coronal laterally, and the frontal. One can easily develop skill at identifying these landmarks on the fetal skull by palpating the skull of the newborn after delivery, first, with eyes closed, and then confirming their location visually.

Figure 22-6.
Vaginal examination. *(A)* Determining the station and palpating the sagittal suture. *(B)* Identifying the posterior fontanel. *(C)* Identifying the anterior fontanel.

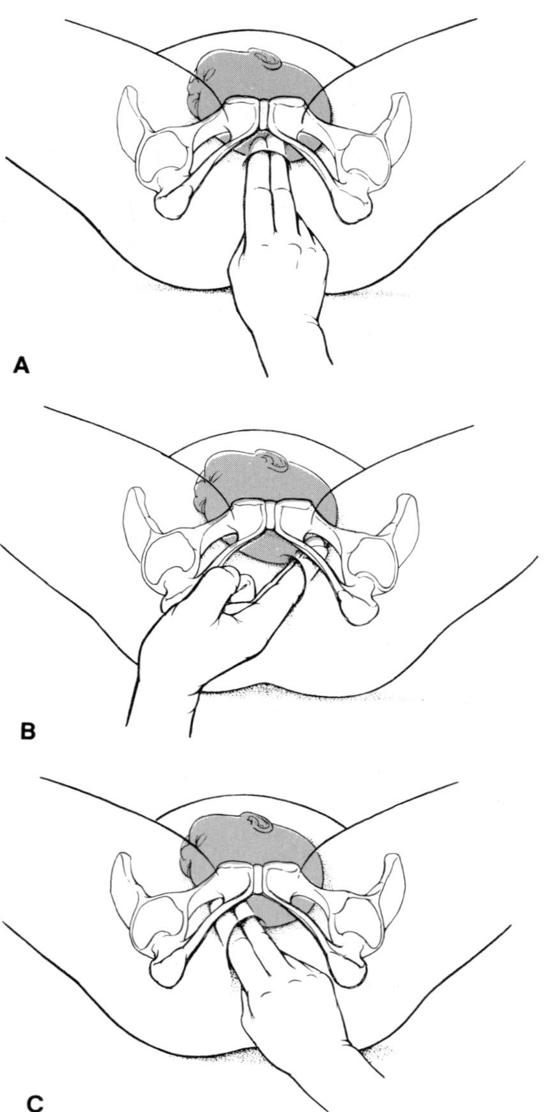

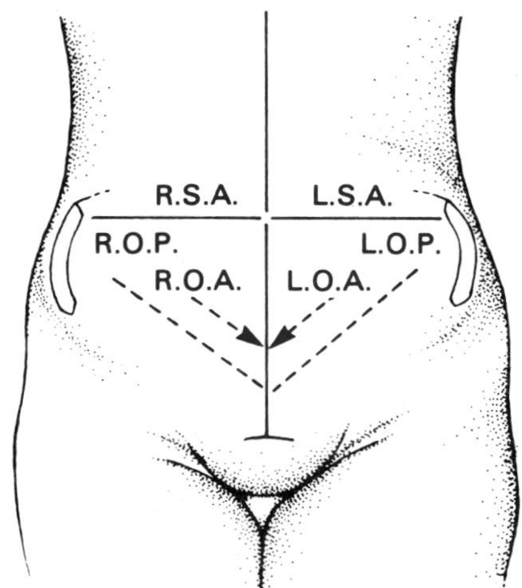

Figure 22-7.
Fetal heart tone locations on the abdominal wall indicate possible corresponding fetal positions and the effects of the internal rotation of the fetus.

Auscultation

The location of the fetal heart sounds, as heard through the stethoscope, yields helpful information about fetal position, but it is not wholly dependable. Certainly, it never should be relied on as the sole means of diagnosing fetal position. Ordinarily, the heart sounds are transmitted through the convex portion of the fetus, which lies in intimate contact with the uterine wall, so that they are heard best through the infant's back in vertex and breech presentations, and through the thorax in face presentation.

In cephalic presentations the fetal heart sounds are heard loudest midway between the umbilicus and the anterosuperior spine of the ilium (Fig. 22-7). In general, in L.O.A. and L.O.P. positions the fetal heart sounds are heard loudest in the left lower quadrant. A similar situation applies to the R.O.A. and R.O.P. positions. In posterior positions of the occiput (L.O.P. and R.O.P.) often the sounds are heard loudest well down in the flank toward the anterosuperior spine. In breech presentation the fetal heart sounds usually are heard loudest at the level of the umbilicus or above.

Suggested Reading

Pritchard JA, MacDonald PC: Williams Obstetrics, 16th ed. New York, Appleton–Century–Crofts, 1980

CHAPTER

23

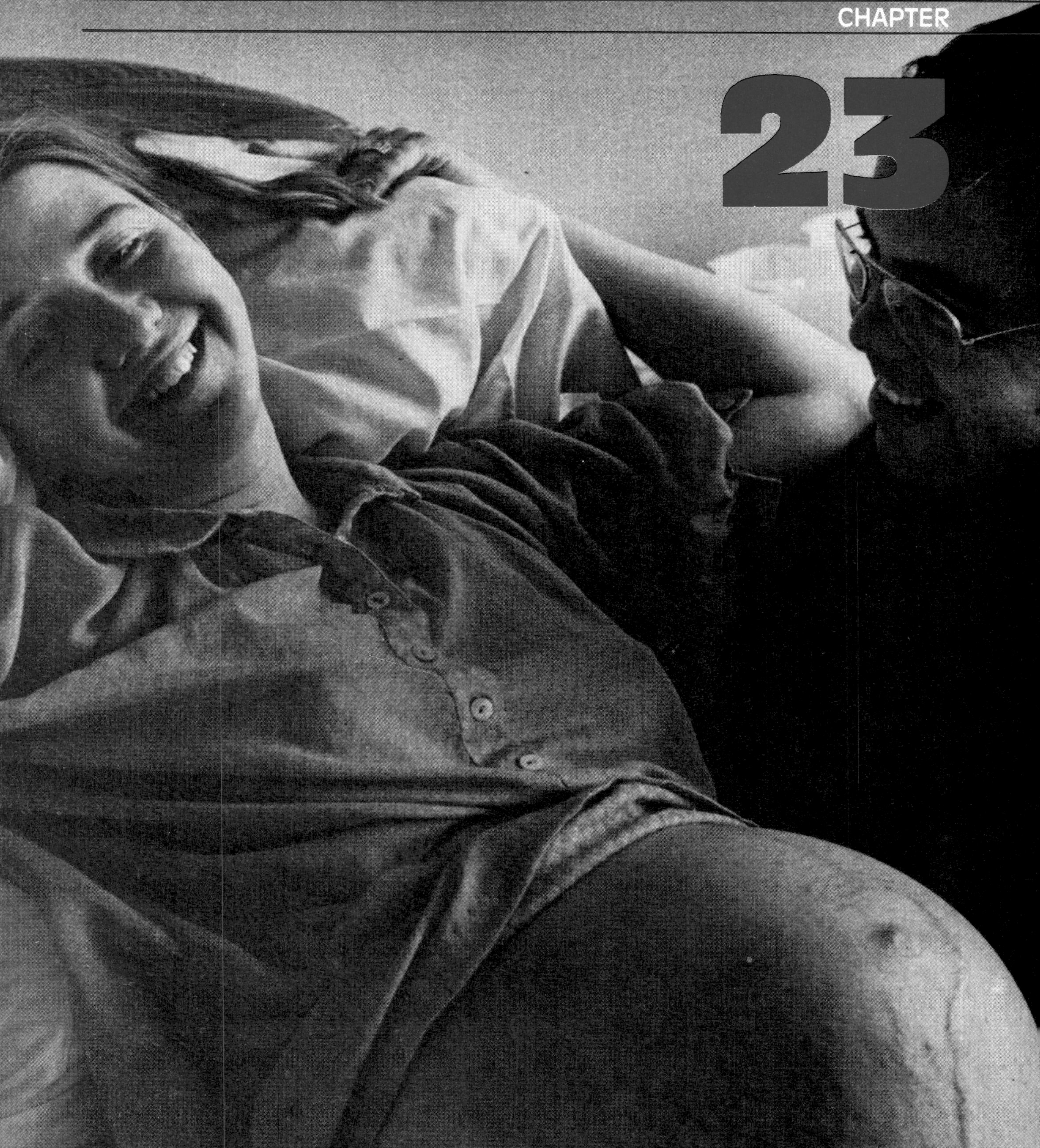

CHAPTER 23

Phenomena of Labor

Labor refers to the series of processes by which the products of conception are expelled by the mother. Childbirth, parturition, accouchement, and confinement are also terms for these processes. The actual birth of the baby is called delivery.

Premonitory Signs of Labor

During the last few weeks of pregnancy a number of changes indicate that the time of labor is approaching. "Lightening" occurs about 10 to 14 days before delivery, particularly in primigravidas. This alteration is brought about by a settling of the fetal head into the pelvis. This may occur at any time during the last four weeks, but occasionally does not occur until labor actually begins. Lightening may take place suddenly, so that the expectant mother arises one morning entirely relieved of the abdominal tightness and diaphragmatic pressure that she had experienced previously.

But the relief in one direction often is followed by signs of greater pressure below, such as shooting pains down the legs from pressure on the sciatic nerves, an increase in the amount of vaginal discharge, and greater frequency of urination due to pressure on the bladder. In mothers who have had previous children, lightening is more likely to occur after labor begins.

True Labor Versus False Labor

For a varying period before true labor begins, women often experience "false labor." The nurse can distinguish between this and effective uterine contractions, as true labor contractions will produce a demonstrable degree of dilatation of the cervix in the course of a few hours, while false labor contractions do not affect the cervix. The crux of the matter, then, between true and false labor is whether or not the uterine contractions affect cervical effacement and dilatation.

False contractions may begin as early as three or four weeks before the termination of pregnancy. They are merely an exaggeration of the intermittent uterine contractions which have occurred throughout the entire period of gestation but now may be accompanied by discomfort. They are confined chiefly to the lower part of the abdomen and the groin and do not increase in intensity, frequency, or duration. The discomfort is rarely intensified if the mother walks about, and may even be relieved if she is on her feet. Examination reveals no changes in the cervix.

The signs that accompany true labor contractions present a contrasting picture. True labor contractions usually are felt in the lower back and extend in girdlelike fashion from the back to the front of the abdomen. They have a definite rhythm and gradually increase in frequency, intensity, and duration. In the course of a few hours of true labor contractions, a progressive effacement and dilatation of the cervix is apparent.

Premonitory Signs of Labor

"Lightening" or descent of fetal head into pelvis
Sciatic nerve pressure
Increased vaginal discharge
Greater frequency of urination

False Labor	True Labor
No change in cervix	Progressive cervical dilatation
Discomfort, usually in low abdomen and groin	Discomfort in back and abdomen
Contractions occur at irregular intervals	Contractions occur at regular intervals
No increase in frequency and intensity of contractions	Progressive increase in frequency and intensity of contractions

Show

Another sign of impending labor is pink "show." After the discharge of the mucous plug that has filled the cervical canal during pregnancy, the pressure of the descending presenting part of the fetus causes the minute capillaries in the cervix to rupture. This blood is mixed with mucus and therefore has the pink tinge. It must be differentiated from substantial discharge of blood, which may indicate an obstetrical complication.

Rupture of the Membranes

Occasionally, rupture of the membranes is the first indication of approaching labor. It used to be thought that this was a grave sign, heralding a long and difficult dry labor, but present-day statistics show that this is not true. Nevertheless, the physician must be notified at once; under these circumstances, the patient may be advised to enter the hospital immediately.

After the membranes rupture there is always the possibility of a prolapsed cord if the presenting part does not adequately fill the pelvic inlet. This is more likely if the infant presents as a footling breech, or by the shoulder, or in the vertex presentation when the fetal head has not descended far enough into the true pelvis prior to the rupture of the membranes.

Cause of Onset of Labor

In mammalian species, whether the fetus weighs 2 g at the end of a 21-day pregnancy, as with the mouse, or whether it weighs 200 pounds at the end of a 640-day pregnancy, as with the elephant, labor usually begins at the right time for that particular species, namely, when the fetus is mature enough to cope with extrauterine conditions but not yet large enough to cause mechanical difficulties in labor. The process responsible for this beautifully synchronized and salutary achievement has not yet been clearly identified.

During pregnancy the uterus consists of a large number of greatly hypertrophied smooth muscle cells. Each cell is activated by a series of chemical reactions to begin rhythmic contractions in a highly coordinated way, and with such force that the cervix is dilated and the baby is expelled. The fundamental question is what stimulates these uterine cells, at a precise time in most pregnancies, to begin labor contractions. Various theories have been advanced to explain the onset of labor. It appears that several mechanisms are involved in initiating and maintaining labor, each having varying importance depending upon individual circumstances.

Progesterone Deprivation Theory

Progesterone, secreted first by the corpus luteum, and then by the placenta, is essential in maintaining pregnancy. Since the uterus is composed of smooth muscle, and most smooth muscle organs will contract when stretched, it is significant that the uterus remains quiescent throughout the greater part of pregnancy. This suggests that some substance, most likely progesterone, is acting to inhibit uterine contractility. The role of a "progesterone block" in the maintenance and termination of pregnancy has been upheld by some investigators for many years. In several animal species, this theory is well supported by studies that show a drop in maternal progesterone with a rise in estrogen, which has opposite effects on uterine musculature, before labor begins. This could not be documented in humans until recently, when new methodology was able to identify a fall in circulating progesterone with a continuing increase of estrogen in a study population of women during the five weeks preceding labor. The onset of labor in humans is felt to result from withdrawal of progesterone at a time of relative estrogen dominance.

Oxytocin Theory

It has been clearly demonstrated that the human uterus is increasingly sensitive to oxytocin as pregnancy advances. Oxytocin is an effective stimulant of uterine contractions in late pregnancy and is commonly used to induce or augment labor. Although oxytocinlike activity in the blood has been found in women during labor, with the highest concentration during the second stage, it is also present in both males and females having surgery. It is possible that any stress may release this hypophyseal hormone. Also, blood contains an enzyme which promptly inactivates oxytocin. Humans as well as several other mammals still go into labor normally when the hypophysis has been removed or destroyed. While oxytocin alone seems unlikely as initiator of the labor process, it may well be significant in combination with other substances.

Fetal Endocrine Control Theory

At the appropriate time of fetal maturity, it appears that the fetal adrenals secrete cortical steroids which are felt to trigger the mechanisms leading to labor. Shortly before labor, the sensitivity of the fetal adrenal to ACTH, produced by the pituitary, increases. As a result, the production of cortisol increases. In laboratory studies with sheep, destruction of the fetal pituitary or hypothalamus (which would interfere with

ACTH production) leads to prolonged pregnancy. In contrast, administration of ACTH or cortisol directly to the fetus leads to premature labor.

Corticosteroids are released during periods of stress, which suggests one cause of premature labor in the instance when the fetus is compromised. Conditions that cause decreased blood flow to the uterus, such as toxemia or uterine overdistention due to multiple pregnancy or polyhydramnios, are known to be related to premature labor. These conditions also compromise the fetus, and thus could be implicated in fetal release of corticosteroids. The suggested mechanism of action is that fetal steroids stimulate the release of precursors to prostaglandins which in turn produce uterine labor contractions.

Prostaglandin Theory

Research has shown prostaglandins to be very effective in inducing uterine contractions at any stage of gestation. Prostaglandins are formed by the uterine decidua, and their concentration in the amniotic fluid and blood of women increases during labor. Study of the mechanisms of prostaglandin synthesis has shown that arachidonic acid, the obligatory precursor to prostaglandin, increases markedly in comparison to the other fatty acids in the amniotic fluid of women in labor. Arachidonic acid injected into the amniotic sac during the second trimester is highly effective in producing abortion, while other fatty acids do not induce labor. It is hypothesized that initiation of human labor results from a sequence of events including the release of lipid precursors possibly triggered by steroid action, release of arachidonic acid from these precursors perhaps at the site of the fetal membranes, increased prostaglandin synthesis from the arachidonic acid, and increased uterine contractions as a consequence of prostaglandin action on the uterine muscle.

Uterine Contractions

The degree of discomfort during labor varies considerably from patient to patient. The patient who anticipates a painful experience generally has more pain than the patient who is properly prepared for what can be a good experience. To allay preexisting fear, one should refer to uterine contractions as *contractions,* not *pains.* The duration of these contractions ranges from 45 seconds to 90 seconds, averaging about one minute.

Each contraction presents three phases—a period during which the intensity of the contraction increases (increment), a period during which the contraction is at its height (acme), and a period of diminishing intensity (decrement). The increment, or crescendo phase, is longer than the other two combined.

The contractions of the uterus during labor are intermittent, with periods of relaxation between, resembling, in this respect, the systole and the diastole of the heart. The interval between contractions diminishes gradually from about ten minutes early in labor to about two or three minutes in the second stage. These periods of relaxation not only provide rest for the uterine muscles and for the mother, but are also essential to the welfare of the fetus because unremitting contractions may so interfere with placental functions that the resulting lack of oxygen produces fetal distress.

Another characteristic of labor contractions is that they are quite involuntary; their action is not only independent of the mother's will but also of extrauterine nervous control.

During labor, the uterus is soon differentiated into two identifiable portions—the upper and lower uterine segments. The upper segment is the active, contractile portion of the uterus. Its function is to expel the uterine contents. It displays a decreasing gradient of intensity of contractions from the fundus downward. As labor progresses, a passive lower segment is developed. With each contraction, the muscle fibers of the upper segment retract, becoming shorter as the fetus descends. The upper segment, therefore, becomes thicker. Fibers of the lower segment stretch and, consequently, it becomes thinner. The distinct boundary between the upper and lower uterine segments is called a physiological retraction ring.

Duration of Labor

Although there is usually some degree of variation in all labors, an estimate of the average length of labor can be based on studies of records of some several thousand primigravidas and multiparas.

The average duration of first labors is about 14 hours, approximately 12½ hours in the first stage, 1 hour and 20 minutes in the second stage, and 10 minutes in the third stage.

The average duration of multiparous labors is approximately six hours shorter than for first labors, for example, 7 hours and 20 minutes in the first stage, ½ hour in the second stage, and 10 minutes in the third stage.

During the first stage of labor full dilatation of the cervix (10 cm) is accomplished, but for the greater part of this time the progress of cervical dilatation is slow (Fig. 23-1). This has been clearly demonstrated in Friedman's study of 500 labors of primigravidas. From his study, the first stage of labor is divided into the latent phase and the active phase. The *latent phase,* from the onset of uterine contractions, takes many hours and accomplishes little cervical dilatation. But with the beginning of the *active phase,* cervical dilatation proceeds at an accelerated rate and then reaches a deceleration phase shortly before the second stage of labor.

The first 4 cm of cervical dilatation occurs during the slow, latent phase. The remainder of cervical dilatation is accomplished much more rapidly in the active phase. Hence, 5 cm of dilatation has taken the patient well past the halfway point in labor, even though 10 cm represents full dilatation. In fact, at that point the average labor is more than two thirds over.

The Three Stages of Labor

The process of labor is divided into three distinct stages.

The *first stage of labor,* or the dilating stage, begins with the first true labor contraction and ends with the complete dilatation of the cervix. This stage may be further subdivided into the latent phase and the active phase.

The *second stage of labor,* or the stage of expulsion, begins with the complete dilatation of the cervix and ends with the delivery of the baby.

The *third stage of labor,* or the placental stage, begins with the delivery of the baby and terminates with the birth of the placenta.

The First Stage of Labor

At the beginning of the first stage the contractions are short, slight, 10 minutes or 15 minutes or more apart and may not cause the woman any particular discomfort. She may be walking about and is generally quite comfortable between contractions. Early in the first stage the sensation is usually located in the small of the back, but, as time goes on, it sweeps around, girdlelike, to the anterior part of the abdomen. The contractions recur at shortening intervals, every three minutes to five minutes, and become stronger and last longer.

When labor has progressed to the active phase, the woman usually prefers to remain in bed as ambulation is no longer comfortable. She becomes intensely involved in the sensations within her body and tends to withdraw from the surrounding environment.

As cervical dilatation progresses to 8 cm to 9 cm, the contractions reach peak intensity. This phase, between 8 cm to 10 cm dilatation, is called *transition,* and is frequently the most difficult and painful time for the woman. At this time, there is usually a marked increase in the amount of show due to rupture of capillary vessels in the cervix and the lower uterine segment.

As the result of uterine contractions, two important changes occur in the cervix during the first stage of labor—*effacement* and *dilatation.*

Cervical Effacement

Cervical effacement is the shortening of the cervical canal from a structure 1 cm or 2 cm in length to one in which no canal at all exists, except a circular orifice with almost paper-thin edges. As may be seen in Figure 23-2, the edges of the internal os are drawn

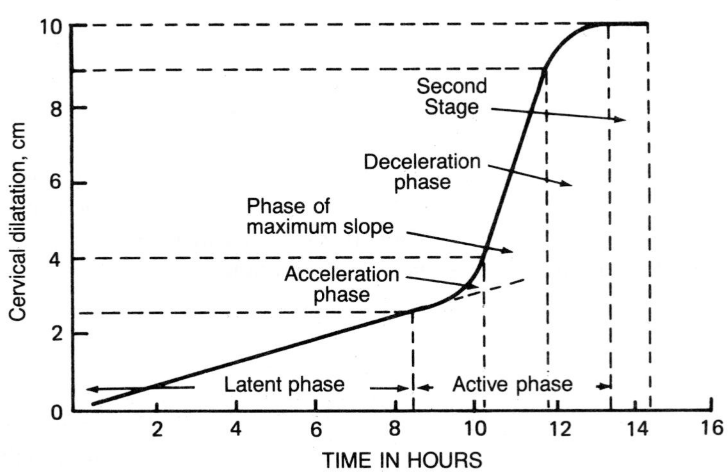

Figure 23-1.
Composite of the average dilatation curve for nulliparous labor. The first stage is divided into a relatively flat latent phase and a rapidly progressive active phase. The active phase has three identifiable component parts—an acceleration phase, a linear phase of maximum slope, and a deceleration phase (Friedman: Labor and Clinical Evaluation and Management, 2nd ed. New York, Appleton–Century–Crofts, 1978).

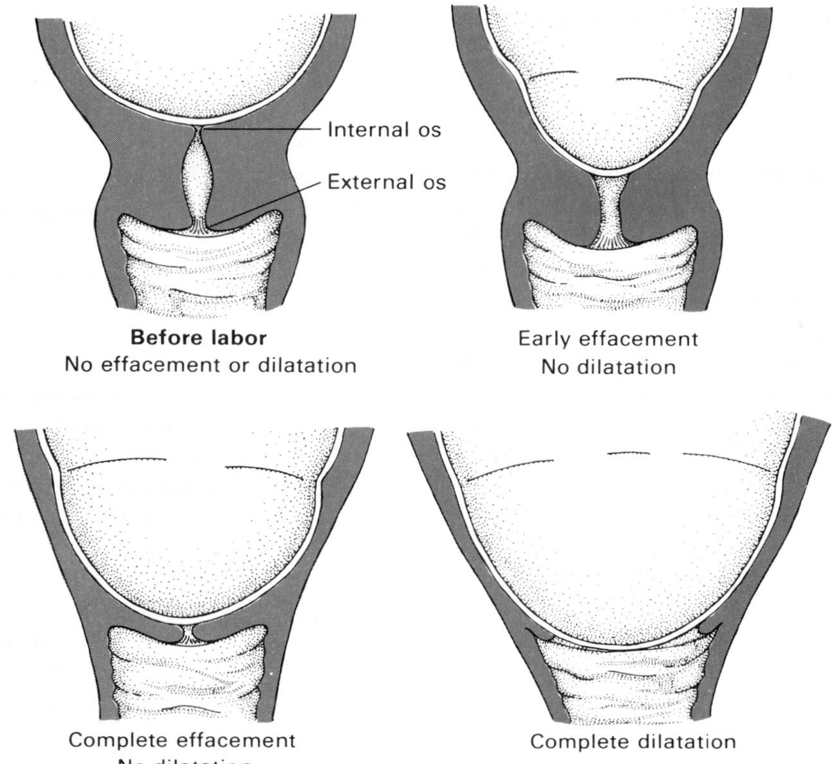

Figure 23-2.
Stages in cervical effacement and dilatation.

several centimeters upward, so that the former endocervical canal becomes part of the lower uterine segment. In primigravidas, effacement is usually complete before dilatation begins, but in multiparas it is rarely complete; dilatation proceeds with rather thick cervical edges.

The terms *obliteration* and *taking up* of the cervix are synonymous with effacement. Effacement is measured during pelvic examination by estimating the percentage by which the cervical canal has shortened. For example, in a cervix 2 cm long before labor, 50% effacement has occurred when the cervix measures 1 cm in length.

Dilatation of the Cervix

This means the enlargement of the cervical os from an orifice a few millimeters in size to an aperture large enough to permit the passage of the fetus, that is, to a diameter of about 10 cm. When the cervix can no longer be felt, dilatation is said to be complete.

Although the forces concerned in dilatation are not well understood, several factors appear to be involved. The muscle fibers about the cervix are so arranged that they pull upon its edges and tend to draw it open. The uterine contractions cause pressure on the amniotic sac and this, in turn, burrows into the cervix in pouchlike fashion, exerting a dilating action. In the absence of the membranes, the pressure of the presenting part against the cervix and the lower uterine segment has a similar effect.

Measurement of cervical dilatation is done during pelvic examination through digital estimation of the diameter of the cervical opening. It is expressed in centimeters, and often tactile charts are available in labor rooms to help the examiner translate the mental picture obtained during this "blind" examination into centimeters.

Dilatation of the cervix in the first stage of labor is solely the result of involuntary uterine contractions. In other words, there is nothing that the mother can do, such as bearing down, which can help to expedite this period of labor. Indeed, bearing-down efforts at this stage serve only to exhaust the mother and cause the cervix to become edematous.

The Second Stage of Labor

The contractions are now strong and long, last 50 seconds to 70 seconds, and occur at intervals of two minutes or three minutes. Rupture of the membranes usually occurs during the early part of this stage of labor, with a gush of amniotic fluid from the vagina.

Sometimes, however, membranes rupture during the first stage and occasionally before labor begins. In rare cases the baby is born in a "caul," which is a piece of the amnion that sometimes envelops the baby's head. According to superstitious beliefs this is considered to be a good omen.

During this stage, as if by reflex action, the muscles of the abdomen are brought into play; and when the contractions are in progress the woman strains, or "bears down," with all her strength so that her face becomes flushed and the large vessels in her neck distended. As a result of this exertion she may perspire profusely. During this stage the mother directs all her energy toward expelling the contents of the uterus. There is a marked pressure in the area of the perineum and rectum, and the urge to bear down is usually beyond her control.

Toward the end of the second stage, when the head is well down in the vagina, its pressure causes the anus to become patulous and everted (Fig. 23-3), and often small particles of fecal material may be expelled from the rectum with each contraction. This should receive careful attention to avoid contamination. As the head descends still further, the perineal region begins to bulge, and the skin over it becomes tense and glistening. At this time the scalp of the fetus may be detected through a slitlike vulvar opening. With each subsequent contraction the perineum bulges more and more, and the vulva becomes more dilated and distended by the head, so that the opening is gradually converted into an ovoid and at last into a circle. With the cessation of each contraction the opening becomes smaller, and the head recedes from it until it advances again with the next contraction.

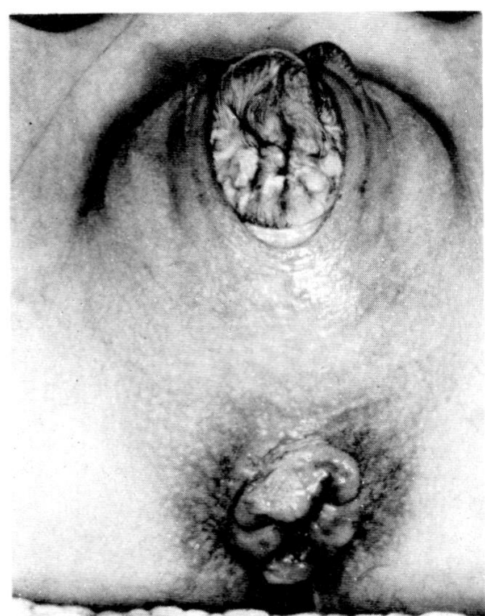

Figure 23-3.
Extreme bulging of perineum showing patulous and everted anus.

The contractions now occur very rapidly, with scarcely any interval between. As the head becomes increasingly visible, the vulva is stretched further and finally encircles the largest diameter of the baby's head. This encirclement of the largest diameter of the baby's head by the vulvar ring is known as "crowning." An episiotomy is usually done at this time, while the tissues surrounding the perineum are supported and the head is delivered. One or two more contractions are normally enough to effect the birth of the baby.

Whereas in the first stage of labor the forces are limited to uterine action, during the second stage two forces are essential, namely, uterine contractions and intraabdominal pressure, the latter being brought about by the bearing-down efforts of the mother. (The force exerted by the mother's bearing down can be likened to that used in forcing an evacuation of the bowels.) Both forces are essential to the successful spontaneous outcome of the second stage of labor, for uterine contractions without bearing-down efforts are of little avail in expelling the infant, while, conversely, bearing-down efforts in the absence of uterine contractions are futile. As explained in Chapter 24, The Conduct of Normal Labor, these facts have most important practical implications.

The Mechanism of Labor

In its passage through the birth canal, the presenting part of the fetus undergoes certain positional changes which constitute the mechanism of labor. These movements are designed to present the smallest possible diameters of the presenting part to the irregular shape of the pelvic canal, so that it will encounter as little resistance as possible.

The mechanism of labor consists of a combination of movements, several of which may be going on at the same time. As they occur, the uterine contractions bring about important modifications in the attitude or habitus of the fetus, especially after the head has descended into the pelvis. This adaptation of the baby to the birth canal involves four processes—flexion, internal rotation, extension, and external rotation (Fig. 23-4).

For purposes of instruction, the various movements are described as if they occurred independently.

Figure 23-4.
Mechanism of delivery for a vertex presentation (Whitley N: A Manual of Clinical Obstetrics. Philadelphia, JB Lippincott. In preparation).

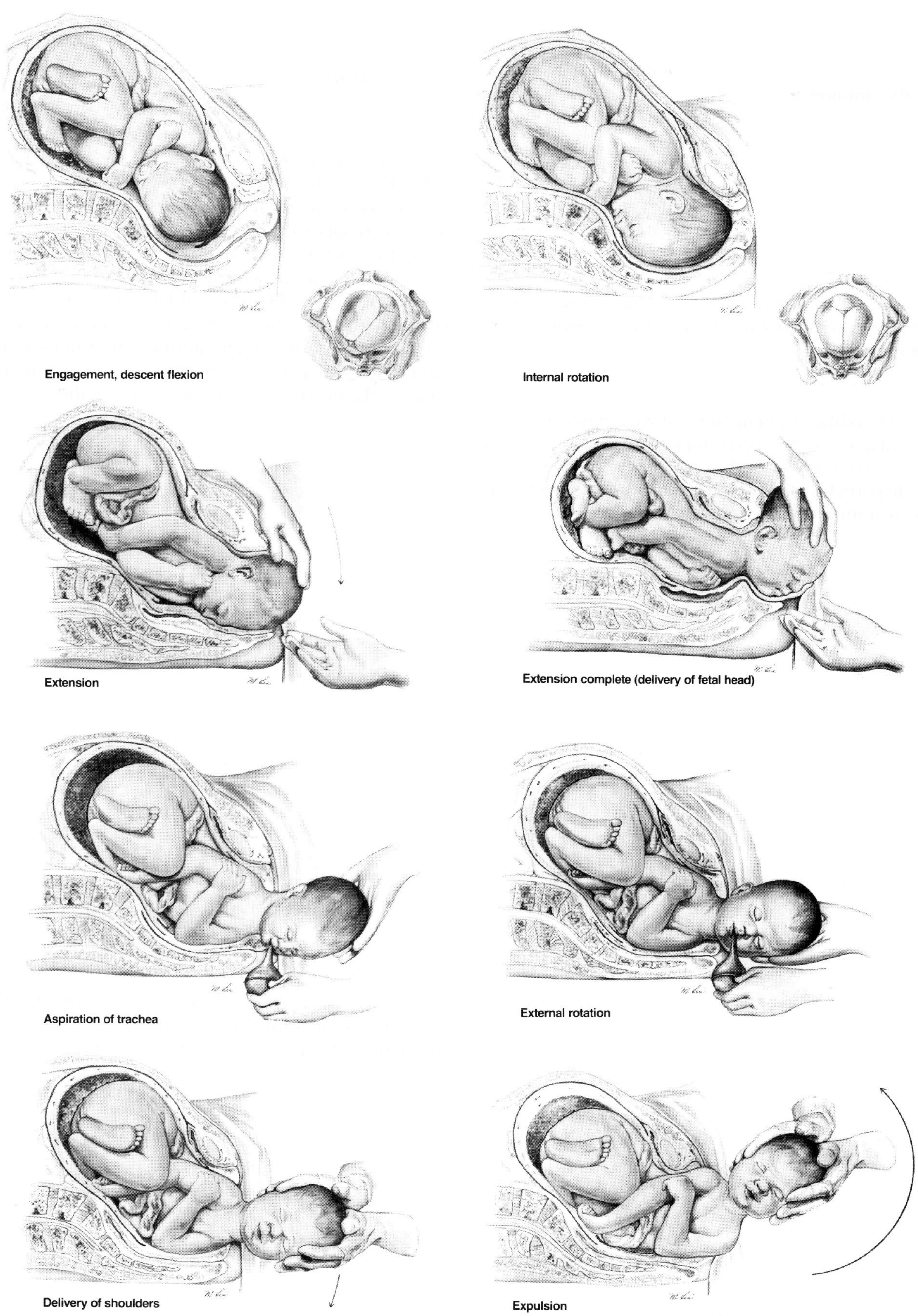
Engagement, descent flexion
Internal rotation
Extension
Extension complete (delivery of fetal head)
Aspiration of trachea
External rotation
Delivery of shoulders
Expulsion

Descent. The first requisite for the birth of the infant is descent. When the fetal head has descended such that its greatest biparietal diameter is at, or has passed, the pelvic inlet, the head is said to be *engaged.* This provides a clear indication that the pelvic inlet is large enough to accommodate the widest portion of the fetal head and is, therefore, of adequate size. For the average fetal head, the linear distance between the occiput and the plane of the biparietal diameter is less than the distance between the pelvic inlet and the ischial spines. Thus, when the occiput is at the level of the spines, its biparietal diameter has usually passed the pelvic inlet, and the vertex is therefore engaged. However, one cannot assume that engagement has occurred simply because the vertex is at the spines. When the fetal head has been molded markedly, with consequent increase in the distance between the occiput and the biparietal diameter, the vertex may be felt at the spines, but its greatest diameter may still be above the pelvic inlet.

The ischial spines are used as a landmark to describe the relative position of the fetal head in the pelvis (Fig. 23-5). When the vertex is at the level of the spines, it is at 0 station. One cm below is a +1 station; 2 cm below is a +2 station; 3 cm below is a +3 station. When the vertex is 1 cm above the spines, it is a −1 station; 2 cm above is a −2 station; 3 cm above is a −3 station. This relationship is evaluated during the course of each pelvic examination and recorded, along with the assessment of cervical dilatation and effacement.

With primigravidas, engagement often precedes the onset of labor. This is the process of "lightening" described earlier. Because the vertex is frequently deep in the pelvis at the onset of labor, further descent does not necessarily begin until the second stage of labor. In multiparas, on the other hand, descent often begins with engagement. Once having been inaugurated, descent is inevitably associated with the various movements of the mechanism of labor.

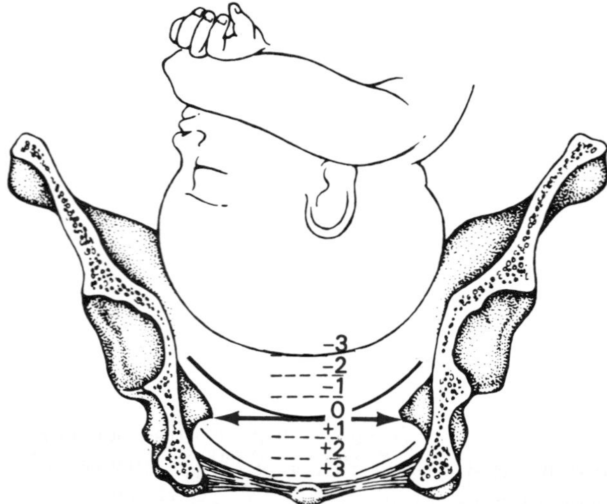

Figure 23-5.
Stations of the fetal head.

Flexion. Very early in the process of descent the head becomes so flexed that the chin is in contact with the sternum, and, as a consequence, the very smallest anteroposterior diameter (the suboccipitobregmatic plane) is presented to the pelvis.

Internal Rotation. The head enters the pelvis in the transverse or diagonal position. When it reaches the pelvic floor, the occiput is rotated and comes to lie beneath the symphysis pubis. In other words, the sagittal suture is now in the anteroposterior diameter of the outlet. Although the occiput usually rotates to the front, on occasion it may turn toward the hollow of the sacrum. If anterior rotation does not take place at all, the occiput usually rotates to the direct occiput posterior position, a condition known as persistent occiput posterior. Because this represents a deviation from the normal mechanism of labor, it will be considered in Chapter 36, under Abnormal Fetal Positions.

Extension. After the occiput emerges from the pelvis, the nape of the neck becomes arrested beneath the pubic arch and acts as a pivotal point for the rest of the head. Extension of the head now ensues, and the frontal portion of the head, the face, and the chin are born.

External Rotation. After the birth of the head, it remains in the anteroposterior position only a very short time, then turns to one or another side of its own accord—*restitution.* When the occiput originally has been directed toward the left of the mother's pelvis, it then rotates toward the left and to the right when it originally has been toward the right. This is known as external rotation and is due to the fact that the shoulders having entered the pelvis in the transverse position, undergo internal rotation to the anteroposterior position, as did the head; this brings about a corresponding rotation of the head, which is now on the outside.

The shoulders are born in a manner somewhat similar to that of the head. Almost immediately after the occurrence of external rotation, the anterior shoulder appears under the symphysis pubis and becomes arrested temporarily beneath the pubic arch

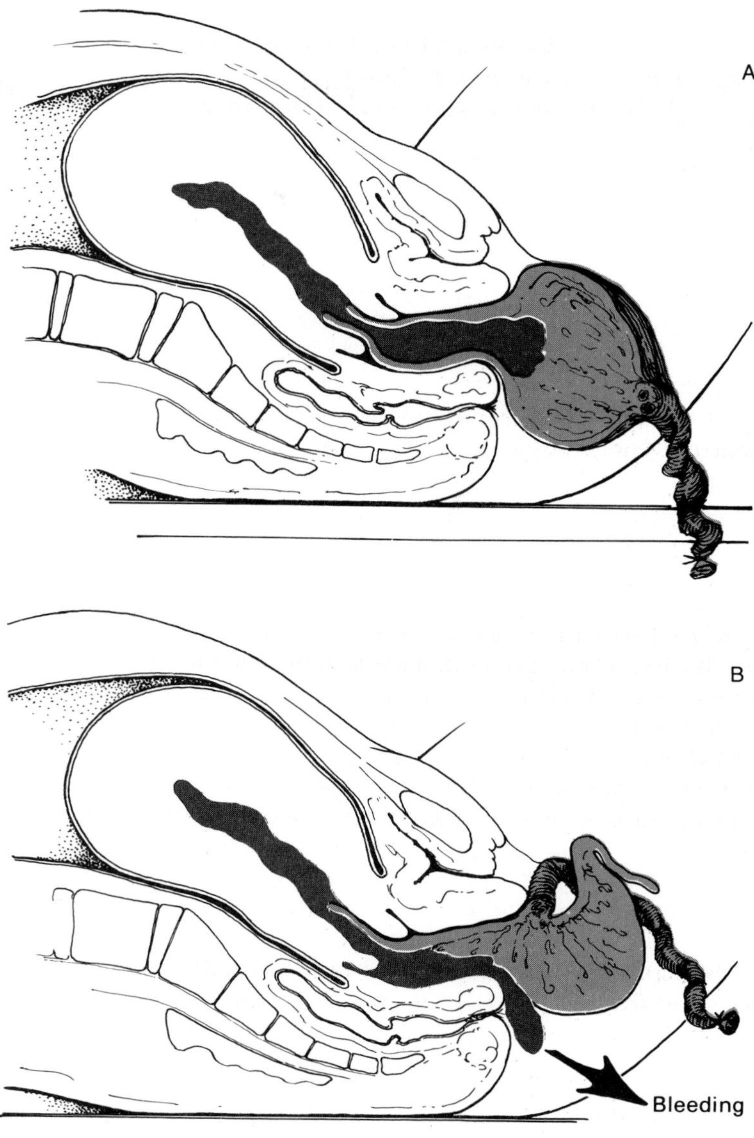

Figure 23-6.
Expulsion of the placenta by *(A)* Schultze's mechanism whereby the placenta is turned inside-out within the vagina and is delivered with the glistening fetal surfaces to the outside; and *(B)* by the Duncan mechanism whereby the placenta is rolled up in the vagina and is delivered with the maternal surface to the outside.

to act as a pivotal point for the other shoulder. As the anterior margin of the perineum becomes distended, the posterior shoulder is born, assisted by an upward lateral flexion of the infant's body. Once the shoulders are delivered, the infant's body is quickly extruded *(expulsion)*.

The Third Stage of Labor

The third stage of labor is made up of two phases—*the phase of placental separation* and *the phase of placental expulsion*.

Immediately following the birth of the infant, the remainder of the amniotic fluid escapes, after which there is usually a slight flow of blood. The uterus can be felt as a firm globular mass just below the level of the umbilicus. Shortly thereafter, the uterus relaxes and assumes a discoid shape. With each subsequent contraction or relaxation the uterus changes from globular to discoid shape until the placenta has separated, after which time the globular shape persists.

Placental Separation

As the uterus contracts down at regular intervals on its diminishing content, the area of placental attachment is greatly reduced. The great disproportion between the reduced size of the placental site and that of the placenta brings about a folding or festooning of the maternal surface of the placenta, and separation takes place. Meanwhile, bleeding takes place within these

Signs of Placental Separation

Globular and firmer uterus
Rise of uterus in abdomen
Descent of umbilical cord
Sudden gush of blood

placental folds, which expedites separation of the organ. The placenta now sinks into the lower uterine segment or upper vagina as an unattached body. The following are signs which indicate that placental separation has occurred:

1. the uterus becomes globular in shape and firmer;
2. it rises upward in the abdomen;
3. the umbilical cord descends 3 inches or more farther out of the vagina;
4. a sudden gush of blood often occurs.

These signs usually occur within five minutes after the delivery of the infant.

Placental Expulsion

Actual expulsion of the placenta may be brought about by the mother bearing down if she is not anesthetized. If this cannot be accomplished, it is usually effected through gentle pressure on the uterine fundus. Excessive pressure should be avoided to obviate the rare possibility of "inversion" of the uterus (see Chap. 36).

The extrusion of the placenta may take place by one of two mechanisms. First, it may become turned inside-out within the vagina and be born like an inverted umbrella with the glistening fetal surfaces presenting. This is known as Schultze's mechanism and occurs in about 80% of cases. Second, it may become somewhat rolled up in the vagina, with the maternal surface outermost, and be born edgewise. This is known as the Duncan mechanism and is seen in about 20% of deliveries. It is believed that Schultze's mechanism signifies that the placenta has become detached first at its center, and usually a collection of blood and clots is found in the sac of membranes. The Duncan mechanism, on the other hand, suggests that the placenta has separated first at its edges, and it is in this type that bleeding usually occurs at the time of separation (Fig. 23-6).

The contraction of the uterus following delivery serves not only to produce placental separation but also to control uterine hemorrhage. As the result of this contraction of the uterine muscle fibers, the countless blood vessels within their interstices are clamped shut. Even then, a certain amount of blood loss in the third stage is unavoidable, commonly amounting to 500 ml or more. It is one of the aims of the conduct of labor to reduce this bleeding to a minimum.

The Fourth Stage of Labor

The first hour postpartum is sometimes referred to as the fourth stage of labor. During this time *restoration of physiological stability occurs,* following the tumultuous events of labor. It is a period of potential crisis, with increased incidence of hemorrhage, urinary retention, hypotension, and side-effects of anesthesia; it requires careful monitoring of uterine contraction, vital signs, and other physiological indices.

The first hour after the baby's birth is also considered critical for initial formation of the mother–child

Summary of Stages of Labor

First Stage—Dilating Stage

Definition—Period from first true labor contraction to complete dilatation of cervix

What Is Accomplished—Effacement and dilatation of cervix

Forces Involved—Uterine contractions

Second Stage—Expulsive Stage

Definition—Period from complete dilatation of cervix to birth of baby

What Is Accomplished—Expulsion of baby from birth canal; facilitated by certain positional changes of fetus—descent, flexion, internal rotation, extension, external rotation, and expulsion

Forces Involved—Uterine contractions plus intraabdominal pressure

Third Stage—Placental Stage

Definition—Period from birth of baby through birth of placenta

What Is Accomplished—Separation of placenta; expulsion of placenta

Forces Involved—Uterine contractions; intraabdominal pressure

relationship and consolidation of the family unit. The process of maternal–child attachment is still under study, but it is possible that early parental interactions with the new baby and each other set the tone for the quality of their relationships later. If so, this is a key time for nursing care which includes assessment of potential problems and support of satisfying interactions for the new family.

Suggested Reading

Friedman EA: Labor and Clinical Evaluation and Management, 2nd ed. New York, Appleton–Century–Crofts, 1978

Pritchard JA, MacDonald RC: Williams Obstetrics, 16th ed. New York, Appleton–Century–Crofts, 1980

Taylor ES: Obstetrics and Fetal Medicine. Baltimore, Williams & Wilkins, 1977

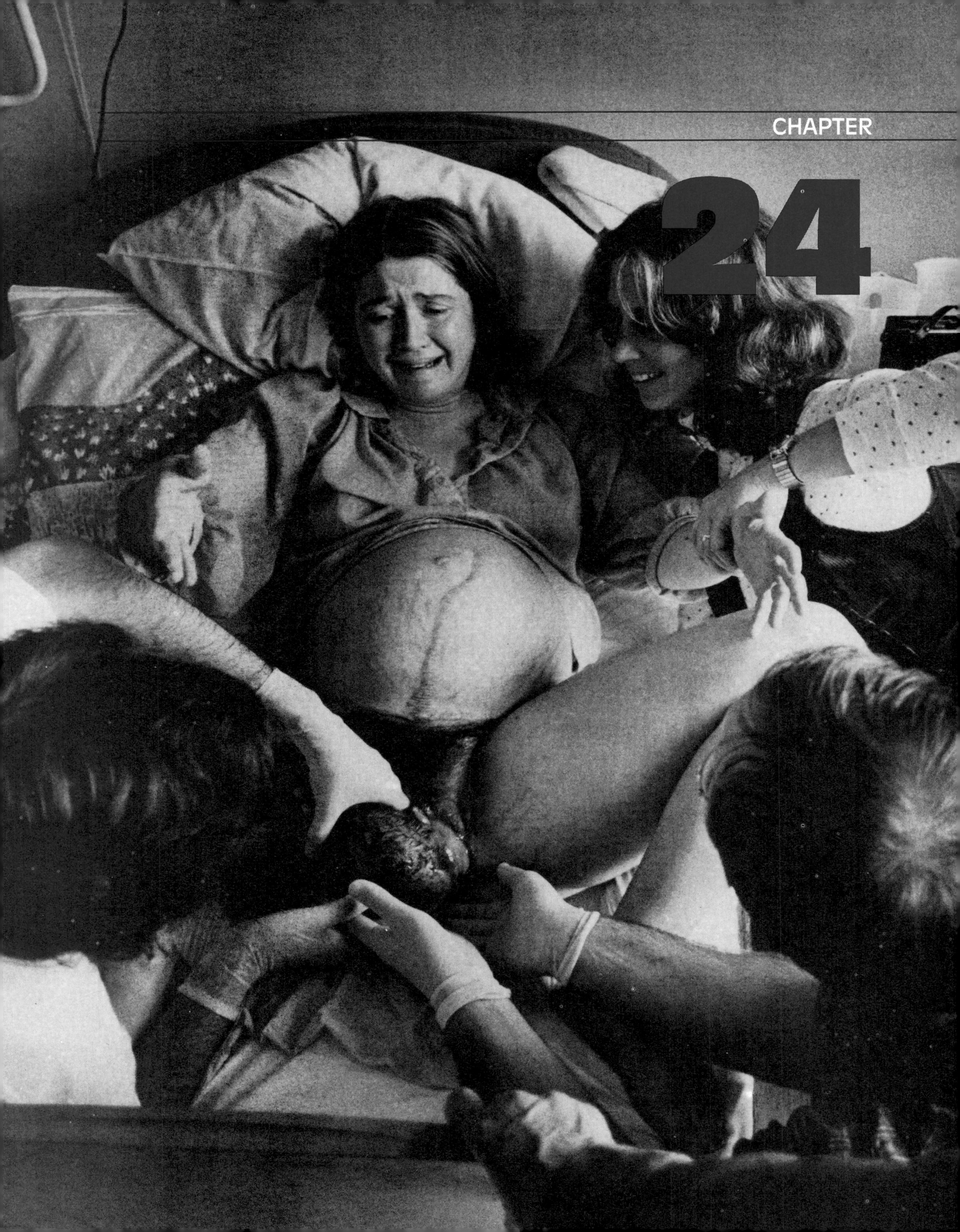

CHAPTER 24

CHAPTER 24

The Conduct of Normal Labor

Dimensions of Effective Nursing Care

Perhaps at no other time during the maternity cycle is the nurse in such an advantageous position to give nursing care as during the time of parturition. It is a unique and humbling experience, this miracle of giving birth, not only for the mother and the father, the main participants, but also for the physician and the nurse who share this experience, and upon whom so much depends.

From the parents' point of view, labor looms as a critical period in the process of childbearing; often it is considered by them, and especially by the mother, as the end of a long-drawn-out process rather than the beginning of a new role. Hence, they attribute enormous significance to events and people who are necessary and helpful to them at this time. They indicate repeatedly that they consider the nurse in particular to be one of the necessary, helpful people.

Effective nursing care during labor provides for maximum well-being and comfort for both mother and infant and at the same time allows the father to participate in the process, insofar as he is able, and to derive a sense of satisfaction from that participation. The nursing intervention is purposeful but flexible and is based always on the needs of each individual patient, infant, and father.

To execute such care, the nurse must have the knowledge and understanding of the course of normal labor, the ability to recognize deviations from the normal, and the judgment and ability to cope with stressful and emergency conditions. Additional attributes include a mastery of certain technical and communicative skills, which can be applied appropriately to meet the exigencies of the situation. The importance of teamwork between physician and nurse should not be overlooked, and it is especially important to keep the physician informed through accurate reporting and recording of the progress of the mother in labor.

However, knowledge and technical ability are not sufficient in themselves, for the nurse must also be able to convey warmth and empathy if nursing care is to be really effective. The empathic nurse is able to enter into the feelings of the patient and at the same time to retain a sense of separateness. Thus, objectivity is maintained, which contributes to more effective care. Yet the worth and the individuality of each mother always are recognized.

In addition, the nurse ought to be accepting and nonjudgmental regarding the behavior of the mother or the father, realizing that this is a stressful period, and that their usual behavior may be drastically different. Sustaining the patient and reinforcing her confidence whenever necessary can help the mother attain the greatest amount of comfort and satisfaction from the labor experience. By assisting the woman and her husband mobilize their resources and strengths, the nurse is able to work with them in a positive way and to reinforce their concept of themselves as adequate people.

The mind of the nurse boggles a bit in the face of this considerable responsibility; certainly the young student has some trepidation when called upon to assume these duties. Yet with competent guidance and instruction, efficient means of fulfilling this role can be learned. To help the student or young graduate prepare for these responsibilities, we focus on both the woman and the nurse as they move through the successive stages of labor. Although it is the mother who truly delivers her infant, the other important people in this event—the husband, the nurse, the physician, and ancillary personnel—are not to be forgotten, for they also play important roles.

Prelude to Labor

The prodromal signs that herald the onset of labor begin several weeks before true labor commences. As indicated in Chapter 23, lightening may occur any time during the last four weeks of pregnancy; in primigravidas it usually occurs about ten days to two weeks prior to labor. This phenomenon causes a sensation of decreased abdominal distention produced by the descent of the presenting part of the baby into the pelvis. In multigravidae, this may not occur until the labor has begun. The usually painless Braxton Hicks contractions which have occurred intermittently throughout the latter part of pregnancy may increase so much that they become annoying. They may cause the mother many restless or sleepless nights that contribute to her gradually increasing tension and fatigue. Since the rise in the anxiety level contributes to heightened awareness, the mother becomes more sensitive to various stimuli—if the fetus is generally less active, she may worry; if the baby moves more than usual, she may worry. She wonders about the 2- to 3-pound weight loss that may occur three to four days before the onset of labor. Ordinarily this might be an occasion of great rejoicing, but now it may give her some concern. Even the increased vaginal mucous discharge may have an ominous significance for her. The spurt of energy that may occur one to two days before labor begins often leads her into activities that are overfatiguing. She needs anticipatory guidance from the nurse and the physician to help her to set limits on activity.

This is the time to finish packing her suitcase and to simplify her housekeeping duties. She may want to complete meal preparations for the family's use when she is in the hospital; if this is done daily little by little, then it should not become bothersome. Last-minute details for the care of the other children or the functioning of the household can be taken care of at this time. Walks in the fresh air are a good way to release extra tension without overfatigue. The mother should be encouraged to achieve a happy balance between activity and rest.

During the latter part of pregnancy the mother is instructed about what to do when she thinks labor has begun. As term approaches, it is wise for the nurse to explore with the mother her preparations for coming to the hospital. The parents should know approximately how long it takes them to reach the hospital and what alternate means of transportation are available if the father is not able to take her. What entrance to the hospital they should use and what admission procedures they must go through also are important. A tour of the ward for the parents can be arranged during the antepartal period so that they can become more familiar with the surroundings.

The Onset of Labor

Most physicians instruct their patients to notify them if the labor contractions become rhythmic and regular or if the water bag breaks. To adequately prepare the patient for what to expect, and to instruct her on an appropriate course of action, it is necessary that the nurse have an understanding of the physiology of labor as well as other factors.

The nurse, as the person who spends a great deal of time with the patient after admission, is expected to report on the general character of the labor contractions as well as the other manifestations of labor. First, it must be determined whether the patient is actually in labor. Friedman has pointed out that there are no fixed or uniformly applicable rules that can be used at the bedside. We can assume that the patient is in true labor if her contractions continue uninterruptedly and result in dilatation of the cervix.[1] In practice, however, a variety of types of contractions may be apparent; thus, the following differential points between true and false labor are to be used only as *guidelines* for assessing the state of the mother's labor (Table 24-1).

Psychosocial Considerations

Because contact with the patient during the labor and delivery process is very short term, the nurse is faced with the problem of providing high quality care in a short space of time. The key to the problem appears to lie in the ability to use whatever time is available, whether it be five minutes or an hour, to provide an atmosphere of receptivity to the patients' needs. The ability to determine needs lies in the perceptions that underlie the collection and diagnosis portions of the nursing process. When effective care is implemented, the nurse's facility with therapeutic communication plus technical understanding and skill are key issues.

There has been a good deal of time and effort spent in nursing research to determine the needs of patients, especially the needs above and beyond those related directly to physiological and pathological conditions. These needs have generally been classified as "emotional" or "psychosocial." Whatever their label they are especially important for consideration in the maternity patient.

Table 24-1.
Differential Factors in True and False Labor

True Labor	False Labor
Contractions	**Contractions**
Occur at regular intervals	Occur at irregular intervals
Intervals gradually shorten	Intervals remain long
Intensity gradually increases	Intensity remains the same
Located chiefly in back	Located chiefly in abdomen
Intensified by walking	Walking has no effect; often gives relief
Not stopped by walking	Relieved by sedation
Show	**Show**
Usually present	None
Cervix	**Cervix**
Becomes effaced and dilated (this can be determined by digital examination)	Usually uneffaced and closed

Newman's study has indicated that patients who were questioned expressed a preponderance of needs that were emotional in origin. These fell into the following general areas: the need to have one's *identity* recognized and maintained in the face of disability; the need to have some *control* over events relating to oneself; and needs deriving from *fear*, *anxiety*, and *loneliness* which become translated into concern for *safety* and *comfort*.[2]

Aiken and Aiken point out that if we as nurses look at patients' behavior as a probable consequence of our own behavior, and if we then view our own behavior as a force to facilitate patients' behavior, we will be in a better position to understand our patients' behavior. Moreover, we will then be better able to devise specific approaches to facilitate change.[3]

Encouragement

Accordingly, one of the first responsibilities of the nurse is to recognize that, in addition to the physical manifestations, there are psychosocial factors which influence each mother's pregnancy and have a bearing on her individual needs for care (see Chap. 18). Therefore, every mother deserves encouragement that tends to inspire assurance during her labor. Her discomfort never should be minimized, and an effort can be made to help her to keep in control when her labor is painful. Attention can be directed to the fact that progress is being made and that her efforts to work cooperatively with her labor are helpful and necessary.

We would like to make the point that one of the most important aspects of care that the nurse can deliver is in the area of helping the mother feel as if she has control of her body and environment during parturition. Recent research has indicated that there are two separate but related dimensions of a woman's birth experience—pain and enjoyment. Feelings of being able to remain in control are heightened by preparation for childbirth but it is the *social support* given by the partner and attendants at the time of birthing that also increases feelings of control and is significantly related to expanding the enjoyment dimension.[4–6]

Establishment of the Nurse–Patient Relationship

For many young women in labor, admission to the maternity unit may mark her first acquaintance with hospitals as a patient. Her immediate reaction may be one of strangeness, loneliness, and homesickness, particularly if the father is not permitted to stay with her in the labor room. Regardless of the amount of preparation for this event, whether she is happy or unhappy, whether she wants the baby or not, every mother enters labor with a certain amount of normal tension and anxiety. Moreover, some mothers are thoroughly afraid of the whole process. This may be attributed in part to the fact that the mother's preparation for childbearing has been limited, or she may have been reared in an environment fraught with mysteries and old wives' tales about childbirth. If she has had children previously, she may have had unfortunate and fear-producing experiences. All these factors make her fear understandable.

Rapport, Empathy, and Identification

Rapport. One of the most often talked about, yet not well understood, concepts deemed essential to an effective nurse–patient relationship is *rapport*. Rapport may be thought of as a relationship consisting of interrelated thoughts and feelings that include empathy, compassion, interest, and respect for each individual as a unique human being.

Empathy. One of the crucial components of this type of relationship is *empathy*; that is, the ability to enter into the life of another person, to accurately perceive her *current* feelings and their meanings.[7] The idea of currency is an important one here. Empathy must involve understanding the current feelings of a patient, not her feelings of sometime in the past. Previous perceptions based on earlier experiences with a patient or patients similar to her can be misleading if they block understanding of what the patient is currently experiencing.

Identification. Perhaps the most important quality necessary for the nurse to begin to empathize with the patient is the ability to identify with the patient. Identification has been described as the mechanism which enables a person to take up any attitude toward another's mental life. Certain changes take place in the ego structure when this mechanism is employed, resulting in an expansion of ego boundaries to include the attitude once observed in the other and now made a part of one's self. This type of identification is seen in children as they learn their various social roles.

However, in the therapeutic relationship, the altered ego structure is only a temporary experience and remains "ego segregated" but available for reality testing and further thought. Certainly to be able to identify and share with another and then revert to one's own identity requires flexibility of the ego boundaries, and this flexibility can become enhanced with repeated use of the mechanism.

After attempting to experience the patient's feelings, the nurse must be able to step back, that is, reestablish normal ego boundaries related to reality. Intellectual processes can then be used to review what has occurred from three perspectives—what is known about the patient, what is known about herself, and what is known from theory. Thus, subjectivity is converted into objectivity and permits valid assessment of needs and problems.

In order for effective nursing therapy to be instituted, empathy must operate within a sound conceptual framework, backed by theoretical knowledge and clinical experience. It is a valuable aid in designing and implementing care, but is not to be considered a substitute for careful planning and rational evaluation. Unfortunately, we do not know if and how empathy can be taught or learned. We do know that the ability to use the identification mechanism has something very vital to do with the empathy process. More research needs to be directed to the identification-empathy-rapport linkage.[7]

Positive Communication

In addition to the notion of empathy, the concept of rapport also involves positive communication that contributes to mutual understanding and acceptance. While no "method" or "rules" have yet been determined to establish this positive, therapeutic communication, the student may find the following general behavioral principles useful when attempting to institute an effective relationship.

1. The nurse's verbalization regarding an aspect of the patient's behavior or appearance confronts the patient with the nurse's perception of the immediate situation. This tends to elicit the patient's agreement or disagreement and any subsequent explanation, especially when nondirective probes are used. Here the nurse indicates attention and concern and the patient has the option of responding.
2. By being alert to the patient's cues regarding her various social roles (*e.g.*, mother, wife, possible breadwinner, career woman) and by demonstrating a genuine interest in her roles, the nurse can collect more data upon which an evaluation of her immediate and future needs can be based. This allows the patient to keep her identity and gives her some feeling of control in the situation.
3. Communication can be facilitated when the nurse acknowledges an understanding of what the mother is saying and asks for further clarification.
4. All members of the health team (and family also, if appropriate) ought to be informed of any needs of the patient that cannot be handled by the nurse alone; moreover, subsequent actions by personnel (and family) are to be communicated to the patient so that she may recognize that communication lines are open and her needs and problems are recognized and attended to as they arise. This retards feelings of helplessness and loss of control.
5. Therapeutic communication is more likely to be initiated and facilitated if the nurse assumes a relaxed or sitting position, *close* to the patient if possible. Standing at the foot of the bed or in the doorway is not conducive to satisfying conversation. In the hustle and bustle of the labor and delivery suite, the nurse often falls into the habit of "popping in and out" with the result that the mother may never have a chance for more than a routine answer to "How are you coming along?" This, of course, obstructs any attempts at positive communication and promotes the feelings that many mothers have of the delivery staff as being "too busy to care."

The nurse who establishes rapport with the patient demonstrates understanding and acceptance of the mother. The mother, in turn, is able to trust the nurse, and an effective nurse–patient relationship is facilitated.

Admission to the Hospital

As previously stated, the mother who has been given adequate antepartal care has also received instruction on what to anticipate when she comes to the hospital to have her baby. If this is the mother's first hospital experience, it will be much easier for her if she has been told about the necessary preliminary procedures, such as any vulvar and perineal preparation, the methods of examination employed to ascertain the progress of labor, and the usual routines exercised for her care in the course of labor.

If the mother has not had adequate antepartal care to prepare her, her labor may be rather advanced upon admission and she may not know what to expect. It then falls to the nurse to reassure this mother and orient her as quickly as possible to the process of labor and the physical environment. In these instances, the ability to make decisive clinical judgments, especially with regard to establishing priorities of care, is extremely helpful and necessary.

The preparation for delivery varies in different hospitals, since every hospital has its own admission procedure. Many of the details of management may be accomplished in a number of ways. Very few institutions employ precisely the same technique in preparing a mother for delivery. Actually, the differences are in details only, for the principles are the same everywhere—namely, asepsis and antisepsis, together with careful observation of the mother for any deviations from the normal, and meticulous supportive care.

First Impressions

The kind of greeting that the patient receives as she enters the delivery suite is extremely important and sets the tone for future interaction with the health team. Some institutions permit the father or significant other to accompany the mother to the area; others prefer to admit the mother first and then let the father or companion remain with her. When the father or companion is present, the nurse should be mindful that he or she is to be considered and welcomed in an appropriate way, as is the mother.

The mother can be made to feel welcome, expected, and necessary (remember that she is the one who delivers the baby). More hospitals are allowing not only the father to accompany the mother to the delivery suite, but also other significant persons whom the mother may want to have with her during her labor. Thus, the mother and her companion can be shown to the labor room. She can then be helped, if necessary, to change to the hospital gown and can be made comfortable in a chair or, if she wishes, she can get into bed.

In this chapter we will describe the environment and care that accompany a labor and delivery that is carried out in a conventional labor and delivery suite. A discussion of the environment and care found in alternate birth centers and facilities will be given in Chapter 44. The care given in a conventional setting tends to be accompanied by more technological intervention and more restriction on the patient's activity. However, even in these environments the nurse can still devise ways to maximize the mother's comfort and assist her in carrying out her prepared childbirth techniques.

Orientation

The mother and the father need to know some of what is to be expected of them, and what they in turn can expect as participants in this new situation. Hence, the nurse can begin an orientation to the process of labor as well as to the general environment. It is to be remembered that there is no set form or content for this orientation and no set time for the introduction and the continuation of this process; rather the nurse must first explore what the parents do know about the environment and the labor process, in order to judge what needs to be introduced, reinforced, and so on, and when the most appropriate time to do this would be. An easy conversational manner may be employed rather than a rapid-fire explanation of dos and don'ts.

The rationale for any procedures or restrictions is always given. The patient must not be overloaded with too many stimuli at one time and should be allowed to absorb any new information and explanation before additional material is presented. The nurse can structure the situation to allow the patient to "feed back" information, so as to reveal how much the mother really understands.

Generally, the mother and the father need to know what procedures and activities will be performed and the reason for them. In addition, the couple should know the limits of the mother's activity and what restrictions of food and fluids there will be. What the patient and the father can expect regarding the progress of labor should be included also (*i.e.*, what will be happening physically, how the mother will be feeling, and how she and her mate can participate in the labor experience). See Participation in Labor: Guidelines to Parents for what the nurse can tell parents about these experiences. The father, if present, can be included in any explanations or information since he may be participating in the care of his mate.

As implied, this orientation continues throughout the entire course of labor and possibly delivery. The nurse determines when and how each phase is to be instituted, according to the cues given by the mother and father.

Admission Information

After making the mother comfortable in the labor room, the nurse needs to find out some rather specific information regarding the mother's general condition (*i.e.*, the frequency, the duration, and the intensity of her contractions, the amount and the character of show, and whether the membranes have ruptured or are intact). At this point it is expedient to learn when the first signs of labor became apparent to the mother and the nature and timing of the uterine contractions from that time.

Since the mother's emotional status often has bearing on her physical labor, it is wise to be continuously alert to her behavior—whether she seems *unduly* apprehensive, or whether she is relatively relaxed or calm. Restlessness, excessive conversation, rapid, darting eye movements, arm and body rigidity, and plucking at the bedclothes are all signs of apprehension. The nurse reports all findings as soon as possible.

Although the nurse wants to avoid any outward display of rush or hurry, she should proceed with the admission as quickly as possible. It must be remembered that the mother's labor usually becomes progressively stronger; hence, the more procedures,

(Text continued on page 492)

PE Participation in Labor: Guidelines to Parents

What is happening	Helping yourself
Prelude to Labor	
Lightening (2–4 weeks before first baby comes)	Simplify housekeeping
Braxton Hicks contractions may increase	Have hospital suitcase packed
Increased vaginal discharge	Conserve energy
Baby less active	Try different relaxation positions
Excitement about labor may make sleeping difficult	
Spurt of energy (1–2 days before labor)	
Onset of Labor	
Regular contractions (felt as backache, pelvic pressure, gas, menstrual cramp, etc.)	Check signs; time contractions
"Show"—vaginal discharge with pink or red tinge	Call doctor; he will advise you when to go to the hospital
Leaking of fluid	Continue usual activity as long as comfortable
You may feel excited and relieved that labor has begun and yet somewhat apprehensive	
Early First Stage	
Cervix effacing, dilatation begins	When contraction starts, take complete breath and try to relax; continue slow deep breathing through contraction
Contractions become strong enough so that you feel need to do something	Between contractions rest, read, watch TV, etc.
Dilatation continuing; contractions becoming somewhat closer and stronger	Relax as much as possible in sitting or lying positions
Contractions consume your attention	Lie on side, breathe deeply and slowly while rocking pelvis very gently throughout contraction
Contractions may cause backache	
Late First Stage	
Dilatation continuing; contractions becoming closer, markedly stronger, and of longer duration	Assume comfortable position
May worry about ability to see labor through	Switch to modified breathing pattern if desired
	Rest between contractions
Transition	
10–20 strong, long contractions, close together but may be somewhat irregular; these contractions complete dilatation	Concentrate on breathing control
Rectal pressure may cause desire to bear down	Use modified breathing
Possible tremors, nausea, heavy perspiration, hiccoughs, sense of panic	Puff out occasionally if there is urge to push
	Don't hold breath; don't push
Second Stage	
Contractions change in character, remaining very strong but slightly further apart	Push toward vaginal opening as directed, relaxing pelvic floor and steadily reinforcing work of uterus
Continuing strong contractions pushing baby down against pelvic floor and causing stretching, perhaps burning sensation	Relax completely between contractions
	While being moved to delivery room, pant deeply through contractions

Breathing pattern in contraction	Other support
	Husband can encourage continued practice of breathing and relaxation techniques
	Husband can assist with timing of contractions Husband or other companion offers diversion and relieves possible tension-producing situations in the home
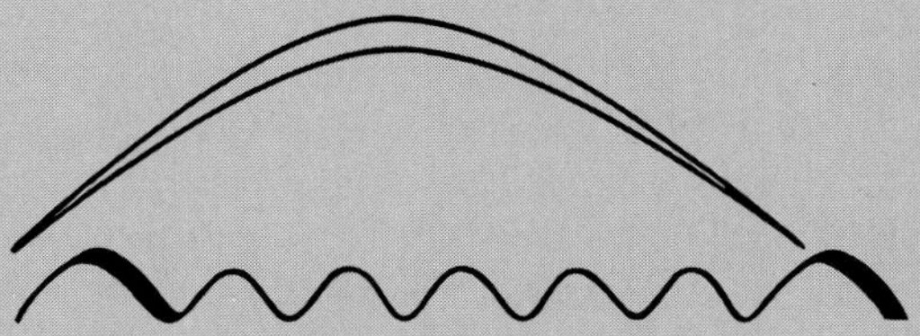	No distracting conversation during contractions Firm pressure against lower back or slow deep massage during contractions
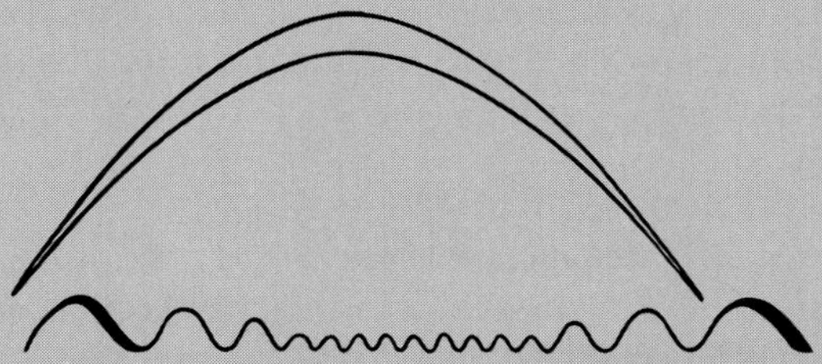	Direction in control of relaxation and of breathing rhythm and depth Face sponged with cool cloth; lips moistened Use effleurage (Medication as indicated)
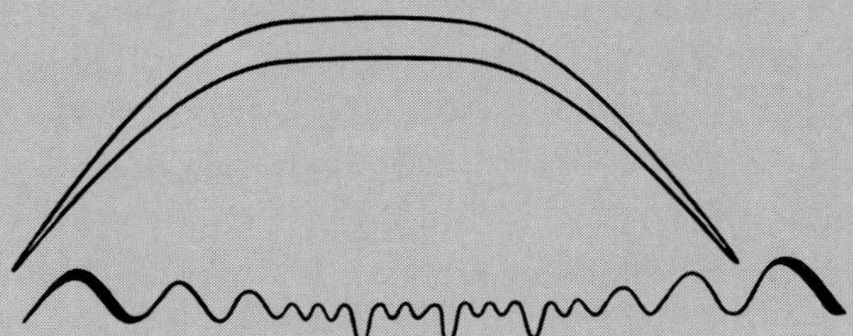	Reassurance about normality of sensations and probable limit of their duration Remind patient that this is transition; contractions not endless Understanding acceptance of possible expressions of irritability Do not leave patient alone at this point
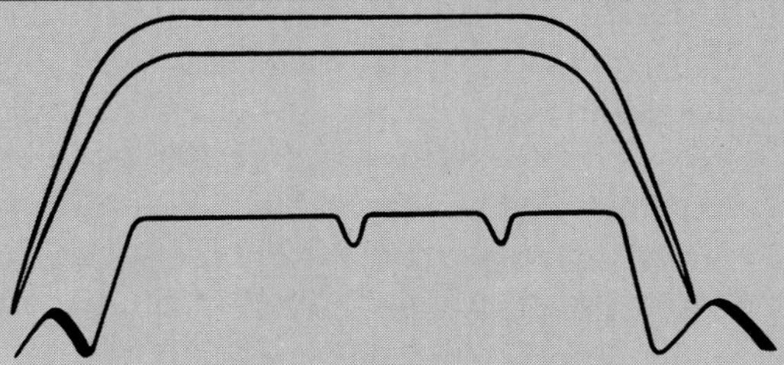	Pillows arranged to support mother in comfortable position for pushing Direction of pushing effort and encouragement of relaxation between contractions; reassurance that progress is continuing

(Continued)

Participation in Labor: Guidelines to Parents (Continued)

What is happening	Helping yourself
Second Stage (Continued)	
May be afraid to push despite desire	When settled on delivery table, push as directed through contractions, remembering to relax pelvic floor and thighs
Baby's head seen at vaginal opening	
As doctor slowly delivers head, there may be strong desire to push	Rest completely between contractions
	Pant to control pushing urge; relax thighs
Shoulders are born one at a time. Relief is experienced as birth of baby is completed	If requested to push, push very gently
Third Stage	
Rhythmical contraction, less intense	Push as directed
Abdomen sensitive	Lie back and enjoy baby
Placenta delivered	

(Maternity Center Association: Preparation for Childbearing, 5th ed. New York, 1980, pp 38–39)

orientation, and so on, that can be accomplished early in labor, while she can be more responsive with relative ease, enhances the patient's comfort and well-being. Also, there generally are several other people concerned with the care of the mother—the physician, the intern, and the laboratory technician—and they often cannot carry out their activities until the patient is fully admitted. Finally, an expeditious completion of the admission procedures leaves more time for the mother and father to be together before the actual delivery.

Awareness of Physical and Behavioral Signs.

The nurse should be constantly alert to the physical and behavioral signs associated with the progress of normal labor. She can be extremely helpful by giving the couple anticipatory guidance in this respect so that they will know what to expect during this experience. At the same time, she watches vigilantly for any sign that may point to abnormal developments. For instance, an increase in pulse rate, a rise in temperature, excessive bleeding, changes in the character of uterine contractions, passage of meconium with a vertex presentation, or alterations in the fetal heart sounds are changes which may have profound implications for the mother's welfare.

Initial Assessment

Initially, the nurse takes the mother's temperature, pulse, respiration and blood pressure, and listens to the fetal heart tones. A voided urine specimen is obtained for the admission specimen and is examined for protein and glucose content. If the patient is allowed to use the bathroom, a receptacle is placed under the toilet seat because whatever material may be passed through vagina should be examined along with the urine specimen. As soon as possible, a blood specimen is taken to check the hemoglobin or hematocrit concentration. Often the routine serologic testing is done and an additional tube of clotted blood is kept available for use by the blood bank to crossmatch a donor if the occasion occurs. If the patient is in labor, the pubic hair may be clipped and the vulva cleansed as prescribed.

Detection of Ruptured Membranes

It is very important to establish whether the mother's membranes are intact or not. Ruptured membranes are significant for the following three reasons: (1) if the presenting part is not fixed in the pelvis, the possibility of prolapse of the cord and consequent cord compression is maximized; (2) labor is likely to occur quite soon after rupture if the pregnancy is at or near term; and (3) if the fetus remains in the uterus 24 hours or more after the membranes rupture, there is an increased probability of intrauterine infection that is especially harmful to the fetus even though the mother is given antibiotics.

Ruptured membranes are often difficult to diagnose unless the fluid is seen or felt escaping through the vagina. Moreover, there are no tests that are completely reliable. Those most widely employed involve testing the acidity or alkalinity of the vaginal fluid. The *p*H amniotic fluid is generally 7 to 7.5 whereas vaginal secretions are in the range of 4.5 to 5.5. The nitrazine tests use test papers similar to the clinitest. These

Breathing pattern in contraction	Other support
	Keep her informed of downward progress baby is making (Transfer to delivery room) (Anesthesia as indicated) (Episiotomy as indicated) Direction for controlled pushing and panting

papers are impregnated with a dye which reacts with the vaginal material and can be compared to a standard color chart. A sterile cotton swab is inserted deep into the vagina, and vaginal secretions are obtained. The swab is then touched to the nitrazine paper and a color estimate is obtained. Color changes can be interpreted as in the chart below.

Bloody show can confound the reading, giving a false reading of ruptured membranes when in fact the membranes are intact, since blood, like amniotic fluid, is not acidic.[8]

Enema

Until recently, an enema was a routine admission procedure. It was deemed a necessity to prevent the presence of stool in the rectum which might impede the descent of the presenting part and also to ensure that no stool would be expelled during delivery which might contaminate the sterile field. It was also thought to enhance the strength of the contractions. However, experience and research indicate that the enema is not so necessary as once believed. In some institutions, the decision to give an enema is left to the nurses on the basis of their clinical judgment. In other hospitals an enema is still required as prescribed. In any case, it is wise for the nurse to ascertain, during the history taking, the state of the mother's bowels. If she has had a normal evacuation that day, an enema is probably not necessary. If the mother is constipated, an enema can be helpful. However, if she is having diarrhea, the procedure is certainly not necessary and the possibility of an infection must be considered.

If an enema is ordered, the cleansing type is given. It may be a disposable type with a prelubricated tube which does not usually cause discomfort if care is taken on insertion and the contents are squeezed in gently. If a water enema is used by way of the more traditional enema can or bag with tubing, the nurse would use the same principles in administering it as for any other patient. However, it may be more difficult to insert the tube because of the pressure of the presenting part of the fetus or because of hemorrhoids that may accompany pregnancy. Hemorrhoids or the strength of the contractions may make the enema uncomfortable for the patient. It is essential that the mother be informed that the nurse is aware of the possible discomfort and that everything will be done to carry out the procedure carefully and comfortably. Giving a step-by-step explanation of the procedure goes far to alleviate the discomfort.

Nitrazine Test Color Interpretations

Membranes Probably Intact	
Yellow	*p*H 5.0
Olive–yellow	*p*H 5.5
Olive–green	*p*H 6.0
Ruptured Membranes	
Blue–green	*p*H 6.5
Blue–gray	*p*H 7.0
Deep blue	*p*H 7.5

Vulvar and Perineal Preparation

The aim in shaving or clipping and washing the vulva is to cleanse and disinfect the immediate area about the vagina, to visualize the perineal area better and to prevent any contamination from entering the birth canal. During labor, pathogenic bacteria can ascend the birth canal and thus every effort is made to protect the mother from intrapartal infection. Interestingly, research over the years has demonstrated that shaving the perineum actually enhances the possibility of infection, probably owing to the myriad of nicks that can occur in the shaving process. Even when clipping the hair is compared with not clipping, data indicate no difference in infection rates.[9–14] Nevertheless, in many institutions, shaving or clipping the perineal hair continues in one form or another.

Some physicians do not require that the mons pubis be shaved because of its distance from the episiotomy area and because of the discomfort that the regrowth of the hair causes; clipping the hair suffices they feel. Some physicians do not wish the perineum shaved and simply have the area washed well with a bacteriostatic soap.

When the perineum is prepared, the woman is generally placed on a bedpan. A sterile gauze sponge is placed against the introitus to prevent contaminated matter, such as hair or soapy fluid, from entering the vagina during the clipping or washing preparation.

If the area is to be shaved, the vulvar hair is lathered prior to shaving to facilitate the procedure and to make it more confortable for the mother. An ordinary safety razor is used. The shave is started at the top of the labia majora. The direction of the stroke goes from above downward as the area of the vulva and the perineal body is shaved. The skin can be stretched above each downward stroke and the razor permitted to move smoothly over the skin without undue pressure.

When the entire area anterior to an imaginary line drawn through the base of the perineal body has been shaved, the patient can be turned to her side to allow the anal area to be completely shaved. With the upper leg well flexed, the anal area is lathered and shaved, again with a front-to-back stroke. It must always be remembered that anything which has passed over the anal region must not be returned near the vulvar orifice.

The solutions as well as the techniques used in cleansing the genitals vary in different hospitals, but warm water with soap is probably the most common one used.

In washing the genitals, the nurse first thoroughly cleanses the surrounding areas, using sterile sponges or disposable washclothes for each area, and gradually works in toward the vestibule. The strokes must be from above downward and away from the introitus. Special attention should be paid to separating the vulvar folds in order to remove the smegma which may have accumulated in the folds of the labia minora or at the base of the clitoris.

Finally, the region around the anus is cleansed. It should be emphasized here again that a sponge which has passed over the anal area must not be returned near the vulvar orifice but should be discarded immediately. The patient is instructed not to touch the genitals after they have been cleaned.

Examinations in Labor

General

The pulse, respiration, and temperature are taken, as previously stated, and are repeated every four hours. In cases in which there is fever, or in which labor has lasted more than 24 hours, it is desirable to repeat these observations every two hours. The blood pressure is recorded and is repeated every hour; in cases of toxemia of pregnancy, this may be done more frequently, according to the physician's instructions. As soon as possible after admission, a complete examination of the heart and the lungs is carried out by the physician to make certain that there are no conditions present which might contraindicate the type of analgesia or anesthesia to be used.

Abdominal

The abdominal examination is similar to that carried out in the antepartal period. The fetal size and position are estimated and the fetal heart sounds are checked.

Rectal and Vaginal Examinations

Both rectal and vaginal examinations may be performed during labor. They are generally done by the physician, although in some institutions, nurses are given this responsibility. It was previously thought that rectal examinations were much safer than vaginal examinations because they reduce the risk of carrying pathogenic bacteria from the introitus and the lower vagina to the region of the cervix and the lower uterine segment. Studies and general experience show that this supposed advantage of rectal examinations over vaginal examinations has been exaggerated. Nevertheless, rectal examinations do have the advantage of not requiring preliminary disinfection on the part of the examiner or the patient.

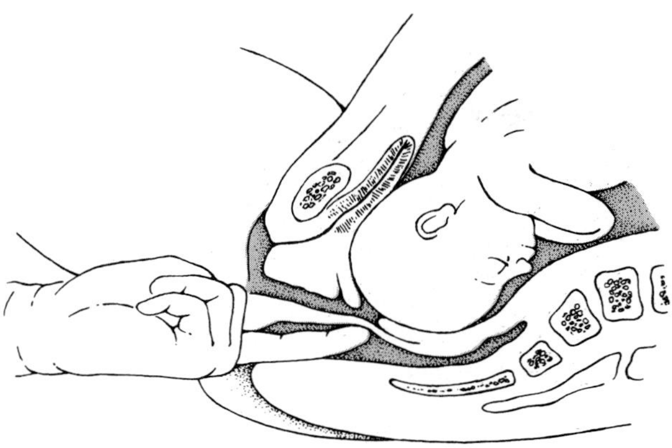

Figure 24-1.
Rectal examination, showing how the examining finger palpates the cervix and the infant's head through the rectovaginal septum.

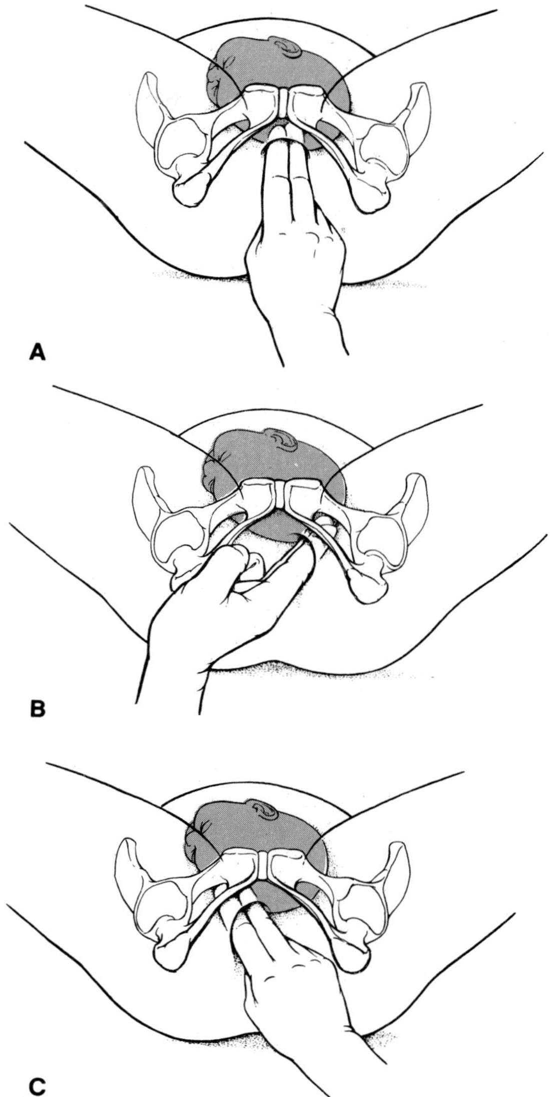

Figure 24-2.
Vaginal examination. *(A)* Determining the station and palpating the sagittal suture. *(B)* Identifying the posterior fontanel. *(C)* Identifying the anterior fontanel.

For either rectal or vaginal examination the patient lies on her back with her knees flexed. The nurse should drape the patient so that she is well protected, but the perineal region is exposed. In making a rectal examination the index finger is used, the hand being covered by a clean but not necessarily sterile rubber glove. As shown in Fig. 24-1, the thumb should be fixed into the palm of the hand, otherwise it may enter the vagina and introduce infection. The finger is anointed liberally with a lubricating jelly and introduced slowly into the rectum. The cervical opening usually can be felt as a depression surrounded by a circular ridge. The degree of dilatation and the amount of effacement are noted. Very often the membranes can be felt bulging into the cervix, particularly during a contraction. The level of the fetal head is now ascertained and correlated with the level of the ischial spines as being a certain number of centimeters above or below the ischial spines. After the completion of the examination the patient's perineum is wiped, and the examiner's hands are washed. The rectal glove is discarded.

The frequency with which rectal or vaginal examinations are required during labor depends on the individual case; often one or two such examinations are sufficient, while in some instances more are required. The nurse who stays with the mother constantly becomes increasingly skillful in the ability to follow the progress of labor to a great extent by careful evaluation of subjective and objective symptoms of the mother (*e.g.,* the character of the uterine contractions and the show, the progressive descent of the area on the abdomen where fetal heart sounds are heard, and the mother's overall response to her physical labor).

If the mother is to have a vaginal examination, she may be prepared by cleansing the vulvar and the perineal region in a manner similar to that used in preparation for delivery. Sterile gloves are donned by the examiner. Before the fingers are introduced into the vagina, the labia are opened widely in order to minimize possible contamination of the examining fingers if they should come in contact with the inner surfaces of the labia and the margins of the hymen. Then the index and the second fingers of the examining hand are gently introduced into the vagina (Fig. 24-2). Vaginal examination is more reliable than rectal because the cervix, the fontanels, and other structures can be palpated directly with no intervening rectovaginal septum to interfere with the tactile sense. Some physicians feel that the danger of introducing infection into the birth canal is increased with repeated vaginal examinations and thus attempt to limit the number of times the examination is repeated, using it only as necessary.

Conduct of the First Stage

The first stage of labor (dilating stage) begins with the first symptoms of true labor and ends with the complete dilatation of the cervix. The physician examines the patient early in labor and sees her from time to time throughout the first stage but may not be in constant attendance at this time.

In normal labor, examination (fetal heart, vagina, and so on) shows that the baby is in good condition and that steady progress is being made. Furthermore, the rate of progress often gives some indication as to when delivery is to be expected. During this stage, the nurse is in constant attendance, safeguarding the welfare of the mother and fetus and notifying the physician of the progress of labor.

Support During Labor

As already emphasized, it is important for the nurse to have an empathic supportive attitude toward the mother in order to interpret the progress of labor and perform certain technical procedures skillfully. It should be pointed out that "supportive care" includes not only emotional support but also aspects of physical care which, in the total context of care, contribute to the well-being and the comfort of the mother and hence to her emotional equilibrium. Thus, a sponge bath, oral hygiene, a backrub, an explanation before a procedure, and so on all enhance the mother's comfort and help her to feel that she is a special, worthwhile person.

The Effective Use of Touch

Many of the physical care activities that nurses perform consist, in part at least, of "laying on of hands," which is known to be necessary and helpful to patients in maintaining or reachieving good health. These activities can be valuable entrées in establishing and maintaining rapport and an effective relationship. Even the intrusive procedures which are so often painful or distasteful, if done with gentleness and skill, show the patient that her dignity and integrity are respected.

Related to this "laying on of hands" is the effectiveness of the use of touch. Although this has not been explored to any great degree scientifically, its importance was recognized as far back as the mid-19th century. More recently, research indicates that the patient's ability to work effectively with her labor contractions increased when extensive physical contact was introduced and then decreased when physical contact was withdrawn.[15] This contact can take the form of a backrub, allowing the patient to grasp the nurse's hand, stroking the patient's brow, and so on. Indeed, many of the relaxation techniques practiced in the prepared childbirth classes rely on the use of this sense.

However, touch need not be used indiscriminately, as excessive or inappropriate touching is offensive to many people. The need varies from patient to patient, and the woman indicates which type of touch is helpful and who is the most appropriate person to give it. The nurse must use professional judgment regarding its use, and rapport with the patient helps to indicate a correct decision. This type of communication can be a way of demonstrating the nurse's concern and empathy, especially when verbal communication is difficult or impossible. It is also an effective means of incorporating the partner into the care and the support of his mate.

Providing Assurance

Once labor is well established, the mother should not be left alone. The morale of women in labor is sometimes hopelessly shattered, regardless of whether or not they have been prepared for labor during pregnancy, when they are left by themselves over long periods of time. During labor the mother is more sensitive to the behavior of those about her, particularly in relation to her perception of how much concern the personnel about her show for her safety and well-being. As labor progresses, there is a normal narrowing of the phenomenal field, an "inward turning," which results in easy distortion of stimuli and perception. For instance, careless remarks dropped in conversation often are misinterpreted as indicative of negligence or lack of feeling. It is important to remember that comments and laughter overheard in the corridor outside the patient's room may contribute to her uneasiness. Therefore, the nurse must be on guard against unfortunate happenings of this kind.

The nurse will want to be aware that her own anxieties in the situation may be communicated to the patient. The process of labor and the forthcoming delivery produce normal anxieties which are no more than a healthy anticipation of the events to come (in both patient and nurse). Thus, most patients tolerate their labor much better if they are told the kind of progress that is being made and assured that they are doing a good job working with their contractions. This is part and parcel of the continuing orientation to the labor process that was mentioned earlier.

Another point that is apropos here is the usefulness and the effectiveness of suggestion for the mother in labor. The nurse can use this suggestibility to great advantage in her supportive care, since the mother responds very readily to suggestions, especially in early labor. The groundwork can be laid at this time for the more complicated instructions that may be necessary later in labor concerning relaxation, breathing techniques, and the management of pain.

The mother who has attended antepartal classes that have included exercise and relaxation techniques is usually better prepared for labor, but nevertheless she needs to be coached in using the techniques which enable her to cooperate with the natural forces of labor. During early labor the patient usually prefers to move about the room and frequently is more at ease sitting in a comfortable chair. She can be permitted and encouraged to do this and whatever else seems to be most relaxing and pleasant to her. If hospital policy permits the father to be in the labor room, his presence can be a valuable asset because of the support that it gives the mother. Research indicates that the presence of the father during labor is a major source of support for the mother.[5] This not only benefits the mother but also helps the father to feel that he has a more vital role in participating with her in the birth of their child.

Positioning

Since the introduction of the electronic fetal monitors (see Chap. 40) many hospitals now attach the monitors to mothers routinely even if there is no high-risk condition present. The mother must be in bed for this equipment to function appropriately. This, of course, limits the mother's mobility. The reason for the use of the monitor needs to be explained to the patient so that she can understand why her activity is restricted and will not become unduly alarmed.

It is important to remember that the usual comfort measures, including backrubs and position changes, need not be slighted if the mother has either an internal or external monitor attached. Very often patients are reluctant to move lest they disturb the monitor; the nurse can assure the patient that she may move and can see to it that the mother does, in fact, assume comfortable positions other than supine. Changes in position and transducer repositioning are to be noted on the graph paper.

If no monitors are employed, the patient can be encouraged to assume any position which is comfortable for her—side, squatting, all fours, sitting, and so on. A mother needn't labor on her back. These other positions have been found to enhance the efficacy of the labor contractions and do not predispose to maternal hypotension as the supine position does.[16,17]

Progression of Active Phase of Labor

When the mother begins to be bothered by labor, she may need help to get into a comfortable position and to relax. During the contractions she can be coached as necessary in the application of the slow deep-breathing technique described in Chapter 26. Regardless of how diligently the mother has practiced the various breathing and relaxing techniques during pregnancy, or the level of her understanding about the physiology of labor, the situation is changed somewhat for her by active labor. Each mother may react in a slightly different way. Some analgesic medication may be required for the mother's comfort after good labor is established. The nurse may observe in time that as the active phase progresses (*i.e.,* 7 cm–10 cm dilatation) slow deep breathing becomes difficult for the patient. The mother herself is aware that "her diaphragm won't cooperate." Rapid, shallow breathing (accelerated breathing) with the contractions is usually easier and more effective at this time.

Uterine Contractions

Dealing with Discomfort

The term "pains" has been associated with uterine contractions of childbirth since time immemorial. One finds this term still in common usage, so that even today many young women approach childbirth with fear of pain. It is no easy task to dispel this age-old fear, but throughout the childbirth experience a conscious effort must be made to instill a wholesome point of view in the mother. The nurse will want to avoid the use of the word "pain" whenever possible because of the very connotation of the word. It is important to remember, however, that as labor progresses, the contractions often do become painful. This is not just a figment of the patient's imagination. Therefore, it is the nurse's responsibility to help the mother to distinguish between the *fear and anticipation* of pain and the *discomfort or actual pain* that she may be experiencing, and to help her cope effectively.

The contribution that the nurse can make in the management of pain during labor and delivery is discussed in Chapter 26. However, we would like to reiterate a few of the major points here in order to reinforce them. We know that studies of pain have demonstrated that the anticipation of pain can raise the anxiety level significantly so as to lower pain tolerance. Thus, the patient reacts sooner to even minimal pain stimuli. The pain is subjectively intensified and even a slight amount of pain seems to be much greater. Furthermore, other sensations may be misinterpreted as pain (*e.g.*, pressure, stretching), which explains why the digital examinations and even the pressure of the nurse's fingers on the abdomen as she manually times contractions "hurt." Therefore, "everything" is painful, and the heightening of the anticipation of pain in turn increases the response to pain, and soon a vicious cycle is established.

The nurse can help to break this cycle or prevent it from becoming established by intervening at the anticipation–anxiety junction. This is done by reminding the patient when a contraction is over (and the pain is gone) and that another contraction is not expected for several minutes: thus, this is the time for the mother to rest and to relax. The anxiety related to the anticipation of pain is then lowered or eliminated (the mother knows that she will be free from pain for several minutes and can rest), and the subjective intensification is diminished. It is obvious that the nurse or some other reliable person must be in continuous attendance in order to do this.

Moreover, sociocultural factors play an important part in the meaning and interpretation and expression of pain for patients. While pain is basically a physiological phenomenon, the meaning pain has and the kinds of responses to pain that are deemed appropriate are partly matters of cultural prescription. Cultural orientations, social conditioning, and sociocultural sanctioning play a large part in molding patterns of response to painful experiences which are modal (*i.e.,* occur most frequently) in a group, and these modal patterns are meaningful in terms of the values and beliefs of a particular group. Therefore, a culture or subculture from which a person comes conditions the formation of her particular reaction patterns to pain, and a knowledge of a group's attitudes toward pain is extremely important to the understanding of the reaction of a particular member of that group.

Characteristics of Contractions

The frequency, duration and intensity of the contractions should be watched closely and recorded whether a monitor is used or not.

The *frequency* of contractions is timed from the beginning of one contraction to the beginning of the next.

The *duration* of a contraction is timed from the moment the uterus first begins to tighten until it relaxes again (Fig. 24-3).

The *intensity* of a contraction may be mild, moderate, or strong at its acme. Since this is a relative factor, measured without the aid of the monitor, intensity is difficult to interpret unless one is at the mother's bedside. For the sake of description, one might say the following:

> During a *mild* contraction, the uterine muscle becomes somewhat tense. During a *moderate* contraction the uterus becomes moderately firm. During a *strong* contraction, the uterus becomes so firm that it has the feel of woody hardness, and at the height of the contraction, the uterus cannot be indented when pressure is applied by the examiner's finger.

When the mother first becomes aware of the contractions, they may be 15 minutes to 20 minutes apart

Figure 24-3.
The interval and the duration of uterine contractions. The frequency of contractions is the interval timed from the beginning of one contraction to the beginning of the next contraction. The interval consists of two parts—*(A)* the duration of the contraction and *(B)* the period of relaxation. The broken line indicates an indeterminate period, because the time *(B)* is usually of longer duration than the actual contraction *(A)*.

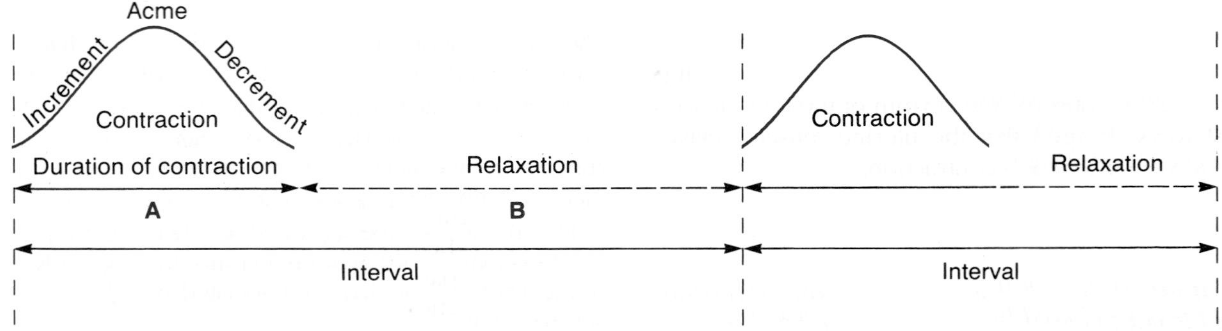

and may last perhaps 20 seconds to 25 seconds. Since these are of mild intensity, she usually can continue with whatever she is doing, except that she must be alert to time the subsequent contractions (to have specific information to report when she calls the physician). If this is her first pregnancy, she may be advised to wait until the contractions are five minutes to ten minutes apart before coming to the hospital (depending on the other signs of labor). However, if she is a multipara, she is more than likely told to come to the hospital as soon as a regular pattern of contractions is established (again, depending on other criteria).

Timing the Contractions

As labor progresses, the character of the contractions changes. They become stronger in intensity, last longer (a duration of 30 sec–60 sec) and come closer together (at a frequency of every two min–three min). If the monitor is not being used, one effective method the nurse can employ to time contractions is to keep her fingers lightly on the fundus. The fingers are recommended because they are more sensitive than the palm. However, for some people the whole hand is helpful. It should be emphasized that enough of the fingers should be used to ensure adequate contact with the abdomen; too slight a contact does not enable the nurse to ascertain the contractions accurately.

Assessing contractions in this manner enables the nurse to detect the contraction, as it begins, by the gradual tensing and rising forward of the fundus, and to feel the contraction through its three phases until the uterus relaxes again. The inexperienced nurse can get some idea of how a contraction feels under her fingertips by contracting her own biceps. First, the forearm should be extended and the fingertips of the hand on the opposite side placed on the biceps. Then the arm is gradually flexed until the muscle becomes very hard, held a few seconds, and gradually extended. This should take about 30 seconds to simulate a uterine contraction.

It is not reliable to rely on the mother to indicate when a contraction begins, because often she is unaware of it for perhaps five or ten seconds, sometimes even until the contraction reaches its acme. It is important to observe the rhythm of the contractions and to be assured that the uterine muscle relaxes completely after each contraction.

As the labor approaches the transition, the contractions become very strong, last for about 60 seconds and occur at two- to three-minute intervals.

If any contraction lasts longer than 90 seconds and is not followed by a rest interval with complete relaxation of the uterine muscle, this should be reported to the physician immediately. The implications for both the mother and her infant can be severe (see Chap. 36).

Psychosocial Support During Contractions

Particularly during the late active phase there is a need for human contact—someone to hold on to—during the severe contractions. The mother responds less well to other physical contact, stroking, sponging, and so on; she may even say, “Leave me alone,” meaning, of course, “Don’t disturb me.” However, if it is helpful for her to have someone’s hand to hold, she should be allowed to do this if she indicates the need.

Since during the first stage of labor the uterine contractions are involuntary and uncontrolled by the patient, it is futile for her to “bear down” with her abdominal muscles, because this only leads to exhaustion. The mother who has been prepared for childbirth has been schooled in breathing techniques, such as diaphragmatic breathing or rapid shallow costal breathing, and with coaching from her partner or her nurse is usually able to accomplish conscious relaxation.

A different situation exists with the unprepared mother. These mothers are often best helped to relax by encouraging and coaching them to keep breathing slowly and evenly during the early contractions and then to assume a pattern of more rapid and shallow breathing that is most comfortable to them during the late active phase. They very often need to be reminded not to hold their breath during the contractions.

One cannot expect perfection in breathing techniques with these patients; however, this activity gives the inexperienced mother a point of concentration, and her feeling that she is actually participating and “controlling” her labor to some degree is helpful to her. Most mothers in labor, whether they are “prepared” or not, want to cooperate, and the calm, kind, firm guidance of an interested nurse can do much to help the mother use her contractions effectively.

Show

Show is a mucoid discharge from the cervix that is present after the mucous plug has been dislodged. As progressive effacement and dilatation of the cervix occur, the show becomes blood tinged due to the rupture of superficial capillaries. The presence of an increased amount of bloody show (*i.e.,* blood-stained mucus, not actual bleeding) suggests that rather rapid progress may be taking place and should be reported immediately, particularly if associated with frequent severe contractions.

A perineal pad is not to be worn during labor because of the nature of the vaginal discharge. The tenacious mucoid discharge frequently comes in contact with the anus and could easily be smeared about the external genitalia and vaginal orifice when the patient moves about the bed or adjusts the pads. A quilted pad or disposable pad placed under the mother's buttocks serves very well to absorb material discharged from the vagina. This pad can be changed frequently and the perineum cleansed as necessary to keep the mother clean and dry.

Evaluation of the Fetal Heart Rate

The behavior of the fetal heartbeat in labor is of great importance. The heart rate can be monitored in a number of ways. The simplest, and still an effective method, is by frequent auscultation using a specialized head stethoscope (Fig. 24-4). The widely used DeLee–Hillis stethoscope or the Leff fetal heart stethoscope are satisfactory for this purpose.

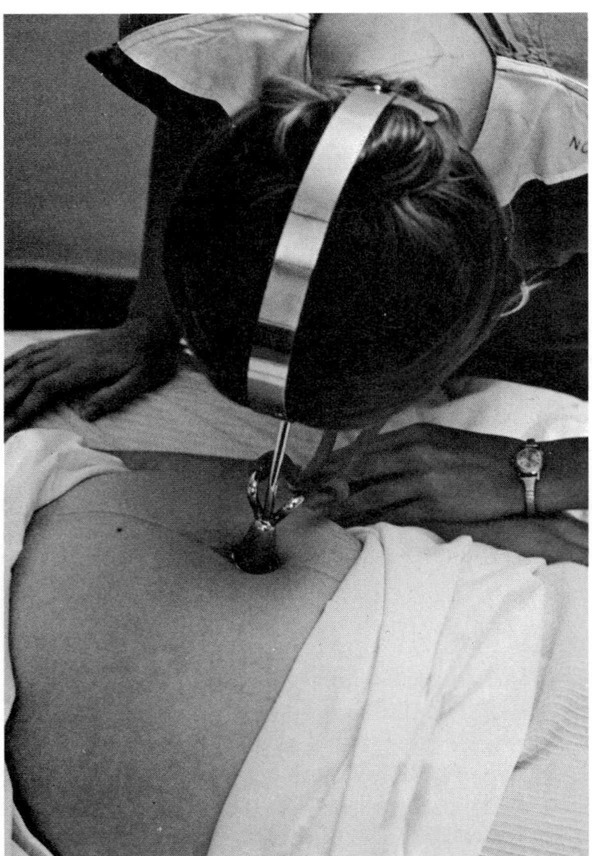

Figure 24-4.
Auscultation of the fetal heartbeat using the fetoscope.

When checking the fetal heart sounds with a head fetascope, the nurse listens and counts the rate for one full minute. Checking the rate before, during, and after a contraction is important so that any slowing or irregularities may be detected.

As previously explained, the fetal heart rate is normally between 120 beats per minute and 160 beats per minute, except during and immediately after a uterine contraction, when it may fall to as low as 70 beats per minute to 110 beats per minute. Hon found that in multigravidas the fetal heart rate might fall from 140 beats per minute to 110–120 beats per minute at the acme of a contraction. In primigravidas the drop is greater, at times reaching 60 beats per minute to 70 beats per minute (Fig. 24-5). This physiological bradycardia begins after the onset of a contraction and ends 10 seconds to 15 seconds prior to its end. It is believed to result from compression of the fetal skull by the partially dilated cervix rather than from fetal hypoxia. It appears to occur most commonly between 4 cm and 8 cm of cervical dilatation.

It may be difficult to hear the sounds during a contraction because the uterine wall is tense, and, in addition, it is more difficult for the mother to lie still during this period. But it is particularly important to listen at this time because these observations inform the listener on how the fetus reacts to the contraction.

From a clinical standpoint, any prolonged slowing should be reported to the obstetrician. *Should the slowing of the fetal heart rate be below 100 beats per minute, and should it last more than 30 seconds after the termination of a contraction, it is no longer considered to be physiological and is taken as a sign of fetal distress.*

Occasionally, this prolonged slow rate is accompanied by the passage of meconium. It must be remembered that unless the membranes have ruptured, the meconium will not be apparent. Therefore, the passage of meconium is another sign of fetal distress if it occurs in a vertex presentation.

Any other unusual observations must be reported to the physician promptly so that measures can be instituted before permanent damage is done to the infant.

Repeated auscultation of the fetal heart sounds constitutes one of the most important responsibilities in the conduct of the first and the second stage of labor when the monitor is not used. During the early period of the first stage of labor, the nurse records the fetal heart rate every hour and, once good labor is established, every half hour or even more often if indicated. During the second stage, the fetal heart rate is checked every five minutes and recorded. The fetal

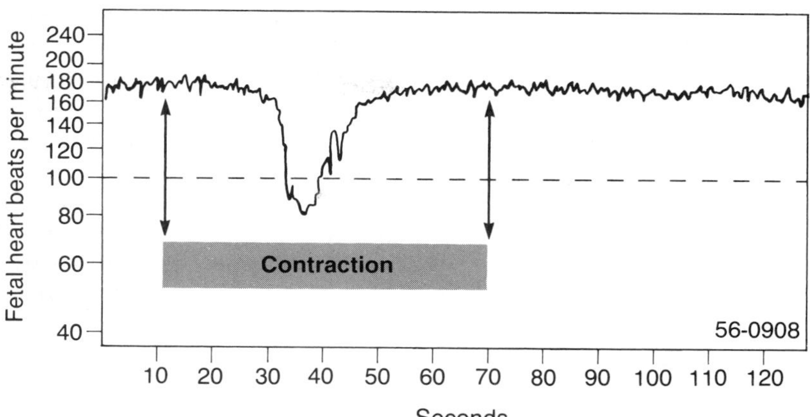

Figure 24-5.
Electronic evaluation of fetal heart rates, showing normal slowing of the fetal heart rate during uterine contraction. (Hon EH: Observations on "pathologic" fetal bradycardia. Am J Obstet Gynecol 77:1084, 1959)

heart rate is checked immediately following the rupture of membranes, regardless of whether they rupture spontaneously or are artificially ruptured by the physician. With the gush of water that ensues, there is a possibility that the cord may be prolapsed, and any indication of fetal distress from pressure on the umbilical cord can thereby be detected. In the last decade, the electronic fetal monitor has been introduced and is often the method of choice for use in fetal auscultation and evaluation of contractions. A thorough discussion of this device can be found in Chapter 41.

Other Aspects of Care

Temperature, Pulse, and Respiration

The pulse in normal labor is usually in the 70s or the 80s and rarely exceeds 100. Sometimes the pulse rate on admission is slightly increased because of the excitement of coming to the hospital, but this returns to normal shortly thereafter. A persistent pulse rate over 100 suggests exhaustion or dehydration.

The temperature and respiration should also be normal. If there is an elevation of temperature over 37.2°C or 99°F (orally), or the pulse and respiration become rapid, the physician is to be notified. The temperature is recorded every four hours, or more frequently if indicated. The pulse and respiration are taken every hour.

Blood Pressure

The blood pressure is recorded every hour during labor. During the first stage of labor there is little change in blood pressure between contractions, but during contractions an average increase of 5 torr to 10 torr may be expected. For this reason the blood pressure readings are taken between the contractions. Any unusual recordings of either systolic or diastolic pressure are reported immediately.

Fluid and Food Intake

The practice here varies greatly. Therefore, the wishes of the physician in charge need to be ascertained before proceeding. In general, it is customary to urge the mother to take water or clear fluids, such as tea with sugar, during the early phase of the first stage of labor, but she is not given solid or liquid foods because digestion is delayed during labor.

It may be necessary to administer a general anesthetic for the delivery; therefore, if the patient takes fluid or food shortly before delivery, vomiting and consequent aspiration may occur. On the other hand, in a prolonged labor, it is most important to maintain adequate fluid and caloric intake in order to forestall dehydration and exhaustion, in the event of which the physician may find it desirable to administer intravenous glucose solutions.

Bladder

The patient can be asked to void at least every three or four hours. The mother laboring often attributes all of her discomfort to the intensity of uterine contractions and therefore is unaware that it is the pressure of a full bladder which has increased her discomfort. In addition to causing unnecessary discomfort, a full bladder may be a serious impediment to labor or the cause of urinary retention in the puerperium. If the distended bladder can be palpated above the symphysis pubis and the patient is unable to void, the physician is to be so informed. Catheterization may be prescribed in such cases. Various techniques are used, all designed to maintain strict asepsis.

Analgesia

Before administering the medication prescribed to promote analgesia, the nurse informs the mother that she is about to receive medication which will make her more comfortable and help her in labor. The mother should be encouraged to rest and should be given reassurance that she will not be left alone. It may also be wise to remain quietly at the bedside and keep conversation to the very minimum to allow the medication to take maximum effect.

The mother may be asked to empty her bladder prior to receiving the drug, and the fetal heart tones and the mother's vital signs recorded before and after such medication is given. Once analgesic therapy has been instituted, the mother should not receive fluids or food by mouth and should remain in bed. The environment needs to be conducive to rest. Most institutions require that side rails be applied when the patient is medicated, even though there is someone in attendance. The necessity of this can be explained to both the patient and her partner to avoid any undue fears or misinterpretations. The father, especially, can be alerted to the importance of keeping the rails up if he is attending to any of his mate's needs.

If the mother has received scopolamine or other drugs in dosage sufficient to cause her to be heavily sedated, she is *never* left unattended. See Chapter 27 for further discussion on analgesia.

Signs of Second Stage

There are certain signs and symptoms, both behavioral and physical, which herald the onset of the second stage of labor. These signs and symptoms, as listed below, are to be watched for carefully.

1. The patient begins to bear down of her own accord; this is caused by a reflex when the head begins to press on the perineal floor.
2. Her mood of increasing apprehension, which has been building since the contractions began, deepens; she becomes more serious and may appear bewildered by the force of the contractions.
3. There is usually a sudden increase in show that is more blood tinged.
4. The patient may become increasingly irritable and unwilling to be touched; she may cry if disturbed.
5. The mother thinks that she needs to defecate. This symptom is due to pressure of the head on the perineal floor and consequently against the rectum.
6. Although she has been "working" successfully with her contractions during most of her labor, the uncertainty that she has been experiencing (since 6 cm to 8 cm cervical dilatation) as to her ability to cope with the contractions may become overwhelming; she is frustrated and feels unable to manage if left alone.
7. The membranes may rupture, with discharge of amniotic fluid. This, of course, may take place any time but occurs most frequently at the beginning of the second stage.
8. The mother may be eager to be "put to sleep"; or if she is given appropriate help, she may narrow her concentration to trying to cope with the contractions or pushing according to instructions. It is important to remember that the mother's consciousness is somewhat altered because of the pain, her enforced concentration, and possibly medication; therefore, any coaching needs to be short and explicit and may need to be repeated with each contraction. The nurse also must be firm but gentle in setting limits with the mother, so that she can conserve her energy for the second stage. Thrashing about and continued crying only lead to exhaustion, and the mother needs the firm guidance of a skillful person to help her to maintain control.
9. The perineum begins to bulge and the anal orifice begins to dilate. This is a late sign, but if signs numbered 1, 3, 5, and 7 occur, it should be watched for with every contraction. Only rectal or vaginal examination (or the appearance of the head) can definitely confirm the suspicion. Emesis at this time is not unusual.

Reporting any or all of these signs promptly allows enough time to transport the mother to the delivery room without a sense of rush and provides an opportunity to cleanse and drape the mother properly. If these signs are overlooked, a precipitate delivery may occur without benefit of medical attention. In general, primigravidas are usually taken to the delivery room when the cervix is fully dilated and multiparas when it is 7 cm or 8 cm dilated.

Conduct of the Second Stage

The second stage of labor (expulsion stage) begins with the complete dilatation of the cervix and ends with delivery of the baby. The complete dilatation of the cervix can be confirmed definitely only by rectal or vaginal examination. However, the nurse often is able to make a nursing diagnosis on the basis of her observations of the progress of labor, particularly if these findings are correlated with knowledge of the mother's parity, the speed of any previous labors, the pelvic measurements, and so on, noted in the antepartal record.

Although the general rule regarding the optimal time for taking a mother to the delivery room has been stated, it must be remembered that, in addition, the physician is guided by such factors as the station of the presenting part and the speed with which labor is progressing. If on examination of a primigravida, the cervix is found to be fully dilated but the presenting part of the fetus has only descended to the level of the ischial spines, the mother most likely will remain in the labor room to permit the forces of labor to bring about further descent of the fetus before she is taken to the delivery room.

Method for Bearing Down

During this period the patient may be requested to exert her abdominal forces and "bear down." In most cases bearing-down efforts are reflexive and spontaneous in the second stage of labor, but occasionally, the mother does not employ her expulsive forces to good advantage, particularly if she has had epidural analgesia.

The nurse is asked to coach and encourage the mother in this procedure as follows:

1. The mother's head and shoulders can be raised to a 45° angle and supported firmly during the contraction. The father is of great help in this regard and can provide the strength needed for this physical support.
2. The mother's thighs are then flexed on the abdomen, with hands grasped just below the knees when a contraction begins.
3. She should be instructed to take a deep breath as soon as the contraction begins and, holding her breath or with gently expelling the breath, to exert downward pressure exactly as if she were straining at stool.
4. Pulling on the knees at this time, as well as flexing the chin on the chest, is a helpful adjunct to maintain downward pressure of the diaphragm and to stabilize the chest and the abdominal musculature.
5. In addition, maintaining the legs flexed as for the "push" position deters the mother from pushing her feet against the table or bed. Avoiding such pressure on the feet is important because it discourages tensing of the gluteal muscles and contributes to further relaxation of the pelvic floor. The bearing-down effort should be as long and sustained as possible, since short "grunty" endeavors are of little avail.

If at this time the mother is in the delivery room, but her legs as yet have not been put up in stirrups or leg holders, she can be coached in the same manner. In most hospitals the delivery tables have firmly attached hand grips which can be adjusted in position so that the mother can reach them comfortably to pull against, if she wishes.

However, in doing so her hands are not free to pull up on her knees with the contraction, so that the nurse or other person in attendance needs to assist her. This can be accomplished by assisting the mother to bring her legs up into position and exerting proper pressure against her knees as she bears down with the contraction. Care should be exercised to grasp the mother's knees from above, since doing so under the knees could exert undesirable pressure on the popliteal veins.

At the end of each contraction the mother is assisted to put her legs down and encouraged to rest until the next contraction begins. Usually, these bearing-down efforts are rewarded by increased bulging of the perineum, that is, by further descent of the head. The patient should be informed of such progress, for encouragement is very important.

In certain instances it may not be desirable for the mother to bear down. In these cases, if the mother has an urge to bear down, she can be instructed to pant during each contraction, since it is impossible to push while panting.

Psychosocial Support

When the mother is ready to be transferred to the delivery room, it is more helpful if the same nurse who has been attending her in labor accompanies her to the delivery room. This transfer means a new environment for the patient to cope with under very stressful circumstances. Great physical and mental exertion may be called for with little preparation or practice. To the mother in labor who is unfamiliar with such surroundings, the "sterile" atmosphere of the delivery room can be strange, cold, and uninviting, with its obstetrical furnishings and supplies that become even more foreboding as they reflect the glittering lights of the room. Under such circumstances the sight of familiar faces and the sound of familiar voices, even though partially concealed and muffled by the surgical caps, masks, and gowns, do give the patient some sense of continuity and security. Furthermore, by this time the nurse and the patient have established a communication pattern, each able to pick up the other's more covert cues. Thus, the coaching, guidance, and follow-through necessary in the second stage of labor is expedited if the same person continues with the care even though the father may be the primary coach.

The nurse will notice that the mother has become increasingly involved in the whole birth process. The seemingly panicky frustration of the late active phase subsides a bit (with appropriate coaching and reassurance), and the patient may experience a sense of relief that the expulsive stage has begun. The desire to push and to bear down is very strong now—uncontrollable, in fact—and the patient generally gets enormous satisfaction with each push. Some patients, however, experience acute pain and need all available help and encouragement to continue bearing down. The nurse will note that in most instances there is complete exhaustion after each expulsive effort, and the mother often drops off to sleep, only to be roused by the next contraction. Because consciousness is still altered, it may be difficult for the mother to follow directions readily even though she may want to. Again, repeated, short, explicit directions are required to encourage her to rest or to work, but especially to prepare the mother for the expulsive effort if she is sleeping between contractions and awakens abruptly.

Muscular cramps in the legs are common in the second stage because of pressure exerted by the baby's head on certain nerves in the pelvis. To relieve these cramps, the leg can be straightened and the ankle dorsiflexed by exerting pressure upward against the ball of the foot until the cramp subsides. Meanwhile, the knee is stabilized with the other hand. These cramps cause excruciating pain and must never be ignored.

Preparation for Delivery

Good obstetrical care during the second stage of labor demands the closest teamwork among the patient, physician, nurse, and anesthetist. By previous understanding, or more often by established hospital routine, each has his or her own responsibilities in the delivery room, and, if the best interests of the mother and her infant are to be fulfilled, the responsibilities of each must be carried out smoothly and efficiently.

Up to now, the primary focus for the nurse has been on direct patient care. Now she must enlarge her focus to include the obstetrician and other allied professionals; that is, there will be more activities which will require the actual assistance of these persons than was necessary during the first stage of labor. Thus, the nurse must be sensitive not only to the cues sent by the mother but also to those relayed by the other personnel.

Preparation of the Delivery Room

There are no two hospitals in which the delivery room setup or the procedure for delivery is precisely the same. Therefore observation and experience in a particular institution serves as the basis for becoming acquainted with the physical layout and the method of care offered.

The following, however, gives a general idea of the equipment and materials used in the typical setting.

The delivery table is designed so that its surface is actually composed of two adjoining sections, each covered with its own mattress. This permits the patient to lie in the supine position (or be propped up at a 30° angle with pillows) until it is desired to put her legs up into stirrups, that is, put her in the lithotomy position. At this time the table is "broken" by a mechanical device. The retractable or lower end of the table drops and is rolled under the main section of the table. Thus, ready access is given to the perineal region. Or, if it is desired to deliver the patient in the dorsal recumbent position, the lower portion of the table can remain in place.

The instrument table opposite the foot of the delivery table contains the principal sterile supplies and instruments needed for normal delivery, including, among other articles, towels, sponges, catheter, solutions, basins, and the "cord set." The cord set is a group of instruments used for clamping and cutting the umbilical cord—two hemostats, a pair of scissors, and a cord clamp. Other instruments often are included because it may be necessary for the physician to perform an episiotomy or to repair lacerations. Other instruments frequently included are two hemostats, two Allis clamps, one mouse-tooth tissue forceps, two sponge sticks, one vaginal retractor, two tenaculae, one needle holder, assorted needles, and a pair of obstetrical forceps.

A double-bowl solution stand or basin rack generally is used to hold the basins, one for wet sponges and the other to receive the placenta. Emergency instruments, a crib, and a radiant warmer and resuscitator (Fig. 24-6) are part of standard delivery room equipment and should be in readiness at all times.

Asepsis and Antisepsis

Persons who have a communicable disease or persons who have been in contact with a communicable disease should be excluded from maternity service

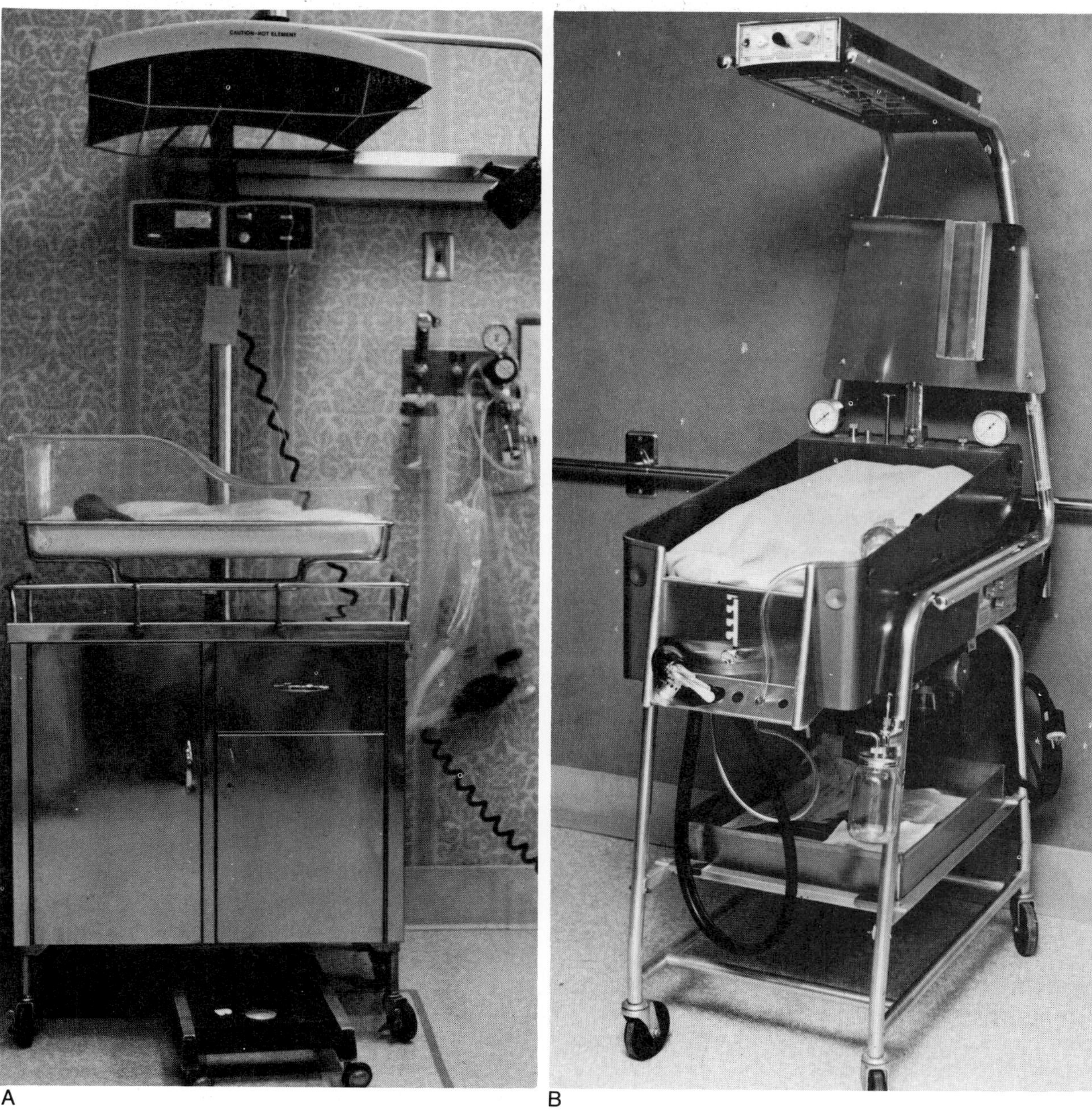

A B

Figure 24-6.
(A) Radiant warmer. *(B)* Resuscitation unit.

until examined by a physician. Only after a physician has certified that the employee is free from infections should he or she be allowed to return to duty. Personnel with evidence of upper respiratory infections or open skin lesions, diarrhea, or any other infectious disease also should be excluded. Furthermore, it is recommended that all persons working in the maternity area should have a preemployment physical examination and rubella titers, and such interim examinations as may be required by the hospital.

Of prime importance in the conduct of the second stage of labor are strict asepsis and antisepsis throughout the entire delivery. To this end everyone in the delivery room wears a clean scrubdress, cap and mask, and those actually participating in the delivery are in sterile attire. Masking must include both nose and mouth. Caps are to be adjusted to keep *all* hair covered. If the nurse scrubs to assist the doctor, the strict aseptic technique is observed. The hands are scrubbed as carefully as for a major surgical operation. Scrubbing the hands should be started sufficiently early to allot full time for the scrub, as well as to don gown and gloves.

Transfer of the Mother to the Delivery Room

When birth appears imminent, the mother is transferred to the delivery room and prepared for delivery. If the father is not accompanying the mother to the delivery room, then time is allowed for them to bid each other a temporary goodbye. This kind of planning not only is supportive but also enables both to cooperate more fully. Care should be taken to have only one person instruct or coach the mother at any one time. When delivery is imminent, her attention is limited, as already illustrated, and the sound of several voices at one time is confusing.

Prior to the actual transfer to the delivery room, the nurse finds out what type of anesthesia will be used. Since the immediate positioning of the patient in the delivery room depends on the type of anesthesia used, this preplanning expedites activities during delivery and promotes smoother functioning of the team.

Delivery

Positioning

If regional anesthesia is to be administered, the patient is usually turned on her side. If she is given a saddle block, she may be placed on her side or assisted to a sitting position on the side of the delivery table, with her feet supported on a stool and her body leaning forward against the nurse. Her back should be toward the operator and bowed (the position requires flexion of the neck and the lumbar spine). This principle of cervical and lumbar flexion is used also in the side lying position (see Chap. 27). A caudal or epidural anesthesia may be started in the labor room.

Although the positioning and the administration of the anesthesia take only a few minutes, the mother may be extremely uncomfortable due to the severity of the contractions at this time; she can be assured that this discomfort is only temporary. The fetal heart rate and the maternal blood pressure are checked frequently—every five minutes or so. In addition, the mother's head should be elevated with at least two pillows to help prevent the anesthetic level from rising beyond the desired height. To allow the anesthetic level to stabilize, the nurse waits for instructions from the anesthetist before putting the mother's legs in stirrups or performing any other manipulations. If the mother is to receive general anesthesia, she lies supine on the table. Local or pudendal anesthesia is administered with the mother in the lithotomy position.

As previously stated, anesthesia should be administered by a qualified physician or a nurse anesthetist. This entire subject is discussed in more detail in Chapter 27.

During the time that the anesthesia is being administered, the circulating nurse can uncover the sterile tables, check the resuscitator, and attach a sterile suction catheter and oxygen mask, and perform other duties for which she is responsible. Once the anesthesia has been administered, the nurse resumes recording the FHR every five minutes.

Some hospitals and physicians do not require that the mother be placed in the lithotomy position for delivery. She simply grasps her legs at the knees as she did during the pushing phase of the second stage. This position allows visualization of the perineum and adequate prepping and draping of the area. Before the mother's legs are placed in stirrups or leg holders of some type, cotton flannel boots which cover the entire leg are put on. When the legs are placed in the stirrups or holders, care is taken not to separate the legs too widely or to have one leg higher than the other. Both legs are raised or lowered at the same time, with a nurse supporting each leg if the mother is unable to help in the positioning. Failure to observe these principles may strain the ligaments of the pelvis, with consequent discomfort in the puerperium. Care should be taken to avoid pressure on the popliteal space, and to angle the stirrups so that the feet are not dependent.

If stirrups are used during the delivery, the mother can be given handles to grip and pull on, which aid her in her bearing-down efforts. Wrist straps which may be secure about the wrist allow some limited movement but prevent the mother from reaching up to touch the sterile drapes. The purpose of the handles and the cuffs should be explained to the mother, since many patients often complain about being "strapped down."

Preparing the Perineum

After the patient is placed in the lithotomy position, the nurse carries out the procedure for cleansing the vulva and the surrounding area. If the delivery is to be conducted with the mother in the recumbent position, this may be carried out with the knees drawn up slightly and the legs separated. Once the physician has scrubbed and donned sterile gown and gloves, the patient is draped with towels and sheets appropriate for the purpose.

After the patient has been prepared for delivery,

catheterization, if needed, is carried out by the physician. Sometimes it is difficult to catheterize a patient in the second stage of labor because the fetus's head may compress the urethra. If the catheter does not pass easily, never force it. Whenever it is possible and appropriate, all procedures, of course, should be explained to the mother as they occur.

The Delivery Process

As the infant descends the birth canal, pressure against the rectum may cause fecal material to be expelled. Sponges (as a rule with saline solution) may be used to remove any fecal material which may escape from the rectum.

Fundal pressure should not be used to accomplish spontaneous delivery or to bring the head deeper into the birth canal. Severe fundal pressure may cause uterine damage or rupture of the uterus.

As soon as the head distends the perineum to a diameter of 6 cm or 8 cm, a towel may be placed over the rectum while forward pressure is exerted on the baby's chin with one hand, at the same time that downward pressure is applied to the occiput by the other hand. This technique, called the Ritgen's maneuver (Fig. 24-7), provides control of the head as it is emerging and directs the extension phase of delivery so that the head is born with the smallest diameter presenting. The head is usually delivered between contractions and as slowly as possible. At this time the mother may complain about a "splitting" sensation caused by the extreme vaginal stretching as the head is born. All these measures (control of head by Ritgen's maneuver, extension and slow delivery between contractions) help to prevent lacerations. If a tear seems to be inevitable, an incision which is called an episiotomy may be made in the perineum. This not only prevents lacerations but also facilitates the delivery.

Immediately after the birth of the infant's head a finger is passed along the occiput to the infant's neck in order to feel whether a loop or more of umbilical cord encircles it. If such a coil is felt, it should be gently drawn down and, if loose enough, slipped over the infant's head (Fig. 24-8). This is done to prevent interference with the infant's oxygen supply, which could result from pressure of its shoulder on the umbilical cord. If the cord is too tightly coiled to permit this procedure, it must be clamped and cut before the shoulders are delivered; then the infant must be extracted immediately before asphyxiation results. The anterior shoulder is usually brought under the symphysis pubis first and then the posterior shoulder is delivered, after which the remainder of the body follows without particular mechanism. The exact time of the baby's birth should be noted. The infant usually cries immediately, and the lungs gradually become expanded. The pulsations in the umbilical cord begin to diminish about this time.

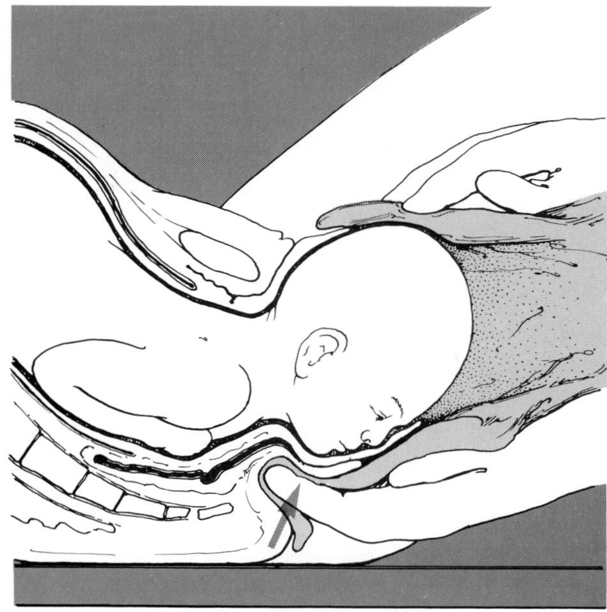

Figure 24-7.
Ritgen's maneuver as it appears in median section. Arrow shows direction of pressure.

Clamping the Cord

The cord usually is clamped before pulsations cease to prevent transfusion from the placenta and, consequently, hyperviscosity in the infant. The cord is then cut between the two Kelly clamps, which have been placed a few inches from the umbilicus; then the umbilical clamp or tie is applied (Figs. 24-9 and 24-10). If a tie is used, it is a sterilized linen tape ligature, usually applied about an inch from the abdomen, with care to secure it tightly enough to prevent bleeding without its cutting into the cord (Fig. 24-11). A second ligature may be applied for further protection if it is desired or if it is necessary because of any bleeding. There are several types of umbilical clamps, such as the Kane, the Hollister, and the Hesseltine, which are used extensively in many institutions (see Fig. 24-9). With these the possibility of hemorrhage is minimized.

Psychosocial Considerations

If the mother is awake, she is usually eager to have a closer look at her baby and hold it. The nurse should remember that, although she is quite tired, she is usually elated, proud of her accomplishment of giving

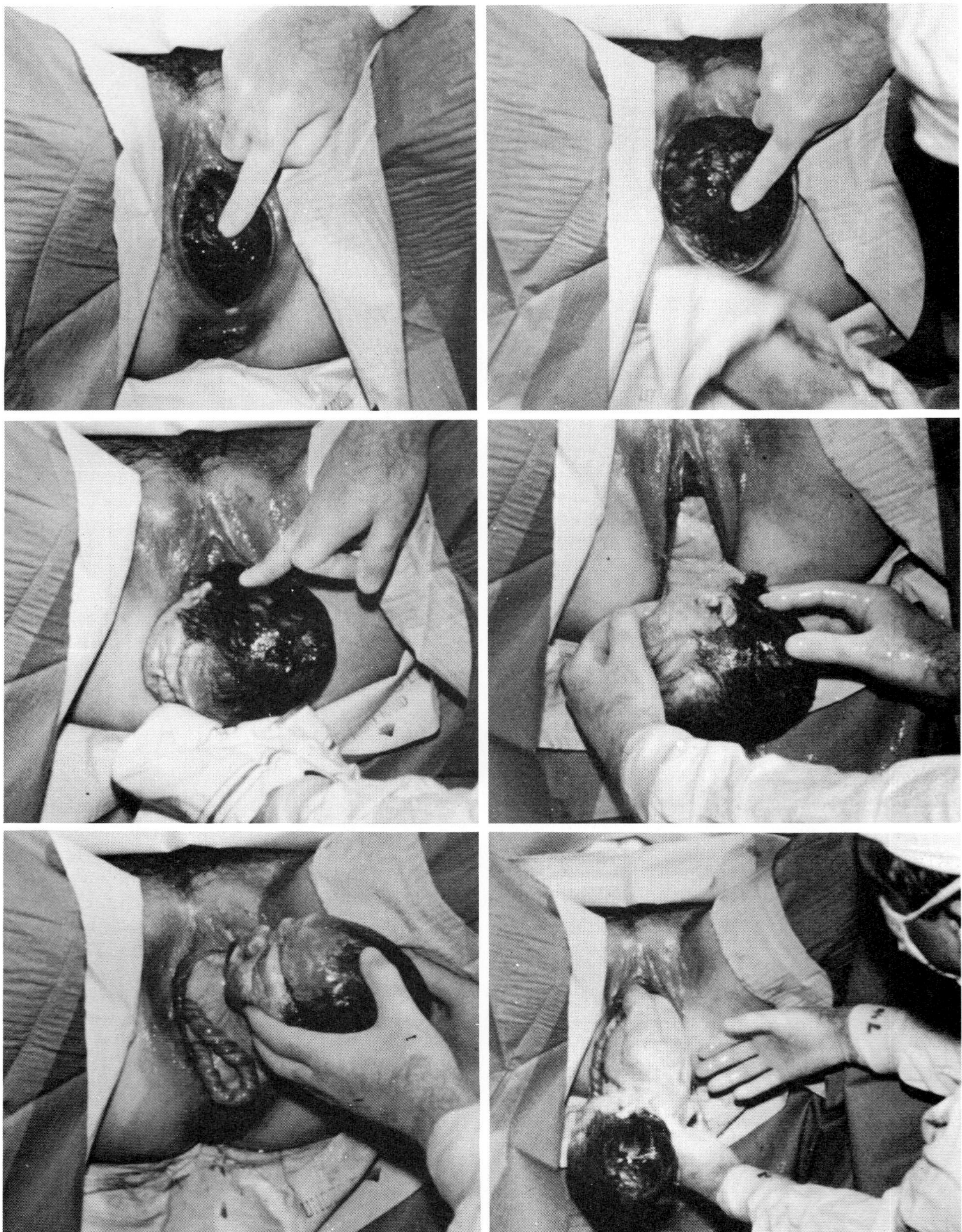

Figure 24-8.
The normal birth process. (From the film Human Birth, published by J. B. Lippincott, Philadelphia.)

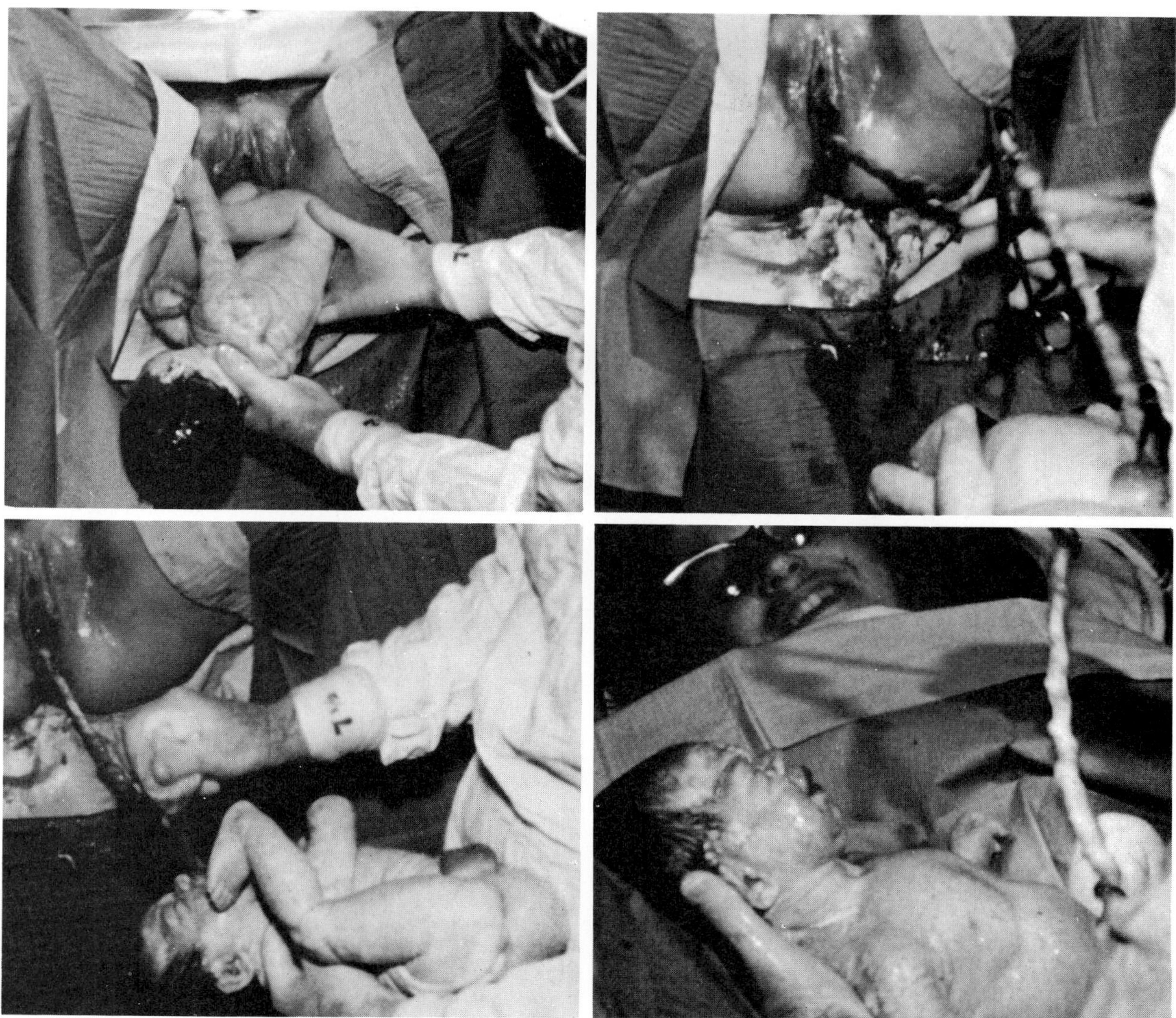

birth and eager to share this with the baby's father. Whenever possible, all efforts should be made to allow the father, the mother, and the infant to share this momentous time together if they so desire. More hospitals are allowing the mother to hold her infant immediately after delivery and put it to breast if she is breast-feeding. Other institutions have the mother wait to hold the infant or nurse it until she has been transferred to the recovery room. These kinds of arrangements provide more opportunities for the parents to have a close, thorough look at their baby and to let the triad begin the necessary process of bonding and integrating the new member into the family constellation.

The Leboyer Method of Delivery

In recent years a newer method of delivery has been advocated by a French obstetrician, Frederick Leboyer, who suggests that delivery room procedures be changed to make birth less of a traumatic event for the newborn. In his book and lectures he has described a method of handling infants during birth which includes a dimly lit and quiet delivery room, placing the infant on the mother's abdomen and stroking (massaging) it gently, delaying the clamping of the cord, and immersing the infant in a warm bath until it is relaxed and quiet.[18,19] Leboyer contends that the traditional method of delivery with all of its harsh, sudden sensory stimulation can be detrimental to the infant. The shock of birth produces jitteriness, interferes with eye contact between mother and infant, and may even prevent optimal bonding with the mother given the other restrictive practices followed in some hospitals.

There has been some controversy about this type of "gentle" birth mainly because of questions concerning possible threats to infant safety from undue chilling, placental transfusion, and possible infection.

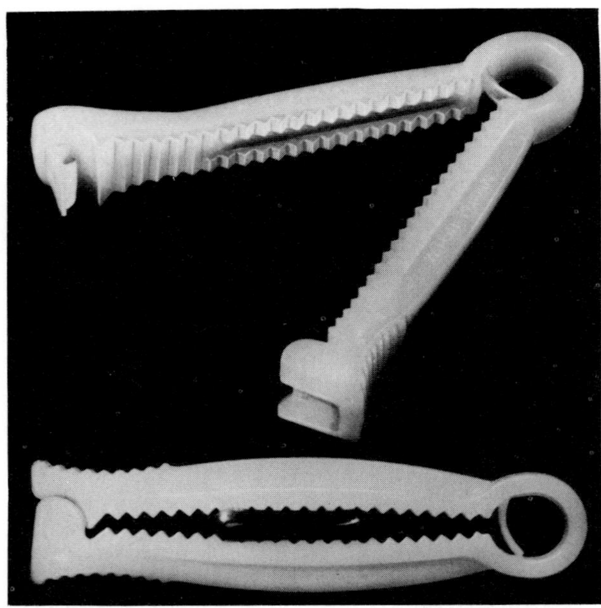

Figure 24-9.
Umbilical cord clamp. A double-grip cord clamp in the opened and closed positions. (Courtesy of Hollister, Inc., Chicago, Ill)

There has been no definitive research to either prove or disprove the efficacy of this method. Preliminary data do indicate that infants delivered by this technique do not tend to tremble or shudder as much and have more relaxed hand muscles than other infants. Moreover, they spend more time with their eyes open in the period immediately subsequent to delivery. In addition, no greater risk for mother or infant of infection or chilling was found.[20] Many hospitals are offering at least a modified version of this technique and more parents are requesting it.

Conduct of the Third Stage

Delivery of the Placenta

The third stage of labor, placental stage, begins after the delivery of the baby and terminates with the birth of the placenta. Immediately after delivery of the infant the height of the uterine fundus and its consistency are ascertained by palpating the uterus through a sterile towel placed on the lower abdomen. A hand is placed on the abdomen *under* the sterile drape and the uterus is held very gently with the fingers behind the fundus and the thumb in front. So long as the uterus remains hard, and there is no bleeding, the policy is ordinarily one of watchful waiting until the placenta is separated; no massage is practiced—the hand simply resting on the fundus to make certain that the organ does not balloon out with blood.

Since attempts to deliver the placenta prior to its separation from the uterine wall are not only futile but may be dangerous, it is most important that the signs of placental separation be well understood. The signs which suggest that the placenta has separated are as follows:

1. The uterus rises upward in the abdomen because the placenta, having been separated, passes downward into the lower uterine segment and the vagina, where its bulk pushes the uterus upward.
2. The umbilical cord protrudes 3 inches or more farther out of the vagina, indicating that the placenta also has descended.
3. The uterus changes from a discoid to a globular shape and becomes, as a rule, more firm.
4. A sudden trickle or spurt of blood often occurs.

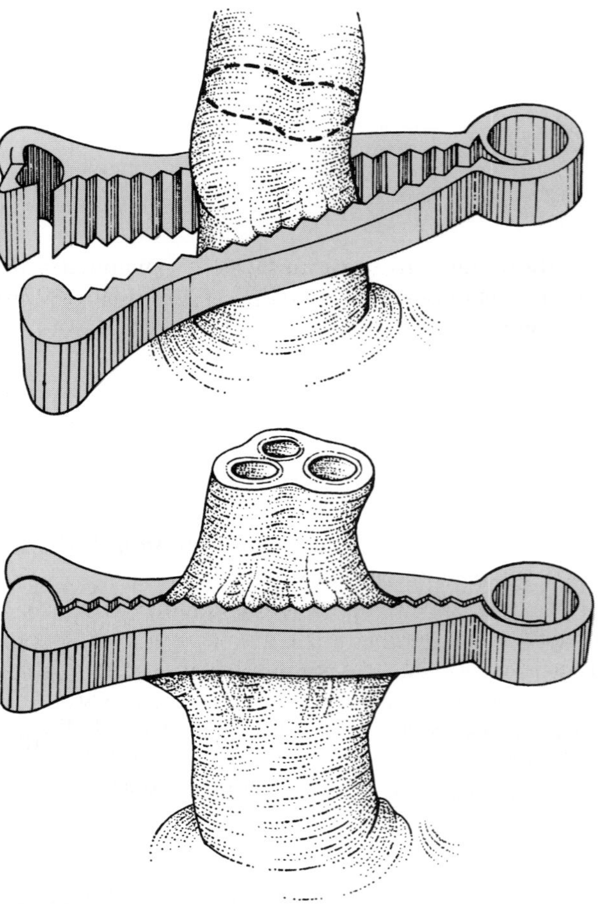

Figure 24-10.
Clamp.

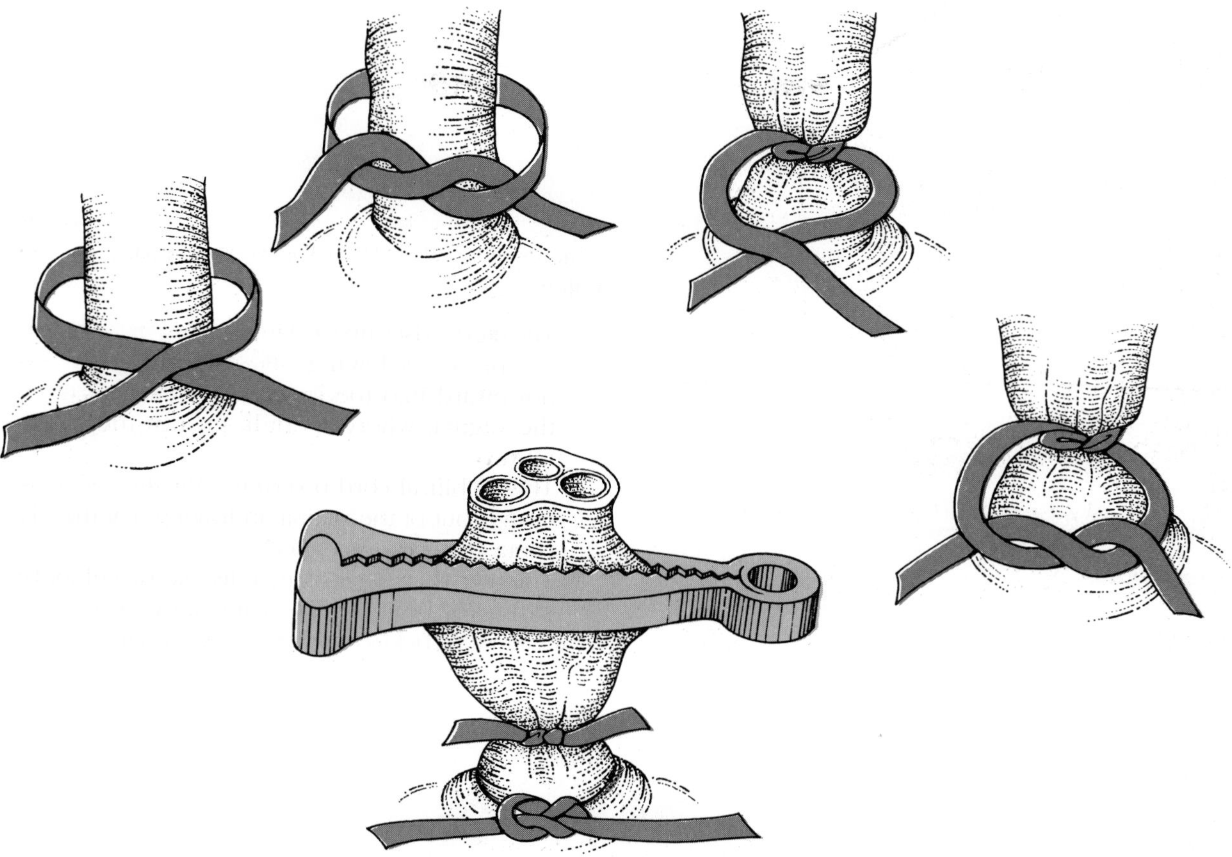

Figure 24-11.
Tying off cord.

These signs are apparent sometimes within a minute or so after delivery of the infant and usually within five minutes. When the placenta has separated and the uterus is firmly contracted, the patient is asked to bear down so that the intraabdominal pressure so produced may expel the placenta. If this fails, or if it is not practicable because of anesthesia, gentle pressure is exerted downward with the hand on the fundus and the placenta is gently guided out of the vagina. This procedure, known as placental *expression,* must be done gently and without squeezing (Figs. 24-12 and 24-13). It never should be attempted unless the uterus is hard; otherwise the organ may be turned inside out. This is one of the gravest complications of obstetrics and is known as "inversion" of the uterus. Once the placenta is expelled, it is carefully inspected to make sure that it is intact (Fig. 24-14); if a piece is left in the uterus, it may cause subsequent hemorrhage.

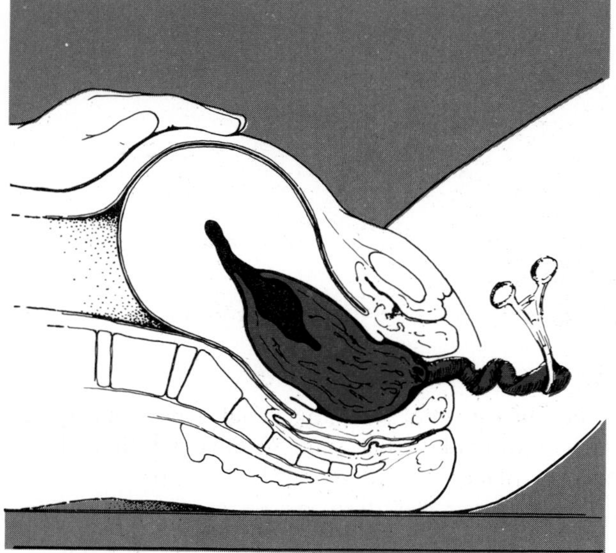

Figure 24-12.
Expression of placenta is usually done by the physician, if necessary, but *on his instructions* may be done by an assistant. The *uterus must be hard* if this is attempted. Note that the uterus is not squeezed.

Use of Oxytocics

Oxytocin or ergonovine, or their derivatives, may be administered at the physician's request to increase uterine contractions and thereby to minimize bleed-

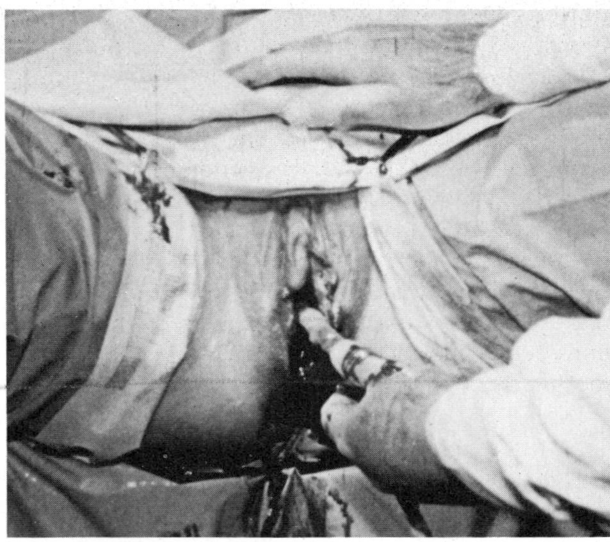
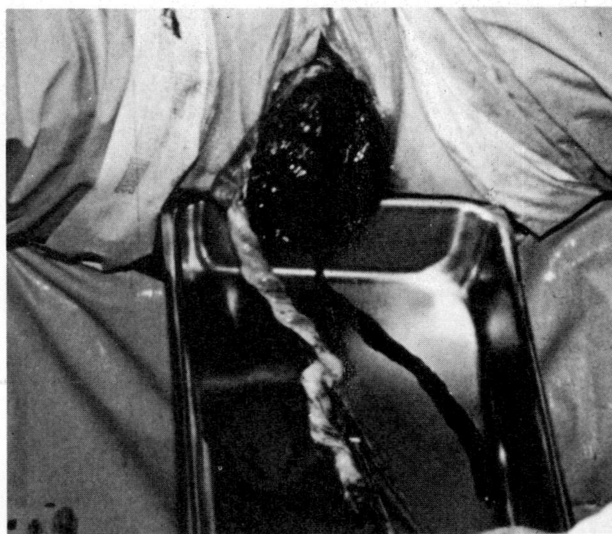

Figure 24-13.
Third stage of labor; the delivery of the placenta. (From the film, Human Birth, published by J. B. Lippincott, Philadelphia.)

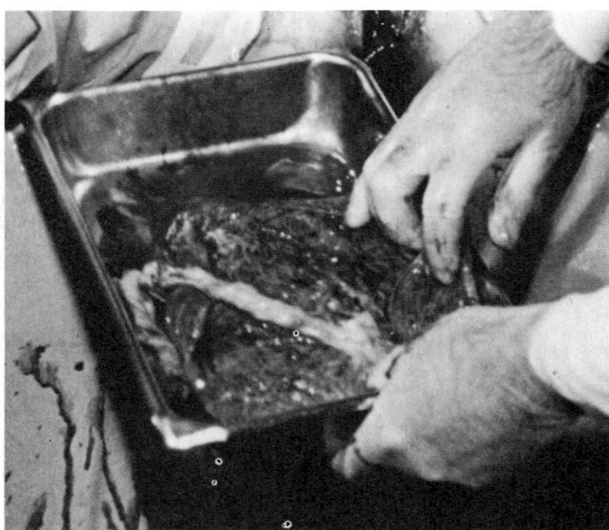
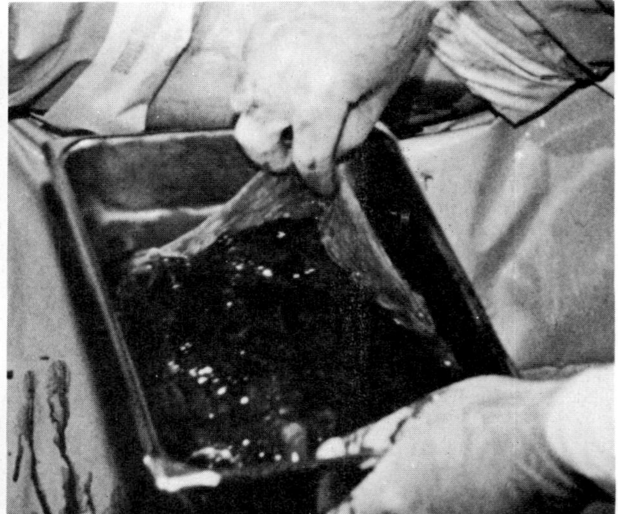

Figure 24-14.
Inspecting the placenta. (From the film, Human Birth, published by J. B. Lippincott, Philadelphia.)

ing. These agents are employed widely in the conduct of the normal third stage of labor, but the timing of their administration differs greatly in various hospitals. These oxytocics are not necessary in most cases, but their use is considered ideal from the viewpoint of minimizing blood loss and the general safety of the mother.

Ergonovine is an alkaloid of ergot and is a powerful oxytocic; it stimulates uterine contractions and exerts an effect which may persist for several hours. When it is administered intravenously, the uterine response is almost immediate, within a few minutes of intramuscular or oral administration. This response is sustained in character with no tendency toward relaxation. *However, this drug does cause an elevation of blood pressure.*

More recently a semisynthetic derivative of ergonovine, *methylergonovine maleate* (Methergine) has been employed. It is thought to cause less elevation of blood pressure when given parentally.

Both drugs when given intravenously may cause transient headache and, to a lesser extent, temporary chest pain, palpitation, and dyspnea. These side-effects are less likely to occur with intramuscular administration of the drugs.

Oxytocin (Pitocin) is another agent which, like ergonovine, causes a marked contraction of the uterus. However, the response of the uterus to oxytocin resembles the response to ergonovine for only the first five to ten minutes; then normal rhythmic contractions of amplified degree return, with intermittent periods of relaxation.

The oxytocic fraction separated from posterior pituitary extract is called oxytocin; it is widely used because it does not possess the strong vasopressor effects of Pituitrin, which was used more extensively in former years.

Oxytocin's most important side-effect is its antidiuretic effect which can cause water intoxication if administered intravenously in a large volume of electrolyte-free aqueous dextrose solution. Fortunately, the antidiuretic effect disappears within a few minutes after the infusion is discontinued.

On the obstetrician's order the nurse administers the oxytocic intramuscularly; or adds the medication to the intravenous fluid. The average doses of the drugs are as follows: oxytocin, 10 units (1 nl) IM or IV, 10 units (1 nl) IM or IV; ergonovine, 0.2 mg ($^1/_{320}$ gr) or 1 nl, IM or IV; and Methergine, 0.2 mg ($^1/_{320}$ gr) or 1 nl, IM or IV. Various institutions use the drugs separately or in conjunction as is necessary to produce the desired results. The choice of the oxytocic usually depends on the anesthetic agent administered. Oxytocin is contraindicated for use with drugs that have a sympathomimetic action.

Lacerations of the Birth Canal

During the process of a normal delivery lacerations of the perineum and the vagina may be caused by rapid and sudden expulsion of the head (particularly when it "pops" out), excessive size of the infant, and very friable maternal tissues. In other circumstances they may be caused by difficult forceps deliveries, breech extractions, or contraction of the pelvic outlet in which the head is forced posteriorly. Some tears are unavoidable, even in the most skilled hands.

Perineal lacerations usually are classified in three degrees, according to the extent of the tear.

First-degree lacerations are those which involve the fourchet, the perineal skin, and the vaginal mucous membrane without involving any of the muscles.

Second-degree lacerations are those which involve (in addition to skin and mucous membrane) the muscles of the perineal body but not the rectal sphincter. These tears usually extend upward on one or both sides of the vagina, making a triangular injury.

Third-degree lacerations are those which extend completely through the skin, the mucous membrane, the perineal body, and the rectal sphincter. This type is often referred to as a complete tear. Frequently these third-degree lacerations extend a certain distance up the anterior wall of the rectum.

First- and second-degree lacerations are extremely common in primigravidas; their high incidence is one of the reasons that episiotomy is widely employed. Fortunately, third-degree lacerations are far less common. All three types of lacerations are repaired by the physician immediately after the delivery to ensure that the perineal structures are returned approximately to their former condition. The technique employed for the repair of a laceration is virtually the same as that used for episiotomy incisions, although the former is more difficult to do because of the irregular lines of tissue which must be approximated.

Episiotomy and Repair

An episiotomy is an incision of the perineum made to facilitate delivery. The incision is made with blunt-pointed straight scissors about the time that the head distends the vulva and is visible to a diameter of several centimeters. The incision may be made in the midline of the perineum—a median episiotomy (Fig. 24-15). Or it may be begun in the midline and directed downward and laterally away from the rectum—a mediolateral episiotomy. In the latter instance the incision may be directed to either the right or to the left side of the mother's pelvis (Fig. 24-16).

If a laceration seems to be inevitable as the infant's head distends the vulva, the physician undoubtedly chooses to incise the perineum rather than allow that structure to sustain a traumatic tear. This operation serves the following purposes:

1. It substitutes a straight, clean-cut surgical incision for the ragged, contused laceration which otherwise may ensue; such an incision is easier to repair and heals better than a tear.
2. The direction of the episiotomy can be controlled, whereas a tear may extend in any direc-

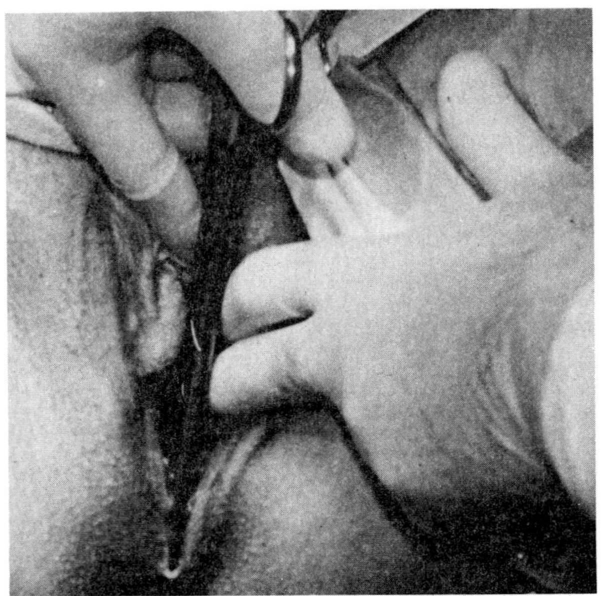

Figure 24-15.
Median episiotomy. (From the film, Human Birth, published by J. B. Lippincott, Philadelphia.)

tion, sometimes involving the anal sphincter and the rectum.

3. Inordinate stretching and tearing of the perineal musculature is avoided and the incidence of subsequent perineal relaxation with cystocele-rectocele may be reduced.
4. The operation shortens the duration of the second stage of labor.

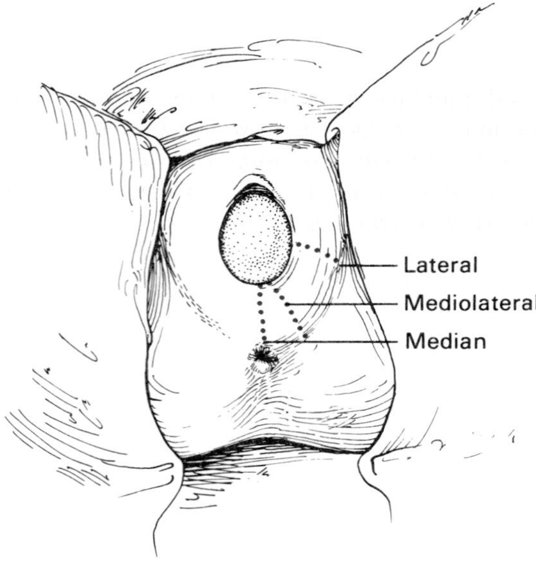

Figure 24-16.
Types of episiotomies.

In view of these advantages many physicians employ episiotomy routinely in the delivery of the primigravida.

There are many equally satisfactory methods that are used for episiotomy repair (Fig. 24-17). The suture material ordinarily used is a fine chromic catgut, either 00 or 000.

A round needle and continuous suture is used to close the vaginal mucosa and fourchet and is then set aside while several interrupted sutures are placed in the levator ani muscle and the fascia. Then the continuous suture is again picked up and used to unite the subcutaneous fascia. Finally, the round needle is replaced by a large, straight cutting needle, and the running suture is continued upward as a subcuticular stitch.

Conduct of the Fourth Stage

Physiological Considerations

These first hours after delivery have been described aptly as the "fourth stage of labor." The wearying work of labor per se is completed and the mother and father can look forward to a brief respite before assuming the forthcoming responsibilities of parenthood. This is truly a transition period and many important physical and psychosocial tasks begin at this time.

After the delivery has been completed and the episiotomy has been repaired, the drapes and the soiled linen under the mother's buttocks are removed, and the lower end of the delivery table is replaced. If stirrups have been used, the mother's legs are lowered *simultaneously* to prevent cramping or twisting of the extremities. A sterile perineal pad is applied and the mother is given a clean, warm gown and covered with a blanket to avoid chilling. Usually she and the infant are then transferred to the postpartum recovery area. Some institutions still require that the infant be transferred immediately to the newborn nursery.

Management of Potential Complications

Hypothermic Reactions. Chilling accompanied by uncontrollable shaking often occurs in this early period after delivery. It is uncomfortable and sometimes embarrassing or frightening for the patient, but it is self-limiting (usually not over 15 minutes) and is not considered an ominous sign. The exact etiology of this chilling has not been determined, although several explanations have been offered, which include

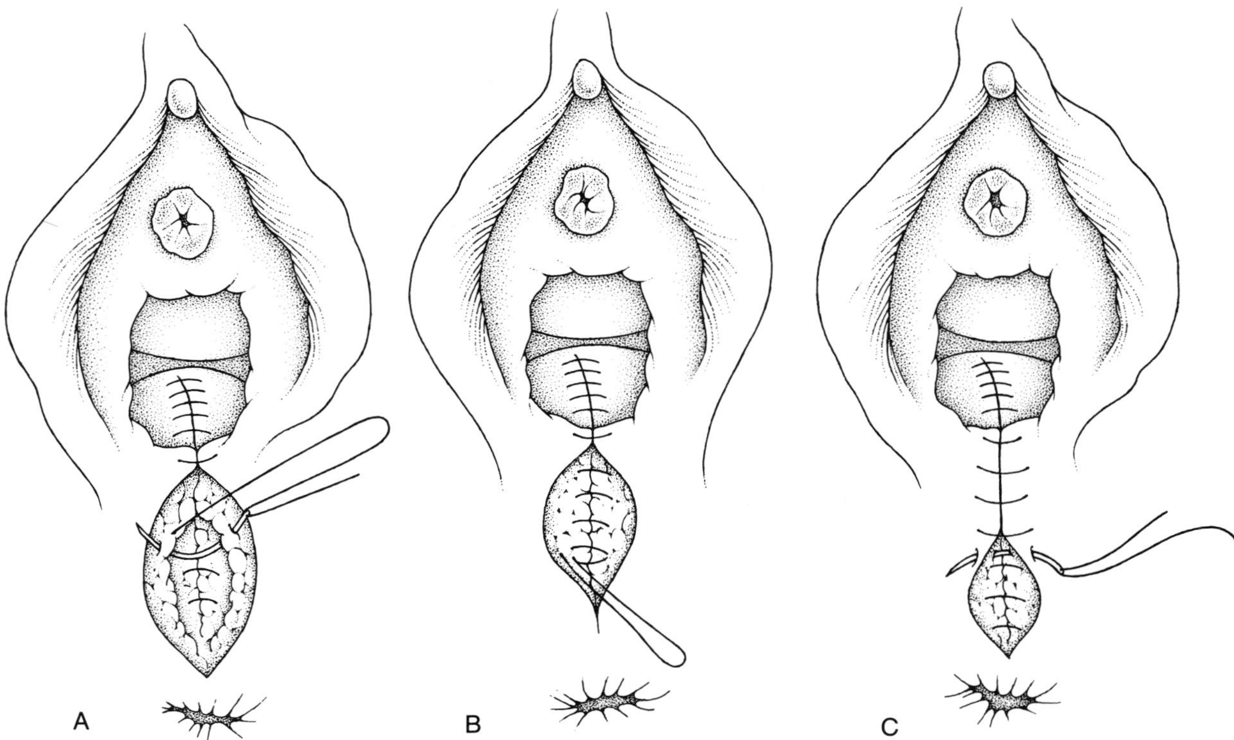

Figure 24-17.
Repair of median episiotomy. *(A)* Chromic catgut 00, or preferably 000, is used as a continuous suture to close the vaginal mucosa and submucosa. *(B)* After closing the vaginal incision and reapproximating the cut margins of the hymeneal ring, the suture is tied and cut. Next three or four interrupted sutures of 00 or 000 catgut are placed in the fascia and muscle of the incised perineum. *(C)* Repair of complete perineal tear. The rectal mucosa has been repaired with interrupted, fine chromic catgut sutures. The torn ends of the sphincter ani are next approximated with two or three interrupted chromic catgut sutures. The wound is then repaired, as in a second-degree laceration or an episiotomy.

sudden release of intraabdominal pressure after delivery, nervous and exhaustion responses related to the stress of childbirth, disequilibrium in the internal and external body temperature resulting from the waste products of muscular exertion, break in aseptic technique which predisposes to infection, minute circulatory amniotic fluid emboli, and previous maternal sensitization to elements of fetal blood.

Clean, dry, warm gowns and blankets as well as a warm nondrafty environment help in the prevention and control of this phenomenon. Warm fluids by mouth can be given and are much appreciated for their hydrating and energy-giving effects.

Postpartum Hemorrhage. Constant massage of the uterus during this period immediately after delivery is unnecessary and undesirable. However, if the organ shows any tendency to relax, it is to be massaged immediately with firm but gentle circular strokes until it contracts effectively. *Relaxation of the uterus is a prime cause of postpartum hemorrhage, and surveillance of the uterus and the amount of bleeding is of extreme importance at this time.*

Since the prevention of postpartum hemorrhage is such a crucial factor in the health and well-being of the mother, those patients at risk (most likely) to develop this condition should be identified quickly. The following are the most predictive factors associated with postpartum bleeding:

Older age and high parity
Rapid labor
Prolonged first and second stages of labor
Operative delivery, that is, forceps extraction
Overdistention of the uterus—polyhydramnios, multiple pregnancy, overly large infant

Previous uterine atony or associated previous postpartal hemorrhage
Other hemorrhagic complications such as abruptio placentae or placenta previa
Induced labor
Heavy medication during labor or general anesthesia
Preeclampsia and eclampsia

The nurse will have an intravenous infusion with an oxytocin for immediate administration ready in the event that the attendants suspect hemorrhage is imminent.

Vital Signs. Thus, the first hour following the delivery is a most critical one for the mother, because it is at this time that postpartal hemorrhage is most likely to occur. *The fundus is to be checked every five minutes or so and massaged as necessary to ensure continued firmness and to prevent its ballooning with blood* (Fig. 24-18).

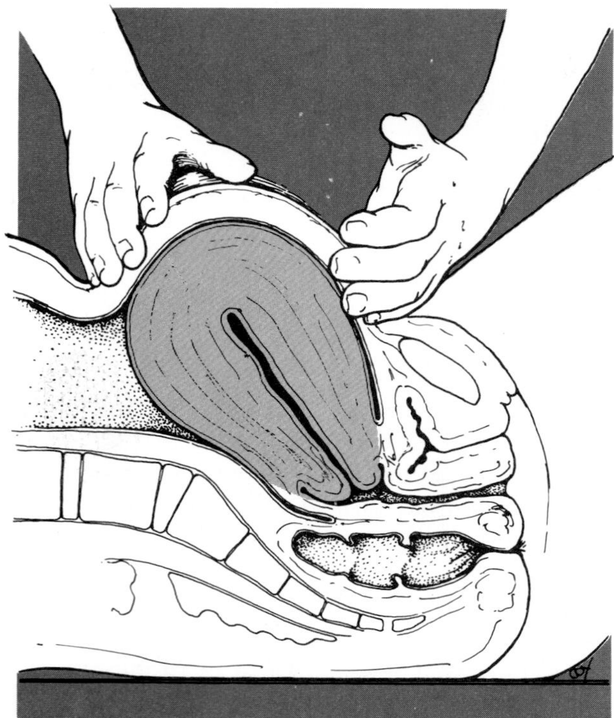

Figure 24-18.
Proper method of palpating fundus of uterus during first hour after delivery to guard against relaxation and hemorrhage. The right hand is placed just above the symphysis pubis to act as a guard; meanwhile the other hand is cupped around the fundus of the uterus.

It is also important to be alert not only to the condition of the mother's uterus but also to any abnormal symptoms relating to her general condition. Thus, checking the maternal vital signs is included in the nursing interventions.

Blood pressure and pulse are generally checked every 15 minutes until stable and then every half hour for one hour. Thereafter, they are continued every hour for several hours until the mother is definitely stabilized.

The flow is also checked about every half hour and the number of pads saturated is recorded.

Psychosocial Considerations

Emotional Reactions

Immediately after delivery, or perhaps later, the parents, particularly the mother, may relieve tension by giving way to some emotional displays such as laughing, crying, talking incessantly, or expressing anger (if all has not gone well or as expected). These emotions often are quite unexpected and may shock and embarrass those involved. A calm, accepting, nonjudgmental attitude on the part of the nurse is very effective in allaying any embarrassment and in helping the patient to gain control.

The nurse must remember that the patient is beginning a period that is enormously important; she is, in fact, now a "mother" with all its concomitant responsibilities; glimmerings of this already are reaching the consciousness. This is not the "end" but only the beginning of a whole new role. In addition, she is physically and emotionally exhausted from the great effort she has put forth; thus, there may be a temporary emotional upheaval.

Several comfort measures can be employed to restore calm and to help the mother relax enough to get some much-needed rest and sleep. A soothing backrub, change of gown and linen, a quiet conversation with the nurse or the father in which the patient is allowed to ventilate her feelings, an environment conducive to rest—all are helpful. In addition, a warm beverage can be offered to help relaxation. Since the mother is apt to be extremely hungry and thirsty, this is welcome nourishment as well as a therapeutic soporific.

Many mothers do not have an emotional outburst per se, although the majority do experience some degree of excitement and elation when the delivery is accomplished. Any of the above nursing activities are also suitable for them. Some patients experience a great need for sleep and drop off as soon as they

(Text continues on page 520)

NC Nursing Care: During Labor

Assessment	Intervention	Evaluation
First Stage Orientation Assessment of knowledge Orientation to unit Orientation to labor	Convey that the couple is expected and welcome After finding out what they know, explain the expectations and restrictions (food, fluids, activity) of the environment and what will be happening during the labor process	Couple becomes familiar with the new environment and settles in Couple verbalizes understanding of equipment, procedures, and expectations
Labor History When labor became apparent Frequency, duration, and intensity of contractions Condition of the BOW Character and amount of show Vital signs—TPR and BP Bowel and bladder patterns	Interview and record and report information as appropriate	Mother and nurse begin to establish rapport
Admission Procedures Enema Perineal clip Abdominal exam Vaginal exam General exam	Explain the intended procedures to the couple Administer enema if necessary Complete perineal prep Palpate abdomen to ascertain presenting part Do or assist with remainder of examinations; record and report information	Couple has an understanding of the upcoming events. Mother assists examiners appropriately Nurse–patient relationship continues to be built
Monitor Labor Contractions, FHR, vital signs, bladder distension, fluid intake, and show Determine need for electronic monitor Determine which comfort measures are necessary (back rub, oral hygiene, clean linen) Determine support person's ability to coach and support the mother Determine mother's need for explanations and emotional support as indicated as labor progresses	Attach electronic monitor if necessary or time contractions, check FHR as indicated Record and report information Encourage voiding Other fluids if ordered early in labor Rub back and change mother's position and linen as necessary Allow couple some time together; encourage support person's participation in mother's care Explain labor process as indicated and help mother change breathing patterns as indicated with onset of transition Keep explanations and instructions short and simple	Labor progresses; mother works with her contractions; bladder does not become distended, fluid intake is appropriate Mother relaxes between contractions Support person feels a part of the labor process; mother benefits by coach's presence and support Support person assists mother in coping with labor Changes to shallow breathing with transition Follows instructions with minimum of difficulty

(Continued)

Assessment	Intervention	Evaluation
Continue to Monitor Labor	**Second Stage**	
Determine appropriateness of bearing down	Record and report as before; monitor FHR every 5 min during delivery Monitor maternal BP Position mother correctly for "pushing"; coach as necessary	Physician has a clear picture of mother's progress—infant's vital signs stable; mother's BP stable; mother works with contractions to enable delivery
Transfer to delivery room	Instruct support person in delivery room procedures and policies if he or she is accompanying the mother	Support person verbalizes understanding of delivery room procedures and policies and coaches mother appropriately
Assist with anesthesia	Help with positioning for anesthesia if necessary; assist with supplies, vital signs monitoring, and intravenous infusions	Anesthesia given on time and appropriately
Assist with delivery	Continue coaching of mother in pushing and panting; do perineal prep and draping as indicated; check FHR and maternal BP as indicated	A healthy infant delivered under aseptic conditions
Postdelivery	**Third Stage**	
Postdelivery observations Fundus Flow Bladder Vital signs Perineum	Administer oxytocin after delivery of placenta as needed Gently massage fundus, if boggy, express clots as necessary; record and report amount and character of flow, vital signs, hematoma/bleeding from episiotomy	Uterus contracts after placental separation Flow moderates Vital signs stable Bladder nondistended Perineum without hematoma; minimal swelling
Determine need for comfort and rest	Reposition mother as needed; give warm, dry gown and blanket; provide adequate explanations, answers to questions; provide quiet environment for rest; provide light nourishment as indicated	Mother warm and comfortable
Postdelivery Observations	**Fourth Stage** Continue as before	Mother and infant's conditions stable
Family interaction	See Chapter 25	Interaction mutually satisfactory

AT Observations of Responses of the Mother During Fourth Stage of Labor

Patient's Name: ______________________________

Please circle appropriate responses.

Verbal Responses

1. Calls baby by name
2. Calls baby affectionate terms
3. Comments on beauty of baby and on realistic defects
4. Voices unhappiness over sex of baby
5. Calls baby "it"
6. Uses unhappy or scolding inflections
7. Asks husband or nurse if baby is all right
8. Talks about baby
9. Answers in monosyllables
10. Complains of difficult labor and delivery
11. Doesn't talk about baby
12. Requests that baby be taken to nursery
13. Seeks considerable support for own discomfort

Nonverbal Responses

1. Looks at the baby and reaches out to it
2. Hugs, touches baby
3. Smiles at baby
4. Kisses baby
5. Undresses baby
6. Doesn't touch baby
7. Doesn't look at baby
8. Pushes baby away
9. Tenses face, arms
10. Sleepy, not drug induced
11. Turns away from baby
12. Turns away from husband, nurse, visitor
13. Positive eye contact, emotional feeling with husband
14. Unresponsive to husband, nurse, visitor
15. Cries unhappily
16. Holds husband's hand
17. Breast-feeds baby

First comments made in delivery room by mother about baby:
____

Visitor with mother during fourth stage: ______________________________

Involvement of husband or visitor: ______________________________

Problems with baby: ______________________________

Subjective opinion of response of mother:
____

Analgesia within last 4 hrs: ______________________________

Anesthesia: ______________________________

Complications: ______________________________

Significant social history: ______________________________
____

Parity: ______________

Age: ______________

Marital status: ______________

Feeding method: ______________

Service: ______________

Race: ______________

Behavior of baby

Crying: None—periodic—almost continuous

Affect: Difficult to arouse—dozes—eyes open—very alert

This form helped nurses at Yale focus their observations of mothers and infants the first one or two hours after delivery. (Rising S: The fourth stage of labor: Family integration. Am J Nurs 74:873, May 1974) ascertain that the baby is "all right." If the patient is sleeping continuously or intermittently, she should be allowed to do so, being disturbed only for those nursing observations which are necessary. When she indicates readiness, her baby can be presented, and she can be allowed to examine and to explore it to her heart's content.

Mothers who have not been conscious during the delivery may have rather different reactions from those patients who have participated in the birth process. Often they do not seem to believe that delivery has taken place or that the baby shown to them is really theirs. They question again and again, "Is it really all over?" "Tell me again, is it a boy or a girl?" "Did I have the baby?" The apparent alteration in awareness seems to be related to the anesthesia and the unconsciousness. These patients may need more firm reassurance and contact with their infants to help them realize that they have had a baby.

The Symbiotic Relationship and Mother–Infant Bonding

Even though the repeated questioning may become annoying, the nurse must recognize that this is necessary for the mother in order to begin the important process of disengagement from the symbiotic relationship that she had with her infant during pregnancy. She must now establish the baby as a real entity outside her body rather than inside. All mothers have this task to perform, but it may be harder for the mother who has been delivered under heavy anesthesia, for as far as she is concerned, she was not "there" when it all happened.

Maternal attachment feelings, as we know, do not spring unbound at the time of delivery. Rather, they are developed, often slowly, as in any other developmental process. It is now recognized that the early encounters the mother has with her newborn, which often begin immediately after delivery, pave the way for later maternal responses in the postpartal period and, indeed, throughout life.[21]

Maternal attachment behavior has been defined as the extent to which a mother feels that her infant occupies an essential position in her life. Components of this phenomenon are feelings of warmth or love, a sense of possession, devotion, protectiveness and concern for the infant's well-being, positive anticipation of prolonged contact, and a need for and pleasure in continuing transactions. As in other meaningful relationships, there is an acceptance of impositions and obligations intolerable with less important objects and a sense of loss experienced with the infant's actual or imagined absence.[21] (See chart on p. 519.)

Assessment of Family Integration

Rising has pointed out that there is a certain openness about the fourth stage of labor that may not occur again during the postpartum period. This openness allows the nurse to make assessments regarding the couple's ability to proceed with integrating the infant smoothly into the family. She and other practitioners have suggested that it may be helpful to use a form to systematically record observations of the family unit during the fourth stage of labor.[22] Such an assessment tool is invaluable in providing a focus for observations of behavior and can be further developed as a predictive tool to help determine those couples who may have difficulty in integration.

If family units are identified as potentially at risk of maladaptive integration, the nurse will want to set aside more time to be with the couple to reinforce any positive responses that they might demonstrate and to give as much encouragement as possible. Listening attentively as the couple relive their recent experiences (and perhaps their disappointments) and encouraging verbalization of these feelings, and at the same time pointing out to them whatever positive realities did occur in the recent event, can prove helpful. Most important, the nurse will pass on her observations and interventions to the postpartum personnel so that they may continue with positive interventions. These personnel, in turn, can work closely with community-health nurses or arrange for other follow-up care to encourage subsequent adjustment. This is a time when the nurse needs to use all the observational skills, time, and "laying on of the hands" to foster initial integration and to begin prescribing future care aimed at consolidating the family unit. The topic of parent–infant attachment is discussed more thoroughly in Chapter 29, Psychosocial Aspects of the Postpartum Period.

References

1. Friedman EA: Labor, Clinical Evaluation and Management, 2nd ed. New York, Appleton–Century–Crofts, 1978

2. Newman MA: Identifying and meeting patients' needs in short-span nurse–patient relationships. Nurs Form 5, 1:76–86, 1966

3. Aiken L, Aiken J: A systematic approach to the evaluation of interpersonal relationships. Am J Nurs 73:863–867, May 1973

4. Doering SG, Entwisle D, Quinlin D: Modeling the quality of women's birth experience. J Health and Soc Behav 21:12–21, March 1980

5. Norr KL, Block C, Charles A: Explaining pain and enjoyment in childbirth. J Health and Soc Behav 18:260–275, September 1977

6. Highley BL, Mercer RT: Safeguarding the laboring woman's sense of control. MCN 3, 1:38–41, January/February 1978

7. Kalisch BJ: What is empathy? Am J Nurs 73:1548–1552, September 1973

8. Pritchard SA, McDonald PC: Williams Obstetrics Chapter 17, pp 473–486. New York, Appleton–Century–Crofts, 1980

9. Kantor HI, et al: Value of shaving the pudendal-perineal area in delivery preparation. Obstet Gynecol 25:509–512, April 1965

10. Johston RA, Sidall RS: Is the usual method of preparing patients for delivery beneficial or necessary? Am J Obstet Gynecol 4:645–650, December 1922

11. Sweeney WJ, III: Perineal shaves and bladder catheterization: Necessary and benign or unnecessary and potentially injurious. Obstet Gynecol 21:291–294, March 1963

12. Long AE: Unshaved perineum at parturition. Am J Obstet Gynecol 99:333–336, October 1, 1967

13. Seropian R, Reynolds BM: Wound infections after preoperative depilatory versus razor preparation. Am J Surg 121:251–254, March 1971

14. Landry KE, Kilpatrick DM: Why shave a mother before she gives birth? MCN 2, 3:189–190, May/June 1977

15. Saltenes SJ: Physical touch and nursing support in labor. Unpublished Master's Thesis. Yale University, 1962

16. Liu YC: Effects of the upright position during labor. Am J Nurs 74:2202–2205, December 1974

17. Roberts JE: Maternal positions for childbirth: A historical review of nursing care practices. JOGN Nurs 8:24–32, January/February 1979

18. Leboyer F: Birth without Violence. New York, Alfred A. Knopf, 1975

19. Oliver M, Oliver GM: Gentle birth, its safety and effect on neonatal behavior. JOGN Nurs 7:35–40, September/October 1978

20. Barnett CR, Leiderman H, Grobestein R, Klaus M et al: The maternal side of interactional deprivation. Pediatrics, 45:197, 1970

21. Robson DS, Moss HA: Patterns and determinants of maternal attachment. Pediatrics, 77:976–985, December 1970

22. Rising S: The fourth stage of labor: Family integration. Am J Nurs 74:870–874, May 1974

Suggested Reading

Chagnon LJ and Heldenbrand CL: Nurses undertake direct and indirect fetal monitoring at a community hospital. JOGN Nurs 3, 4:41–46, September/October 1974

Cronenwett LR, Newmark LL: Fathers' responses to childbirth. Nurs Res 23:210–217, May/June 1974

Henson D: Natural childbirth in the year, O. Nurs For 17, 3:228–244, 1978

Highley BL, Mercer RT: Safeguarding the laboring woman's sense of control. MCN 3, 1:39–41, January/February 1978

Huprich PA: Assisting the couple through a Lamaze labor and delivery. MCN 2, 4:245–253, July/August 1977

McDonough M, Sheriff D, Zimmel P: Parents' responses to fetal monitoring. MCN 6, 1:32–34, January/February 1981

Roberts JE: Maternal positions for childbirth: A historical review of nursing care practices. JOGN Nurs 8:24–32, January/February 1979

Shannon–Babitz M: Addressing the needs of fathers during labor and delivery. MCN 4, 6:378–382. November/December 1979

Shields D: Maternal reactions to fetal monitoring. Am J Nurs 78:2110–2112, December 1978

Yunek MJ, Lojek M: Intrapartal fetal monitoring. Am J Nurs 78:2106–2190, December 1978

CHAPTER 25

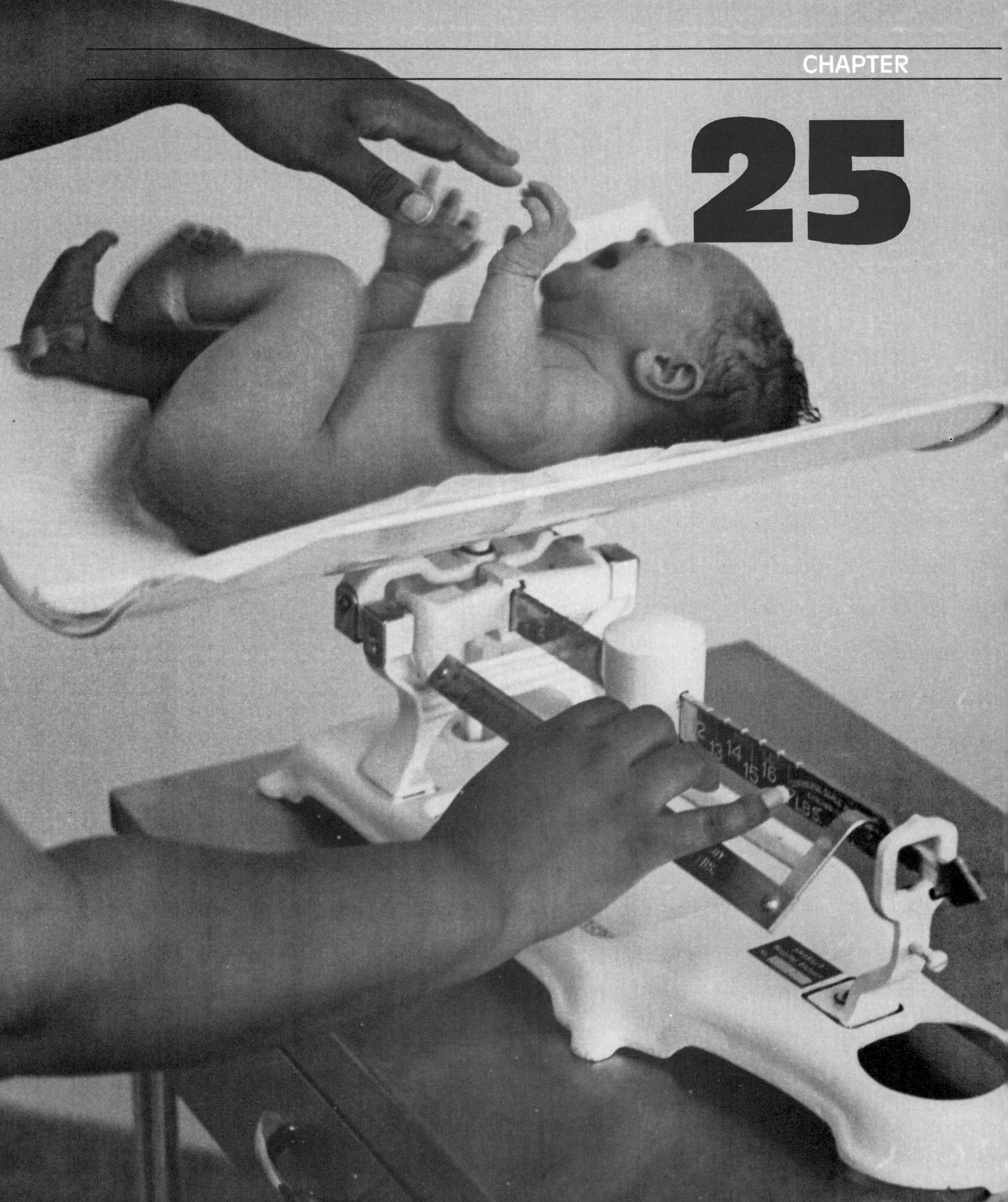

CHAPTER 25

Immediate Care of the Newborn

- **Suctioning the Airway**
  - Resuscitation
- **Stimulating Crying**
- **Preventing Hypothermia**
- **Assessment of the Newborn Infant**
  - The Apgar Scoring System
    - Heart Rate
    - Respiratory Effort
    - Muscle Tone
    - Reflex Irritability
    - Color
    - Interpretation
- **Other Aspects of Care**
  - Care of the Cord

AT **Guide for Perinatal Assessment of the Newborn**

- Care of the Eyes
- Hypoprothrombinemia Prophylaxis
- Identification Methods
- After the Delivery
- Baptism of Infant

NC **Nursing Care: Immediate Care of the Newborn**

When the infant is born, he or she undergoes a profound and rapid physiological change as the fetoplacental circulation ceases to function. The infant's survival depends upon a rapid and sequential interchange of oxygen and carbon dioxide which comes from both the pulmonary circulation and the new environment. In this exchange, the infant's fluid-filled alveoli of the lungs must fill with air, and that air must be exchanged by vigorous respiratory motion. A microcirculation also needs to be established in close proximity to the alveoli.[1]

Almost immediately after the birth, the shallow episodic breathing that characterizes fetal breathing is replaced by regular deeper breathing.[2–4] As the fluid is replaced by air, the pulmonary vascular compression is reduced and thus, there is a lowered resistance to blood flow, which helps the ductus arteriosus to close.

If conditions are normal, subsequent breathing after the first breath brings about more air that accumulates in the lungs. Hence, with each successive breath, lower pulmonary opening pressure is required and finally, pressure-volume changes are achieved which emulate normal extrauterine breathing.

Suctioning the Airway

As soon as the infant is born, measures are taken to promote a clear air passage. As the head is delivered, the mucus and fluid are wiped from the infant's nose and mouth before it has a chance to gasp and aspirate with the first breath. Babson and Benda recommend that the infant be kept in a face-down position immediately after delivery in order to facilitate the drainage of mucus, blood, and amniotic fluid from the oropharynx.[5] A small rubber bulb syringe or a soft rubber suction catheter attached to a mechanical suction or mouth aspirator can be used promptly to suction the oropharynx and to remove fluids that may be obstructing the airway (Fig. 25-1). If there seems to be much mucus present, the physician will hold the infant up by the ankles to encourage more mucus to drain from the throat. The mucosal surfaces of the palate and the posterior pharynx should not be wiped with gauze because the rough texture can lead to abrasions and thus provide a portal of entry for pathogenic organisms. A flexible rubber catheter may be passed by the physician to suction the larynx if the above measures do not clear the mucus well enough.

It is important *not to oversuction* at any time, because this merely deprives the infant of oxygen and irritates the mucous membrane. If further suctioning is necessary, the nurse may use the suction apparatus on the electric infant resuscitator, a bulb syringe, or a soft rubber catheter attached to a DeLee glass trap, which was designed especially for aspirating mucus in newborn infants (Fig. 25-2). Care should be taken not to traumatize the tissues of the oropharynx with the tip of the catheter or with forceful suction. When the nasopharynx is obstructed by mucus, which must be removed through the nostrils, a small French catheter may be passed into the nostril if force is avoided. The catheter must *not* be inserted far back. If the catheter is directed horizontally, as if passing over the roof of the mouth, instead of directing it upward as for the adult patient, it usually slips into the tiny infant nostril with more ease. If a bulb syringe is used, it should be collapsed before it is inserted in the baby's mouth; otherwise the material in the oropharynx will be forced into the bronchi and lungs when the bulb is collapsed.

Resuscitation

For the majority of normal newborns, there is little need for resuscitative measures beyond clearing the airway and applying warmth and gentle tactile stimulation. There is a small percentage of newborns who do require assistance, and for them it is lifesaving assistance. Successful active resuscitation requires skilled personnel who have been trained in the procedure, a warm well-lighted work area, a means to deliver oxygen by positive pressure, intubation if necessary and, finally, appropriate drug therapy.

Inadequate respirations that persist beyond a minute severely compromise the infant by leading to a falling heart rate, decreased muscle tone, and greater possibility of acidosis (Fig. 25-3). The airway must be cleared and oxygen delivered through a well-fitting mask at a pressure of about 20 cm of water in 1- to 2-second spurts to deliver oxygen into the bronchi. The airway must be cleared well through suctioning, however, because the oxygen delivered under pressure forces any foreign material deep into the infant's lungs. If this procedure (called "bagging") does not promptly stimulate breathing and correct the evidence of hypoxia, endotracheal intubation will be

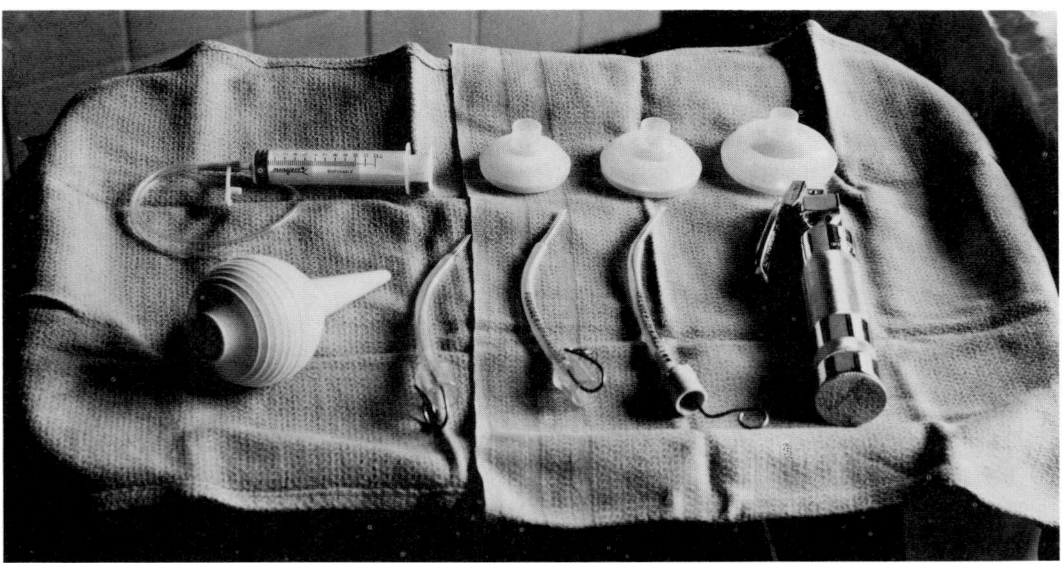

Figure 25-1.
Close-up view of a sterile tray for management of the airway. Counterclockwise from top left are a sterile, disposable syringe and tube for suctioning the stomach; a bulb syringe for suctioning the mouth; Cole endotracheal tubes (three sizes); an infant laryngoscope; and Bennet masks (three sizes).

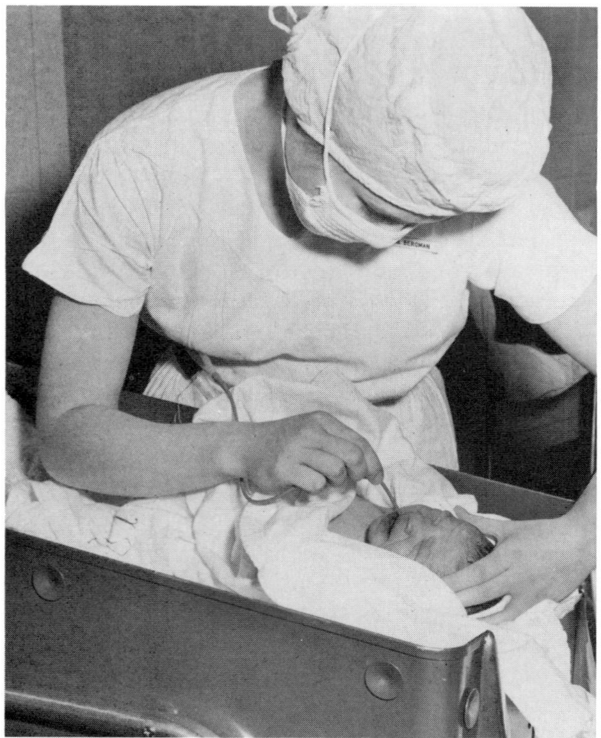

Figure 25-2.
Suctioning the newborn in the delivery room.

necessary under direct visualization with a laryngoscope. Further details of resuscitative measures can be found in Chapter 41.

Stimulating Crying

The baby may not cry at once, but it usually gasps or cries after the mucus has been removed, as oxygen by way of the lungs is now needed, since the accustomed supply was cut off when the placental circulation stopped.

If crying has to be stimulated, it is to be done with extreme care. As the infant is being held in the head-down position to promote the drainage of mucus from the respiratory passages, gentle rubbing of the infant's back is usually sufficient stimulus to initiate crying. And, in the act of crying, mucus is forced from the nose and the throat, thus enabling the infant to be better able to breathe.

Vigorous, external irritants are *unnecessary* and *dangerous* and should not be employed. These include harsh spanking on the soles of the feet or buttocks, forcible rubbing of the skin along the spine,

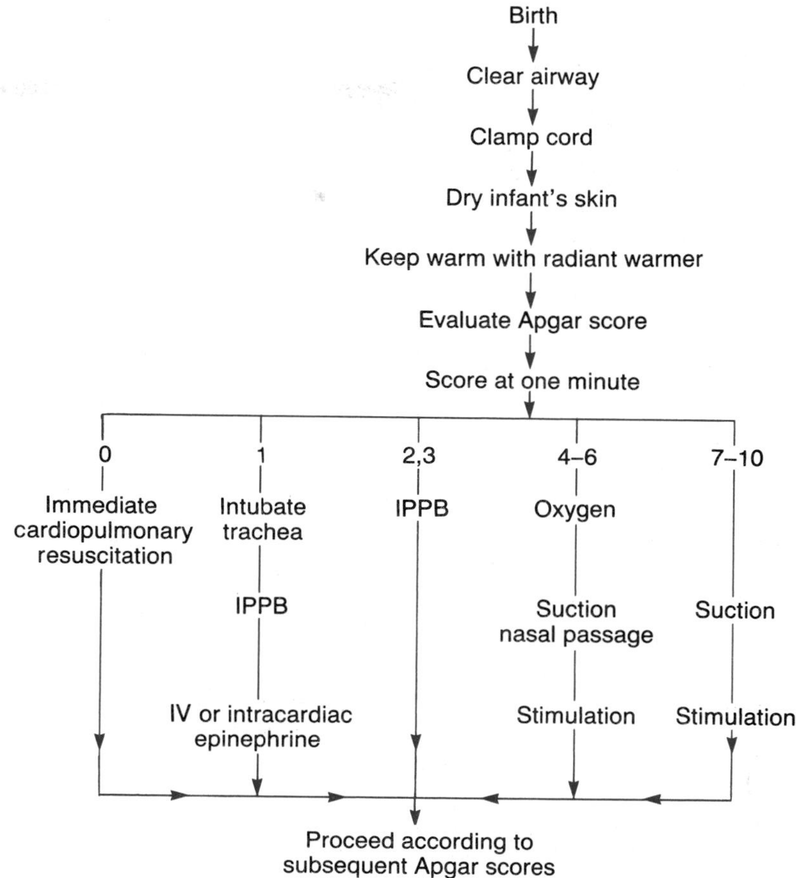

Figure 25-3.
Schematic approach for resuscitation based on the one-minute Apgar score result.

alternate hot and cold tubbing of the infant, and dilatation of the anal sphincter. These obsolete procedures are shocking to the infant.

Preventing Hypothermia

A sterile receiving blanket is made available so that the infant may be wrapped securely to prevent heat loss. It must be remembered that any room, and particularly the delivery room, is much cooler than the mother's body, and if not properly cared for the infant can become dangerously chilled. Korones and others stress the importance of providing environmental warmth to minimize loss of the infant's body heat.[7] At birth, a major cause of heat loss is the evaporation of amniotic fluid from the infant's skin. Thus, the infant is to be dried rapidly by the nurse who takes the infant from the physician as soon as the infant's airway is satisfactorily cleared.

The baby can be placed in a slight Trendelenburg position (15°) or in a supine position for the immediate appraisal. There are various devices for preventing hypothermia in the infant including a warmed incubator, resuscitators that can be warmed, and overhead radiant lights. *The basic principle behind the use of this equipment is the same—to maintain the infant's body temperature which is related to the amount of oxygen needed by the infant, the control of apnea, and finally an acid-base balance.*

Assessment of the Newborn Infant

It cannot be stressed enough that the infant's condition be assessed accurately immediately after birth and that close observations be continued by the nurse. The information that is gathered concerning the baby's responses provides valuable baseline data for subsequent care in the nursery.

The Apgar Scoring System

The Apgar score provides a valuable index for assessing the newborn infant's condition at birth. Every nurse who is responsible for the care of newborn infants, not merely those in the delivery room, should be familiar with the principles set forth by Apgar for infant assessment because they provide a simple, accurate, and safe means of quickly appraising the infant's condition.

The Apgar scoring system is based on the following five signs (ranked in order of importance) each of which is evaluated at one minute of life and repeated again in five minutes. Each sign is evaluated according to the degree to which it is present and is given a score of 0, 1, or 2 (Table 25-1). The scores of each of the signs then are added to give a total score (10 is maximum).

Heart Rate

This sign is the most important and the last to be absent when the infant's condition is grave. It may be evaluated by palpating the pulsation of the cord or by observing the pulsation where the cord joins the abdomen. Listening to the heartbeat with a stethoscope is the most accurate method of ascertaining the beat. The beat may range from 150 beats per minute to 180 beats per minute during the first few minutes of life; later, within the hour, it usually slows to between 130 beats per minute and 140 beats per minute. Crying or increased activity will increase the number of beats. If the rate is 100 per minute or under, asphyxia is present, and resuscitation is indicated.

Respiratory Effort

A baby who is responding well cries vigorously and has no difficulty in breathing. "Regular" respiration usually is established in a minute or so. Depressed, irregular respiration or apnea indicates that respiratory difficulty is present, and these signs should be reported immediately so that prompt treatment may be instituted.

Table 25-1.
The Apgar Scoring Chart

Sign	0	1	2
Heart rate	Absent	Slow (less than 100)	Over 100
Respiratory effort	Absent	Slow, irregular	Good, crying
Muscle tone	Flaccid	Some flexion of extremities	Active motion
Reflex irritability	No response	Weak cry or grimace	Vigorous cry
Color	Blue, pale	Body pink, extremities blue	Completely pink

Muscle Tone

An infant who has excellent tonus will keep his extremities flexed and resist efforts to extend them. A baby who does not keep his extremities flexed consistently usually has only moderate tonus; one who is flaccid is in extremely poor condition.

Reflex Irritability

Although there are several ways to test this sign, the one most frequently used is a gentle slap on the sole of the infant's foot. This sign can be observed when a vigorous infant is suctioned for mucus by the way in which it resists the catheter. A baby who is in excellent condition will respond with a vigorous cry. An infant is judged to have a poor response if it cries weakly or merely makes a grimace. If there is a good deal of central nervous system depression, the infant does not respond at all.

Color

Cyanosis is seen in all infants at the moment of birth. As the infant's circulation makes the change from fetal to extrauterine existence and breathing begins, the body of a healthy infant usually becomes pink within three minutes. Since acrocyanosis usually is present for a short while, even in infants who are in excellent condition, those who have scored 2 for each of the other signs may receive only a score of 1 for this part of the evaluation. This, of course, influences the total score.

Interpretation

An Apgar score of 7 to 10 indicates that the infant's condition is good. If the infant breathes and cries (or coughs) seconds after delivery, there are usually no special procedures necessary other than those of routine close observation, maintaining a clear airway, and supplying warmth as necessary.

A score of 4 to 6 means that the baby is in fair condition. There may be moderate central nervous system depression, some muscle flaccidity, and cyanosis; respiration is not readily established. *These infants must have the air passage cleared and be given oxygen promptly.* Administration of oxygen can best be done by mask, and the flow should not exceed 4 liters. Gentle patting and rubbing with the receiving blanket to dry the infant's body usually acts as an additional stimulus.

A score of 0 to 3 denotes an extremely poor condition. Resuscitation is needed immediately (see Chap. 41).

During the interval following the five-minute Apgar score, the nurse continues to evaluate the infant according to the following:

1. Auscultation of the chest ascertains proper position of the heart and normal air exchange.
2. The head and body surfaces are scrutinized for trauma and for obvious congenital anomalies. These can include caput succedaneum, cephalhematoma, or forceps marks.
3. The anterior fontanel is checked for bulging or sunkenness, and the head circumference is checked for enlargement or smallness.
4. The skin is also checked for scaling or undue wrinkling, which is indicative of the maturity of the infant. Any jaundice is also noted.
5. The abdomen is palpated for masses and for enlargement of the liver, spleen, or kidneys.
6. The genitalia are examined for normal sexuality and the anus for patency.
7. Each of the shoulders is moved while a finger is placed over the clavicle. A crunching sensation (crepitus) indicates a fracture.
8. Before the final clamp is applied to the cord, the physician or nurse examines it closely to see if it contains the normal number of vessels (two arteries and one vein). The presence of only one artery suggests one or more major congenital malformations. The cut edges of the arteries are seen as two white papular structures, which usually stand out slightly from the surface. The vein is larger, often gaping so that the lumen and thin wall are easily seen.

The student is referred to Chapter 32 for details of the physical assessment and the nurse's responsibilities.

One further note of caution is appropriate at this time. Als and Brazelton have made the point that infants whose mothers have been heavily premedicated may respond at delivery with excellent function and optimal Apgar scores. However, these same infants arrive in the neonatal nursery as little as 30 minutes later in a dangerously depressed state of unresponsiveness. Their color, respirations, and muscle tone, as well as their ability to respond to life-threatening mucus in the airway is so depressed that they need constant nursing care for this transient period of depressed function.[7] This fact has special relevance if the baby is to spend some time with the parents before being transferred to the nursery. The nurse should be especially watchful whenever the mother has had a good deal of medication throughout labor or just before delivery.

The Guide for Perinatal Assessment of the Newborn provides a comprehensive assessment form for determining possible perinatal risk factors in the newborn. Although this may appear lengthy, necessary physiological and behavioral data are obtained. The assessment can begin immediately after birth and can be continued during the nursery stay.

Other Aspects of Care

Care of the Cord

In present care no dressing is applied after the cord has been clamped or ligated and cut. It is imperative that frequent inspection be done to note any signs of bleeding. The method of leaving the cord stump exposed has proved to be very satisfactory. If it is left free, it dries because water is lost and separates more quickly than when it is kept covered.

AT **Guide for Perinatal Assessment of the Newborn—Identification of Risk Factors by Neonatal Components**

	Risk
Delivery room assessment	
Apgar score (1 min)	
1–4	3
5–7	2
7–8	1
Apgar score (5 min)	
1–4	3
5–7	3
7–8	2
Temperature regulation (<97°F)	2
Resuscitation measures	
Intubation	3
Sustained O_2	3
Bagging	3
Drug administration	3
Respiratory effort	
See-saw respiration	3
Retractions	3
Chin-tug	3
Expiratory grunt	3
Flaring nares	2
Tachypnea >60	2
Noisy respiration (rales)	1
No initial spontaneous respiration	3
Maternal bonding	
No bonding	2
Inappropriate affect	2
Admission nursery assessment	
Gestational age by dates	
<37 wk	3
>42 wk	2
Gestational age by Dubowitz	
<37 wk	3
>42 wk	2
Variation of Dubowitz from dates >2 wk	2

(Continued)

AT Guide for Perinatal Assessment of the Newborn—Identification of Risk Factors by Neonatal Components (Continued)

Item	Risk
Admission nursery assessment (Continued)	
Size and gestational age	
SGA	2
LGA	2
Measurements	
Weight <5 lb (2000 g)	3
>9 lb (3500 g)	2
Length <18 in (45 cm)	3
Head circumference	
<12½ in (32 cm)	3
>14 in (36 cm)	3
Chest circumference <12 in (30 cm)	3
Head circumference < or > in (2 cm) of chest	3
Dextrostix® ≤30 mg/100 ml	3
Color	
Pale	3
Cyanotic	3
Jaundiced	3
Axillary temperature	
97°F–96°F	2
<96°F	3
Heart rate (<100 or >160)	3
Respiratory rate (<40 or >60)	3
Respiratory effort	
Flaring nares	2
Rales	2
See-saw respiration	3
Retractions	3
Chin-tug	3
Expiratory grunt	3
Cry	
Weak	2
Shrill	3
Umbilical cord	
2 vessels	3
Meconium stained	3
Newborn Physical Examination	
Skin	
Ecchymoses	2
Petechiae	2
Plethoric	2
Pustules	3
Edematous	2
Head	
Circumference <32 cm or >36 cm	3
Enlarged fontanels	2
Bulging fontanels	3
Sunken fontanels	2
Facial asymetry	1
Excessive molding	1
Cephalhematoma	2
Eyes	
Dull	3
Nonreactive	3
Fixed	3
Nose patency (obstruction)	2
Mouth	
Cleft lip or cleft palate	2
Frenulum linguae	1
Chest	
Circumference <12 in (30 cm)	3
Heart rate <100 or >160	3
Heart murmur	3
Respiratory rate <40 or >60	3
Breath sounds (rales)	2
Retractions	3
Abdomen	
Poor muscle tone	2
Distention	3
Enlarged liver	3
Enlarged kidney	3
Enlarged spleen	3
Inguinal hernia	2
Umbilical hernia	1
Omphalocele	3
Urogenital	
Undescended testes	1
Hydrocele	1
Hypospadias	2
Enlarged clitoris	1
Ectopic bladder	3
No voiding	3
Spine	
Curvature	2
Sacral dimple	1
Spina bifida	3
Extremities	
Paralysis	3
Deviation in position and ROM	2
Extra gluteal creases	2
Hip click	2
Club feet	2
Polydactyly	1
Gross malformation	2
Fractured clavicle	1
Reflexes	
Absence of any of the normal reflexes (Moro, sucking, rooting, swallowing, tonic neck, gag, grasp, walking, Babinski)	3
Nursery Activity Patterns (First 24 hours)	
Sleeping pattern	
>20 hr–22 hr	2
No quiet alert states	3
Constantly fussy	3
Flaccid	3
Feeding pattern	
Inability to suck, swallow, or retain	3
Poor intake	2
Voiding pattern (no voiding)	3
Bowel elimination (no stooling)	3
Weight loss 1st day (>4 oz)	2
Temperature regulation	
Axillary temperature <97°F	2
Warming unit necessary to maintain body temperature	2
Color	
Pale	2
Cyanotic	3
Jaundiced	3
Heart rate	
<100 or >160	3
Murmur present	3
Respirations	
Rate <40 or >60	3
Breath sounds (rales)	2
Retractions	3
Flaring nares	2
See-saw respiration	3
Chin-tug	3
Expiratory grunt	3
Parental bonding	
Calling baby "it"	2
Refusal to touch	3
No desire to see	3
No interest in caring for	3
No eye-to-eye contact	3
Disappointment in sex of baby	2
Anxiety about breast-feeding	1

(Risk significance: 3 = High risk, 2 = Moderate risk, 1 = Slight risk)
(Brodish M: Perinatal assessment, 42–46 JOGN Nurse, 1981)

Care of the Eyes

As soon as the cord is cared for and the infant's respiration is well established, the eyes receive prophylactic treatment for protection against ophthalmia neonatorum (see Chap. 43). This treatment is so important that at the present time the use of some antibacterial agent is mandatory by statute in all states.

Penicillin and silver nitrate are the usual agents employed, although tetracycline (1%) is preferred by some physicians. When silver nitrate is used, it is supplied in wax ampuls containing a 1 percent solution especially prepared for eye instillation (Fig. 25-4).

Instilling drops in the infant's eyes is more easily accomplished if the infant's eyes are shaded from the light while the drops are put first in one eye, allowing time for the baby to recover from the shock and the discomfort before the drops are put in the other eye. One of the best methods is to draw down the lower lid gently and carefully instill two drops of the solution in the conjunctival sac, using great care not to drop it on the cornea. After two minutes, when it will have diffused itself over the entire conjunctiva, the lids should again be held apart and the conjunctival sac of each eye flushed gently with sterile distilled water (Fig. 25-5). Prompt irrigation of the eyes following instillation of silver nitrate drops is said to reduce the incidence of chemical conjunctivitis without affecting prophylaxis, although there remains disagreement on the efficacy of this. Special precautions should be taken to avoid contaminating the eyes or dropping any silver solution upon the face. Silver nitrate prophylaxis may cause signs of irritation, such as redness, edema, or discharge, however, these manifestations are transient and in no way cause permanent damage if the silver nitrate solution used is in correct concentration. Pritchard and McDonald state that silver nitrate instillation should be replaced with tetracycline.[1]

Recently there has been some discussion concerning the timing of the silver nitrate instillation. Research has indicated that the instillation tends to blur the infant's vision temporarily and would thus interfere with the focusing and eye-to-eye contact deemed necessary for maternal–infant bonding in the first hours of life. Klaus and his coworkers have delayed the instillation for one to two hours after birth until the infant has had time to interact with the parents. They report that there has been no increase in infection as a result of this delay.[8,9]

If penicillin is to be used, it can be obtained in ophthalmic drops or ointment. The technique for instillation is similar to that for silver nitrate, except that there is no flushing with water. Penicillin is also given intramuscularly for both prophylaxis and treatment of ophthalmia neonatorum. When gonorrheal ophthalmia does develop, it can be cured by penicillin within a few hours, whereas silver nitrate has long since been abandoned for treatment of this disorder. The incidence of chemical irritation with penicillin ointment or intramuscular injection is much less than with silver nitrate, and the irritation is generally milder. However, some sensitivity reactions have been reported; thus silver nitrate continues to be used.

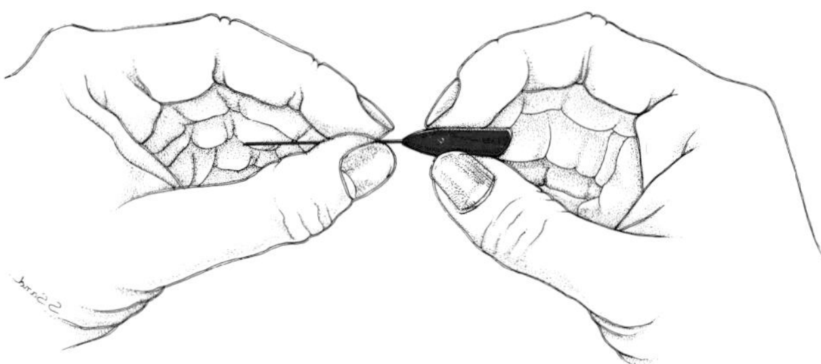

Figure 25-4.
Needle puncture of wax ampule that contains silver nitrate 1% solution for the care of the newborn's eyes.

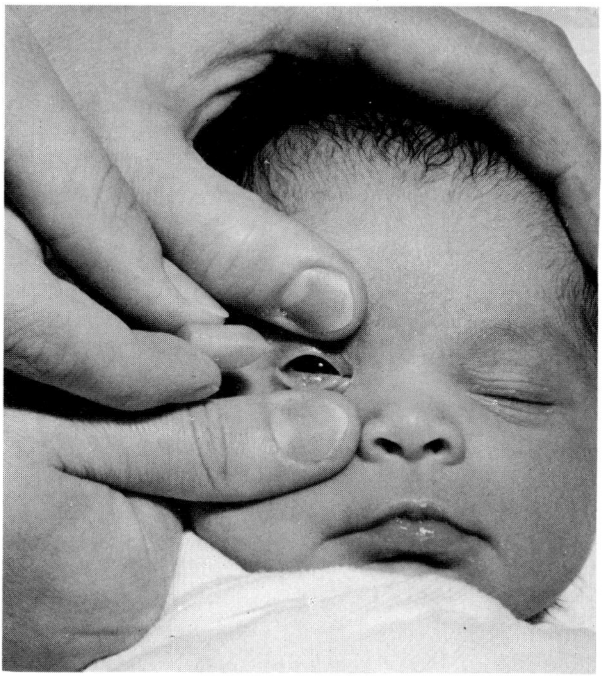

Figure 25-5.
Silver nitrate prophylaxis. Instillation of two drops of silver nitrate 1% solution from a wax ampule into the conjunctival sac of each eye.

Hypoprothrombinemia Prophylaxis

Many physicians prescribe a single dose (1 mg, 0.5 ml) of phytonadione solution (AquaMEPHYTON) 1.0 mg (0.5 ml) to be administered intramuscularly during the course of the immediate care of the newborn after delivery. This water-soluble form of vitamin K_1 acts as a preventative measure against neonatal hemorrhagic disease. Amounts of the medication in excess of 1 mg may predispose to the development of hyperbilirubinemia and are to be avoided.

Identification Methods

Some method of identification of the newborn is applied before the cord is cut or before the baby is removed from the delivery room. Most hospitals use pliable plastic tapes which are applied to the infant's wrist and ankle. These contain the mother's name, physician's name, date, time of birth, and sex of the infant, and often the mother's hospital number. The baby's identification is checked against the mother's each time the baby is brought to her.

In addition, palmprints or footprints may be taken. This method of identification consists of a stainless procedure made on chemically treated, sensitized paper. It is designed to take the palmprints or footprints of the baby and the thumbprint of the mother at the time of delivery and may be repeated at the time of discharge from the hospital. It is a simple, quick, and permanent method.

Current practice emphasizes that the newborn should be discharged without removing the identification band. Several states now have laws making it mandatory not to remove the identification bands on hospital premises. The mother should be taught how to remove the band as part of the discharge instructions.

As already discussed in Chapter 2, the registration of the infant's birth is a legal responsibility. It is mandatory that a birth certificate be filled out on every birth and submitted promptly to the local registrar.

After the Delivery

If the mother is awake after delivery, she may be anxious to have her baby brought near so that she may see it at close range. If she is drowsy, it may be better to wait until she is more alert. The nurse is governed by each mother's response at this time.

If the infant is well wrapped and warm, it may be kept in a crib at the mother's side until placed in her arms or leaves the delivery room. The infant should be kept in a slight Trendelenburg position (at an angle of 15°) to promote drainage of mucus, and on his side to avoid aspiration of this mucus.

Care should be taken to avoid placing the infant in an exaggerated Trendelenburg position (almost directly downward) because the relatively large amount of abdominal contents will press against the diaphragm and the partially expanded lungs and may impede the infant's respiratory efforts.

The nurse observes the infant at frequent intervals to make sure that he is breathing properly, that the mouth and the nose are free from mucus, and that there is no bleeding from the cord. Because this period may be a critical one for the infant, many hospitals have facilities, such as a receiving nursery on the labor and delivery division, where the infant is transferred at this time. It is felt that this provides closer supervision for the infant and permits the nurse in the delivery room to devote her undivided attention to the mother. However, more institutions are letting the infant remain in the bed with the mother and are finding that the infant fares just as well, and there is more opportunity for bonding. (See Nursing Care: Immediate Care of the Newborn.)

Baptism of Infant

If there is any probability that the infant is in imminent danger and may not live, the question of baptism should be considered if the family is Roman Catholic; this also applies to some of the other denominations of the Christian church. This is an essential duty and means a great deal to the families concerned, and thoughtfulness in this matter will never be forgotten by them. (It is to be understood that such baptism would be reported to the family.)

The following simple instructions, issued by a member of the clergy, may be followed:

> The Catholic Church teaches that in case of emergency, anyone may and should baptize. It is important to make the intention of doing what the Church wishes to do and then to pour the water on the child (preferably the head) saying at the same time, "I baptize thee in the name of the Father and of the Son and of the Holy Ghost." The water may be warmed if necessary but it must be pure water and care should be taken to make it flow. If there is any doubt whether the child is alive or dead, it should be baptized, but conditionally (*i.e.,* "If thou art alive, I baptize thee . . .").

In the Book of Common Prayer of the protestant Episcopal church, it is stated, "In cases of extreme sickness, or any imminent peril, if a Minister cannot be procured, then any baptized person present may administer holy Baptism, using the foregoing form" (*i.e.,* the form given above).

NC Nursing Care: Immediate Care of the Newborn*

Assessment	Intervention	Evaluation
Determine general status	Apgar score at 1 min and 5 min Provide for warmth with radiant heat, blanket Monitor airway and breathing Eye prophylaxis Weigh and measure height and head circumference Examine body systems by thorough observation, inspection, palpation, and auscultation Record, report as appropriate	Infant adapts to extrauterine life with minimal trauma Respirations stable, color and muscle tone good No abnormalities or anomalies
Assess family interaction	Allow father or support person to be with mother Allow couple to hold and explore infant as soon as possible Point out features of infant; explain any deviations that are normal (*eg.*, caput, molding, milia) Identify the phase of maternal behavior the client is in (*eg.*, taking-in, taking-hold, letting-go) Observe for any inappropriate behaviors; identify causes (*eg.*, won't touch baby; cold, hateful remarks, no eye contact)	Appropriate family interaction evident
Postdelivery observation	Fourth stage	Mother's condition and infant's condition stable

*Care plan revised by Cheryl Hayes R.N., M.N.

References

1. Pritchard JA, McDonald PC: Williams Obstetrics, pp 473–486. New York, Appleton–Century–Crofts, 1980
2. Dawes GS: Breathing before birth in animals or man. New Engl J Med 290:557–67, 1974
3. Duenhoelter JH, Pritchard SA: Human fetal respiration. Obstet Gynecol 42:746–55, 1973
4. Duenhoelter JH, Pritchard SA: Fetal respiration: Quantitative measurements of amniotic fluid inspired near term by human and rhesus fetuses. Am J Obstet Gynecol 125:306–320, 1976
5. Babson S, Pernoll ML, Benda C: Diagnosis and Management of the Fetus & Neonate at Risk, 4th ed. St Louis, CV Mosby, 1980
6. Korones SB: High Risk Newborn Infants: The Basis for Intensive Nursing Care, 3rd ed. St Louis, CV Mosby, 1981
7. Als H, Brazelton TB: Comprehensive neonatal assessment. Birth and the Family Journal 2:3–9, Winter 1974–1975
8. Lum Sister B, Lartz R, Barnett E: Reappraising newborn eye care. Am J Nurs 80, 9:1602–1603, September 1980
9. Klaus MH: The biology of parent-to-infant attachment. Paper and discussion presented at the meeting: Technological Approaches to Obstetrics: Benefits, Risks, Alternatives. San Francisco, February 3–4, 1979

Suggested Reading

Auld PA: Resuscitation of the newborn infant. Am J Nurs 74:68–70, January 1974

Brodish MS: Perinatal assessment. JOGN Nurs 10, 1:42–46, January/February 1981

Korones SB: High Risk Newborn Infants: The Basis for Intensive Nursing Care, 3rd ed. St Louis, CV Mosby, 1981

Lum Sister B, Lartz R, Barnett E: Reappraising newborn eye care. AJN 80, 9:1602–1603, September 1980

Taylor PM, Hall BL: Parent–infant bonding: Problems and opportunities in a perinatal center. Seminars in Perinatology 3, 1:73–84, January 1979

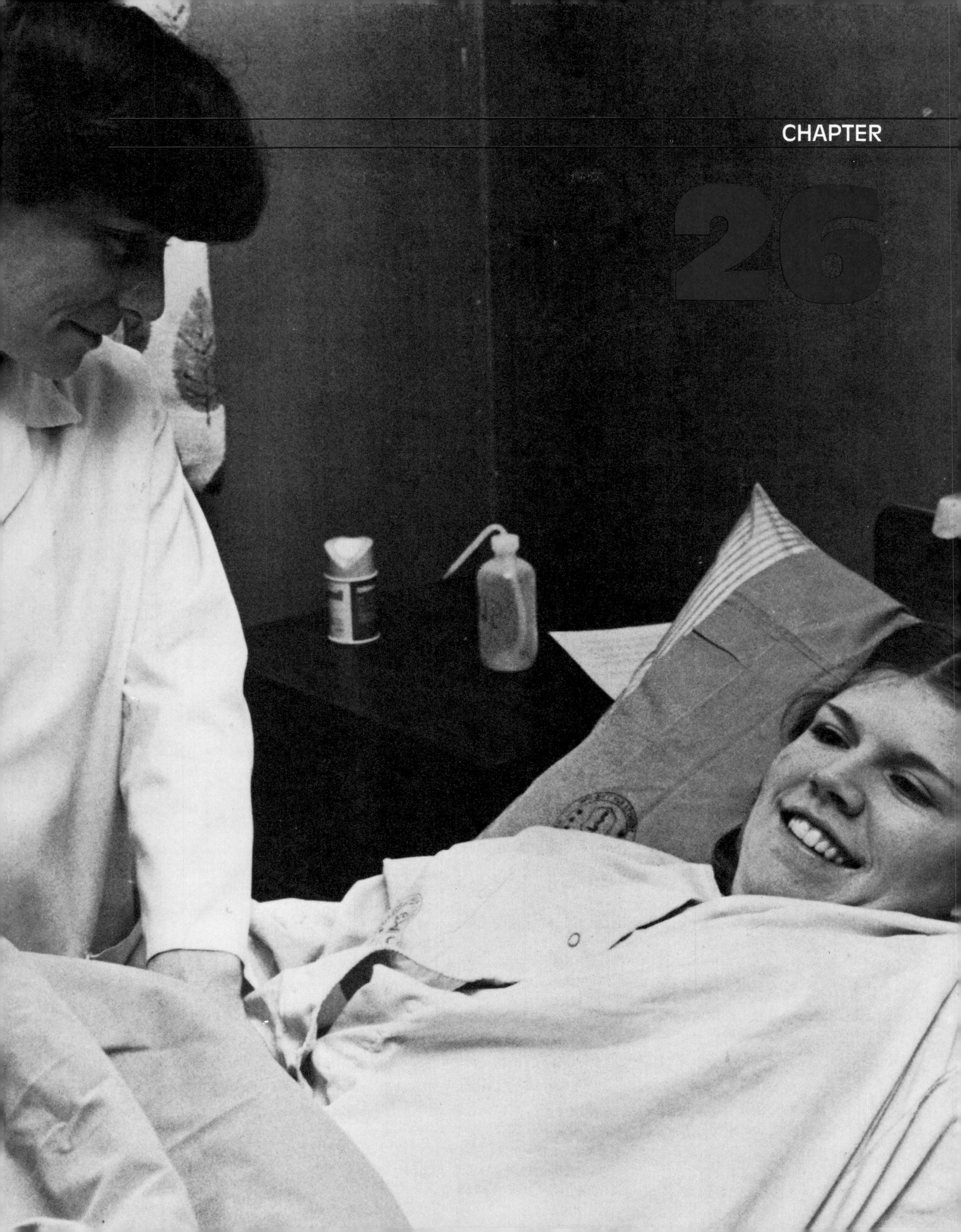

CHAPTER

26

CHAPTER 26

The Nurse's Contribution to Pain Relief During Labor

■ ■ ■

Nature of the Pain Experience During Labor

Beliefs About Pain During Labor

Is childbirth painful or painless? Most laypeople expect pain to occur during childbirth. This expectation may evolve from a variety of sources, such as television, movies, books, comments from one's own parents, and reports from friends who have had babies. However, information about childbirth in general may be incomplete, if not inaccurate. Hence, fear of pain may be anticipated by expectant parents as a result of their overall lack of knowledge about labor.

The fear of pain is second only to the fear of death. Understandably, then, some expectant parents are eager to examine and accept any information suggesting that childbirth need not be associated with pain. Such information may be forthcoming from several sources.

Reports of how childbirth is handled in some other cultures, especially the more primitive ones, often emphasize the lack of any expression of pain. In other words, there is a lack of the overt behavioral responses usually associated with pain, such as crying and moaning, inactivity or fatigue following pain, or requests for pain relief. Some women are noted to have their babies in the fields and resume work immediately following delivery. Other women are observed to remain quiet with relaxed facial expressions during childbirth.

From this information some people erroneously conclude that these women experience no pain and, therefore, the pain results *only* from anxiety or cultural expectations. However, *lack of expression of pain does not necessarily mean that pain is absent.* Indeed, a study of Samoan women revealed that while their expressions of pain were minimal during labor, they admitted afterward in interviews that they did experience pain or discomfort.[1]

Some methods of prepared childbirth may also suggest that labor is painless. One paperback book about a method of childbirth uses the phrase "painless childbirth" in the title.[2] Currently most methods of prepared childbirth do not purport to be painless, but they seem inadvertently to insinuate lack of pain in their films on childbirth and in the written narratives of couples who use the organization's particular method of childbirth. These films and reports focus on the techniques of a particular method and on the "peak experience" or ecstasy of giving birth while fully conscious. Expressions of pain are notably absent, often giving expectant parents the impression that childbirth is painless.

In answer to the question of whether childbirth is painful or painless, one must simply conclude that there are a number of very different responses to the event of childbirth. While some responses entail minimal expression of pain, this does not mean that pain is absent. Certainly there are reports of painless labors, but these are infrequent. Untreated labors that are painless or minimally uncomfortable are certainly no higher than 14%.[3] In one study of both multiparae and primiparae, the women were asked how painful childbirth was in comparison to other pain they had experienced. Ninety-seven percent said it was the most painful experience they had ever had.[4] In another study of both multiparae and primiparae using the McGill Pain Questionnaire, the intensity of labor pain showed a wide variation but was found to rank among the most intense of pains. Further, pain intensity was significantly higher for primiparae than multiparae.[5] In a study of primiparae only, 35% rated their pain as intolerable; 37% rated it as severe; and 28% rated it as moderate. Various studies of both primiparae and multiparae reveal that between 35% and 58% of the women report pain that is intolerable or severe.[6]

Importance of Pain Control During Labor

The relief of pain and suffering is traditionally a humane and moral act. However, pain relief is often given a low priority by health team members, especially in regard to childbirth. It has been pointed out that during childbirth the two primary tasks of the mother and the staff are "to deliver a 'good' baby and to conclude that process with an unimpaired mother . . . each takes precedence over the relief of pain."[7] However, an analysis of the situation reveals that pain relief results in certain emotional and physiological benefits that contribute to the health of the mother and baby (see Table 26-1). Information about nonpharmacological pain relief measures is now more readily available to parents and health professionals. Thus, pain relief can be a priority without harming the mother or child. In fact, pain relief may contribute to their physical and emotional well-being.

Emotional Advantages

Control or relief of pain potentially allows the significant step toward becoming parents to be a positive experience for the mother and father. Ultimately one

Table 26-1.
Importance of Pain Control in Labor and Delivery

Emotional Advantages	Physiological Advantages
Positive experience with a significant step toward parenthood	Mother can cooperate with examinations
Feeling of actual participation in birth of own child	Mother can work with contractions
Fostering growth of relationship between parent and child	Mother is less fatigued after labor and delivery
Fostering growth of relationship between parents	Successful use of nonpharmacological pain relief reduces risk to infant

or both parents may be able to witness that moment which remains miraculous and awesome even to many obstetricians—the emergence of a new human being into the world. Even when the parents do not observe the delivery, there are other desirable outcomes. If the mother and father can handle the discomforts during childbirth, they can feel they are active participants in the actual birth of their own child. When people jointly plan for an event such as childbirth and are then able to carry through with these plans, the event will probably foster growth in the relationship between them. In the case of childbirth, a satisfying labor experience for both parents probably also fosters their relationship with their baby (Fig. 26-1).

At least a childbirth experience in which pain is adequately controlled does not impede these relationships. Pain has the potential for eliciting anger and aggression, often referred to as the fight or flight response. Such feelings resulting from a miserably painful childbirth experience sometimes are projected onto the infant or the father. The mother temporarily may express hatred toward the infant or father, and she may withdraw from these relationships for a while. During and following very painful labors mothers have been quoted as saying they despise their partners. Fathers have been known to say they felt angry toward the baby because its birth caused the mother pain. One mother even commented that her labor was so painful it took her a year to forgive her child and establish a warm relationship with him.

It does not seem likely, however, that pain and suffering during labor could be the sole reason for permanent or prolonged impairment of mother–father–child relationships. Labor may be a convenient scapegoat. Other more significant factors operating over a long period of time have probably affected the relationships.

Physiological Advantages

The adequate relief of pain also results in physiological benefits. The mother who experiences tolerable discomforts in labor is able to cooperate with examinations and to work with her contractions. Consequently, she facilitates efforts of the health team members to obtain information and she avoids prolongation of labor. After childbirth she is less fatigued.

If she is able to use pain relief measures other than medication, she may eliminate the need for medication or reduce the amount necessary. This is of enormous physiological benefit to the infant because many analgesics and anesthetics, including regional anesthesia, have untoward effects on the fetus, such as respiratory depression and bradycardia. There simply is no drug that has been proven entirely safe for the unborn child.

Definitions

Pain

Pain defies definition. It is always a personal and subjective experience, differing from one person to another and varying within the same person from one time to the next. Quite simply, pain is a localized sensation of hurt. But, for both the nurse and patient who work together to relieve pain, it seems more productive for the nurse to adopt the patient's definition of pain.

The nursing definition of pain may then be stated as whatever the experiencing person says it is, existing whenever he or she says it does.[8] A crucial aspect of this definition is that the nurse believes what the patient tells her. And, of course, the patient may com-

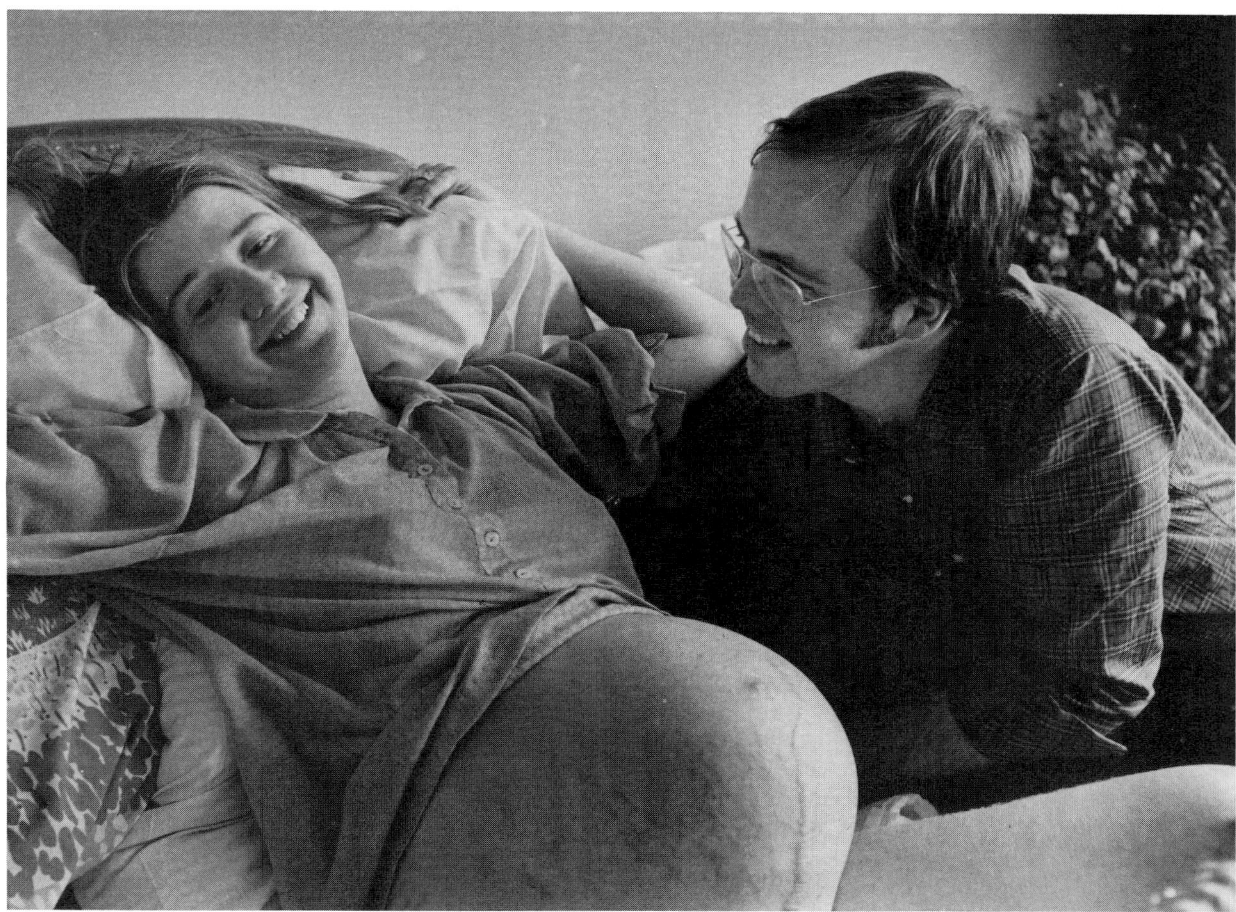

Figure 26-1.
This mother and father work together throughout labor and delivery in an alternative birthing center. Such experiences can foster a closer relationship between the parents and contribute significantly to successful parental–infant attachment.

municate the pain experience in any number of ways besides verbalization. For example, in some patients a marked increase in rate and depth of respirations may alert the nurse to the intensification of discomfort.

Pain Experience

The phrase "pain experience" encompasses all the patient's sensations, feelings, and behavioral responses, including physiological activities such as blood pressure changes. The pain experience may also refer to any or all of the three phases of pain—anticipation, presence, aftermath. And it may include not only the patient's actions, but also the impact that others have upon the patient during the pain experience.

Pain Expressions

People respond to pain in many ways. The manner in which an individual responds to pain is dependent upon numerous and varied factors such as the culture in which the person lives, the personal meaning of the pain, and the intensity of the pain. Hence, pain expressions may be absent or minimal or not easily observed. For example, a slight and momentary frown may be the only sign that the patient is experiencing pain. Or the patient may be more expressive and engage in prolonged moaning.

Expressions of pain are usually observed in one or more of the following categories of behavioral response: physiological, verbal, vocal, facial, body movement, physical contact with others, and general response to the environment.[8]

Definitions

Pain—a localized sensation of hurt; whatever the experiencing person says it is, existing whenever he or she says it does

Pain experience—all aspects surrounding the sensation of pain, before, during, and after it is felt, including the patient's responses and external events of which the patient is aware

Pain expressions—the patient's observable responses to pain, both behavioral and physiological

Pain intensity—the severity of the pain sensation

Pain tolerance—the intensity or duration of pain the patient is willing to endure without making further efforts to relieve it

Suffering—the agonizing or bothersome component of pain

Pain Intensity

The intensity of pain refers to the severity of the sensation itself. To determine this the patient may be asked to rate the intensity of pain on a numerical scale such as zero to ten, with zero being no pain at all and ten being the worst possible pain. An alternative is a series of words for rating pain intensity such as none, mild, moderate, severe, and very severe.

When a patient does not exhibit many expressions of pain, it is very helpful to ask the patient to use a rating scale to convey the intensity of pain since it cannot be easily observed. If this is explained early in labor, the patient may be able to use the scale throughout labor and delivery whenever she is requested to do so.

Pain Tolerance

It is very important to differentiate between the presence and intensity of a pain sensation, as indicated by expressions of pain, and the patient's tolerance for that pain. Pain tolerance may be defined as the amount of pain that the patient is willing to endure without pain relief.

Pain tolerance differs markedly from one person to another. Some patients state that the pain sensation is severe, yet they are willing to tolerate the pain and do not request pain relief. Other patients request pain relief measures when they rate the pain as mild. The latter group may be said to have a low tolerance for pain. While a high pain tolerance is valued by many people, the nurse should realize that a patient's tolerance for pain is not a matter of good or bad, or right or wrong. Indeed, none of the patient's responses to pain are to be judged in this way.

During childbirth, the mother is expected to endure or tolerate a certain amount of pain to ensure her own and her baby's good health.[7] However, some mothers have a low pain tolerance, and it is especially important for the nurse to help these mothers find a way to cope with their discomfort. Admonishing the mother to cope with the discomfort or leaving the room when she complains certainly is not helpful. Other techniques can be called upon in such instances. The nonpharmacological measures discussed in this chapter are especially appropriate for the mother with a low pain tolerance.

Suffering

Suffering is an affective state that may accompany pain. Copp, a nurse-researcher in the field of pain, pointedly uses the term suffering in reference to pain and defines it as "the state of anguish of one who bears pain, injury, or loss."[9] When pain cannot be eliminated, it is imperative that the patient receive whatever assistance is necessary to prevent or diminish feelings of suffering. While a painful experience is at best only unpleasant, in most cases it need not be unrelenting agony.

Pain Mechanisms

Gate Control Theory

The mystery and complexity of pain are especially well demonstrated by the fact that no one really knows what neurophysiological mechanism underlies the sensation of pain. Through the ages a number of theories have been advanced, and among the more recent of these is the *gate control theory.* It was first proposed in 1965 by Melzack and Wall, and has since been debated and expanded.[10–13] Like all theories, it is not absolute truth. Rather, it uses available information to explain the phenomenon of pain, suggesting reasons for known facts and offering possibilities where facts are absent.

There are numerous facets to the theory and many ways to categorize them. The following discussion focuses only on those aspects which seem most pertinent to a basic understanding of the mechanisms of pain and its relief in childbirth.

As its name implies, the gate control theory proposes that there is a gating mechanism involved in the transmission of pain impulses. A closed gate results in no pain; an open gate results in pain; and a partially open gate results in less pain. This gating mechanism is probably located in various places throughout the central nervous system. When the gate is closed, the transmission of pain impulses is stopped and pain does not reach the level of awareness.

The transmission of pain impulses to the level of cortical awareness can be affected in the following three ways:

1. *The activity in large and small sensory nerve fibers.* The gate is opened by excitation of small-diameter fibers that carry pain impulses. However, these pain signals can be blocked (*i.e.,* the gate can be closed to prevent or decrease their transmission to the cortex) by stimulation of large-diameter fibers. Since many cutaneous fibers are large-diameter fibers, stimulation of the skin by rubbing or other means may result in pain relief (Fig. 26-2).

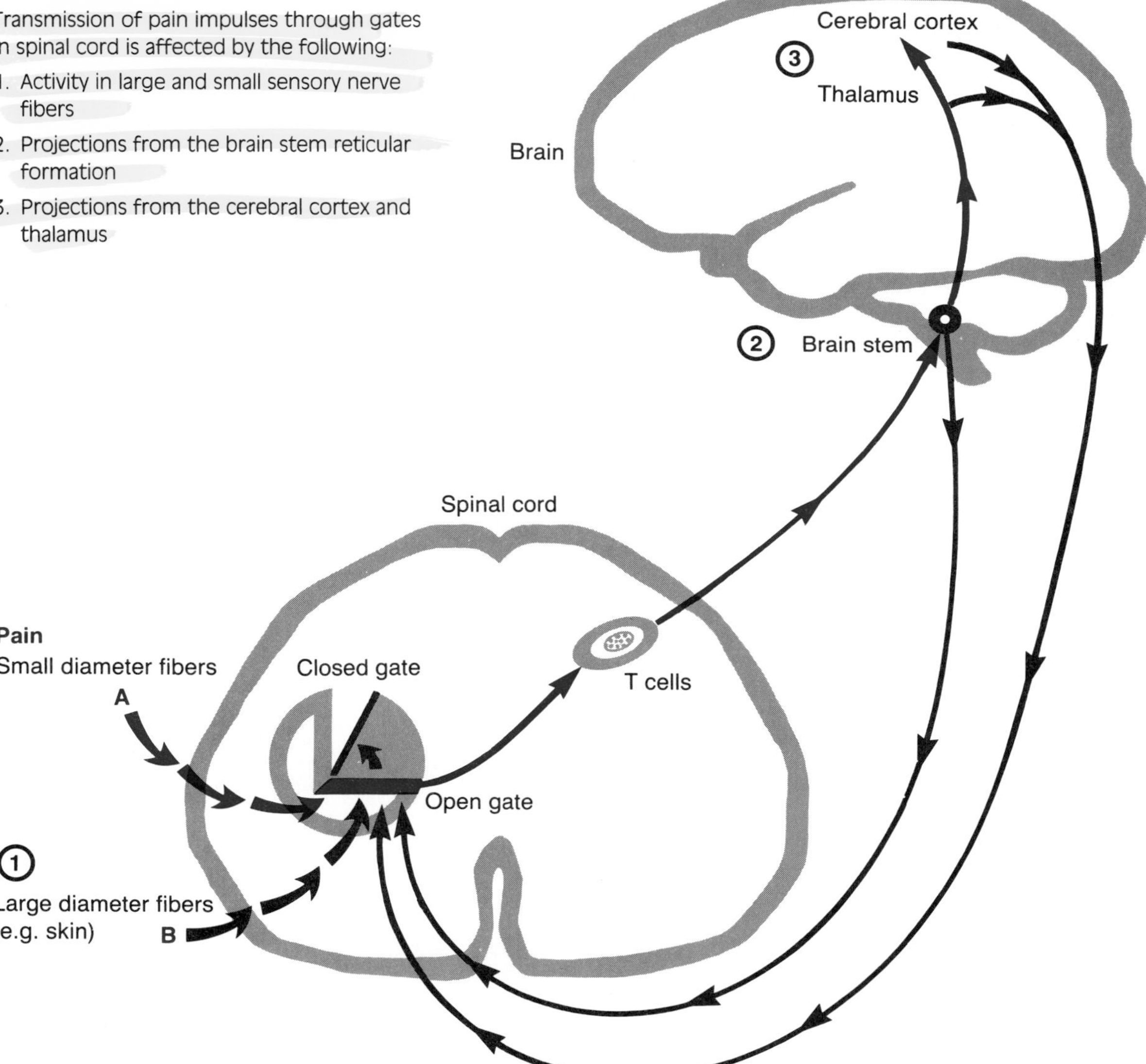

Figure 26-2.
One influence on the gating mechanism is the ratio of large/small fibers activated. *(A)* Impulses traveling on small-diameter nerve fibers cause the gate to be held open. *(B)* Impulses traveling on large-diameter fibers generate feedback to the gate, almost closing it. (Hassid P: Textbook for Childbirth Educators. New York, Harper & Row, 1978)

2. *Projections from the brain stem reticular formation.* The reticular activating system regulates or adjusts incoming and outgoing signals, including the amount of sensory input. Somatic inputs from all parts of the body, as well as visual and auditory inputs, are monitored by the reticular system. Although it is not well understood, it appears that a sufficient amount of sensory input may cause the reticular system to project inhibitory signals to the gate; that is, the reticular formation may cause the gate to be closed to the transmission of pain impulses. Hence, pain signals would not reach the level of cortical awareness (no pain), or fewer pain signals would reach the brain (less intense pain). Thus, distraction, for example, may inhibit pain impulses whereas monotony (unvarying sensory input) would increase pain.
3. *Projections from the cerebral cortex and thalamus.* Signals from the cortex or thalamus can open or close the gate to transmission of pain impulses, either indirectly by projecting through the reticular formation or directly by projecting to the gate. Cognitive and affective processes are subserved at least in part by neural activity in the cortex and thalamus. Therefore, the individual's own unique thoughts and feelings can influence the transmission of pain impulses from the gate to the level of cortical awareness. Such thoughts and feelings may include the meaning of the pain, the person's beliefs, anxieties, memories of past painful experiences, and any number of other factors. Thus, input to the gating mechanism is evaluated by the individual *before* it is felt as a sensation as well as afterward.

Perhaps the most important contribution of the gate control theory is the possible explanation it offers for the individuality of the pain experience (Table

Table 26-2.
Nursing Practice Aspects of the Gate Control Theory of Pain

Major contributions

1. An integrated conceptual model for appreciating the many factors that contribute to individual differences in the experience of pain
2. Conceptualization of categories of activity that may form a theoretical base for developing various pain relief measures

Nature of the gate

The transmission of potentially painful impulses to the level of conscious awareness may be affected by a gating mechanism, possibly located at the spinal cord level of the CNS.

Structures Involved	No Pain or Decreased Intensity of Pain	Pain
Spinal cord (?)	Results from closing the gate in one of the following ways:	Results from opening the gate in one of the following ways:
Nerve fibers	1. Activity in the *large-diameter nerve fibers* (*e.g.,* caused by skin stimulation)	1. Activity in the *small-diameter nerve fibers* (*e.g.,* caused by tissue damage)
Brain stem	2. Inhibitory impulses from the *brain stem* (*e.g.,* caused by sufficient or maximum sensory input arriving through distraction or guided imagery)	2. Facilitory impulses from the *brain stem* (*e.g.,* caused by insufficient input from a monotonous environment)
Cerebral cortex and thalamus	3. Inhibitory impulses from the *cerebral cortex and thalamus* (*e.g.,* caused by anxiety reduction based on learning when the pain will end and how to relieve it)	3. Facilitory impulses from the *cerebral cortex* and *thalamus* (*e.g.,* caused by fear that the intensity of pain will escalate and will be associated with death)

(McCaffery M: Nursing Management of the Patient with Pain, 2nd ed. JB Lippincott, Philadelphia, 1979)

26-2). One thing has been clear for many years—comparable stimuli (or lesions) in different people do not produce comparable sensations of pain. In other words, when comparable stimuli are applied to several people, one person may perceive intense pain, another moderate pain, and still another no pain at all. The gate control theory suggests mechanisms by which a myriad of factors may determine the existence of pain and influence the nature of a painful experience. In summary, these factors may include not only stimulation of pain fibers but also cutaneous stimulation, other sensory input, thoughts, and feelings.

The gate control theory also provides a basis for understanding and devising pain relief measures.

Endorphins

It has recently been discovered that opiatelike substances occur naturally within the body.[14] These substances have been called endorphins, a combination of the words endogenous and morphine. To date several have been isolated, but it is clear that many more exist. Their role in the cause and alleviation of pain has not yet been clarified. An overview of the possible ways endorphins affect pain such as that felt in labor and delivery follows.

Endorphins influence the transmission of impulses interpreted as painful. Endorphins may possibly act as either neurotransmitters or neuromodulators that inhibit the transmission of pain messages. Thus, the presence of endorphin at the synapse of nerve cells results in a decrease in the sensation of pain. Failure to release endorphin allows pain to occur.

Endorphin levels differ from one individual to another, explaining in part why some people feel more pain than others. Persons with high endorphin level obviously feel less pain. Also, it has been found, for example, that persons with low endorphin level prior to surgery require more analgesia postoperatively than persons with a higher level of endorphin. Differences in endorphin levels may be inherited and may thereby explain cultural differences in pain sensitivity.[15]

Certain situations such as stress and pregnancy cause an increase in endorphin levels. Therefore, the endorphin level varies within the individual from one situation to another. During pregnancy and birth both mother and infant may have a decreased sensitivity to pain because of increased endorphin levels.[15]

Various pain relief measures may be dependent upon the endorphin systems. For example, it is possible that certain kinds of patient teaching or stimulation of the skin, such as massage, can cause an increase in endorphin, which in turn relieves pain.[16]

Descriptions of Painful Sensations of Normal Labor

Uterine Contractions

During the first stage of normal labor, pain or discomfort may result from the involuntary contraction of the uterine muscle. The contraction tends to be felt in the lower back at the beginning of labor. As labor progresses the sensation encircles the lower torso, covering both back and abdomen.

Contractions are frequently described as wavelike—they come and go rhythmically, each one increasing to a certain height or intensity and then decreasing, and finally disappearing. Contractions last from about 45 seconds to 90 seconds. In early labor the contractions are not necessarily uncomfortable. As labor progresses the intensity of each contraction increases, resulting in a greater possibility or intensity of discomfort.

The quality of the discomfort is difficult to describe and certainly is varied. Basically there appear to be three possible qualities to any painful sensation—burning, pricking, and aching. Also, pain can be either deep or superficial. Consequently, one may say that a labor contraction is felt as deep aching.

The intervals between contractions shorten as labor proceeds. Early labor contractions are about 20 minutes apart. Then for several hours they occur 3 minutes to 5 minutes apart. During about the last hour prior to delivery the intervals between contractions may be only a few seconds long. This period, when the cervix is dilating from about 7 cm to 10 cm, is referred to as transition.

Uterine contractions are at their highest intensity and greatest frequency during transition. This is usually when the mother experiences the most discomfort and has the most difficulty handling her discomfort.

Back Labor

In addition to uterine contractions, approximately 25% of women in labor also have to cope with the discomfort of *back labor.* This occurs when the fetus is in an occipitoposterior position (see Chap. 34). With each contraction the occiput presses on the mother's sacrum, causing extreme discomfort as the intensity of contractions increases. Back labor is considerably more painful for the mother than labor in which there is an anterior occipital position.

Delivery

A common but false assumption about labor is that the most painful part is the expulsive stage. However, mothers report a decrease in pain during this stage. Apparently the mother's more noisy behavior during expulsion efforts has been interpreted by observers as indicative of more pain.[17]

Of course, the mother certainly may experience discomfort during delivery but it is generally much less intense than what she felt during transition.

The predominant sensations during delivery occur in the vaginal and perineal area and can be described as pressure, stretching or splitting, and sometimes burning. Most of the time the mother has an overwhelming desire to push. Pushing may relieve whatever discomfort is felt. Also, the pressure of the baby's head causes a degree of numbness in the perineum. If desired, the physician can take advantage of this numbness during a contraction and perform a painless episiotomy.

The foregoing is a description of the painful or uncomfortable sensations often felt during normal labor (Table 26-3). Considerably more pain may be experienced with certain complications of labor, such as hypertonic uterine dysfunction, delivery of an oversized baby, or a contracted pelvis.

Uniqueness of Pain During Childbirth

Most of the pain experienced by the general patient population is characterized by one or more of the following anxiety-producing factors. The patient may not know what causes the pain, may not have expected pain to occur, and may not know how to predict the course of the pain (*e.g.,* how long it will last, how severe it will become). Pain may cause the patient to fear some dreaded illness or a long-term change in lifestyle.

The discomfort and pain of childbirth are unique in that in most cases these common sources of anxiety need not be present. In fact, there are elements inherent in childbirth that are just the opposite of these sources of anxiety. Hence, the childbirth experience has a high potential for the achievement of satisfactory pain relief. Following is a brief discussion of those elements which render childbirth a more manageable pain experience.

Anxiety-Reducing Knowledge

Studies suggest that anxiety is reduced if the person knows when a painful event will occur and how long the discomfort will last.[18] Ordinarily the mother knows the approximate date of confinement and she has some idea of the approximate length of labor. In other words, she knows labor will occur, she knows the expected date within a few weeks, and she knows labor usually lasts a matter of hours, not days.

Even more helpful is the information the mother has once labor has actually begun. With the assistance of a watch she can determine the usual length of her contractions and predict when the next one will

Table 26-3.
Painful Sensations in Normal Labor

	Uterine Contractions	Back Labor	Delivery
Site	Initially, lower back; as labor progresses, encircles lower torso	Lower back	Vagina, perineum
Pain Intensity	Progresses throughout labor from no discomfort to mild to moderate, perhaps severe; may be severe, especially during transition	Severe	Less than during transition
Quality of Pain	"Wavelike," each one increases to a certain intensity and decreases, usually over a 45- to 90-second period	Deep pressure, aching	Pressure, stretching, splitting, sometimes burning

occur. In addition, she knows that contractions generally become more intense and more frequent as labor progresses. And although her discomfort may increase in intensity, she is not usually in constant discomfort. Between contractions there are periods of relative comfort even during the final phase of labor contractions.

The mother also knows the cause of her discomfort. At least she knows it is a normal process that has something to do with the expulsion of her baby and that parts of her body are contracting and stretching to accomplish this event. This is quite different from the knowledge possessed by the person who suddenly experiences his first myocardial infarction. Most mothers recognize the onset of labor and do not fear that something harmful or life threatening is happening.

An End Product

The discomfort of labor is also unique in that there is a tangible end product—the baby. The birth of the baby is something in which there has been deep personal involvement, both emotional and physiological. The involvement may have been positive and desirable or unpleasant and unwanted. Nevertheless, when the baby is born, the discomfort of labor subsides markedly and the event is characterized by physical and psychological closure. Few episodes of pain end so dramatically.

Assessment of Labor Pain

Prejudices that Hamper Assessment of Pain

Signs of Acute Pain

Precautions must be taken to avoid certain prejudices that may hamper the nurse's assessment of the pain experience. There is a tendency to recognize the existence of pain only in those patients who show signs of acute pain, such as perspiration, muscle tension, or moaning. The absence of these expressions of pain, as noted previously, does not necessarily mean the patient is not in pain. In fact, the patient may suffer greatly but exhibit only minimal pain expression.[8]

In childbirth there appear to be two major reasons for minimal pain expressions—(1) the mother may have learned that minimal pain expressions are the expectations of the culture, or (2) activities learned from a method of prepared childbirth may preclude expressions of pain. For example, practicing relaxation techniques may preclude muscle tension as a sign of acute pain; use of a breathing pattern or mouthing the words of a song may preclude the behavior of moaning.

It is often quite difficult, if not impossible, to rely upon signs of acute pain in assessing the laboring mother who is using one of the methods of prepared childbirth. Usually she simply is too busy to show signs of acute pain.

Physical Cause of Pain

We also tend to be prejudiced in favor of believing patients only when we know the physical cause of pain.[8] This hampers our understanding of the subjective pain experience. Hence, when the mother states, for instance, that she feels severe pain, her statement must be believed even if there seems to be no physical cause for such a painful labor. The temptation to judge the mother's discomfort by the results of electronic monitoring of intrauterine pressure must also be avoided.

Values of Mother or Father

The mother or father may also harbor prejudices or values that make it difficult for the nurse to assess the pain experience. Either or both of the parents may feel that responses to pain should be minimized. The only appropriate response may be a verbal description of the pain. Some mothers may not even volunteer this much, so they have to be questioned directly and at regular intervals. Still other mothers may want to avoid using the word pain or resist any tendency to say they feel pain. They may prefer to use other terms, which may be deceptive if taken at face value. For example, the mother may verbalize feeling "enormous pressure" but refuse to call it painful. Yet the mother may need assistance in coping with this sensation, so that measures designed to relieve severe pain may be very appropriate.

Still another type of problem may arise with a father who forcefully tries to impose his own goals upon the mother who does not share his values. In the situation where the father does not want the mother to admit pain or to seek assistance with pain relief measures, the nurse may find that she obtains more accurate information when the father is absent from the room. She may also discover that the mother asks the father to get the nurse, but the father merely stands in the hall and then reports to the mother that the nurse is not available. Of course, the opposite type of situation may exist. The mother may feel perfectly capable of handling the pain and discomforts of labor, but the father may become insistent that she be "put out of this misery."

Agreement Between Health Team Members

There is a tendency for health team members to rate the mother's pain as less intense than the mother rates her pain. This is particularly true of the first stage of labor. Health team members also tend to agree with each other about the degree of the mother's pain.[6,19] In other words, the staff observing the patient may agree with one another that the patient's pain is not as severe as the patient actually experiences it. We must guard against letting agreement among ourselves about the patient's pain cause or reinforce any doubts about the intensity of the mother's pain.

Table 26-4.
Tools for Assessing the Pain Experience During Labor

I. Contractions
  - Onset
  - Frequency
  - Duration
  - Intensity
  - Description of sensation
  - Attitude toward contractions

II. Pain Relief Methods Employed by Parents for Labor
  - Persons to assist or be present during labor
  - Positioning
  - Relaxation techniques
  - Distraction (or concentration) methods
  - Breathing patterns
  - Physical activities
  - Medication

III. Current Discomforts of Mother Other than Labor
  - Pregnancy
  - Chronic illness
  - Recent illness or injury
  - Methods of handling above; effectiveness of methods

IV. Parents' Current Concerns Other than Labor
  - Activities or plans interrupted by labor
  - Care of children at home
  - Financial arrangements
  - Condition of mother or unborn child
  - Plans for care of infant
  - Unexpected change in childbirth plans
  - Plans and needs for assistance regarding above

V. Parents' Goals and Expectations Regarding Labor
  - Presence and intensity of pain
  - Provisions for pain relief (if any)
  - Father's (coach's) presence
  - Episiotomy
  - Differences between mother and father regarding above
  - Which of the above not possible or not discussed with physician

Nursing Assessment of Pain and Pain Relief Measures

When the laboring mother is admitted to the hospital, the nurse identifies several factors important to the management of pain (Table 26-4). Since a thorough assessment is inextricably related to intervention, some pain relief measures will be mentioned in the discussion of assessment. Actually, the manner in which the nurse assesses the patient often contributes to pain relief. When the nurse conveys to the mother that she believes her and that she desires to understand the mother's experience as completely as possible, anxiety may be reduced and the pain thereby relieved.

Contractions

When labor is discussed with the mother, the sensations should be referred to as contractions, not pains. Although many laypeople continue to use the term pains, the nurse should attempt to help the parents substitute the word contractions, because the word pain tends to suggest not just discomfort but an unbearable sensation. The initial contractions are not necessarily uncomfortable, and pain is usually a misnomer. Later in labor the contractions may be uncomfortable but not unbearable. Most mothers probably are not so suggestible that they would actually feel unbearable pain during contractions simply because the nurse used the term pains rather than contractions. But the use of the term pains may generate needless anxiety about the sensations of labor.

When assessing the characteristics of uterine contractions (onset, frequency, duration, intensity, description of sensation, and attitude toward contractions) it is important to note the time when labor begins *(onset)* since prolonged labor intensifies the painful experience. Not only is a longer time spent in discomfort, but a lengthy labor often fatigues and discourages the parents, making it more difficult to cope with labor (see Part I of Table 26-4).

Regularity and increasing *frequency* of contractions along with increasing intensity of contractions indicate a normal labor. Such information can be used to assure the parents that progress is being made.

To obtain more detailed and useful information about *intensity of contraction,* the nurse may ask the mother to rate the contraction on a scale of mild, moderate, intense (strong), or very intense (very strong).

It is also helpful to encourage the mother to *describe* other characteristics of the contraction, such as where the sensation begins and where it is felt most intensely. This information often suggests the need for specific pain relief measures. For example, if the contraction begins in the lower back and is felt most intensely there, rubbing that area and applying pressure may provide considerable comfort.

At the same time that the mother is discussing her contractions she may reveal her *attitude* toward labor in general. The degree of fear or anxiety experienced is of special importance as these feelings have a profound effect upon pain. They decrease pain tolerance and increase the perceived intensity of pain. Anxiety or fear also increases muscle tension and may increase painful stimuli during labor by interfering with contractions.

Anxiety or fear during labor may be related to worry about how pain will be managed and how labor is progressing. To alleviate such anxiety, the nurse may inform the mother of the various pain relief measures that may be employed. Concern over the progression of labor, or the effectiveness of the contractions, may be partially diminished if the nurse keeps the mother informed of signs of progress such as increasing cervical dilatation or regularity of contractions. It is sometimes helpful to assure the mother that it is possible to stop or correct ineffective or dysfunctional uterine contractions.

Pain Relief Methods Employed by Parents for Labor

Whether or not the parents have any special or well-defined method of handling childbirth (*e.g.,* Lamaze method), the nurse questions them about how they have handled the discomforts of labor thus far and what their plans are for the remainder of labor. In the United States there are many methods of preparation for childbirth, based on different techniques and philosophies. Some of the techniques and pain relief methods employed in prepared childbirth may seem odd. Sometimes mothers feel foolish doing them and nurses may be surprised to observe such techniques. However, a woman should be encouraged to use whatever method works for her. Some mothers intuitively devise their own special way of handling childbirth.

It is difficult to keep abreast of the constant changes taking place within each method, but the nurse can be reassured by the fact that in any single hospital labor suite one or two basic methods are used. This is partially because physicians using one particular method of childbirth tend to congregate at the same hospital where they can share ideas and know that the nursing staff is reasonably familiar with the method. Also, certain methods tend to be popular only in certain geographical areas. Thus, the nurse is likely to be able to quickly identify which methods are most common and can then study them in greater depth.

Part II of Table 26-4 lists some common pain relief methods employed during childbirth, such as comfortable positioning, relaxation techniques, and awareness of the persons who will be in attendance during labor. They are discussed briefly below and additional examples are given under Nonpharmacological Pain Relief.

Persons Present During Labor

With regard to the *person or persons to assist or be present during labor,* the father is almost always included if the couple has attended classes on one of the methods of prepared childbirth. Sometimes the couple's children are allowed an occasional and brief visit to the labor room. When the father is absent or does not want to attend labor, or when the mother is unwed, the person in attendance may be a childbirth educator, the mother's friend, or a relative.

After identifying this person the nurse finds out if that person has been with the mother prior to hospital admission and if the mother wants that person to remain with her in the labor and delivery rooms. She also assesses the attending person's attitude and desires. It is possible, for instance, that the mother might want the father to remain with her, but the father may be quite reluctant and fearful. (For convenience, the person the mother brings to the hospital to be with her during labor henceforth will be referred to as the father.)

In addition, the nurse determines what the father has done for the mother prior to admission, what is planned for the remainder of labor, what (if any) preparation the mother and father have had, and whether they have practiced what they plan to do. Sometimes the father simply stays near the mother, touching her gently and offering verbal encouragement. In other cases the father is expected to take a very active role in the following pain relief measures, such as massaging the back or abdomen or applying counterpressure.

Positioning

A variety of *positions* may be assumed during the course of normal labor. At the beginning of labor the mother may walk around between contractions, and during a contraction she may remain standing but bend forward, leaning on her husband's arms or back for support. As labor progresses she may be more comfortable sitting or lying in bed.

When the mother is admitted to the labor room the nurse asks her which positions have been comfortable and which have not and which positions she may wish to consider later in labor. Some positions require additional pillows which the nurse can then obtain in advance.

Relaxation

Numerous techniques are used to achieve and maintain total skeletal muscle *relaxation*. A pillow may be placed between the mother's legs when she is on her side to support the limbs. For general relaxation, the mother may smile, yawn, or take deep breaths at regular intervals. The father may aid by giving tactile or verbal cues to induce relaxation.

Again, the nurse finds out what techniques are used for relaxation so she can accurately interpret the mother's behavior. Knowing that the mother intends to keep her eyes closed, for example, prevents the nurse from mistakenly concluding that this laboring mother is sleeping most of the time.

Distraction

Distraction and concentration are frequently used for coping with pain. Distraction techniques are also the most individualized and therefore the most varied of all the techniques a mother may employ during childbirth. For example, some women bring with them a personal "concentration point"—an object to be stared at during a contraction. Other examples of distraction are breathing patterns, which are discussed below (see also Distraction, pp 557–559).

Breathing Patterns

Controversy and change are characteristic of many of the *breathing patterns* employed in the various methods of prepared childbirth. The two basic types of breathing are chest breathing and abdominal or diaphragmatic breathing.

Some childbirth educators feel that abdominal breathing places more pressure on the uterus by forcing the diaphragm down and the abdomen out. However, other educators feel that abdominal breathing prevents pressure on the uterus by relaxing and lifting the abdominal wall off the uterus. They also feel that it enhances relaxation because it is the type of breathing used during sleep. Some mothers tend to find it difficult to breath abdominally as labor progresses, while others find it comfortable throughout labor.

Chest breathing with panting and rapid breathing is also a subject of controversy. Some instructors are modifying the panting or rapid superficial breathing because it is difficult to learn or because it may become fatiguing during labor and has caused hyperventilation in a few mothers during labor.[20,21] Hence, some childbirth educators have abandoned panting and substituted another breathing rhythm, while others have simply solved the problem by teaching a more moderate rate of shallow breathing.

Mothers may be taught to use either abdominal breathing only, chest breathing only, a combination of both, or simply a pattern of breaths with no special attention directed at either abdominal or chest breathing. In general, the rate of breathing increases as labor progresses. Also, during a contraction the rate of breathing may accelerate as the contraction intensifies and decelerate as the contraction subsides.

The mother may breathe only through the mouth or she may inhale through the nose and exhale through the mouth. Any number of combinations of this technique may be used by any one mother. In addition, breathing may be accompanied by body movement or sounds such as a whisper.

The nurse may be able to obtain information about the breathing patterns from some mothers simply by asking. Others may not be aware of the breathing pattern they are using. In such cases the mother should be observed closely to ascertain the breathing patterns being used. A thorough assessment of breathing patterns helps the nurse anticipate the needs of the mother. If a breathing pattern is not helpful, the nurse can suggest another. If the mother will be breathing through her mouth, the nurse can obtain ice chips or a damp cloth to alleviate dry lips and mouth. Some mothers are taught to use a lollipop for this purpose. If the mother uses rapid breathing, the nurse can remind her to report any tingling in the hands and other initial signs of hyperventilation (carbon dioxide insufficiency). In anticipation of these signs, the nurse can have a paper bag available. The patient can breathe in and out of the paper bag to inhale enough carbon dioxide to reverse the hyperventilation.

Physical Activities

Physical activities other than those which fall into the above categories may be used during labor. During a contraction the mother or father may rhythmically massage the abdomen, using some preparation such as talcum powder to keep the skin smooth. The father may rub her lower back between and during contractions. The mother may rock her pelvis while standing or lying on her side. The latter appears to be particularly helpful during back labor. Counterpressure is also useful. To achieve this the father may place tennis balls, a rolling pin, his knee, or his fist against the lower back.

Medications

When the mother is admitted, the nurse also asks whether or not she has taken medication or any other substance for pain relief, such as aspirin, codeine, an alcoholic beverage, or even paregoric, which is prescribed for false labor. If medication was taken, the nurse notes the time, type, and amount.

It is always possible that the mother has taken some illegal drug such as marijuana, heroin, or a black market drug of unknown composition. The mother who uses illegal drugs may fear legal action against her or disdain from the health team. Therefore, to increase the likelihood of obtaining an honest answer from a mother who has used an illegal drug, the nurse should always stress that the questions about medication are asked for important reasons, such as determining what other medication can be used safely.

It is also important to inquire about what analgesics and anesthetics are being considered for use during labor. The mother may have no knowledge at all about medication, or she and the father may have discussed several possibilities with the obstetrician.

Current Discomforts Other than Labor

The process of labor may not be the only source of discomfort for the mother. Indeed, there are other diseases or symptoms that may be much more irritating and painful than the concurrent labor. Such discomforts may be associated with the pregnancy itself or may represent a chronic illness or a recent illness or injury (see Part III of Table 26-4). For example, pregnancy may cause or increase heartburn, hemorrhoids, or varicose veins in the legs or vagina, all of which can be extremely uncomfortable.

As for chronic illness, any one of a number of disorders (*e.g.*, arthritis, allergy) may result in pain and discomfort. The same is true of a recent illness or injury, such as influenza or an accident resulting in a broken bone, lacerations, or sprained ankle.

The nurse assesses sources of discomfort extraneous to labor so that appropriate actions can be taken to provide relief. For example, if a mother is experiencing heartburn, the simple administration of an antacid may enable her to devote her attention and energy to the process of childbirth. At the same time, any treatment instituted prior to the onset of labor should be identified. If the mother has found effective means of handling discomforts, it obviously is expedient for her to use the same methods during labor whenever possible.

Current Concerns Other than Labor

Since the precise time for the onset of labor is rarely predictable, significant activities or plans may be interrupted by labor (see Part IV of Table 26-4). For example, the onset of labor may interfere with the requirements of the father's occupation and cause him to worry over the possibility of losing his job if he does not report to work. If the parents have other children, they may be anxious about what will happen to them during their absence.

The parents may also be concerned about financial arrangements related to hospitalization and the physician's fee, particularly if complications arise such as prematurity or if there is an unexpected multiple birth. More simply, perhaps the parents failed to make recommended financial payments to the hospital during the weeks prior to admission and are now afraid the hospital will not allow them to stay.

For some reason, realistic or not, the parents may be fearful about the condition of the mother or the unborn infant.

The mother or father may be considering giving up the baby for adoption. Onset of labor may precipitate many feelings about this.

There may have been an unexpected change in some aspect of the parents' plans for childbirth. Their obstetrician may be out of town, or labor may have progressed so rapidly that they were unable to reach the hospital of their choice.

It is important for the nurse to realize that such concerns can stir anxiety and interfere with the parents' ability to concentrate on handling discomforts, responding to directions, cooperating with examinations, and dealing with all the other aspects of labor. The nurse is frequently in a position to assist the parents in solving the problem or directing them to obtain appropriate assistance.

Goals and Expectations Regarding Labor

Parents generally have certain expectations regarding labor (Table 26-4). The nurse may encounter extremes in parents' expectations related to pain and pain relief. One mother may expect severe pain and desire that the physician render her practically unconscious throughout labor. Another mother may expect no pain at all and, therefore, no pain relief measures. When discomfort and pain are expected, the parents may believe that the techniques they have been taught to use during labor, such as breathing patterns, are sufficient assistance for the mother. Their goal may be a completely unmedicated labor. Or, the parents may expect to use the methods they were taught in combination with some type of medication if they desire it.

In some cases the father remains with the mother from the beginning of labor, during delivery, and through the recovery period following delivery. In other instances the mother does not want the father present. Parents' expectations of the nurse and physician also need to be determined.

Some parents, particularly mothers, want very much to observe the effects of their pushing and the delivery of the baby. Many delivery rooms have mirrors for this purpose. The parents may have brought a camera to take pictures in the labor room and in the delivery room. They may also want someone to take a picture of them with their baby immediately after delivery. Some parents want to tape record the delivery.

An episiotomy is done in most deliveries, but some parents hope for or expect no episiotomy. The mother may have done certain exercises daily for weeks prior to labor to achieve this.

A fully conscious mother almost always wants to touch the newborn as soon as possible. The mother may plan on holding the baby before the cord is cut. She may also expect to be allowed to breast-feed the baby on the delivery table.

In helping the parents express their goals and expectations the nurse is alert to differences between the desires of the mother and father. For example, the father may not want to witness the delivery although the mother wants him in the delivery room. Or, the father may think the mother is unrealistic in her plans for little or no medication. When the nurse observes such differences she helps the parents become aware of them and hopefully formulate compatible goals.

In her assessment of the parents' goals the nurse also notes whether or not these goals have been discussed with the physician. Some goals may be contraindicated for medical reasons. Other goals may require the awareness and cooperation of the physician. In addition, hospital policy sometimes places limitations on the parents. For instance, some delivery rooms are so small that the hospital must have a policy of excluding the father.

As labor progresses the nurse continues to monitor the patient for any changes in the items listed in Table 26-4. Some aspects of the labor situation may change dramatically, such as the nature of the contractions. There may be a sudden need for modification of pain relief methods. Also, the discomforts and concerns extraneous to labor may be resolved or suddenly may appear when none had existed before.

Nonpharmacologic Pain Relief During Labor

This discussion of pain relief measures is focused on those other than medication. These pain relief methods may be used either instead of or in addition to analgesics and anesthetics. The focus is purposefully limited to what the nurse may do for the mother or what she may assist the mother or father to do. Nursing activities related to the use of pharmacological agents are discussed elsewhere.

Methods of Prepared Childbirth

Methods of prepared childbirth do not necessarily have the management of pain during labor as their primary objective. They encompass preparation for and assistance with much more than labor.

Nevertheless, pain management is inherent in the preparation of the mother or father if other objectives are to be met. These objectives may be reduced need for analgesia and anesthesia, an awareness of the birth, or simply a personally satisfying experience for the parents. In any event, each method takes into account that some control of pain is essential. Hence, it behooves the nurse to be acquainted with the nature of preparation. Many methods of prepared childbirth require a considerable investment of time and energy on the part of the parents.

The particular method of prepared childbirth used by a mother during labor may have been recommended by her physician, or she may have chosen it herself. Typically, the mother and father attend a series of six or more two-hour classes during the last trimester of pregnancy. The classes usually include about ten couples, and they are taught by an instructor specially trained in that method. In addition to attending classes and performing other related tasks, the mother and father practice certain activities that are to be used during labor daily. Some of these activities assist the mother to tolerate pain or reduce the intensity of pain. Information about the processes of labor is also given in the classes. This tends to reduce anxiety in the mother and father and thereby assist them to cope with pain.

The number of parents seeking childbirth education is increasing. In a 1973–1974 survey of 54 university hospitals in the United States, almost three fourths reported that some form of psychoprophylaxis or natural childbirth was practiced during labor for the purpose of relieving pain. Most of the time these methods were used in combination with other techniques, such as regional anesthesia.[22] The method of prepared childbirth growing most rapidly throughout the United States is the psychoprophylactic method (PPM) or Lamaze. In 1966 there were 77 Lamaze childbirth educators nationwide.[23] That number increased to 2500 in 1976.[24] In 1975 more than 190,000 couples were trained in the Lamaze method of childbirth. This represented 7% of the pregnant population in the United States.[25]

Because of the growing popularity of the Lamaze method among laypeople, Table 26-5 summarizes those activities the nurse generally might expect to be used by Lamaze-trained couples during labor for the purpose of handling discomfort or pain. The nurse encounters variations in these activities because instructors are always making efforts to improve the method and because each mother may adapt the method to her own particular needs.

Sometimes the nursing staff tends to spend very little time with Lamaze-trained or otherwise prepared couples. While it is true that some couples may manage quite well on their own, most couples need some type of assistance. Knowledge of how a mother and father may attempt to cope with pain and discomfort enables the nurse to provide appropriate help. For example, when a breathing pattern has ceased to be effective, the Lamaze-trained mother may need assurance that labor has progressed sufficiently to warrant changing to the next breathing pattern. Or when the father must leave the labor room the nurse knows how to assume some of his responsibilities, such as counting or breathing with the mother.

Goals and Principles of Pain Relief

Good pain relief does not necessarily mean the total elimination of painful sensations. In fact, complete abolition of pain in rarely a realistic goal. It is significantly helpful to the patient and often more reasonable to aim at a decrease in the intensity of pain or a decrease in the degree to which pain bothers the patient. The latter is closely related to another possible goal of increasing the patient's tolerance for pain.

Two important principles that underlie the accomplishment of these goals are decreasing the pain impulses that reach the cortex of the brain, and managing anxiety. The transmission of pain signals may be interrupted in a number of ways such as decreasing the source of noxious stimuli or closing the gate (see Gate Control Theory, pp 540–543). Likewise, there are numerous ways of managing anxiety.

It has long been recognized that most types of pain cause some degree of anxiety or fear, which increases the intensity of pain, or at least renders pain less tolerable and more bothersome. The gate control theory suggests that anxiety opens the gate to pain impulses, thereby actually increasing the intensity of pain. Anxiety may also increase the intensity of pain directly by causing muscle tension. During labor it is obvious that tension in the muscles of the abdomen, perineum, and lower back increases discomfort.

The interaction between anxiety and pain may become a spiraling process. Pain may cause anxiety, which may increase the intensity of pain by causing muscle tension or by opening the gate to pain impulses. In this way mild pain and anxiety can eventually become severe pain and panic.

Pain Relief Measures During Labor

Pain relief measures are aimed at reducing either anxiety or pain impulses. Some guidelines to the effective use of these pain relief measures are as follows:

1. Use a variety of pain relief measures.
2. Use pain relief measures *before* pain becomes severe. (It is easier to prevent severe pain and panic than to alleviate them once they occur.)
3. Include those pain relief measures which the patient believes will be effective.
4. Take into account the patient's ability to be active or passive in the application of the pain relief measure.
5. Regarding the potency of the pain relief measure needed, rely on the patient's experience of the severity of pain rather than the known physical stimuli.
6. If a pain relief measure is ineffective the first time it is used during a contraction, encourage the mother to try it at least one or two more times before abandoning it.

Some of the pain relief methods discussed later are not possible or acceptable in conventional labor rooms or when external monitoring is used. However, there is growing public demand for more natural childbirth and nonpharmacological methods of pain relief during childbirth. Alternative Birth Centers (ABCs) are one response to that demand. Thus, in the future the following low-risk, nonpharmacological pain relief measures may be increasingly acceptable to both health professionals and expectant parents.

Table 26-5.
Summary of Pain Relief Measures Used by Lamaze-Trained Parents During Labor

Approximate Progress of Labor	Position	Relaxation	Mother's Activities During Massage
Onset to 3 cm, or contractions 5 min–20 min apart	Supported comfortably sitting or lying on side; may walk between contractions; may stand and lean on object during contractions	Inhales deeply at beginning of contraction and relaxes totally upon exhalation; takes a deep breath at end of each contraction	Hands move slowly from pubic area up to umbilicus and out around abdomen down to pubic area; or, other body areas such as thighs may be massaged
Dilates from 4 cm–7 cm, or contractions 2 min–4 min apart	Same as above	Same as above	Same as above
Dilates from 8 cm–10 cm, or contractions 1 min apart	Same as above	Same as above	Omitted

Eye Focus	Each Contraction in Relation to Breathing Pattern	Thoughts	Father's Activities Either During or Between Contractions
Eyes open and focused on one particular object ("concentration point," "focal point")	Slow chest breathing (6 min–9 min), inhale through nose, exhale through mouth	On inhalation, "In, 1, 2" On exhalation, "Out, 1, 2"	Times frequency of each contraction Helps her get in comfortable positions Checks for state of relaxation by moving parts of her body As need arises, may give signals to help increase relaxation, do abdominal massage for her, or rub her lower back
Same as above	Shallow chest breathing through mouth; begin slowly, accelerates as contraction intensifies, decelerates as contraction subsides; breathing is 4/4 rhythm	Counts each breath in 4/4 rhythm emphasizing count of one (*e.g.*, "1, 2, 3, 4, 1, 2, 3, 4," etc., or silently sings Yankee Doodle, a 4/4 song)	Same as above plus the following: During contractions—at 15-sec intervals he calls off time that elapses, that is, "15 sec, 30 sec, 45 sec, 60 sec" until contraction is over As need arises, may breathe in rhythm with her, count aloud in rhythm to her breathing or sing song in rhythm, remind her of eye focus, remind her to breathe deeply at end of contraction. If "back labor," may try deep counterpressure to lower back
Same as above or focuses eyes on father	Shallow chest breathing through mouth (rhythm of 4, 6, or 8 breaths and then one blow); begins slowly, accelerates and decelerates with intensity of contraction; if not allowed to push but feels urge to push, blows repeatedly If uncomfortable between contractions, uses slow chest breathing	Counts each breath according to rhythm selected (*e.g.*, "1, 2, 3, 4, 5, 6, blow")	Between contractions—offers encouragement; wipes face with cool wet cloth, moistens lips and mouth with water, ice chips, or lollipop. Reminds her to void q2h

(Continued)

Table 26-5.
Summary of Pain Relief Measures Used by Lamaze-Trained Parents During Labor (Continued)

Approximate Progress of Labor	Position	Relaxation	Mother's Activities During Massage
Delivery (fully dilated)	Same as above, except when pushing For pushing in labor room—may conserve energy during pushing by elevating and supporting legs on pillows, or by lying on side with back curved and top knee pulled up For pushing in delivery room—semipropped position with back curved, head and shoulders supported by pillows, head forward; if legs not in stirrups, she holds legs under knees with elbows out and brings knees as close to shoulders as possible	Same as above, except omitted when pushing	Omitted

Support During Labor

From the beginning of labor the mother needs to have someone with her at increasingly frequent intervals and to know that someone is available at all times. Toward the end of labor she needs to have someone with her constantly. The presence, actions, and words of this person can be very supportive to the mother. This person may be the nurse, the father, or someone else. At times the nurse's greatest contribution is to support the father so that he can in turn support the mother. Specific ways the mother may be supported during labor are discussed on pages 554–560.

Support during labor lowers anxiety and increases the mother's ability to handle discomforts. It also enhances the effectiveness of other pain relief methods.

Giving Information

As mentioned previously, part of the uniqueness of labor pain is that the mother may possess anxiety-reducing knowledge. If the mother does not obtain this information for herself, the nurse can supply it. For example, the nurse may tell the mother approximately how long it will be before the next contraction and how long that contraction will last. During intense contractions the nurse may "count down" at 15-second intervals until the end of the contraction, telling the mother how long it will be until the contraction is over. Or the nurse may time the contraction so she can reassure the mother by telling her when the contraction has reached its peak and will begin to subside. Information about the progress of labor, such as cervical dilatation and descent of the baby, is also important. It serves as a reminder that there is a purpose to labor, that labor does end, and that the end is getting closer and closer.

Such information not only reduces anxiety but may also motivate the mother to tolerate pain. Especially toward the end of labor when discomfort increases, the knowledge that the ordeal is almost over may enable the mother to tolerate an intensity of pain that she would otherwise find unbearable.

Knowing that she and her baby are not in danger also reduces anxiety. Sometimes the mother finds the forces of labor so unexpectedly powerful that she is fearful of harm. The nurse should periodically reassure the mother that she and her baby are doing well (provided, of course, that this is true). She may say, for example, that the baby's heartbeat is strong and regular. Remembering that discomfort is associated with a normal process and not a life-threatening illness may be helpful to the mother. Briefly and in simple terms the nurse can remind the mother of what is happening, for example, that each contraction enlarges the opening for the baby.

Understanding what is happening during labor seems to increase the mother's sense of control over

Eye Focus	Each Contraction in Relation to Breathing Pattern	Thoughts	Father's Activities Either During or Between Contractions
Same as above, except when pushing; then may focus on mirror or perineum, if visible, to see results of pushing	Same as above, except when pushing For pushing—2 or 3 deep breaths, inhale, hold breath, lean forward, slowly count to 10, release breath; repeat inhalation and hold to count of 10 until contraction is over or until instructed to stop pushing Alternate method—2 deep breaths, on 3rd breath blow out slowly and bear down; repeat as necessary	Same as above, except when pushing For pushing—slowly counts to 10 during each breath holding	Same as above, except when pushing For pushing—stands at mother's back to support her in pushing position Counts aloud to 10 during each breath holding, tells her to take a deep breath and hold it, then counts to 10 again Reminds her to relax pelvic floor and "push through vagina"

the event. Feelings of powerlessness can provoke anxiety, so it is important to further feelings of control. This may be done through instructions and explanations that help the mother cooperate with examinations and with the process of labor such as effective pushing. In particular the mother's feelings of control can be strengthened by teaching her about pain relief measures as early as possible. When this has not been done prior to labor the nurse can begin in early labor to explain certain of the following pain relief measures. The mother then knows that pain relief is available, that there are several possibilities, and that to some extent she may choose from among them.

Decreasing Sources of Noxious Stimuli

One source of noxious, or painful, stimuli is abdominal pressure on the contracting uterus. Total skeletal muscle relaxation, discussed in more detail later, relaxes the abdominal muscles and contributes to relieving pressure on the uterus.

Breathing Methods

Pressure may also be prevented by either abdominal breathing or chest breathing. While there is controversy as to which breathing method best relaxes abdominal muscles, the fact seems to be that it depends largely upon the individual mother. Hence, regardless of the breathing method the mother may be using, if she feels it is exerting uncomfortable pressure on her uterus, it seems wise for the nurse to help her learn the other method.

Between contractions the nurse can assist the mother to differentiate between abdominal and chest breathing and learn to use one or the other of the methods. While the mother is lying on her back, she places one hand on her chest, the other on her abdomen. The nurse points out that during an abdominal breath, the abdomen rises as air is inhaled. During a chest breath, the chest rises as air is inhaled. The nurse can have the mother practice each breathing method several times. Then the mother can choose the method that seems the most comfortable or the easiest. However, there may be no need for the nurse to assist the mother to differentiate between chest and abdominal breathing as long as the abdominal muscles are not contracted and the mother finds breathing easy and comfortable.

Abdominal Lifting

Another obvious method of reducing abdominal pressure is simply to lift the abdominal wall (see Fig. 26-3). The nurse may do this for the mother, or the father may be taught how to do this maneuver. A hand must be kept on the uterus to identify the beginning of the contraction. The instant the uterus begins to contract, the nurse places both hands at waist level with

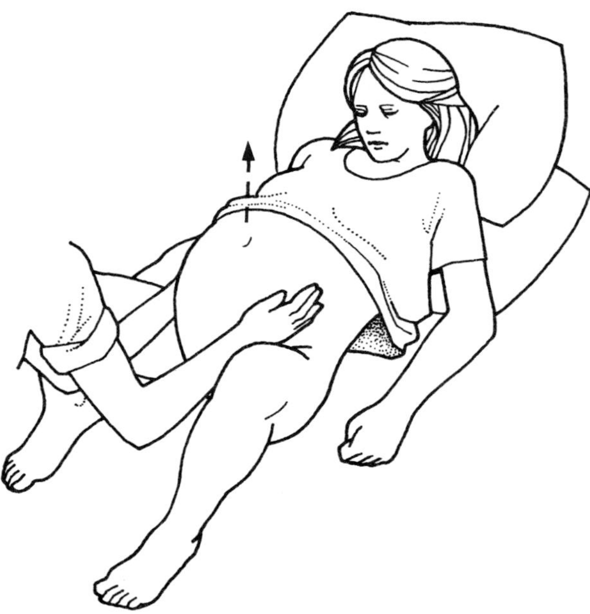

Figure 26-3.
Abdominal lifting. One approach to lifting the abdominal wall begins at the onset of the contraction with hands on the back at waist level, fingers pointing toward the spine. Firmly and gently turn hands and bring to the position shown here with pressure that lifts. Use no inward pressure.

the fingers pointing toward the spine. She quickly slides her hands down and under the mother's back until the fingertips meet at the spine. The nurse then firmly and gently *lifts* until her hands rest between the pelvic bone and rib cage. As the hands are drawn from underneath the back, the hands are turned gradually (without releasing the upward lift) until the fingertips point toward the rib cage. The upward lift must be completed before the contraction reaches its peak. There should be lifting only and *no inward pressure.* When the contraction is over, the upward lift is released slowly.[26]

A more simple method of abdominal lifting is possible, but it is equally strenuous for the nurse or father. At the beginning of the contraction the fingers are hooked under the ribs and the distended abdomen lifted as the mother inhales. In both methods of abdominal lifting it is important that the mother not arch her back, since this would cause discomfort. Depending upon the amount of pressure exerted by the hand, the latter method may also result in lifting the baby, thus removing the pressure of the uterus on the back.[27]

Position

Decreasing the weight of the uterus and baby on the muscles and bones of the mother's back can lessen the amount of noxious stimuli considerably. This is an especially important and effective pain relief measure when the mother experiences "back labor," that is, when the occiput of the fetus presses on the mother's sacrum. Regardless of the position of the fetus, a mother in normal labor is probably more comfortable if she avoids the supine position.

One study compared the 30° upright position with the recumbent position during labor. The upright position was recommended for several reasons. Although the intensity of contractions was higher in this position, the contractions did not last any longer, the uterus relaxed more completely between contractions, and the first two stages of labor were shorter.[28] Thus, the duration of discomfort may be shortened by the upright position. In another study ambulation shortened labor and reduced the mother's discomfort.[29]

Unless there are complications such as a prolapsed cord, the mother should be allowed to choose the position she finds most comfortable. However, if she wants to lie on her back, the head of the bed should be somewhat elevated and her thighs slightly flexed.

Besides the 30° upright or semisitting position, other positions which may provide comfort during labor are the lateral Sims's and the tailor-sitting position. An unusual but increasingly popular position for mothers with back labor is the up-on-all-fours position. This position may even succeed in rotating the baby's head to an anterior position. If the baby's head is not in the posterior position, this crawl position may still relieve pain, especially during transition, when labor is so often felt in the back.

Pushing

As delivery approaches, most mothers feel the urge to push. However, unnecessary noxious stimuli can be eliminated if the mother understands that it is futile to push early in labor. Painful stimuli may also be avoided during delivery if the mother obeys instructions as to when she should and should not push. The urge to push can be almost irresistible. Thus, the mother may need some techniques such as blowing or rapid breathing to help her refrain from pushing.

Relieving External Pressure

When external electronic monitoring is used, the transducer may be a source of discomfort if it is secured in the same position over a period of time.

The sensations of discomfort or heaviness may be decreased by moving the transducer as little as ¾ inch.

Distraction

Research studies as well as personal experiences comfirm that distraction is an effective method of pain relief. As indicated earlier, the gate control theory provides some possible explanation. When the cerebral cortex is involved in activity (cortical excitation), the gate may be closed to pain. The cortex may signal a decreased attention to pain impulses. Or the reticular system in the brain stem may register that there is sufficient incoming stimuli and therefore signal the gate to be closed to further stimuli—painful stimuli in this case.

Regardless of the theoretical mechanism, common sense suggests that pain is more tolerable if the patient becomes less aware of it—in short, distracted from it. Distraction places pain on the periphery of awareness. A person may be distracted from pain in an almost limitless variety of ways.

Instructors of methods of prepared childbirth have devised and taught many means of distraction for use during contractions. It is interesting to note that a large number of these are rhythmic in nature, such as "riding the wave," tapping out the rhythm of a song, rhythmic head movements, and rhythmic breathing.

The method of distraction tends to change as labor progresses, seemingly taking into account the increasing intensity of pain and the increasing effort the mother must exert to engage in any activity not related to labor. Thus, as demonstrated by the Lamaze method (see Table 26-5), abdominal massage is eliminated and a relatively more easy breathing pattern is adopted during transition. As a rule, the more intense the pain, the more involved the patient must become in the distraction to achieve pain relief. However, the involvement must be compatible with the patient's ability.

Table 26-5 provides examples from the Lamaze method of activities that may serve as distracters. Many of these activities have other purposes as well. The breathing rhythms and purposeful thoughts undoubtedly serve as distracters, but maintenance of rhythmic breathing is also thought to relieve pain by providing adequate oxygenation of the uterus.

While relaxation also serves other purposes such as anxiety reduction and prevention of abdominal pressure, the mother may find that her concentrated efforts to relax provide a significant distraction. Changing positions and massaging the abdomen require both motor and cognitive effort, and therefore may be distracting. Keeping the eyes open and focused on a particular point is perhaps the purest and simplest distracter. Altogether, the Lamaze-trained mother consciously performs several varied activities with the end result of distraction from pain.

Other breathing patterns for use during contractions are suggested by the Maternity Center Association (MCA) and are described in Chapter 19.

A brief comparison of the Lamaze method and the MCA method reveals some of the ideas common to most methods of prepared childbirth—concentration on relaxation and a rhythmic breathing pattern during contractions.

The nurse needs to be familiar with a variety of distracters that she may suggest to the mother. What is sufficiently distracting for one mother may not be for another. And a mother may need assistance with distracters even if she has attended prepared childbirth classes.

Emphasis is placed on distracters that are of some proven effectiveness and also relatively easy to teach the mother. Most of the techniques taught in the MCA method and the Lamaze method meet these criteria. (A review of the information in Chapter 19 and Table 26-5 will assist the reader in the following discussion of these distracters.) Some distracters used in the various methods of prepared childbirth are extremely distracting but difficult to teach quickly once labor is in progress.

Early in labor the mother may be able to distract herself by "walking and talking" through a contraction. As labor progresses, some form of rhythmic breathing pattern is usually helpful. Slow rhythmic breathing is both relaxing and distracting, examples being either the "complete breathing" of the MCA or the "slow chest breathing" of Lamaze. If this is not effective, the nurse may suggest adding some of the distracters of the Lamaze method, such as a concentration point, counting during inhalation and exhalation, and abdominal massage.

When discomfort intensifies and a more powerful form of distraction is needed, the nurse may teach the mother the "modified complete breathing" of MCA or the accelerating and decelerating "shallow chest breathing" of the Lamaze method. Either of these may result in hyperventilation, so the nurse should caution the mother to inform her of any dizziness or tingling. Hyperventilation may be treated by having the mother breathe into a paper bag and suggesting that henceforth she breathe more slowly. Again, more distraction may be added to these breathing patterns by incorporating one or more of the distracters of the

Lamaze method—the concentration point, abdominal massage, silent counting, or singing in rhythm with breathing. Another effective and relatively easy distracter to employ is finger tapping the rhythm to a 4/4 song, coordinating the rhythm with breathing.

Of all the breathing patterns suggested here, the one most likely to be difficult for the mother to learn during labor is the accelerated and decelerated aspect of the Lamaze "shallow chest breathing." If the mother finds this or any other distracter too difficult or fatiguing, it should be abandoned.

During transition the mother's focus tends to become extremely narrow because of the great increase in the intensity of contractions. Whereas earlier in labor the distracters could be suggested and taught between contractions, there is little time now and it is difficult for the mother to focus on anything but labor. Therefore, distracters used during transition should be more simple and must be taught prior to the onset of transition. The Lamaze method suggests rhythmic, shallow chest breathing with blowing. Although this breathing pattern includes acceleration and deceleration with the intensity of the contraction, it is an easy breathing pattern to learn and to use. The MCA suggests "modified complete breathing" with the further modification of puffing out gently upon exhalation of every third or fourth breath. Simple additions to these breathing rhythms include coordinated and silent counting and use of a concentration point.

When the nurse wishes to assist the laboring mother with pain relief measures in the form of distracters, it is only reasonable to approach the mother between, not during, contractions. The nurse can describe briefly one or two possibilities. This needs to be accompanied by some explanation, such as, "It may seem silly at first, but many mothers find that it makes the contractions less bothersome because it forces them to think of something else." The mother should be asked to decide which one she would like to try first. It usually is most helpful if the nurse first demonstrates the pattern and then has the mother do it. If a song or counting is to be used, it is often much easier for the mother if the nurse counts or sings for her during the first contractions in which the pattern is used.

Certainly not everyone deals with pain in the same way. That is why it is so necessary to involve the mother in a decision about which distracters she would like to use. If the mother does not like any of the distracters discussed in this section, the nurse may creatively invent some others or simply ask the mother for suggestions. Some mothers prefer a form of distraction that involves an inward focus rather than the outward focus of the distracters described here. For example, the mother may stare into space or close her eyes and focus on the forces of her body, concentrating on the contraction being a wavelike force, which she envisions herself on top of.

We have not yet begun to uncover and understand fully the various strategies people use to cope with pain. These strategies include much more than distraction, but within the area of distraction there are numerous approaches.

Whatever type of distracters the mother may choose to use during a contraction, the nurse and others must take care not to prevent her from using them. Early in labor it may be a helpful distraction to

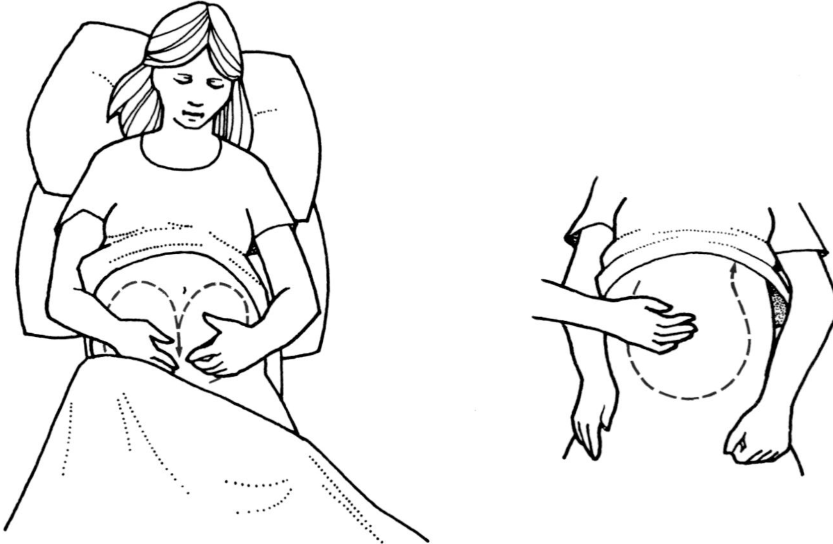

Figure 26-4.
Two types of effleurage or abdominal massage.

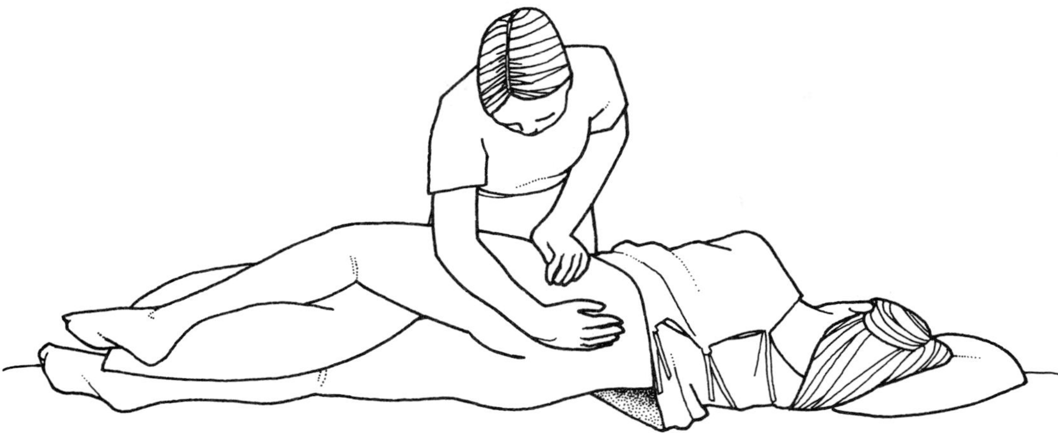

Figure 26-5.
Deep back massage, while the mother lies on her side, relieves back pain between contractions.

the mother to have someone to talk with during a contraction, but later she may find this irritating because it interferes with other strategies for coping with pain. In any event, the nurse needs to find out from the mother what, if anything, she wants the nurse to do for her during a contraction.

Cutaneous Stimulation

Rubbing a painful body part is a universal means of relieving pain. The gate control theory provides a possible reason for the effectiveness of this and other forms of cutaneous stimulation. As discussed previously, the theory suggests that stimulation of large-diameter nerve fibers may partially or completely close the gate to the transmission of pain impulses to the cortex. Because many cutaneous (skin) fibers are large-diameter fibers, stimulation of the skin may result in pain relief.

Several types of cutaneous stimulation may be used during labor and may prove to be effective pain relief measures. One of the more common of these is effleurage, or abdominal massage (Fig. 26-4). Rubbing the lower back is also common (Fig. 26-5). The Lamaze method describes a type of abdominal massage. The application of heat or cold (with the physician's permission) may be especially comforting to the patient with "back labor."

Creams or gels containing menthol may also be rubbed on the lower back for pain relief.

The above are examples of relatively moderate stimulation of cutaneous fibers. Mild to moderate stimulation is ordinarily more effective than intense stimulation. However, one notable exception is the use of intense pressure over the sacrum during a contraction. The pressure may be applied with the knee or fist, or the mother may lean back (in a semisitting position) on a tennis ball or rolling pin (Fig. 26-6). It has been estimated that applying pressure during a contraction is equivalent to the pain relief potential of 50 mg to 100 mg of meperidine.[30]

Rubbing of any part of the body, even between contractions, possibly may contribute to pain relief. This not only encourages relaxation, but experimentation with cutaneous stimulation shows that it may help close the gate to painful impulses long after its

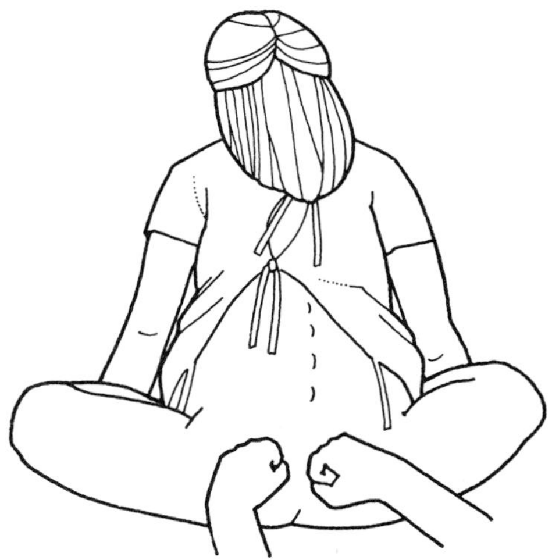

Figure 26-6.
Firm counterpressure of the fists on the lower back, while the mother is in the tailor sitting position, effectively relieves back labor.

usage and that the painful area need not always be the area of stimulation.[8] For example, if an external monitor prevents abdominal massage, the thighs may be massaged instead. Some mothers find that foot massage by the father or nurse brings considerable comfort.

Transcutaneous electric nerve stimulation (TENS) is a newer form of cutaneous stimulation that has been used successfully for pain relief during the first stage of labor. A mild electric current is applied to the skin by way of electrodes connected to a battery-operated device with controls to regulate the sensation. The patient usually feels a buzzing, tingling, or vibrating sensation. In one study of labor pain, two pairs of electrodes were placed on either side of the spinal column over the sacral and thoracic regions. Low-intensity stimulation was provided continuously, and the mother increased the stimulation during a contraction. Of the 147 women treated, 44% considered TENS pain relief to be good to very good. No complications occurred except that in a few cases sacral stimulation interfered with monitoring the fetal heart rate. These researchers recommended TENS as a primary method of pain relief during labor, noting that it is low-risk, nonpharmacological method, and can be interrupted at any moment.[31] Comparable results have been obtained in studies of Egyptian and Italian mothers during childbirth.[32,33]

Nursing responsibilities when TENS is used might include placing and securing the electrodes, explaining the use of the controls to the mother, and evaluating the effectiveness of TENS in relieving pain.

Relaxation

Virtually every method of prepared childbirth heavily emphasizes total skeletal muscle relaxation during labor. Relaxation contributes to pain relief in a variety of ways. Some of these have already been mentioned, such as relaxing the abdominal muscles to decrease the noxious stimuli of pressure on the uterus.

But even when noxious stimuli are not affected directly, skeletal muscle relaxation itself may be a pain relief measure. It relieves pain by interrupting the spiraling process of pain and anxiety. Muscle tension is a response to pain and anxiety. Since relaxation is the opposite of muscle tension, it prevents or diminishes tension. The behavioral response of relaxation, therefore, is incompatible with pain–anxiety responses. Some research suggests that a person's evaluation of the intensity of pain is in part a function of her evaluation of her own overt behavioral response to pain.[34] Possibly, when the patient observes herself relaxed instead of tense, she evaluates her pain as less intense. Or, relaxation may cause the cortex to send signals to close the gate to the transmission of pain impulses.

Relaxation undoubtedly provides pain relief for other reasons, depending upon the individual patient. For some patients efforts to relax can serve as a distraction from pain. In other patients a state of relaxation may increase suggestibility, causing the patient to accept explicit and implicit suggestions of comfort.[35]

How can the patient achieve total skeletal muscle relaxation? Possibly, the most frequently used but most unproductive method is for the nurse to say, "Relax." The verbal cue "relax" may be used effectively with patients who have been trained in relaxation, but to the untrained patient such a command often sounds impossible, if not absurd. The patient's inability to follow such an instruction may engender feelings of powerlessness, failure, and more tension.

People may be trained in relaxation techniques in many different ways and for many reasons besides childbirth, such as handling the tensions of daily living.

When the nurse encounters a mother who has been trained in relaxation techniques, she simply finds out how best to assist her. It is particularly helpful to identify cues that will encourage relaxation if the mother becomes tense. These cues may be verbal, such as "relax," or tactile-kinesthetic, such as touching or moving the tense body part.

If the mother has not been trained in relaxation, the nurse may use some simple techniques that can make a significant difference in the mother's level of relaxation. The nurse first explains to the mother that relaxing during a contraction is very important because it can decrease abdominal pressure on the uterus and also help her feel more calm and generally comfortable. The quickest and easiest ways to promote relaxation are to instruct the mother to take a deep breath or to yawn and to "go limp" or relax as she exhales. The nurse suggests that the mother try one or both of these at the beginning and end of contractions and anytime during contractions that she feels the need to relax. (The patient who chooses to yawn may find it becomes spontaneous and more frequent.)

These techniques are effective because they take advantage of conditioned responses. Both a big sigh (deep breath) and a yawn are associated with relaxation.

Relaxation may be furthered by providing support to comfortably positioned and slightly flexed extremities. Also, the nurse may gently move extremities and the head to test for the degree of relaxation. This slight movement enables the mother to feel tense muscles and helps her to relax them.

Assistance with Change in Expectations and Goals

During the relatively brief and rapidly moving events of labor, any unexpected change in the parent's goals or expectations must be handled quickly. Otherwise anxiety may persist or increase, resulting in an increased intensity of pain. Some items listed in Part V of Table 26-4 are examples of areas in which a disturbing change may occur.

Sometimes the mother's personal obstetrician is not available, and a physician unknown to the parents must manage labor and delivery. Or the mother and father may have expected to be together throughout labor, but perhaps the father cannot be located or is unable to get to the hospital. In some instances the labor suite is too crowded to accommodate the father. Parents may have planned to use the ABC but the facilities may be occupied.

If external or internal electronic monitoring of the fetus is used, this may be disconcerting to parents for several reasons. The parents may be very fearful if they associate its usage with possible complications. Some hospitals monitor only high-risk situations, but others routinely monitor all patients. Regardless of the reason for electronic monitoring, the parents may strongly object to the use of such equipment because it renders childbirth a less natural experience. In addition, external monitoring in particular makes it difficult for the parents to use certain pain relief measures such as abdominal lifting, abdominal massage, and some positioning. Often external monitoring requires that the mother lie quietly on her back. If this is disturbing to the parents, the nurse should, if possible, remove the external monitoring equipment for a few contractions so that the parents can employ some of their pain relief activities.

When a situation occurs that disturbs the parents, the nurse encourages them to express their feelings and indicates an appreciation of their disappointment. She then explains the reasons for any rules, policies, or circumstances that prevent them from achieving their goals or expectations.

One of the more difficult problems is assisting the parents who are not able to achieve their "ideal" of labor and delivery. This ideal may vary considerably from one couple to another and may consist of any one or a combination of goals referred to previously. Inability to achieve this ideal labor may cause profound feelings of failure in the mother or father. Also, they may refuse or be very reluctant to accept measures incompatible with their ideal.

Patients who have specific expectations or goals associated with an ideal labor may have arrived at these in a number of ways. But these parents seem most often to be a product of classes that prepare them in a specific method of childbirth. One of the most common criticisms of methods of prepared childbirth is that the mother and father are taught to strive for a particular kind of labor and delivery experience, such as medication-free delivery or ecstasy over the delivery. Not all childbirth educators state such goals. Yet parents, especially mothers, tend to adopt these goals and feel a sense of failure if they are not achieved. The reason for this is not necessarily related to what the childbirth educator says. Rather, the goals are implicit in personal narratives and films to which the mother is exposed.

Written personal labor experiences are found in books and may be available from the childbirth educator's collections from former students. Some methods of childbirth use their own particular film to introduce their method to the parents. Examples are "The Story of Eric," showing the use of the Lamaze method, and "Childbirth for the Joy of It," showing the use of husband-coached childbirth. In viewing these films, it is easy to understand why the mother or father would desire the same "ideal" experience. The films do not focus on pain but on the techniques of the particular method of childbirth and on the parents' extreme happiness immediately following delivery. These films are emotionally appealing and very persuasive.

At the end of the film, with tears of joy in her eyes, the pregnant woman is not likely to want to settle for less than what she has just seen. She may reason, "If those women can give birth that way, I should be able to do it, too." Hence, the feeling of failure or not being "good at childbirth" may result if the mother finds that she is unable to go through her own labor as she saw it portrayed in film or in written narratives.

How does the nurse help the mother and father minimize feelings of failure and accept a change in their goals? Throughout childbirth, and particularly when goals must change, the nurse praises the mother and father for their efforts and abilities to handle labor. This promotes feelings of success. For example, the mother may have the goal of an unmedicated labor, but she may find the discomfort intolerable and request medication. If medication is given, the nurse can say that she knows medication was not planned. She can allow the mother to express her feelings and then praise the mother for the success of her efforts up to now and for the length of time medication was not necessary. She may add that the mother's continuing efforts may reduce the amount of medication required. She may also stress to the father that his approval and support are extremely valuable.

The mother may, however, choose to handle the

above situation in a different manner. She may decide it is in the best interests of herself and her baby for her not to request medication, in spite of how intolerable she finds the pain. Such pain may cause her to become extremely tense and unable to cooperate with examinations or the forces of labor. This may prolong labor and increase the possibility of complications. If medication seems highly desirable, the nurse may find it necessary to use a direct approach with the mother to modify her perceptions of the situation. This may be accomplished by stating how the health team views the situation and pointing out differences in this view and the mother's perceptions. One thing the nurse may point out is that the mother wants to avoid both medication and complications, but the two goals are now incompatible.

This direct approach tends to cause unpleasant psychological tension, called cognitive dissonance. In other words, the mother's goals are at odds with one another and with the knowledge received from the nurse. Cognitive dissonance may motivate a person to change. One way the mother may reduce dissonance in this case is to adjust her thinking so that she accepts other pain relief measures.[36]

Another approach to this type of situation is to employ analogy. This may disrupt the mother's denial of what is actually happening, assist her with a clearer understanding of the situation, or foster feelings of normality about her childbirth experience. Explaining the situation by comparing it with something else allows the mother to distance herself from the actual situation. She is able to understand the problem but avoid the anxiety associated with looking directly at the problem.[37] For example, the nurse may compare labor to a menstrual cycle. She may say that no two labors are exactly alike, just as no two women have exactly the same menstrual cycle. She may add that some women normally experience more pain than others. Or, she may cite some other symptom or sign that explains the need for a change in the mother's goal.

Aftermath Assimilation

After anticipation of pain and the presence of pain, a third and final phase of the pain experience occurs—the aftermath. The pain experience does not end with the cessation of the painful sensations. The patient does not necessarily immediately forget about the pain, especially if it was severe, frightening, or in any way disconcerting.

On the maternity unit it is a common observation that mothers talk a great deal about their childbirth experiences. It is a frequent topic of conversation regardless of whether the mother experienced "ecstasy," "failure," or simply relief mixed with satisfaction. Not only may the mother want to talk about the pain, but a variety of feelings resulting from the pain may be present, such as nausea, vomiting, chills, anger, or embarrassment. The mother may even have nightmares about the pain.

Clearly, at least some mothers need assistance during the aftermath phase of the pain experience. The most appropriate nursing action may be to assist the mother with the intellectual and emotional assimilation of her childbirth experience. In a sense the nurse helps the mother relive her labor. The nurse can ask the mother questions that help her discuss her discomforts, emotions, thoughts, overt responses, and the reactions of others during her labor. The nurse needs to be particularly alert and responsive to the mother's needs for support, such as praise, confirmation that her perceptions of discomfort are believed by others, or reassurance that her behavior was acceptable. Some patients need information to help them fill in memory gaps or to correct understandings that are inaccurate and anxiety provoking.[8]

It is particularly important to encourage assimilation in mothers who may harbor feelings of failure about childbirth. But assimilation may help maintain or restore a positive self-concept for any mother and aid in her ability to deal with mothering and other impending tasks.

References

1. Clark AL, Howland R, Affonso D, Uyehara J: MCH in American Samoa. Am J Nurs 74:700–702, April 1974
2. Lamaze F: Painless Childbirth: The Lamaze Method. Chicago, Henry Regnery, 1970
3. Potter H, Macdonald RD: Obstetric consequences of epidural analgesia in nulliparous patients. Lancet 1:1031–1034, 1971
4. Davenport-Slack B, Boylan CH: Psychological correlates of childbirth pain. Psychosom Med 36:215–223, May/June 1974
5. Melzack R, Taenzer P, Kinch RA: Labor pain: Nature of the experience and the role of prepared childbirth training. Pain (Suppl) 1:S271, 1981
6. Nettelbladt P, Fagerstrom C-F, Uddenberg N: The significance of reported childbirth pain. J Psychosom Res 20:215–221, 1976
7. Fagerhaugh SY, Strauss A: Politics of Pain: Staff-Patient Interaction, pp 223–224. Menlo Park, CA, Addison–Wesley, 1977
8. McCaffery M: Nursing Management of the Patient with Pain, 2nd ed. Philadelphia, JB Lippincott, 1979
9. Copp LA: The spectrum of suffering. Am J Nurs 74:491, March 1974
10. Melzack R, Wall PD: Pain mechanisms: A new theory. Science 150:971–979, 1965

11. Melzack R: The Puzzle of Pain, pp 153–190. New York, Basic Books, 1973

12. Nathan PW: The gate-control theory of pain: A critical review. Brain 99:213–258, 1976

13. Wall PD: Modulation of pain by nonpainful events. In Bonica JJ, Albe–Fessard D (eds): Advances in Pain Research and Therapy, Vol 1, pp 1–16. New York, Raven Press, 1976

14. Snyder SH: Opiate receptors and internal opiates. Scientific Am 236:44–56, March 1977

15. Terenius L: Endorphins and Pain. Front Horm Res 8:162–177, 1981

16. West A: Understanding endorphins: Our natural pain relief system. Nursing 81 11:50–53, February 1981

17. Cogan R: Comfort during prepared childbirth as a function of parity, reported by four classes of participant observers. J Psychosom Res 19:33–37, July 1975

18. Jones A, Bentler PM, Petry G: The reduction of uncertainty concerned future pain. J Abnorm Psychol 71:87–94, April 1966

19. Winsberg B, Greenlick M: Pain response in Negro and white obstetrical patients. J Health Soc Behav 8:222–227, September 1967

20. Sasmor JL, Castor CR, Hassid P: The chilbirth team during labor. Am J Nurs 73:444–447, March 1973

21. Ulin PR: Changing techniques in psychoprophylactic preparation for childbirth. Am J Nurs 68:2586–2591, December 1968

22. Osanai K, Nishijima M: Comparison of analgesia and anesthesia for labor between the university hospitals of the U.S.A. and Japan, including our own. Acta Obstetrica et Gynaecologica 21:76–85, 1974

23. Gandy M: Ten years ago in ASPO. Conceptions, Fall 1976

24. Stotland N: What has ASPO done for me? Conceptions, Winter 1976–77

25. Declerck E: National Teachers Survey. The American Society of Psychoprophylaxis in Obstetrics, Washington, D.C., 1977

26. Gamper M: Preparation for the Heir Minded, p 48. Illinois, Margaret Gamper, 1971

27. Bean CA: Methods of Childbirth, pp 103–104. New York, Dolphin Books, 1974

28. Liu YC: Effects of an upright position during labor. Am J Nurs 74:2202–2205, December 1974

29. Flynn AM, Kelly J, Hollins G: Ambulation in Labor. Br Med J 2:591–593, August 1978

30. Pace JB: Psychophysiology of pain: Diagnostic and therapeutic implications. J Fam Pract 1:4, May 1974

31. Augustinsson L-E, Bohlin P, Bundsen P, Carlsson CA, et al: Pain relief during delivery by transcutaneous electrical nerve stimulation. Pain 4:59–65, October 1977

32. Tawfik MO, Badraoui MHH: The value of transcutaneous nerve stimulation (TNS) during labour in Egyptian mothers. Pain (Suppl) 1:S146, 1981

33. Piva L et al: Transcutaneous electrical stimulation as a safe and useful method for pain relief in labour. Pain (Supp) 1:S142, 1981

34. Bandler RJ Jr, Madaras GR, Bem DJ: Self-observation as a source of pain perception. J Pers Soc Psychol 9:205–209, July 1968

35. Chertok L: Motherhood and Personality: Psychosomatic Aspects of Childbirth, pp 13–16. Philadelphia, Tavistock Publications and JB Lippincott, 1969

36. Miller J: Cognitive dissonance in modifying families' perceptions. Am J Nurs 74:1468–1470, August 1974

37. Wacker MS: Analogy: Weapon against denial. Am J Nurs 74:71–73, January 1974

Suggested Reading

Abouleish E, Depp R: Acupuncture in obstetrics. Current Research 54:83–88, 1975

Aleksandrowicz MK, Aleksandrowicz DR: Obstetrical pain-relieving drugs as predictors of infant behavior variability. Child Dev 47:294–296, 1974

Aleksandrowicz MK, Aleksandrowicz DR: Obstetrical pain-relieving drugs as predictors of infant behavior variability: A reply to Federman and Yang's critique. Child Dev 47:297–298, 1976

Angelini DJ: Nonverbal communication in labor. Am J Nurs 78:1220–1222, July 1978

Augustinsson L-E, Bohlin P, Bundsen P, Carlsson CA et al: Pain relief during delivery by transcutaneous electrical nerve stimulation. Pain 4:59–65, October 1977

Baer E, Davitz LJ, Lieb R: Inferences of physical pain and psychological distress. I. In relation to verbal and nonverbal patient communication. Nurs Res 19:388–392, September/October 1970

Bean CA: Methods of Childbirth. New York, Dolphin Books, 1974

Benson H, Beary JF, Carol MP: The relaxation response. Psychiatry 37:37–46, February 1974

Bing E: Six Practical Lessons for Easier Childbirth. New York, Grosset and Dunlap, 1967

Bonica JJ: The nature of pain in parturition. Clin Obstet Gynecol 2:499–516, 1975

Bonica JJ: Principles and Practice of Obstetric Analgesia and Anesthesia, Vol I. Philadelphia, FA Davis, 1967

Bonica JJ: Principles and Practice of Obstetric Analgesia and Anesthesia, Vol II. Philadelphia, FA Davis, 1969

Bowes WA, et al: The effects of obstetrical medication on fetus and infant. Monogr Soc Res Child Dev 35:1–55, 1970

Bradley RA: Husband-Coached Childbirth. New York, Harper & Row, 1974

Chertok L: Motherhood and Personality: Psychosomatic Aspects of Childbirth. Philadelphia, JB Lippincott, 1969

Clark AL, Howland R, Affonso D, Uyehare J: MCH in American Samoa. Am J Nurs 74:700–702, April 1974

Cogan R: Comfort during prepared childbirth as a function of parity, reported by four classes of participant observers. J Psychosom Res 19:33–37, 1975

Corah NL, Boffa J: Perceived control, self-observation, and response to aversive stimulation. J Pers Soc Psychol 16:1–4, September 1970

Cronenwett LR, Newmark LL: Fathers' responses to childbirth. Nurs Res 23:210–217, May/June 1974

Davenport–Slack B, Boylan CH: Psychological correlates of childbirth pain. Psychosom Med 36:215–223, May/June 1974

DeLyser F: A Professional's Guide to Prepared Childbirth. American Society for Psycho-Prophylaxis in Obstetrics, Washington, D.C., November 1973

Dick–Read G: Childbirth Without Fear. New York, Harper & Row, 1972

Diers D, Schmidt RL, McBride MA, Davis BL: The effect of nursing interaction on patients in pain. Nurs Res 21:419–428, September/October 1972

Dooher ME: Lamaze method of childbirth. Nurs Res 29:220–224, July/August 1980

Eppink H: Catheterizing the maternity patient. Am J Nurs 76:829, May 1975

Fagerhaugh SY, Strauss A: Politics of Pain Management: Staff-Patient Interaction. Menlo Park, CA, Addison–Wesley, 1977

Federman EJ, Yang RK: A critique of 'obstetrical pain-relieving drugs as predictors of infant behavior variability.' Child Dev 47:294–296, 1976

Field P-A: Relief of pain in labor. In Jacox, AK (ed): Pain: A Source Book for Nurses and Other Health Professionals, pp 427–434. Boston, Little, Brown, 1977

Fisher DE, Paton JB: The effect of maternal anesthetic and analgesic drugs on the fetus and newborn. Clin Obstet Gynecol 17:275–287, 1974

Gamper M: Preparation for the Heir Minded. Illinois, Margaret Gamper, 1971

Grad RK, Woodside J: Obstetrical analgesics and anesthesia: Methods of relief for the patient in labor. Am J Nurs 77:242–245, February 1977

Hackett TP: Pain and prejudice: Why do we doubt that the patient is in pain? Research Staff Physician 18:100–109, May 1972

Haire D: The Cultural Warping of Childbirth. International Childbirth Education Association Supplies Center, Seattle, Wash, 1974

Hassid P: Focus . . . on the behavioral responses. Am J Nurs 76:1244, August 1976

Hassid P: Textbook for Childbirth Educators. New York, Harper & Row, 1978

Henneborn WJ, Cogan R: The effect of husband participation on reported pain and probability of medication during labor and birth. J Psychosom Res 19:215–222, 1975

Hill SY, Schwin R, Goodwin DW, Powell BJ: Marihuana and pain. J Pharmacol Exp Ther 188:415–418, 1974

Hollingsworth AO, Brown LP, Brooten DA: The refugees and childbearing: What to expect. RN 43:44–48, November 1980

Hunter M, Philips C, Rachman S: Memory for pain. Pain 6:35–46, 1979

Johnson JE, Rice VH: Sensory and distress components of pain: Implications for the study of clinical pain. Nurs Res 23:203–209, May/June 1974

Johnson JM: Teaching self-hypnosis in pregnancy, labor, and delivery. American Journal of Maternal Child Nursing 5:98–101, March/April 1980

Joseph SS: Whatever happened to prepared childbirth? JOGN Nurs, pp 48–49, January/February 1975

Karmel M: Thank You, Doctor Lamaze. Philadelphia, JB Lippincott, 1959

Kitzinger S: Experience of Childbirth. London, Victor Gollancz, 1972

Kroger WS: Childbirth with Hypnosis. Hollywood, Wilshire Book, 1965

Lennane KJ, Lennane RJ: Alleged psychogenic disorders in women—A possible manifestation of sexual prejudice. N Eng J Med 288:288–292, February 1973

Leppert P, Williams B: Birth films may miscarry. Am J Nurs 68:2181–2183, October 1968

Liu YC: Effects of an upright position during labor. Am J Nurs 74:2202–2205, December 1974

Lubic RW, Ernst EKM: Psychological analgesia: Natural childbirth and psychoprophylaxis. Clin Obstet Gynecol 2:2–16, December 1975

Maternity Center Association: Preparation for Childbearing. New York, The Association, 1972

McCaffery M: Nursing Management of the Patient with Pain, 2nd ed. Philadelphia, JB Lippincott, 1979

McCaffery M: Relieving pain with noninvasive techniques. Nurs 80 10:55–57, December 1980

McCaffery M: When your patient's still in pain don't just do something: Sit there. Nurs 81 11:58–61, June 1981

McDonough M, Sheriff D, Zimmel P: Parents' responses to fetal monitoring. Journal of Maternal Child Nursing 6:32–34, January/February 1981

Melzack R: The Puzzle of Pain. New York, Basic Books, 1973

Nettelbladt P, Fagerstrom C-F, Uddenberg N: The significance of reported childbirth pain. J Psychosom Res 20:215–221, 1976

Neufeld RWJ, Davidson PO: The effects of vicarious and cognitive rehearsal on pain tolerance. J Psychosom Res 15:329–335, September 1971

The Pregnant Patient's Bill of Rights. Distributed by Committee on Patient's Rights, Box 1900, New York, NY 10001, ND

Redland A: Perineal splinting. Am J Nurs 76:1258, August 1976

Rowbotham CJF: Obstetric pain. Physiotherapy 60:103–106, April 1974

Sasmor JL, Castor CR, Hassid D: The child-birth team during labor. Am J Nurs 73:444–447, March 1973

Scott JS: Patient-controlled intravenous narcotic administration during labour. Lancet 1:251, January 1976

Shealy CN, Maurer D: Transcutaneous nerve stimulation for control of pain—A preliminary technical note. Surg Neurol 2:45–47, 1974

Shannon–Babitz M: Addressing the needs of fathers during labor and delivery. Am J of Maternal Child Nurs 4:378–382, November/December 1979

Siegele DS: The gate control theory. Am J Nurs 74:498–502, March 1974

Smith BA, Priore RM, Stern MK: The transition phase of labor. Am J Nurs 73:448–450, March 1973

Stevens RJ: Psychological strategies for management of pain in prepared childbirth: A study of psychoanalgesia in prepared childbirth. Birth and the Family Journal 4:4–9, Spring 1977

Swartz R: A father's view. Children Today 6:14–17, March/April 1977

Tanzer D: Natural childbirth: Pain or peak experience. Psychology Today 2:17–21, 69, October 1968

Ulin PR: Changing techniques in psychoprophylactic preparation for childbirth. Am J Nurs 68:2586–2591, December 1968

White JR: Effects of a counterirritant on perceived pain and hand movement in patients with arthritis. Phys Ther 53:956–960, September 1973

Williamson J: Hypnosis in obstetrics. Nursing Times 71:1895–1897, November 1975

Winsberg B, Greenlick M: Pain response in Negro and white obstetrical patients. J Health Soc Behav 8:222–227, September 1967

Wright E: The New Childbirth. New York, Hart Publishing, 1966

CHAPTER

27

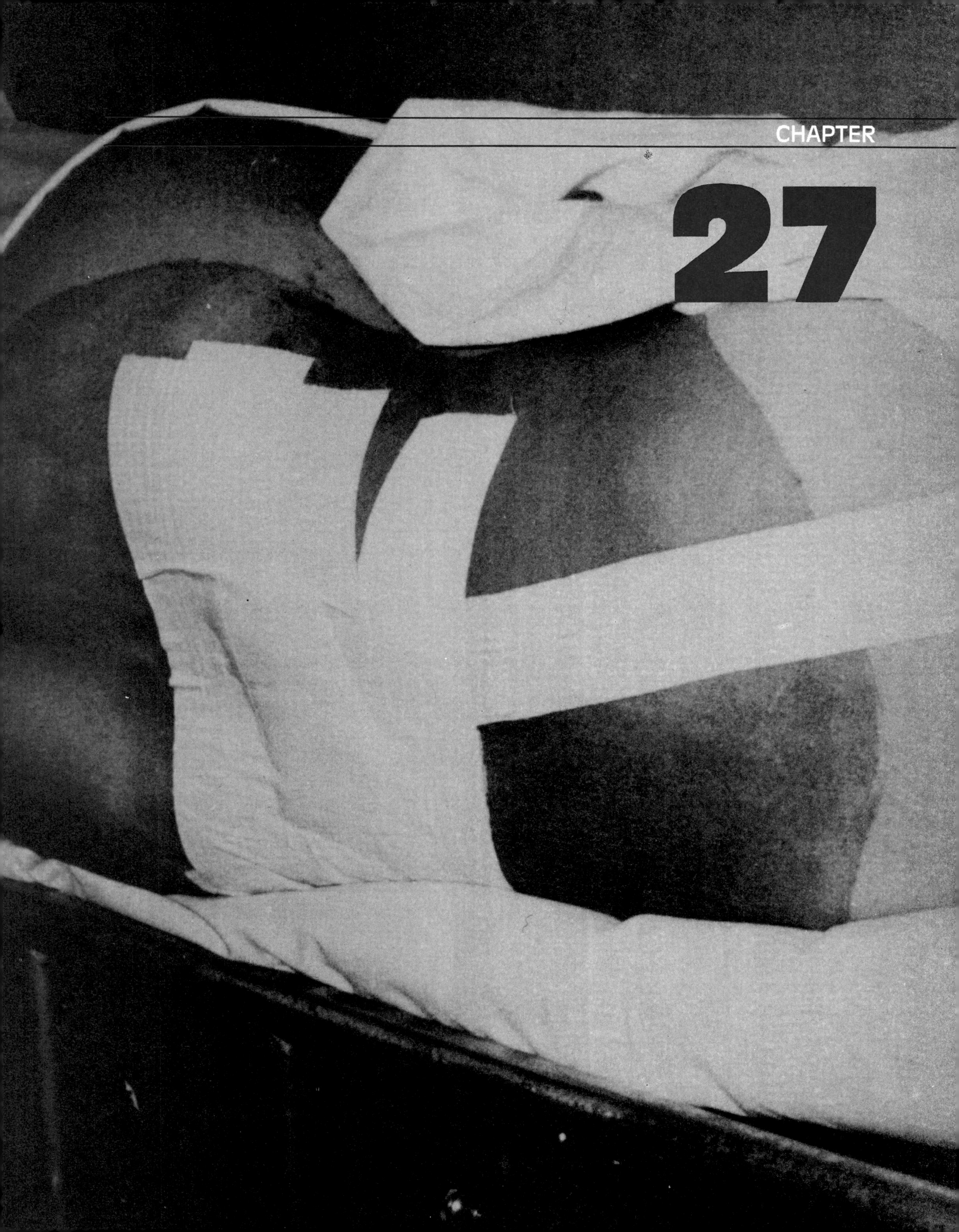

CHAPTER 27

Analgesia and Anesthesia for Childbirth

The discomfort and suffering endured by women during childbirth has been recounted in historical records since early civilizations. In Europe and in colonial America, women were imprisoned and even put to death for either seeking or providing pain relief during parturition. It was not until November 8, 1847, that James Young Simpson, a courageous 36-year-old obstetrician reported to the Edinburgh Medical and Chirurgical Society on the efficacy of chloroform to alleviate the pain associated with childbirth. Simpson was harshly criticized on theological grounds based on the Bible passage, Genesis 3:16:

> Unto the woman He said, I will greatly multiply thy sorrow and thy conception; in sorrow thou shalt bring forth children. . . .

It was not until six years later that obstetrical anesthesia was accepted and respectable. In 1853, the first fulltime physician anesthetist, John Snow, introduced "chloroform à la reine" when he attended the birth of Queen Victoria's eighth child, Prince Leopold, and administered chloroform analgesia for 53 minutes during labor. Snow again used chloroform for the anesthetic needs of his queen at the birth of Princess Beatrice in 1857. The monarch herself ended the need for women to suffer in childbirth by saying, "Dr. Snow gave that blessed chloroform and the effect was soothing, quieting and delightful beyond measure."

Despite the acceptance of obstetrical anesthesia, pain relief during childbirth was administered by persons untrained in the art and science of anesthesia. Anesthetic practices varied tremendously from area to area. Little thought was given to tailoring the anesthesia or analgesia to the specific needs of the laboring mother and the welfare of the fetus. New drugs producing analgesia, sedation, and anesthesia were often used for the first time in the parturient after few, if any, controlled studies. The concept of "twilight sleep," in which the mother was drugged to the state of oblivion (oftentimes lasting hours if not days into the postpartum period), came into vogue. To this, general anesthesia was frequently added at the time of delivery, primarily for the convenience of the obstetrician. The labor floor nurse or the nearest medical student, who was completely untrained and unaware of the dangers associated with general anesthesia, usually administered it. In some more "enlightened" centers, conduction or regional anesthesia was used by farsighted obstetricians who lacked training and support from their colleagues in anesthesia. Indeed, as late as 1962, it was estimated that in the United States 100 women died each year from pulmonary aspiration of stomach contents during the administration of general anesthesia for childbirth.

In the early 1950s, Dr. Virginia Apgar, then the Director of Anesthesia at Columbia Presbyterian Hospital in New York City, effectively addressed this problem. Although Apgar is better known for her evaluation of the newborn with the Apgar score, her realization that trained anesthesia personnel had as important a role to play on the labor floor as in the operating room is a greater contribution. Apgar's labors resulted in the first effective multidisciplinary teaching and research program devoted to obstetrical anesthesia. Her program encouraged the interest of many young anesthesiologists in the neglected area of obstetrical anesthesia. The program also provided the impetus for other well-known teaching institutes to establish similar fulltime anesthesia coverage for the labor floor and adequate training in obstetrical anesthesia for both nurses and physicians specializing in anesthesia.

In the past two decades there have been great improvements and advances in the field of obstetrical anesthesia. The Joint Commission on Accreditation of Hospitals has come to require that adequate and competent anesthesia coverage be available at all times on the labor floor. The American Board of Anesthesiology requires all residents to have adequate exposure to obstetrical anesthesia in order for a residency program to gain approval. Obstetricians and patients alike are recognizing the desirability of fulltime anesthesia coverage for parturition. Yet, we still have a long way to go before anesthesia on the labor floor is on a par with that in the operating room.

General Principles

> . . . The application of anesthesia to midwifery involves many more delicate problems than its mere applications to surgery. New rules must be established for its use, its effects upon the action of the uterus, upon the state of the child and on the puerperal state of the mother. These and other questions all require to be accurately studied and to be duly answered.

These words were spoken over a century ago by Sir James Y. Simpson. Many of the guidelines covering anesthesia for the surgical patient have little place on the labor floor. The psychological status of the obstetrical patient is usually different from her surgical counterpart's. Furthermore, unlike the surgical patient, the parturient is an active participant and her cooperation is needed in a vaginal delivery.

The administration of anesthetic and analgesic drugs affects not only the mother, but also the fetus and the newborn.

Despite the fact that pregnancy, labor, and delivery are considered normal physiological processes, the changes wrought by these physiological processes have the following profound implications for anesthetic techniques:

1. Pregnancy is associated with an increased sensitivity to most anesthetics, analgesics, and tranquilizers, which makes overdose more likely.
2. Because of the edema of the upper airway normally present in late pregnancy, the possibility of airway obstruction is increased.
3. Changes in pulmonary function and an increased oxygen requirement predispose the parturient to the rapid development of hypoxia, particularly in the second stage of labor or during induction of anesthesia. A 40% increase in pulmonary minute ventilation at term, which may increase further to 300% in the second stage of labor, makes induction of anesthesia with inhalation drugs rapid.
4. The effects of the use of medications during labor, and the fact that the maternity patient may have recently eaten, subject her to an increased risk of pulmonary aspiration of gastric contents with its devastating morbidity and mortality.
5. Changes in the cardiovascular system, particularly those associated with aorta caval compression by the gravid uterus, predispose the obstetrical patient to sudden hypotension and cardiovascular collapse and her fetus to hypoxia and acidosis at the time of general or major conduction anesthesia.

Pregnancy alters, and often exacerbates, the pathophysiology of many disease states, particularly those involving the cardiovascular and endocrine systems. Obstetrical emergencies, especially fetal distress and maternal hemorrhage, demand the rapid induction of anesthesia. Thus, although the parturient is usually considered a healthy young female undergoing a physiological process, she becomes a high anesthetic risk requiring markedly different considerations from those applied to the surgical patient. Failure to take these factors into account can result in a disaster for the mother and her fetus.

Cause of Discomfort During Labor and Delivery

The discomfort experienced during labor and delivery comes from two distinct sources. The pain associated with the first stage of labor is visceral and results from uterine contractions. As the uterus contracts, it causes dilatation (stretching) and effacement (thinning) of the cervix by the presenting part. In addition, uterine contractions constrict the arterial blood supply to the myometrium, causing uterine ischemia. It is the stretching of the cervix and uterine ischemia that cause discomfort. The pain is experienced over the lower abdomen and the lumbar area of the back and it may radiate into the thighs. Between contractions, the mother is pain-free.

In the second, or expulsive, stage of labor, uterine or *visceral* pain decreases as the cervix is completely dilated and effaced and is overshadowed by perineal or *somatic* pain. As the presenting part navigates the birth canal, it causes stretching of the vagina and perineum. When the uterus contracts in the second stage, forcing the presenting part down the birth canal, the mother has a reflex urge to bear down, bringing into play the secondary or ancillary forces of labor necessary to propel the fetus down the birth canal for a vaginal delivery.

Oversedation, general anesthesia or regional anesthesia of the perineum may delay or even prohibit vaginal delivery by abolishing the bearing-down reflex.

Selection of Anesthesia and Analgesia

Three factors should play a major role in deciding the anesthetic management of labor and delivery—the desires of the mother, the amount of discomfort experienced during labor and delivery, and the anesthesia personnel and facilities at hand. Ideally, the most appropriate form of pain relief should be available for each individual parturient.

Anesthesia is best tailored to the conditions surrounding the labor of each individual parturient. However, it is unwise for the obstetrician or the delivery room nurse to promise any particular type of analgesia. Furthermore, the mother should approach her labor with an open mind toward anesthesia. The patient should be aware that intervention with pharmacologic analgesia at times may be necessary in the best interest of both her and her fetus. She can be reassured that there is *no* evidence that modern tech-

Conditions of Ideal Obstetrical Analgesia and Anesthesia

Satisfactory alleviation of pain
No interference with normal labor or delivery
No undue risk to mother
Absent or minimal fetal and newborn depression
Safe conditions for delivery
Mother alert to allow early interaction with newborn

niques of analgesia and anesthesia have any prolonged or deleterious effects on the newborn, if they are administered properly. To the contrary, there is much evidence that properly conducted analgesia throughout labor may help to maintain a better respiratory, cardiovascular, and metabolic status for the mother. Routine use of any particular type of pain relief is also to be discouraged. When the woman arrives on the labor floor in early labor, she should be visited by those who will administer anesthesia and given further counseling and reassurance that her anesthetic needs will be met, as much in accordance with her own desires as possible. Only when this approach is used by all involved will optimal anesthesia be employed and contribute to a successful and fulfilling outcome.

Ideal analgesia or anesthesia for labor and delivery satisfies the following conditions:

1. It provides satisfactory alleviation of pain for the individual parturient.
2. It does not interfere significantly with the normal mechanics or progress of labor and delivery.
3. It is not associated with undue risk to the mother.
4. It is associated with minimal fetal and newborn depression.
5. It provides safe and satisfactory conditions for the delivery.
6. It allows early interaction between the mother and her newborn, preferably in the delivery room.

No single technique of pain relief fulfills all of the above objectives for every mother.

Nonpharmacologic Methods

Natural Childbirth

This term applies to a rather broad and general philosophy of labor management. Such methods are based upon the principle that, with careful prenatal education, along with support from the father and those attending the delivery, and the application of controlled breathing and voluntary muscle relaxation, the need for anesthesia and analgesia can be minimized or eliminated. The effectiveness of these methods is not based primarily on the physical techniques employed, but rather on the total involvement and acquired knowledge of the patient and the father, and the interest of the people supporting her.

The methods outlined by the British obstetrician Grantly Dick–Read have more recently been replaced in popularity by the Lamaze method, or psychoprophylaxis, an approach involving controlled breathing and active participation by the husband. Instructions in the use of such an approach are available in most areas through registered instructors. If such instruction is not available, there are a number of books which may be used. Such an approach is not applicable to all patients, and the key to a successful application of the technique is motivation. Those interested only because of intellectual curiosity and those who are talked into the idea generally do poorly.

In recent years, prepared or natural childbirth has become increasingly popular in the United States. Much of this growth is due to the desire of mothers to experience birth and to be able to relate to their newborn shortly after birth. In addition, both the medical profession and the lay public have come to realize that heavy sedation and narcosis used during labor may have prolonged and pronounced deleterious effects on the neonate.

Childbirth classes vary in emphasis and the material taught, but despite their diversity they have certain basic principles in common. The father or a trusted companion attends the classes with the mother. During labor and delivery this companion is with the mother to encourage and coach her. The mother is taught certain exercises, usually related to breathing and to bearing down, which she uses during contractions and delivery. The specific exercises and conditioning vary and, in general, serve to distract her from the painful aspects of childbirth. In the classes, which are usually attended during the latter half of pregnancy, the mother and her companion are taught the principles of labor and delivery. Attempts are made to correct misconceptions, to allay fears, and to make childbirth a fulfilling experience for both the mother and father. Finally, the prepared childbirth classes seek to minimize the need for the use of medications which can decrease the mother's awareness and cause newborn depression. Patients who select this approach should understand that, even though they may fail to get through their entire labor without anesthesia, they have still accomplished something and should not feel guilty. When used successfully, this approach can be a very rewarding experience for all concerned (see Chaps. 19 and 26).

Hypnosis

Hypnosis has been used sporadically for pain relief in both obstetrical and surgical patients. Hypnosis per se is not associated with maternal and neonatal depression. Enthusiasts claim that its use results in better maternal cooperation, reduces or eliminates the need for depressant drugs, decreases blood loss, provides postpartum analgesia, and aids in milk letdown in nursing mothers. The use of formal hypnosis requires that the subject enter a state of trance which is essentially a state of altered and focused attention and hypersuggestibility. The trance state is not associated with sleep but rather with increased attention. Narcotics, sedatives, and tranquilizers decrease the ability to reach a state of trance by decreasing the ability to concentrate. The depth of the hypnotic or trance state varies tremendously from individual to individual. A rare individual may be placed sufficiently deep to allow surgery with no other anesthesia. In others, the depth of trance state is minimal or nonexistent. The use of formal hypnosis requires preparation by a medical hypnotist well before the onset of labor and may require his or her presence throughout parturition. Some patients may be taught autohypnosis or self-induction of trance.

While formal hypnosis may not be available, informal hypnosis or hypnoidal techniques involving suggestion, encouragement, and reassurance are most valuable and can be safely used by both the nurses and physicians responsible for the care of the parturient. Examples of such techniques include using the term uterine "contractions" rather than uterine "pains," reassuring the mother that she can relax and rest between contractions, and having concerned and experienced medical personnel present throughout labor and delivery. The injection of one's understanding presence and encouragement may do far more than the injection of pharmacologic substances to alleviate anxiety and pain.

■■■

Pharmacologic Analgesia and Anesthesia

The pharmacologic techniques that are used to relieve pain during labor and delivery fall into four general categories—(1) systemic medication with narcotics, sedatives, tranquilizers, and amnestics; (2) inhalation analgesia with subanesthetic concentrations of inhalation drugs; (3) general anesthesia; and (4) regional or conduction anesthesia (*i.e.,* nerve block with local anesthetics).

Systemic Medication

Systemic medications, given intravenously or intramuscularly, are frequently used to decrease the pain and anxiety of the first stage of labor. In the past, this form of pain relief was selected because it is simple to administer. Small doses of systemic medications can be used with relative safety for the mother, although certain aspects of newborn neurobehavior may be modified for several days following their use in labor.

Narcotics or analgesics are the keystone of systemic medications. In general, equal analgesic doses of various narcotics produce equal amounts of depression in both mother and newborn. The major difference among the various narcotics is in the duration of their action. Knowledge of the duration of action allows the rational selection of the appropriate narcotic. If prolonged duration is desired, for example, in early labor, narcotics such as meperidine (Demerol) or morphine are indicated. If the narcotics are administered late in labor, when only a short duration of action is desired, short-acting narcotics such as fentanyl (Sublimaze) or alphaprodine (Nisentil) are appropriate.

Both the analgesic and the depressant properties of all the narcotics can be rapidly antagonized in mother and newborn by the use of naloxone (Narcan), a specific narcotic antagonist. Unlike the previous narcotic antagonists, nalorphine (Nalline) and levallorphan (Lorfan), naloxone has no narcotic or depressive activity of its own. It is useless in antagonizing depression from causes other than narcotics. The effective duration of naloxone is only about one hour. After its use, both the newborn and the mother must be carefully observed for signs of renarcotization, which can be treated with additional doses of the drug.

Naloxone should not be used in the mother to treat narcotic depression in the fetus shortly before birth unless another form of analgesia is first instituted because it rapidly antagonizes the analgesic activity of the narcotic. Furthermore, the effects of its use in a patient who has received a narcotic are unpleasant; its use is often associated with dyspnea as well as nausea and vomiting. It must be used with great caution in mothers who take narcotics chronically or habitually and in their newborns, as it can cause sudden and severe narcotic withdrawal. The usual dose of naloxone in the adult is 0.4 mg intramuscularly or intravenously and, in the newborn, 0.01 mg/kg similarly given.

Frequently a tranquilizer or sedative is administered with a narcotic. These drugs may produce sedation and alleviate anxiety. However, they add little, if any, analgesia and, if given in the presence of pain without adequate alternative analgesia, they produce confusion, disorientation, delirium, and uncontrollable behavior during contractions. Tranquilizers and sedatives also add to the depressant effects of narcotics in both mother and newborn. Finally, many of the commonly used tranquilizers, particularly the phenothiazines such as promethazine (Phenergan), have a long duration of action (6 hr–8 hr) and should not be repeated each time a narcotic is used. Scopolamine, a belladonna alkaloid and an anticholinergic, may be used in labor to produce sedation and amnesia. In the past, the desire for amnesia was common, but it is much less popular with maternity patients today. If administered in the presence of pain without adequate analgesia, scopolamine frequently produces delirium, excitement, and even hallucinations. When it is used, precautions must be taken to prevent patient injury. Scopolamine, while not associated with newborn depression, may cause fetal tachycardia, decreased fetal heart rate, beat-to-beat variability and may modify certain fetal heart rate decelerations. The anticholinesterase, physostigmine, antagonizes the maternal sedation and delirium associated with the use of scopolamine. It has also been claimed to antagonize these effects associated with the use of other tranquilizers such as the phenothiazines (*e.g.*, promethazine) and diazepam. Physostigmine is usually administered to the mother intravenously in 1-mg doses until the desired effect is obtained or the maternal heart rate falls below 70 beats per minute. Its efficacy and safety in the newborn have as yet to be determined.

In recent years the use of ketamine, a dissociative intravenous anesthetic, has found its way into obstetric anesthesia. Given in intravenous doses of 0.25 mg/kg (10 mg–15 mg), it produces profound analgesia lasting for 2 minutes to 5 minutes. Used in these quantities, the dosage may be repeated as needed, but not exceeding 1 mg/kg total before the birth of the baby. It is associated with minimal newborn depression, no appreciable effects on uterine activity, and few bad dreams or hallucinations. When ketamine is given alone or in combination with inhalation analgesia in doses of 0.25 mg/kg, the mother remains awake with upper airway reflexes intact. Larger doses are associated with newborn depression and loss of maternal consciousness, which predisposes the mother to the catastrophe of pulmonary aspiration of gastric contents unless her airway is protected with a cuffed endotracheal tube. Ketamine in analgesic doses is most often indicated at the time of delivery. Its use in combination with a pudendal block frequently allows the obstetrician to employ low forceps without the use of general anesthesia.

Inhalation Analgesia

Inhalation analgesia requires that the mother breathe subanesthetic concentrations of inhalation anesthetics. If the analgesia is administered properly, the mother remains conscious, yet has profound analgesia. Numerous inhalation anesthetic drugs have been used, including chloroform, ether, nitrous oxide, ethylene, cyclopropane, trichloroethylene (Trilene), methoxyflurane (Penthrane), and, more recently in this country, enflurane (Ethrane). Today in the United States, the two most commonly used inhalation drugs to produce analgesia in obstetrics are nitrous oxide and methoxyflurane.

Methoxyflurane

Inhalation analgesia may be administered in the first stage of labor. Because of its potency, methoxyflurane is usually administered in air in concentrations between 0.2% to 0.6%. The drug may be self-administered through a calibrated vaporizer such as the Duke Inhalor or the Cyprane Inhalor, held in the mother's hand and set at the desired concentration. A disposable inhalor, the Penthrane Analgizer, is also available for use with methoxyflurane. When the contraction begins, the mother breathes through the vaporizer until the contraction ends. After two or three contractions an adequate blood level is maintained to provide profound analgesia in a conscious patient who remains responsive and cooperative. This analgesia may be continued through delivery of the newborn, delivery of the placenta, and the immediate postpartum examination. The total amount of methoxyflurane administered throughout labor and delivery should not exceed 15 ml of liquid to avoid renal toxicity secondary to its breakdown in both mother and newborn to inorganic fluoride.

Nitrous Oxide

Since nitrous oxide is a gas at atmospheric conditions, it is stored under pressure in steel gas cylinders and must be administered through a calibrated anesthesia machine with oxygen by a trained physician or nurse. As 30% to 50% nitrous oxide is required to produce analgesia, it is given in a mixture of 50% to 70% oxygen. In the United Kingdom (during labor and delivery) midwives often give a 50% nitrous oxide,

50% oxygen mixture called Entonox that has been premixed in cylinders. In the United States, nitrous oxide analgesia is usually administered in the delivery room by a nurse or physician during the latter part of the first stage of labor and for delivery of the baby, the placenta and the immediate postpartum examination. While intermittent administration of nitrous oxide analgesia during contractions is still used, it is more effective when administered continuously in 30% to 50% concentration with oxygen.

Advantages and Disadvantages

Inhalation analgesia provides profound but not complete analgesia for labor and delivery. Used alone, it often produces adequate pain relief for labor and uncomplicated vaginal delivery without episiotomy. If an episiotomy is to be performed and repaired or use of forceps is anticipated, the obstetrician should supplement inhalation analgesia with local infiltration of the perineum, or better still a bilateral pudendal block. In addition to analgesia, inhalation analgesia often provides amnesia, particularly for painful events.

If inhalation analgesia is properly administered, it has many advantages and is extremely safe for mother and newborn. Maternal and newborn depression is not produced in measurable degree by subanesthetic concentrations of inhalation drugs, regardless of the duration of their administration. The mother remains awake with upper airway reflexes intact and is protected from catastrophe of pulmonary aspiration of gastric contents without the need for intubation. The mother's reflex urge and ability to bear down in the second stage of labor are little affected. The onset of inhalation analgesia is rapid and the degree of analgesia can be altered quickly by changing the inspired concentration of the inhalation drug. It can be given safely to nearly every parturient and may be used to supplement other forms of analgesia, particularly regional or conduction anesthesia.

Despite its advantages, however, inhalation analgesia does have drawbacks. The amount of inhalation drug required for adequate analgesia varies from mother to mother and indeed for the same mother throughout the various phases of labor. She may pass from the stage of analgesia and amnesia (first stage anesthesia) into the stage of delirium and excitement (second stage of anesthesia) or even into the stage of surgical anesthesia (third stage of anesthesia), with loss of protective airway reflexes, subjecting her to the danger of pulmonary aspiration and her fetus to newborn anesthetic depression. *It is imperative that a fully trained nurse or physician always be present when inhalation analgesia is used.*

Inhalation analgesia does not produce complete analgesia. Except for the uncomplicated vaginal delivery, it must be supplemented. Even then, adequate analgesia and patient cooperation may not be satisfactory. Increasing the concentration of the inhalation drug often results in excitement and activity or general anesthesia with its attendant problems. When a patient receiving inhalation analgesia is delirious and uncooperative, this is often an indication that too much inhalation drug is being administered; this can be corrected rapidly by decreasing the concentration of the inhalation drug.

General Anesthesia

General anesthesia is rarely, if ever, indicated for uncomplicated vaginal delivery. Indeed most vaginal deliveries are more safely performed with other forms of analgesia or anesthesia. Obstetricians today are coming to realize that vaginal delivery with general anesthesia is fraught with many serious complications. Fortunately, women of the childbearing age are now less inclined to request that they be "put under" for delivery. Rather, they want to take part in the delivery and frequently wish the baby's father to be present in the delivery room to share the joy of birth. These changing attitudes deserve to be encouraged and supported by all those involved in the care of the mother-to-be.

Disadvantages

The disadvantages of general anesthesia in obstetrics are many. General anesthesia prevents the mother from participating in the birth of her baby and relating with her newborn at birth. When used for vaginal delivery, it cannot be administered until the baby is deliverable because it immediately stops the bearing down reflex of the second stage of labor. In addition, the newborn, like the mother, is depressed by the anesthetic. Despite occasional statements to the contrary, controlled studies indicate that neonatal depression following general anesthesia for delivery is directly proportional to the depth of anesthesia and the length of the interval from induction of anesthesia to the delivery of the baby. While this depression from general anesthesia is usually rapidly overcome by ventilatory support of the newborn, it may compound depression from other sources. If the interval from induction of anesthesia to the delivery of the newborn is kept to less than 10 minutes with "light anesthesia," newborn depression from well administered general anesthesia is minimal.

General anesthesia predisposes the parturient to the dreadful complication of pulmonary aspiration of gastric contents. Every parturient is at risk of this catastrophe because her stomach is rarely empty, the gastroesophageal junction may not function as a result of changes in gastric position caused by the gravid uterus, and the gravid uterus and lithotomy position increase intragastric pressure.

General anesthesia for any woman in the third trimester of pregnancy necessitates intubation with a cuffed endotracheal tube. The endotracheal tube should be inserted either before induction or immediately after a rapid induction during which cricoid pressure (Sellick's maneuver) is applied from the time of the loss of consciousness until intubation (Fig. 27-1). General anesthesia for the parturient without endotracheal intubation is unacceptable anesthetic practice today.

Indication for General Anesthesia

Despite the numerous disadvantages and problems associated with the use of general anesthesia for delivery, its proper use with rapid induction by a skilled anesthetist may result in the delivery of a healthy baby and the prevention of maternal morbidity and mortality. In certain circumstances, general anesthesia is the only form of anesthesia that can provide adequate conditions for the obstetrician to deliver the newborn rapidly and safely. The immediate availability of a skilled anesthetist who is provided with proper equipment and assistance in the obstetrical suite is a primary requirement for good obstetrical care.

The indications for general anesthesia for vaginal delivery include the following:

1. Fetal distress, which demands immediate delivery and which can be safely accomplished by the vaginal route; often the use of inhalation analgesia supplemented by local infiltration of the perineum or pudendal block provides satisfactory conditions for such a delivery
2. When a parturient becomes uncontrollable during delivery
3. When a parturient refuses regional or other forms of analgesia or anesthesia, or when these forms of pain relief are contraindicated
4. The need for rapid depression of uterine activity

Indications for General Anesthesia

- Fetal distress, which demands immediate delivery
- Uncontrollable parturient during delivery
- Patient's preference for general anesthesia and refusal of alternative methods
- Tetanic uterine contractions that require depression

Depression of uterine activity may be indicated to abolish a tetanic uterine contraction, which is usually the result of too large a dose of oxytocin given during induction or augmentation of labor. It may also be required to allow intrauterine manipulation for the extraction of a distressed second twin or removal of a retained placenta. Although ether and all of the halogenated inhalation anesthetic drugs can depress uterine activity, halothane, given initially in a 2% concentration, or enflurane, given initially in a 3% concentration, is usually favored because the onset of its effect is rapid and its action is predictable.

Techniques for General Anesthesia

While the scope of this chapter does not allow a discussion of techniques of general anesthesia, the following points concerning its use should be emphasized.

1. Patients in the third trimester of pregnancy who require general anesthesia need to be intubated

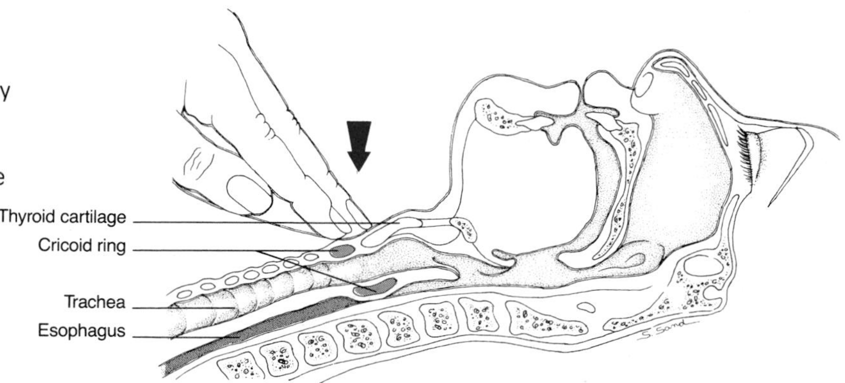

Figure 27-1.
The technique of cricoid pressure (Sellick's maneuver) prevents pulmonary aspiration of gastric contents during anesthesia induction. The esophagus is compressed and occluded between the cricoid ring of the trachea and the bodies of the cervical vertebrae. Pressure is applied as soon as the patient loses consciousness and is maintained until the trachea is intubated with a cuffed endotracheal tube.

during anesthesia to protect against the risk of pulmonary aspiration of gastric contents. The time interval from the last ingestion of food or the onset of labor to the time of induction of general anesthesia is of no value in determining the risk of aspiration. The use of oral antacids during labor does not lessen the need for intubation when general anesthesia is used.

2. The extent of newborn depression is directly proportional to the induction-to-delivery interval. General anesthesia is induced only when the obstetrician is ready. Delivery should be accomplished as rapidly thereafter as is in keeping with good obstetrical principles. Nothing is gained by delaying delivery after induction to allow the drug to be removed from the fetus. Such delay only exposes the fetus to more depressant anesthetic drug.
3. The plane of anesthesia sought before delivery is that which provides maternal analgesia and amnesia. Favorable surgical conditions and prevention of movement are provided by the use of minimal amounts of skeletal muscle relaxants such as succinylcholine and curare. If used in large doses, nondepolarizing relaxants such as curare may cross the placenta in amounts sufficient to depress newborn skeletal muscle activity.
4. Oxygen should make up more than 50% of the inspired maternal anesthetic mixture before birth to assure more vigorous and better oxygenated newborns. To ensure maternal analgesia and amnesia, the addition of low concentrations of potent inhalation drugs such as 0.5% halothane, 0.75% to 1% enflurane or 0.2% to 0.5% methoxyflurane added to 30% to 40% nitrous oxide is required.
5. While adequate maternal ventilation is to be assured, marked maternal hyperventilation as regulated by the anesthetist must be avoided until birth of the newborn, since hyperventilation is associated with decreased uterine blood flow and fetal acidosis.
6. Left uterine displacement must be maintained at all times until the birth of the newborn to avoid aorta-caval compression with its associated decreased maternal cardiac output and hence depressed uterine blood flow.
7. Following delivery, the depth of maternal anesthesia may be increased by increasing the concentration of nitrous oxide and giving narcotics. The concentration of the potent inhalation drugs should not be increased because this may cause depressed uterine contraction and may be associated with increased maternal blood loss.
8. The same quality of anesthetic care must be available to the parturient as it is to the surgical patient. This includes adequate monitoring during anesthesia and adequate postoperative observation.
9. When general anesthesia is required in an emergency, it is usually in the mother's interest to wait until qualified anesthesia personnel are available or to proceed with an alternative form of anesthesia. Nurses and physicians who are not fully trained and competent in anesthesia should not attempt to administer general anesthesia.

Regional Anesthesia

Regional or conduction anesthesia is ideally suited to vaginal delivery. If the complications of hypotension and local anesthetic toxicity are avoided, it is associated with minimal newborn depression and a mother who is awake and free from pain and capable of relating to her newborn baby immediately following birth. Awake, she is unlikely to aspirate gastric contents and can cooperate with the obstetrician. Except when uterine relaxation is required, regional analgesia can provide complete pain relief and suitable conditions for both vaginal and abdominal delivery.

The primary neuropathways of pain and methods of effectively blocking them with local anesthetics are illustrated in Fig. 27-2. Uterine pain, resulting from dilatation and effacement of the cervix and from uterine contractions, is conveyed by small nerve fibers which pass from the cervix diffusely through the pelvis, join the sympathetic chain at L2 to L5 and enter the spinal cord at T10 to T12. These pain fibers can be blocked effectively by a paracervical block at the cervix, by a bilateral lumbar sympathetic block at L2 or by a segmental lumbar epidural block from T10 to T12. Vaginal and perineal pain, associated with the second and third stages of labor, is mediated primarily through the pudendal nerve originating from S2 to S4. There is additional perineal innervation from the genitofemoral, ilioinguinal, and lateral femoral cutaneous nerves. Pudendal nerve block, true "saddle block" (subarachnoid or "spinal" block), (S1 to S5) and low caudal epidural block (S1 to S5) alleviates most of the vaginal and perineal pain. A combination of blocks or a subarachnoid, lumbar epidural, or caudal epidural block from T10 to S5 provides relief of all pain during labor and delivery.

Disadvantage

Despite its many advantages, regional anesthesia has disadvantages and requires constant observation of the mother if it is to be safe and effective. Recent work has suggested that both the local anesthetics lidocaine (Xylocaine) and mepivacaine (Carbocaine) may be associated with minimally depressed neonatal tone at birth which resolves rapidly. This has not been observed with the use of the local anesthetics bupivacaine (Marcaine) and chloroprocaine hydrochloride (Nesacaine).

The newer amide local anesthetics lidocaine, mepivacaine, and bupivacaine have a prolonged half-life in maternal and neonatal blood due to their slow metabolism by the liver. This causes no difficulty in routine use, as levels usually remain well below toxic levels. However, repeated injection of these drugs, as in the case of continuous lumbar and caudal epidural anesthesia, can result in increasing blood levels in both mother and fetus. This is not a problem with the older ester type local anesthetics, such as procaine and chloroprocaine hydrochloride, which are rapidly metabolized to nontoxic products by the enzyme pseudocholinesterase, normally found in both maternal and fetal blood.

Local anesthetics administered during labor may decrease fetal heart rate beat-to-beat variability, making fetal heart rate evaluation more difficult. This action of local anesthetics has not been associated with deleterious effects on the newborn and is shared by other drugs including the narcotics, tranquilizers, and anticholinergics.

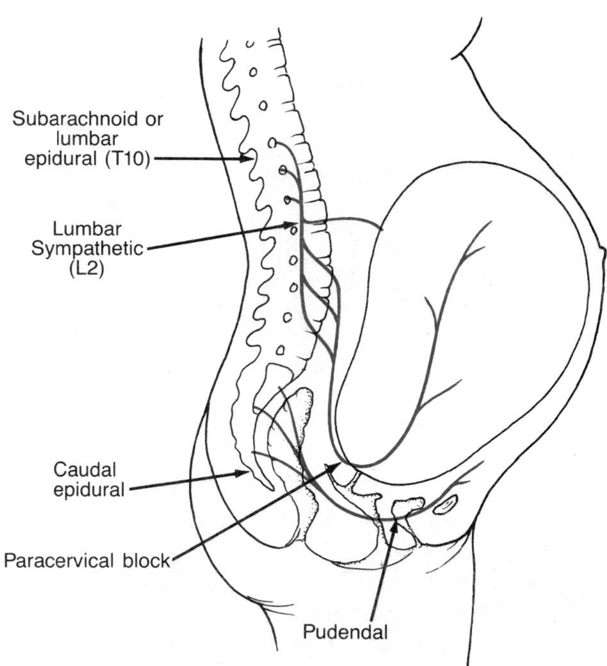

Figure 27-2.
Pain pathways during labor and appropriate techniques of nerve block. (After Bonica J J: Principle and Practice of Obstetric Analgesia and Anesthesia. Philadelphia, F A Davis, 1967)

Nursing Implications

The use of regional anesthesia in the obstetrical patient requires constant monitoring during labor, delivery and in the postpartum period by a trained maternity nurse. An accurate record of maternal vital signs must be kept (Fig. 27–3). A reliable intravenous infusion must be maintained at all times. The personnel and means to assure a clear airway and apply positive pressure ventilation with oxygen and the ability to treat local anesthetic reactions, high levels of block, and maternal hypotension must be immediately available if serious problems to both mother and fetus are to be avoided. Continuous recorded electronic monitoring of fetal heart rate and uterine contractions should be considered when regional anesthesia is used in the first stage of labor. Such monitoring is indicated in the high-risk pregnancy or when regional anesthesia is used for the mother receiving oxytocin stimulation.

Paracervical Block

Paracervical block is produced by injection of small quantities of dilute local anesthetic solution into the parametrium at sites in the cervix of 3 o'clock and 9 o'clock or 4 o'clock and 8 o'clock (Fig. 27–4). It provides rapid complete relief of uterine pain with minimal maternal side-effects. Paracervical block does not affect vaginal and perineal sensation and therefore does not interfere with the bearing-down reflex of the second stage of labor. Unfortunately, paracervical block has been associated with fetal bradycardia, fetal acidosis, and even fetal death. These untoward fetal effects are thought to be caused by the local anesthetic passing rapidly through the placenta to the fetus secondary to absorption through the uterine artery. There is also evidence that proximity of the local anesthetic to the uterine artery may result in vasoconstriction of the uterine artery with decreased uteroplacental perfusion. The danger to the fetus can be minimized by using minimal doses of the less toxic local anesthetics such as 2-chloroprocaine and by injecting them superficially and laterally in the parametrium.

The use of paracervical block is a good indication for continuous electronic fetal heart monitoring. Paracervical block is best avoided in the premature fetus and in the fetus at high risk.

Lumbar Sympathetic Block

Like paracervical block, a bilateral lumbar sympathetic block at L2 abolishes uterine pain only. While this mode of anesthesia is associated with maternal hypotension, such a reaction is usually minimal and can be avoided by providing adequate hydration and left

SEEN 7³⁰/AM – D.D.

20868 **HOSPITAL OF THE UNIVERSITY OF PENNSYLVANIA – OBSTETRIC ANESTHESIA RECORD**

Patient's Name: M B	B. P.: 110/70 - 120/80	Pulse: 88	Temp.: 99 4/0 F	Drug Reactions: NONE
History No. 335726 - 2111	Race: BLACK	Height: 5' 8"	Weight: 193 lbs.	Consent: SELF
Age 24 Date NOV. 22, 1982	Hct. or Hgb.: – 34%	Rh. Factor: O+	Grav.: III	Para.: I
Procedure: OUTLET FORCEPS DELIV. EPLS REPAIR	Time and Nature of Last Oral Intake: SOLIDS 7⁰⁰AM NOV. 22		E. D. C.: NOV. 20, 1982	
Anesthetists: D.D. / BBG	Location: DR #2	Onset of Labor: 5⁰⁰AM NOV. 22	Signif. Meds.: AEP. ASTHMA	

Physical Status: I Emergency: NO

Times: X 9⁴⁵/AM ⊙ 11³⁴/PM ⊗ 12⁰⁵/PM

Obstetricians: R.R. / R.P.

Obstetric Diagnosis: TERM INTRAUTERINE PREG.

Pre-Anesthetic Condition: HISTORY OF SEASONAL ASTHMA Rx c̄ A.E.P. LAST ATTACK SEPT. '82. MODERATE OBESITY – 30 Lb. WT. GAIN c̄ PREGNANCY

Time	45	10⁰⁰AM	30	11⁰⁰AM	30	12⁰⁰N	30
Cervical Dilatation	5	6	8	10			
O2	10 LIT – NRB MASK						
Anesthetics m/ 1/4% MAR	2+8						
Anesthetics m/ 1/2% MAR				2+10			
Fluids D5½ NS	500		1000				1300
Level of Block		T10		T9-S5			T9
Maternal Position	(L.U.D)						
Monitoring	EXT UC	INT EHR					

Blood Pressure V Λ; Mat. Pulse Rate •; Fetal Heart Rate; Start Stop Anes. X; Start Surgery ⊙; End ⊗

Scale: 180, 160, 140, 120, 100, 80, 60, 40, 20, 0

Chart markers: X 1 2 ⊙ ⊗ 3 RR

Medications During Labor

Drug and Dose	Route	Time
DEMEROL 50	IV	8³⁰/A
PHENERGAN 25	IV	8³⁰/A

Infant Data	Infant #1		Infant #2	
Weight (GM)	3090			
Sex	MALE			
Time of Delivery	11³⁴/AM			
Time To Sust. Resp.	< 30 SEC.			
Apgar	1 Min.	5 Min.	1 Min.	5 Min.
Heart Rate	2	2		
Respiration	2	2		
Reflex	2	2		
Muscle Tone	1	2		
Color	1	1		
Total (0 - 10)	8	9		

Time Placenta Expressed

Abnormalities NONE

Manual Spont. 11³⁸/A

N.B. Resuscitation, Methods, Drugs, Congenital Abnormalities: SUCTION, O_2 BY FACE MASK, STIMULATION

Condition on Leaving O.R. GOOD (REG. NUR.)

OXYTOCICS	Dose	Rte.	Time
PITOCIN	5U	IV PUSH	11³⁹
PITOCIN	15U	IV BOT	11³⁹

Agents	1/4% MARCAINE	1/2% MARCAINE	EPHEDRINE
	10 CC TOTAL	12 ml TOTAL	10 MG IV
Tech.	VIA EPIDURAL CATH.		HYPOTENSION

Remarks: X BEGIN CONTINUOUS EPIDURAL I2 & ALCOHOL PREP LOC INFILT 5mg MARCAINE. ENTER EPIDURAL SPACE c̄ EASE AT L3-4 18g HUSTEAD NEEDLE, INSERT CATH. REMOVE NEEDLE. NO HEME. OR CSF ASPIRATED.

1) EPHEDRINE 10mg IV FOR MAT. HYPOTENSION

2) COMPLETE DILITATION – SITTING DOSE – TAKE TO DEL. RM.

3) REMOVE EPIDURAL CATH. INTACT

Airway Nat.	OP.	NP.
Intub.	OT	NT
Blade	CR	ST

Complications of Labor & Delivery: NONE

Est. Bl. Loss .350 Ml.

Length of Labor Stages 6 1st (Hr) 19 2nd (Min) 4 3rd (Min)

Obstetric Complications: NONE

Form 055095 2/78

STUDY COPY

Figure 27-3.
Obstetric anesthesia record during the course of continuous epidural anesthesia for labor and delivery. Note frequency of recordings of maternal vital signs.

uterine displacement. Lumbar sympathetic block is associated with minimal, if any, fetal and newborn depression, which makes its use acceptable in the high-risk pregnancy. Bilateral sympathetic block may result in improved uterine contraction because it interrupts the sympathetic innervation of the uterus which inhibits uterine activity. Since the block is rather complicated and somewhat painful to administer, it is not widely used.

Pudendal Block

Of all the regional anesthetic blocks for vaginal delivery, bilateral pudendal nerve block is perhaps the safest and one of the most useful available. Although pudendal block provides no relief of uterine pain and no analgesia for cervical or uterine manipulations, it does alleviate most of the vaginal and perineal pain associated with delivery. It produces adequate analgesia for episiotomy and repair and allows most uncomplicated outlet forceps deliveries. When supplemented with inhalation analgesia, it usually produces adequate analgesia for other types of forceps deliveries. Since pudendal block does not completely anesthetize the perineum, it does not completely abolish the bearing-down reflex of the second stage of labor. It is relatively painless to administer and when local anesthetic toxicity is avoided, it has essentially no ill effects on the mother or her newborn. Pudendal block is not associated with maternal hypotension and is the only technique of conduction anesthesia that does not affect autonomic innervation of the uterus.

The pudendal nerve runs just lateral to the tips of the ischial spines, the obstetric landmarks which determine the station of the presenting part. It may be blocked from either the transvaginal approach (Fig. 27–5), most commonly used in obstetrics, or from the transcutaneous route. A bilateral block requires only 10 ml to 20 ml of a dilute local anesthetic solution, such as 1% lidocaine or 1% chloroprocaine hydrochloride, and is usually administered by the obstetrician or midwife who is delivering the baby.

Spinal Anesthesia

Subarachnoid or "spinal" block is one of the most useful blocks for obstetrics and is technically easy to administer (Fig. 27–6). The amount of drug needed is less than that required for any other block used in obstetrics—about one fifth that required to produce the same level of anesthesia by the epidural route. Thus, local anesthetic toxicity in both mother and fetus is not a problem. Onset of anesthesia is very rapid, usually complete within 5 minutes. Essentially every obstetric procedure not requiring depression of uterine activity can be accomplished with subarachnoid block. Late in labor a true saddle block of the perineum (S1 to S5) allows forceps delivery and repair of episiotomy. If a modified saddle block (T10 to S5) is produced, both uterine as well as perineal discomfort are completely abolished. Long-acting local anesthetics such as tetracaine (Pontocaine) with epinephrine produce 3 hours of pain relief when injected into the subarachnoid space, permitting elimination of all pain in the latter part of labor and for delivery. Increasing the level of block to T4 or higher produces satisfactory anesthesia for cesarean birth.

Disadvantages. The major disadvantages of subarachnoid block are its potential for causing maternal hypotension, total spinal block, postspinal headache, the abolishment of the reflex urge to bear down in the

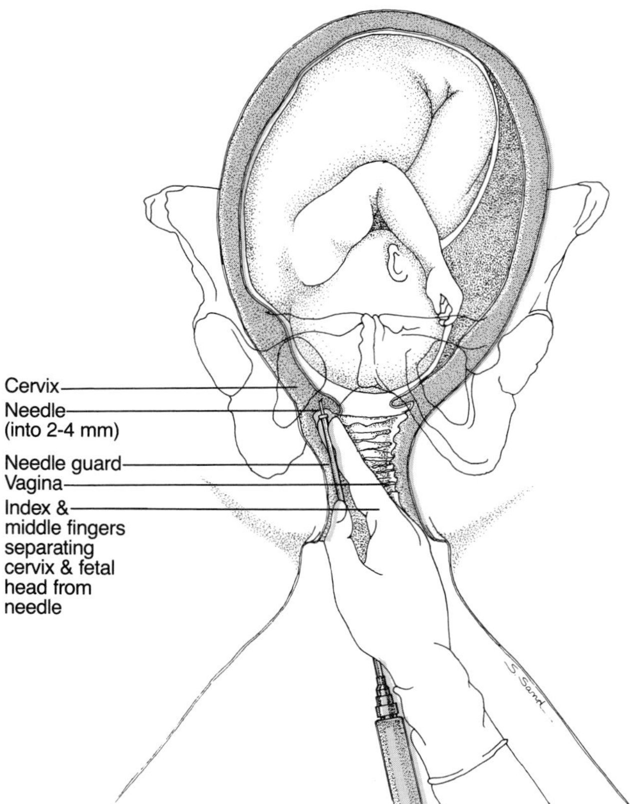

Figure 27-4.
Technique of paracervical block. Five ml of dilute local anesthetic solution is injected superficially into the vaginal fornix at 3 and 9 o'clock *or* at 4 and 8 o'clock.

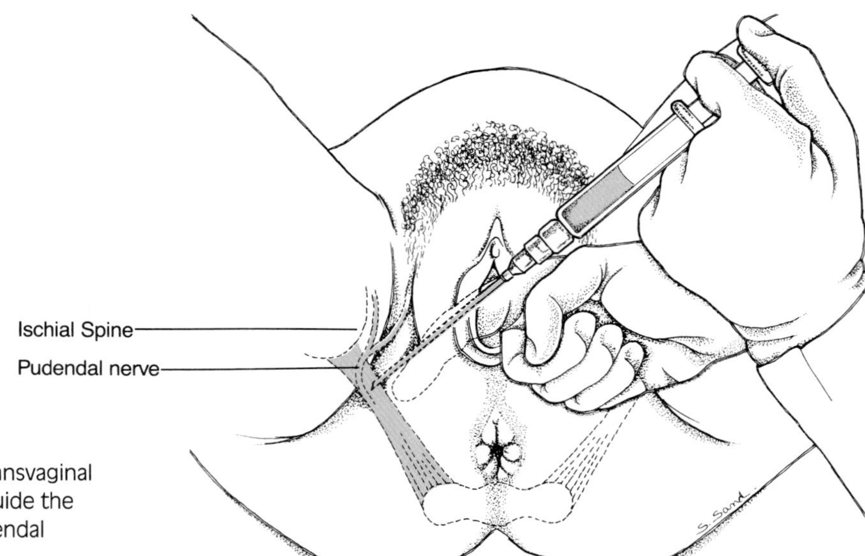

Figure 27-5.
Pudendal block technique by the transvaginal approach. The examiner's fingers guide the needle to the ischial spine; the pudendal nerve is lateral to the spine at its tip.

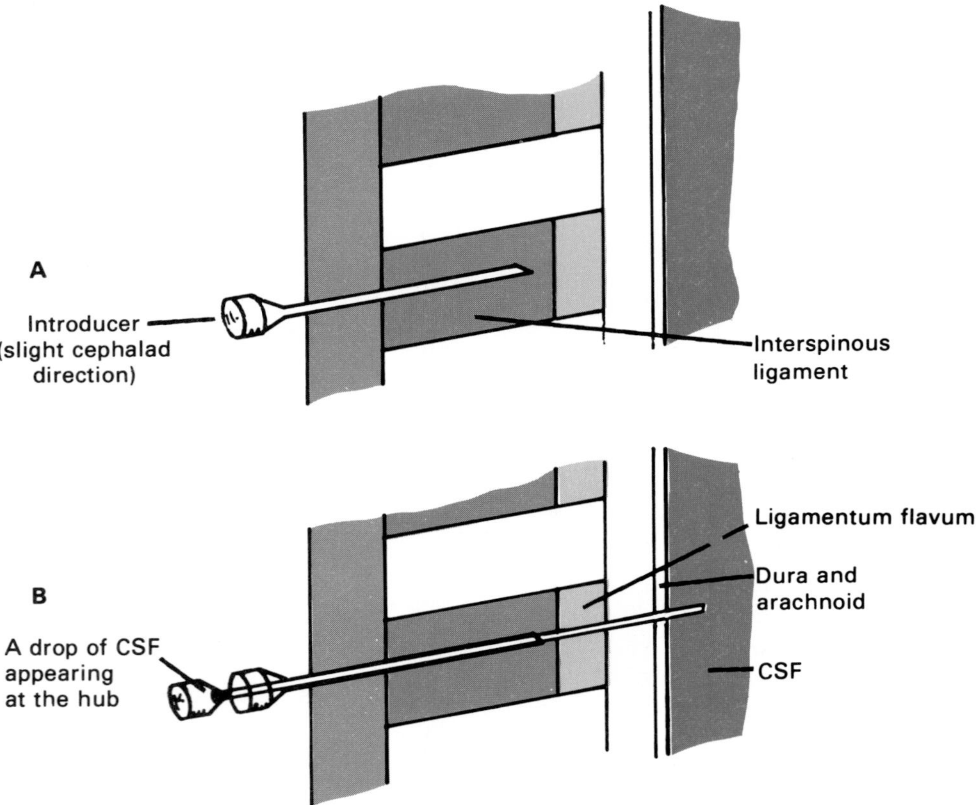

Figure 27-6.
Technique of subarachnoid (spinal) block. The small 25- or 26-gauge spinal needle transverses the epidural space and pierces the dura and arachnoid to enter the subarachnoid space that contains the cerebral spinal fluid. Local anesthetic injected subarachnoid acts on the spinal nerve roots within the subarachnoid space.

second stage of labor, and early relaxation of the perineal musculature, which can result in persistent occiput posterior presentation.

Severe and sudden maternal hypotension which leads to fetal distress and maternal cardiovascular collapse due to vasodilatation, secondary to sympathetic block, is still a significant cause of maternal mortality. Prophylaxis includes left uterine displacement and hydration with a liter or more of balanced salt solution administered intravenously 15 minutes to 30 minutes before the block is instituted. Treatment of hypotension includes these two steps as well as the use of a central acting vasopressor, such as ephedrine (10 mg–25 mg given intravenously), and the administration of high concentrations of oxygen. Potent peripheral vasoconstrictors such as norepinephrine (Levophed), phenylephrine (Neo-Synephrine), and methoxamine (Vasoxyl) rapidly correct maternal hypotension but are to be avoided because they cause further decline in uterine perfusion, resulting in additional fetal distress.

Total or dangerously high levels of subarachnoid block usually result when the subarachnoid injection is made just before or during a uterine contraction or when too larger a dose of local anesthetic is used. The same level of block can be obtained in the obstetric patient with only two thirds of the amount of drug required to produce a given level in her nonpregnant counterpart. Treatment of a high block consists of immediate correction of hypotension, support of maternal ventilation with positive pressure oxygen and, if necessary, protection of the upper airway with a cuffed endotracheal tube. With proper therapy a high or total spinal need not delay delivery and should not be associated with increased maternal or fetal morbidity or mortality.

The incidence of postspinal headache is highest in the postpartum patient. An incidence of over 40% can be expected when the subarachnoid space is entered with a 20-gauge or larger bore needle. The headache usually occurs within 24 hours to 72 hours of the subarachnoid block, may last a few days to several weeks, and can be mild to incapacitating. The headache inevitably resolves. It is positional and is characteristically exacerbated in the upright position and relieved by assuming the supine position or by increasing abdominal pressure. It is caused by loss of cerebral spinal fluid through the hole made in the dura mater and pia-arachnoid by the spinal needle. Steps to prevent post spinal headaches include using small-gauge needles (25-gauge or less), adequate hydration during the postpartum, and using a tight abdominal binder when the patient is in the upright position. Treatment consists of appropriate analgesics, bedrest, preferably in the prone position with the head down, hydration, a tight abdominal binder, and reassurance. When the headache is incapacitating, "epidural blood patch," which consists of sealing the hole in the dura by injecting the patient's own non-anticoagulated blood into the epidural space, can result in a dramatic cure.

Abolishment of the reflex urge to bear down in the second stage of labor results from the complete perineal analgesia produced by subarachnoid block. It does not prevent the parturient from bearing down voluntarily with each contraction. In cases of occiput posterior presentation, the tone in the muscles of the perineum causes the occiput to rotate to the anterior presentation. As subarachnoid block does produce profound relaxation of the perineum, an increased incidence of persistent occiput posterior presentations can be expected with its use. Since perineal relaxation occurs, the occiput can usually be easily rotated manually or delivery can be accomplished in the occiput posterior position.

Epidural Anesthesia

Epidural anesthesia is carried out by introducing anesthetic agent into the epidural space.

The epidural space (Fig. 27-7) is a potential space filled with loose fatty tissue and a marked plexus of veins. It is the space in the vertebral canal that is surrounded by the ligamentous and bony structure of the vertebral canal on the outside and the dura containing the cerebrospinal fluid and the spinal cord on the inside. The uppermost limit of the epidural space is the foramen magnum at the base of the skull; interiorly it ends at the sacral hiatus at the base of the sacrum. It may be entered at any of the intervertebral spaces from the cervical area C1–2 to the L1–S1 interspace or through the sacral hiatus. As the nerve roots leave the spinal cord, they pass through the epidural space and hence are exposed to a local anesthetic injected in the epidural space.

Injection of local anesthetic through the sacral hiatus is referred to as caudal epidural block. Because the sacral hiatus is located low in the vertebral column, the anesthetic agent reaches the sacral nerves first, resulting in perineal anesthesia initially. In order to provide relief during contractions, additional amounts of agent must be introduced at the level of the lumbar and low thoracic nerves.

When the anesthetic agent is introduced at the lumbar level, the technique is referred to as a lumbar epidural anesthesia. Lumbar epidural anesthesia has largely replaced caudal epidural anesthesia in obstetrics. The latter is technically more difficult to perform, requires three to four times as much anes-

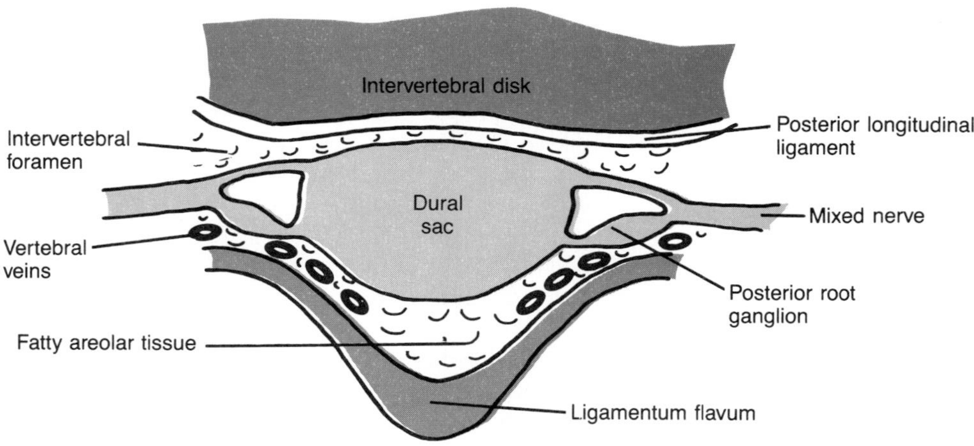

Figure 27-7.
Diagrammatic cross section of the vertebral canal showing the contents of the epidural space. Note the prominent epidural veins. Local anesthetic injected into the epidural space primarily blocks conduction of nerve roots as they transverse the epidural space.

thetic agent, and cannot reliably be extended to provide adequate analgesia for cesarean birth. Using a continuous catheter technique, a segmental block with an upper level of T10 can be established with the onset of painful contractions and then maintained throughout the first stage of labor. In the second stage of labor, the block can be extended to give perineal analgesia. If a cesarean section becomes necessary, the level of the block can be elevated to T4. Thus, as with subarachnoid block, lumbar epidural block can provide adequate anesthesia for all obstetrical procedures not requiring depression of uterine activity. Its use allows a pain-free labor in an alert and cooperative mother who will require no additional medications for pain.

Advantages and Disadvantages. There are two primary advantages of lumbar epidural anesthesia over subarachnoid anesthesia. Since the dura is normally not entered, the problem of postspinal headache is avoided. Second, the epidural technique allows the placement of a catheter for reinjection of local anesthetic drug as required.

The major drawback of epidural block as compared with subarachnoid block is that close to five times the amount of drug is required with the epidural technique. As an example, 150 mg to 200 mg of lidocaine are required by epidural injection to provide complete anesthesia for vaginal delivery, whereas by the subarachnoid route only 40 mg to 50 mg of lidocaine are needed. Epidural anesthesia necessitates careful control of the amount of local anesthetic drug used, particularly when the slowly metabolized amide-type drugs are employed, to avoid local anesthetic toxicity. When it is necessary to use large amounts of local anesthetic drug with epidural technique, one can employ the rapidly metabolized ester-type local anesthetics, such as procaine and 2-chloroprocaine.

Like subarachnoid block, epidural block blocks sympathetic outflow and can result in vasodilatation and maternal hypotension. Although the onset of hypotension is slower with the epidural technique, it can be as serious as with subarachnoid block if unrecognized and untreated. Prevention and treatment of hypotension resulting from epidural block is the same as with subarachnoid block and includes left uterine displacement, intravenous hydration with balanced salt solutions, the use of small intravenous doses of ephedrine and oxygen administration. As the onset of hypotension is slower with epidural block, so also is the onset of analgesia. The onset of analgesia following subarachnoid injection occurs within a minute and is usually complete in 5 minutes, whereas the onset of analgesia with epidural block requires about 5 minutes and is not complete for 15 minutes to 20 minutes. This slow onset of block can be partially overcome by initiating the block with a short-acting rapid onset local anesthetic such as 2-chloroprocaine, then using longer acting local anesthetics such as bupivacaine through the epidural catheter for later injections. Like subarachnoid block, epidural block, by providing complete perineal analgesia, eliminates the urge to bear down in the second stage of labor.

Since the amount of local anesthetic required for epidural block is five times greater than that required

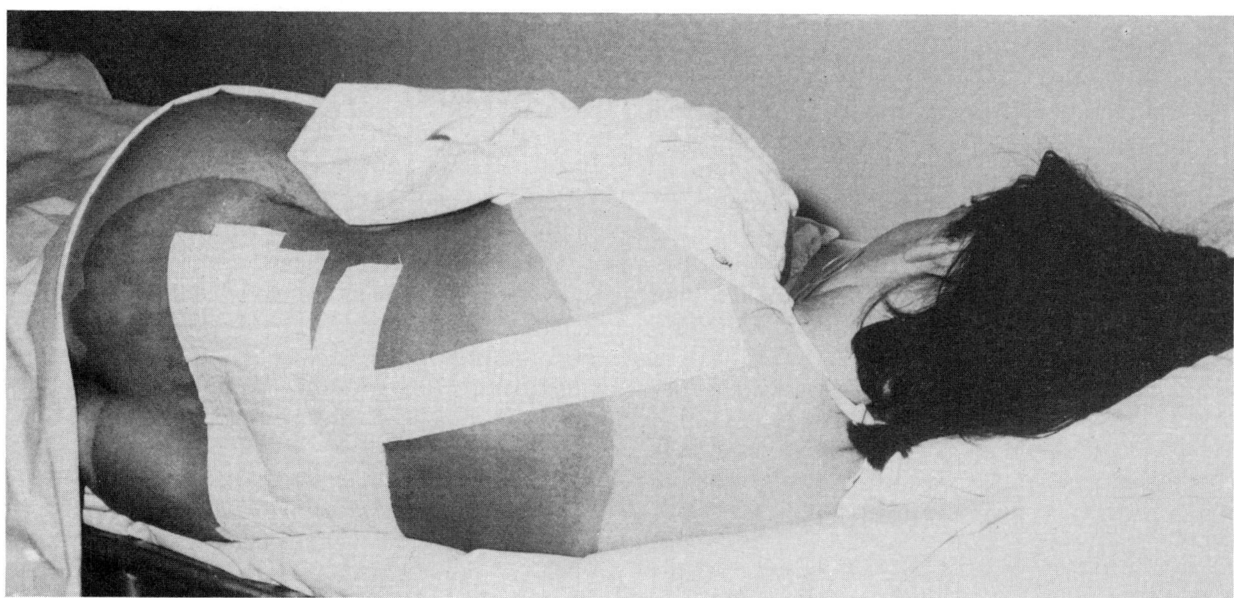

Figure 27-8.
Lumbar epidural block.

for subarachnoid block, accidental subarachnoid injection of the epidural drug will produce a sudden, extremely high or total spinal block. This is avoided by always preceding each epidural injection with a small test dose and waiting a minute or two to ascertain that a subarachnoid block does not ensue before completing the injection. In pregnancy the epidural veins are markedly dilated and can easily be entered by the epidural needle or catheter. Due to the nature of these veins, blood frequently cannot be aspirated. Injection of local anesthetic into the veins in a dose needed for epidural analgesia could produce sudden local anesthetic toxicity in the mother with the onset of grand mal convulsions. This complication is avoided by injecting the first 4 ml or 5 ml of local anesthetic slowly, and then waiting a minute while observing for signs and symptoms of toxicity. These include ringing or buzzing in the ears, a metallic taste, perioral numbness, tremor, and a feeling of lightheadedness or discomfort by the patient. If any of these signs or symptoms occur, no further injection is made, the needle or catheter is withdrawn and the procedure is repeated. With a small dose, the signs and symptoms of toxicity rapidly abate and no further problems arise. The anesthesiologist administering epidural analgesia in the labor room must have immediately available the equipment and drugs necessary to treat the patient should these complications of high block or local anesthetic toxicity occur. Failure to be so prepared can rapidly result in the unnecessary death of the mother and her fetus.

Since epidural block is frequently started during the first stage of labor, its effect on the progress of labor must be assessed. While there is great debate on this issue, it is generally felt that once active labor is achieved, epidural anesthesia does not slow its progress. In the primigravida active labor is usually present when the cervix is 5 cm to 6 cm dilated. In the multipara active labor is usually present when the cervix is 4 cm to 5 cm dilated.

Lumbar epidural anesthesia has revolutionized the field of obstetrical anesthesia. In hospitals with adequate personnel, its use has become widespread because of its ability to alleviate all maternal pain associated with labor and delivery in an alert, cooperative mother with minimal danger of neonatal depression. If complications are to be avoided, the same expertise in both administration and peripartum care as would be afforded the surgical patient is required. If this care is not available, epidural anesthesia should not be used (Fig. 27-8).

Anesthesia for Cesarean Birth

Cesarean delivery can be performed under local infiltration, major conduction anesthesia (subarachnoid or epidural block), or general anesthesia.

Local infiltration was used widely in the past because of the apparent lack of depression in the newborn. Unfortunately, local infiltration seldom produces complete and satisfactory maternal anesthesia, and frequently the mother required supplemental general anesthesia following delivery. Other problems with local infiltration include the time required to produce analgesia and the large amount of local anesthetic drug required. With the refinements in major conduction anesthesia and general anesthesia, there is seldom justification for using local infiltration unless no skilled anesthetist is available.

Major conduction anesthesia is now widely used for cesarean birth, particularly when trained anesthesiologists are available. The advantage of this type of anesthesia is the absence of associated newborn depression. In addition, there is evidence that the induction-to-delivery interval is not as important with conduction anesthesia in causing newborn depression, provided normal maternal physiology is maintained. The pressure for a quick delivery is eliminated. Major conduction anesthesia allows the mother to be wide awake, to be comfortable, and to see and relate early with her baby. Provided hypotension and local anesthetic toxicity are avoided, the risk of pulmonary aspiration is minimal.

The disadvantages of conduction anesthesia for cesarean birth include the following: (1) it provides inadequate analgesia, (2) it involves the risk of maternal hypotension, (3) the time required for its onset may delay urgent surgical intervention, and (4) it is contraindicated in certain maternal conditions. Inadequate analgesia is usually the result of low level of block, compounded by traction on the perineum. A minimum of solid T4 sensory block is required to avoid maternal discomfort unless the obstetrician is extremely gentle and quick. Sensory levels of less than T4 frequently allow delivery, but then general anesthesia or heavy sedation is required for closure. Without proper prophylaxis, such high levels of block, particularly in the parturient, will uniformly result in significant maternal hypotension that will be associated with fetal and newborn acidosis secondary to a depressed uterine perfusion. The prevention and treatment of this hypotension has been dealt with in the section concerned with regional anesthesia.

Despite the fact that subarachnoid block produces complete analgesia in less than 5 minutes, performing the block requires several minutes even in the most skilled hands. General anesthesia can be induced in less than 1 minute. The minimal time required to induce general anesthesia is extremely important when an emergency cesarean section is indicated. As the anesthetist is preparing the patient for general anesthesia, the obstetrician can be preparing and draping the abdomen. In patients who have a functioning epidural catheter in place with a T10 sensory, injection of a rapid-acting local anesthetic such as 2-chloroprocaine usually produces an adequate level of sensory block in about 3 minutes to 5 minutes. Thus, if the mother's condition is stable, an epidural can often be used for emergency c-section. However, in a true emergency situation, one should not delay the cesarean section while waiting for the onset of adequate epidural analgesia.

There are several conditions which contraindicate major conduction anesthesia. An unstable maternal personality or cases in which the newborn is to be given up for adoption constitute relative contraindications. Maternal fear of or refusal to have major conduction anesthesia is an absolute contraindication. Maternal hypovolemia or shock from any cause is a contraindication because these conditions are exacerbated by the sympathetic block associated with subarachnoid or epidural anesthesia. Sepsis or localized infection at or near the site of injection is an absolute contraindication because of the danger of causing an epidural abscess or arachnoiditis. Abnormal coagulation of maternal blood contraindicates the use of conduction anesthesia because of the risk of forming an epidural hematoma. Certain neurologic conditions, such as multiple sclerosis, meningomyelocele, and spina bifida, contraindicate the use of major conduction anesthesia.

In general, major conduction anesthesia is ideal for elective cesarean section or cesarean section that is urgent but not emergent. It provides ideal conditions for the father to be present with the mother in the delivery room. If an adequate level of block is obtained, ensuring freedom from pain, nearly all mothers opt for major conduction anesthesia for repeat cesarean birth.

General anesthesia, properly administered, can be used safely for almost every cesarean birth. Unlike major conduction anesthesia, there are few absolute contraindications for its use. It is possible to induce anesthesia and to allow the obstetrician to commence surgery in less than 1 minute if the mother has a functioning intravenous and the anesthetist has drugs and equipment ready. It is the method of choice in cases of hypovolemia, shock, abnormal blood coagulation, septicemia, and a fearful mother or mother who refuses major conduction anesthesia. For anesthetists not trained or allowed to use major conduction anesthesia, it is the method of choice for cesarean birth anesthesia.

General anesthesia for cesarean section has three major disadvantages. It denies the mother immediate contact with her baby at birth. Second, it is associated with a higher incidence of newborn depression. With modern techniques of light balanced general anesthesia, however, the obstetrician usually has at least 10 minutes from induction to delivery of the baby before depression from anesthesia is significant. And even when the baby is depressed from general anesthesia alone, there is no associated acidosis, provided that the mother has been maintained in good physiological balance during the anesthesia. Resuscitation of anesthetic-depressed babies is usually easy and consists largely of support of the respirations and maintenance of the airway until the anesthetic gases and vapors can be eliminated through the newborn's lungs.

The third disadvantage is that general anesthesia exposes the mother to the potentially lethal complication of pulmonary aspiration of gastric contents. However, proper protection of the airway with cricoid pressure (Sellick's maneuver, see Fig. 27-1) from the time consciousness is lost until the trachea can be intubated with a cuffed endotracheal tube essentially eliminates this catastrophe.

The Role of the Maternity Nurse in the Safe Practice of Obstetrical Anesthesia

For safe and effective analgesia or anesthesia to be available to all parturients, the maternity nurse is required to play an active role. Unfortunately, it is impracticable today to have qualified anesthesiologists or nurse anesthetists remain in the labor room with the parturient throughout labor. However, the parturient deserves to have constant, competent observation and support throughout labor, delivery, and in the immediate postdelivery period. The administration of any form of anesthesia or analgesia during parturition demands constant observation if anesthetic morbidity and mortality are to be minimized.

It is usually the responsibility of the maternity nurse to adequately monitor and record important observations of the patient receiving analgesia in labor. While generally not responsible for administering most forms of analgesia or anesthesia, the maternity nurse must appreciate the complications of various techniques of pain relief, be able to recognize the signs and symptoms of the complications early, and know what action to take until an anesthesiologist or anesthetist is available. Without this kind of support, conduction anesthesia cannot be safely used during labor.

The maternity nurse may have to assist the anesthesiologist in the performance of regional anesthetic techniques. The nurse may be asked to administer various drugs under supervision, to apply cricoid pressure for the intubation of a mother who requires general anesthesia, and to evaluate the newborn and take initial appropriate steps in its resuscitation in the delivery room. Postpartum, the maternity nurse may have to observe and support the patient until the effects of anesthesia have dissipated.

> To help women through childbirth is to share a mystery and a miracle. . . . It is also to touch life at a key point. . . . There the opportunity is taken to grow in understanding and in love. There is more to having a baby than simply pushing an occiput-anterior out into the world. Birth is also implicitly an assent to life. Those who help women in childbirth have the privilege of sharing that act of assent.*

*Kitzinger S: Education and Counseling for Childbirth. London, Balliere Tindall, 1977, p xii

Suggested Reading

Abouleish E: Pain Control in Obstetrics. Philadelphia, J B Lippincott, 1977 (An excellent and recent text on obstetric anesthesia with emphasis on the indications, advantages, disadvantages and complications of obstetric anesthesia.)

Albright GA: Anesthesia in Obstetrics, Maternal, Fetal and Neonatal Aspects. Menlo Park, CA, Addison–Wesley, 1978 (Another recent text devoted to the problems in obstetric anesthesia and their solutions. Has a good chapter on psychoanalgesia.)

Hartland J: Medical and Dental Hypnosis and Its Clinical Applications, 2nd ed, pp 305–325. Baltimore, Williams & Wilkins, 1971 (A good description of hypnosis for obstetrics.)

Heardman H, Ebner M: Relaxation and Exercise for Natural Childbirth, 4th ed. New York, Churchill Livingston, 1975

Shnider SM, Moya F: The Anesthesiologist, Mother, and Newborn. Baltimore, Williams & Wilkins, 1974 (A well-written short book dealing with many aspects of obstetric anesthesia, fetal and newborn evaluation and newborn care.)

Wylie G: Psychological analgesia. In Shnider, SM (ed): Obstetrical Anesthesia, Current Concepts and Practice, pp 57–59. Baltimore, Williams & Wilkins, 1970

Study Aids for Unit V: Intrapartal Assessment and Management

Conference Material

1. A patient who is contemplating the delivery of her first child is worried for fear that she may not get her own baby if another infant is born at the same time she is delivered. How would you reassure this patient concerning the identification methods for newborn infants?

2. An 18-year-old woman who is having her first baby is admitted to the hospital in early labor. It is obvious from her behavior that she has had no preparation for this experience and is frightened and apprehensive. What specific measures would you include in your nursing plan for her care?

3. An unwed mother goes into labor, having made no arrangement for the care of her 2-year-old girl and her 12-year-old boy. What resources could you suggest in this situation? What is the responsibility of hospital and community agencies in this case?

4. A couple who have attended Lamaze childbirth education classes find that all patients must be monitored externally during labor at the hospital they have chosen for delivery. What explanation would you give the couple for this practice? What specific measures would you include in your care plan to help the couple practice their relaxation and concentration, and still maintain monitoring?

5. Why is prophylaxis for the eyes of the newborn required by law in all states? How would you go about securing the desired information concerning such legislation in the various states of the United States?

6. A 21-year-old mother at term, who has attended "natural childbirth" classes for a previous pregnancy, comes to the hospital on her physician's instructions because her membranes have ruptured. She is apologetic because her contractions are only 10 minutes to 12 minutes apart, of mild intensity, lasting about 35 seconds and "not really good enough yet to come to the hospital." On examination, her cervix is found to be 2 cm dilated and 10% effaced. Discuss the nursing care you would plan for this mother if she were assigned to your care.

7. Your hospital does not permit the infant to be placed in the mother's arms after delivery. What specific steps might you take to help get this policy changed. Who would you have to talk to?

8. What arguments might you put forth to institute a policy of putting the newborn to breast immediately after birth?

9. You are attending a mother in the recovery room who was heavily medicated immediately before delivery. She has her infant in the bed with her. What precautions should you take to insure the safety of *both* the mother and infant? What signs should you be especially alert for in the couple?

10. A mother is dilated 6 cm and states that she is experiencing severe discomfort in the lower back during contractions and some discomfort in that area between contractions. What noninvasive methods can you consider using to relieve this discomfort?

Multiple Choice

Read through the entire question and place your answer on the line to the right.

1. After a protracted labor and a difficult delivery, the mother, upon seeing her baby, was shocked at the elongated appearance of the infant's head. The nurse could correctly reassure the patient by saying
   A. "The baby's head is molded during delivery and will return to normal in a few days."
   B. "All newborn babies' heads are shaped this way."
   C. "The child's head shape was changed during delivery, and it will take 6 months for it to return to normal."
   D. "After the 'soft spot' closes, the head will return to normal." _____

2. Indicate the abbreviations that might be used on a patient's chart to represent each of the positions and the presentations described:
   A. Back of head directed straight to the left _____
   B. Back of head directed toward the left side and the front quadrant of the pelvis _____
   C. Back of head directed toward the right side and the back quadrant of the pelvis _____
   D. Breech presentation, buttocks at the left back quadrant _____
   E. Face presentation, chin at the right front quadrant _____
   F. Traverse lie, shoulder is to the right of mother's pelvis, back is posterior _____

3. Give the term or the phrase which best fits each of the following statements:
   A. Enlargement of the external os to 10 cm in diameter _____
   B. Maximum shortening of the cervical canal _____
   C. A condition caused by failure of the uterine muscle to stay contracted after delivery _____
   D. A surgical incision of the perineum during second stage of labor _____
   E. Settling of the baby's head into the brim of the true pelvis _____

4. The character and the frequency of uterine contractions and the location of the discomfort experienced by the mother during labor often provide pertinent information regarding the labor.

   Situation No. 1: In the case of a multipara who is having discomfort but is not in real labor, which of these symptoms would most probably serve to identify false labor contractions?
   A. Discomfort may begin as early as 3 weeks or 4 weeks before the onset of true labor.

Multiple Choice
(continued)

B. Discomfort occurs 3 days or 4 days before the onset of true labor.
C. Contractions occur at regular intervals.
D. Contractions occur at irregular intervals.
E. Discomfort is confined to the lower abdomen and the groin.
F. Discomfort is felt in the upper abdomen and the back.

Select the number corresponding to the correct letter or letters.
1. A only
2. A and C
3. A, D, and E
4. All of the above _____

Situation No. 2: In the case of a primigravida in the beginning of the first stage of labor, which of the following symptoms would most probably describe her labor contractions?
A. Contractions occur at regular intervals.
B. Contractions occur at irregular intervals.
C. Discomfort is confined to the lower abdomen and the groin.
D. Discomfort is located in the lower back and the abdomen.
E. Contractions occur at intervals of from 2 minutes to 3 minutes.
F. Contractions occur at intervals of from 10 minutes to 15 minutes.

Select the number corresponding to the correct letters.
1. A and C
2. A, D, and F
3. B, C, and E
4. All of the above _____

Situation No. 3: In the case of a primigravida approaching the end of the first stage of labor, which of the following symptoms would most probably give an accurate description of her labor?
A. Contractions occur at regular intervals.
B. Contractions occur at irregular intervals.
C. Contractions occur at 1-minute to 1½-minute intervals.
D. Contractions occur at 2-minute to 3-minute intervals.
E. Duration of contraction is from 35 seconds to 50 seconds.
F. Duration of contraction is from 50 seconds to 70 seconds.

Select the number corresponding to the correct letters.
1. A, C, and E
2. A, D, and F
3. B, D, and E
4. All of the above _____

5. Labor is divided into the first, the second, and the third stages.
A. When is the first stage of labor considered to be terminated?
   1. When contractions occur at 10-minute to 15-minute intervals.
   2. When the cervix is completely dilated.
   3. When the baby is delivered. _____

B. When is the second stage of labor considered to be terminated?
   1. When the cervix is completely dilated.
   2. When contractions occur at 2-minute to 3-minute intervals.
   3. When the baby is delivered. _____

C. When is the third stage of labor considered to be terminated?
   1. When the baby is delivered.
   2. When the placenta is delivered.
   3. After the uterus has remained firm for 1 hour. _____

6. In the typical vertex presentation, the sequence of events by which the fetal head adapts to the birth canal during descent are:
   A. Flexion, external rotation, internal rotation, and extension
   B. External rotation, internal rotation, extension, and flexion
   C. Flexion, internal rotation, extension, and external rotation
   D. External rotation, extension, flexion, and internal rotation _____

7. The signs which suggest that the placenta has separated include
   A. The uterus becomes firmer and globular in shape
   B. The umbilical cord descends further out of the vagina
   C. There is often a sudden gush of blood
   D. The mother exhibits deep respirations

   1. A only
   2. A and D
   3. A, B, and C
   4. All of the above _____

8. Give the term or the phrase which best fits each of the following statements:
   A. Enlargement of the external os to 10 cm in diameter _____
   B. Maximum shortening of the cervical canal _____
   C. A type of drug used in obstetrics which blots out memory of whatever occurs under its influence
   D. A condition caused by failure of the uterine muscle to stay contracted after delivery
   E. A surgical incision of the perineum during second-stage labor
   F. Settling of the baby's head into the brim of the pelvis.

9. The nurse is caring for a mother in the accelerated phase of labor who is being monitored internally because of suspected fetal distress. Which of the following observations would you report promptly to the physician?
   A. A silent FHR baseline for 15 minutes
   B. A consistent reactive FHR baseline that is fluctuating more than five beats per minute
   C. Moderate amount of bright blood in the vaginal discharge
   D. Plugs of blood-streaked mucus in the vaginal discharge
   E. FHR rate that slows during a contraction but returns to its usual rate of 10 seconds to 15 seconds following contractions

Multiple Choice (continued)

Select the number corresponding to the correct letters.
1. A and C
2. A, C, and E
3. B, D, and E
4. All of the above ____

10. On admission of the mother to the labor suite, which of the following procedures are usually carried out routinely?
   - **A.** Check mother's temperature, pulse, respirations and blood pressure.
   - **B.** Take the mother to the bathroom and have her void.
   - **C.** Cleanse the vulvar and perineal area.
   - **D.** Listen to the fetal heart sounds.
   - **E.** Prepare the mother for vaginal examination.
   - **F.** Give a cleansing enema.

Select the number corresponding to the correct letter or letters.
1. A and F
2. A, E, and F
3. A, C, and D
4. All of the above ____

11. Why is an enema sometimes ordered for a mother during the early part of the first stage of labor?
   - **A.** To obtain a stool specimen
   - **B.** To avoid straining as the mother bears down with contractions
   - **C.** To cleanse the lower bowel ____

12. If the baby's head is not engaged, the cervix is dilated, and the membranes have ruptured, what facilities would provide the mother with the greatest degree of comfort and safety to expel an enema?
   - **A.** Use the toilet facilities in bathroom.
   - **B.** Remain in bed and use the bedpan.
   - **C.** Use the bedpan on a chair close to the bed. ____

13. Often it is the nurse's responsibility to decide when the mother is ready to be moved from the labor room to the delivery room. Which of the following signs would signify to the nurse that the time of delivery is near?
   - **A.** Mother has a desire to defecate
   - **B.** Increase in frequency, duration, and intensity of uterine contractions
   - **C.** Mother begins to bear down spontaneously with uterine contractions
   - **D.** Bulging of the perineum
   - **E.** Increase in amount of blood-stained mucus from the vagina

Select the number corresponding to the correct letter or letters.
1. D only
2. A, C, and E

3. B, D, and E
4. All of the above ____

14. A physician was busy suctioning mucus from the mouth of the baby immediately after its birth and asked the nurse to let him know as soon as the placenta seemed to be separating. Which of the following would indicate that it was separated?

A. Gradual descent of the uterus farther into the pelvis
B. Protrusion of several more inches of umbilical cord
C. Uterus becomes more firm and rounded
D. A sudden gush of blood from the vagina
E. Large clots of blood coming out of the vagina

Select the number corresponding to the correct letters.
1. A and C
2. B, C, and D
3. B, C, and E
4. All of the above ____

15. The nurse who is caring for the mother during the fourth stage of labor would include which of the following in her nursing care plan?

A. Keep the mother warm and out of drafts.
B. Massage the uterus from time to time to keep it contracted.
C. Massage the fundus continuously.
D. Administer 0.2 mg ergotrate intramuscularly.
E. Check the mother's vital signs at frequent intervals.

Select the number corresponding to the correct letter or letters.
1. B only
2. A and C
3. A, B, and E
4. All of the above ____

16. The most common cause of postpartal hemorrhage is atony of the uterus. What is the first thing to do as a preventive measure if the uterus appears to be atonic?

A. Take a firm grasp on the uterus.
B. Massage the uterus firmly.
C. Administer an oxytocic drug. ____

17. The physician told the nurse to watch a mother during labor for evidence of a prolapsed cord which he feared might occur.

A. What type of FHR pattern would be most likely to appear if the cord prolapses?
   1. Combined acceleration waveform
   2. Isolated acceleration waveform
   3. Severe variable deceleration waveform
   4. Late deceleration waveform
   5. Early deceleration waveform ____

Multiple Choice (continued)

B. If the nurse did suspect the cord to be prolapsed, what position should she put the mother in, with the hope of relieving the pressure on the cord?
1. Knee–chest position
2. Fowler's position
3. Sims's position
4. A prone position _____

C. In addition to changing the mother's position to relieve pressure on the cord, what other measures may the nurse employ if she observes the umbilical cord prolapsed out of the vagina?
1. Immediately wash the cord with warm antiseptic solution and replace in vagina.
2. Cover the cord with a wet sponge.
3. Apply a clamp to the exposed cord and cover with a sterile towel.
4. Keep the cord warm and moist by continuous applications of sterile saline compresses. _____

D. What are the chief objectives of the emergency care given when prolapsed cord occurs?
1. To prevent cold air from prematurely stimulating respiration
2. To prevent drying of the cord while it is still pulsating
3. To stimulate and restore circulation in the cord by vasodilatation
4. To prevent or relieve pressure on the cord _____

18. Soon after the mother was normally delivered, she complained of feeling chilly. The nurse observed that she was having a chill. In addition to reporting this to the physician, which of the following measures would the nurse carry out?

A. Provide external warmth to the mother with blankets.
B. Give a heart stimulant.
C. Prepare to give oxygen.
D. Give a hot drink.
E. Place the mother in shock position.

Select the number corresponding to the correct letter or letters.
1. A only
2. A and C
3. A and D
4. B and E _____

19. If a mother making satisfactory progress has a pulse rate of 90 immediately before delivery, what average rate or rates would be considered to be favorable soon after delivery?

A. 60
B. 70
C. 80
D. 90
E. 100

Select the number corresponding to the correct letter or letters.
1. C only
2. A, B, and C
3. C, D, and E
4. All of the above ____

20. Which of the following are reasons to place the infant in the mother's arms right after delivery:

A. Prevent chilling in the infant
B. Allow the bonding process to begin in the sensitive period
C. Prevent infection in the mother and infant
D. Allow the mother to begin identifying her infant

Select the number corresponding to the correct letter or letters.
1. A, C, and D
2. A and B
3. B and D
4. B, C, and D
5. All of the above ____

21. As soon as the physician had clamped and cut the umbilical cord, he handed the infant over to the nurse to care for. Which of the following acts would the nurse perform in the immediate care of the infant?

A. Place the infant so that he lies skin-to-skin with the mother and cover the couple with warm blankets.
B. Wipe the mucus out of the infant's mouth with sterile gauze.
C. Slap the infant's back and soles of the feet sharply to stimulate crying.
D. Gently remove all vernix caseosa and blood in drying the infant's body with the receiving blanket.
E. "Label" infant with required item of identification before he is transferred to the nursery.

Select the number corresponding to the correct letter or letters.
1. A only
2. A and C
3. A and E
4. B, D, and E
5. B, C, and D ____

22. All of the following may be used to relieve discomfort during labor. Which is especially effective in relieving back labor?

A. Abdominal lifting
B. Shallow chest breathing
C. Abdominal massage
D. Relaxation ____

23. Which of the following may relieve pain during labor contractions by distracting the mother from pain?

A. Walking and talking

Multiple Choice
(continued)

B. Slow rhythmic breathing
C. Focusing eyes on an object
D. Firm pressure to the lower back.

Select the number corresponding to the correct letter or letters.
1. A only
2. B only
3. A, B, and C
4. D only ____

24. One method of helping a mother who is untrained in relaxation to relax quickly at the beginning or end of a contraction is to suggest that she
A. Stare at an object.
B. Count backwards from 100.
C. Take a slow, deep breath.
D. Massage her abdomen. ____

25. What is the main objective in prophylactic eye care in the newborn?
A. To enhance and protect the infant's vision in the immediate period after birth
B. To prevent candidiasis neonatorum
C. To prevent ophthalmia neonatorum
D. To prevent staphylococcus colonization

Select the number corresponding to the correct letter or letters.
1. A only
2. B only
3. C only
4. A, B, C
5. B, C, D
6. All of the above ____

26. Which of the following are needed for successful resuscitation of the newborn immediately after birth?
A. Skilled personnel trained in resuscitation
B. Well lighted area
C. Equipment to deliver O_2 by positive pressure
D. Drug therapy
E. Intubation as necessary

Select the number corresponding to the correct letter or letters.
1. A, C, E
2. A, B, C, and D
3. A, C, D
4. C only
5. All of the above ____

27. The factors which should be considered in selection of an anesthetic for labor and delivery include:

A. The amount of discomfort experienced
B. Experience of the personnel available and the facilities available
C. The desires of the mother
D. The dictum that no anesthesia is the safer course of action in all circumstances

Select the number corresponding to the correct letter or letters.
1. A and B
2. A, B, and C
3. A and D
4. All of the above ____

28. The discomfort caused by uterine contractions and cervical dilatation is conveyed to the spinal cord
A. At levels T10 to T12
B. At L3 to L5
C. At S1 to S4
D. At T8 to T10 ____

29. Identify and match the most important risks of the various methods of obstetrical anesthesia listed below:
A. General anesthesia ____
B. Conduction anesthesia ____
C. Paracervical block ____
1. Aspiration of stomach contents
2. Fetal bradycardia
3. Maternal hypotension

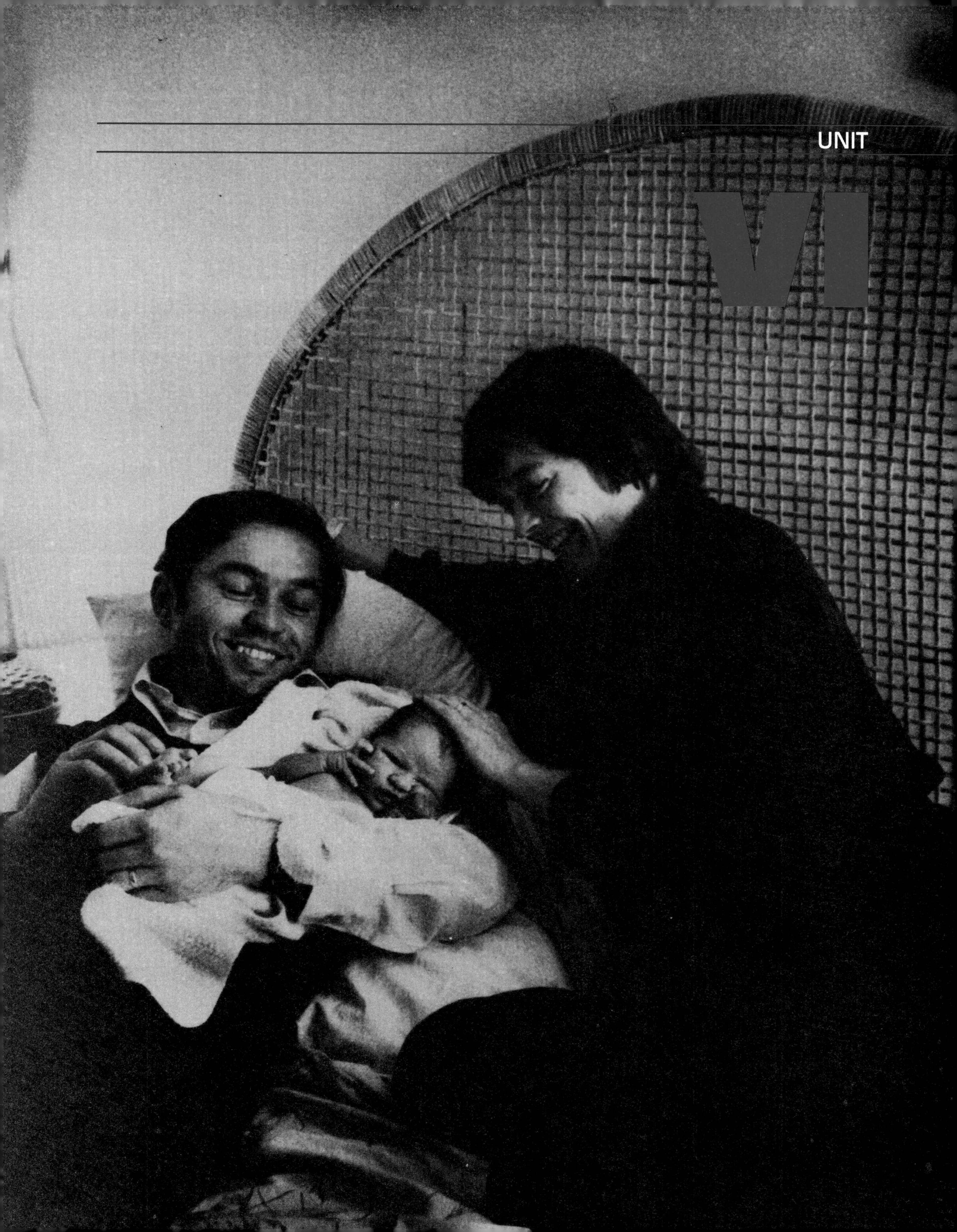

UNIT VI

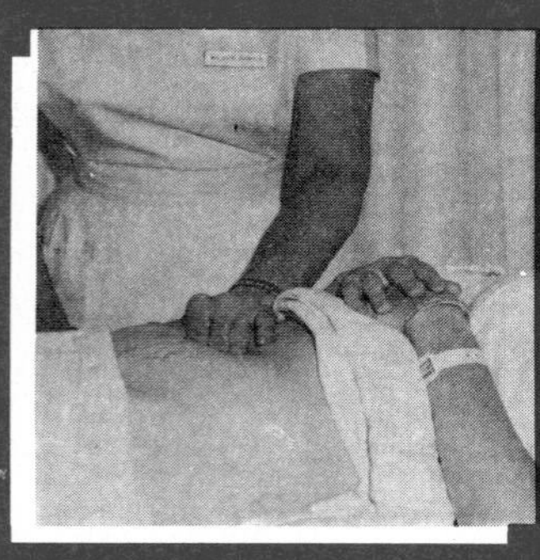

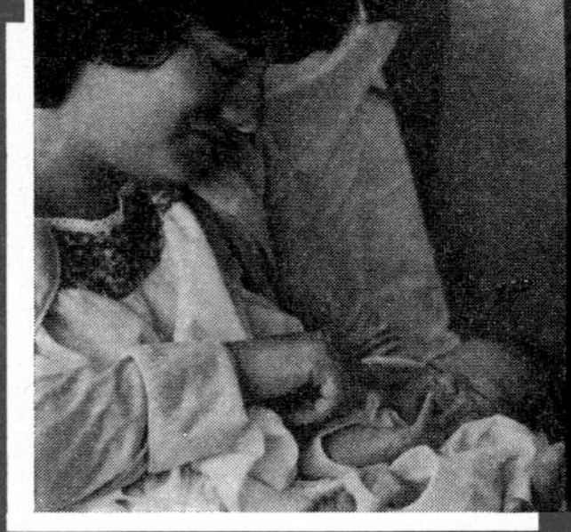

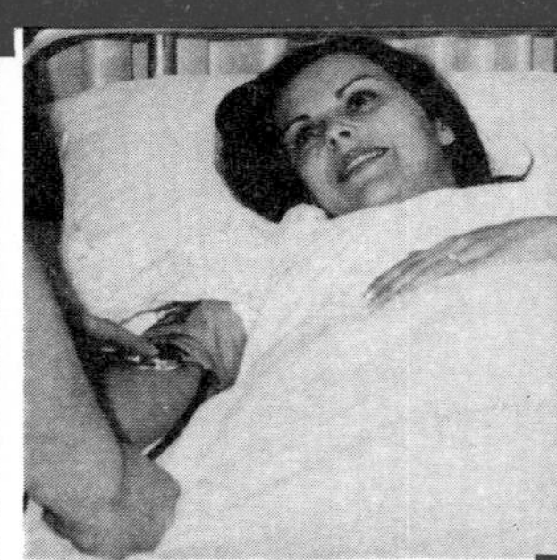

Postpartal Assessment and Management of the New Family

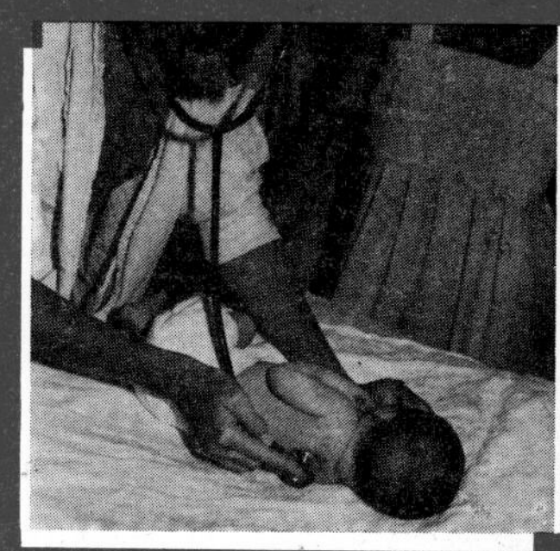

31 Assessment of the Newborn Infant

Physiological Basis of Assessment

Physical Assessment

Assessment of Body

Neurologic Assessment

Behavioral Assessment

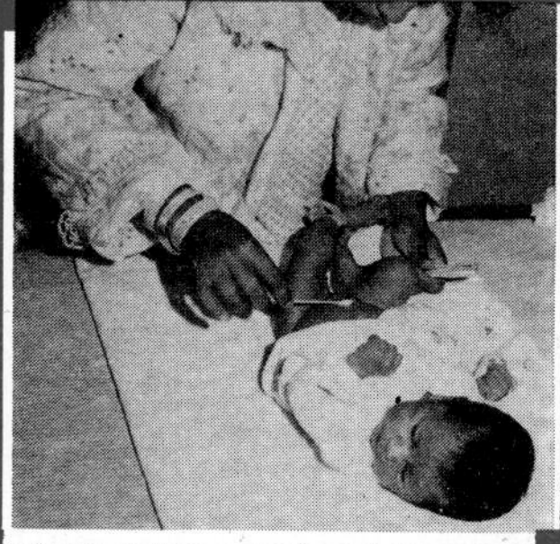

32 Care of the Newborn Infant

Providing a Safe Environment

Nursing During the Transition Period

Continuing Care and Parent Teaching

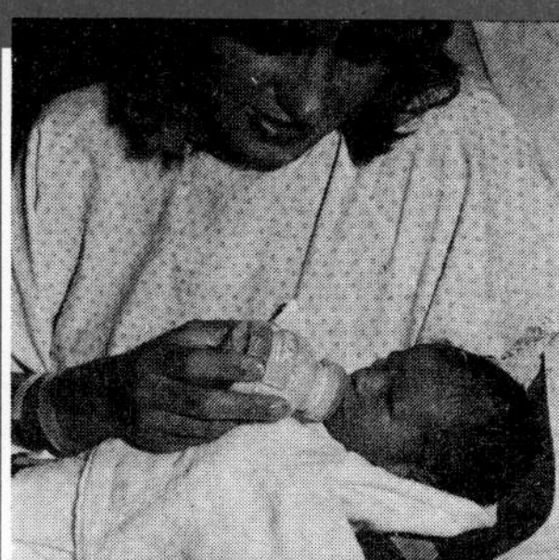

33 Infant Nutrition

The Newborn's Ability to Handle Food

Methods of Feeding—Making the Decision

Breast-Feeding

Artificial Feeding

Common Concerns in Infant Feeding

Nutritional Considerations During the First Year

CHAPTER

28

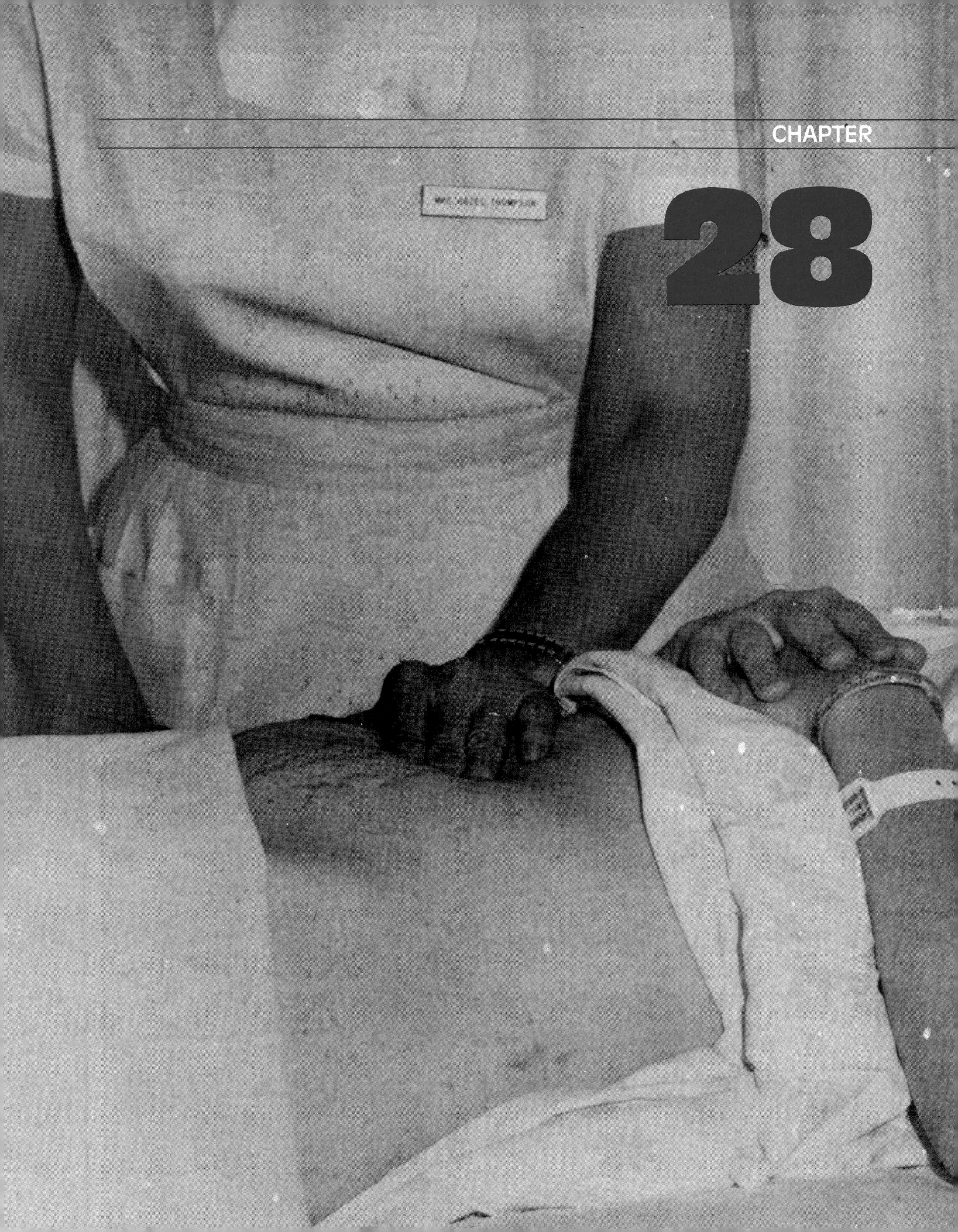

CHAPTER 28

Biophysical Aspects of the Postpartum Period

The postpartum period encompasses the time between delivery until the reproductive organs have returned to their prepregnant state. Marked anatomical and physiological changes occur during this period, as the processes undergone during pregnancy are reversed. Knowledge of the reproductive process in pregnancy and labor serves as a basis for understanding how the generative organs and the various systems of the human body adapt following the delivery.

The term puerperium (from *puer,* a child; and *parere,* to bring forth) refers to the six-week period elapsing between the termination of labor and the return of the reproductive organs to their normal condition. This includes both the *progressive changes* in the breasts for lactation and *involution* of the internal reproductive organs. Although the changes brought about by involution are considered normal physiological processes, they are remarkable in that under no other circumstances does such marked and rapid involution of tissues occur without a departure from a state of health. For this reason, the quality of the mother's care at this time is important to ensure her immediate as well as her future health.

Anatomical and Physiological Changes

Involution of the Uterus

Immediately following the delivery of the placenta the uterus becomes an almost solid mass of tissue. Its thick anterior and posterior walls lie in close opposition, leaving the center cavity flattened. The uterus remains about the same size for the first two days after delivery but then rapidly decreases in size by a process called involution. This is effected partly by the contraction of the uterus, with decrease in size of individual myometrial cells, and partly by autolytic processes in which some of the protein material of the uterine wall is broken down into simpler components which then are absorbed.

Constriction and occlusion of underlying blood vessels occurs at the placental site. This accomplishes hemostasis (to control postpartal bleeding) and causes some endometrial necrosis. Involution occurs by the extension and downward growth of marginal endometrium and by endometrial regeneration from the glands and stroma in the decidua basalis. Except for the placental site, where involution is not complete until 6 weeks after delivery, the process is completed in the remainder of the uterine cavity by the end of the third postpartum week.

The Process of Involution

The separation of the placenta and the membranes from the uterine wall takes place in the outer portion of the spongy layer of the decidua, and, therefore, a remnant of this layer remains in the uterus to be partly cast off in a vaginal discharge called the lochia. Within 2 days or 3 days after labor, this remaining portion of decidua becomes differentiated into two layers, leaving the deeper or unaltered layer attached to the muscular wall from which the new endometrial lining is generated. The layer adjoining the uterine cavity becomes necrotic and is cast off in the lochia. The process is very like the healing of any surface; blood oozes from the small vessels on this surface. The bleeding from the larger vessels is controlled by compression of the retracted uterine muscle fibers.

The process of regeneration is rapid, except at the site of former placental attachment, which requires 6 weeks or 7 weeks to heal completely. Elsewhere, the free surface of the endometrium is restored in half that time.

The Progress of Involution

The normal process of involution requires 5 weeks or 6 weeks, and at the end of that time the uterus regains its normal size, although it never returns exactly to its nulliparous state.

One can realize more fully the rapidity of this process by comparing the changes that occur in the weight of this organ. Immediately following the delivery the uterus weighs approximately 1 kg (2 lb); at the end of the first week, about 500 g (1 lb); at the end of the second week, about 350 g (12 oz); and by the time involution is complete, it should weigh only about 40 g to 60 g (1½ oz–2 oz).

By observing the height of the fundus, which may be felt through the abdominal wall, the nurse is able to appreciate more fully these remarkable changes. Immediately after the delivery of the placenta the uterus sinks into the pelvis, and the fundus is felt midway between the umbilicus and the symphysis, but it soon rises to the level of the umbilicus (13 cm–14 cm, 5 in–5½ in, above the pubes); and 12 hours later, it

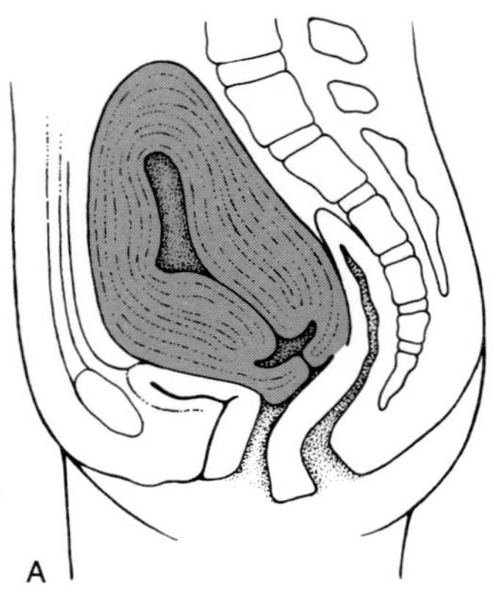

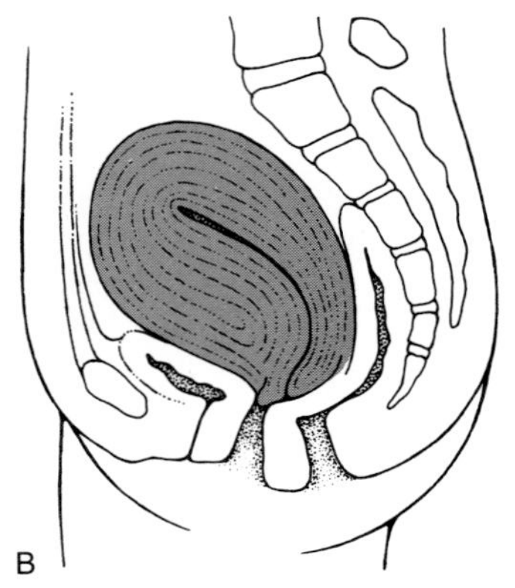

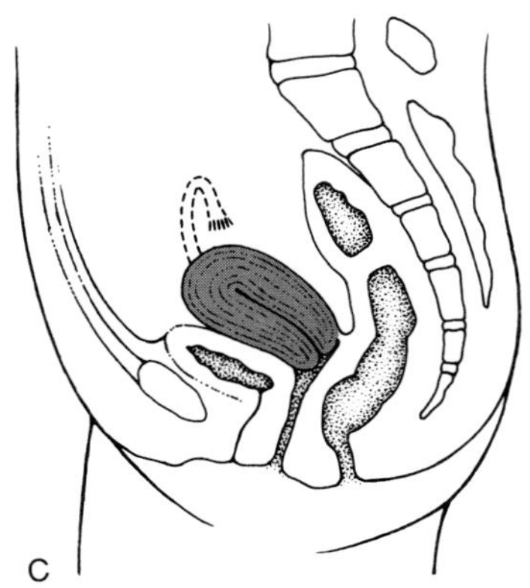

Figure 28-1.
Changes of uterus size and shape following delivery. *(A)* Uterus after delivery, *(B)* uterus at 6th day, *(C)* nongravid uterus.

is probably found a little higher. Day-by-day careful measurements show that it diminishes in size, so that at the end of 10 days or so it cannot be detected by abdominal palpation (Figs. 28-1 and 28-2).

The approximate rate of decrease in the height of the fundus is a little over a centimeter (½ in) or one fingerbreadth a day. Observation of this rate of involution is very important; the physician should be kept informed about any marked delay, especially if it is accompanied by suppression of the lochia or retention of clots. In measuring the height of the uterus, care should be taken that the observations are made after the bladder is emptied, as a full bladder raises the height of the fundus.

The following are indications that involution is not occurring satisfactorily: the uterus fails to decrease progressively in size, and it remains "flabby" and causes the mother much discomfort (see Subinvolution in Chap. 38).

The Lochia

A knowledge of the healing process by which the lining of the uterus becomes regenerated is valuable in understanding and interpreting the lochial discharge. At first the discharge consists almost entirely of blood with a small amount of mucus, particles of decidua and cellular debris that escape from the placental site. It should not contain large clots or mem-

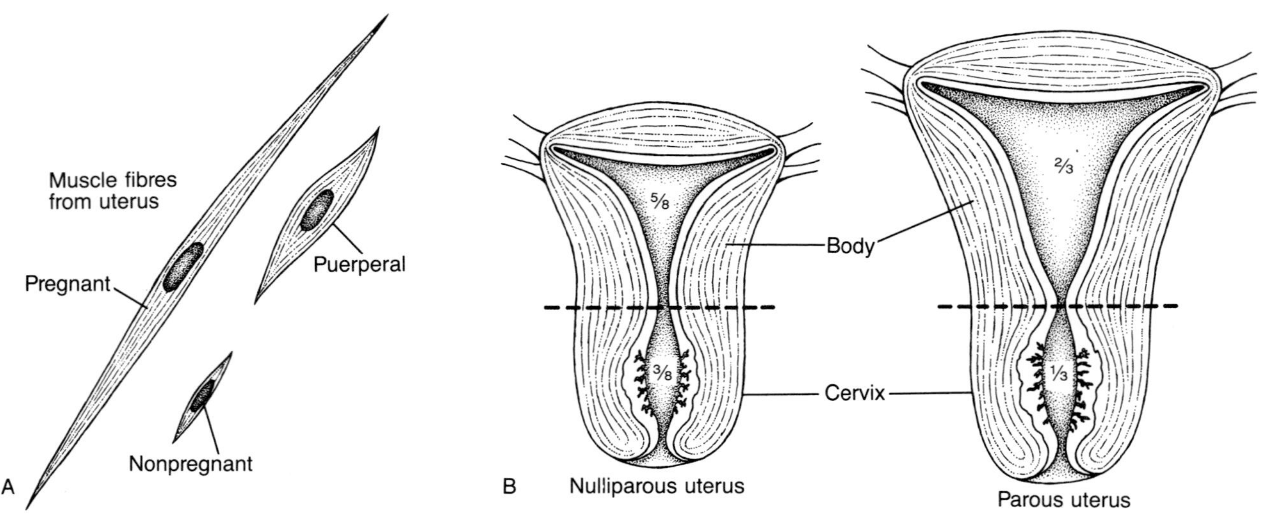

Figure 28-2.
(A) Changes in the size and shape of myometrial cells during the nonpregnant, pregnant, and puerperal states. *(B)* Size and relationship of the cervix and fundus in the nulliparous and parous uterus.

brane or be excessive in amount. The discharge lasts about three days and is called *lochia rubra.*

As the oozing of blood from the healing surface diminishes, the discharge becomes more serous or watery and gradually changes to a pinkish color, called *lochia serosa.* Toward the tenth day the lochia is thinner, greatly decreased in amount, and almost colorless, and is called *lochia alba.* By the end of the third week the discharge usually disappears, though a brownish mucoid discharge may persist a little longer. Lochia possesses a peculiar animal scent which is quite characteristic and should never, at any time, have an offensive odor.

Assessment. The quantity of lochia varies with individuals, but generally it is more profuse in multiparas. It is to be expected that when a mother is out of bed for the first time there may be a definite increase in the amount of discharge. *Nevertheless, the recurrence of fresh bleeding after the discharge has become dark and diminished in amount, or the persistence of bright blood in the lochia or the suppression of the discharge should be reported to the obstetrician.* The daily observation of the amount and the character of the lochia is of the greatest importance as an index of the progress of healing of the endometrial surface.

The Cervix

Immediately following delivery the cervix collapses and has little tone; it appears soft, edematous, and has multiple small lacerations. It can admit two fingers and is about 1 cm thick. Within 24 hours it rapidly shortens and becomes firmer and thicker. The cervical os closes gradually to 2 cm to 3 cm after a few days, and by 1 week is only about 1 cm dilated. Histological examination immediately after birth reveals almost universal edema and hemorrhage. The endocervical epithelium remains generally intact, with occasional areas of partial denudation. As early as the fourth day, there is regression of glandular hypertrophy and hyperplasia seen during pregnancy, and reabsorption of interstitial hemorrhage. Cervical involution is still proceeding beyond 6 weeks, however, with edema and round cell infiltration persisting as long as 3 months to 4 months.

Examination of the cervix with a colposcope (a viewing instrument similar to a microscope, with low magnification and binocular viewing, designed to fit a speculum for close viewing of the cervix) shows ulceration, laceration, bruising, and yellow areas within several days of delivery. These lesions, which are usually smaller than 4 mm, are seen more often in primiparas. Repeat examination 6 weeks to 12 weeks later usually shows complete healing; this indicates rapid reepithelialization of the injured tissue.[1] There is variable retraction of everted columnar epithelium (ectropion) beginning early in the postpartum period. Not every cervix regains its prepregnant appearance; some have more ectropion, and the os is generally wider, shaped in a transverse slit, and may gape if there have been lacerations of clinical significance (Fig. 28-3).

The Vagina

The vagina is smooth and swollen and has poor tone following delivery. After 3 weeks the vascularity, edema, and hypertrophy resulting from pregnancy and birth are markedly decreased. Rugations first reappear at about 3 weeks. When vaginal cells are examined microscopically on a smear, the epithelium appears atrophic by the third week to the fourth week, but regains its proper estrogen index by 6 weeks to 10 weeks postpartum. This relative estrogen deficiency contributes to poor vaginal lubrication and vasocongestion, which leads to a diminished sexual response in the weeks following delivery. The lower vagina usually has multiple superficial lacerations after birth, but these are resolved by 6 weeks postpartum. There may be varying degrees of muscular-fascial relaxation, causing cystocele, rectocele, or gaping of the introitus. Regular postpartal exercises, particularly Kegel's exercises (see Chap. 21), help to restore vaginal muscle tone.

Other Pelvic Organs

Histological changes in the *fallopian tubes* reveal reduction in the size of secretory cells, decrease in size and number of ciliated cells, and atrophy of the tubal epithelium. After 6 weeks to 8 weeks, the epithelium reaches the condition of the early follicular

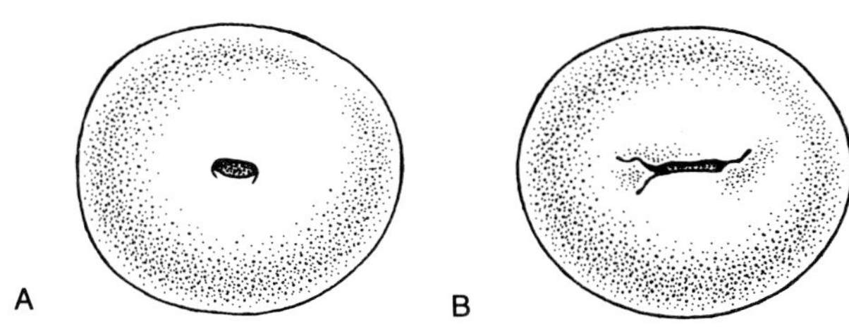

Figure 28-3.
The perfectly round os of the nulliparous cervix becomes elongated after childbirth. The cervical os may gape if there have been significant lacerations during delivery. *(A)* Round os of nulliparous cervix, *(B)* Transverse slit of os in parous cervix.

phase of the menstrual cycle. There is transient nonbacterial inflammation of the tubal lumina appearing about the fourth day.

The *ligaments* that support the uterus, the ovaries, and the tubes, which have also undergone great tension and stretching, are now relaxed, but it takes them a considerable amount of time to return almost to their normal size and position.

Abdominal Wall

The abdominal wall recovers partially from the overstretching but remains soft and flabby for some time. The striae, due to the rupture of the elastic fibers of the cutis, usually remain but become less conspicuous because of their silvery appearance. The process of involution in the abdominal structures requires at least 6 weeks. Provided that the abdominal walls have retained their muscle tone, they gradually return to their original condition. However, if these muscles are relaxed because they have lost their tone, there may be a marked separation or *diastasis of the recti muscles,* so that the abdominal organs are not properly supported. Rest, diet, prescribed exercises, good body mechanics, and good posture may do much to restore the tone of these muscles.

Cardiovascular System

After delivery there often is a transient bradycardia, with a pulse rate as low as 40 beats per minute to 50 beats per minute, lasting for 24 hours to 48 hours. This is caused by hemodynamic changes and a vagal hyperreactivity in response to the increased sympathetic nervous system activity during labor. The 40% increase in blood volume that occurs during pregnancy gradually undergoes reduction until it reaches normal levels by about 2 weeks postpartum. However, it is important to note that there is an increase of 15% to 30% in circulating blood volume in the first 2 to 3 postpartal days, due to the elimination of placental circulation and an increase in venous return. This process is responsible for the profound diuresis that occurs in the early puerperium. It also explains the fall in hematocrit, which is a hemodilutional phenomenon. Cardiac output increases by 35% as a result of these combined hemodynamic changes, making the early postpartum period the time of greatest risk of heart failure in women with heart disease and limited cardiac reserve.[2]

The pregnant total blood volume of 5 liters to 6 liters decreases to 4 liters by the fourth postpartum week. There is a loss of about 400 ml of blood in a normal vaginal delivery, although this varies considerably. By the third to seventh postpartal day, the hematocrit usually rises unless there has been substantial blood loss at delivery. The leukocytosis that occurs during pregnancy and labor continues for the first several post delivery days, with values up to 20,000 WBC/ml to 25,000 WBC/ml, and is characterized by increased neutrophils and eosinophils and decreased lymphocytes. There is a rapid but short-lived reticulocytosis as a result of sudden blood loss. Sedimentation rate, fibrinogen, and thromboplastic factors remain elevated after delivery and return to normal in 2 weeks to 3 weeks. These increased clotting factors may interact with immobility, sepsis, or trauma to predispose women to postpartum thrombosis.

Heart rate, systolic and diastolic blood pressures, oxygen consumption, and total body water return to prepregnant levels in the early postpartum period. The rate of return of cardiovascular changes follows a hyperbolic curve, with most of the regression occurring early, and return to basal levels accomplished by 6 weeks postpartum.

Urinary System

The bladder mucosa following delivery shows varying degrees of edema and hyperemia, with diminished bladder tone. This results in decreased sensation to increased pressure, increased capacity, overdistention with overflow incontinence, and incomplete emptying of the bladder. It is important that postpartum nursing care include careful monitoring of the condition of the bladder, as distention and urinary retention are common occurrences and can cause discomfort as well as predispose to infection. With adequate emptying of the bladder, tone is usually restored within 5 days to 7 days.

The glomerular filtration rate (GFR) remains elevated during the first postpartum week, and combined with increased blood volume, it causes marked diuresis of up to 3000 ml/day for the first 4 days to 5 days. Fluid is lost from the body tissues, and combined with involutional changes, it contributes to a loss of about 9 lb of weight during the puerperium. Glycosuria occurs about 20% of the time, and proteinuria for a day or two occurs up to 50% of the time. The ureters and renal pelvis of the kidneys remain dilated after delivery and return to normal in 3 weeks to 6 weeks, although this may occasionally take as long as 8 weeks to 12 weeks. This must be kept in mind in interpreting intravenous pyelography (IVP) during this time. By 6 weeks postpartum, the renal plasma flow, GFR, plasma creatinine, and nitrogen usually return to nonpregnant levels.

Ovulation and Menstruation

Circulating levels of *estrogen* and *progesterone* decline rapidly after delivery. Follicle stimulating hormone levels are low in postpartum women for 10 days to 12 days, then increase to follicular phase concentrations by the third week. Estrogen reaches follicular phase levels in about 3 weeks in nonlactating women, and it takes longer in those who are lactating. Ovulation and menstruation following childbirth are influenced by whether or not the woman is breast-feeding. Menses that occur within the first 6 weeks are rarely ovulatory; the longer after delivery the first menses occur, the greater the likelihood that they will be ovulatory. Once menstruation begins, the percentage of subsequent menses that are ovulatory rises rapidly.

The first ovulation after delivery in nonlactating women occurs, on an average, at 10.2 weeks. Among women lactating for at least 3 months, the first ovulation occurs at 17.0 weeks, on an average. With increased duration of lactation, the average time of ovulation rises, and among women lactating for 6 months, ovulation occurred at 28 weeks. Nonlactating women may ovulate as early as 27 days after delivery.

The return of menstruation after delivery follows a linear pattern. By 12 weeks postpartum, 70% of nonlactating women will have their first menses; over the next 24 weeks this rises to 80%. In lactating women menses return more gradually, with 55% to 75% menstruating by 36 weeks. The average time until the first menses in nonlactating women is 7 weeks to 9 weeks, and in women who breast-feed the average time until menstruation is greater than in women who are not breast-feeding, depending upon the length of nursing (Table 28-1).

The basis for postdelivery amenorrhea is not completely understood. The hormone *prolactin* (associated with lactation) reaches peak concentration around delivery, then declines erratically over the next 2 weeks in nonlactating women. In nursing mothers it increases in early puerperium, then diminishes. Levels of LH and HCG decline rapidly after delivery to low follicular phase by 2 weeks and do not change again until ovulation occurs. *FSH* levels are low until they reach normal levels by 3 weeks. This return of gonadotropins occurs whether or not the woman is lactating, although return to normal estrogen levels is delayed by lactation. This is interpreted to mean that lactation causes a temporary refractory state of the ovaries to pituitary gonadotropins.

Intestinal System and Weight Loss

The motility and tone of the gastrointestinal system usually returns to normal within 2 weeks after delivery. Most women are quite thirsty the first 2 days to 3 days, probably because fluids are restricted during labor, and because fluid shifts within the body are associated with diuresis. Constipation is common during the early postpartum period. Physiological processes are exacerbated by effects of the predelivery enema, restriction of fluids during labor, and drugs given during labor and delivery. Pain from the episiotomy and from hemorrhoids may further deter defecation. Most postpartum patients are given stool softeners or laxatives such as DOSS, Dulcolax, or Milk of magnesia to aid elimination.

Weight loss after delivery totals about 22 lb; this is composed of loss from the fetus and placenta, amniotic fluid, and blood at the time of delivery; perspiration and diuresis during the first postpartum week; and involution of the uterus as well as lochial discharge (Table 28-2).

The Breasts

During pregnancy, progressive changes occur in the breasts in preparation for lactation. The breast lobules have developed under the stimulation of the estrogen

Table 28-1.
Return of Menstruation

	Average Time of First Ovulation	Average Time of First Menstruation
Nonlactating women	10.2 weeks	7–9 weeks††
Lactating women	17.0 weeks* 28.0 weeks†	30–36 weeks§

*Lactating for 3 months
†Lactating for 6 months
††First menses usually anovulatory
§Depends upon duration of lactation

Table 28-2.
Sources and Amount of Weight Loss During the Postpartum Period

Source of Weight Loss	Amount of Weight Loss: Pounds	Kilograms
Fetus and placenta; amniotic fluid and blood loss at delivery	12–13	5.5–6
Perspiration and diuresis during the first postpartal week	5–8	2.5–4
Uterine involution and lochia	2–3	1
Total weight loss	19–24	9–10

and progesterone produced by the placenta while the lactiferous ducts have undergone further branching and elongation. Prolactin, released from the anterior pituitary, cortisol from the maternal adrenal, and insulin, all of which appear in increasing amounts during gestation, also contribute to breast changes. Although all of the essential factors are more and more available as gestation progresses, milk production per se is held in abeyance. Its appearance is delayed until 3 days or 4 days after delivery, when estrogen and progesterone levels have decreased.

Physiology of Lactation

At least six pituitary hormones play a role in mammary development and lactation. These include prolactin, adrenocorticotropic hormone (ACTH), human growth hormone (HGH), thyroid stimulating hormone (TSH), FHS, and LH. In addition, human chorionic somatotropin (HCS), human placental lactogen (HPL), and steroid hormones secreted by the adrenal glands, the ovaries, and placenta play a part, as does pancreatic insulin. Prolactin has a central role in preparation of the breasts for lactation. It is involved in the increase in breast size and in the number and complexity of the ducts and alveoli which occur during pregnancy. As pregnancy progresses, prolactin stimulates secretion by mammary alveolar cells, and estrogen and progesterone stimulate ductal and alveolar growth, but these latter two paradoxically inhibit milk secretion.

With the delivery of the placenta, the source of most estrogen and progesterone during pregnancy, as well as of all HPL, is suddenly removed. The blood levels of these hormones falls rapidly, but the secretion of prolactin by the anterior pituitary gland continues. The appearance of milk postpartally has been demonstrated to coincide with falling estrogen and progesterone levels in the presence of elevated prolactin. The synthesis and secretion of milk is thus initiated when the inhibitory effects of estrogen and progesterone are removed, and under the continuing effects of prolactin.

The secretion of milk begins at the base of the alveolar cells, where small droplets are formed and migrate to the cell membrane, then they are extruded into the alveolar ducts for storage. Milk ejection is the process by which contraction of myoepithelial cells in the breasts propels milk along the ducts into the lactiferous sinuses. These sinuses are located beneath the areola, and milk is removed from them by infant suckling. A neurohormonal reflex controls milk ejection and works through afferent nerve pathways to the hypothalamus. Suckling is the primary afferent stimulus, but the ejection reflex can be activated by auditory (infant crying) and visual (seeing the infant) stimuli. The efferent limb of this pathway is clearly hormonal, as oxytocin that is released from the posterior pituitary causes contraction of the myoepithelial cells of the breasts.[3]

The importance of higher cortical centers in the brain is demonstrated by the sensitivity of the ejection reflex to various noxious stimuli. Anxiety and tension, severe cold, and pain inhibit the ejection reflex and decrease milk ejection. This points to the need for the mother to have a comfortable, relaxed setting in which to breast-feed her infant. Chronic stress in life situations contributes to an ineffective lactation response. The nurse needs to assess the mother's psychosocial situation carefully and to plan approaches to alleviate factors which increase stress if successful breast-feeding is to be accomplished.

Prolactin appears to be more critical for initiation of lactation than for its maintenance once it is established. With continued nursing, levels of prolactin released in response to suckling increase less dramatically than in the beginning. Eventually prolactin levels may not rise at all with suckling. Figure 28-4 illustrates the pathways by which lactation and milk ejection are brought about.

Lactation Suppression

The production and ejection of milk may be suppressed at the level of the breast, the pituitary, or the hypothalamus. The most simple, natural method is to avoid stimulation of the breast, which reduces the milk ejection reflex and decreases the stimulation of prolactin required for continuation of milk production. When the milk ejection reflex is inhibited in this way, over the course of several days the distended alveoli suppress lactation. However, some women experience engorged breasts during this time and have considerable discomfort. Lactation can be suppressed with natural methods in about 60% to 70% of postpartum women by wearing a tight brassiere and avoiding stimulation of the nipples and breast.

Hormonal methods are also frequently used to suppress lactation. Estrogens can successfully inhibit milk production in another 10% of women. Adding an androgen to the estrogen increases the success rate of hormonal suppression of lactation to about 90%. However, the use of these hormones is not infrequently associated with rebound lactation (resurgence of milk production some time after administration of hormones) and is implicated in postpartum thromboembolic disorders. Inhibiting prolactin secretion with synthetic ergot alkaloids, such as bromocriptine, is a safe and highly effective approach to lactation suppression, but the drug must be admin-

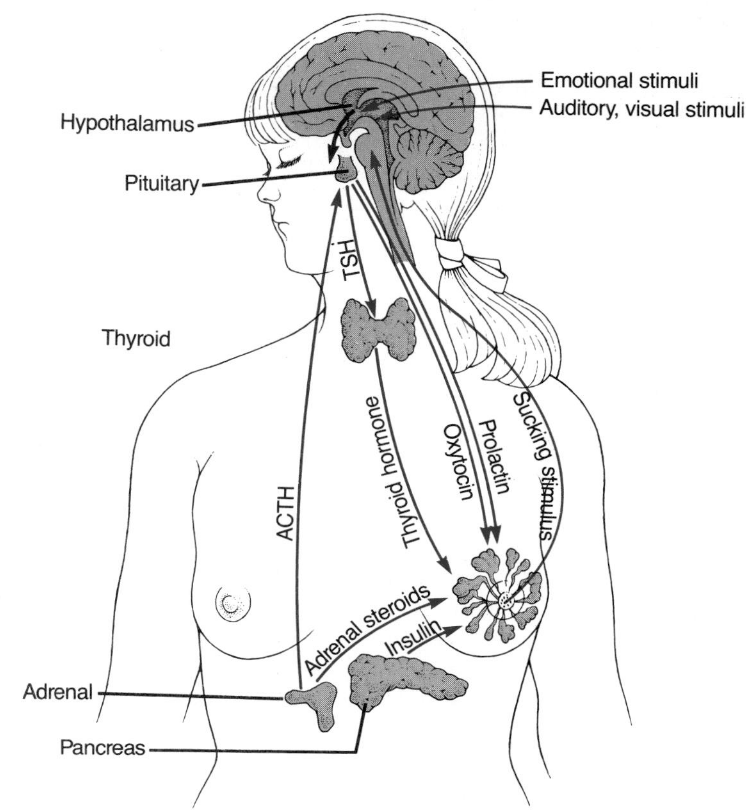

Figure 28-4.
Neurohormonal pathways influencing lactation and milk ejection. (Redrawn from Hytten FE, Leitch I: The Physiology of Human Pregnancy, 2nd ed. Oxford, Blackwell Scientific Publications, 1971)

istered for a 2-week period. A single injection of testosterone enanthate and estradiol valerate is equally effective, and it is not associated with significant risk in young women with normal vaginal deliveries.

Colostrum

On delivery, the breast produces increased amounts of a thin yellow fluid, colostrum. Women who carry out special breast care preparation during the last weeks of pregnancy often are able to express manually small amounts of it before birth. Colostrum contains more protein and inorganic salts, but less fat and carbohydrate than breast milk. It also contains demonstrable levels of antibodies, and its immunoglobulin content (IgA) may offer the newborn protection against enteric infections. The nutritive value of colostrum is lower than that of breast milk.

Lactation

On the third or fourth day postpartum the breast milk usually "comes in." There is an obvious change in the color of the secretion from the nipples; it becomes bluish white, the usual color of normal breast milk. At this time the breasts suddenly become larger, firmer, and more tender as lacteal secretion is established, causing the mother to experience throbbing pains in the breasts that extend into the axillae. This congestion, which usually subsides in one or two days, is caused in part by pressure from the increased amounts of milk in the lobules and the ducts but even more by the increased circulation of blood and lymph in the mammary gland, producing tension on the very sensitive surrounding tissues. This is sometimes referred to as *primary engorgement* (see Chap. 33).

The efficiency and maintenance of milk production is, in large measure, controlled by the stimulus of repetitive nursing. The neurohormonal mechanism involving prolactin and oxytocin release, which triggers the milk ejection reflex, has been discussed previously. The oxytocin released by suckling also stimulates uterine contractions, which explains the mild abdominal cramps often associated with the initiation of breast-feeding.

Supply of Breast Milk

Breast milk varies markedly in its quality and quantity, not only in different individuals, but also in the same individual at various times. In general, the amount of breast milk increases as the infant's need for it increases. Nature seems to have carefully coordinated the mother's need for rest and the infant's need for food during the first two days, when only colostrum is secreted. But during this time, lactation is definitely stimulated by the infant's sucking, and, although the secretion of breast milk would occur naturally, without this stimulation and the complete emptying of the breasts the secretion of breast milk would not continue for more than a few days.

If the infant is put to breast consistently, by the end of the first week a healthy mother usually has about 200 ml to 300 ml (6 oz–10 oz) of breast milk a day. By the end of 4 weeks this amount almost doubles, so that she produces about 600 ml (20 oz) a day. Breast milk is produced on the basis of "supply and demand" (*i.e.,* the amount secreted gradually adjusts in relation to what the baby takes at an average feeding). In time, as the baby grows, the mother may have about 900 ml (30 oz) of breast milk a day.

The supply of breast milk is dependent on several factors, such as the mother's diet, the amount of exercise and rest she gets, and her level of contentment. An adequate diet for lactation requires increased amounts of protein, calcium, iron, and vitamins as well as an ample fluid intake. The mother who is breast-feeding needs a good night's sleep, a rest period in the middle of the day, and normal exercise. Worry, emotional tension, and too much activity (overexertion and fatigue) have an adverse effect on lactation (see Chap. 33).

In relation to lactation, the actual size of the breast is not as important as the amount of glandular tissue, since the secreting tissues of the mammary gland produce the breast milk and not the fat. It has been verified that if large doses of salicylates, certain cathartics, iodides, bromides, quinine, atropine, or opium are administered to the lactating mother, they are excreted in the breast milk.

Clinical Considerations

Early Ambulation

The normal patient should be encouraged to get out of bed as soon as practical, and certainly within the first 24 hours postpartum. In general, patients feel stronger and psychologically better as a result of early limited activity, and constipation and bladder complications are less frequent. Most important, the incidence of thrombophlebitis and pulmonary embolus has been decreased materially in recent years as a result of early ambulation.

Temperature

Slight rises in temperature may occur without apparent cause following the delivery, but, in general, the mother's temperature should remain within normal limits during the puerperium, that is, below 38°C. (100.4°F.) when taken orally. Any mother whose temperature exceeds this limit in any two consecutive 24-hour periods of the puerperium (excluding the first 24 hours postpartum) is considered to be febrile.

It was formerly believed that an elevation of temperature naturally occurred with the establishment of lactation on the third or the fourth day after delivery; the so-called *milk-fever* was considered a normal accompaniment of this proces. At the present time this is considered to be a fallacy. On rare occasions a sharp peak of fever for several hours may be caused by extreme vascular and lymphatic engorgement of the breasts, but this does not last longer than 12 hours at the most.

In judging the significance of a rise in temperature, the pulse rate is a helpful guide because a puerperal patient with a slow pulse or a slightly elevated temperature is not likely to signify a complication. Nevertheless, any rise of temperature in the puerperium should excite the suspicion of endometritis (see Chap. 38).

Pulse

In the early puerperium a pulse rate somewhat slower than normal is a favorable sign. The rate usually averages between 60 and 70 but may even become a little slower than this (*e.g.,* 40–50) in one or two days after the delivery. This is merely a transient phenomenon, so that by the end of the first week or 10 days the pulse returns to its normal rate. On the other hand, a rapid pulse after labor, unless the mother has cardiac disease, may be an indication of shock or hemorrhage.

Blood

Most of the blood and metabolic alterations characteristic of normal pregnancy disappear within the first two weeks of the puerperium.

Afterpains

Normally, after the delivery of the first child, the uterine muscle tends to remain in a state of tonic contraction and retraction. But if the uterus has been subjected to any marked distention, or if tissue or blood clots have been retained in the cavity, then active contractions occur in an effort to expel them, and these contractions may be painful. In multiparas a certain amount of the initial tonicity of the uterine muscle has been lost, and these contractions and retractions cannot be sustained. Consequently, the muscle contracts and relaxes at intervals, and these contractions give rise to the sensation of pain, called "afterpains."

These afterpains are more noticeable after a pregnancy in which the uterus has been greatly distended, as with multiple births or hydramnios. They are particularly noticeable in the breast-feeding mother when the infant is put to breast (because sucking causes release of oxytocin from the posterior pituitary which stimulates the uterus to contract), and they may last for days, although ordinarily they become almost unoticeable in about 48 hours after delivery. They also occur with increased intensity, following the administration of oxytocic agents such as ergotrate. Often afterpains become so sharp that the administration of a sedative is necessary. Any time that they are severe enough to disturb the mother's rest and peace of mind, the physician should be notified.

Digestion

Although the mother's appetite may be diminished the first few days after labor, the digestive tract functions normally early in the puerperium. Thirst is considerably increased at this time due to the marked diuresis and diaphoresis associated with puerperium. Moreover, the fact that the mother may have gone without fluids for some hours in labor undoubtedly increases her thirst.

Kidneys

The amount of urine excreted by the kidneys in the puerperium is of particular significance. During pregnancy there is an increased tendency of the body to retain water, so that now the tremendous output of urine represents the body's effort to return its water metabolism to normal. Diuresis regularly occurs between the second day and the fifth day after delivery, sometimes reaching a daily output of 3000 ml as discussed previously. After the delivery, in particular, the bladder may distend without any awareness on the part of the mother, especially if she has received any form of analgesia. *Therefore, it becomes a major responsibility of the nurse to be alert to signs of a full bladder and thus to prevent distention from occurring.*

During the first few days after labor there may be an increase in the amount of nitrogen in the urine. This excretion is due to the breakdown of protein material of the uterine wall during involution. The presence of acetone in the urine, related to the incomplete metabolism of body fat, occurs when the woman has gone a long period without food. Occasionally, during the first weeks of the puerperium the urine contains substantial amounts of sugar, which is due to the presence of lactose (milk sugar) in the circulation. This glycosuria has no relationship to diabetes.

Intestinal Elimination

The mother is nearly always constipated during the first few days of the puerperium. This is because of the relaxed condition of the intestinal and the abdominal muscles, in particular, and to the inability of the abdominal wall to aid in the evacuation of the intestinal contents. In addition, if hemorrhoids are present, the mother often is afraid to have a stool because of the discomfort these varicosities cause during elimination.

Skin

It is to be expected that elimination of waste products by way of the skin is accelerated in the early puerperium, often to such a degree that the mother is drenched with perspiration. These episodes of profuse sweating, which frequently occur in the night, gradually subside and do not require any specific treatment aside from protecting the mother from chilling when they occur.

Postpartal Examinations

The condition of the mother is confirmed before she is discharged from the hospital to make sure that her progress has been satisfactory during the early puerperium. In addition to verifying her vital signs and present weight, observations are made to determine the condition of her breasts, the progress of involution, and the healing of the episiotomy. A pelvic examination is deferred, since findings made by palpation of the uterus and inspection of the lochia give satisfactory evidence as to the progress of involution at this time.

Follow-Up Examinations

As has been mentioned previously, the reproductive tract should return to its normal condition by the end of the puerperium. In order to investigate the general physical condition of the mother and determine with what normality she has completed her maternity experience, she should return for examination about 6 weeks postpartum.

During the visit the weight and the blood pressure are taken, the urine is examined for albumin, and a blood count may be done. The condition of the abdominal walls is observed, and the breasts are inspected. If the mother is breast-feeding, the condition of the nipples and the degree of lacteal secretion are a significant part of the observation. If the mother is not breast-feeding, the breasts should be observed to see that physiological readjustments have occurred.

A thorough pelvic examination is carried out to investigate the position of the uterus, the healing of the episiotomy or perineal lacerations, the support of the pelvic floor, and whether involution is complete.

In addition, this return examination provides an opportunity to discuss any other problems relating to this maternity experience and to discuss methods of family planning (see Chap. 30). If abnormalities are found, they may be treated at this time and arrangements are made for further examinations and treatments as necessary.

The postpartal visit is an ideal time to emphasize the importance of periodic examinations at 6-month to yearly intervals for continued health care and advice on family planning.

References

1. Monheit AG, Cousins L, Resnik R: The puerperium: Anatomic and physiologic readjustments. Clinical Obstetrics and Gynecology 23/4:973–984, December 1980

2. Frisoli G: Physiology and pathology of the puerperium. In: Iffy L, Kaminetzky HA (eds): Principles and Practice of Obstetrics and Perinatology, p 1659. John Wiley & Sons. New York, 1981

3. Kochenour NK: Lactation suppression. Clinical Obstetrics and Gynecology 23/4:1045–1059, December 1980

Suggested Reading

Barden TP: Perinatal care. In Romney SL, Gray MJ, Little AB, Merrill JA et al (eds): Gynecology and Obstetrics, The Health Care of Women, pp 657–712. New York, McGraw–Hill, 1975

Willson JR, Carrington ER: Obstetrics and Gynecology, 6th ed. St. Louis, CV Mosby, 1979

Larson BL, Smith VR (eds): Lactation: A Comprehensive Treatise. Academic Press, New York, 1974

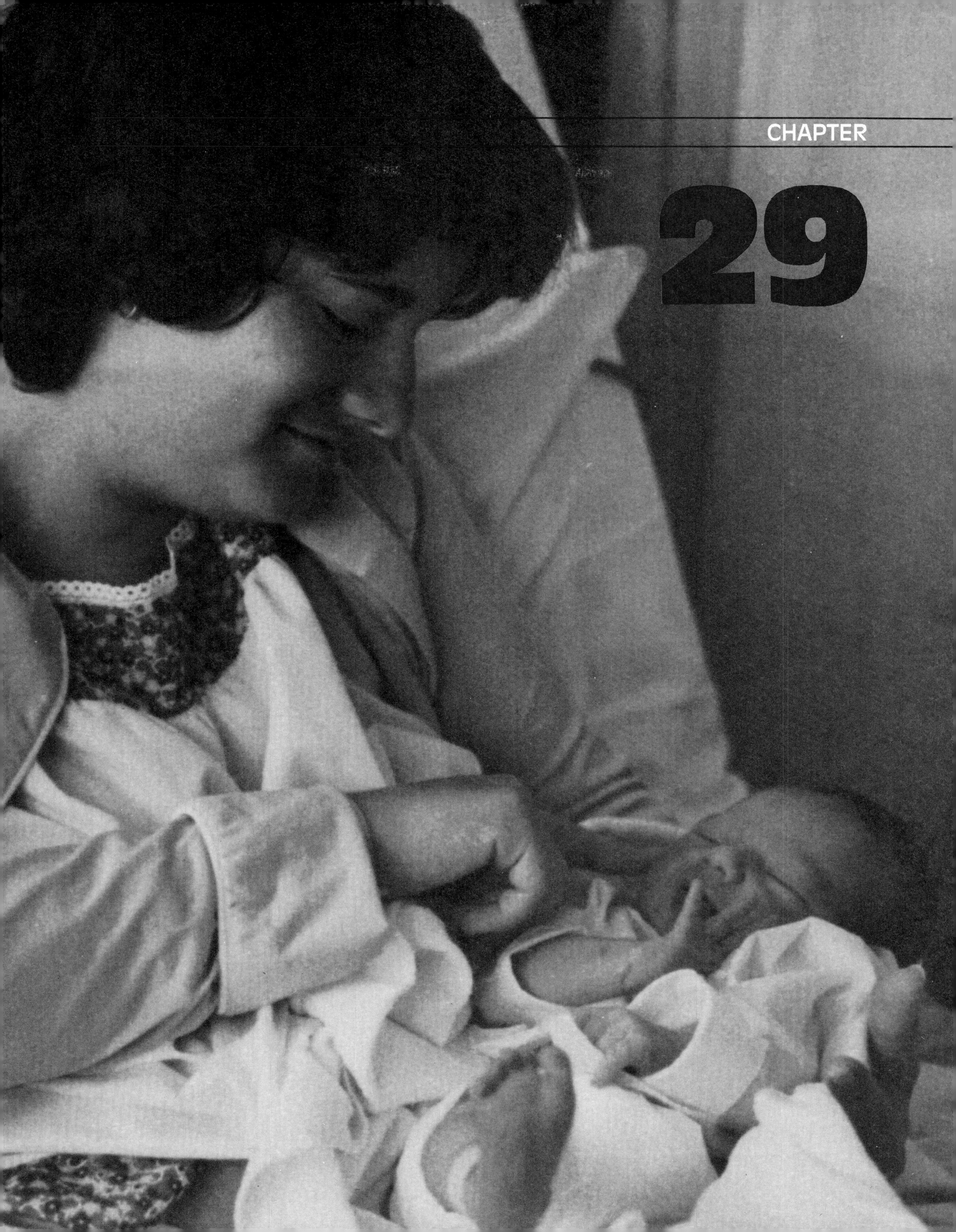

CHAPTER

29

CHAPTER 29

Psychosocial Aspects of the Postpartum Period

In discussing psychosocial aspects of pregnancy in Chapter 18, we made the point that pregnancy and parenthood can be thought of as a role transition. We noted the tremendous change that comes with childbirth and the assumption of the new role, and the concomitant instability that can occur until new roles are allocated and the new member is integrated. In this chapter we continue our exploration of the psychosocial needs of the new, expanded family as they assume their responsibilities as parents.

The present discussion is based on the underlying assumption that the degree of ease and satisfaction with which individuals make the transition to parenthood is directly affected by how successfully they have defined and accepted their relationship with each other. If they have developed an ability to see each other as they are (not as they ought to be), if they can allow for divergence of values and behaviors, work collaboratively toward a flexible power base for each and develop norms that allow for mutual growth, then they are more likely to move smoothly into the new role.

This assumption is identified specifically here because much of the literature on parenting singles out either the content of the parent–child relationship per se or the parents' own childhood relationships as the primary determinants of the family's progression through this phase. This neglects two other vital areas—(1) the needs of each person within the system as an individual and (2) the needs of the parents as a couple. Use of this assumption does not negate the importance of the parent–child relationship or the parents' own background, but it does provide some focus on the marital couple as an entity. In reality it is the balancing of the three areas of needs within the family that is the ultimate task of the new family. Moreover, it is these areas that the nurse must be aware of and respect when working with families undergoing the transition to parenthood.[1]

According to Meleis, one integrative conceptual framework for the care and support of couples experiencing role transition to parenthood is role supplementation.[2,3] By using this framework health providers can help the parents and their significant others gain the necessary information or experience to bring them to a full awareness of the anticipated behavior patterns, sensations, and goals involved in the complementary roles of mother and father. In essence, this approach assists the parents-to-be in moving to role mastery of parenthood. The student will recall that we previously said that pregnancy is the anticipatory phase of the transition to parenthood. The impending role must be at least partly rehearsed, modeled, and clarified through a process of communication with significant others. In so doing, the role expectations become clearer and the couple begin to put themselves into the role of parents (role take). As this is done, there is a better "fit" to the impending role with increased confidence leading to role mastery. See Figure 29-1 for a schematic drawing of the role mastery process. Ideally this process should be begun during pregnancy. However, a similar modified process can be instituted or reinforced in the crucial early postpartum period. Thus, the parents are not entirely separated from providers during this critical fourth period in their reproductive cycle. The student is referred to the article by Swendsen, Meleis, and Jones in the Suggested Reading for details in the implementation of the process.

Transition to Parenthood

The student will recall that we have used Rossi's formulation of phases in the process of role transition. Specifically, these were the anticipatory phase, the honeymoon phase, the plateau phase, and the disengagement phase (see Chap. 18). In the puerperium, it is the honeymoon phase of the transition that has the most bearing on the nursing care that the maternity nurse must render. However, we shall also review briefly the anticipatory phase since we previously focused primarily on its relevance to pregnancy rather than to parenthood.

Anticipatory Phase

We noted previously that pregnancy is an anticipatory stage to becoming a parent and we outlined tasks that the parents must accomplish during this time. We spoke of decision making and expectations which have bearing on later parenting. Another aspect is the division of labor in the family. This becomes extremely crucial when the baby arrives. The mundane activities of family maintenance are often indicative of how comfortable the parents are in accepting their changing roles. This also gives a clue as to what later role assignments the child may have in the family. It is important that the nurse note whether there is any negotiation for task assignment or some indication of a flexible allocation and sharing of tasks. If one part-

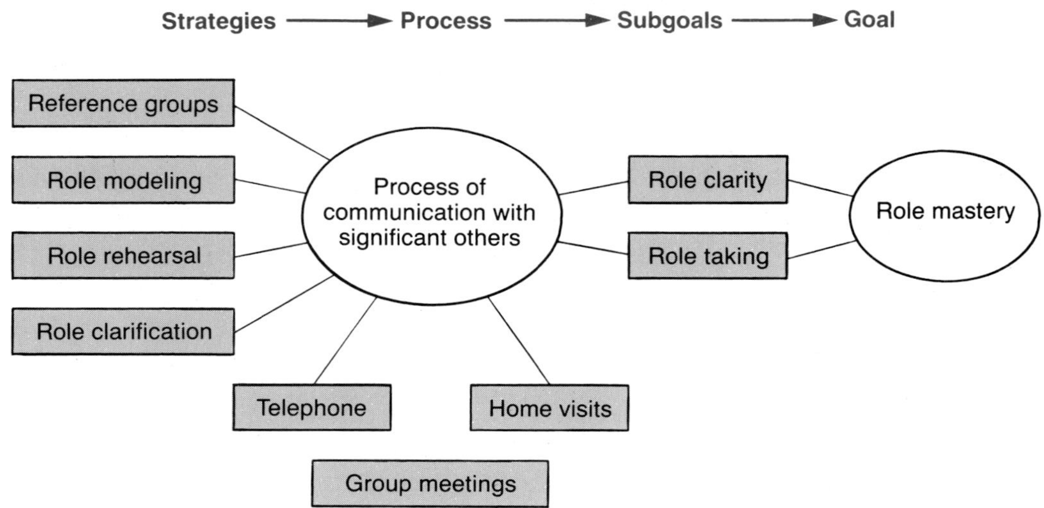

Figure 29-1.
A conceptual framework of preventive role supplementation leading to role mastery. (After Swendsen LA, Meleis A, Jones D: Role supplementation for new parents—A role mastery plan. MCN 3, 2:84–91, March/April 1978)

ner unilaterally appoints the other to a responsibility or if there is a rigid "his work, her work" attitude, there may be subtle sabotage or task overload as responsibilities mount with the addition of the infant.[4] Thus, how the family uses the time of pregnancy to work out or rework their division of labor in the family has a large impact on their transition.

Overall, couples in the anticipatory phase experience many intense feelings, challenges, and responsibilities. If used correctly, this can be an opportune time to test skills in preparing to accept and integrate the new family member into the system. The nurse can be very helpful in aiding the couple to examine and understand what they are experiencing by providing accurate information and feedback of perceptions and offering validation of the dynamics that are emerging.[1]

Honeymoon Phase

This phase refers to the postchildbirth period during which, through prolonged contact and intimacy, an attachment between the parents and child is achieved.[5] It should be noted that this is a "psychic honeymoon" and not necessarily a time of romanticized peace and joy. Rather, it is a period of intensity when both the mother and the father are exploring the new family member and where they stand in relation to him or her. The couple's personal relationship is no less important at this time, but with the limited energy, emphasis is often placed on development of the new relationship.

Bonding and Attachment

Much has appeared in the literature regarding the fourth stage of labor—the time immediately after delivery when there appears to be an optimum time for close contact between parents and child to initiate the process of bonding the trio together. The terms "bonding" and "attachment" are often used interchangeably to describe this process of parent–child affiliation. Brazelton has pointed out, however, that there is a difference in the connotation of these terms. Bonding refers to the initial attraction and desire to "make it" with another person. Attachment, on the other hand, is the long, hard work of staying in love.[6] Thus, bonding can be thought of as the initial step in a process, the mutual attractiveness and response *between parents and child* that paves the way for the later development of love and affiliation. In everyday usage, however, the two terms are interchangeable.

Until quite recently health providers and the public in general have viewed the newborn as essentially passive. Many medical schools still teach that the newborn infant has limited perceptual abilities, as if only the midbrain is functioning. This misconception has directly and indirectly affected the delivery of maternity care at all levels. If, instead of using the "lump of clay" model of the infant, we think of the child as organizing around various positive stimuli and experiences, we can readily see that the present tendency toward overstimulating and noncontingent care (caretaking timed *asynchronously* with the infant's responses) is not conducive to the organization of the infant's central nervous system and hence to expeditious positive parent–infant interaction. Care for the newborn needs to be timed to his activity and responses, not to schedules preordained by professionals.[6]

As we explore more carefully the amazing newborn, research indicates that neonates are very adaptive, not only able to survive in an often unwelcoming or uncomfortable environment but also to capture the important adults around them. For instance, they demonstrate a marked ability to habituate to different stimuli. If a light is flashed repeatedly into the eyes, the baby startles the first two or three times, then gradually settles down and no longer responds. The same response occurs with the stimuli of a rattle, bell, and pinprick. Moreover, there are definite auditory and visual orienting responses. If one talks and begins to play with the baby, he becomes alert and searches for a face (Fig. 29-2). When he finds it, he softens, and as long as the face moves, the baby follows it. If it becomes still, however, the infant frowns and averts his face. The immobile face has no attraction for the newborn.[6]

Responses to auditory stimuli also demonstrate the ability of the neonate to make choices. If a man and woman stand on opposite sides of the baby and begin to talk, the infant stops moving, his face knits, and he turns toward the female's voice again and again. There is also a differential response to human and nonhuman, machine sounds even if their qualities are exactly alike. When you present a baby who is sucking with a nonhuman sound, he stops sucking and then quickly resumes. If, however, he is offered a human sound, he stops, and then resumes with a pattern of suck, suck, pause, suck, suck, pause, indicating by this different, complex pattern a preference for the human sound.[6]

These manifestations of the infant's ability to con-

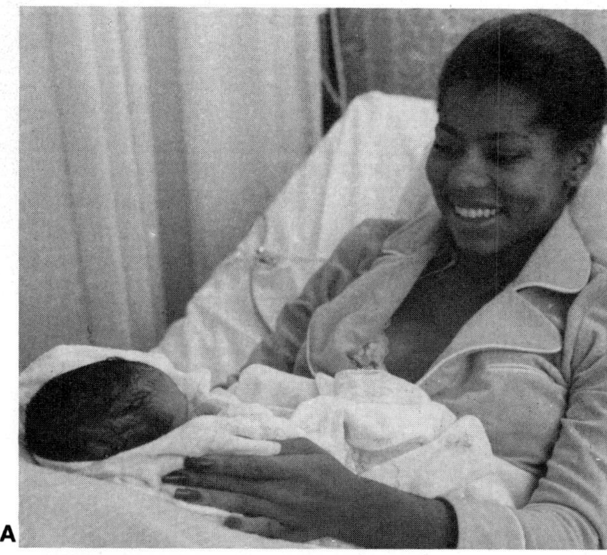

A

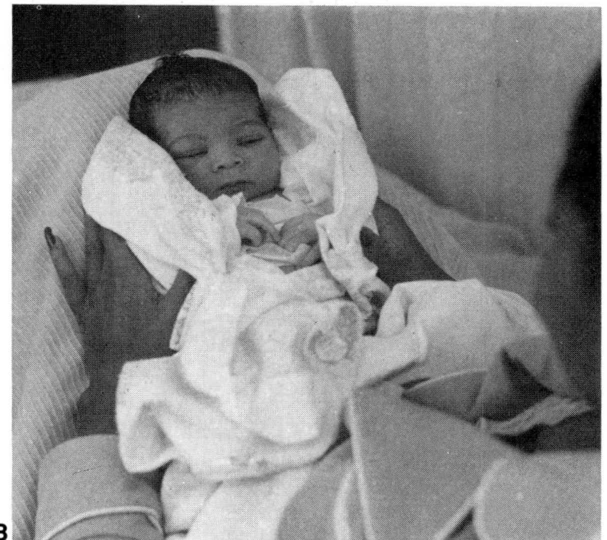

B

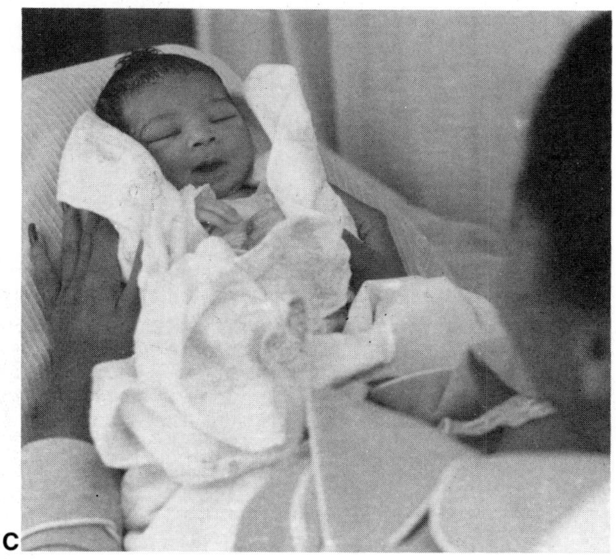

C

Figure 29-2.
(A). An infant responds to an animated smiling face. Note the infant's different expressions as the mother smiles and talks and the manner in which he moves his mouth in response to the mother's voice and smile.
(B). The infant establishes eye contact with the mother.
(C). The infant begins to move his mouth as the mother smiles and talks.

trol and console himself are powerful reinforcers for parents who are ready to move beyond the initial bonding and continue their attachment. The nurse, during both the immediate and later postpartum period, can be very helpful to parents and facilitate bonding by pointing out and *reinforcing parents' perceptions* of their infant's ability to interact with them. One reinforcer to attachment that can be shown to the mother and father is the manner of consoling the baby. When a baby is crying, even at the top of his voice, he can be quieted by insistently saying "baby, baby, baby. . . ." Simply by using the voice, one can get the infant to turn his head, put his fist in his mouth and start looking for you. When this and other behaviors we have mentioned are shown to parents, they usually react by saying such things as "Now I know what I must do to mother," or "You have shown me how to father!" Parents also turn to the nurse for validation of their impressions. "Do you think she really sees (or hears) me?" When you confirm this impression, their faces light up and another link is forged in the bond.[6]

Principles of Bonding

The work of Robson, Rubin, Moss, Brazelton, Klaus, Kennell, Bowlby and many others has begun to shed light on the fascinating subject of how infants and parents first develop their acquaintance. While we still do not have many of the answers and some of the information that we do have must still be considered tentative, there appear to be several vital principles of the bonding process. Again, these are not to be regarded as definitive; rather they reflect the state of the art in thinking and research in the area. Based on their work, Klaus and Kennell specify the following crucial principles:

1. There appears to be a sensitive period in the first minutes and hours after birth when it seems necessary for the mother and father to have close contact with their infant for later development to be optimal.
2. There appear to be species-specific responses to the infant in the human mother and father when the infant is first given to them.
3. The attachment process seems to be structured so that the parents become attached to only one infant at a time. In 1958, Bowlby stated this principle as *monotropy*.
4. For attachment to occur appropriately, it is necessary for the infant to respond to the mother and father by some signal such as body or eye movements. This principle has been called the "You can't love a dishrag" phenomenon.
5. Individuals who witness the birth process become strongly attached to the infant.
6. It is difficult (but not impossible) to simultaneously go through the processes of attachment and detachment. Thus, it is difficult (but not impossible) for parents to attach to an infant while mourning the loss or threatened loss of another person.
7. Some early events may have a long-lasting effect. For instance, anxiety over an infant with a temporary disorder in his or her early days may result in long-term concerns or behavior that will have implications for future development.[7]

Assumption of the Parental Role

As the parents continue in their transition, certain behaviors become apparent. It is important to note that there is much more information on maternal behavior than on paternal behavior.

Paternal Behavior

While most researchers agree that more studies need to be done regarding paternal behavior, we are still in the very early stages of this type of research. Parke, a pioneer in this area, has concluded in his studies that there are no significant behavioral differences between fathers alone with their infants and mothers alone with their infants. If, however, the trio are together, the father tends to hold the infant twice as much as the mother, he vocalizes more, touches the infant slightly more but smiles significantly less. Thus, the father plays a far more active role than the passive cultural stereotype suggests.[8,9] The term *engrossment* has been used by Greenberg and Morris to describe the behavior pattern noted in fathers when they are involved and interacting with their newborn (Fig. 29-3). They conclude that there are identifiable aspects of paternal bonding similar to maternal bonding that are enhanced by newborn behavior and normal reflex activity.[10] A study by Bowen and Miller tends to substantiate this contention. These researchers compared three groups of fathers—those who had attended childbirth classes and were present during delivery, those who were present at delivery but had not attended childbirth classes, and those who did not attend either childbirth classes or delivery. Fathers who attended the birth demonstrated significantly more attachment behavior to their infants than fathers who were not present. Interestingly, attendance at childbirth education classes was not correlated with better attachment scores. Moreover, sleeping infants elicited significantly less attachment behavior from the father than did alert infants. These results lend support for the theory of a sensitive period shortly after birth in the development of parental bonding for the father as well as the mother.[11]

Lamb and Howells, on the other hand, contend that mothering and fathering are separate entities and may be dissimilar. Lamb proposes the following thesis: (1) the mother–child relationship is originally based on the infant's dependence and helplessness and gradually diminishes in importance as the child becomes older and more independent and (2) the father–child relationship revolves around not only caretaking activities but also many outside enjoyable activities. Hence, the father introduces and socializes the child to the world outside the home. Female parents could function in the paternal role but would have to dissociate from the mothering and nurturing tasks. This, therefore, is the reason for the dissimilarity of the two roles.[12] Why the father can caretake and socialize outside the home at the same time and the mother cannot is not clear in Lamb's formulation.

Howells also believes that both fathering and mothering are equally important but may have dissimilar components. According to his formulation, the relationship of both parents to a child is unique and is dependent on the sum total of the variables that make up the psychosocial dynamics of each family.[13]

In view of the similarities found in the better research studies and society's recent trend toward a more flexible masculine-feminine role definition, the utility of breaking apart maternal and paternal behavior may well be called into question.

Maternal Behavior

A pioneer in delineating parental behavior was Reva Rubin, who focused on the mother and identified various phases of maternal behavior, particularly relating to maternal touch and the infant. She contends that mothering is composed of a set of interpersonal and production skills designed to foster the emotional, intellectual, and physical development of the child. Thus, Rubin described the tasks of mothering as (1) identifying the new child, (2) determining one's relationship to the child, and (3) guiding and reconstructing the family constellation to include a new member. In general, this formulation is still accepted.[14]

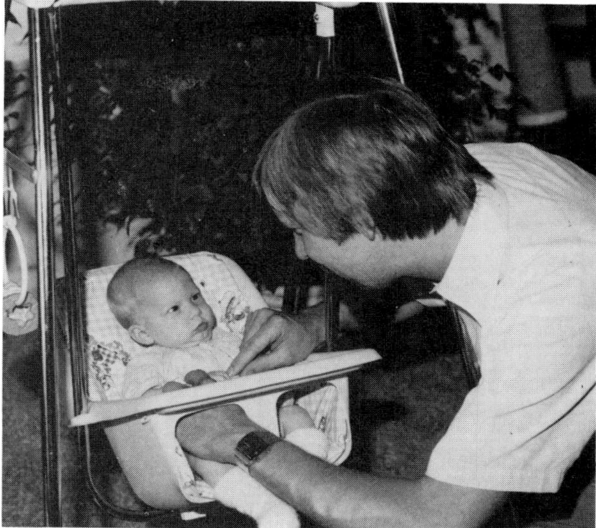

Figure 29-3.
Fathering. Paternal involvement is engrossing and can be satisfying to everyone.

Certain behaviors have been found to accompany these various tasks and the assumption of the maternal role. These behaviors have also been found to be specific to three phases which Rubin also classified. The time spans for these phases may vary, particularly if the parents are permitted immediate contact with the newborn. The following discussion derives primarily from Rubin's classification.[15]

Taking-In Phase

In this phase the mother is oriented primarily to her own needs. She may be quite passive and dependent. This phase may last a day or two and it is important that the nurse try to help meet the mother's dependency needs so that she can move into more complex mothering tasks. The mother does not usually initiate contact with the infant. This is not out of disinterest, but rather because of her own immediate dependency. Although she is not indicating much interest in assuming responsibility for the baby's care, she is taking in information which helps her identify the infant. In this phase *finger-tip touch* with the infant can be observed (Fig. 29-4). The mother may lay the infant on her lap or bed and gently explore him or her with her fingers. This is one of the first steps in the identification process and an indication of awakening interest in the newborn. One may also note that she holds the baby facing her, so that they mutually explore each other's faces. This has been called the *en face* position.

Gottlieb has pointed out that beginning attachment is accompanied by a *discovery* process. The

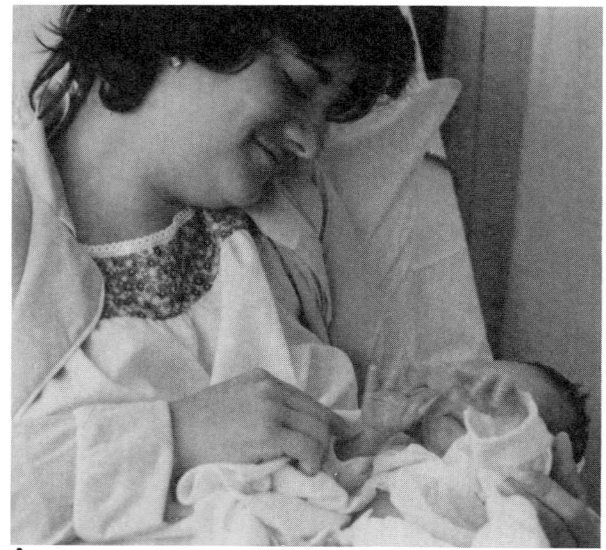
A

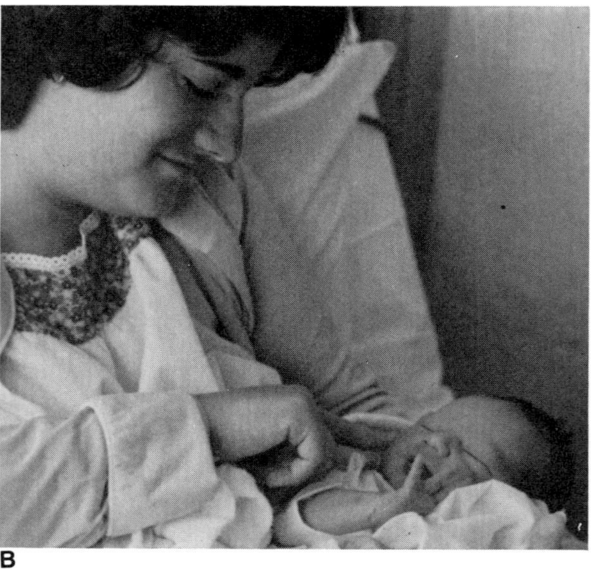
B

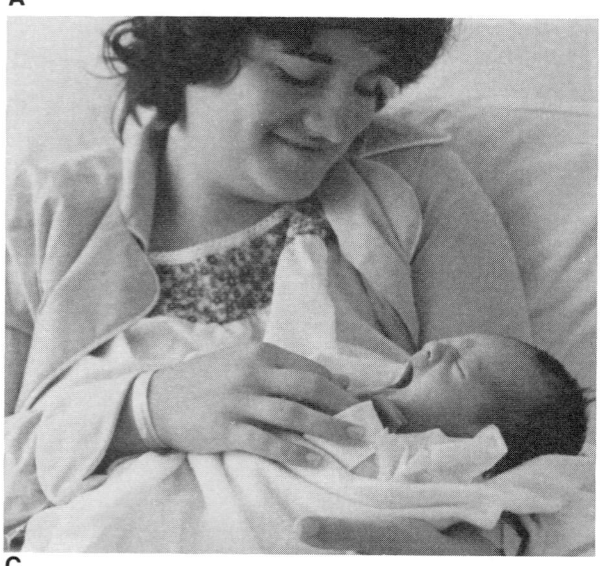
C

Figure 29-4.
Identification process through maternal touch.
(A). Exploring the infant with fingertip touch.
(B). The mother continues her exploration progressing to the infant's face.
*(C).*The baby is finally enfolded by the mother.

mother must ask herself, "Who is this infant? What is he able to do?" and so on. She accomplishes this discovery during the taking-in phase by means of *identification, relating,* and *interpreting* with the infant.[16] In *identification* she points out various physical aspects or features of the infant so as to have a frame of reference. From there she *relates* actions and characteristics to some familiar person, object, or fantasy (*e.g.,* "Face like daddy; hiccups like I used to have.") Finally, in *interpreting* she gives a meaning to the infant's actions and perceived needs. For instance, if the infant is crying and is difficult to quiet, she may say, "He's going to be a holy terror, I just know it." All of these behaviors help the mother realize the infant as a separate entity.[16]

Sleep and Food. Sleep and food play an important part during this phase. The mother is far more able to begin the activities required of her if she is allowed to have a well-earned refreshing sleep. If this necessary rest is disrupted, the mother may experience a "sleep hunger" which may last for several days; this results in irritability, fatigue, and general interference with the normal restorative process. Thus, the necessity of appropriate intervention by the nurse to allow the mother to get adequate sleep cannot be stressed enough.

The nurse should also note if the mother usually has a good appetite and, in fact, may talk a good deal about either the adequacy or the inadequacy of her meals. Between-meal nourishment is appreciated and needed, especially by nursing mothers. The concern about food seems to be a part of the mother's general need to be restored. Food, as we know, has tremendous psychological significance for care-asking and care-giving. The nurse should be especially cognizant of the mother's need for hearty meals and should expedite extra nourishment whenever possible. Moreover, she should be aware that a poor appetite often is one of the first symptoms that all is not proceeding normally in the puerperal period.

Integrating the Experience. During the taking-in phase the mother begins to relive the delivery experience in order to integrate it fully into reality. She is apt to be very talkative at this time, and she may want to know certain specifics and details so that she can form a total picture of what "really happened" during delivery. As she obtains this information, she is able to realize more fully that the pregnancy and the delivery are truly over and that her baby now is born and is an individual outside of and separate from herself. This is a considerable task and involves rather profound changes in attitudes and feelings. The symbiotic relationship between mother and infant during pregnancy is at an end, and the mother now must identify her child as a separate individual.

Taking-Hold Phase

The second phase in the puerperal period has been described as a "taking-hold" phase; that is, the mother strives for independence and autonomy and finally begins to be the initiator. One of her main concerns at this point seems to be her ability to control her bodily functions; her bowels and bladder must perform well, and she takes an active part in seeing that they do. If she is nursing her infant, she is concerned about producing an acceptable quantity and quality of milk. She often asks the nurses and the doctors anxiously (referring to the milk), "Has it come in yet?" And later she wants to know: "Do you think I have enough?" She cannot have enough explanation and reassurance that she is "performing" well at this time. She wants to walk, to sit, to move as she did before delivery and is very anxious and impatient if she cannot make her body behave as it once did. It is as though she is thinking, "How can I possibly assume all my responsibilities for others if I cannot control my own body?"

Her first mothering tasks are especially important to her, and "failures" (inability to elicit a bubble from her infant, poor sucking response on the part of the baby, her awkwardness in handling her child), no matter how small and expected (by the staff), can send her to the depths of despair. Even the skillful intervention of the nurse seems only to point up her "inadequacy" as a mother. She often voices her feelings with an "Oh, I'll never be able to bathe her as easily as you do." Or another mother may say, "He always seems to take his milk better when *you* feed him." Conversely, when she succeeds at a task, her delight and relief are wonderful to behold. It is difficult to imagine (for anyone other than a new mother) how thrilling a hearty bubble from a small infant can be.

Since there is a good deal of anxiety as well as activity in this phase, fatigue and exhaustion may occur if the mother is not helped to set realistic expectations and limits for herself. Since this "taking-hold" phase lasts about ten days, much of it takes place at home.

The nurse can be invaluable in giving the mother, as she appears able and ready to accept it, anticipatory guidance about what to expect and how to manage. During the hospital stay the mother profits greatly from reassurance and explanation regarding the various processes and hour-by-hour events. She finds guidance and reinforcement of appropriate behavior particularly helpful when she attempts to perform her mothering tasks.

When assisting the mother, the nurse must be careful not to impose herself between the mother and her baby (no matter how awkward or maladroit the mother seems). Rather, the nurse should allow the mother to perform the actual task (after necessary demonstration or instruction) and then encourage or reinforce whatever behavior was appropriate. This is one way of demonstrating confidence in the mother's ability to cope with new tasks. In order to gain skill and confidence in her mothering ability, the mother needs the opportunity to make decisions about the baby's needs as well as guidance regarding his or her physical care. When she is allowed to find answers to her questions (again with guidance as necessary) and is reassured that her judgment is correct, she is able to feel confident in her ability to perceive needs accurately and to make decisions. Thus, she is better able to meet problems in the future.

As the mother becomes more comfortable with her infant, she moves to the second stage of maternal touch, *total hand contact,* and finally the third stage, *enfolding* (Fig. 29-4B, C). In general, the more competent she feels and the more satisfying her relationship with the infant, the greater the enfolding. These touching behaviors can be observed in fathers also if they are given the opportunity to handle and care for the infant. They, too, can be observed placing the infant in the *en face* position.

The mother who remains distant and aloof may not be attaching to her infant as optimally as she should. The nurse will want to be alert for such signs.

Letting-Go Phase

As her mothering functions become more established, the mother enters the "letting-go" phase. This generally occurs when the mother returns home. In this phase there are two separations that the mother must accomplish. One is to realize and accept the physical separation from the baby and the other is to relinquish her former role of childless person. As we pointed out in Chapter 18, she will never again be childless until the death of those whom she has borne. The implications are enormous. She must now adjust her life to the relative dependency and helplessness of her child. If she stops working, she must adapt, at least temporarily, to less freedom, autonomy, and social stimulation. If she does continue working, she and the father will have to handle the complex details of

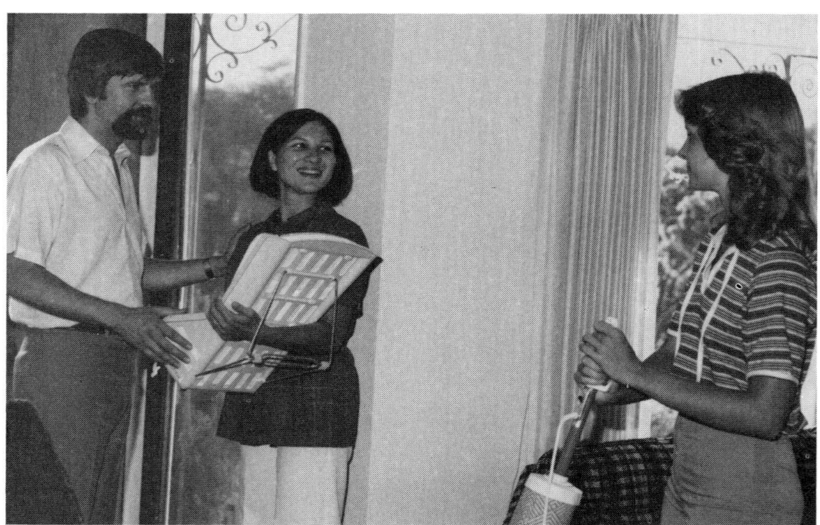

Figure 29-5.
Teenaged "mother's helpers" allow parents more time to enjoy an outing with their infant.

finding mother substitutes and other household caretakers (Fig. 29-5). Her work load is such that there is almost always some role strain and overload even when the father is helpful or outside help is found. This can be managed by appropriate anticipatory guidance from the nurse, but nearly all mothers find the adjustment at least somewhat difficult.

Thus, during the puerperium (for no apparent reason, the mother thinks) she may experience a letdown feeling accompanied by irritability and tears. Occasionally her appetite and sleep patterns are disturbed. These are the usual manifestations of the postpartal or "baby" blues. This depression is usually temporary and may occur in the hospital. It is thought to be related in part to hormonal changes and in part to the ego adjustment that accompanies role transition. Discomfort, fatigue, and exhaustion certainly contribute to this condition if not cause it. Crying often relieves the tension, but if the parents are not knowledgeable about the condition, the mother, especially, may feel rather guilty for being depressed. Understanding and anticipatory guidance help the parents become aware that these feelings are a normal accompaniment to this role transition. (This aspect of postpartal care is explored more extensively in Chap. 30.)

Influences on Parental Behavior

Figure 29-6 presents a schematic diagram of the major influences on parental behavior and their outcomes, including some disorders that have been hypothesized to arise from them. The diagram has been adapted from the earlier work of Klaus and Kennell.[7] We note that, at the time of the infant's birth, some of the influences or determinants are felt to be fixed (less changeable = black line), such as the genetic endowment of the parents, the type of mothering they received, previous pregnancies, and the like. Other determinants are more alterable, however (blue line), such as practices of hospital personnel, separation of infant and mother, and future parental relations. Klaus and Kennell felt that many of the disturbances and disorders could be directly attributed to separation of the infant from the mother after birth and the consequent interference with the bonding process. They point out that the separation of mother and infant is the one variable that is most easily manipulated and urge that hospitals reexamine their policies to bring them in line with more current findings regarding bonding and attachment.[7] In a later work Klaus and Kennell state that the "fixed" determinants may, in fact, be mutable and can be influenced by positive life experiences. We show them here as "alterable with positive life experiences" to indicate to the student that these may be a little more difficult to change and not easily attained in the first days postpartum.[17]

Once again, it is important to note that new parents face a major decision regarding the enactment of their sex roles in addition to the myriad of other large and small decisions they must make. For instance, will the woman assume the more traditional role of total homemaker/mother or will she attempt to combine a career with parenthood? Similarly, will the father extend his role to active involvement in homemaking and childrearing or choose the traditional "breadwinner" role (Fig. 29-7)? The choice of either of the nontraditional parental roles is accompanied by a

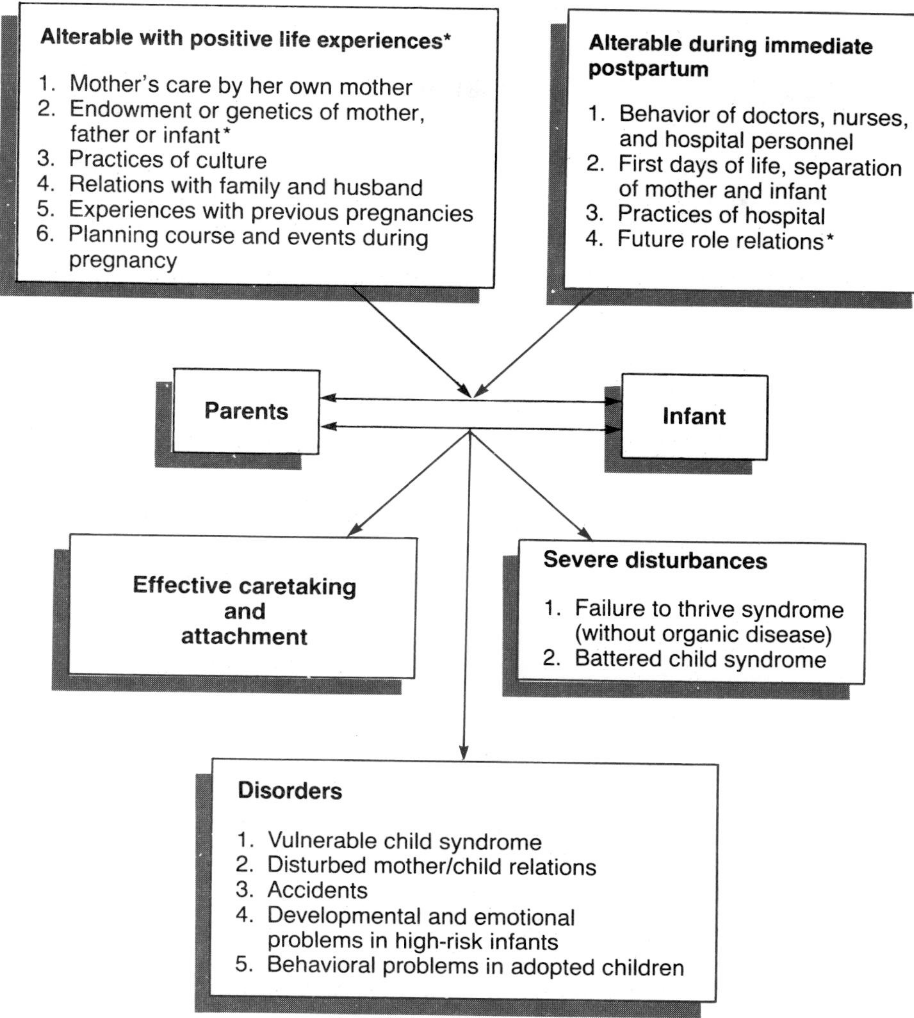

Figure 29-6.
Hypothetical diagram of the major influences on maternal behavior and the resulting disturbances. (After Klaus MH, Kennell JH: Maternal-Infant Bonding. St Louis, CV Mosby, 1976)

certain amount of stress. There is little support for either mother or father from employers, and there may be little support from significant others. On the other hand, assuming the traditional parental roles can also be stressful because this course of action may be thwarting the potential and actualization of the parents.[18] Zaslow and Pedersen found that in the case of fathers' adjustment to parenthood, it does not matter so much whether they choose a traditional fathering role or nontraditional fathering role, but rather whether they assume the role in a consistent and coherent manner.[18] As more research is done on this fascinating topic, we should gain more insight into how we can better help the family make the parental role transition more smoothly.

Responding to Family Developmental Changes—Nursing Implications

One key element of nursing intervention with the expanding family is the teaching of parenting skills that promote the child's maturity, autonomy, and competence. If the parents have a realistic conception of the infant's needs and their resources, they need not expend all their energy on their parenting responsibilities at the expense of their own personal needs and growth.

We have seen that skill in task performance is a cornerstone in both the mothering and fathering.

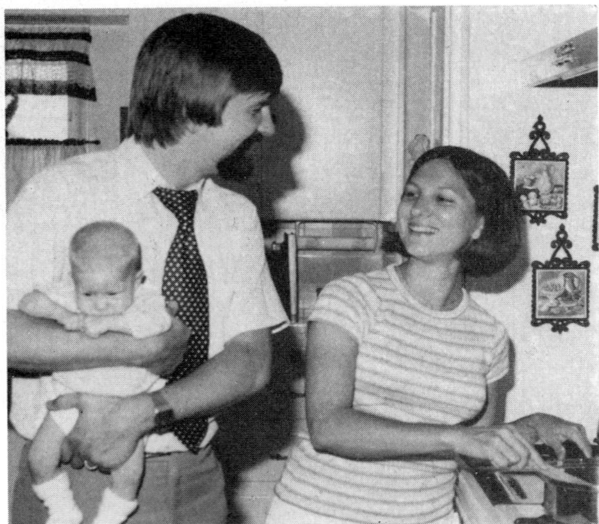

Figure 29-7.
The extension of the paternal role is often helpful for new parents.

Thus, promoting the development of infant-care skills is a vital aspect of the nurse's teaching role. Heretofore, we have focused on coaching parents about childbirth and we have found that planned learning has value. Similarly, nursing's involvement in the recent trend toward health maintenance and promotion has set the stage for an expansion of these types of classes to include information and skill development needed after the infant is born. Teaching styles and format for parenting classes resemble those in prenatal instruction.[19]

Learning needs of the parents can be determined by assessing the following areas: expectations of children's performance ability, lags in development task fulfillment, social isolation, immobilization due to role overload, and ability to set limits and carry them out. When these learning needs are diagnosed, the nurse can develop a teaching plan aimed at preventing and alleviating problems in these areas. Active participation by the parents enhances the learning process and a variety of activities such as role playing, group discussions, and readings enhance the movement of the class. Strengths of the couple should always be delineated and worked with. When deficits are found, verbal and behavioral skills can be developed to cope with the problem. If the deficit is related to outside institutions, the nurse will want to be aware of community insitutions and agencies to which she can refer the parents.[19]

The nurse must recognize that it is impossible to teach all of the skills necessary to parenting. However, if she can help parents sort out problems, examine options and resources, and negotiate outcomes, she has accomplished a great deal for her patients and has been instrumental in this momentous role transition.

References

1. Hrobsky DM: Transition to parenthood: A balancing of needs. Nurs Clin North Am 12:457–468, September 1977
2. Meleis AI: Role insufficiency and role supplementation: A conceptual framework. Nurs Res 24:264–271, July/August 1975
3. Swendsen LA, Meleis À, Jones D: Role supplementation for new parents. MCN 3, 2:84–91, March/April 1978
4. Turner RH: Family Interaction. New York, John Wiley & Sons, 1970
5. Rossi A: Transition to parenthood. Journal of Marriage and Family 30:26–39, February 1968
6. Brazelton TB: The remarkable talents of the newborn. Birth and the Family Journal 5:187–191, Winter 1978
7. Klaus MH, Kennell JH: Maternal-Infant Bonding, St Louis, CV Mosby, 1976
8. Parke R: Father–infant interaction. In Klaus M et al (eds): Maternal Attachment and Mothering Disorders, A Roundtable. Sausalito, CA, Johnson & Johnson Co., 1974
9. Parke R: The father's role in infancy: A re-evaluation. Birth and the Family Journal. 5:211–213, Winter 1978
10. Greenberg M, Morris N: Engrossment: The newborn's impact upon the father. Am J Orthopsychiatry 44:520–531, July 1974
11. Bowen SM, Miller BC: Paternal attachment behavior as related to presence at delivery and preparenthood classes: A pilot study. Nurs Res 29, 5:307–311, September/October 1980
12. Lamb ME: Fathers: Forgotten contributors to child development. Human Development 18:245–266, 1975
13. Howells JG: Fathering. In Howells JG (ed): Modern Perspective in International Child Psychiatry, pp 125–156. Edinburgh, Oliver and Boyd, 1969
14. Rubin R: Basic maternal behavior. Nursing Outlook, 683–686, November 1961
15. Rubin R: Puerperal change. Nursing Outlook, 753–755, December 1961
16. Gottlieb L: Maternal attachment in primiparas. JOGN Nurs 7, 1:39–44, January/February 1978
17. Klaus MH, Kennell JH: Parent–Infant Bonding, 2nd ed. St Louis, CV Mosby, 1982
18. Zaslow MJ, Pedersen FA: Sex role conflict and the experience of childbearing. Prof Psych 12, 1:47–55, February 1981
19. Perdue BJ et al: Mothering. Nurs Clin North Am 12:491–503, September 1977

Suggested Reading

Anderson CJ: Enhancing reciprocity between mother and neonate. Nurs Res 30, 2:89–93, March/April 1981

Hrobsky D: Transition to parenthood: A balancing of needs. Nurs Clin North Am 12:457–468, September 1977

Kiernan B, Scoloveno MA: Fathering. Nurs Clin North Am 12:481–489, September 1977

Lazoff B et al: The mother-newborn relationship: Limits of adaptability. J Pediatr 91:1–13, July 1977

Parent to infant attachment, Special Issue. Birth and the Family Journal 5:4, Winter 1978

Riesch S: Enhancement of the mother-infant social interaction. JOGN Nurs 8, 4:242–246, July/August 1979

Swendsen LA, Meleis A, Jones D: Role supplementation for new parents. MCN 3, 2:84–91, March/April 1978

Zaslow MS, Pedersen FA: Sex role conflict and the experience of childbearing. Prof Psychol 12, 1:47–55, February 1981

CHAPTER

30

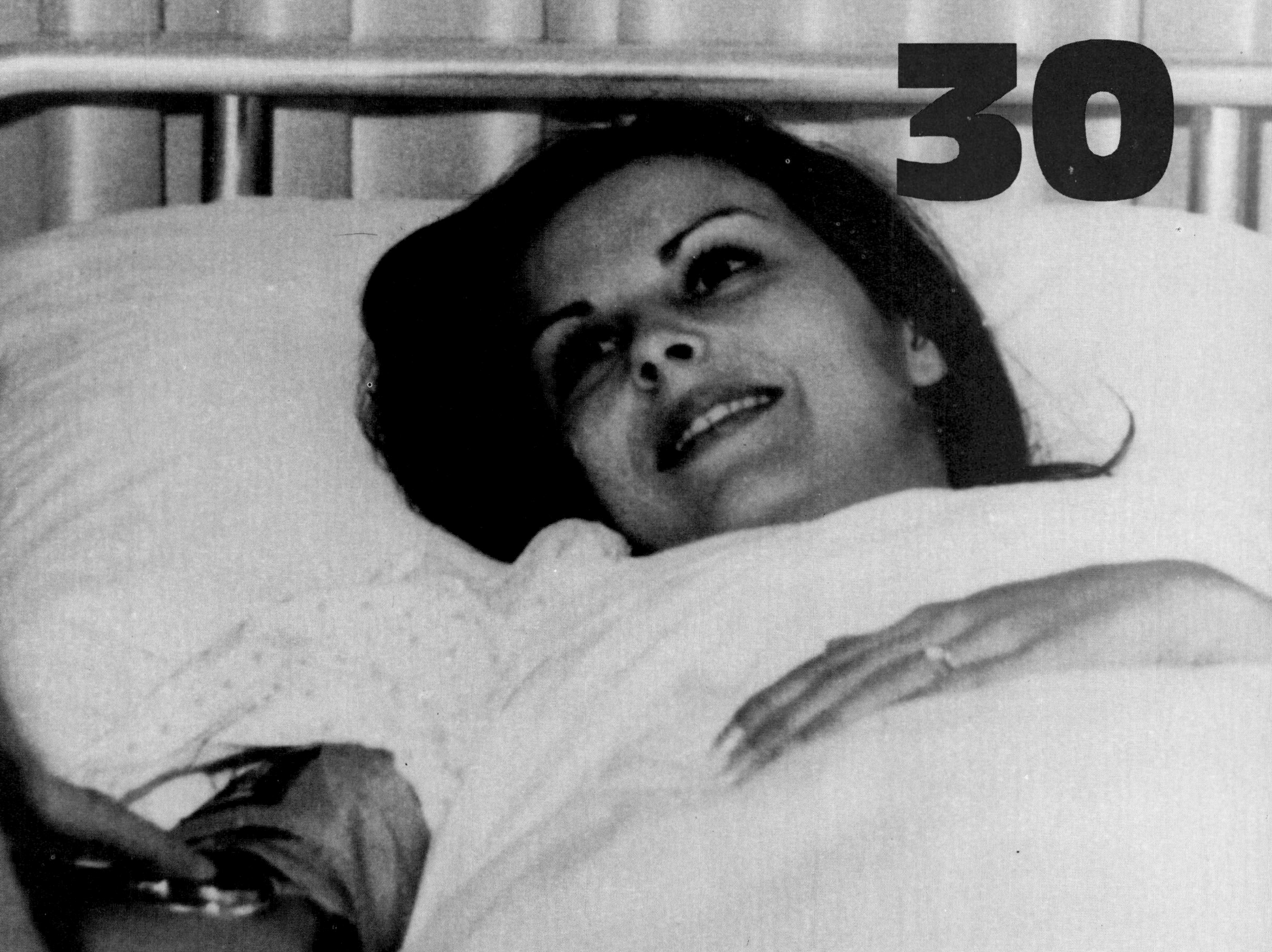

CHAPTER 30

Postpartal Care

The postpartal period is a time of major physical and psychological transition for the new mother. During the 6 weeks postdelivery, her body undergoes restoration as involution of the reproductive organs returns them to their nonpregnant condition. If the mother is breast-feeding, progressive changes occur with the beginning of lactation. The new mother also experiences psychological processes related to the ending of pregnancy, separation from the fetus, and development of a caretaking relationship with the infant, as discussed in Chapter 29. The father experiences similar psychological processes in initiating and developing his relationship with the infant. Both parents must adapt to a new family structure, integrate the infant into their family, and develop different interactional patterns within the family unit. The postpartum period is usually stressful, and sensitive professional care can be very helpful to new parents.

Providing optimal maternal care requires a thoughtful approach to the many facets and factors responsible for the health and the well-being of the maternity patient. Her needs for physical care have been greatly modified by the advent of early ambulation following delivery and the subsequent evolution of more simplified maternity nursing procedures. Newly delivered mothers need physical care related to evaluating the progressive changes which occur in the breasts prior to lactation, as well as the involutional changes of the internal reproductive organs (Fig. 30-1). New mothers need nourishment, rest and sleep, and activity balanced with purposeful use of early ambulation.

Increased insight into the psychosocial needs of the newly delivered mother has resulted in greater attention to the emotional aspects of her care. This does not in any sense negate the need for physical care. As has been emphasized previously, the mother, the infant, the father, and other children are considered as a family unit.

A very important consideration is the need that the mother and her newly born infant have for each other; and in today's highly organized hospitals, such needs do not always coincide with hospital policy or routine. Increased awareness of the importance of the first few days after birth for development of appropriate bonding and attachment between mother and baby has led many hospitals to alter routines. Modified rooming-in procedures and other family-centered approaches generally provide mother and infant with longer time periods together, during which the identification and claiming phases of maternal–infant attachment may occur. Progressive policies for visits by fathers and other family members in many hospitals encourage integration of the new infant into the family.

Nursing care takes the physical and psychological needs of mothers and families into consideration during the postpartum period. The mother's physiological functioning must be observed accurately, her dependency needs must be met, anticipatory guidance and health teachings must be given according to the mother's readiness to learn, and the developing relationship between the mother and infant should be appropriately observed, guided, and nurtured.

Immediate Postpartum Care

Immediately after labor, the mother usually experiences a sense of complete fatigue comparable to that which would normally follow any strenuous muscular activity. At the same time, she may be so exhilarated by the experience and the feeling of relief which accom-

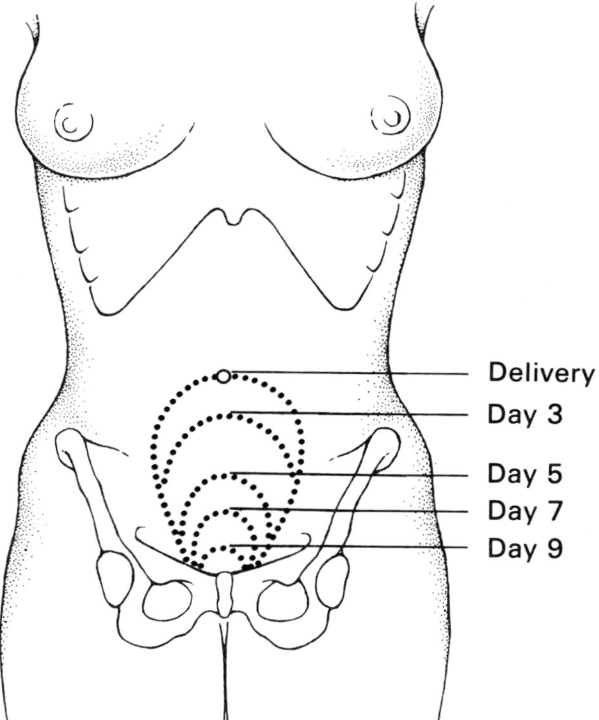

Figure 30-1.
Involution of the uterus.

panies it that she is not aware of being exhausted. She is interested in seeing and holding her baby and visiting with the father. Within the first hour of delivery, the mother, the father, and the infant ideally should be provided the opportunity for a private session together, in which the parents can get to know the infant by holding and exploring the nude infant in skin-to-skin contact. As the infant is in the quiet, alert state for 45 minutes to 60 minutes following birth, his eyes are generally wide open and he can respond to his environment. He is ideally equipped for the critical first encounter with parents, an important phase in bonding and attachment (see Chap. 29). Silver nitrate eye drops can be withheld while the baby is in this alert state and can visually relate to his parents.[1] Following the parents' session with their newborn baby, every effort should be made to help the mother rest. With a little encouragement she usually falls into a sound natural sleep. The discomforts and activities which may interfere with sleep, such as soreness of the vulva, hemorrhoids, "afterpains," and frequent postpartal observations, should be expedited or mitigated as much as possible.

Many mothers complain of feeling chilled immediately after labor; some actually shake with the chill. Such chills may be due in part to neurologic excitation and exhaustion. There is some disturbance of equilibrium between internal and external temperature caused by excessive perspiration during the muscular exertion of labor. Some authorities believe that the "chill" may be due partly to the sudden release of intraabdominal pressure which results as the uterus is emptied at delivery. This reaction may be alleviated if the mother is made comfortable in a warm bed and given a warm beverage when possible. If her body does begin to quiver, an extra cotton blanket should be placed over her or tucked close around her body for comfort. Many mothers (and their partners) are frightened or disturbed by the chill; thus, reassurance by the nurse that this is not an unusual occurrence following delivery is extremely helpful.

Postdelivery Observations

During the first few hours after birth, nursing care focuses on evaluating the mother's physical condition because the risk of complications is greatest at this time. Hemorrhage is the major danger to the mother, and the condition of the uterus must be carefully monitored and bleeding assessed. Observations of vital signs and the condition of the bladder are also part of postdelivery care.

Considerable information can be gained by palpating the fundus through the abdominal wall to be assured that the uterus remains firm, round, and well contracted. At the same time it is also important to inspect the perineal pad for obvious signs of bleeding, as well as to take the pulse and the blood pressure. During the first hour these observations should be made at least every 15 minutes, or more often if indicated.

As long as the bleeding is minimal and the uterus remains firm, well contracted, and does not increase in size, it is neither necessary nor desirable to stimulate it. However, if the uterus becomes soft and boggy because of relaxation, the fundus should be massaged immediately until it becomes contracted again. This can be best accomplished by placing one hand just above the symphysis pubis to act as a guard, as the other hand is cupped around the fundus and rotated gently. It should be remembered that the uterus is a sensitive organ that, under normal circumstances, responds quickly to tactile stimulation.

Care must be taken to avoid overmassage, because, in addition to causing the mother considerable pain, this may stimulate premature uterine contractions and thereby cause undue muscle fatigue. Such a condition would further encourage uterine relaxation and hemorrhage.

If the uterus is atonic, blood that collects in the cavity should be expressed with firm but gentle force in the direction of the outlet, but only after the fundus has been first massaged (Fig. 30-2). Failure to see that the uterus is contracted before pushing downward against it could result in inversion of the uterus, which is an extremely serious complication.

Although excessive postpartum bleeding can happen to any mother, the nurse can identify those at increased risk as evidenced by factors related to their pregnancy or labor. A multipara who has had several deliveries has an increased tendency for heavy postpartum bleeding, as does the woman whose uterus was excessively distended by hydramnios, multiple pregnancy, or a large infant. Operative deliveries

Postpartum Recovery Checklist

After postdelivery observations, the following items are checked before transferring the patient to the postpartum unit from the recovery area:

Vital signs

Condition of the uterus (fundus)

Amount of blood lost; pad count

Care and condition of bladder and rectum

Inspection of vulva and perineum for hematomas

Intravenous fluids and medications administered

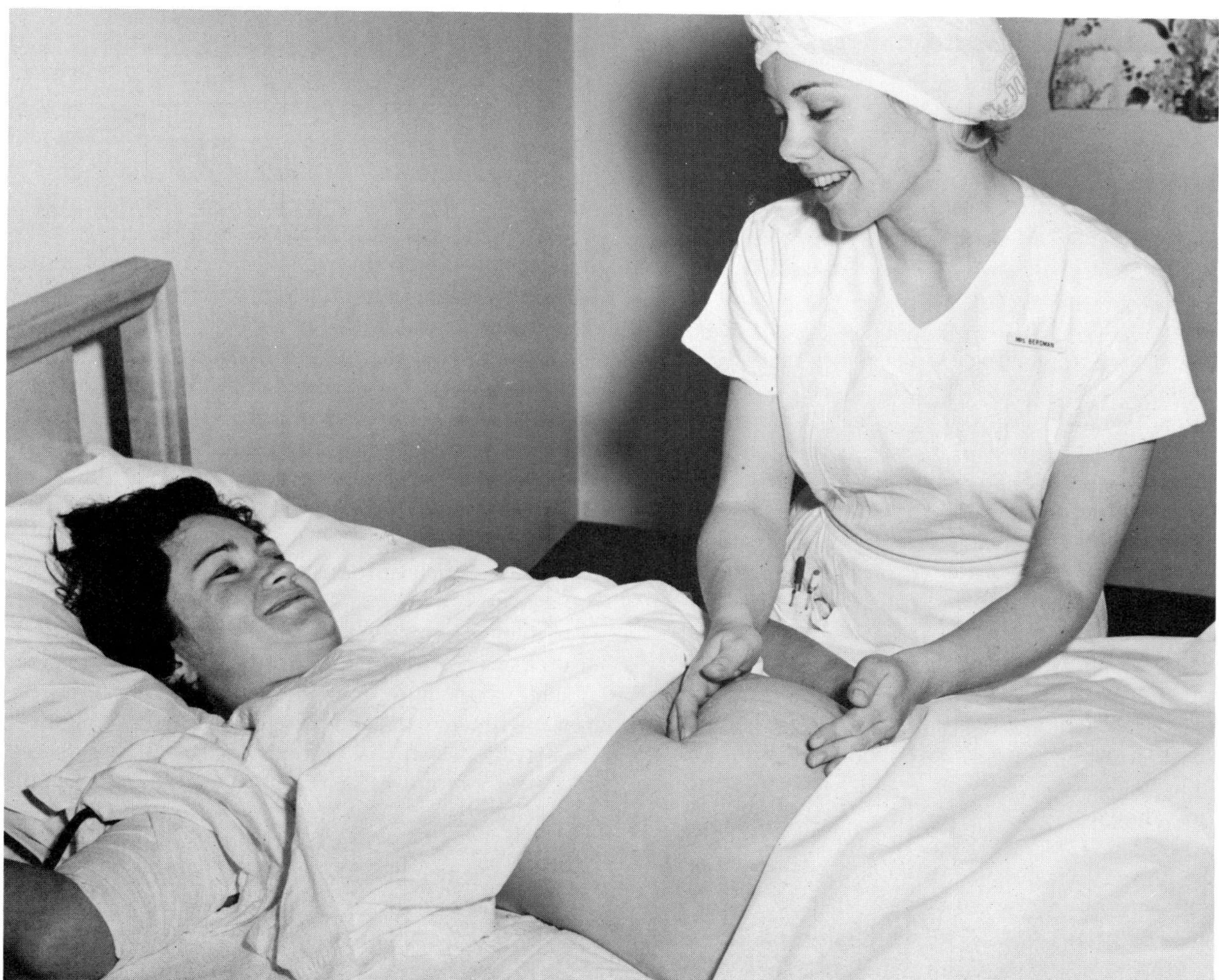

Figure 30-2.
Uterine massage.

with lacerations of the cervix, vagina, or perineum also predispose toward hemorrhage. Patients with a history indicating increased risk require more frequent observation for bleeding.

If the mother's bladder becomes distended, this can interfere with uterine contraction and produce atony, which leads to heavy bleeding. With each 15-minute check of the condition of the uterus, the bladder should also be assessed. It is not unusual for the mother to need to void within the first 4 hours after delivery. If she is unable to void spontaneously and there is bladder distention, catheterization is necessary to prevent both bladder and uterine atony.

Observations of the perineum and vulva are made to detect hematomas or continued bleeding from lacerations. As perineal pads are changed, the amount of saturation is noted and a careful pad count is kept to estimate blood loss.

At the end of the first hour after delivery, if the uterus remains well contracted, bleeding is normal and vital signs are stable, observations can be made less frequently, usually every 4 hours. Temperature is taken at this time also. The mother is allowed to rest as much as possible and kept comfortable. Liquids are usually provided if the mother's condition is stable.

Family Interactions

The immediate postpartum period, also called the fourth stage of labor (see Chap. 24), is important for the development of parent–infant relations as well as for the mother's physiological status. When there is no contraindication due to the infant's condition, the infant is usually placed in the mother's arms, and the two are allowed to visit with the father in a private area. The infant's state of alertness immediately after

Procedure for Fundus Check

1. Explain procedure and rationale to patient.
2. Position patient on back, with feet together and knees apart.
3. Remove perineal pad, note amount of saturation, and record pad count.
4. Have patient empty bladder if necessary.
5. With one hand supporting the lower fundus just above the symphysis pubis, cup the other hand around the fundus and rotate gently.
6. If the uterus is boggy (atonic), blood that has collected in the cavity is expressed with firm but gentle pressure downward. Only do this procedure to express blood *after* the fundus has been first massaged to increase its contraction.
7. Observe the vulva for passage of blood clots and for development of hematomas or bleeding from lacerations.
8. Remove bloody pads, cleanse perineum, and apply fresh perineal pad.
9. Provide comfort, such as sips of water and helping the patient find a comfortable position.
10. Record findings related to fundus, bleeding, and perineum.

birth facilitates eye contact with parents and is felt to be important in establishing the parental bond.[2]

After the excitement and strain of labor and delivery, the parents also appreciate this quiet time together. Needs for information or support vary during this time, and care must be individualized. People of various cultural backgrounds respond differently during the immediate postdelivery period. In some cultures, the mother's female relatives assume the major supportive role during childbirth and thus want to be with her after delivery. The extent of the father's involvement can vary considerably even among families where fathers have a significant part in the childbearing process. Flexible policies in hospitals permit the nurse to respond individually to these different cultural practices and family structures.

Ongoing Care in the Hospital

The daily routine procedures for the postpartal patient vary in different hospitals, but the principles of care are essentially the same. Certain observations should be made and recorded daily. These would include such findings as temperature, pulse, and respiration; urinary and intestinal elimination; the physical changes which occur normally in the puerperium. One should note the changes in the breasts, the height and consistency of the fundus, the character, the amount and the color of the lochial discharge, and the condition of the perineum and episiotomy. Furthermore, it is equally important for the nurse to be alert to the mother's general comfort and well-being—how she rests and sleeps, her activity, her appetite, her emotional status, and particularly, because of its vast influence, how she is adjusting to her role as a new mother.

Temperature, Pulse, and Respiration

The temperature is carefully observed during the first few days of the puerperium, since fever is usually the first symptom of an infectious process. The pulse rate provides a helpful guide in determining the significance of a rise in temperature. These observations are usually made and recorded every 4 hours to 8 hours for the first few days after delivery, omitting the 2 A.M. observations, which would disturb the mother's sleep. If the temperature rises above 37.8°C (100°F) or if the pulse rate rises above 100, the physician should be notified immediately. Usually, the blood pressure is checked daily unless there has been some abnormality. Then observations and recordings are made every two to four hours or more frequently, as indicated.

Nutrition

Very shortly following the delivery, after having gone without food or fluids for some hours, the mother may express a desire for something to eat. Unless she has received a general anesthetic or is nauseated, there is usually no contraindication to giving her some nourishment. She usually enjoys a normal diet.

The two factors to bear in mind when considering the mother's diet are as follows: (1) providing for her general nutrition and (2) providing enough nourishing foods to supply the additional calories and nutrients required during lactation. If these nutritional requirements are provided for, the mother's convalescence is more rapid, her strength is recovered more quickly, and the quality and quantity of her milk is better. She is also more able to resist infections.

Mothers in general, and particularly mothers who are breast-feeding, usually have good appetites and become hungry between meals. For this reason it is advisable to see that they receive intermediate nourishment consisting of a nourishing beverage or a snack three times a day. If the nourishment is in the form of a glass of milk or some milk product, this helps to incorporate the additional milk requirement for the nursing mother (see Chap. 33).

Rest and Sleep

During the puerperium the mother needs an abundance of rest and can be encouraged to relax and sleep whenever possible. This can best be accomplished if she is comfortable and free from worry and other anxiety-producing situations. The need for rest has even more significance for the mother who is breast-feeding, because worry and fatigue inhibit her milk supply. With the exception of the father, visitors should be limited during the first few days because they can be tiring. A mother who is not getting sufficient rest is usually anxious, and worries over minor things that otherwise might cause her little concern. Furthermore, many emotional problems are often precipitated by sleeplessness and fatigue.

It becomes the nurse's responsibility to adjust the hospital routine whenever possible to provide the mother with uninterrupted periods of rest. Routine procedures can be delayed or rearranged to meet the mother's needs. A bottle-fed infant may be fed occasionally by the nurse if the mother is sleeping and does not want to be awakened. If the mother is unable to nap during the day (and she may not, due to excitement and fatigue), she can be encouraged to rest as quietly as possible for certain periods. The need for rest and sleep may have to be explained and reiterated, especially during the "taking-hold" phase, as she is eager to be up and about and may tend to overdo things.

Early Ambulation

Early ambulation has intrinsic health-promoting value for the newly delivered mother. With this increase in exercise, circulation is stimulated, and there are fewer complications of thrombophlebitis. Moreover, bladder and bowel functions are improved, therefore, bladder complications leading to catheterization are greatly reduced. Abdominal distention and constipation occur less frequently. The majority of healthy mothers are encouraged to be out of bed in four to eight hours.

If the patient has had a conduction anesthesia that involves entering the dura, she may be kept in a recumbent position for about the first eight hours. Many physicians feel that keeping the patient flat in bed for this time helps to prevent the occurrence of a postspinal headache, since headache is precipitated and aggravated when the head is elevated. Postspinal headache is thought to be caused by a leakage of the spinal fluid through the puncture hole of the dura, with subsequent decrease in cerebrospinal fluid volume and pressure. Therefore, having the patient in a recumbent position while the puncture hole is sealing, and encouraging the patient to force fluids (to hasten fluid replacement) may help this condition.

The first time that any mother is out of bed she can "dangle" for a short time before actually getting up. Then usually she can walk a few steps from the bed and sit in a chair for a brief period. On succeeding times up, she can increase her activity gradually. The newly delivered mother needs someone to assist her in and out of bed and to go with her when she walks to the bathroom. The nurse should remain close at hand while the mother is in the bathroom so that she can give immediate assistance if the mother becomes weak or faint.

It is important that the nurse explain the purposes of early ambulation to the mother and help her to learn how she can achieve an effective combination of sitting, walking, and lying in bed. All too many mothers feel that once they are out of bed they are "on their own," and expected to take care of themselves entirely. Most of them are afraid of being a nuisance and hesitate to ask for help, whereas others do not realize that help is available. The nurse's attitude is important. Acting interested in the mother and demonstrating a desire to help her and making her feel comfortable encourages the mother to ask for help. New mothers, in particular, are sensitive to the attitudes of those responsible for their care. Many of them are experiencing an enforced dependency for the first time in their adult lives and find this difficult. Others become anxious because they feel that they are being forced toward independence too quickly. By recognizing each patient as an individual the nurse is able to gain insight in providing for the mother's total nursing needs.

Although it is customary for mothers to be discharged home on the second or third day (or after 24 hours in some hospitals, when mother and infant are considered low risk), it should be remembered that early ambulation and the duration of the hospital stay are two entirely different matters. Regardless of the day of discharge, mothers need to be cautioned to proceed slowly at home during the puerperium, resting a large part of the time. If teaching about "getting back to routine gradually" was begun early in the antepartal period, the mother is better prepared during the puerperium.

Bathing

The mother is prone to have marked diaphoresis in the early puerperium, so that a daily shower is refreshing and a source of comfort. When the mother showers for the first time, the nurse usually gives the self-care instructions for breast care, perineal care, and other aspects of physical care. The nurse is guided by the mother's readiness to learn as well as by the realization that the mother can absorb only so much information at one time. Subsequently, when the mother is able to absorb the information, the nurse can explain about breast care, perineal hygiene, elimination, general activity and hospital routines.

Showers usually are permitted as soon as the patient becomes ambulatory. The first time or two that the mother takes a shower, the nurse or the attendant should remain nearby for safety. It is particularly important that a patient who has had a cesarean birth be instructed regarding her bathing. Usually, these patients are not allowed to shower even though they are ambulatory, because the incision should be kept dry until it has closed and the sutures have been removed. Tub baths usually are allowed in two weeks.

Urinary Elimination

The newly delivered mother may not express a desire to void, in part because the bladder capacity is increased as a result of reduced interabdominal pressure. In addition, if the mother has received analgesia or anesthesia during labor, the sensation of a full bladder may be further diminished. The mother should be encouraged to void within the first 6 hours to 8 hours following the delivery. It is not prudent, however, to adhere to a designated time for the mother to empty her bladder, but rather on evidence indicating the degree of bladder distention. It is important to keep in mind that there is an increased urinary output during the early puerperium. Moreover, mothers who have received intravenous fluids are very likely to develop a full bladder. As the bladder fills with urine, it gradually protrudes above the symphysis pubis and can be observed bulging in front of the uterus (Fig. 30-3). If the bladder is markedly distended, the uterus may be pushed upward and to the side and may become relaxed. When a hand is cupped over the fundus to massage it and to bring the uterus back to its midline position, the bladder protrudes further. When the hand is removed, the uterus returns to its displaced position.

Further evidence of bladder distention can be gained by palpation and percussion of the lower abdomen, which reveals a difference in consistency between the uterus and the bladder. The latter is ballotable and filled with liquid in contrast with the uterus, which has a firm tone. Such observations are of extreme importance and demand immediate attention.

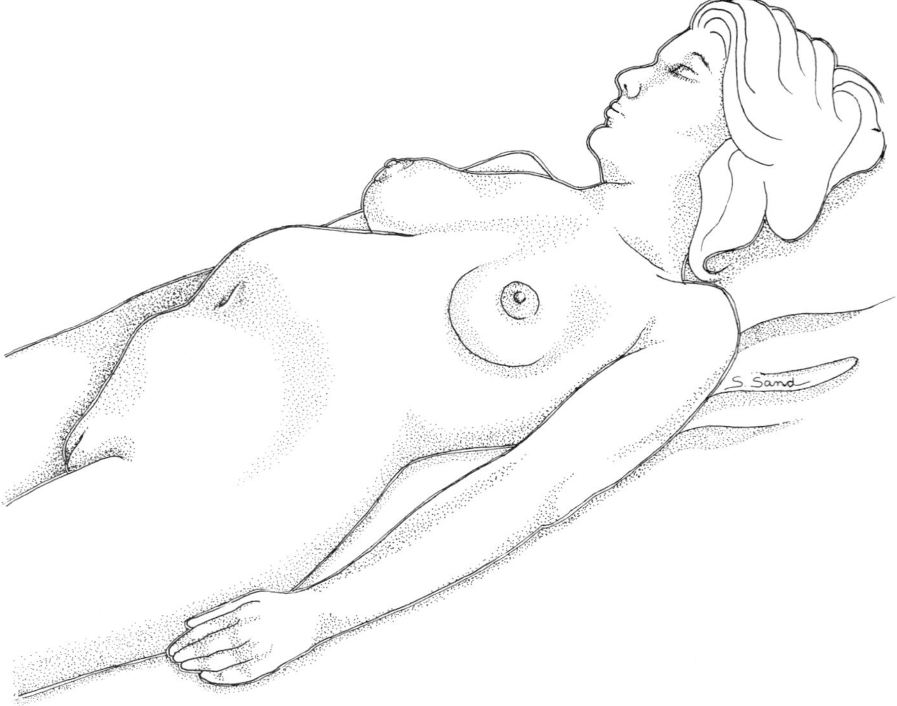

Figure 30-3.
Full bladder displacing uterine fundus. (Redrawn from Ruben D: De Lee's Obstetrics for Nurses, 18th ed. Philadelphia, WB Saunders, 1966)

A full bladder is considered to be one of the causes of postpartal hemorrhage, and if the bladder is permitted to become distended, urinary retention will inevitably follow.

Some mothers have difficulty in voiding at first. As a result of the labor itself, the tone of the bladder wall may be temporarily impaired, or the tissues at the base of the bladder and around the urethra may be edematous. When the mother is allowed early bathroom privileges, urinary elimination may present no problem. On the other hand, some efforts may be needed to stimulate normal urination. Running water so that the mother can hear it, letting the mother dabble her fingers in water or offering a beverage (preferably warm) may help to initiate voiding.

If the mother must be on bedrest, the nurse can assist the mother in voiding by helping her assume a comfortable position on the bedpan, providing privacy and giving her assurance that she will soon be able to urinate. The nurse should offer the mother a bedpan at two-hour to three-hour intervals at first and measure the urine at each voiding during the first day (or days) until it has been established that the mother is emptying her bladder completely. A voiding must measure 100 ml to be considered satisfactory.

At the first voiding, it may be apparent that the bladder has not been entirely emptied. If the bladder is not distended, the mother may be allowed to wait for an hour or so, as the second voiding usually empties the bladder. If, however, the mother continues to void small amounts frequently, one may suspect that she has residual urine, and these voidings are the result of the overflow of a distended bladder. If all attempts fail and the mother cannot void a sufficient quantity, catheterization is necessary. Because of the risk of hospital-induced infection, it is very important to avoid this procedure unless the mother is absolutely unable to void, despite astute and persistent nursing intervention.

Catheterization

Although the procedure for catheterization varies to some degree in different hospitals, the principles involved are essentially the same. Aseptic technique must be maintained throughout to avoid introducing bacteria into the bladder or contaminating the birth canal. If the mother is given routine perineal care prior to the catheterization procedure, the potential danger of infection is further reduced.

Because there is a certain amount of soreness of the external genitalia, it is important to proceed with extreme gentleness and convey an awareness of the additional tenderness. As the labia are separated to expose the vestibule, care should be exercised so as not to pull on the perineal sutures. The meatus may be difficult to locate due to the edema and consequent distortion of the tissues; therefore, a good light is imperative.

The urinary meatus and surrounding area are cleansed prior to the insertion of the catheter. The cleansing procedure is carried out in a gentle manner with just enough friction to allow proper cleansing of the area. None of the cleansing solution is permitted to run into the vaginal orifice because of the danger of contaminating the birth canal. Immediately following the cleansing, a dry cotton ball can be placed at the introitus to prevent excretion from the vagina (i.e., blood or lochia) from spreading upward to the urinary meatus, from which it can be carried into the bladder when the catheter is inserted.

Intestinal Elimination

Constipation

Because the bowel tends to remain relaxed in the early puerperium (as in pregnancy), intestinal elimination may be somewhat of a problem. In view of the sluggishness of the bowels during this time, constipation can be anticipated unless certain measures are instituted to prevent it. It is common to give a stool softener each night after delivery or a laxative on the evening of the first or second day following delivery. If a bowel evacuation has not occurred by the morning of the second or third day, a cleansing enema or a suppository may be prescribed. The latter is very effective and less traumatic for most patients.

If there has been no elimination and especially if the mother has had more extensive perineal repair done, an oil retention enema, followed some hours later by a cleansing enema, sometimes is prescribed.

The mother who is breast-feeding is advised to follow her physician's prescription if laxatives are required to encourage proper elimination after she is discharged from the hospital. Certain laxatives are excreted in breast milk and therefore affect the infant (see Chap. 33). In addition, the usual measures employed to encourage good bowel habits (*i.e.,* adequate fluid intake, roughage foods in the diet, establishing a habit time, and so on) are to be included in the health teaching. Prevention of constipation is discussed in Chapter 21.

Hemorrhoids

Hemorrhoids are a common problem for women during the postpartal period, as a result of pressure exerted on the pelvic floor by the presenting part and the straining of the expulsive phase of labor. They are most painful during the first two to three days after delivery, then gradually reduce in size and regress.

Painful hemorrhoids are treated with sitz baths, anesthetic sprays, and cool astringent compresses (such as witch hazel or Tucks). Comfort is promoted by wearing perineal pads loosely and lying on the side in Sims's position while in bed. Prevention of constipation is the main measure to relieve ongoing difficulties with hemorrhoids.

Care of the Perineum

Observations of the condition of the vagina, perineum, and perianal area are made regularly. The kind of lochia is noted, whether rubra, serosa, or alba, as well as its odor and whether clots are present. Lochia has a characteristic odor but should not have a foul smell. Presence of clots indicate heavy flow. Observing the lochia provides evidence of the progression of involution and enables the nurse to identify infection, hemorrhage, and other complications. The mother is informed about the changes which should occur in lochia and the signs which would indicate problems. The difference between lochia and a menstrual period is explained.

The perineum is observed for healing and signs of complications, such as hematoma, bruising, swelling, and tenderness. If an episiotomy has been done, the status of the stitches is assessed, particularly for infection and hematoma. The anal area is inspected for hemorrhoids and fissures. Usually some method of perineal cleansing is used after voiding and defecation, with the patient instructed in the method and the proper removal and application of perineal pads. Cotton balls, soap and water, or medicated wipes may be used, or a method employed such as use of the surgitator which directs a spray of solution onto the perineum while the patient sits on the toilet (Fig. 30-4).

The woman is instructed to cleanse and wipe from front to back in one motion, to prevent contamination of the vagina and urinary meatus with fecal material. She should wash her hands before applying a perineal pad and should not touch the inner surface of the pad before applying it from front to back. Pads should also be removed with this motion.

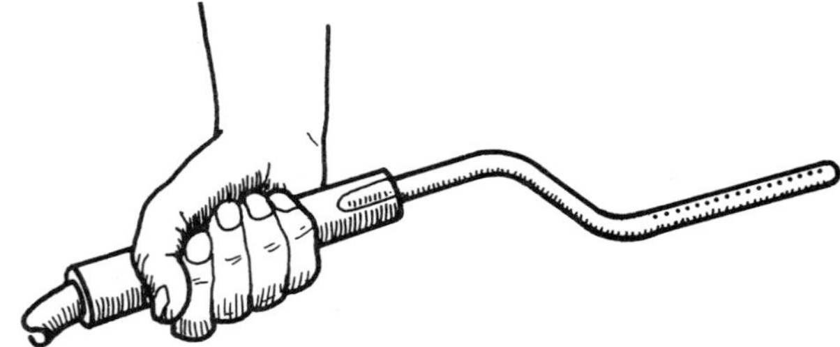

Figure 30-4.
Surgitator for perineal care. With patient seated on toilet, hold nozzle several inches from perineum, start flow and direct against perineum. Do not touch nozzle to perineum; use a new nozzle for each patient. Dry perineum with gentle front-to-back blotting motion.

Perineal Discomfort

Following a spontaneous vaginal delivery without laceration, mothers usually do not experience perineal discomfort. It is most likely to be present if an episiotomy has been performed, or if lacerations have been repaired, particularly if the perineum is edematous and there is tension on the perineal sutures. Almost all primigravidas experience some degree of discomfort from an episiotomy, depending largely on the extent of the wound and the amount of suturing done. For the most part, during the first few days, local treatment in the form of dry heat, analgesic sprays, or ointments is all that is necessary to alleviate the discomfort. But if the pain is more severe in the first day or so, such treatment may not be sufficient, and analgesic medications may have to be administered by mouth or hypodermic injection. Later on, sitz baths may be ordered if the discomfort persists.

A perineal heat lamp may be used for 20 minutes three times per day. When the mother has assumed the dorsal recumbent position, the lamp can be easily

Characteristics of Lochia

Rubra	Serosa	Alba
Bright red, bloody, may have small clots	Pink to pink–brown, serous, no clots	Cream to yellowish, may be brownish
Characteristic fleshy odor (animallike scent)	Usually no odor (unless poor hygiene)	Usually no odor (unless poor hygiene)
1–3 days postpartum	5–7 days postpartum	1–3 weeks postpartum

Perineal Care

The patient is instructed to carry out her own perineal care once she is awake and alert. The following points are generally included:

1. The perineal pad is removed from front to back, to avoid dragging microorganisms from the rectum across the vaginal opening and perineum.
2. The perineal area is flushed with warm water or a mild antiseptic solution, using a pitcher, squeeze bottle, or applicator such as the surgitator (Fig. 30-4).
3. The perineal area is patted dry with clean paper wipes (using a wiping motion should be avoided in order to provide comfort and to prevent contamination).
4. A fresh perineal pad is applied, again using a front to back motion, and secured with a belt to prevent its moving back and forth between the rectum and vaginal opening.

slipped between her legs and placed about 10 in to 12 in from the perineum. After the perineum is exposed, the bulb is adjusted so that the light shines directly on it. The mother can be completely covered during the treatment, because the arch of the lamp frame acts as a cradle to support the top bedclothes.

Mothers who have discomfort from perineal sutures usually find it uncomfortable to sit for the first few days. Many of them are observed sitting in a rigid position, bearing their weight on one side of the buttocks or the other, with obvious discomfort to the back as well as the perineum. Therefore, it is important to teach the mother how to sit comfortably with her body erect.

In the sitting position, the perineum is suspended at the lowermost level of the ischial tuberosities, which bear the weight of the body. Thus, in order to achieve a greater measure of comfort, the mother must bring her buttocks together to relieve pressure and tension on the perineum, in the same manner as that described in the exercise for contraction and relaxation of pelvic floor muscles (Kegel's exercises). After assuming a sitting position the mother is instructed to raise her hips very slightly from the chair, only enough to permit her to squeeze her buttocks together and contract the muscles of the pelvic floor, and hold them this way momentarily until after she has let her full weight down again. This exercise is also helpful to the mother when she is reclining in bed.

Lower Extremities

The lower extremities are observed for varicosities, symmetry, edema, shape, size, temperature and color, and range of motion. Signs of thrombophlebitis include unilateral swelling, erythema, tenderness and pain in the calf when the foot is flexed with the leg extended *(Homan's sign)* (Fig. 30-5). Pulses in the lower extremities may be absent in thrombophlebitis. The mother is advised to avoid constricting garters or clothing that interferes with circulation.

Afterpains

Uterine contractions following delivery continue as part of involution and in some instances are felt as cramps similar to that of a menstrual period. Intermittent uterine contractions with subsequent afterpains occur more frequently in multiparas than in primiparas, because in primiparas the uterus remains tonically contracted. Afterpains are also more common and severe when there has been excessive distention of the uterus due to a large baby, hydramnios, or multiple pregnancy. Breast-feeding mothers notice afterpains occurring when the infant nurses, because suckling stimulates release of oxytocin, which increases uterine contractions. These cramps gradually diminish and are usually quite mild within 48 hours of delivery. Often simply explaining the cause of afterpains and their functional purpose enables the mother to tolerate them. If afterpains are severe, an analgesic is usually ordered to provide relief.

Breast Care

Routine breast care is directed at maintaining cleanliness and adequate breast support necessary for the normal function of the breasts and the comfort of the mother. The breasts should be handled gently and precautions given to avoid rough rubbing, massage, or pressure on these organs.

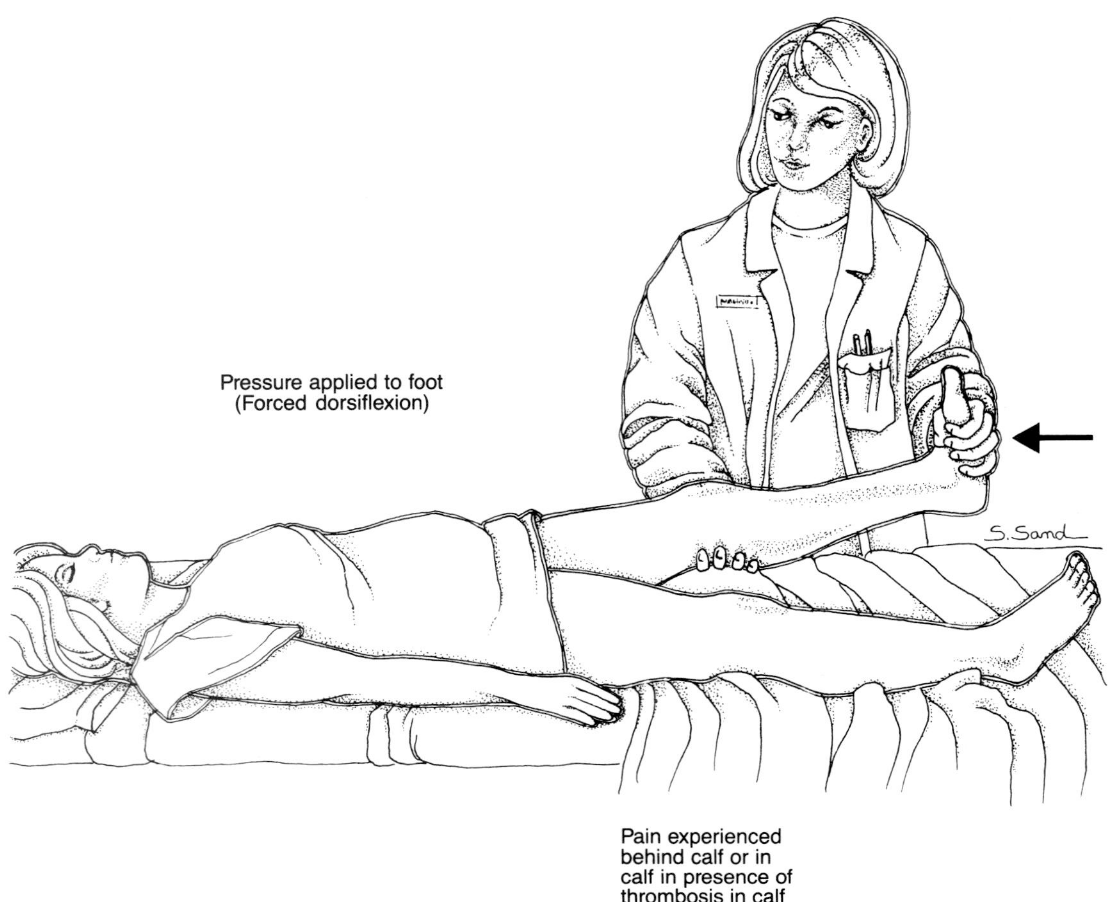

Figure 30-5.
Homan's sign—method to identify presence of thrombosis in the calf.

The mother who is bottle-feeding her infant can bathe her breasts daily with mild soap and water; this is done most conveniently at the time of the daily shower or bath. No other special care need be given.

If the mother is breast-feeding, her nipples may be cleansed with clear water. It is recommended that soap not be used on the nipples; the nipple skin itself is cleansed by the natural antiseptic, lysozyme. It is important to instruct the mother not to use any drying agent, such as alcohol, on her nipples because it tends to remove the secretions of sebum, a physiological emollient. Under normal circumstances, the best nipple care is provided by the body itself, without outside interference.[3] Additional cleansing before each nursing need not be done, but the mother is to be instructed to wash her hands with soap and water, as they come in contact with the nipples and breast during nursing. In this way precautions can be taken against infection.

The mother can be encouraged to wear a well-fitted support nursing brassiere as soon as her milk begins to come (in about the second to fourth day but sometimes earlier). Further care of nipples and breasts in the breast-feeding mother is covered in Chapter 33.

Mothers who are not breast-feeding also need breast support with a well-fitted brassiere. Usually these mothers are given some type of lactation-suppressing hormone to help the breasts dry up, and engorgement is not a problem. Occasionally, however, they do suffer this phenomenon and may experience throbbing pains in the breasts which extend back into the axillae. During this time, analgesic medication may be required for pain relief until the condition subsides in 1 day or 2 days. Ice bags to the breasts and axillae also are often helpful.

Engorgement

Breast discomfort several days after delivery that mothers experience in relation to initiation of lactation is termed engorgement. This postpartal breast discomfort is attributed to venous and lymphatic breast engorgement, and filling of the lobes and ducts of the breasts with milk. Although engorgement usually disappears in 48 hours with regular nursing, it may continue for 4 days to 5 days. The mechanism underlying breast engorgement, and its prevention and management, are fully discussed in Chapter 33.

Postpartum Exercises

Exercises may be initiated postpartally to hasten recovery, prevent complications, and strengthen the muscles of the back, pelvic floor, and abdomen. By toning the muscles, these exercises assist the mother to restore her figure and can be psychologically beneficial. Exercises can be started on the first postpartum day and increased gradually. The mother must take care not to overexercise and to allow slow progression in adding to the routine. A new exercise can be added daily, with each done five to ten times per day for at least 6 weeks after delivery (see Chap. 19, chart on postpartum exercises).

Kegel's exercises can be taught to increase vaginal tone which may be flaccid and distended following delivery. This exercise consists of contracting the muscles of the perineum with enough force to stop a stream of urine. The contraction is held for a few seconds and then released. The exercise is repeated 50 to 100 times and can be done several times per day (see Chap. 21).

Parental Guidance and Instruction

Each mother's understanding and ability in providing infant care varies, depending largely on her background and previous experiences. Undoubtedly, the primipara who has not been accustomed to infants has much to learn about the care and handling of her new baby. On the other hand, the multipara may feel uncertain about the response of an older child to the new baby and thus require guidance in understanding and dealing with sibling rivalry. Many mothers need to know more about their own care; others need to know how to facilitate certain adjustments within the home or the family group. If the mother knows what she can expect and what to do, she usually can handle simple problems that might otherwise cause fear or apprehension.

Proper care for the mother during the puerperium emphasizes the need for rest and nourishing food, and protection from worry. Parents, as a rule, seem to be under the impression that once the delivery is over, things return to "normal," allowing them to resume their usual activities immediately. However, it takes several weeks before the generative organs have returned to normal size and position and the emotional and endocrine adjustments are made.

One of the most important points to be emphasized is that the mother should proceed *as slowly as possible* in the postpartal period at home. The general feeling of well-being and the excitement of having the baby, together with the emotions aroused in the "taking-hold" phase, all too often provide so great a stimulus that the mother has a tendency to overdo things. If there are other children in the household, especially toddlers, the demands on the mother may be considerable.

If it is at all possible, the major responsibilities of housekeeping should be taken over by a "helper," so that the mother can be more relaxed and devote herself primarily to caring for her new infant and spending more time with the immediate family. At this time family relationships can be strengthened if the mother is not overwhelmed with apprehension and fatigue. The subject of household assistance needs to be explored thoroughly with the mother (and if necessary, the father).

The parents may need help in realizing what possibilities and alternatives they have in this matter. Some parents, for instance, manage very nicely when the father takes some vacation time and assumes management of the household. However, it must be remembered that not all fathers are able (or willing) to shoulder this considerable task. Other couples rely on parents, in-laws, or relatives for a time. Still others must hire outside help; in these cases the expense and consequent budgeting may have to be discussed.

If outside help is employed, then the mother may have some question as to whether a housekeeper or a "nurse" (to take care of the baby) would be more desirable. This, of course, depends on many factors. Most mothers find that when they are relieved of the heavy housekeeping chores, the "care" of the baby is relatively easy and provides an opportunity to get thoroughly acquainted with the new addition to the household.

By the time the mother leaves the hospital, she should have at least a basic understanding of her own condition and status, and she ought to know what physical and emotional changes to expect. In addition, she should be familiar with the daily care of her baby and know what to expect of him, as well as any other important details related to infant care. Parents also need to know how and where to contact the physician if any medical problem pertaining to either the mother or the infant should arise before the next scheduled visit.

Since the present-day maternity stay is rather short, some type of follow-up service often is desirable and necessary. Therefore, parents need to be offered information about the services of the public health nursing agency in the community and how they may use these services. In cases of obvious need, a referral to an agency should be instituted before the patient leaves the hospital.

Individual Teaching

Regardless of the fact that a mother may attend all the group classes offered in the maternity hospital, each mother should be given individual help to learn how to handle and care for her infant while she is in the hospital, particularly if this is her first baby. Many new mothers are timid at first because they do not know what to expect of their infants, or they are afraid of what they may do to them because of their own feelings of inadequacy. A mother who has had no previous experience with infants needs some guided practice in changing diapers, dressing her baby, and handling the infant in general (Fig. 30-6). Rooming-in units provide an environment in which the mother can have such an experience over an extended period of time. However, even in situations in which the infants are kept in a central nursery, the nurse should plan to spend some time with the mother, in addition to the regular feeding periods, to help her learn to care for her baby. If hospital staffing permits the time, it may be desirable for some mothers to bathe their own infants at the bedside, under the nurse's guidance, before leaving the hospital. Demonstration of

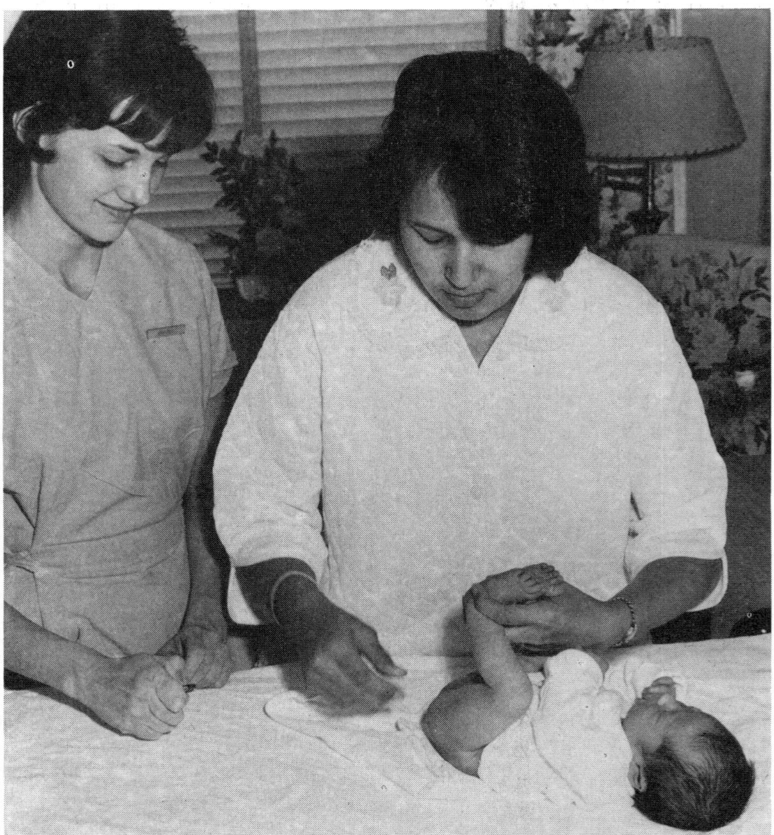

Figure 30-6.
Helping mother to learn how to handle her infant.

the infant bath by the nurse, in the patient's room, is often an important step in the mother's gaining infant care skills.

A rooming-in experience is undoubtedly beneficial for mother, father, and baby. But when this is not possible because of hospital facilities or policies, a daily extended visiting period can be extremely helpful. In this way the parents and the baby can become better acquainted in the security of the maternity division, where experienced personnel are near at hand to answer the parents' questions and to offer advice.

Sexuality and Contraception

Postpartum sexuality is affected by the degree to which the mother's steroid hormones have been depleted following delivery. This is discussed more fully in Chapter 12. Postpartum instructions are given regarding resumption of intercourse, with the couple advised that sex is appropriate after lochia has ceased and the perineum has healed to the point that intercourse is not painful, and as long as there are no contraindicating factors such as hematoma or infection.

Sexual adjustment following birth of a baby is a major concern of new parents, and it is often a source of conflict and confusion. The mother's interest in intercourse is usually less than her partner's in the first month or so after delivery, and her physiological responses diminish[4] because of low hormonal levels, the adjustment to the maternal role, and fatigue due to lack of sleep and rest. Lochia has generally ceased or progressed to the alba stage by 2 weeks to 4 weeks postpartum, and the perineal area and episiotomy are well healed and not painful. If intercourse causes discomfort, the couple is advised to wait somewhat longer or use noncoital sexual practices if they find this acceptable. Positions for intercourse which avoid the penile shaft pressing posteriorly on the perineum can also alleviate discomfort. In addition to the emotional benefits to the parents' relationship, intercourse after childbirth can promote perineal healing by softening the episiotomy scar.[5]

For most couples, intercourse is resumed before the 6-week checkup, so it is important to provide contraceptive information before the mother leaves the hospital. Although it is unlikely that she will ovulate and become fertile before 6 weeks, it is possible. Menses usually resume by about 9 weeks in the nonlactating woman, and by 30 weeks to 36 weeks in the lactating woman. However, the time of return of fertility is unpredictable, and all postpartum women are counseled to use contraception if they desire to avoid pregnancy (see Chaps. 13 and 28). Many hospitals provide a supply of contraceptive vaginal cream and condoms and nurses instruct the parents on their use before discharge.

The First Weeks at Home

The process of integration of a new baby into the family is a stressful period and one in which there is little professional help available. Many parents have no contact with health providers during the time between discharge from the hospital and the 6-week checkup, although they are contending with major changes and adjustments in what is often a new experience in their lives. In contrast to the cultural ideals of joyful parenthood and fantasies of blissful motherhood, many women find the first few weeks of their child's life to be extremely disillusioning.[6] The household is often disorganized and untidy, with greatly increased work related to diapers, feeding, and care of the new baby, while the mother copes with fatigue and frustration in trying to learn the baby's patterns and ways of communicating. Within the first 6 weeks, many mothers find that they have yelled at and spanked their infants, that they cannot cope with or understand the baby's crying, that they feel trapped spending the greatest part of their lives caring for the baby, and that they wish they had not had the baby because they feel unsuited for such responsibility.[7]

The concerns of new mothers in the first weeks after delivery cover a wide range, and there seem to be few resources to assist them in coping with problems and providing information and support. The most common concerns expressed by new mothers are in the following areas: changes in their figures, fatigue and lack of sleep, infant care, changing roles and life styles, and nursing care.

Changes in Body Image

One of the most frequently expressed concerns of the postpartum involves return of the figure to normal. This concern appears to be more than just a minor anxiety. Although new mothers are initially delighted when their abdomens decrease in size after delivery, this positive feeling turns to dismay in the days and weeks following when the abdominal wall remains soft and flabby and part of the weight gained during pregnancy is retained, making it impossible to wear clothes that fit before pregnancy. Frequently, the mother feels as though she is still several months pregnant.

Although mothers may want to lose weight and tighten up muscles, they often find that the baby's demands and their own fatigue interfere with these attempts. A flabby postpartum figure, and the feeling that one lacks the control or ability to improve it can be depressing.[8] Fathers, too, are often disappointed because of the time it takes for the figure to become slim again, and both partners may fear that the figure changes are permanent. Another source of concern is the lack of tone in the vaginal introitus which carries many implications for the couple's sexual relationship.

The first few weeks at home can also be a time of continued physical discomfort, much to the woman's dismay, especially if she has anticipated a quick return to normal. Persistent discomforts—from episiotomy pain which lasts about 2 weeks to 3 weeks, breast engorgement, which is a source of discomfort for both breast-feeding and nonbreast-feeding mothers, nipple soreness and the annoyance of leaking milk—all are troubling in themselves and a drain on energy at a time when added strength is needed to respond to the infant's constant demands. The continued discharge of lochia may also be disconcerting, particularly if it is compared to a menstrual period.

Fatigue and Lack of Sleep

Fatigue appears to be a consistent problem for new mothers. Labor and delivery are hard, exhausting work, followed immediately by the demands of caring for a totally dependent infant. The short stay in the hospital is insufficient to restore energy levels, as excitement, the strange environment, and physical discomforts often interfere with rest and sleep. Most women have also not slept well during the last weeks of pregnancy. This leaves them with a tremendous deficit of energy and sleep, which increases sharply during the first weeks at home with the baby.

Sleep deprivation is to some degree a part of living

Factors Related to Transition to Parenthood

Factors Contributing to Difficulty in the Transition to Parenthood in Contemporary United States Society

1. Minimal role preparation—few American parents enter parenthood with sufficient previous child care experience to give them a comfort level with care of their infant
2. Limited role preparation during pregnancy—there is little opportunity to develop skills and make adjustments to ease transition to parenthood during pregnancy when the focus of education is on childbearing
3. Abruptness of transition—there is no gradual taking on of responsibility for the infant, as there is in assuming a work role
4. Lack of guidelines for successful parenthood—childrearing advice can include general recommendations, but it is not possible to tell new parents exactly what they must do to achieve a specific end result with their infant

Factors Positively Related to Adaptation to Motherhood in Women

1. The capacity to visualize oneself as a mother in the first and second trimesters of pregnancy
2. The personality characteristics of being high in nurturance and having ego strength
3. A retrospective recall of one's own mother as being warm, empathetic, close, and happy with her role
4. Having interest in and experience with children
5. The existence of a high-quality marital relationship
6. Physical health during pregnancy

Factors Positively Related to Adaptation to Fatherhood in Men

1. Previous experience with children
2. Enjoyment of taking care of young children in the past
3. Knowledge of baby care
4. Knowing the number of children desired before marriage
5. Knowing number of children desired after baby's arrival
6. Planning this pregnancy

(After Jennings B, Edmundson M: The postpartum period: After confinement: The fourth trimester. Clin Obstet Gynecol 23,4:1093–1103, December 1980) for all new mothers, and it can be severe. The mother's sleep needs are curtailed by the baby's needs for food and attention. It may be difficult for new mothers to obtain more than 30 minutes to 45 minutes of uninterrupted sleep per night, particularly if there are other small children who frequently need attention at night. Increased bodily tension as a result can lead to insomnia when there is the opportunity to sleep. Mothers may find themselves resenting their partner's ability to sleep uninterrupted. Sleep deprivation can also produce changes in mood and mental functioning, with the mother experiencing increased anxiety, apathy, depression, withdrawal, irritability, illogical thought patterns, mental confusion and aggression and decreased sociability.[6]

Infant Care

Concerns about caretaking activities for the infant vary. Many primiparae have had little previous contact with infants and possess little knowledge of procedures and the common behaviors expected. Often care is learned by trial and error because there are few sources of expert advice. Infants are quite different in their patterns, so even multiparae may find that their prior experience does not apply to the new infant. Babies range from quiet to active and respond in different ways to attempts to console and comfort them. A new mother must learn her baby's particular patterns and why he cries and fusses at various times. The greatest part of this learning occurs during the first few weeks after birth, and the difficulty is compounded by such concerns and problems as fatigue, discomforts, and worries about restoration of the figure.

Mothers are concerned about how normal their infant's behaviors are, particularly in the areas of weight gain and loss, crying, bowel movements, feedings, and sleeping patterns.[9] There is little written information which can help identify "normal" ranges, and health professionals often do not discuss specific changes that may occur during the first months of life. Parents are often surprised at the range of behaviors among infants. Conflicting advice regarding how frequently the baby should be fed, when to add solid food, when to pick up a crying baby, what clothes to put on the baby, who should be allowed to visit and when, and so forth, leads to further confusion.

The processes for successful mothering have apparently been set in motion by the end of the first month following birth. The way a mother perceives her one-month-old infant is an indication of the child's subsequent growth and development and reflects the degree to which the mother is satisfied with her interaction with the infant. If she feels rewarded, she has a more positive perception of the infant and reinforcement of her own identity as a mother. This, in turn, fosters a nurturing relationship.[7] Clearly, nursing intervention before maternal perception is set should be aimed at increasing the mother's sense of mastery and satisfaction in infant care, thereby promoting healthier infant development.

Changing Roles and Lifestyles

Few parents are prepared for the amount of change required in their roles, relationships, and lifestyles as the infant is integrated into the family. Many parents may actually "grieve" over the passing of former life patterns. The mother particularly may have to make major changes in career and other activities, although the gratifications of motherhood may be enough to compensate for these relinquishments. Changes occur in the family constellation, with problems related to jealousy among the other children and marital problems between spouses arising from relative neglect of their relationship. With less time for each other, and possible strain in their sexual relations, many couples report stress in their relationship following the birth of a new baby. Social isolation, lack of recreational activities, and financial concerns can compound family stresses.

Nursing Care

The structure of the health care provided during childbearing makes it difficult to respond appropriately to concerns and problems which can occur during the first few weeks at home. This period represents a gap in health care services, with limited resources available to patients and families. However, the nurse can provide some anticipatory care during that phase of the prenatal period when the mother is most responsive to this type of information. Prenatally, the woman primarily focuses attention on the pregnancy and preparation for labor and delivery. During the third trimester, however, there is increased interest in caretaking activities, so that teaching related to infant behavior and infant care can be productive at this time. As the mother expresses some anticipated concern, the nurse can discuss these problem areas with the prenatal patient, including such topics as preparing other children for the new baby, exploring ways to meet the increased demands of a new baby for attention and continuous care, considering sources of potential stress to the marital and family relations and ways of coping with these problems.

Reinforcing the importance of some kind of help with household tasks during the first few postpartal weeks at home may encourage the mother to arrange for such help to alleviate fatigue and sleep deprivation. If the mother can appreciate that she will need time to regain her energy levels to compensate for the numerous drains that will occur in late pregnancy and postpartally, she may be more realistic in her expectations. Also knowing that her figure will take time to return to its prepregnant form and that physical discomforts will exist for a time after delivery will prepare the parents and reduce the dissonance which occurs when expectations are not borne out by reality.

Postpartally, there is limited time for teaching and providing supportive care in the aforementioned areas of concern. Priorities must be set, and focus set on information concerning bodily changes and methods for relieving physical discomforts. Exercises and diet assume an important place and specific instruction is helpful. During hospitalization, the mother may not be very receptive to learning about infant care, as her needs are directed more toward identification and claiming, or getting to know her baby than toward details of caretaking. The best time to instruct and reinforce specific techniques in infant care is when the mother is engaged in feeding her infant and attending to his needs. Providing the mother with written brochures and instructions in infant care procedures is another effective way of offering information at a time when she is more receptive and feels the need directly.

Most women can benefit from professional contact within the first week to 2 weeks after leaving the hospital. By this time, they have experienced most of the demands and difficulties in integrating the new baby into the family and have specific questions and concerns. Mothers can be assisted to recognize and respond appropriately to their baby's unique patterns and ways of communicating and to identify various states of consciousness of the infant and its particular needs for stimulation, sleep, and feeding. When able to respond more smoothly to her infant, the mother's satisfactions are increased and the development of a healthy relationship is encouraged.[10]

Community health nurses may be available to visit new mothers and provide this teaching and support during the first few weeks at home. For many others, however, there is no clearly identifiable resource and they are often reluctant to call the hospital or physician's office with these kinds of concerns. Even provision of such contact by telephone as part of postdischarge care would be helpful.[9]

The Six-Week Checkup

A follow-up visit in the physician's office or clinic is scheduled for 6 weeks after delivery to evaluate the process of involution and the woman's and family's adaptation to the new baby. At this visit, weight, blood pressure, breast, pelvic, and perineal examinations are done. The amount and character of lochia is assessed, along with the size and position of the uterus and cervix and the condition of the breasts and nipples, especially if the mother is breast-feeding. Problems with healing or infection are treated if present. The family's response to the new baby is discussed, and questions related to behavior, patterns of feeding, sleep and elimination, crying, weight gain and so forth are explored. The need for further care or referrals is identified.

Contraception is discussed at this visit, and a suitable method decided upon if the parents wish to prevent another pregnancy. The method is instituted at this time, and the couple is instructed in its uses and risks. The mother's concerns about rest and exercise, weight, diet, her energy level, household tasks, relations with relatives and friends, sexual relations, and physical needs or discomforts are discussed. If weight continues to be a problem, a suitable weight reduction diet and other measures can be started. If desired, the woman can resume full employment or activities at this time, if there are no complications and she feels psychologically ready.

Content of the Six-Week Postdelivery Checkup

- Vital signs and weight
- Perineal examination
  - Amount and character of lochia
  - Condition of episiotomy or lacerations
  - Condition of anus, hemorrhoids
- Pelvic examination
  - Size and position of uterus and cervix
  - Condition of vagina (musculature, lacerations)
  - Pap smear
- Breast examination
  - Condition of breasts and nipples
  - Whether lactating or not
- Growth and development of baby
  - Infant behavior
  - Patterns of feeding, sleep, and elimination
  - Crying
  - Weight gain
- Family response to new baby
  - Father's response and involvement in care
  - Reactions of siblings
  - Relatives' and friends' visits or assistance
  - Mother's response to caretaking, feeding, and reactions of others
- Mother's physical condition and recovery
  - Rest and exercise
  - Weight loss
  - Diet
  - Energy level
  - Recreation and activities
  - Returning to work
  - Physical discomforts and remedies
- Sexual relations
  - Resumption of intercourse
  - Concerns or difficulties
  - Responses of father
  - Responses of mother
- Contraception
  - Current contraceptive practice (if any)
  - Desires for regulating fertility and family planning
  - Contraceptive methods and selection of best suited method for couple

NC Nursing Care: Postpartum Care

Assessment	Intervention	Evaluation
Postdelivery observations		
Fundal checks Bleeding Status of bladder Vital signs Condition of perineum	Give gentle massage of fundus if boggy Express clots from fundus Report and record amount and character of bleeding Report and record increase in pulse rate or decrease in blood pressure and elevation of temperature Encourage voiding if bladder becomes filled; catheterize if distended and unable to void Report development of hematoma or bleeding from episiotomy	Fundus maintained well contracted Bleeding normal amount without clots Vital signs stable Bladder emptied as needed Episiotomy remains intact
Family interactions		
Comfort and rest Mother–infant contact Contact with partner or companion	Comfort measures (position, keep clean and dry, provide fluids as appropriate, encourage rest by doing observations efficiently) Enable mother to hold and explore infant if condition permits Enable partner or companion to visit mother and infant Respond to questions about labor and delivery, status of infant, postpartum status	Mother rests well between observations Mother holds and explores infant Partner or companion visits, able to interact satisfactorily Questions answered adequately
Hospital postpartum observations		
Vital signs Fundal checks Lochia Condition of perineum Elimination Ambulation and rest Nutrition Comfort Breast care	Record progress of involution, report signs of hemorrhage, infection, hematoma, thrombophlebitis Instruct in perineal and breast care Administer stool softeners and laxatives as needed Provide supportive measures to enjoy nutritious diet, snacks Measure first voiding, check for bladder residual, catheterize as needed Assist patient to ambulate and shower first time Plan procedures to provide rest times without interruptions	Involution progresses normally without complications Bowel and bladder elimination maintained Patient able to do perineal and breast care Patient's appetite good Ambulates without tiring Able to rest and sleep well

NC Nursing Care: Postpartum Care

Assessment	Intervention	Evaluation
Development of mothering relation	Provide opportunity for extended mother–infant contact Answer questions about infant behavior and care, and feeding Provide specific instruction in areas of infant care as needed	Able to feed and care for infant satisfactorily No further questions
Integration of infant into family	Discuss family adaptation to new baby, changes in routines, response of father and other children Provide information, referrals as appropriate to individual needs Assist in planning for care of infant at home, management of tasks and sources of assistance	Mother's questions are answered and concerns responded to Expresses comfort with family's ability to adapt to new baby Identifies specific sources of help Follows through on referrals
Sexuality and contraception	Discuss postpartum sexual responses and alterations Instruct on when to resume intercourse, signs of problems Advise on contraceptive method until 6-week checkup	Validates understanding of changes in sexual response, when to resume intercourse, use of contraception Uses contraceptive measure successfully
6-week checkup		
Progress of involution Family adaptation to new baby Contraception	Examine reproductive organs, provide specific treatment for problems Discuss routines of infant care, responses of family, concerns and problems, resumption of activities Discuss contraceptive methods, benefits and risks	Involution complete, reproductive organs returned to prepregnant condition Family adaptation and routines are stable and functional Contraceptive method instituted and used successfully

References

1. Jenkins RL, Westhus NK: The Nurse Role in Parent-Infant Bonding. JOGN Nurs 10:114–118, March/April 1981

2. Klaus MH, Kennell JH: Maternal–Infant Bonding, pp 12–14, 50–66. St Louis, CV Mosby, 1976

3. Countryman B: Breast care in the early puerperium. JOGN Nurs 2:36–40, September/October 1973

4. Kyndely K: The sexuality of women in pregnancy and postpartum: A review. JOGN Nurs 7:28–31, January/February, 1978

5. Clark AL, Hale RW: Sex during and after pregnancy. Am J Nurs 74:1430, 1974

6. Roberts F: Perinatal Nursing, pp. 165–167. New York, McGraw-Hill, 1977

7. Clark AL: Recognizing discord between mother and child and changing it to harmony. MCN 1:100–106, March/April 1976

8. Gruis M: Beyond maternity: Postpartum concerns of mothers. MCN 2:182–188, May/June 1977

9. Brown MS, Hurlock JT: Mothering the mother. Am J Nurs 77:439–441, March 1977

10. Clark AL, Affonseo DD: Infant behavior and maternal attachment: Two sides to the coin. MCN 1:95–99, March/April 1976

Suggested Reading

Ludington–Hoe SM: Postpartum: Development of maternicity. Am J Nurs 77:1171–1179, July 1977

Smith D, Smith HL: Toward improvements in parenting. JOGN Nurs 7:22–27, November/December 1978

Rubin R: Binding-in in the postpartum period. Matern Child Nurs J 6, 2:67–75, Summer 1977

Barnard MA: Supportive nursing care for the mother and newborn who are separated from each other. MCN 1:107–110, March/April 1976

Weir R, Feldman W: A study of infant feeding practices. Birth and the Family Journal 2:64–65, Spring 1975

Sheehan F: Assessing postpartum adjustment: A pilot study. JOGN Nurs 10:19–23, January/February 1981

CHAPTER 31

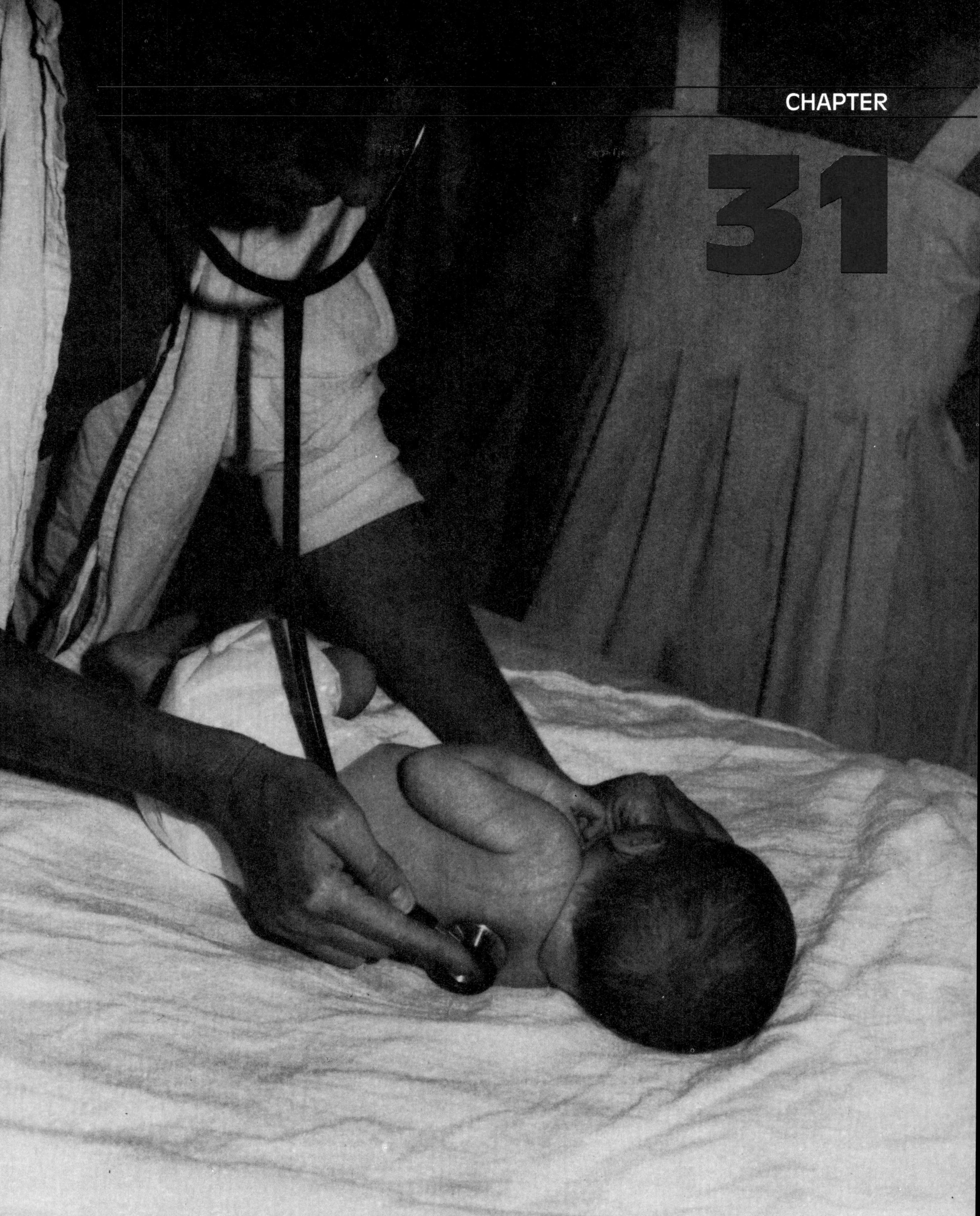

CHAPTER 31

Assessment of the Newborn Infant

During the first few days of life, the newborn undergoes more profound physiological changes than at any other time in his life. Frequent assessments of the infant help to determine how well he is coping with all the changes that are occurring. The types of assessments that are done, and who does them, depend on the setting and the infant's condition. The registered nurse is usually the health-care professional who has closest contact with the newborn during this period of transition to extrauterine life. She needs to possess the knowledge and skills to comprehensively evaluate the newborn's status during this period.

Assessments continue to be made throughout the infant's hospital stay. Vital signs, general activity, color changes, feeding status, elimination, and condition of skin, eyes, and cord are usually checked at least once each shift, and the infant is usually weighed daily. Although the infant's physical condition is most important, increasing attention is now placed on assessment of other areas, such as the infant's behavior and the interaction between the parents and the infant.

Physiological Basis of Assessment

While undergoing the changes that lead to adaptation to extrauterine life, the infant passes through several phases. This transitional period must be negotiated successfully if the infant is to survive and develop normally. The transition begins with labor when the fetus is stimulated by uterine contractions and pressure changes due to the rupture of the membranes. At birth a variety of foreign stimuli are encountered, such as light, sound, heat, cold, and gravitation. Breathing then must start and profound changes and reorganization in the functioning of the organ systems and metabolic processes begin (Fig. 31-1). Respiration must be initiated, circulation must shift from fetal to neonatal, hepatic and renal function must be altered, and meconium must be passed. The final phase of the transition involves further reorganization of the metabolic processes to achieve a viable, steady state. This includes changes in blood oxygen saturation, reduc-

Figure 31-1.
Periods of reactivity. (After Arnold HW, Putman NJ, Barnard BL, Desmond MM et al: Transition to extrauterine life. Am J Nurs, 65, 10:78, 1965)

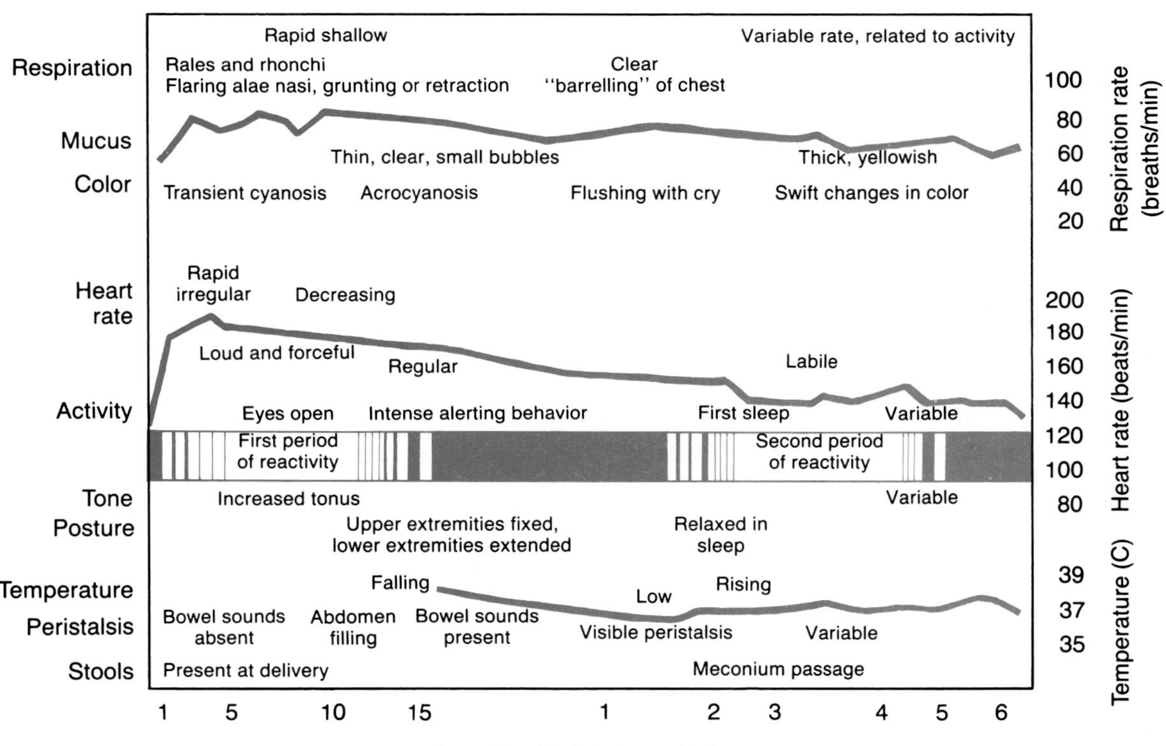

tion of enzymes, diminution in postnatal acidosis, and recovery of the neurologic tissues from the trauma of labor and delivery. Since these changes take time, it is no wonder that the infant's natal day is so crucial to his life and future well-being.

Respiratory Changes

Prior to birth, the oxygen needs of the fetus are met by the placenta. While the fetal lungs do not function as organs of respiration, it has been confirmed in recent years that respiratorylike movements do occur. The function of this "fetal breathing" is not known, but some of the hypotheses are that it is "prenatal practice" for later breathing; may aid in the development of alveolar and bronchial structures; or might have some relationship to the synthesis, release, and distribution of surfactant.[1]

For the newborn to survive extrauterine life, adequate maturation of the lungs is essential. The lungs are in a continuous state of development structurally throughout fetal life and early childhood. About the twentieth week of gestation, canals begin to develop in the bronchial tree and primitive air sacs begin to form. By the twenty-eighth week, these are in close enough proximity to the developing blood vessel structures for gas exchange to be possible and surface-active lipoproteins (surfactant) to be detected for the first time, so there is a potential for independent survival. However, if the infant is born this early, he is at high risk for respiratory problems as a result of the limited amount of surfactant and the incomplete development of the alveoli.[2] (See Chap. 41 for discussion of respiratory problems of the preterm infant.)

At the time of birth, the normal, full-term fetus is ready for the initiation of effective breathing. For example, fetal respiratory movements have prepared the lungs for this activity and the complex interrelationships of swallowing and breathing have been developed. With everything in readiness, the question is often asked, "What keeps the fetus from taking real breaths before it is born?" Some important inhibitory mechanisms have been identified. One of these is facial immersion. Another is the inhibition of respiration by the presence of fluid in the laryngeal area. This emphasizes the importance of clearing fluid from this area after birth. Also, the fetal lungs are constantly filled with fluid that is thought to be secreted by the alveolar cells, and this fluid in the deep respiratory tracts stimulates inhibitory stretch receptors.[2]

Initiation of Respiration

A multiplicity of factors is probably involved in stimulating the infant's initial respirations. This would seem to provide a margin of safety for the infant. Physical, sensory, and chemical factors are involved, but precisely how each of these influences the other and to what degree is not known exactly. There is some evidence to indicate that the change in pressure from intrauterine to extrauterine life may produce enough physical stimulation to prompt respiration.

Of the sensory stimuli that have been thought to play a role, such as cold, pain, touch, light, sound and gravity, cold seems to be the most important. In animal studies, cold stimulation has induced breathing in fetal sheep.[2] This should not be taken to mean that the infant needs to be in a cold environment. Just being in normal room air of about 22°C (72°F) is a drop of more than 15°C (25°F) below the mother's normal body temperature which the neonate has been used to.

The chemical changes that occur in the blood as a result of the transitory asphyxia during delivery seem to be of paramount importance. These include a lowered oxygen level, an increased carbon dioxide level, and a lowered *p*H. If the asphyxia is prolonged, depression of the respiratory center ensues rather than stimulation, and resuscitation is usually necessary (see Chap. 41). A vigorous infant often breathes seconds after birth and certainly within one minute of delivery.

A great effort is required to expand the lungs and to fill the collapsed alveoli. Surface tension in the respiratory tract, as well as resistance in the lung tissue itself, the thorax, the diaphragm, and the respiratory muscles must be overcome. Moreover, any obstruction (*i.e.,* mucus, and so on) in the air passages has to be cleared. The first active inspiration comes from a powerful contraction of the diaphragm, which creates a high negative intrathoracic pressure, causing a marked retraction of the ribs because of the pliability of the baby's thorax.

This first inspiration distends the alveolar spaces and on expiration a residual volume of nearly 20 ml of air remains as molecules of pulmonary surfactant diminish surface tension. Therefore, the second breath takes less effort than the first, and the third breath even less, since by this time most of the small airways are open. Fluid is rapidly removed from the lungs by drainage, swallowing, evaporation, and pulmonary, capillary, and lymphatic circulation. After several minutes of breathing, lung expansion is usually complete.[3]

Respiration in First and Second Periods of Reactivity

A healthy infant begins life with intense activity. This phase has been designated by some authorities as the first period of reactivity. In this phase the infant exhibits outbursts of diffuse, purposeless movements

Initiation of Respiration

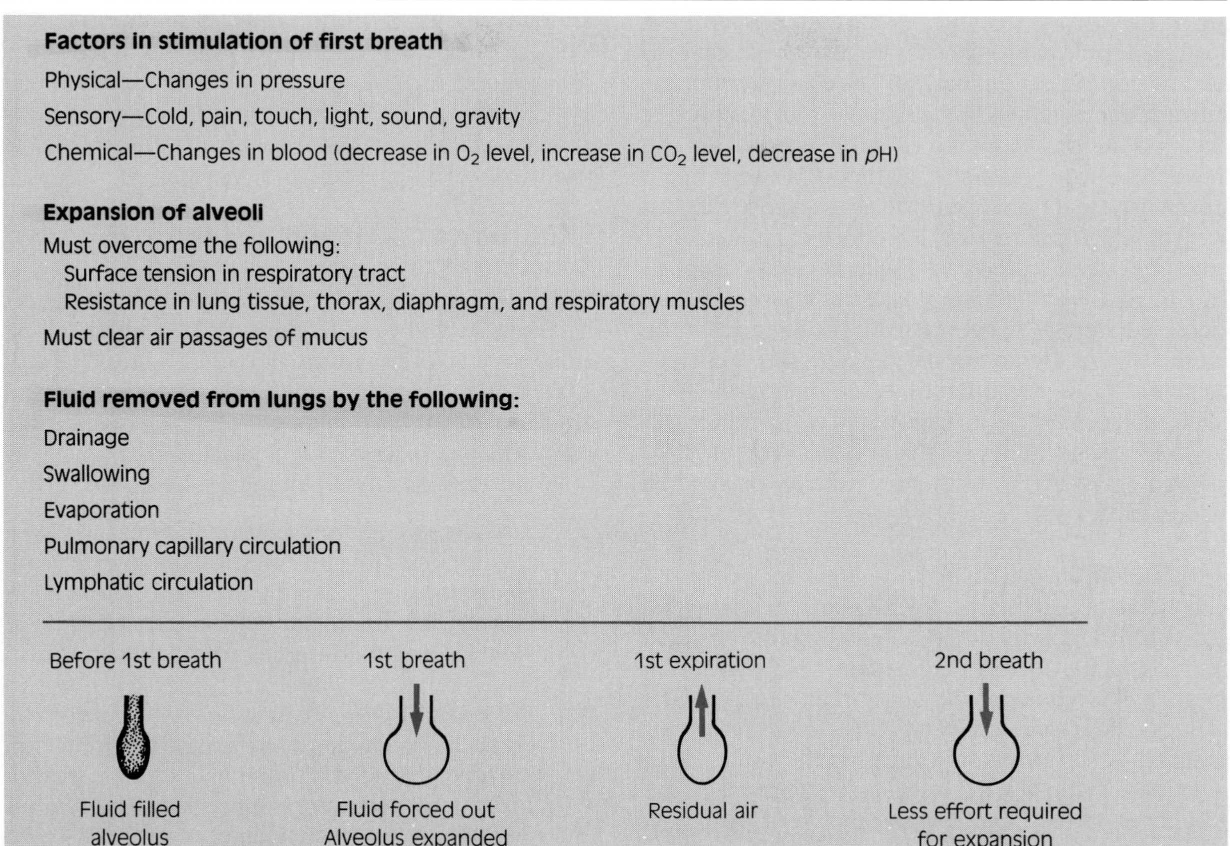

Factors in stimulation of first breath

Physical—Changes in pressure

Sensory—Cold, pain, touch, light, sound, gravity

Chemical—Changes in blood (decrease in O_2 level, increase in CO_2 level, decrease in *p*H)

Expansion of alveoli

Must overcome the following:
- Surface tension in respiratory tract
- Resistance in lung tissue, thorax, diaphragm, and respiratory muscles

Must clear air passages of mucus

Fluid removed from lungs by the following:

Drainage

Swallowing

Evaporation

Pulmonary capillary circulation

Lymphatic circulation

which alternate with periods of relative immobility. At this time respiration is rapid (reaching as high as 80 breaths per minute), and there may be *transient* flaring of the alae nasi; retraction of the chest and grunting are not uncommon. Tachycardia also is present at times, and the heart rate may reach 180 beats per minute in the first minutes of life. Thereafter it falls to an average of 120 to 140 beats per minute.

After this initial response, the baby becomes relatively quiet and does not respond intensely to either internal or external stimuli. He relaxes and may fall asleep. His first sleep occurs, on an average, at 2 hours after birth and may last anywhere from a few minutes to several hours.

When he awakes, he is again hyperresponsive to stimuli, and he begins his second period of reactivity. His color may change rapidly (from pink to moderately cyanotic), and his heart rate responds to stimulation and becomes rapid. Oral mucus may be a major problem in respiration during this period. Choking, gagging, and regurgitation alert the nurse to the presence of mucus, and appropriate intervention must be taken (see Chap. 41). Since the length of the second period of reactivity is variable, the nurse must be particularly alert for the first 12 hours to 18 hours of the infant's life[4] (see Fig. 31-1).

Circulatory Changes

The anatomical changes that occur with birth have been discussed previously in Chapter 11. It will be recalled that a rapid change takes place with closure of several fetal structures and with the redistribution of oxygenated blood to a circulation similar to that of an adult. Since all changes are not immediately complete, this time of conversion may be called a period of *transitional circulation*.

Total Blood Volume

It is difficult to give accurate values for the total blood volume of the newborn because of the variables involved, such as time of clamping the umbilical cord, weight and gestational age of the infant, type of delivery (vaginal or cesarean), and the time after delivery the determination is made.

For example, an additional 50 ml to 100 ml of

blood may be added to the circulation if the infant is placed below the level of the placenta and the clamping of the cord is delayed several minutes until the cord stops pulsating. Many studies have been done to help decide the issue of early or late clamping, but it is still unclear whether this placental transfusion that occurs with late clamping is advantageous for the infant. The rapid increase in blood volume might stress the heart and pulmonary vasculature, but according to some reports, incidence of neonatal respiratory distress is decreased with delayed clamping. The infants who receive this extra blood gain an increased storage supply of iron, resulting from the breakdown of the additional hemoglobin. This may contribute to hyperbilirubinemia during the first week of life, but the iron stores may be utilized to good advantage later when iron is needed for rapid growth or when the dietary intake of iron is inadequate.[5]

Peripheral Circulation

Peripheral circulation in the newborn is somewhat sluggish. It is felt that this accounts for the residual cyanosis of the infant's hands, feet, and circumoral area. These areas often remain mildly cyanotic for 1 hour or 2 hours after delivery. The general circulatory lability probably accounts for the mottled appearance of the baby's skin when it is exposed to air and for the "chilliness" of the infant's hands and feet.

Pulse Rate

Like the rate of respiration, the pulse rate also is labile and generally follows a pattern similar to that of the respiration. When the respiration is rapid, the pulse tends to be rapid; similarly, when the respiration slows down, so does the pulse. Since the pulse is affected by both internal and external stimuli, taking the *apical* pulse rate while the baby is quiet provides a more accurate evaluation of the infant's pulse rate. The normal rate is usually 120 beats per minute to 150 beats per minute, but it may rise to 180 beats per minute for short periods with crying and other intense activity, or drop to 100 beats per minute during deep sleep.

Blood Pressure

The blood pressure is not routinely checked on term newborns in most nurseries. It is difficult to get accurate blood pressure readings on newborn infants for several reasons. When the palpation method is used or auscultation with a stethoscope, only the systolic pressure is obtained. With the color change (flush) method, the result is the midpoint between the systolic and the diastolic pressure. Direct recording through an arterial catheter is more accurate, but usually is only used when there is reason to have an arterial catheter in place. A newer method using a Doppler-shift ultrasonic device for auscultation has shown good correlation with the direct method and has confirmed that the newborn's blood pressure is characteristically low, with a mean value of 71/49 at birth, and rises slowly for the first week.[6]

Erythrocyte Count and Hemoglobin Concentration

The newborn infant has a much higher erythrocyte, hemoglobin and hematocrit level than an adult. The erythrocyte level ranges between 5,000,000 and 7,000,000 per microliter, the hemoglobin level is usually 15 to 20 gm per 100 ml of blood, and the hematocrit values average about 55 percent.[5]

The following factors influence these values:

1. *Duration of gestation.* During the final weeks of intrauterine life, hemoglobin concentration rapidly increases. The infant born before term does not have the benefit of this increase and has a low concentration compared to the full-term infant.
2. *Time of cord clamping.* In infants who receive the additional blood that is added to the circulation with delayed cord clamping, increased hemoglobin and hematocrit levels can be demonstrated for at least 3 or 4 days.
3. *Site of blood sample.* In the first week, capillary blood samples usually show higher hemoglobin values than venous samples drawn at the same time. The venous samples are considered to be more accurate.[5]

The higher blood values are needed by the fetus *in utero* for adequate oxygenation. After birth, the need no longer exists, since the lungs are functioning, and a gradual decrease takes place. Immediately after birth there is an increase in erythrocyte count from cord blood levels because of a decrease in plasma volume. This reaches a maximum level 2 hours to 6 hours after birth. Then it decreases to cord blood levels when the infant is about 1 week of age. Red blood cell production (erythropoiesis) is suppressed for several months after birth and this, added to the increased blood volume caused by the infant's rapid growth, results in a progressive decline in the hemoglobin concentration. A low point of 10 g/100 ml to 11 g/100 ml may be reached after 2 months to 3 months, producing a physiological anemia which does not represent any abnormality or nutritional deficiency in the infant and is not affected by giving iron or other hematinics. Active erythropoiesis resumes about this time and, if the iron supply is adequate, the hemoglobin concentration gradually increases to an average of 12.5 g/100 ml, where it stays during early childhood.

Physiologic Jaundice

In the newborn period there is a rise in the serum concentration of unconjugated bilirubin from approximately 2 mg/100 ml in cord blood to a mean peak of 6 mg/100 ml between 60 hours of age and 72 hours of age. Then there is usually a rapid decline to 2 mg/100 ml by the fifth day of life and a slower decline until normal adult levels of less than 1 mg/100 ml are reached by about the tenth day. Jaundice is the visible evidence of this rise in serum concentration of unconjugated bilirubin to levels of 5 mg/100 ml to 7 mg/100 ml or above.[7] Approximately 40% to 60% of full-term newborns (and a higher number of preterm infants) develop jaundice between the second and fourth days of life, and in the absence of disease or specific causes, this has been called "physiologic" jaundice. Appearance during the first 24 hours or levels greater than 12 mg/100 ml are two indications for considering jaundice "pathologic." (See Chap. 43 for discussion of pathologic jaundice and treatment.)

The etiology of physiologic jaundice is not fully understood, nor are the hypotheses agreed upon. The following are possible mechanisms in the development of this condition: (1) The newborn's high erythrocyte count and the shorter mean red cell life span lead to an increased breakdown of red blood cells, which contributes to the increased bilirubin load presented to the liver in the first days of life. Bilirubin from other sources such as myoglobin, a protein found in muscle, is also produced in increased amounts in the newborn. (2) The unconjugated, fat-soluble form of bilirubin that is produced when hemoglobin is broken down is usually changed in the liver to the conjugated, water-soluble form which can be excreted. In the newborn, there is interference with this conjugation, possibly owing to inhibition of the activity of the enzyme glucuronyl transferase. (3) Uptake of bilirubin from the plasma by the liver cells may be decreased because of immaturity of the liver. (4) Due to the lack of intestinal bacterial flora in the newborn, bilirubin may be reabsorbed from the intestine and recirculated to the liver, rather than being excreted. Retention of meconium, which has a high bilirubin content, may add to the amount of bilirubin reabsorbed.[8]

There seem to be some genetic and ethnic influences on the incidence of physiologic jaundice. Oriental infants and some other isolated groups have mean maximal serum unconjugated bilirubin levels between 10 mg/100 ml and 14 mg/100 ml, which is approximately double that of nonoriental populations. Kernicterus is also significantly increased in oriental neonates. The reasons for these increases are not known, but there may be a genetic predisposition to slower maturation of hepatic bilirubin metabolism

Course of Hyperbilirubinemia in Normal Newborn

Unconjugated bilirubin in cord blood = approximately 2 mg/100 ml
Mean peak between 60 hours and 72 hours = 6 mg/100 ml
Rapid decline by 5th day to 2 mg/100 ml to 3 mg/100 ml
Slower decline by about 10th day to <1 mg/100 ml

Possible Mechanisms Related to Development of Physiologic Jaundice

- Increased production of bilirubin due to increased breakdown of red blood cells
- Decreased clearance of bilirubin by the liver cells probably secondary to inhibition of glucuronyl transferase
- Immaturity of the liver
- Recirculation of increased amounts of bilirubin reabsorbed from the intestine

or a possible relationship to ethnic food or herbal medicines.[7]

The nurse should not be lulled into a false sense of security by the term "physiologic." Any baby who develops observable jaundice should be closely watched for symptoms of other possible problems.

Blood Coagulation

Immediately after birth the intestinal tract of the infant does not harbor the bacteria necessary to help to synthesize the very important substance, vitamin K. Other substances important in blood coagulation are manufactured in the liver and are under the influence of vitamin K; these substances are temporarily diminished. Thus, the infant suffers from a transitory deficiency in blood coagulation. This condition occurs between the second and the fifth postnatal days and returns to normal spontaneously in several more days.

This deficiency can often be minimized or prevented by administration of water-soluble vitamin K to the infant on the day of birth. This is now done routinely in most nurseries.

White Blood Cells

The normal newborn has a wide range in the total number of white blood cells. A leukocytosis (15,000–45,000 cells per microliter) is present at birth, with polymorphonuclear cells accounting for a large percentage of the total count. During the first few days after delivery there is a considerable decrease in the total count, as well as a shift in the type of predominating cell. The polymorphonuclear neutrophils decrease, and the lymphocytes increase, so that by the end of the first week the lymphocytes predominate.

Temperature Regulation and Metabolic Changes

The infant is born into an environment that is considerably cooler than the one encountered in the uterus. Because of this rapid change in environmental conditions, the newborn's temperature may drop several degrees after birth. In recent years attention has been focused on the effects of hypothermia on the newborn and increasing efforts have been made to prevent this temperature drop in the delivery room and in the nursery. Neonates are predisposed to heat transfer between themselves and the environment because they have a limited supply of subcutaneous fat and a large surface area in relation to body weight.

Heat Loss

Evaporation, conduction, convection, and radiation are four ways in which the newborn can lose body heat to the environment. Excessive loss by *evaporation* occurs most often in the delivery room when the infant is wet (see Chap. 24), but it can also occur when the infant is being bathed. Heat evaporation may also occur from the lungs if the infant has tachypnea or if the humidity is low. Heat loss by *conduction* involves the transfer of heat from a warm object to a cooler one by direct contact and can occur when the infant is placed on a cold surface, or when cool blankets or clothing are used. Through *convection,* the transference of heat is from a body to the surrounding air, the infant's temperature is affected by the air currents in the environment, such as those caused by air conditioners. The fourth mechanism, *radiation,* occurs when heat is transferred from a warm object to a cooler one when the objects are not in direct contact (Table 31-1). This type of heat loss can occur in infants if the walls of an incubator are cool or if the crib is placed close to a cool outside wall or window. Each of these mechanisms with the exception of evaporation can be responsible for an increase in the infant's temperature as well as the losses described.

Heat Production

To maintain a normal temperature when exposed to a cool environment the newborn increases his rate of heat production in an attempt to replace what is lost (see Table 31-1). Shivering is the most common mechanism of heat production in an adult, but the neonate rarely shivers although there may be an increase in voluntary muscular activity. The primary mechanism of heat production in the newborn is nonshivering thermogenesis whereby a chemical reaction occurs in brown fat, which breaks down triglycerides into glycerol and fatty acids and thereby produces heat. Brown fat cells contain many small fat vacuoles in contrast to the single large vacuole of white fat. There is also a richer blood supply which helps to account for its darker color and aids in the distribution of the heat produced. Brown fat is usually not found in adults, but in the newborn it accounts for 2% to 6% of the total weight and can be found between the scapulae, at the nape of the neck, in the axillae, in the mediastinum, and around the kidneys and adrenals.[9]

Heat Conservation

Conservation of body heat in the infant occurs through peripheral vasoconstriction and through assumption of a flexed or fetal position which decreases the surface area from which heat may be lost.

Effects of Cold Stress on the Newborn

The increased metabolic rate associated with nonshivering thermogenesis necessitates an increase in both oxygen and calorie consumption. To replace the

Table 31-1.
Thermal Regulation in the Newborn

Mechanisms of Heat Loss	Prevention
Evaporation—loss of heat to air by way of moisture from skin or lungs	Dry well after delivery, especially head; protect from exposure while wet during bath; avoid very low humidity
Radiation—loss of heat to cool objects not in contact with infant	Avoid placing infant near cold outside walls or windows
Conduction—Loss of heat from infant to cold surface	Do not place on cold surface; use warmed blankets in delivery room
Convection—loss of heat to air by way of drafts	Keep infant out of air flow currents

Mechanisms of Heat Production and Conservation	Effects
Nonshivering thermogenesis (metabolism of brown fat)	Increased metabolic consumption of calories Increased oxygen consumption
Increase in voluntary muscular activity (shivering is rare in the newborn)	Increased glucose consumption
Peripheral vasoconstriction	Conserve heat for body core Hands and feet may be blue, mottled, or cold to touch.
Assumption of fetal position	Decreased surface area for loss of heat

heat lost during a temperature drop of 3.5°C (6.3°F), it has been found that the infant requires a 100% increase in oxygen consumption for more than one and one-half hours.[10] Even vigorous full-term infants may develop metabolic acidosis if allowed to become hypothermic. It is obvious that cold stress can be detrimental or even fatal to an infant who is having difficulty with metabolism or oxygenation.

Efforts should be made to keep an infant in a neutral thermal environment, which means an environment where the infant's metabolic rate, and therefore oxygen consumption, is minimal but the body temperature remains within the normal range.

Neurologic Changes

The nervous system of the newborn is immature; that is, it is neither anatomically nor physiologically fully developed. Although all neurons are present, many remain immature for several months and some for years. Thus, the infant is uncoordinated in his movements, is labile in his temperature regulation, and has poor control over his musculature—he "startles" easily, is subject to tremors of the extremities, and so on. However, during the neonatal period, development is rapid, and as the various nerve pathways controlling the muscles are used, the nerve fibers connect with one another. Gradually, more complex patterns of behavior emerge, and the higher cerebral levels begin to function.

Reflexes

The reflexes are important indices of the baby's normal development, for their presence or absence at certain times reflects the extent of normality in the functioning of the central nervous system. (Individual reflexes will be discussed in the section on Neurological Assessment.)

Gastrointestinal Changes

The gastrointestinal (GI) tract functions in a very limited capacity during fetal life. The fetus is known to swallow amniotic fluid and a fecal material called meconium is formed, but the GI tract is not responsible for the digestion or absorption of nutrients. By 36 weeks to 38 weeks, though, it is mature enough to adapt readily to extrauterine life. The various enzymes necessary for digestion are active and the muscular and reflex development provide the capability of transporting the food.

In order for the infant to swallow, food must be placed well back on the tongue, since the infant does not have the ability to transfer food from the lips to the pharynx. This means that the nipple should be placed well inside the infant's mouth. Sucking is facilitated by strong sucking muscles and ridges or corrugations in the anterior portion of the mouth. In addition, the *sucking pads* (deposits of fatty tissue in each cheek) prevent the collapse of the cheeks during nursing and further make sucking effective. This fatty tissue remains (even when fat is lost from the rest of the body) until sucking is no longer essential to the baby's getting food. The salivary glands are immature at birth and manufacture little saliva until the infant is about 3 months old.

The newborn's intestinal tract is proportionately longer than that of an adult. Although it contains a large number of secretory glands and a large surface for absorption, its elastic tissue and supporting musculature are poor and not fully developed. This increases the likelihood of distention. Furthermore, nervous control is variable and inadequate. Nevertheless, the infant digests and absorbs a tremendous amount of food in proportion to body weight.

Most of the digestive enzymes seem to be present and adequate, with the exception of pancreatic amylase and lipase, which are somewhat deficient for several months but eventually reach a normal amount. The infant can digest simple foods easily, but has a difficult time with the more complex starches. Protein and carbohydrates are easily absorbed but fat absorption is poor.

Changes in Kidney Function and Urinary Excretion

The kidneys become functional during fetal life, as evidenced by the presence of urine in the bladder as early as the fourth month of gestation. However, kidney function is fairly low until immediately after birth when the kidneys must replace the placenta as the organ responsible for excretory and regulatory functions. Due to the relatively low rate of glomerular filtration at birth, excess water and solute cannot be disposed of rapidly and efficiently. The limitations in tubular reabsorption that are also present may cause inappropriate substances from the glomerular filtrate, such as certain amino acids and bicarbonate, to appear in the urine.[11] In the healthy neonate these limitations do not have a detrimental effect, but they do restrict the ability of the newborn to respond to stress. As the kidneys grow and mature, function increases.

Ninety-two percent of healthy infants void within 24 hours, but the first voiding may occur shortly after delivery and not be noticed. Voidings during the first days after birth may be scanty and somewhat infrequent unless the infant was edematous at birth, but as the fluid intake increases so does the output. Frequency usually increases from 2 times to 6 times on the first and second day to 5 times to 20 times per 24 hours after that until the infant begins to develop bladder control and the number of voidings per day decreases.

The urine of the newborn may appear cloudy due to high mucus and urate content, but with increased fluid intake the urine becomes clear, straw-colored and nearly odorless. Uric acid crystals in the urine may cause a reddish "brick-dust" stain on the diaper that is sometimes confused with blood in the urine.

Changes in Hepatic Function

During fetal life, the liver performs an important role in blood formation, and it is thought that it continues this function to some degree after birth. Later in the neonatal period the liver produces substances that are essential in the coagulation of the blood. If the mother's iron intake has been adequate during pregnancy, enough iron is stored in the infant's liver to carry him over the first months of life when his diet (primarily milk) is iron deficient. About the fifth month, however, the baby's iron reserve is depleted, and unless foods containing iron are given, a deficiency will ensue.

Physical Assessment

The physical examination has traditionally been done by the physician. In recent years many nurses have learned physical assessment skills and in some hospitals a pediatric nurse practitioner has the responsibility for part of the newborn physical examinations. Although all nurses do not possess practitioner skills, they should be able to do a basic assessment and recognize deviations from normal.

The Newborn Physical Assessment Guide on pages 662 to 664 can be used in learning to assess the newborn infant. The discussion of newborn characteristics that follows and Table 31-2 are helpful in using the guide. Practice and experience also improve the nurse's ability to recognize the range of normal. Discussion of abnormalities is found in Chapters 41 to 43.

The format of the Newborn Physical Assessment Guide can be used for an admitting assessment, or a later one. It is not intended to be a complete physical examination, but should give the nurse a good idea of the status of the infant. The examiner can use any system of notation that is helpful to fill in the spaces on the form. A suggestion is to use a "check" to indicate

(Text continued on page 661)

TABLE 31-2.
Summary of Newborn Physical Assessment

Assessment Area	Usual Findings	Deviations
General observations		
Muscle tone	Flexed position; good tone	"Floppy"; rigid or tense
Skin		
Color	Pink tone to ruddy when crying; appropriate to ethnic origin; acrocyanosis	Pallor; cyanosis; jaundice; ecchymosis; petechiae
Texture	Smooth; dryness with some peeling; lanugo on back; vernix	Excessive peeling or cracking; roughness
Rashes and pigmentation	Erythema toxicum; milia; mongolian spots	Impetigo; hemangiomas; nevus flammeus (port wine stain)
Hydration	Skin pinch over abdomen immediately returns to original state	Skin maintains "tent" shape after pinch
Cry	Lusty	Shrill; weak; grunty
Measurements		
Weight	2700 g–4000 g (6 lb–9 lb)	
Length	48 cm–53 cm (19 in–21 in)	
Head circumference	33 cm–37 cm (13 in–14.5 in)	
Chest circumference	31 cm–35 cm (12.5 in–14 in)	
Vital signs		
Temperature	Axillary (preferred method)—36.5°C–37°C (97.7°F–98.6°F) Rectal—36.5°C–37.2°C (97.7°F–99°F)	Hypothermia; fever
Respirations	40 respirations/min–60 respirations/min; quiet and shallow; diaphragmatic; occasional periods of rapid breathing, alternating with short periods of apnea	Prolonged rapid breathing; apnea lasting longer than 10 sec; grunting; retractions; persistent slow rate
Heart rate (apical pulse)	120 beats/min–160 beats/min; faster when crying (up to 180 beats/min); slower when sleeping (down to 100 beats/min)	Tachycardia—greater than 160 beats/min at rest Bradycardia—less than 120 beats/min when awake
Head	Vaginal delivery—elongated (molding) Breech or cesarean birth—round, symmetrical Size within normal range	Caput succedaneum; cephalhematoma; hydrocephaly; microcephaly
Fontanels	Flat; soft; firm	Bulging; sunken
Anterior	Diamond shaped; 2 cm–3 cm wide; 3 cm–4 cm long; smaller at birth with molding	Small; almost closed; closed (craniostenosis); widened
Posterior	Triangular shape; small; almost closed	Enlarged
Face	Small; round; symmetrical; fat pads in cheeks; receding chin	Asymmetrical; distorted
Eyes	Edematous lids; usually closed; blue or slate gray color; no tears; red reflex present; pupils equal, round, react to light	Elevation or ptosis of lids; epicanthal folds; absence of red reflex; unequal, dilated, or constricted pupils
	Common variations—subconjunctival hemorrhages; chemical conjunctivitis; occasional slight nystagmus or convergent strabismus	Purulent discharge; frequent nystagmus; constant, divergent, or unilateral strabismus

(Continued)

Table 31-2.
Summary of Newborn Physical Assessment (continued)

Assessment Area	Usual Findings	Deviations
Mouth	Intact lips, gums, palate; epithelial pearls; "sucking blisters" on lips; tongue midline, mobile, appropriate size for mouth; can extend to alveolar ridge	Cleft lip or palate; white, cheesy patches on tongue, gums, or mucus membrane; large or protruding tongue
Nose	In midline; even placement in relation to eyes and mouth; nares patent; septum intact, midline	Flattened or bruised; unusual placement or configuration; obstructed nares; deviated or perforated septum
Ears	Well formed cartilage; appropriate size for head; upper attachment on line extended through inner and outer canthus of eye; external auditory canal patent	Floppy; large and protruding; malformed; low set; obstruction of canal
Neck	Short; thick; full range of motion; no masses	Webbing; abnormal shortening; limitation of motion; torticollis; masses
Clavicles	Straight; smooth; intact	Knot or lump; decreased movement of extremity on one side
Thorax	Round; symmetrical; protruding xiphoid process	Asymmetrical; funnel chest
Breath sounds	Loud; bronchial; bilaterally equal	Decreased breath sounds; increased breath sounds
Heart sounds	Regular rate and rhythm; first and second sounds clear and distinct	Murmurs; arrhythmias
Breasts	Symmetrical; flat with erect nipples; engorgement 2nd or 3rd day not unusual	Redness and firmness around nipple
Abdomen	Symmetrical; slightly protuberant; no masses	Scaphoid or concave shape; distention; palpable masses
Liver	Palpable 2 cm–3 cm below right costal margin	Enlargement
Spleen	Tip may be palpable in left upper quadrant	Enlargement
Kidneys	May be palpable at level of umbilicus	Enlargement
Femoral pulses	Bilaterally equal	Unequal or absent
Umbilicus	No extensive protrusion or herniation; no signs of infection	Umbilical hernia; omphalocele; redness; induration; foul-smelling discharge
	Cord—bluish white, moist → black, dry; 3 vessels; no oozing or bleeding	Two vessels; bleeding or oozing from stump
Genitalia	Appropriate for gender	Ambiguous genitalia
Female Labia	Edematous; labia majora cover labia minora; vernix in creases	Hematoma; lesions; fusion of labia
Vagina	Mucus discharge, possibly blood tinged	
Male Foreskin	Adherent to glans penis	
Urethra	Opening at tip of penis	Opening below tip of penis (hypospadias) Opening above tip of penis (epispadias)
Testes	Palpable in each scrotal sac	Palpable in inguinal canal; not palpable

(Continued)

Table 31-2.
Summary of Newborn Physical Assessment (continued)

Assessment Area	Usual Findings	Deviations
Posterior of body		
Spinal column	Straight; flexible; intact; no masses	Exaggerated curves; spina bifida; any masses; pilonidal cyst
Anus	Patent	Imperforate anus; anal fissures
Extremities	Symmetrical in size, shape, and movement	Unequal or abnormal size or shape; asymmetrical or limited movement of one or more extremities
Digits	Five on each hand and foot; appropriate size and shape	Missing digits; syndactyly (webbing); polydactyly (extra digits)
Hips	Even leg length, knee height, gluteal folds; no resistance or limitation to abduction	Uneven leg length, knee height, or gluteal folds; uneven or limited abduction; hip "click" or "clunk" on abduction
Feet	Straight, or postural deviation easily corrected with gentle pressure	Structural deformities—talipes equinovarus (clubfoot); metatarsus adductus
Reflexes		
Rooting and sucking	Turns toward object touching cheek, lips or corner of mouth; opens mouth; begins sucking movements; strong suck, pulls object into mouth May be diminished or absent after eating	No rooting; weak, ineffective or absent suck
Grasp		
Palmar	Fingers grasp object when palm stimulated and hang on briefly	Weak or absent
Plantar	Toes curl downward when soles of feet are stimulated	Weak or absent
Moro	Symmetrical response to sudden stimulus—lateral extension of arms with opening of hands, followed by flexion and adduction	Asymmetrical; absent; incomplete
Stepping	Stepping movements when infant held upright with sole of foot touching surface	Asymmetrical or absent

"within normal limits" and a "plus" or "minus" to indicate whether something is present or absent. When appropriate, descriptions can be written in the spaces or under "comments."

Methods used in physical examination are inspection, auscultation, palpation, and percussion, usually in that order. Percussion is not specifically used in this form. The examination is written for use in evaluating the infant in a cephalocaudal direction, but it may be best to begin with items, such as auscultation of the chest, which require the infant to be quiet, before performing procedures that might cause the infant to cry. Each examiner should establish a definite pattern and follow it each time so that nothing is missed.

When any assessment of the newborn is carried out, the parents should be included as much as possible. If they cannot be present for the examination it should at least be discussed with them. Being there, though, is a good way to help them get better acquainted with their infant (see Fig. 31-7). Also, it is important for the nurse to look at the baby from the parents' viewpoint. The healthy newborn infant has many characteristics which momentarily may look unusual to them. The nurse should be ready to talk with the parents about their baby and to answer their questions.

Physical assessment begins with the Apgar scoring in the delivery room (see Chap. 25). When the infant is brought to the nursery, the delivery room nurse reports pertinent information on the mother's ante-

(Text continued on page 664)

AT Newborn Physical Assessment Guide

Baby's Name ____________ Date and Time of Birth ____________

Mother's Name ____________ Date and Time of Exam ____________

Initial Evaluation

1. General Appearance: Color ____________ Muscle tone ____________
2. Respiratory Effort: Retractions ____________ Gasping ____________
   Grunting ____________ Quality of cry ____________
3. Temperature: ____________

Comments: ____________

Assessment of Head and Neck

1. Observe and palpate the infant's head for symmetry; note absence or presence of:
   Molding ____________ Caput succedaneum ____________ Cephalhematoma ____________
2. Palpate the fontanels and sutures for: Fullness ____________ Depression ____________
   Overriding ____________ Shape ____________ Size ____________
3. Measure circumference of head: ____________
4. Evaluate ears: Position ____________ Shape ____________ Location ____________
5. Evaluate symmetry of face: ____________
6. Observe eyes for: Shape ____________ Position ____________ Size ____________
   Appearance of pupils ____________ Presence of hemorrhage ____________ Red reflex ____________
7. Evaluate mouth for: Clefts ____________ Teeth ____________ Frenulum linguae ____________
8. Observe neck for: Length ____________ Relationship to body ____________
   Mobility ____________ Presence of webbing or fat pad ____________
9. Observe skin of scalp, face and neck for: Abrasions or contusions ____________
   Other breaks or marks ____________
10. Observe nose for: Symmetry ____________ Septum ____________ Flaring ____________

Comments: ____________

Assessment of Body

General Appearance

1. Measurements: Weight ____________ Length ____________ Circumference of chest ____________
2. Observe throughout evaluation for: General activity ____________
   Posture ____________ Responsiveness ____________
3. Observe skin for: Lanugo ____________ Vernix ____________ Meconium staining ____________
   Texture ____________ Hydration ____________ Color ____________ Rashes ____________
   Pigmentation ____________ Lesions ____________

Comments: ____________

Thorax

1. Palpate clavicles for masses and intactness: ____________
2. Inspect thorax for: Size ____________ Symmetry ____________ Shape ____________

3. Auscultate for: Breath sounds ____ Heart sounds ____ Rhythm ____
4. Count: Respiratory rate ____ Apical pulse ____

Comments: ____

Abdomen

1. Inspect shape of abdomen: ____
2. Palpate: Liver ____ Spleen ____ Kidneys ____
3. Observe cord for number of vessels: ____
4. Palpate: Femoral pulses ____

Comments: ____

Genitals

1. Observe visible genitals for: Appropriateness with stated sex ____
2. Observe female infant for: Maturation of labia ____ Vaginal discharge ____
3. Observe male infant for: Position of urethral opening ____
   Maturation of scrotum ____ Presence of testes ____
4. Note elimination: (should occur within 24 hours)
   Urine ____ Color ____ Amount/24 hours ____
   Stool ____ Color ____ Type ____ Number/24 hours ____

Comments: ____

Posterior of Body

1. Palpate and inspect spinal column for: Masses ____
   Symmetry of vertebrae ____ Intactness ____
2. Determine patency of anus: ____
3. Observe pilonidal dimple for intactness: ____

Comments: ____

Extremities

1. Note for all extremities: Symmetry ____ Abnormalities ____
   Ability to move ____
2. Count digits on: Hands ____ Feet ____
   Observe for polydactyly ____ Syndactyly ____
3. Evaluate rotation of hips: Abduct thighs to bed ____
   Rotate hips through full range of motion ____
   Observe leg length, front and back (Are they equal?) ____ Knee height ____
   Observe symmetry of leg creases ____
4. Note position of feet ____
   Can they passively be returned to normal? ____

Comments: ____

(Continued)

AT **Newborn Physical Assessment Guide (continued)**

Assessment of Neurologic Function—Reflexes—Elicit and Evaluate:

1. Rooting and sucking: ______
2. Grasp: Palmar ______ Plantar ______
3. Traction: (Pull to sitting position, note head and arm position) ______
4. Moro: ______
5. Stepping: ______

Comments: ______

Items that require manipulation, such as palpation of the abdomen and abduction of the hips, require care in performance to avoid injury to the infant and should not be attempted for the first time without supervision by a trained examiner.

(After NAACOG Technical Bulletin Number 2, "Physical Assessment of the Neonate")

partum history, labor and delivery course, condition of the infant, and care given while in the delivery room.

The next step is an initial evaluation of the infant's general condition by the nursery nurse, which includes the following:

1. Observe the infant's appearance. Is the color ruddy, pale, cyanotic, or jaundiced? Is the color evenly distributed? The infant usually is in a flexed position with good muscle tone. A "floppy" baby or a very tense baby needs careful observation.
2. The infant's cry can also be an indicator of general condition. A lusty cry is usually a good sign, but a weak or shrill cry can be indicative of central nervous system problems, and grunting sounds mean that the infant is having to work harder to get oxygen.
3. Other signs of increased respiratory effort such as retractions, gasping or flaring of the nostrils should also be noted.
4. The vital signs should be taken.

From the foregoing observations the nurse can make a decision about whether the infant needs some immediate treatment, needs time for the temperature to stabilize, or if the assessment can continue.

It is important to remember that certain symptoms which might be cause for concern in an older child (*e.g.*, rapid rate and rhythm of respiration), may merely represent normal neonatal physiology in a newborn. (See Newborn Physical Assessment Guide.)

Assessment of Head and Neck

The infant's head is large, comprising about one quarter of his size, and with cephalic presentations may initially appear to be asymmetrical because of the molding of the skull bones during labor (Fig. 31-2). If there has been extended pressure on the head, caput succedaneum (a swelling of the soft tissues) or cephalhematoma (an accumulation of blood between the bone and the periosteum) might be present (see Chap. 43).

The suture lines between the skull bones and the anterior and the posterior fontanels can usually be palpated easily (see Fig. 22-7). When the hand is passed over the fontanels, the areas should feel soft but neither bulged nor depressed. The anterior fontanel, the diamond-shaped and larger of the two (normally 2 cm–3 cm wide and 3 cm–4 cm long), may feel smaller for the first several days when there is marked overriding of the skull bones. It usually closes by 12 months to 18 months. The posterior fontanel is triangular and is located between the occipital and the parietal bones. It is smaller than the anterior fontanel and may be almost closed at birth, and completely closed by the end of the second month.

The circumference of the head is measured by placing a nonstretchable tape measure just above the eyebrows and over the most prominent part of the occiput (Fig. 31-3). Normally the head circumference is 2 cm larger than the chest circumference, but an accurate measurement may not be obtained at first if molding is present. The normal range is 33 cm to 37 cm (13 in–14½ in), depending on the general size of the infant.

The face is small and round, and the lower jaw appears to recede. Facial asymmetry is sometimes seen, especially of the chin and mandible. This can be the result of posture *in utero* when the flexed head is tilted to one side and presses against the shoulder. The nose may also be asymmetrical or have a deviated septum from intrauterine pressure. It is important that the nose not be obstructed, since infants are nose breathers and have difficulty breathing through their mouths.

The scalp, face, and neck should be observed carefully for any abrasions, contusions, or breaks in the skin. These can result from application of internal fetal monitor electrodes, forceps, or other instruments used in delivery. Any opening in the skin is a potential site for bacterial invasion and should be watched for signs of infection.

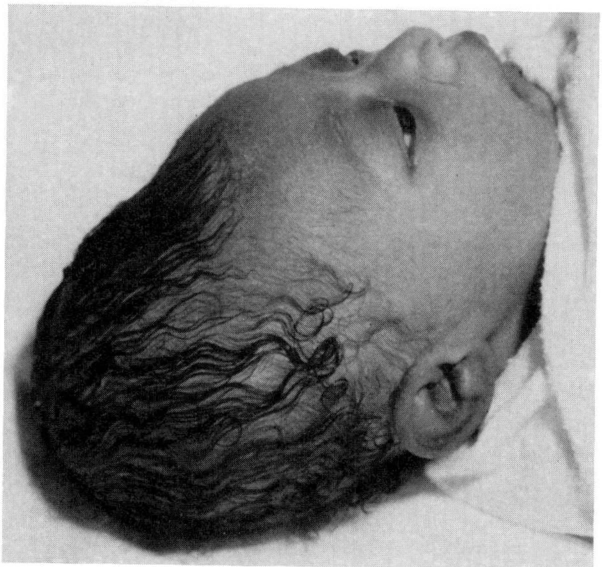

Figure 31-2.
Molding of the head.

Eyes

The eyes are closed much of the time but may open spontaneously if the infant's head is lifted or rocked gently (a valuable point to remember when one wants to inspect the eyes). From birth the infant can see and discriminate patterns as the basis for form perception. This capacity is rather limited by imperfect oculomotor coordination and inability to accommodate for varying distances. Moreover, the eye, the visual pathways, and the visual part of the brain are poorly developed at birth. Nevertheless, although the baby's vision is much less acute than an adult's, a good deal of visual experience is possible for him.

Most mothers do not realize that their infants can see as well as they do, and they appreciate being informed of this fact. In addition, some mothers become exceedingly anxious when they observe strabismus or nystagmus in their infants, but they should be reassured that this lack of coordination is normal during the first few months of life.

Most babies' eyes are blue or a slate-gray color at birth. By the time the infant is 3 months old, most have achieved their permanent color, although complete pigmentation of the iris does not occur until the infant is about a year old. Since the lacrimal glands may not be functioning at birth, the baby does not usually shed tears when he cries. Tears may not appear for several weeks and sometimes for several months. There may be some edema of the lids or purulent discharge caused by the silver nitrate. The changes in the vascu-

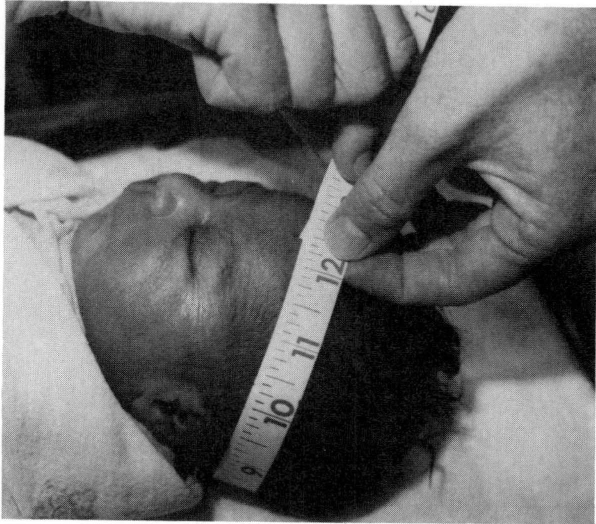

Figure 31-3.
Measuring the circumference of the head. Place a nonstretchable tape just above the eyebrows and over the most prominent part of the occiput.

lar tension of the eyes during delivery sometimes cause small areas of subconjunctival hemorrhage. These areas disappear spontaneously in 1 week or 2 weeks and are not significant.

If an ophthalmoscope is used in examining the eyes, the pupil should appear as a small red–orange circular spot when the light is directed at it. This is the red reflex, which is caused by the light shining on the retina, and any opacities of the lens or other obstructions would be visible if present.

Ears and Hearing

The ears should be inspected for size, shape, position, and anomaly. The point where the top of the ear is attached to the scalp should fall on or above an imaginary line drawn from the inner through the outer canthus of the eye (Fig. 31-4). Abnormal positioning of the ears is frequently associated with kidney or extensive chromosomal abnormalities.

Otoscopic examination of the ear establishes the patency of the external auditory canal, but the tympanic membranes are usually difficult to visualize for the first 2 days or 3 days of life due to accumulated vernix caseosa. Phibbs suggests, however, that visualization should be attempted in the infant suspected of having an infection because otitis media can occur during these first days.[12] During the first few months the light reflex is diffuse, rather than cone shaped as it is later.

The ear and the nerve tracts for hearing are anatomically mature at birth, and the newborn can hear after his first cry. Hearing apparently becomes acute within several days as the eustachian tubes become aerated, and the mucus in the middle ear disappears.

Hearing can be tested by sounding a bell or rattle near the baby's head but out of eyesight. Hearing the sound causes blinking of the eyes, momentary cessation of activity, or a startle response. This is not an accurate test, but it may be helpful in alerting the examiner to a possible problem.

Neck

The newborn infant generally appears to have a short neck, which sometimes makes it difficult to tell if webbing or other problems are present. The head should be gently rotated to determine the range of motion of the neck and the muscles should be palpated for any masses.

Lips, Mouth, and Cheeks

The rounded, thickened areas often present on the lips (particularly on the center of the upper lip) are known as labial tubercles or "sucking blisters," although they are not true blisters since there is no fluid in them. Sucking (fat) pads are usually present in the cheeks. The lips, gums, and palate should be examined to see that they are intact. Epstein's pearls, small white cysts, which may be seen on the hard palate or gums, are not abnormal. Occasionally a tooth is present, which may be pulled to avoid the possibility of its being aspirated.

At this early age, the tongue does not extend far beyond the margin of the gums because the frenulum is normally short. A mother's concern that her baby is tongue-tied is usually unwarranted.

Assessment of Body

General Appearance

The average term infant weighs 3500 g (7½ lb), and 95% weigh between 2500 g (5½ lb) and 4250 g (9½ lb). There is usually some weight loss in the first 3 days to 5 days, possibly as much as 10% of the infant's birth

Figure 31-4.
(A) Normal ear. *(B)* Abnormally angled ear. *(C)* Low-seated ear.

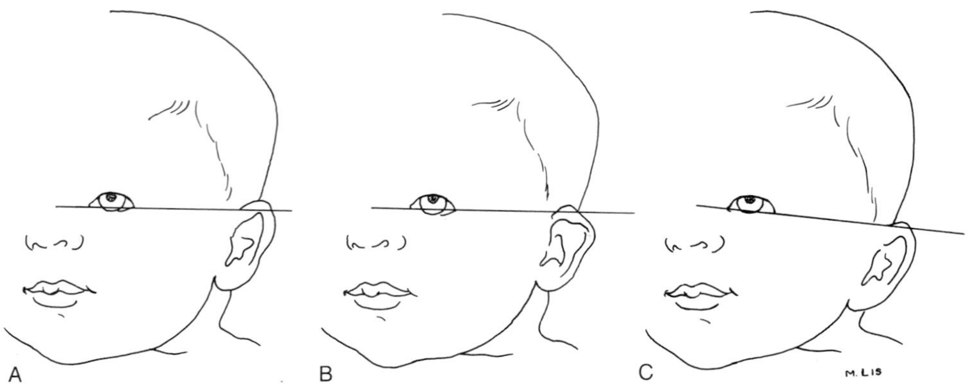

weight. This is usually regained by the eighth to twelfth day.

Length should also be measured soon after birth to serve as a baseline from which to judge future growth. The average length of a full-term infant at birth is 51 cm (20 in), with 95% between 46 cm and 56 cm (18 in and 22 in). Since the newborn infant usually assumes a somewhat flexed position, it can be difficult to get an accurate measurement from the top of the head to the heels. Measurement is more accurate when done on a firm surface, and it is helpful to have an assistant hold the infant's head.

Skin

The infant's skin appears to be thin and delicate and is often dry and peeling. The baby's color may be pink, reddish, or pale, becoming very ruddy when he cries. Initially, the hands and the feet are quite blue (acrocyanosis) due to the sluggish peripheral vascular circulation, but this cyanosis of the extremities soon disappears, often within a few hours.

Careful assessment of the newborn for jaundice is an important part of nursing care. The red color of the blood or the pigment in the skin of dark-complected babies sometimes hides the yellow color. Blanching the skin over a bony area such as the chest or forehead by pressing with a finger and observing the area before the color comes back often allows the yellow to be seen. The sclera or the buccal mucosa are also good places to look.

Vernix caseosa, a white cheesy material that was a protection to the skin while the fetus floated in amniotic fluid in the uterus, may be apparent, particularly in the creases of the body. Also, on the body there may be large areas of fine downy hair called lanugo. Milia may be present on the nose and the forehead and small flat hemangiomas may be apparent on the nape of the neck, the eyelids, or over the bridge of the nose. These so-called stork bites, clusters of small capillaries, usually disappear spontaneously during infancy.

Gray-blue pigmented areas are seen most often in dark-skinned infants, especially in the lumbosacral area, although other sites are not uncommon. These "mongolian spots" have no relationship to mongolism and usually disappear spontaneously during late infancy or early childhood, although some may persist until adulthood.

Erythema Toxicum. Erythema toxicum is a blotchy erythematous rash which may appear in the first few days of life (Fig. 31-5). It is sometimes referred to as the newborn rash, or "flea-bite" dermatitis (although no fleas are involved). The erythematous areas, which develop more frequently on the back, the shoulders and the buttocks, have a small blanched wheal in the center. The cause of this skin disturbance is obscure, and no treatment is necessary. The rash is transient, is likely to change appreciably within a few hours, and may disappear entirely within a day or so.

Milia. Milia are pinpoint-sized, pearly white spots which occur commonly on the nose, forehead, or chin of the newborn infant. When touched gently with the tip of the finger, these spots feel like tiny, firm seeds. They are due to retention of sebaceous material within the sebaceous glands, and if they are left alone, usually disappear spontaneously during the neonatal period. Mothers often mistake milia for "whiteheads" and may attempt to squeeze them if the nurse or the physician has not warned them against such practice.

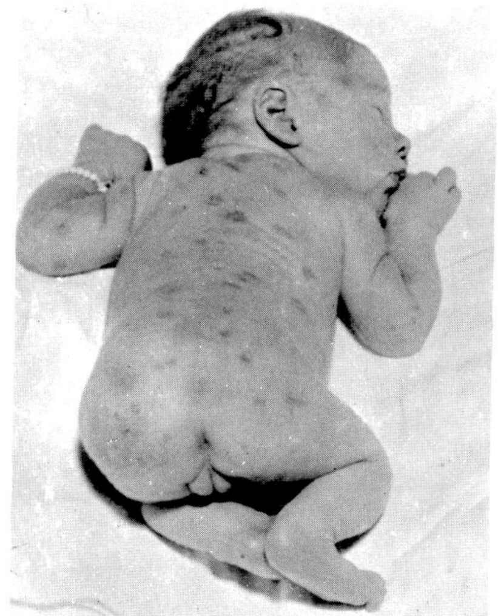

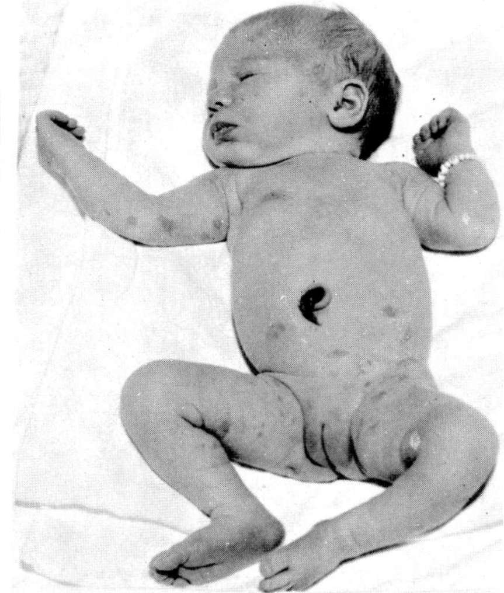

Figure 31-5.
Erythema toxicum. This "newborn rash" develops more frequently on the back, the shoulders, and the buttocks. (Courtesy of MacDonald House, The University Hospitals of Cleveland, Cleveland, Ohio)

Thorax

The infant's chest is round with a transverse diameter that is approximately equal to the anteroposterior diameter, and the circumference, measured just above the nipple line, slightly smaller than the head. The thorax is relatively short compared to the abdomen. The chest wall is thin with little musculature and the rib cage is very soft and pliant. The tip of the xiphoid process often protrudes visibly.

Engorgement of the breasts is common during the neonatal period in both male and female infants (Fig. 31-6). It is due to the same causes that bring about mammary engorgement in the mother—that is, endocrine influence. In the case of the infant, the breasts have been acted on throughout pregnancy by the estrogenic hormone that passes to them through the placenta from the mother. This is the same hormone which prepares the mother's breasts for lactation. When it is withdrawn after birth, changes in the infant's breasts similar to those in the mother take place. Mammary engorgement in the newborn subsides without treatment, but sometimes it persists for 2 weeks or 3 weeks.

Sometimes a small amount of fluid that has been called "witches' milk" is secreted. Mothers should be cautioned against massaging the breasts or trying to express the fluid because handling predisposes to infection such as breast abscess or mastitis.

Assessing Respiration. As the infant adapts successfully to extrauterine life, the respiratory rate usually ranges from 40 breaths per minute to 60 breaths per minute and is easily altered by internal and external stimuli. Counting respirations in the newborn can be very frustrating since the infant may have periods of rapid breathing alternating with short periods of apnea. Intermittent crying may also interfere with counting. Respirations should be counted for one full minute or longer if necessary. Since the infant primarily uses diaphragmatic breathing, it is easier to count abdominal rather than chest excursions. An alternate method is to count respirations by auscultation (Fig. 31-7).

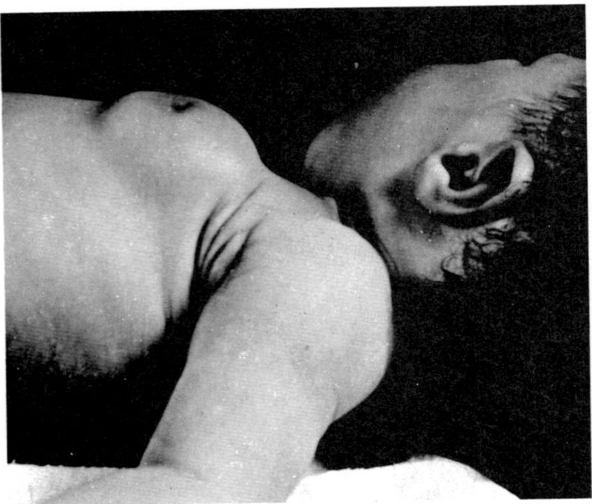

Figure 31-6.
Hypertrophy of breast developing in the neonatal period.

The respiration is normally quiet and shallow with the chest and abdomen moving together. Although retractions, mild expiratory grunting, and nasal flaring may be considered normal during the first few minutes after birth, presence after that time leads one to suspect obstruction or abnormality.

In auscultation of the infant's chest, it is best to use the bell or small diaphragm of the stethoscope, since the adult-sized diaphragm may not make complete contact with the small chest wall. Auscultation should be done in both the upright and supine positions because breath sounds may be altered with changing positions. Bronchial breath sounds are normally heard over most of the chest and sound louder and harsher because they are closer.

Periods of dyspnea and cyanosis may occur suddenly in an infant who is breathing normally, even after the transition period is over. This *may* indicate some anomaly or other pathologic condition and should be reported promptly. Therefore, the nurse should notify the physician if the respiratory rate is persistently below 40 respirations per minute or if it increases beyond 60 respirations per minute when the infant is at rest, or if dyspnea or cyanosis occurs.

Heart. The heart rate is determined by counting the apical pulse (Fig. 31-8). It is normally between 120 beats per minute and 160 beats per minute, and like the respiratory rate, changes with the infant's activity. It beats faster when he is crying, active, or breathing rapidly, and it beats more slowly when he is quiet, especially during the short periods of no breathing.

The first and second heart sounds should be clear and well defined. Murmurs may be present in the newborn period. They may be heard more easily with the bell of the stethoscope held lightly against the chest wall. The areas of cardiac auscultation where murmurs are most likely to be heard are the right sternal border, upper left sternal border, lower left sternal border, and the apex. Any murmurs should be reported, recorded, and followed but may be less significant in the newborn period than at other times since a closing ductus arteriosus may cause a loud murmur that soon disappears, while a serious heart anomaly may cause no murmur at all.

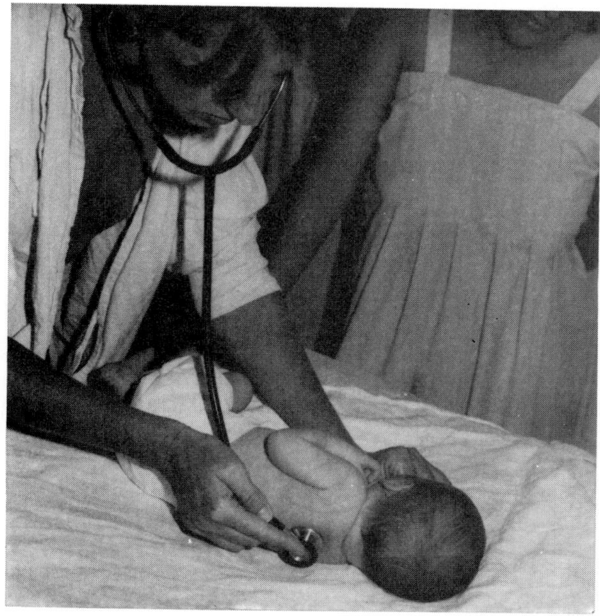

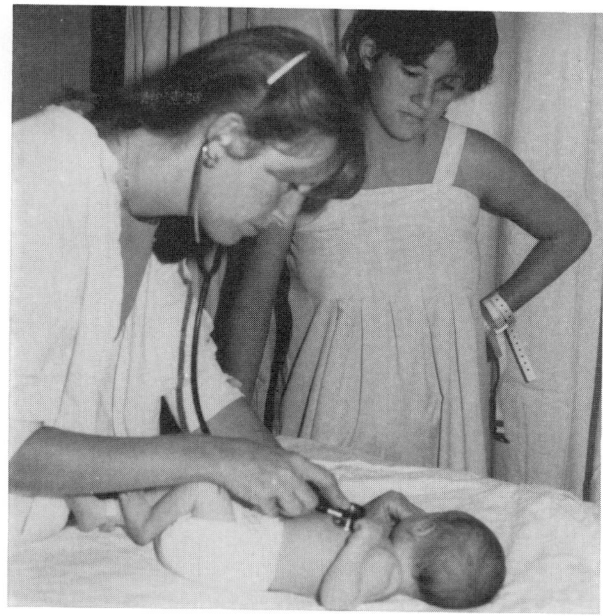

Figure 31-7.
Auscultation of the newborn. Nurse practitioner performs discharge physical exam while mother observes.

Early experiences in listening to the newborn's chest can be confusing because both the heart rate and respirations are so much faster than an adult's and the infant often wiggles and fusses. With practice the student will learn how to quiet the infant and to be able to distinguish between the different sounds.

Abdomen

The abdomen is round and slightly protuberant due to the relative size of the abdominal organs and weak muscular structures. Superficial veins are often visible. Observation can be a valuable part of the examination of the abdomen since outlines of the anterior organs may sometimes be seen and asymmetry suggestive of abnormalities can be noted. Palpation should begin with gentle pressure or stroking of the abdomen upward, then deeper palpation may be done. The liver edge is usually palpable just below the right rib margin, but it is not sharp and may be missed if palpation is too high or too forceful. The tip of the spleen may sometimes be palpated in the left upper quadrant. The kidneys can usually be palpated during the first 4 hours to 6 hours after birth, but they are more difficult to locate after this. If palpable, the lower edges are usually located approximately at the level of the umbilicus, about half way between the infant's side and the midline.

The umbilical cord stump should be checked for bleeding or oozing (Fig. 31-9), and the number of vessels noted if not already recorded (see Chap. 25). The umbilicus and surrounding area should also be inspected carefully. Redness, induration, skin warmth, or foul-smelling discharge are signs of infection which should be reported. Infection in this area is

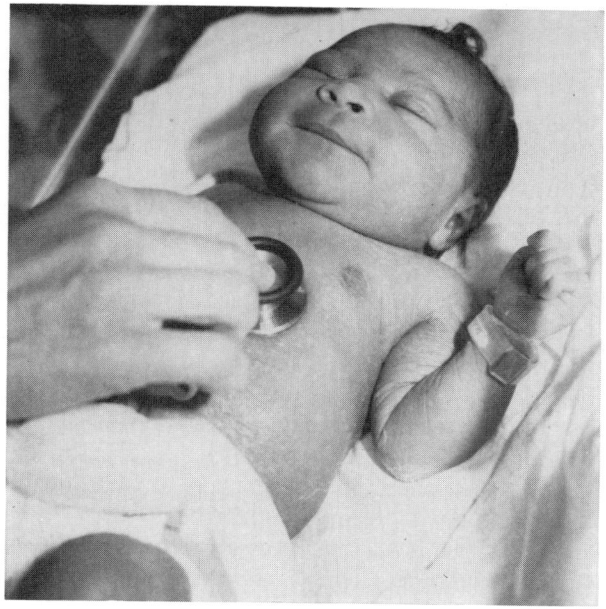

Figure 31-8.
Taking an apical pulse.

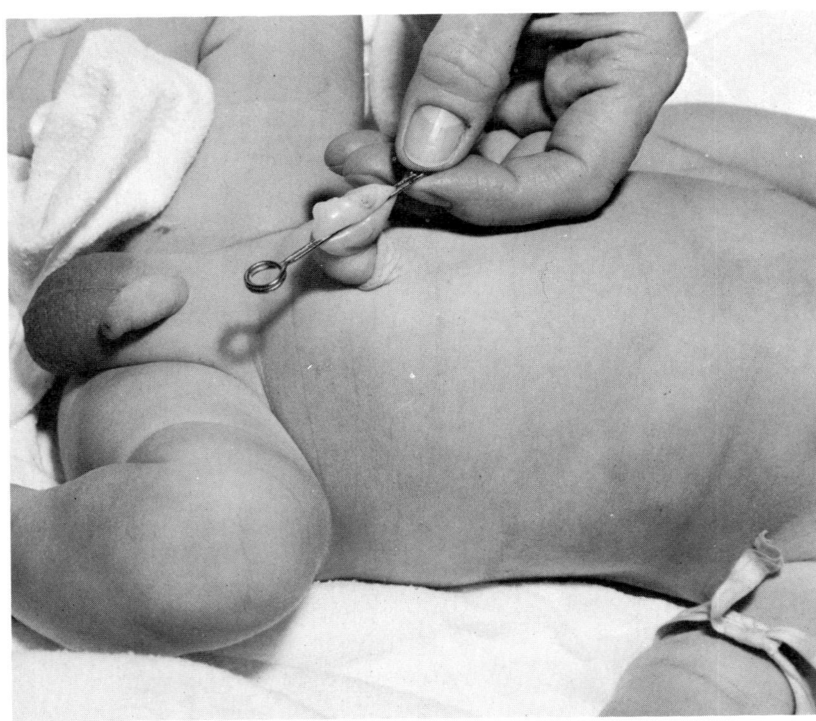

Figure 31-9.
Inspection of cord stump.

potentially dangerous in the newborn infant because it can spread up the open arteries into the peritoneum. Serous or serosanguineous discharge continuing after separation of the cord stump may indicate a granuloma. This has the appearance of a small red button deep in the umbilicus. It can be cauterized by the physician with a silver nitrate stick or borax powder.[13]

Genitals

Female genitalia should be inspected for presence and size of the labia majora, labia minora, clitoris, and vaginal opening. Enlarged labia or vaginal discharge may be present due to *in utero* stimulation by maternal hormones. The discharge is sometimes blood tinged but need cause no special concern. The swelling and discharge disappear spontaneously.

In male babies the scrotum usually appears relatively large. At term in most infants the testes can be palpated in the scrotum or can be easily brought down. The prepuce (foreskin) covers the glans penis and is usually adherent at birth. During the first few months it becomes less adherent and can be manually retracted. When the opening in the foreskin is so small that it cannot be pulled back at all, the condition is called *phimosis.* There is some difference of opinion as to whether this is an indication for circumcision. Many doctors feel that it is, but others feel that as long as urination is not interfered with it is a normal condition of the newborn and the foreskin will gradually become retractable as the child grows.The penis should be inspected to determine the location of the urinary meatus. If the opening is covered by the foreskin, observing the infant while he is voiding helps locate it.

Posterior

With the infant in the prone position, the entire posterior surface of the body should be inspected and palpated. Any masses or abnormal curvatures of the spine should be noted. Tufts of hair or small indentations, especially in the sacral area, may be an indication of spina bifida occulta.

The perineal area should be inspected to determine the patency and location of the anus. A pilonidal "dimple" resulting from an irregular fold of skin is sometimes seen in the midline over the sacrococcygeal area. It should be examined for intactness to make sure no sinus is present.

Extremities

Throughout the exam, the infant's ability to move all four extremities is evaluated, and the limbs are compared as to size, shape, and movement. Webbing (syndactyly) or extra digits (polydactyly) should be noted also.

To check for congenital problems of the hip, the infant is placed in the supine position, the legs are

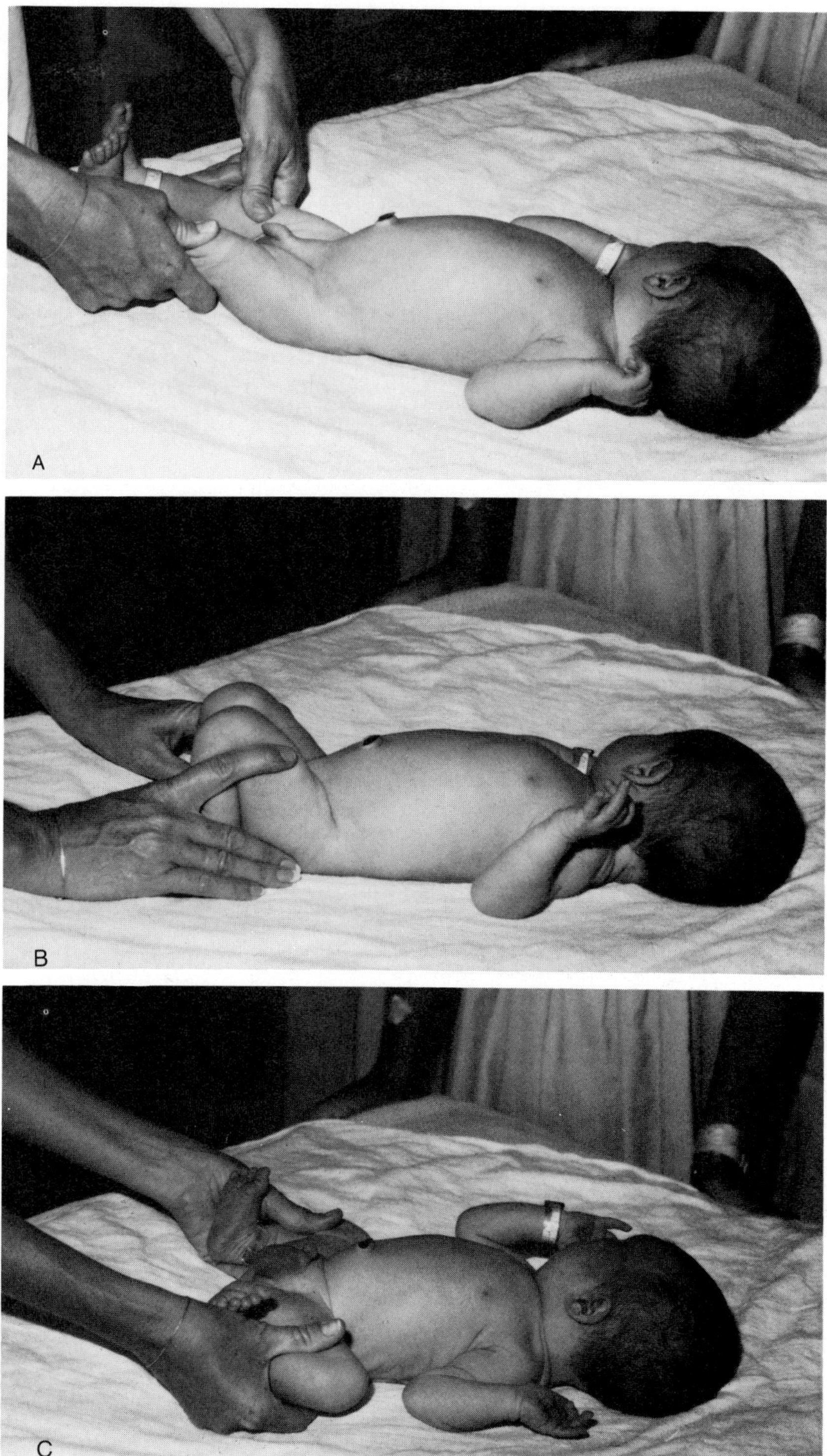

Figure 31-10.
Assessment of the lower extremities. *(A)* Comparing the length of the legs. *(B)* Comparing the height of the knees. *(C)* Hip abduction.

flexed on the abdomen and then abducted laterally toward the bed. With congenital dislocation, there may be uneven or limited abduction, uneven leg length or knee height or a "hip click" might be felt (Fig. 31-10). Unsymmetrical skin folds on the posterior aspect of the thigh are not diagnostic but may alert the examiner to this condition. Unusual positions of the feet can indicate congenital clubfoot or other foot and

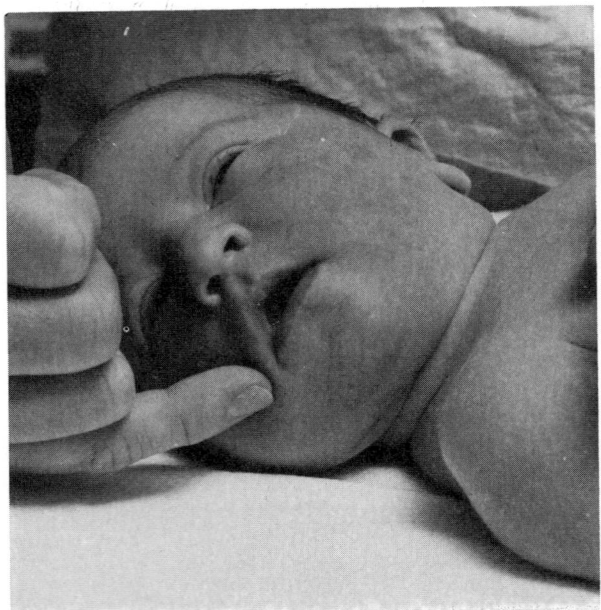

Figure 31-11.
Rooting reflex. (Whitley N: A Manual of Clinical Obstetrics. Philadelphia, JB Lippincott. In preparation.)

ankle deformities. If the foot can be moved to the normal position with ease, the condition may just be due to intrauterine malposition.

Neurologic Assessment

Rooting and Sucking

Gently stroking the infant's cheek or corner of the mouth with a sterile nipple or clean finger causes the baby to open his mouth and turn toward the stimulus (Fig. 31-11). This is known as the *rooting reflex*. The *sucking reflex* can be evaluated by placing the nipple or finger in the baby's mouth and noting the strength of the sucking response. These reflexes may not be too active if the infant has eaten recently.

It is well known that during the first 2 months of life the newborn infant has a great need to suck and usually sucks on anything that comes in contact with his lips. Newborn infants can suck while sleeping and nonnutritive sucking can have a quieting effect on excited babies.

Grasp Reflex

The *grasp reflex* is present at birth in both the hands and the feet (Fig. 31-12). The infant grasps any object placed in his hands, clings briefly, and then lets go.

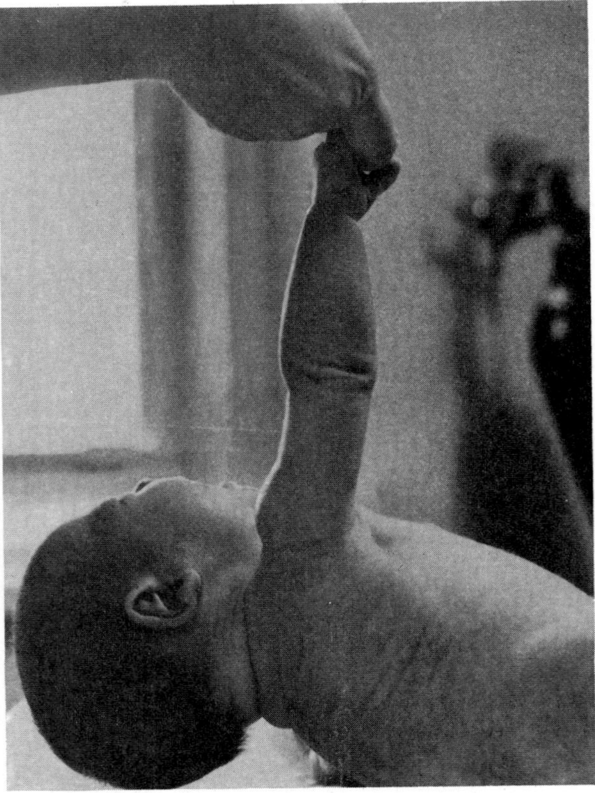

Figure 31-12.
Grasp reflex. (Whitley N: A Manual of Clinical Obstetrics. Philadelphia, JB Lippincott. In preparation. Courtesy of Mead Johnson)

Even at birth he may be able to hold onto an adult's forefinger so securely that he can be lifted to a standing position. Although the baby cannot actually grasp with his feet, stroking the soles causes the toes to turn downward as though trying to grasp. The grasping movements are a reflex action at birth, but with practice and experience the hand grasp soon becomes voluntary and purposeful.

By grasping the infant's hands and arms, the examiner can gently pull the infant to a sitting position. The infant flexes the elbows to resist extension (traction response). The strength of the neck muscles can be assessed by noting the amount of head lag. The normal term newborn is able to support his head momentarily.

Moro Reflex

The *Moro* or *startle reflex* indicates an awareness of equilibrium in the newborn (Fig. 31-13). The preferred method of eliciting this reflex is to hold the infant with his head supported, then allow the head to drop backward a short distance. Alternately, the infant

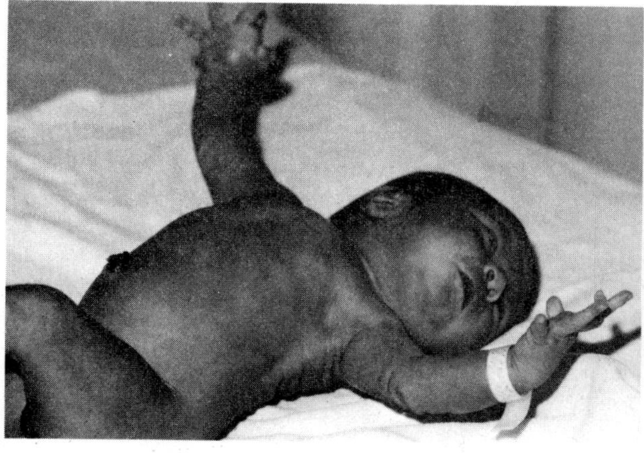

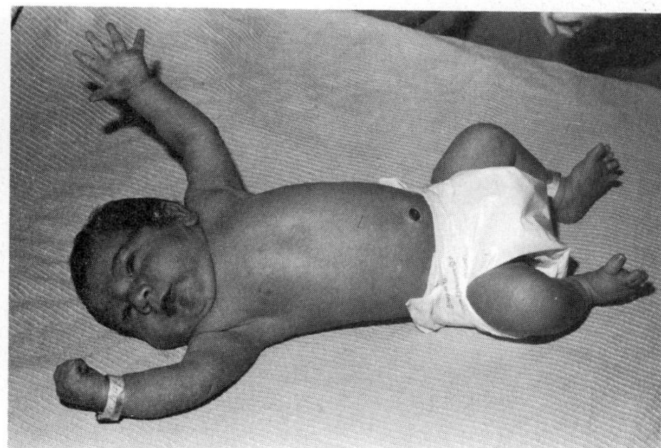

Figure 31-13.
Moro reflex.

can be lying quietly and the mattress struck, or the head lifted a few inches and allowed to drop back. The reaction should consist of lateral extension of the upper extremities and opening of the hands, followed by anterior flexion and adduction of the arms in an embracing motion. The movements should be symmetrical. If they are not, injury to the part that lags should be suspected.

The Moro reflex should be present at birth; normally it disappears by 3 months of age. If it cannot be elicited at birth, edema of or injury to the brain may be present. As the edema subsides, the reflex returns, and it should be demonstrable on the day following delivery. If frank brain damage has occurred, the reflex is absent for several days; if the damage is not too severe, the reflex returns in 3 days or 4 days. Occasionally, the reflex is present at birth but disappears over the first days. Increasing cerebral edema or slow intracranial hemorrhage then is suspected.

Tonic Neck Reflex

When the *tonic neck reflex* is elicited, the infant assumes a "fencing" position; that is, he lies on his back with his head rotated to one side. The arm and the leg on the side to which he is facing are partially or completely extended and the opposite arm and leg are flexed (Fig. 31-14). This reflex also disappears in a few months, since it is another manifestation of the immaturity of the newborn's nervous system.

Stepping Reflex

The *stepping* or *dancing reflex* is another action that is present at birth but soon disappears. This reflex causes the infant to make little stepping or prancing movements when he is held upright with his feet touching a surface (Fig. 31-15). After this reflex diminishes, the infant does not attempt stepping motions until he is ready to stand and walk. However, he does exercise the leg muscles a great deal and seems to derive much enjoyment from waving and kicking his legs about.

Other Reflexes

The next group of reflexes might be termed protective, since they are necessary and at times essential to the preservation of the newborn's safety. The *blinking reflex* occurs when the infant is subjected to a bright light. The *cough* and the *sneeze reflexes* clear his respiratory passages. The *yawn reflex* draws in additional oxygen. These, together with the infant's ability to cry when uncomfortable, to withdraw from painful stimuli, to resist restraint, and so on, are all defensive measures. As the baby grows and develops, these together with the other reflexes mentioned either diminish or become more highly developed according to the need. Thus, the infant's behavior patterns become more complex and highly developed.

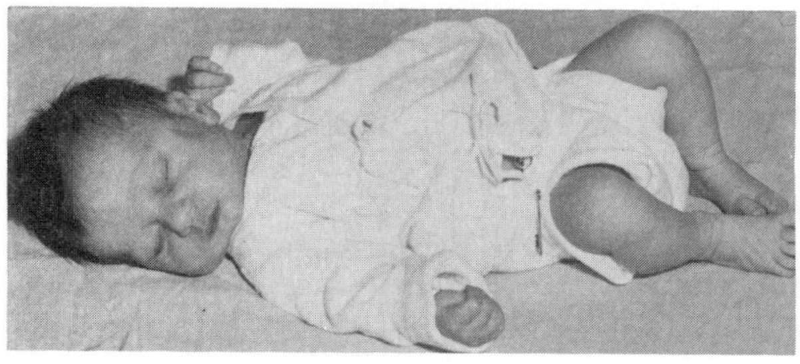

Figure 31-14.
Tonic neck reflex.

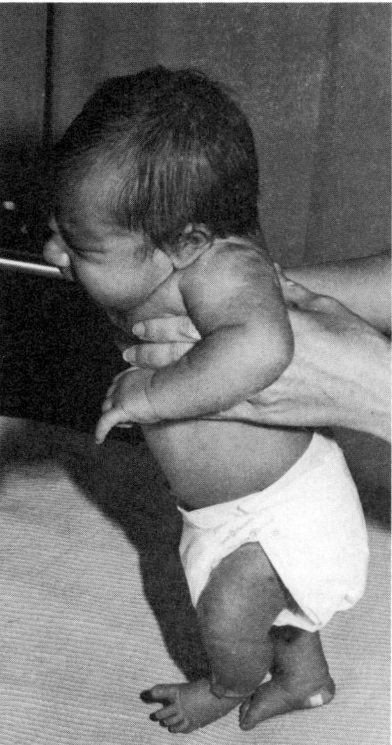
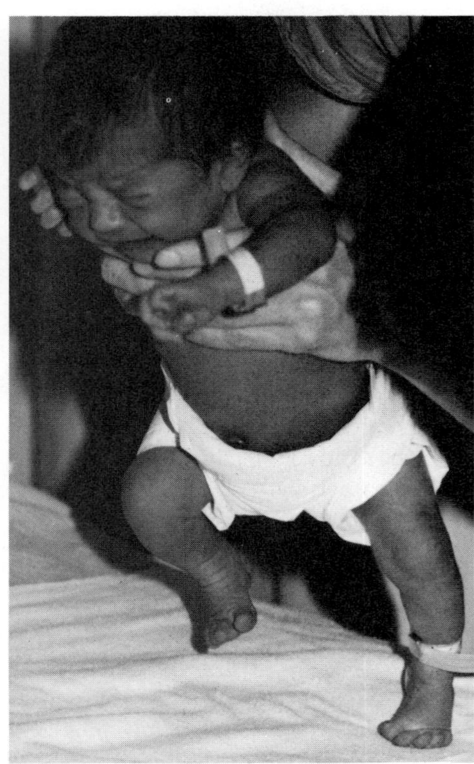

Figure 31-15.
Stepping reflex.

Gestational Age

Evaluation of gestational age may also be included in the nurse's initial examination of the newborn. This will be discussed in Chapter 41.

Behavioral Assessment

Although the newborn used to be thought of as essentially passive, we now recognize that the infant interacts actively with his environment from birth. To evaluate this interaction, a behavioral assessment can be conducted.

The Neonatal Behavioral Assessment Scale, developed by T. Berry Brazelton, includes both physical and behavioral assessment of the newborn.[14] According to Brazelton, the scale can be used both in clinical practice, as a predictive tool, and in research. Use of the scale for its intended purposes requires a trained examiner and considerable time, but some aspects of the scale and some of the findings can be useful to anyone working with newborns.

Essential to an understanding of the infant's behavior is the concept of the state of consciousness or "state." Brazelton recognizes the following six states.[14]

Sleep States

1. Deep sleep—regular breathing, eyes closed, no spontaneous activity except startles or jerky movements at quite regular intervals; external stimuli produce startles with some delay; suppression of startles is rapid, and state changes are less likely than from other states; no eye movements
2. Light sleep—eyes closed, rapid eye movements can be observed under closed lids; low activity level, with random movements and startles or startle equivalents; movements are likely to be smoother and more monitored than in state 1; responds to internal and external stimuli with startle equivalents, often with a resulting change of state; irregular respirations; sucking movements occur off and on

Awake States

3. Drowsy or semidozing; eyes may be open or closed, eyelids fluttering; activity level variable, with interspersed, mild startles from time to time; reactive to sensory stimuli, but response often delayed; state change after stimulation frequently noted; movements are usually smooth
4. Alert, with bright look; seems to focus attention on source of stimulation, such as an object to be sucked, or a visual or auditory stimulus; imping-

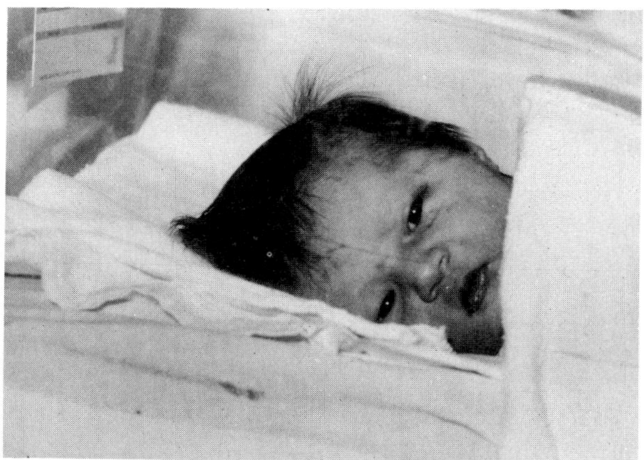

Figure 31-16.
Quiet alert state.

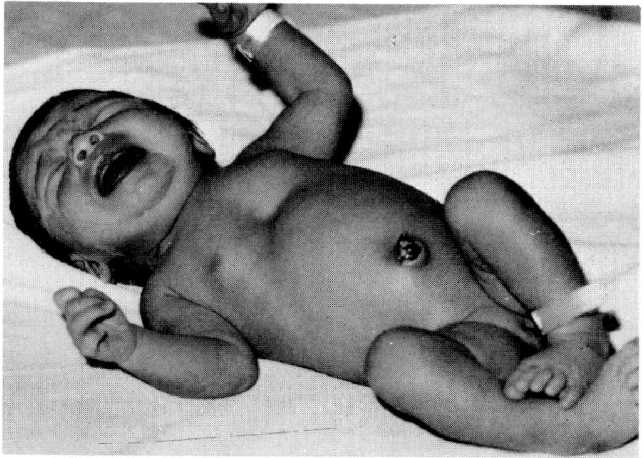

Figure 31-17.
Active crying state.

ing stimuli may break through but with some delay in response; motor activity is minimal (Fig. 31-16)

5. Eyes open; considerable motor activity, with thrusting movements of the extremities, and even a few spontaneous startles; reactive to external stimulation with increase in startles or motor activity, but discrete reactions difficult to distinguish because of general high activity level.
6. Crying; characterized by intense crying which is difficult to break through with stimulation (Fig. 31-17)

Babies vary greatly in the amount of time they spend in the various states and in the ease or difficulty with which they make the transition from one state to another. The concept of state is often helpful to parents in interacting with their baby. If they can learn to recognize the various states and the individuality of their infant, they are better able to use the infant's timetable rather than their own in giving care and have a better understanding of when the infant will respond to them.

The Neonatal Behavioral Assessment Scale measures a total of 27 items (see Brazelton Scale Criteria). Each item is scored on a scale of one to nine and is based on the infant's best rather than his average performance. The infant's state at the time any given item is tested is important. Some items require that the infant be in a certain state for valid testing.

The items can be divided into the following six categories:[15]

1. Habituation—how soon the neonate diminishes his responses to specific repeated stimuli
2. Orientation—how often and when he attends to auditory and visual stimuli

Brazelton Scale Criteria

1. Response decrement to light
2. Response decrement to rattle
3. Response decrement to bell
4. Response decrement to pinprick
5. Orientation response—inanimate visual
6. Orientation response—inanimate auditory
7. Orientation—animate visual
8. Orientation—animate auditory
9. Orientation—animate visual and auditory
10. Alertness
11. General tonus
12. Motor maturity
13. Pull-to-sit
14. Cuddliness
15. Defensive movements
16. Consolability with intervention
17. Peak of excitement
18. Rapidity of buildup
19. Irritability (to aversive stimuli—uncover, undress, pull-to-sit, prone, pinprick, Tonic Neck Response, Moro, defensive reaction)
20. Activity
21. Tremulousness
22. Amount of startle during exam
23. Lability of skin color
24. Lability of states
25. Self-quieting activity
26. Hand to mouth facility
27. Smiles

3. Motor maturity—how well the infant coordinates and controls motor activities
4. Variation—how often he exhibits alertness, state changes, color changes, activity, and peaks of excitement
5. Self-quieting abilities—how often, how soon, and how effectively the neonate can use his own resources to quiet and console himself when upset or distressed
6. Social behaviors—how often and how much the newborn smiles and cuddles

A better understanding of the scale may be obtained from the booklet[14] or the films prepared by Dr. Brazelton. The discussion here is limited to a few items of particular interest.

Most parents are interested in what kinds of stimuli their infant will focus attention on. Some parents discover these things for themselves. Others need to be told that most infants will focus on a bright red ball and follow it briefly when they are in the quiet-alert state (state 4), or that the infant particularly likes to follow a moving human face or a high-pitched voice.

Many people think that all infants are cuddly and that if an infant does not cuddle when held there is either something wrong with them or with the infant. In fact, infants respond in many different ways to being cuddled. Scores on "cuddliness" range from: (1) "Actually resists being held, continuously pushing away, thrashing or stiffening" to (9) Molds into arms and relaxes, turns toward examiner's body when held horizontally, or leans forward when held on the examiner's shoulder, all of the body participates and baby grasps examiner to cling to him.[14]

Infants also vary in their ability to be consoled or to console themselves. These items are scored when the infant is upset (state 6). Some babies only quiet down when they are dressed and left alone. Others need restraint to help them inhibit the startle reflex. These babies are the ones that usually do best when swaddled in a blanket.

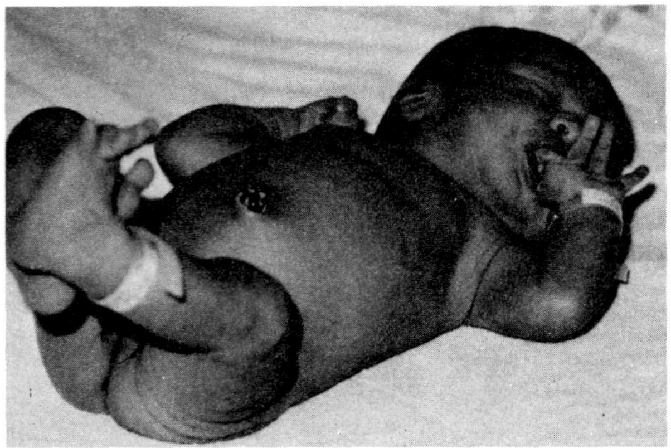

Figure 31-18.
Self-consoling activity according to the Brazelton behavioral assessment scale: hand-to-mouth and sucking activity.

Possible self-consoling activities that are counted in the assessment are hand to mouth efforts, sucking on fist or tongue (Fig. 31-18), or using visual or auditory stimulus from the environment to quiet self. Finding out ways in which their particular infant can console himself or be consoled can be very helpful to the parents.

Babies often smile even in the first days, but the statement is usually made that it is just a reflex or "gas." Brazelton comments that he has "seen close replicas of 'social smiles' in the newborn period" and that, although they are hard to be sure of, "they surely are the precursors of such smiling behavior and a mother reinforces them as such."[14]

References

1. Manning FA, Platt L, LeMay M: Fetal breathing. In McNall L, Galeener J (eds): Current Practice in Obstetric and Gynecologic Nursing, Vol 2 pp 108–119. St. Louis, CV Mosby, 1977

2. Harned Jr H: Respiration and the respiratory system. In Stave U (ed): Perinatal Physiology, pp 53–101. New York, Plenum, 1978

3. Nelson NM: Respiration and circulation after birth. In Smith CA, Nelson NM (eds): The Physiology of the Newborn Infant, 117–262. 4th ed. Springfield, Ill., Charles C Thomas, 1976

4. Arnold HW, Putman NJ, Barnard BL, Desmond MM et al: Transition to extrauterine life. Am J Nurs 65, 10:77–80, October 1965

5. Honig G, Hruby M: Disorders of the blood and hematopoietic system. In Behrman RD (ed): Neonatal-Perinatal Medicine, 2nd ed, pp 345–393. St. Louis, CV Mosby, 1977

6. Hernandez A, Meyer DA, Goldring D: Blood pressure in neonates. Contemporary OB/GYN 5:34–37, March 1975

7. Gartner L, Lee K: Unconjugated hyperbilirubinemia. In Behrman RD (ed): Neonatal-Perinatal Medicine, 2nd ed, pp 395–415. St. Louis, CV Mosby, 1977

8. Gartner LM: Hyperbilirubinemia In Pediatrics, 16th ed, p 1077. Appleton–Century–Crofts, New York, 1977

9. Sinclair JC: Metabolic rate and temperature control. In Smith CA, Nelson NM (ed): The Physiology of the Newborn Infant, 4th ed, pp 354–415. Springfield, Ill, Charles C Thomas, 1976

10. Roberts FB: Perinatal Nursing. New York, McGraw-Hill, 1977

11. Spitzer A, Bernstein J, Edelmann, Jr CM: Diseases of the urinary tract. In Behrman RD (ed): Neonatal-Perinatal Medicine, 2nd ed, pp 650–677. St. Louis, CV Mosby, 1977

12. Phibbs RH: The Newborn Infant. In Rudolph AM (ed): Pediatrics, 16th ed, p 147. Appleton–Century–Crofts, New York, 1977

13. Alexander MM, Brown MS: Pediatric Physical Diagnosis for Nurses, p 156. McGraw–Hill, New York, 1974

14. Brazelton TB: Neonatal Behavioral Assessment Scale. Clinics in Developmental Medicine, No. 50. Philadelphia, JB Lippincott, 1973

15. Erickson MP: Trends in assessing the newborn and his parents. MCN 3, 2:99–103, March/April 1978

Suggested Reading

Als H, Brazelton TB: Comprehensive neonatal assessment. Birth and the Family Journal 2, 1:3–9, Winter 1974–1975

Behrman RD (ed): Neonatal-Perinatal Medicine, 2nd ed. St. Louis, CV Mosby, 1977

Binzley V: State: Overlooked factor in newborn nursing. Am J Nurs 77:102–103, January 1977

Desmond M, Franklin RR, Vallbona C, Hill RM et al: The clinical behavior of the newly born. J Pediatr 62:307–325, March 1963

Faber M: Circumcision revisited. BFJ, 1, 2:19–21, Spring 1974

Hervada A: Nursery evaluation of the newborn. Am J Nurs 67:1669–1671, August 1967

Nalepka CD: Understanding thermoregulation in newborns. JOGN Nurs, 5, 6:17–19, November/December 1976

Pang LM, Mellins RB: Neonatal cardiorespiratory physiology. Anesthesiology 43, 2:171–196, August 1975

Simpkin P, Simpkin PA, Edwards M: Physiologic jaundice of the newborn. BFJ 6, 1:23–40, Spring 1979

Smith AN: Physical examination of the newborn. In Clausen JP, Flook MH, Ford B (eds): Maternity Nursing Today, 2nd ed. New York, McGraw–Hill, 1977

Smith CA, Nelson NM (eds): The Physiology of the Newborn Infant, 4th ed. Springfield, Ill, Charles C Thomas, 1976

Stave U (ed): Perinatal Physiology. New York, Plenum Medical Book, 1978

Williams JK, Lancaster J: Thermoregulation of the newborn. MCN 1, 6:355–360, November/December 1976

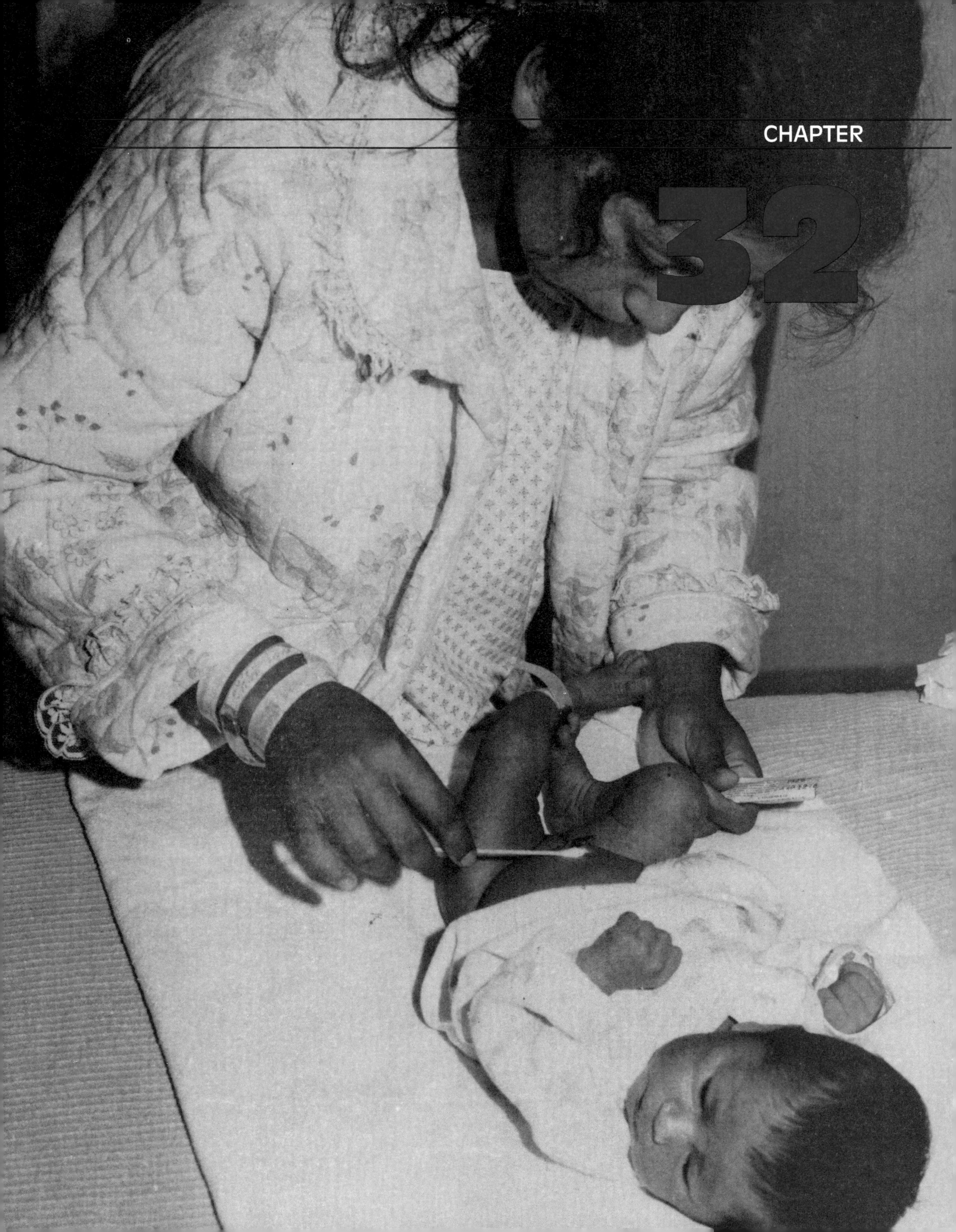

CHAPTER

32

CHAPTER 32

Care of the Newborn Infant

The care of the newborn infant presents an interesting challenge to those in maternity nursing. In a very short period of time, usually a matter of seconds, the fetus, who has been completely dependent on the mother to supply all his physiological needs, suddenly becomes an "independent" being.

Although independent of the mother for vital functions, the new baby is, of course, still very dependent in other ways. He could not survive long without a caretaker. In the immediate postnatal period this caretaker is often the nurse.

Since these first days and weeks are so critical, the care given by the nurse is very important. The nurse must use the utmost care in handling the baby, keeping him warm and protecting him from exposure and injury, at the same time making accurate observations and recording and reporting them. Communication and teaching skills are used in contributing to the infant's future well-being by helping the parents to develop an understanding of their baby's needs and acquire skill in his care. In this way their concept of themselves as adequate parents is reinforced. The nurse must also be aware that some parents need assistance in developing healthy attitudes regarding childrearing practices, so that the infant can make a satisfactory emotional and social adjustment. Opportunity must be provided in the hospital environment for the beginning development of a close parent–infant relationship. Also of importance is the maintenance of communication between the nurse and the parents.

Providing a Safe Environment

Prevention of Infection

The prevention of infection is of paramount importance in caring for the newborn. Everyone who is in contact with the infant, including parents and personnel, must assume this responsibility. Staff should take special care to instruct parents so that their activities conform to the prevention of infection. The basis of "good" technique in handling the infant is thorough handwashing with an antiseptic detergent or soap. Some institutions require that the hands be scrubbed initially with a brush; others feel that detergent, water, and friction are sufficient. Whichever the procedure, meticulous handwashing is essential, whether the infant is cared for in the central or regular nursery or in a rooming-in situation. Staff should be especially careful to wash their hands before a feeding, and after a diaper change, before going from one baby to another, and after touching anything that is not clean to that baby, such as a door, or their own face or hair.

The parents need instruction about the importance (and technique) of proper handwashing, and reinforcement should be given as necessary during the hospital stay.

As with personnel in the delivery room (see Chap. 24), all nursery staff should have a preemployment physical examination and a yearly physical examination thereafter to minimize the possibility of spreading infection from the staff among the newborn. In addition, any staff member who contracts *any* infection (*i.e.,* respiratory, gastrointestinal, skin lesions, and the like) should remain away from the nursery and contact with the newborn until the infection is gone *completely.*

If a mother shows signs of infection, particularly an elevated temperature, diarrhea, or skin lesions, the infant is not brought to her until the infection subsides. The infant who has spent some time with the mother before the symptoms were noticed may be isolated from the other babies. The importance of the precautions should be explained to the mother since she undoubtedly will find it difficult to be separated from her infant. Sometimes arrangements can be made for her to see the baby through the nursery window, but if this is not possible, the nurse should bring her frequent reports about the baby to let her know how he is eating and sleeping, and so on.

The mother who plans to breast-feed her baby should be helped to pump her breasts to ensure stimulation and continued supply of milk. The milk is usually discarded, however, depending on the type of infection and the antibiotic used to treat it.

Babies who are born outside a hospital are often not admitted to the regular newborn nursery. They usually are cared for in the observation nursery or with the mother in a rooming-in situation.

To further protect the infant from outside sources of infection, everyone coming in contact with the infant or his environment is required to change from his or her street clothes or wear a gown over them. For the nursery nurse, the gowns should be short-sleeved so that the hands, forearms, and elbows may be given a thorough scrub or wash. A clean gown should be donned at the beginning of each shift and changed if soiled. Those coming into the patient's room when the baby is there, or into the nursery for shorter periods of time, may wear a long-sleeved cover gown over their clothes. If they are going to touch the baby, their hands and arms should be scrubbed.

Most hospitals limit the number of visitors to the maternity area and exclude visitors from the nursery proper, although sometimes exceptions are made. Children are usually excluded from the maternity unit because various infections and particularly communicable diseases are so prevalent among them. With the increasing emphasis on the total family in maternity care, however, some hospitals are making provision for sibling visitation, usually in special rooms.

Old regulations about wearing masks and hair coverings are being changed. However, the hair should be worn short or pulled back to avoid coming in contact with the infant. Masks are no longer worn, since they must be changed every 20 minutes to 30 minutes to be effective, and, in fact, they can become a reservoir of bacteria when not applied properly or changed regularly.

Occasionally, the mother is instructed to wear a mask in tending the baby if she has had a recent cold or if she develops a cold when she goes home. The nurse should make certain that the mother understands the underlying principles for applying and wearing the mask and especially that she is aware of how her hands can be contaminated in adjusting and tying it. Even at home a clean mask should be worn each time the need arises, and the mother should be instructed to wash her hands each time after she adjusts it.

Hospital Set-Ups for Care of the Newborn

Rooming-In

Rooming-in is a term applied to the plan of having the new infant share the mother's hospital unit so that mother and child may be cared for together. This type of arrangement has come to mean much more than caring for the mother and the infant in the same unit of space. Rather, it implies an attitude in maternal and infant care that supports parental education and is based on recognition and understanding of the needs of each mother, infant, and family. Some authorities feel that the separation of mother and child (and father) results in an unnatural fragmentation of the family at an important time for building family unity.

Rooming-in often is discussed as if it were a modern innovation. Historically, however, all mothers back to Paleolithic times "roomed-in" until the central nursery was instituted during the first two decades of the 20th century. Nevertheless, rooming-in as it is practiced today does represent a departure from the concept of the traditional central nursery.

Attitudes in maternal and infant care have changed, in part because of increased insight into the needs of the mother, her baby, and the family as a unit. Rooming-in plays an important part in the family-centered approach to maternity care, for it not only provides an environment that fosters a wholesome, natural mother–child relationship from the very beginning, but it also affords unlimited opportunities for the parents to learn about the care of their baby (Fig. 32-1).

Some hospitals have special rooming-in units with adjoining nurseries and workrooms. Although this is an ideal arrangement, it is not always possible, and the benefits of rooming-in should not be denied the family because of the physical set-up of the hospital. Many hospitals allow rooming-in if the mother has a private room and keeps the baby in the room all the time. Some women are discouraged by this arrangement because of the expense of a private room or their desire to have more contact with other people. Perhaps a good compromise is the modified program used in many hospitals which allows a mother to have her infant in the room for long periods of time and in the central nursery the rest of the time.

The newborn infant must be protected from sources of infection regardless of where he is cared for. The same basic principles for asepsis employed in the nursery must be followed in infant care in the rooming-in unit.

The Central Nursery System

The central or general newborn nursery on the postpartal division is designed for the care of a variable number of healthy newborn infants (Fig. 32-2). In this system the infants are brought to their mothers at certain specified times during the day, generally for feeding or visiting. The staff assumes the responsibility for all the care of the babies. Some type of central nursery is usually found in most hospitals.

With the emergence of the many drug-resistant organisms that abound in the hospital environment, the danger of epidemics (whenever a large aggregate of persons collect) is enhanced. Control of the physical facilities and stringent personnel policies provide a good deal of protection for the newborn. For instance, cribs should be placed at least 2 feet apart with 3-feet-wide aisles between the cribs. Limiting the number of infants in a nursery to between 8 and 12 is

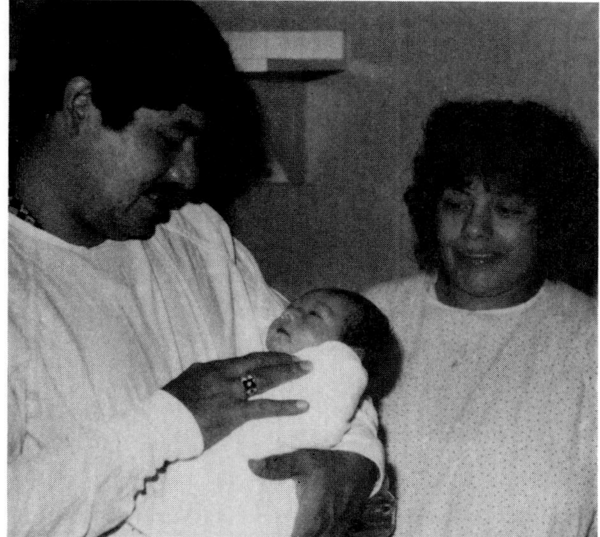

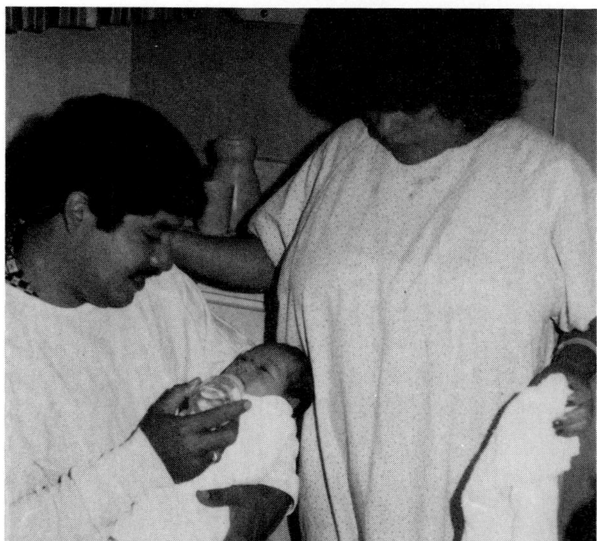

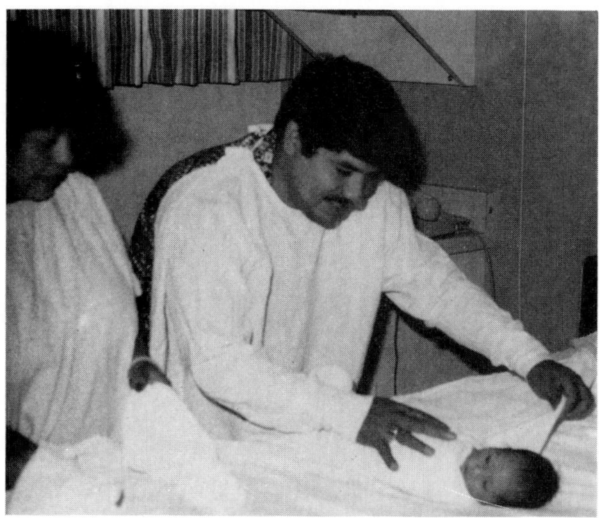

also helpful. The precautions previously mentioned, such as handwashing, wearing scrub clothes, and following other aspects of nursery aseptic technique, afford additional protection.

The central nursery is a so-called clean nursery. But it must be understood that there is a difference in nursery technique between what is considered to be nursery clean and what is considered to be baby clean (*i.e.,* what is clean for an individual baby). There should be no common equipment, such as a common bath table, used in providing care for the babies. There should be provisions in the nursery for individual technique to be followed. Each infant should have his own crib and general supplies, so that he can be given such care as his daily inspection bath or be diapered or dressed in his own bed. Most cribs are constructed with a built-in cabinet for the infant's own supplies (*e.g.,* clean diapers, shirts, and linens) and a drawer to hold the containers for cotton balls, safety pins, thermometers, and so on. When such cribs are not available, improvised units for the infant's crib should be obtained so that individual-care techniques can be carried out.

If there is any evidence of a questionable infection at the time of delivery, if the infant is born on the way to the hospital, or if the infant is suspected of having an infection of the eyes, the skin, the mouth, or the GI tract, the infant should not be admitted to general nursery care, but should be kept in isolette isolation or in a separate isolation nursery.

Observation Nursery

Maternity hospitals should have an observation nursery where infants suspected of developing an infectious condition may be kept until the presence or absence of infection is determined. When a definite diagnosis of infection is made, the infant must be transferred immediately to an isolation nursery away from the maternity division.

Aside from the fact that infants in the suspect or observation nursery must be segregated from others, and naturally require closer supervision and care because of suspected infection, their nursing care otherwise should be like that given a healthy newborn infant.

Figure 32-1.
In the rooming-in unit the father has the opportunity to gain experience holding and caring for the new baby while the mother observes.

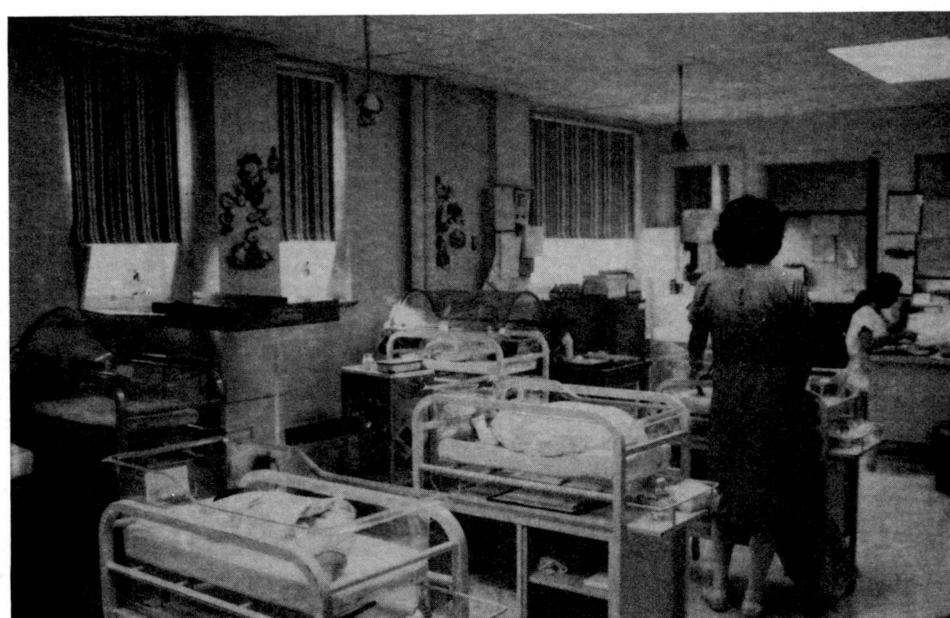

Figure 32-2.
Term newborn nursery.

Nursing Care During the Transition Period

In the delivery room initial care has been given to the infant and any early problems have been dealt with (see Chap. 25). From the delivery room the infant may be taken to the recovery room and remain with the mother and father for a while, go to a transitional nursery, or be admitted directly to the regular nursery. Of course, if the infant has serious problems, a special care nursery is indicated (see Chap. 41).

Since the day of birth is the most hazardous time for the infant, it is important that continuing observations be made during the first 24 hours. A receiving or transition nursery in the labor or nursery section provides an excellent physical environment for the extensive observations that are necessary, similar to that of recovery room care for adults. An infant whose mother has been heavily medicated during labor and delivery is particularly in need of this recovery care. If this kind of set-up is not available, the new babies should be placed in an area of the regular nursery where they can be easily observed. Low-risk babies whose mothers had little or no medication can probably be safely left with their mothers for a time under close supervision of a nurse in case of presence of mucus or other sudden changes in the infant's condition. If the mother plans to have rooming-in, it is often delayed until the infant is 12 hours to 24 hours old.

Initial Assessment and Care

When the infant is admitted to the nursery, the nursery nurse receives a report from the delivery room nurse, checks identification bands according to hospital policy, and does an initial assessment of the infant. If silver nitrate was not placed in the infant's eyes in the delivery room, it is done as soon as possible in the nursery. Also, the vitamin K injection, if ordered, may be given in the nursery. Figure 32-3 shows the injection technique.

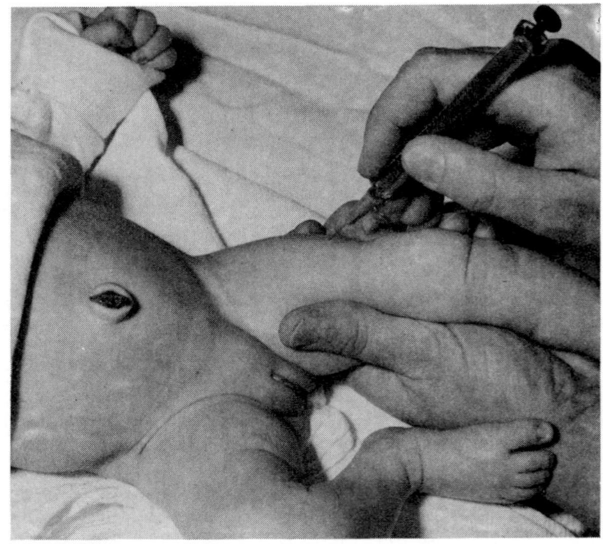

Figure 32-3.
IM injection for infant.

The vital signs should be checked every half hour until they are stable or as indicated by hospital policy. Apical heart rate and respirations should each be counted for a full minute. The pulse, as noted before, varies with the infant's activity, but a persistent rate below 120 beats per minute or above 150 beats per minute should be reported.

Depending on the infant's temperature and the facilities available, he is usually placed under a radiant warmer or in an isolette, until the axillary temperature reaches about 36.6°C (97.8°F). Axillary temperature is preferred because it eliminates the potential danger of perforation of the rectum with the rectal thermometer (Fig. 32-4). The axillary reading is usually lower than the rectal temperature, but occasionally it is higher if brown fat is stimulated.[1]

If a radiant warmer is used, frequent checking of the infant and the placement of the skin probe is essential. A probe not touching the skin causes the warmer to continue to radiate heat after the desired infant temperature is reached and the infant can become overheated or possibly even burned. Hyperthermia, like hypothermia, increases the infant's metabolic requirements and oxygen consumption.[2] The temperature of an isolette being used as a warmer should also be checked periodically because it also can rise higher than expected and cause overheating.

The first bath is usually delayed until after the temperature has stabilized. The temperature should be taken again following the bath, and the infant should be placed back under the warmer if the temperature has dropped.

In a vigorous, normal infant, the cry should be lusty and should occur especially when the baby is handled or moved. If this does not happen, and the infant seems "sleepy" or depressed or if the pulse and respiratory rate are slow, it may be necessary to stimulate him to cry every hour or more frequently, depending on the degree of depression. This response may be aroused by changing his position or rubbing his back, head, or feet.

Brief tremors and twitching are not unusual in the transition period, but if they are prolonged or occur frequently, they may indicate a problem and the doctor should be notified.

Respiration and Color

The infant's color and respiratory pattern are good indices of whether or not the newborn is experiencing respiratory insufficiency. Dyspnea, rapid respiration exceeding 50 breaths per minute, and persistent cyanosis should be reported. Since mucus in the nasopharynx often causes respiratory distress, the nurse should be particularly watchful for its presence. Gagging, vomiting, breath holding, retraction of the head, choking, and cyanosis are all signs of the presence of mucus, which is particularly prone to develop in the second period of reactivity following the first sleep. Postural drainage and the technique for aspirating mucus are explained in Chapter 43.

Skin

The baby's skin should be observed for pallor and jaundice as well as cyanosis. Pressing the skin with a finger often enables clearer visualization of jaundice. The blanching that occurs with the maneuver pro-

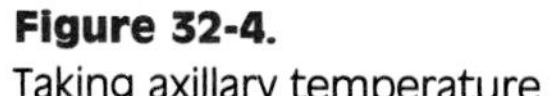

Figure 32-4.
Taking axillary temperature.

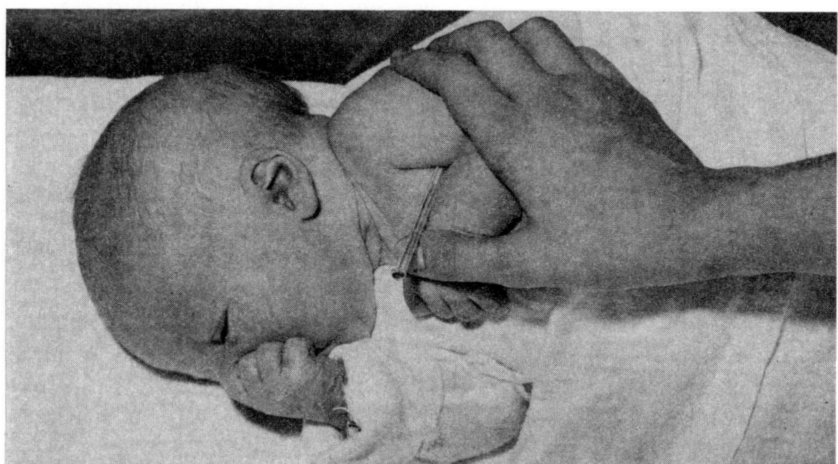

vides a contrast that shows up the icteric color more clearly. The significance of pallor and jaundice in the first 24 hours is explained in Chapter 43.

Stools and Urine

The time of the baby's first stool and voiding should be noted in order to indicate proper excretory function. It is sometimes necessary for the nurse to check with the delivery room records to see whether the infant voided or defecated at delivery.

Condition of the Cord

The cord should be checked periodically; any oozing or hemorrhage should be reported immediately, and the cord should be reclamped or retied as indicated. Oozing occurs most often between the second and the sixth hour of life and is frequently associated with crying or the passage of meconium.

Continuing Care and Parent Teaching

During the infant's hospital stay, the nurse is responsible for providing daily care. The mother should be involved with as much of this care as possible to help her prepare for taking over the responsibility when she gets home. This is easiest if there is a rooming-in or modified rooming-in arrangement, but it is possible even with central nursery care.

It is important that the nurse assess the mother's understanding and her skill in caring for her infant. Any basic principles or procedures related to infant care that the mother finds necessary and useful should be part of the nurse's teaching plan for the mother during her hospital stay. A written plan or check list of what the mother wants to learn and what teaching has been done is helpful in providing continuity between health care providers. Consistency in what is taught is necessary to avoid confusing the parents. The following principles of care can be conveyed easily to the mother (and to the father when he is present).

Handling the Infant

Although they are small, newborns are not as fragile as they sometimes seem. They should be treated gently, of course, but firm, smooth handling helps them feel secure. There is no one right way of turning, lifting, or holding a newborn, but the following points should be kept in mind:

1. The head and buttocks need to be supported.
2. Babies are wiggly and can push themselves out of your grasp.
3. It is easier to pick an infant up from the supine position than from the side-lying or prone position.

A suggested way to lift a baby is to place one hand under the neck to support the head and shoulders and the other hand under the buttocks to grasp the opposite thigh (Fig. 32-5). The baby can then be lifted up to a holding position or moved from one place to another. A useful position for holding or carrying is the "football hold" (Fig. 32-6). Mothers appreciate learning about this position, because, like the nurse, they often have times when they need to hold the baby and still have one hand free.

Feelings of confidence in dressing and undressing the baby come with practice. When putting on a shirt or gown, it is helpful to reach through the sleeve with your fingers and pull the infant's hand through. Diapering is fairly simple if disposable diapers that fasten with tapes are used. If pins are needed they should be inserted pointing toward the infant's back so there is less danger to the infant if they come open. The infant is usually wrapped snugly in a blanket (swaddling) before he is taken to his mother or placed in his crib. Some infants seem happier with their arms inside the blanket, and others like their arms free. Positioning in the crib is usually on the side with a blanket roll at the infant's back for support. This should extend from shoulder to hip. If it is behind the baby's head, it pushes the head forward.

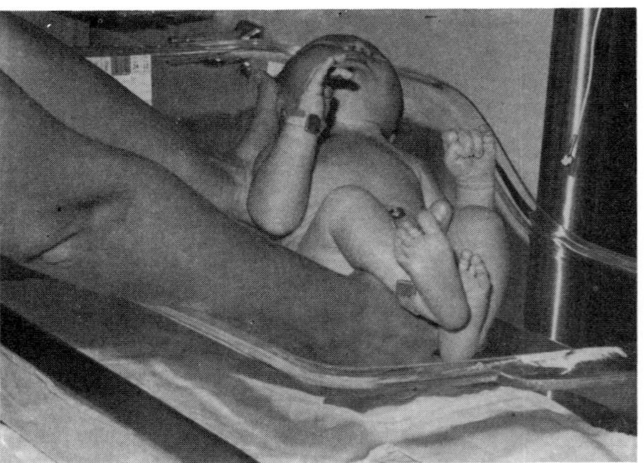

Figure 32-5.
One method of lifting the baby is to place one hand under the infant's neck and the other under the buttocks.

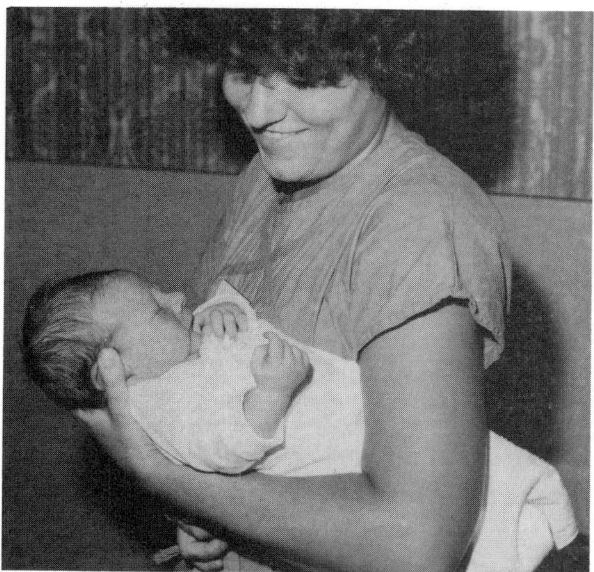

Figure 32-6.
Football hold for carrying the infant.

Bathing and Hygiene

The daily cleansing of the infant affords an excellent opportunity for making the observations that are necessary during the immediate postnatal period. How frequently a bath is given and what materials are used may vary from institution to institution.

Several decades ago the daily soap and water and oil baths were replaced with merely wiping off excess vernix with dry or slightly moist cotton balls. The diaper area was cleansed as necessary. Recently, there has been a return by many hospitals to the practice of bathing the baby daily or every other day while in the hospital. In view of the increase in staphylococcal infections in newborn nurseries, many nurseries give an initial sponge bath with a liquid detergent containing 3% hexachlorophene with special attention to the cord and genital areas. It is particularly important to rinse the baby well after the use of hexachlorophene. Daily use is no longer recommended because of suggestive evidence of CNS damage following prolonged exposure.

For the remainder of the baby's stay in the hospital, a mild soap and plain warm water can be used for cleansing purposes. The use of strong soap, oil, and baby powder is discouraged because of the sensitivity of the newborn's skin.

Blood is removed from the skin after the delivery, but no attempt is made to thoroughly remove the vernix caseosa unless it is stained with blood or meconium. The vernix caseosa serves to protect the skin and disappears spontaneously in about 24 hours. If it remains in the creases and folds of the skin longer than two days, it is apt to cause irritation. In this case gentle wiping usually removes it sufficiently.

Basic Principles

Each nurse and mother develops her own manner of bathing the newborn according to her manual dexterity, the size and the activity of the infant, and the facilities available (Fig. 32-7).

The following basic principles should be observed:

1. First, all equipment, clothing, and supplies should be assembled. Safety pins, if used, should be closed and placed out of the reach of the baby. Receptacles for soiled clothing, cotton balls, and so on should be available.
2. Second, care should be taken so that the environment is free from drafts and warm enough (*i.e.,* 24°C–27°C or 75°F–80°F). The nurse should not have to interrupt the bath to close a door or a window. The water for the bath should be about 37°C to 38°C (98°F–100°F). Water that feels warm to the elbow is approximately that temperature.
3. Third, in giving the bath the nurse should proceed from the "cleanest" areas to those that are "most soiled." Thus, the eyes are bathed first, then the face, ears, scalp, neck, upper extremities, trunk, lower extremities, and finally the buttocks and the genitals. Each of these in turn are washed, *rinsed well,* and dried. Particular attention should be paid to cleansing and drying the scalp and all creases at the neck, behind the ears, under the arms, the palms of the hands and between the fingers and the toes, under the knees, and in the groin, the buttocks, and the genitals.
4. Finally, ***the infant never should be left alone,*** even on a large work area; one hand should be kept on him at all times. If it is necessary to leave the area, even for a second, he should be taken along or placed in the crib.

Bathing Principles

- Have all necessary supplies within reach before beginning.
- Have area free from drafts.
- Have water correct temperature—about 98°F to 100°F (comfortable to your elbow).
- Wash cleanest areas of baby first.
- Never leave infant unattended.

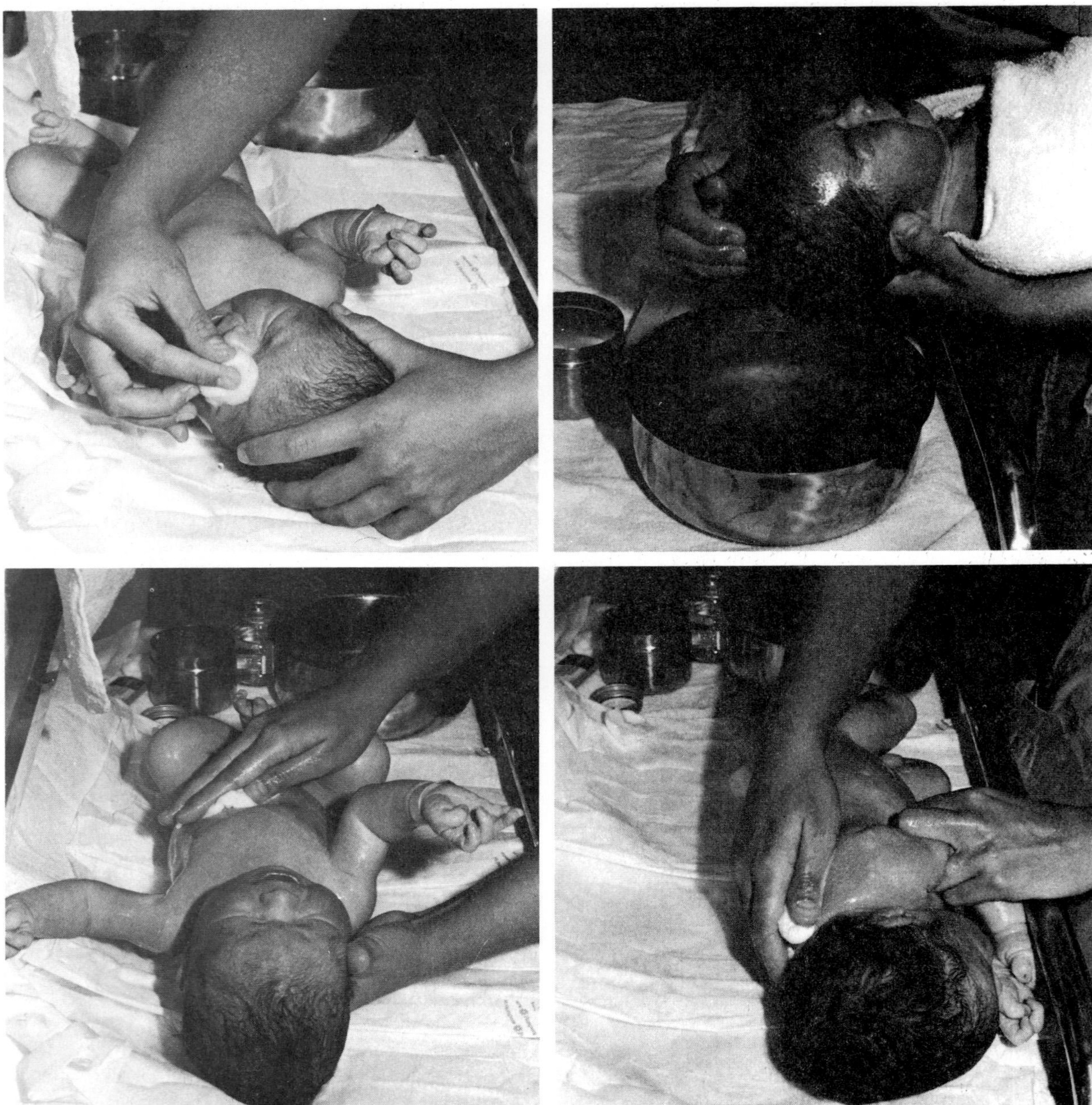

Figure 32-7.
The cleanest areas of the infant are bathed first (eyes, head) before the chest and back.

Demonstration and Practice

Each mother should have an opportunity to observe a demonstration of a sponge bath and, if at all possible, to give a bath to her infant. If there is an opportunity for only one bath with the mother present, the nurse can combine the demonstration and return demonstration by discussing the bath with the mother first and then letting her give the bath with the nurse there for moral support and assistance as necessary. If the father can be present and encouraged to participate, it is an added benefit.

The basic principles of bathing should be conveyed to the mother, for safety's sake, but she should not be made to feel that there is only one way to bathe the baby. By discussing with the mother what she already knows or has heard about bathing the baby, the nurse can make her teaching more meaningful for the individual client.

The nurse should also explore with the mother what equipment and facilities are available in the home, and instruct her in how the use of these might differ from what is available in the hospital. Usually the necessities can be met without undue expense or difficulty. For instance, a large drainboard which can be washed and padded adequately (and is a comfortable height for handling the infant) can be used as the bath area. A large pan or basin serves very well for the bathtub in the early weeks; it should be kept only for the baby's use. Thus, the extra expense of special equipment can be minimized. A soft towel and washcloth, for the baby's use only, and a mild soap is also needed.

A mother should not be made to feel that she has to give the baby a bath at the same time every day, or that she can't skip a day of bathing. Some mothers and babies enjoy the bath as a daily routine, but others do not or can not always find the time. For these, as long as the face, neck creases, and diaper area are washed as needed, giving a bath every other day should be sufficient. The mother should be advised that the sponge bath should continue to be the type of bath given until the cord stump has fallen off and the area has healed. After this, a tub bath can be given.

Suggestions for Care of Specific Areas

Eyes. The eyes should be wiped from the inner corner to the outer corner, using a clean cotton ball or clean area of the washcloth for each eye. No care, other than this cleansing with clean water, is necessary unless there is evidence of inflammation or infection. There may be some reaction from the medication used for prophylaxis against ophthalmia neonatorum beginning in the first few hours and this condition does not usually require treatment. However, any redness, swelling, or discharge should be reported and recorded so that the eyes can be observed more closely and tests to rule out infection can be done if necessary.

Nose and Ears. Cotton-tipped applicators should not be used to clean the infant's nose or ears because of danger of injuring the delicate tissues. The nose usually does not need cleaning because the infant sneezes to clear the nasal passages. If some dried mucus does need to be removed from the nose, a small twisted piece of cotton moistened with water may be used. Only the outer ear should be cleaned. Nothing should be put inside the ear.

Hair. The head should be washed each time the baby is bathed. Swaddling the baby in a blanket or towel and using the "football" hold makes the job easier. The same soap the baby is washed with or any brand of baby shampoo can be used. Oil should not be put on the hair, as it may predispose to "cradle cap."

Skin. The newborn's skin is often dry and peeling within a few days after birth, and dry cracks may appear in the wrist and ankle areas. This is sometimes a cause of concern to mothers and they want to put oil or some other preparation on the skin to get rid of the dryness. They can be reassured that the flakiness and cracks will disappear in a few days and that oil and some lotions may make matters worse by causing a rash.

The skin is thin, delicate, extremely tender, and very easily irritated. Since the skin is a protective covering, breaks in its surface may initiate troublesome infection; hence, skin disturbances constitute an actual threat to the baby's well-being.

The new baby does not usually perspire until after the first month. Warm weather or excessive clothing may cause the infant to develop prickly heat, a closely grouped pinhead-sized rash of papules and vesicles, on the face, the neck, and wherever skin surfaces touch. Fewer clothes and some control over the room temperature help to relieve the discomfort.

Buttocks. Sometimes, despite good nursing care, the infant's buttocks become reddened and sore. A diaper rash that is caused by the reaction of bacteria with the urea in the urine may occur. This in turn causes an ammonia dermatitis. The most important prophylaxis is to keep the diaper area clean and dry. Sometimes petroleum jelly, baby oil, or a bland protective ointment, such as Vitamin A and D ointment, is used to protect the area. Pastes may not be advised, because they are much more adhesive than ointments and thus create cleansing problems.

A simple treatment that is often effective is merely to expose the infant's reddened buttocks to air (Fig. 32-8) and light several times a day, using care to keep the infant covered otherwise. Air may be all that is necessary, although the use of a *lamp* treatment is more effective and at the same time provides a measure of warmth. An ordinary gooseneck lamp with a screened bulb (no stronger than 40 watts) can be placed on the table so that it is a foot or more away from the infant's exposed buttocks. The light may be used for 30 minutes at a time. Because the already irritated skin is very sensitive, care should be exercised so that it is not burned by too strong a bulb or by placing the light too close.

If the condition occurs at home, the treatment

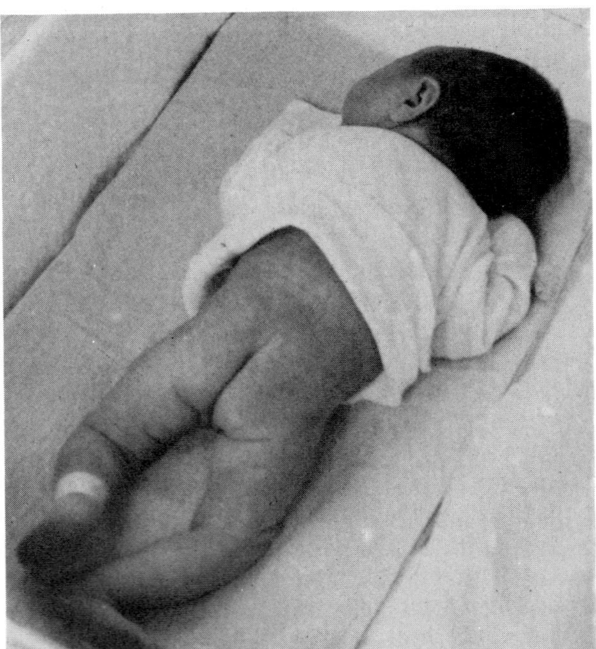

Figure 32-8.
Exposing buttocks to air.

described above also is appropriate, and the mother can be so instructed. Boiling the diapers is another effective measure, since this destroys the bacteria. However, many of the detergents and conditioners used today have antibacterial agents in them, and these may be effective in washing the diapers. Care should be taken to rinse the diapers thoroughly, since the residue of the detergent in itself can be irritating. In this respect, the modern diaper services have very effective facilities; many sterilize diapers and entire layettes as part of the service.

Cord Care. The cord clamp is removed when the umbilical stump has dried sufficiently. This is usually in about 24 hours, but it might take more time for a cord that is cut long or that is thick and gelatinous. Care of the umbilical area usually consists of cleaning around the junction between the cord stump and the skin with alcohol to encourage drying and discourage the possibility of infection. In some hospital settings, an antibiotic ointment is used instead of alcohol (Fig. 32-9).

To further promote drying of the cord, babies do not receive a tub bath until the cord has separated, and the umbilicus has healed. A cord dressing is considered to be unnecessary since exposure to the air enhances drying of the cord.

No attempt should be made to dislodge the cord before it separates completely. If there is a red inflamed area around the stump or any discharge with an odor, this condition should be recorded and reported immediately. The cord usually becomes detached from the body between the fifth and the eighth day after birth, but it may not detach until the twelfth or the fourteenth day. When the cord drops off, the umbilicus is depressed somewhat and usually free from any evidence of inflammation. No further treatment is necessary, except to keep the part clean and dry. When inflammation or discharge is present, the physician gives specific orders for care.

Cleaning Genitalia. In the newborn male infant, adhesions between the prepuce and the glans penis are very common. If a circumcision is not done, it is often recommended that the foreskin be retracted for cleaning purposes beginning a few days after birth. If retracted, it should not be forced, and must be replaced over the glans after cleaning, or edema may occur. Current recommendations are often to wait until separation occurs naturally with further growth and development before trying to retract the fore-

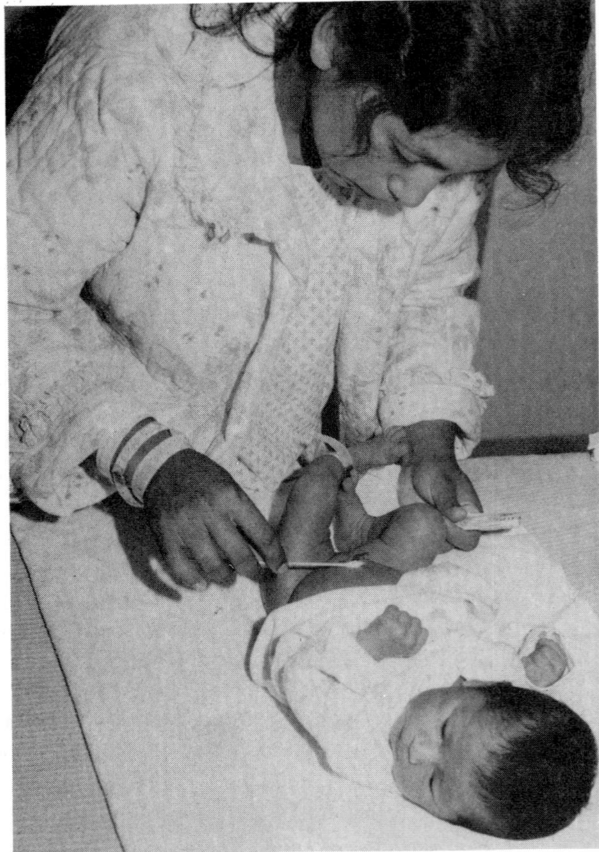

Figure 32-9.
The mother can be encouraged to give cord care to her infant.

skin.[3] Most foreskins are retractable by age three and should be pushed back gently once a week. As the child learns to do more for himself, he should be taught to retract the foreskin and wash his penis, as he is taught to wash other areas of his body. By the time he is ten, this should be done daily.[4]

A curdy secretion, smegma, sometimes forms and collects under the prepuce behind the glans. Also, small amounts of urine may be retained. This condition, which does not usually occur in the newborn period, may lead to infection and necessitate separations of the adhesions or circumcision.

In female infants, smegma may accumulate between the folds of the labia and should be carefully cleansed with moistened cotton balls, using the front-to-back direction and a clean cotton ball for each stroke. When demonstrating this technique to the mother the nurse can underscore the importance of teaching a little girl to wipe herself from front to back to help prevent urinary tract infections.

Circumcision and Care

Whether or not a male infant should be circumcised is an old controversy. The procedure is said by some to promote better hygiene, prevent inflammation and infection, and decrease the incidence of cancer of the penis. Others say that these advantages are also present in uncircumcised males who practice good personal hygiene. The Committee on Fetus and the Newborn of the American Academy of Pediatrics states that there are no valid medical indications for circumcision.[5] Traditional, cultural, and religious factors are all involved in deciding whether or not the procedure is done.

The decision concerning circumcision is becoming more of a dilemma for some parents. When it was a recommended procedure it was easier for the parents to justify the possible risks and discomforts by saying "It's the best thing to do." Now that the procedure is not encouraged by many doctors, the parents have to take more responsibility. The final decision is up to them and a consent must be signed by one of them before the circumcision is done. "Informed consent" often means listening to a long list of possible undesirable side-effects of the procedure. Some mothers feel very guilty after deciding to have it done. It is important for the nurse to give the parents factual answers to their questions, then support them in their decision, whichever it is.

The infant should not be fed for several hours prior to being circumcised, since he will be restrained in a supine position for some time and might regurgitate (Fig. 32-10). Sterile gloves, instruments, and drapes are used by the physician during the procedure. Several methods have been devised, includ-

Figure 32-10.
(A) Plastic restraining form used in many hospitals to restrict the infant's movements during the circumcision procedure. *(B)* Proper positioning of infant for circumcision.

A

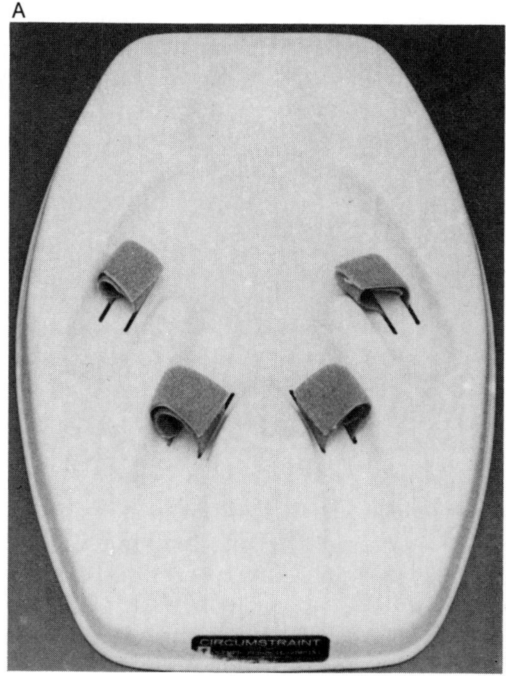

B

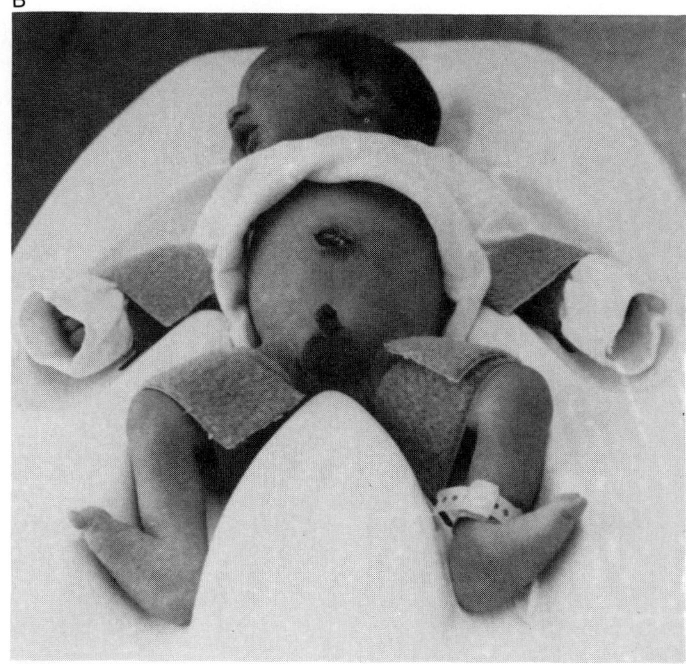

ing the use of the Gomco (Yellen) clamp and the Plastibell.

Care Following Circumcision

When the newborn infant is circumcised, the main principles of postoperative care are to keep the wound clean and to observe it closely for bleeding (see Fig. 32-11). For the first 24 hours the area is covered with a sterile gauze dressing to which a liberal amount of sterile petroleum jelly has been added. If the circumcision is done with the Plastibell, no dressing or petroleum jelly is used.

Mothers are naturally anxious about their babies at this time, so, as soon as it is feasible after the circumcision has been done, the nurse should take the baby to his mother for a brief visit. She can be reassured that the procedure has probably not been very painful for her child. The infant cries during the operation, but this is due as much to the necessary restraints as to the discomfort. It may be helpful to show her what the circumcision looks like and explain how it will look when healing, so that she can recognize any deviations from normal. With the Plastibell, there is a plastic ring and suture in place which drops off with the foreskin in about 7 days to 10 days.

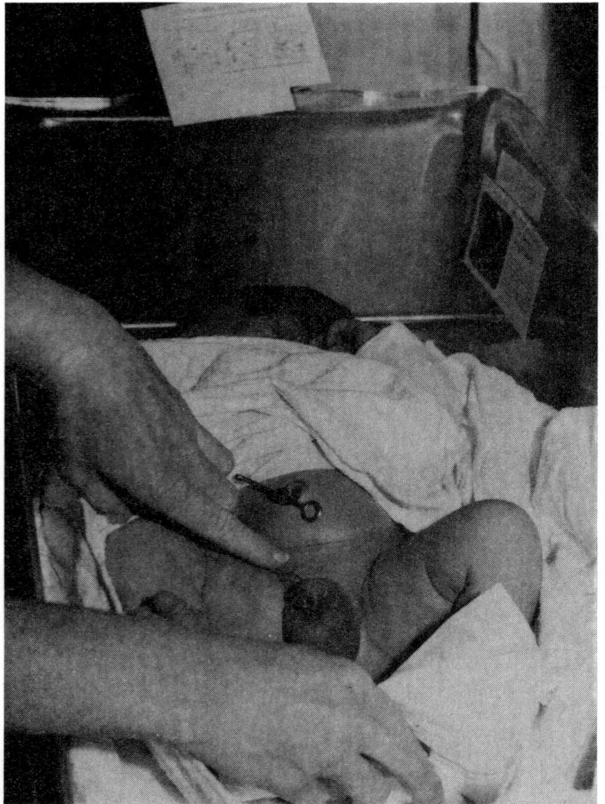

Figure 32-11.
Postcircumcision inspection.

Occasionally, a local anesthetic is used, but generally, the procedure is performed without it. Thus, the infant may be fed immediately after the circumcision, and both mother and baby seem to enjoy the comfort that the feeding and cuddling bring. If the infant is left in the mother's room for an extended length of time, the nurse should go in periodically to check the circumcision for bleeding.

In changing the infant's diaper the nurse should hold his ankles with one hand so that he cannot kick against the operative area. Unless the physician orders otherwise, the circumcision dressing can be removed postoperatively when the infant voids for the first time. Cleansing must be done gently but can be accomplished as necessary with cotton balls moistened with warm tap water. A fresh sterile petroleum jelly dressing usually is applied to the penis each time the diaper is changed for the first day. The penis must be observed closely for bleeding, and during the first 12 hours should be inspected every hour. It is advisable to place the infant's crib where he can be watched conveniently. Moreover, to keep all the nursing personnel alerted, some signal, such as a red tag, can be attached to the identification card on the crib. If bleeding occurs, usually it can be controlled with gentle pressure. If bleeding persists, the physician should be notified immediately.

Since the length of the maternity stay has been considerably shortened, circumcision may be done on the second or the third postnatal day or even before the baby leaves the delivery room. Sometimes the operation is performed on the day preceding or day of discharge; therefore, the nurse should ascertain the physician's wishes for aftercare and make certain that the mother knows how to care for her newly circumcised infant. Generally, the care is the same as that described.

Other Areas of Concern

Weight

The baby should be weighed on the birth date and then daily or every other day while in the hospital. If the infant remains in the hospital longer than five days, he should be weighed at intervals prescribed by the medical staff. His weight should be recorded accurately.

During the first few days after birth the infant may lose 5% to 10% of his birth weight. This is due partly to the minimal intake of nutrients and fluid and partly to the loss of excess fluid.[4] About the time the meconium begins to disappear from his stools, the weight begins to increase, and in normal cases does so regularly until about the tenth day of life, when it may equal the birth weight. Many infants regain their birth weight in a shorter period of time. During the first 5 months, the weight gain should be from 4 oz per week to 6 oz per week. After this time the gain is from 2 oz per week to 4 oz per week. At six months of age, the baby has usually doubled his birth weight, and tripled it by his first birthday.

This is one way to note the baby's condition and progress. When the baby is not gaining weight it should be reported to the physician. Besides gaining regularly in weight and strength, the baby should be happy and good-natured when awake and inclined to sleep a good part of the time between feedings.

Sleeping

The baby needs rest and sleep, with as little handling as possible. If he is well and comfortable, he usually sleeps much of the time and wakes and cries when he is hungry or uncomfortable. He may sleep as much as 20 hours out of 24 hours (although this varies considerably from infant to infant). It is not the sound sleep of the adult; rather, he moves a good deal, stretches, and at intervals awakens momentarily. Since he responds so readily to external stimuli (and this may make him restless), his clothing and coverings are important. They should be light in weight, warm but not too warm, and free from wrinkles. His position should be changed frequently when he is awake. He can be placed on either side or his abdomen, especially when he is ready for sleep. If he is positioned on his back, someone should be present, for if the baby regurgitates, he is more likely to aspirate in this position. The importance of avoiding the back as a sleeping position should be emphasized to parents. As he gets older and learns to roll over, he will assume the position that he likes most for sleep.

Crying

After the baby is dressed and placed in a warm crib he usually does not cry unless he is wet, hungry, ill, uncomfortable for some reason, or is moved. One learns to distinguish an infant's condition and needs from the character of his cry, which may be described as follows:

1. A loud, insistent cry with drawing up and kicking of the legs usually denotes colicky pain.
2. A fretful cry, if due to indigestion, is accompanied by green stools and passing of gas.
3. A whining cry is noticeable when the baby is ill, premature, or very frail.
4. A fretful, hungry cry, with fingers in the mouth and flexed, tense extremities, is easily recognized.
5. A peculiar, shrill, sharp-sounding cry suggests injury, especially CNS.

Every effort should be made to recognize any deviation from the usual manner in which a baby announces his normal requirements. Moreover, this information should be conveyed to the mother, since it is essential that the mother learn to interpret her infant's cues. The newborn has only his posture and his voice at this time to inform others of his needs.

Hypertonic Babies. Occasionally, the nurse finds an infant that seems to be fussy from birth. He appears very active, startles easily, cries readily and more frequently (and apparently for no reason), is alert and awake much of the time, and in general does not fit the usual pattern of activity, feeding, and sleeping described. These babies may be described as *hypertonic,* that is, they do not seem to be able to relax as well as other infants.

The parents of hypertonic babies may find it difficult to adjust to their new baby and may experience a great deal of anxiety until they are informed (or learn by trial and error) that this is "normal behavior" for this child. Too often they assume they must be doing something "wrong," since despite their efforts, their baby remains fussy, tense, and crying. The nurse can be very helpful to the parents in giving them anticipatory guidance about their baby's behavior and helpful ways in which he can be soothed. The physician should also be informed of the nurse's observations in order to give appropriate advice to the parents.

These infants usually respond favorably to being held securely. Thus, wrapping them snugly with a receiving blanket, cuddling them securely and changing their position slowly and surely rather than quickly all help to allay undue tenseness. Rocking the baby and walking with him are particularly successful measures, but no parent can or should do this over protracted periods of time.

Any new activity or procedures should be introduced slowly to this kind of infant. For instance, when a tub bath is given for the first time, the infant should be placed very slowly in a small amount of water, and each lower extremity immersed gradually in order not to frighten or startle the infant too much. The parents should not consider an occasional evening out a luxury; rather it should be considered a necessary item in the care of their baby. These infants do place greater demands on their parents than do infants of a more placid nature, and a short time away from the baby does wonders in restoring the perspective and good humor of the parents.

Urinary Elimination

Urinary activity of the fetus is evidenced by the presence of urine in the amniotic fluid. The baby usually voids during delivery or immediately after birth, but the function may be suppressed for several hours. However, if the baby does not void within 24 hours, the condition should be reported to the physician, as retention of the urine may be due to an imperforate meatus. After the first 2 days or 3 days the baby voids from 10 to 15 times a day. When the urine is concentrated, red or rusty stains on the wet diaper may be due to uric-acid crystals in the urine.

Intestinal Elimination

During fetal life the content of the intestines is made up of greenish black tarlike material called meconium. It is composed of epithelial and epidermal cells and lanugo hair that probably were swallowed with the amniotic fluid. The color of the meconium is due to the bile pigment. Before birth and for the first few hours after birth, the intestinal contents are sterile. Apparently, there is no peristalsis until after birth, because normally there is no discoloration of the amniotic fluid.

The newborn infant passes meconium stools for the first day or two of life (Fig. 32-12). After this, the stools gradually begin to change to greenish brown and then to yellowish brown. These "transitional stools" are less sticky than meconium and contain some milk curds. Following the transitional stools, the characteristics depend on whether the infant is fed breast milk or formula. The stools of the breast-fed infant tend to be a golden yellow color with a distinctive odor, sometimes described as "sweet." Their consistency varies from loose to mushy, and they may be frequent or infrequent. If the infant is formula fed the stools may be pale yellow to light brown, of firmer consistency, and may have a slightly offensive or foul odor.

Most newborns pass the first stool within 12 hours of birth—nearly all have a stool in 24 hours. If an infant has not passed a stool by this time, imperforate anus or intestinal obstruction must be considered as a possible reason for the delay, and the baby must be observed closely.

The daily number of stools on about the fifth day of life is usually four to six. As the infant grows, this number decreases to one or two each day. The type of stool of the breast-fed baby may be influenced by the mother's diet. However, there may be slight variations from the normal, which may have little significance if the baby appears to be comfortable and sleeps and

Figure 32-12.
Stool cycle.

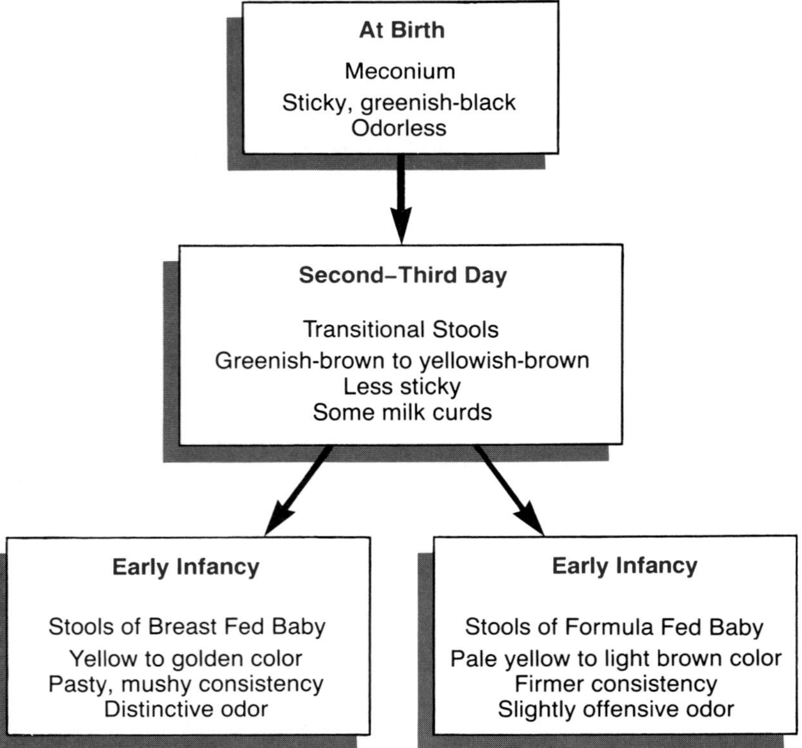

nurses well. If the baby's stools have a watery consistency, are of a green color, contain much mucus, and flatus is being passed, the condition may be evidence of some digestive or intestinal irritation and should be reported to the physician.

The number, color, and consistency of stools should be recorded daily on the baby's record.

Discharge from the Hospital

Discharge planning for a new mother and baby may begin in the prenatal class or clinic, when discussions are held about planning for "What happens after the baby comes?" During the hospital stay the nurse continues to assess the needs of the family in planning for care of the baby at home. Although much teaching can be done in the hospital, for some new mothers, especially the inexperienced, a referral to a community health agency may be appropriate for follow-up. Some families with financial problems may need to be referred to a family service agency.

Plans for health care follow-up of the infant should be discussed with the mother. A follow-up appointment should be made with a private physician or at a well-baby clinic. Most new mothers appreciate an opportunity to talk to the nurse regarding their concerns about taking the baby home. Taking time for such a talk is well worth the nurse's effort, since it can help make those first few days at home less frightening and more enjoyable for the new parents.

Infant Stimulation

Infant stimulation is an important corollary to physical care of the newborn. Infant stimulation is the provision of appropriate sensory stimuli to enhance infant growth and development. Each of the six senses—visual, auditory, tactile, gustatory, olfactory, and vestibular-proprioceptive—is receptive to environmental stimulation and helps the newborn learn from his environment. When an infant is exposed to appropriate sensory stimulation, greater curiosity, improved mental capabilities, accelerated neuromuscular growth, enhanced gastrointestinal functioning, quicker weight gain, and pleasing mother–infant interactions are likely to occur.[7]

Sensory stimulation is the primary source of learning for infants under 6 months. Each sense should be appropriately stimulated to use and expand sensory capabilities. Care-givers may automatically (passively) be providing pleasurable and desired stimulating experiences. If so, these can be observed and positively reinforced by the nurse. If not, instructing the mother and demonstrating easy and suitable stimuli for each sensory modality is indicated for optimal infant growth and development. The parents booklet, *Infant Stimulation for Parents,* can help the nurse in patient education.[8] Other educational materials, such as the "Infant Stimulation Care Plan" are available through the Infant Stimulation Education Association.[9]

Development of the Senses

The senses are known to be functional by 25 weeks gestation. It is not unreasonable to expect that the senses are capable of detecting changes in the intrauterine environment after 17 weeks of gestation. Mothers commonly report that the fetus kicks more when music is played or quiets down when she starts rocking. Verny reports that fetuses behave in a particular manner when classical music is played over the abdomen.[10] Bright lights and sounds induce specific heart rate changes in the fetus as he becomes aware of their presence.[11,12] It is evident that the newborn is capable of perceiving environmental events at birth. The senses may be exquisitely sensitive at birth as in the olfactory sense, or they may be relatively immature as in the visual and auditory senses; however, even the immature senses perform well within their limitations. The full-term newborn is able to see clearly, hear well, respond to very light touch and movement, and has acute taste and smell.

The Importance of Infant Stimulation

Sensory stimulation plays a major role in infant learning. According to Piaget, the first stage of infant development and brain growth is the sensory motor period, which means that the infant learns through stimulation of the senses and responds with movement and development of motor skills. In the first 6 months of life all learning occurs by having a sense stimulated. For example, within the first 2 weeks of life an infant learns who his mother is by learning her smell, sensing her body warmth, and looking at her face. Opportunities to see her, to hear her voice, and to be close teach him to discriminate between mother and all others. The senses then, are the primary source of information for the neonate brain and by 6 months of age the newborn's brain will have attained 50% of its adult size and weight.[13] Sensory stimulation has its greatest influence on brain development during the brain's growth spurt which occurs in the first year of life.

Providing Infant Stimulation

Sensory stimulation may be actively and passively provided by the environment. Active provision means that deliberate efforts to stimulate each sense are being made, as in showing an infant a black and white toy. Passive infant stimulation occurs spontaneously without conscious intent. Fortunately, care-givers offer a plethora of passive stimulation. These instinctual presentations of sensory stimuli are to be encouraged if they are in accordance with principles of infant stimulation.

Briefly, these principles are as follows: (1) all newborns have right-sided preferences during the first 3 months. The infant's right side is more sensitive to touch than his left,[14] conducts messages to the brain faster than the left, and infants turn to the right more reliably than to the left.[15] Stimulating experiences induce more infant attention if they are begun on the infant's right side regardless of the infant's eventual handedness. (2) If newborn attention or concentration is desired, it is best to present the stimulus during periods of alert inactivity when the infant is awake with his eyes open, but his legs and arms are still (see Chap. 31). During this restive phase the newborn can attend to objects for 4 seconds to 10 seconds. Alert inactivity is present for an hour or two immediately after birth and for 5 minutes to 10 minutes before and after feedings. These are the times when eye-to-eye contact should be stressed. (3) Newborns become alert for longer periods if they are in upright positions and being held. Sitting in this manner increases infant gazing by 70%. When an infant looks around he receives visual stimulation which helps him learn how to relate to his environment.[16] (4) Stimulating an infant to the point of agitation may not be wise because agitation causes increased heart rate, increased respiratory rate, and prolonged inspiratory phases which may induce aspiration. Newborns have rhythms and stimulation should be congruent to the rhythm.[17] When an infant demonstrates agitation by crying, restless limb movements, and frustrated head turning, he is reaching the end of his rhythm and point of withdrawal and can handle no more environmental stimulation. These signs indicate that it is time to gradually withdraw the rocking, stroking, talking, and kissing.

Infant Stimulation Interventions

Visual Stimulation

The normal newborn has very good visual abilities. He can see items with great clarity as long as they are within his visual field, which is 20 cm to 22 cm (9 in), the same distance from the breast-feeding infant's eyes to his mother's eyes. Within this visual field, he can see items distinctly, without blurriness, and can search the field to 60 degrees either side of midline before deciding the item of preference on which to gaze.[18] Gazing can be deliberately prolonged, depending upon the amount of interest an item holds for the infant. Newborns do have individual preferences and differences, so allow for variation as you present visual items to the newborn.[19]

Newborns love eyes the most. The newborn prefers visual items that provide contrast between the figure and background.[20] The greatest contrast occurs when black is placed against a white background. Mother's eyes are usually dark centered (pupils) against a white or light background (the sclera). Moving objects are more fascinating to an infant than stationary ones.[21] The eyes move from side to side, up and down, and even get bigger and smaller. The eyes are also circular. Newborns prefer to maintain their gaze (fixate) on circular items because of their immature ocular movement ability. The newborn searches his entire field by moving across it with little jumps (saccades) rather than rolling both eyes simultaneously in the same direction. He normally fixates on the eyes in the human face, as the face is the most attractive visual stimulus for the newborn. Eye-to-eye contact in an enface position facilitates eye fixation for both parent and infant. If the mother's or the father's face is not available, black and white schematic faces on black and white glossy photos are the next best thing.

Infants also like to look at geometric figures, and they prefer cylinders and circles to rectangles and squares.[22] The geometric figures should be sharp rather than blurry and in a black and white configuration to enthrall the newborn. Newborns do not like to look at plain colored walls or walls with little figures on them.[23] Animals and cartoon characters are inappropriate visual stimuli for the full-term newborn. These patterns are not appreciated until the infant is more than one year of age. In the first 6 months of life, infants prefer to look at big geometric figures (2 in by 2 in) rather than small ones (½ in by ½ in).[24] After the first 3 weeks of life, the size of the geometric figures can be decreased to accommodate the newborn's preference for increasing complexity and visual information processing. Stripes (especially good for the first 3 weeks to 4 weeks of life), black and white checkerboards, bulls eyes, dots, and triangles are appealing geometric shapes. Cards containing these items can be used separately as stimuli or used in mobiles and wall decoration.

Auditory Stimulation

Speech Stimulation. The newborn has the capacity to hear all sounds greater than 55 decibels.[25] The infant can learn to discriminate his mother's and father's voices from all others within the first 2 weeks of life, and has at that time a distinct reaction pattern established to the voice he hears.[26] Newborns prefer the female voice to the male voice, based primarily on the pitch, tone, and inflection pattern women demonstrate when speaking to infants. Women tend to exhibit cooing behaviors which are various pitched musical sounds. Instinctual maternal speech uses exaggerated intonation. Higher pitched sounds are preferred to low, bass sounds as they are attention-getting. Monotonous speech and monotone sounds are boring to the newborn who prefers modulating auditory input.[27] The infant accustoms to monotone quickly and does not attend to it. Some fathers have a tendency to speak in bass, monotone speech patterns, and should be encouraged to use more inflection and exaggerated tone. Slow speech at 55 words per minute or less is easier for the infant to discern than faster speech.[28]

Talking to an infant is very important. The more talk he hears, the sooner he will learn language. The more talk he is exposed to, the more likely he is to reach his potential for mental skills, such as math, creative thinking, and reasoning.[29] Gorski and Brazelton have suggested that maternal speech is the singular most important aspect of the newborn's sensory environment, and desirable maternal speech can ameliorate anticipated delays and handicaps in risk infants.[30]

Desirable Characteristics of Maternal and Paternal Speech

- Tone variation
- Higher pitch, rather than lower pitch
- Spoken at a rate of 55 words per minute
- Imitating the infant sounds when infant makes them
- Simple words
- More questions than statements and more statements than commands. (*i.e.*, Don't you want to stop sucking? *vs* You can stop sucking now. *vs* Stop sucking now!)
- Spoken at all waking times. It is advisable to increase the total amount of time spent talking to an infant.[31]

Sound Stimulation. Speech stimulates the development of the left hemisphere of the brain, and music stimulates the right hemisphere.[32] Therefore, parents may provide musical stimulation for their infant also. Newborns have demonstrated a preference for classical music over rock and roll music.[33] However, individual preference may very well be for the music the neonate was exposed to while *in utero*. If mother played jazz during her pregnancy, her newborn will probably enjoy jazz more than unfamiliar classical music.

Tactile Stimulation

Tactile stimulation, or touching, is instrumental in helping the neonate adjust to life outside the womb. Skin-to-skin touch in a rhythmic stroking pattern has been found to reduce the birth weight loss from 10% of birth weight to 3% of birth weight.[34] This is accomplished because skin-to-skin stroking, in a head-to-toe fashion, stimulates the haptic nerve pathways, which in turn stimulate the gastrointestinal and genitourinary systems to function. As a result, feces and urine are passed through the system more quickly, but also with better utilization of digested food.[35]

Skin-to-skin touch is to be encouraged at all times. Newborns cannot be spoiled by too much caressing. The closer they are held and the more often they are patted, the more secure they become.[36] Observe the power of touch on the newborn. It makes him quiescent and can arouse him. Crying subsides, the extremities flex, and the eyes open.

It is wise to provide skin-to-skin stroking in a head-to-toe, central-to-distal fashion. Nerve myelinization occurs in this sequence, and touch can accelerate the process if it is provided in a similar way. Stroking in this manner, at a rate of 12 times per minute to 16 times per minute may decrease the incidence of apnea and encourage even, regular respirations in the neonate.[37] As you stroke, it is wise to give extra strokes of slightly more pressure to the most sensitive tactile areas—the face (especially around the mouth), the palms, the soles, the genital area, and along the spinal column. Stroking that is begun on the right should continue on the infant's left to encourage midline awareness.[38] Stroking the head is very comforting to the neonate, especially if the hand proceeds from the forehead to the occiput.

Many infants become quite fond of stroking and never tire of it. For these infants it becomes a relaxation therapy and is widely used as such in Australia and India. Touch helps relieve the unspent tensions infants develop and also accelerates neuromuscular development.[38] Two tools are available for mothers who desire to continue with a stroking treatment.

Indian Baby Massage has many pictures and is in most bookstores. A scientifically validated stroking protocol called "Loving Touch," which is accompanied by a tape that also provides appropriate music stimulation, is also available.[39]

Vestibular Stimulation

Vestibular stimulation refers to movement. Movement changes pressure in the vestibule of the ear. Rocking is the most common vestibular stimulation given passively, and it provides excellent opportunities for vestibular sensations that aid in weight gain,[40] head growth,[41] improved respiratory status,[42] neuromuscular coordination,[43] and memory development. There is no recommended rate of rocking or frequency, but a minimum of twenty minutes a day can be encouraged.

Parents may prefer to provide vestibular stimulation by carrying infants during the day. No detrimental effects have resulted from this. In fact, infants who accompany their mother in a pouch appear to fall into deep levels of sleep more smoothly and awaken less irritable.

Baby exercises provide opportunities for vestibular stimulation. Extension and flexion of all extremities followed by tummy tickles, pressure against the kicking foot, circular swinging of the well-supported infant, and relaxation techniques are advised. Levy's *Baby Exercise Book* is a useful resource for additional motor games.[44]

Olfactory Stimulation

Olfaction in the newborn is quite sensitive. Within 2 weeks of birth an infant can differentiate the odor of his mother's breast pad from that of a stranger.[45] This ability to perceive maternal odor originates at birth when the infant is held close. At this time he begins his association by detecting his parents' body odors. It is instrumental to the bonding/parental recognition process.

Actively providing various smells such as cherry juice, nutmeg, cinnamon, and honey is not really necessary. The newborn detects these in his environment without special attention to them for the first 6 months of life. After that, smelling can become a stimulating game. Various "smelling" books are available in toy stores.

Gustatory Stimulation

The most prevalent taste sensation the newborn is exposed to is breast milk (or formula). As the nipple is compressed against the hard palate, the milk spurts on to the bitter receptors in the back of the tongue. With repetitive stimulation of the bitter receptors, the infant grows quite fond of the bitter-tasting foods. Yet, they always like sweet tastes as well, and can smile with sweet and frown with sour tastes. Breast milk is the preferred gustatory stimulus for newborns. Mothers should be encouraged to avoid sour tastes that might pass into breast milk (*i.e.,* lemon juice, cranberry juice) so that the newborn does not associate his care-giver with unpleasant stimuli.

References

1. Phibbs RH: The Newborn Infant. In Rudolph AM (ed): Pediatrics, 16th ed, p 153. Appleton–Century–Crofts, New York, 1977

2. Scopes JW: Thermoregulation in the Newborn. In Avery GB (ed): Neonatology, 2nd ed, p 178. JB Lippincott, Philadelphia, 1981

3. Kaplan G: Circumcision, an overview. Current Problems in Pediatrics Vol 7, pp 1–33. March 1977

4. Poole CJ: Neonatal circumcision. JOGN Nursing 5:207–211, July/August 1979

5. Committee on Fetus and Newborn, American Academy of Pediatrics: Report of the ad hoc task force on circumcision. Pediatrics 56:610–611, October 1975

6. Kaplan S: Normal and Abnormal Growth. In Rudolph AM (ed): Pediatrics, 16th ed, p 107. New York, Appleton–Century–Crofts, 1977

7. Gutelius M et al: Promising results from a cognitive stimulation program in infancy. Clin Ped Vol. II, pp 585–593, 1972

8. Wallin C: Infant Stimulation for Parents. Washington, D.C., ISEA Publications, 1982 available through ISEA

9. Infant Stimulation Education Association, UCLA Center for the Health Sciences, Factor 5-942, Los Angeles

10. Verny T: The Secret of Life of the Unborn Child. New York, Simon & Schuster, 1981

11. Grimwade JD, et al: Response of the human fetus to sensory stimulation. Aust NZ J Obstet Gynaecol 10:22, 1970

12. Peleg D, Goldman JA: Fetal heart rate acceleration in response to light stimulation as a clinical measure of fetal well-being. Journal Perinatal Medicine 8:38, 1980

13. Dobbing T: Brain Growth. In Brain Physiology & Development. Marco Island Report, Johnson & Johnson, 1974

14. Turkewitz G: A sensory basis for the lateral difference in the newborn's response to somesthetic stimulation. J Exp Child Psychol 18:304–312, 1974

15. Kavkowicz D: Lateral differences and head turning to somesthetic stimulation in premature infants, Dev Psychobio 12:607–614, 1979

16. Korner A, Grobstein R: Visual alertness as related to soothing in neonates: Implications for maternal stimulation and early deprivation. Child Dev 42:867–876, 1966

17. Ludington–Hoe S: Postpartum: Development of maternicity. Am J Nurs 77:1171–1174, July 1977

18. Maurer D, Maurer C: Newborn babies see better than you think. Psychol Today 85–88, 1976

19. Restak R: Newborn knowledge. Science 82, 59–65, February 1982

20. Apostolakis E, Cha C: Visual preference of preterm and term neonates. Journal of the California Perinatal Association 11, 1:62, May 1982

21. Haith MM: The response of the human newborn to visual movement. J Exp Child Psychol 31:235–243, 1980

22. Fantz RL, Miranda SB: Newborn infant attention to form of contour. Child Dev 46:224, 1975

23. Hershenson M: Visual discrimination in the human newborn. J Comp Physiol Psychol 58:270, 1964

24. Fantz RL, Fagan JF: Visual attention to size and number of pattern details during the first 6 months. Child Dev 46:3, 1975

25. Dunkle T: The Sound of Silence. Science 82, 33:3–12, April 1982

26. Brazelton TB: Maternal-infant interactions. In The Family: Can It Be Saved, pp 133–142. Chicago, Yearbook Medical Publishers, 1975

27. Leventhal SA, Lipsitt LP: Adaptation, pitch discrimination and sound localization in the neonate, Child Dev 35:759–767, 1964

28. Morse PA: The discrimination of speech and nonspeech stimuli in early infancy. J Exp Child Psychol 14:477–492, 1972

29. Ling D, Ling A: Communication development in the first three years of life. Journal Speech & Hearing Res 17:146–159, 1974

30. Gorski P, et al: Neurobehavioral organization of the high risk neonate. Semin Perinatol 3:61–72, 1979

31. Ludington–Hoe S: Summation report: Essential tools and techniques of infant stimulation. Washington, D.C., ISEA Publication, p 35, 1980

32. Morse PA: The discrimination of speech and nonspeech stimuli in early infancy. J Exp Child Psychol 14:477–492, 1972

33. Klaus MM, Fanaroff AA: Bach, Beethoven, or rock—and how much. Journal of Ped 88:300, 1976

34. Ludington SM: Vaginal and Cesarean Infant's Responses to Extra Tactile Stimulation, Ph.D. dissertation, p 74, Texas Woman's University, 1976

35. Rausch P: Effects of tactile and kinesthetic stimulation on premature infants. JOGNurs 34–40, 1981

36. Lamb M: Second thoughts of first touch. Psychol Today 9–11, April 1982

37. Kattwinkel T, et al: Apnea of prematurity and effects on CPAP, cutaneous stimulation and levels of urinary biogenic amines. Ped Res 8:468, April 1974

38. Rice RD: The effects of sensorimotor infant stimulation treatment on the development of high risk infants. Birth Defects 15:7–26, 1979

39. Cradle Care Incorporated, 6455 Meadow Road, Dallas, Texas

40. Frieman DG, et al: Effects of kinesthetic stimulation on weight gain and on smiling in premature infants. Paper read at annual meeting of American Orthopsychiatric Association, San Francisco, April 15, 1979

41. Kramer LJ, Pierpont ME: Rocking waterbeds and auditory stimuli to enhance growth of preterm infants. J Ped 88:297–299, 1976

42. Ludington–Hoe S: Summation report: Essential tools and techniques of infant stimulation. Washington, D.C., ISEA Publication p 35, 1980

43. Porter L: Role of activity in growth and development. Philippine Journal of Nursing 40:91–94, 1971

44. Levy J: The Baby Exercise Book. New York, Pantheon Books, 1975

45. McFarlane G: Breastfood recognition in newborns. In Brazelton TB: Newborn Behavior: Scientific Foundation of Obstetrics and Gynecology, p 556. Englewood Cliffs, Prentice Hall, 1979

CHAPTER 33

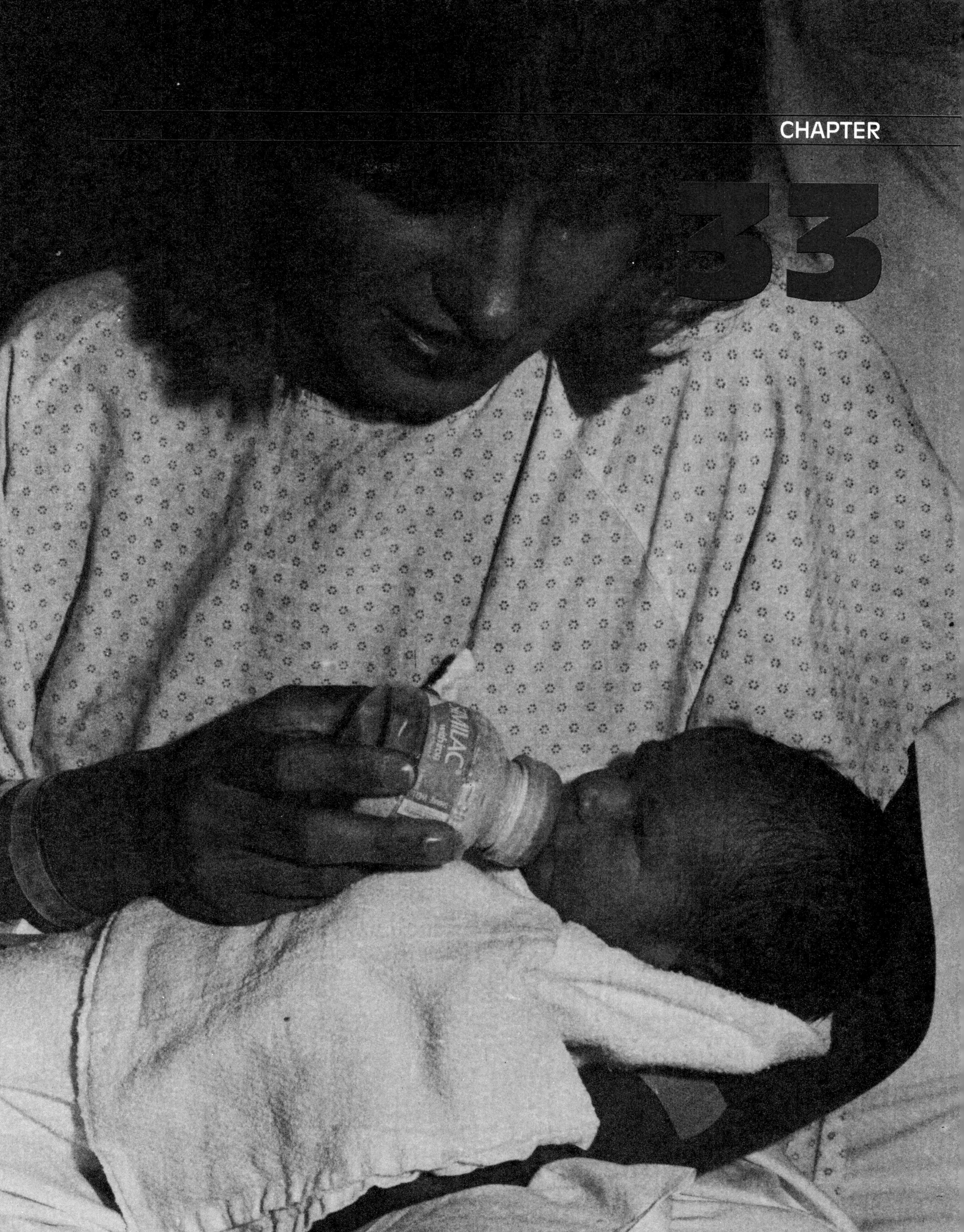

CHAPTER 33

Infant Nutrition

Nutrition is very important in preserving health throughout the life cycle. It is particularly important during the rapid growing phase of infancy. The long-term effects of feeding practices in early infancy are just beginning to be recognized. According to Neumann and Jelliffe, infant feeding is more than just "nutrient refueling"; it is also a "social, psychological and educational interaction between caretaker and baby."[1]

The Newborn's Ability to Handle Food

Up until the time of birth, the nutritional needs of the fetus have been met through placental circulation. One of the major physiological adaptations that the infant must make in the transition from intrauterine to extrauterine life is to adjust to the change in the source of nourishment and to take food into the body orally, digest it, and assimilate it.

Following birth, the gastrointestinal tract begins abruptly to process a rather large amount of food. At the same time the infant must begin to suck and swallow as a means of taking food into the stomach. The sucking and swallowing reflexes are already present at birth and are normally quite strong. In fact, the swallowing reflex, as well as peristaltic movements in the stomach, becomes active during the last two months of fetal development, as noted in the bits of vernix caseosa and lanugo that are found with other debris in the meconium stool. In the delivery room, the infant will often swallow mucus or suck on anything that gets near his mouth.

Another important instinctive reaction is the rooting reflex, which enables the newborn to find food. The human infant does not have to search for its food, but it does turn toward anything that touches its cheeks or lips. This is a help in latching onto the bottle or breast.

At the time of birth, the infant's stomach is small, with a capacity of approximately 50 ml to 60 ml. But it can dilate considerably so that during feeding it stretches to at least three or four times its approximate capacity. Not only is it distended by the amount of food taken in (*i.e.,* milk) but also by the amount of air swallowed as the infant sucks the milk or cries. In the act of crying, the infant tends to gulp in air.

The glandular structures in the gastric mucosa are present at birth, although they are shallow in comparison to those of the adult. The gastric musculature is somewhat deficient. This, plus the relatively greater length of the intestinal tract and the weakness of the abdominal musculature, which serves as a supporting structure, explains in part why considerable distention of the stomach is possible.

Studies on gastric motility have demonstrated wide individual differences in the emptying time of the stomachs of newborn infants. The major portion of the feeding usually leaves the stomach in less than 3 or 4 hours; however, in some instances, the emptying time of an infant's stomach is more than 8 hours. It was found also that the introduction of a second feeding before the stomach was empty caused portions of the first feeding to remain somewhat longer in the stomach than if the stomach was emptied before the next feeding was offered. Another important finding is that human milk leaves the stomach somewhat more rapidly than cow's milk, although a formula made of cow's milk that has been boiled leaves the stomach more rapidly than that which is fed without being boiled.[2]

Methods of Feeding—Making the Decision

Choosing the method of infant feeding is an important decision for parents to make. Their ultimate choice will be influenced by a variety of factors, physical and psychological as well as social. Ideally, the subject of infant feeding will be raised during the antepartal period, thereby providing an opportunity to guide the parents in making a decision that is most suitable for them. It is wise for the physician and the nurse to explore adequately with the mother (and the father, if possible) mutual attitudes concerning this subject.

In the past, breast-feeding, by the mother or a "wet-nurse," was essential for the survival of the infant. This is still true to some extent in underdeveloped countries, but in most of the world modern methods of artificial feeding have offered women an alternative. Although the production of infant formulas has become a big business and the choice of artificial feeding is now safe for the infant and convenient for the mother, there are still many advantages to breast-feeding.

One should avoid being so overzealously in favor of breast-feeding that it is forced on a reluctant mother. Those women who do not want to breast-feed their infants should not be made to feel guilty about their choice. On the other hand, the nurse should not hesitate to inform expectant parents of the differences between the various milks available (including human) and of the advantages of breast-feeding to both mother and infant (see Table 33-1). Many women are uninformed about the differences in the available methods and may base their decision on how their mothers fed them or what a friend has said. For these women, information can be very useful in helping them to make a decision based on facts.

Advantages of Breast-Feeding

For many years, the saying "breast is best" was used when talking about the relative merits of breast- or bottle-feeding. At the same time reassurances were given that formula was also fine for babies. In the past 10 years to 12 years, research studies from many disciplines have focused attention on the uniqueness of human milk and other favorable aspects of breast-feeding. Though knowledge is still incomplete, certain advantages of breast-feeding can be identified.

Biochemical/Nutritional Considerations

Contrary to the idea promoted by some commercial literature that modern formula is "almost like mother's milk," the constituents of cow's milk and human milk are dissimilar in almost every way, except for water and lactose.[3] Even when the formula has been "modified" or "humanized," there are still many differences. For example, whey protein, which accounts for more than 60% of the total protein in human milk, constitutes only 20% of cow's milk. Even

Table 33-1.
Composition of Mature Breast Milk, Cow's Milk, and a Routine Infant Formula*

Composition/dl	Mature Breast Milk	Cow's Milk	Routine Formula with Iron†
Calories	75.0	69.0	67.0
Protein, g	1.1	3.5	1.5
Lactalbumin, %	80	18	
Casein, %	20	82	
Water, ml	87.1	87.3	
Fat, g	4.0	3.5	3.7
CHO, g	9.5	4.9	7.0
Ash, g	0.21	0.72	0.34
Minerals			
Na, mg	16.0	50.0	25.0
K, mg	51.0	144.0	74.0
Ca, mg	33.0	118.0	55.0
P, mg	14.0	93.0	43.0
Mg, mg	4.0	12.0	9.0
Fe, mg	0.1	Tr.	1.2
Zn, mg	0.15	0.1	0.42
Vitamins			
A, IU	240.0	140.0	158.6
C, mg	5.0	1.0	5.3
D, IU	2.2	1.4	42.3
E, IU	0.18	0.04	0.83
Thiamin, mg	0.01	0.03	0.04
Riboflavin, mg	0.04	0.17	0.06
Niacin, mg	0.2	0.1	0.7
Curd size	Soft	Firm	Mod. firm
	Flocculent	Large	Mod. large
*p*H	Alkaline	Acid	Acid
Anti-infective properties	+	±	–
Bacterial content	Sterile	Nonsterile	Sterile
Emptying time	More rapid		

*Composite of a number of sources
†Enfamil
(Avery GB, Fletcher AB: Nutrition. In Avery GB (ed): Neonatology, 2nd ed, p 1020. Philadelphia, JB Lippincott, 1981)

when amounts of a substance are approximately the same, absorption may be different. For instance, similar concentrations of zinc are present in both milks, but the human infant absorbs zinc more effectively from human milk because human milk has a different zinc binding factor than is found in cow's milk.[3] Formulas also have added substances such as emulsifiers, thickening agents, *p*H adjusters, and antioxidants, the effects of which are unknown and which are "not found in the original product for human infants."[3]

Another difference of unknown consequence is the rigidly consistent composition of formula compared to the variability of mother's milk. Besides the changes that occur in the progression from colostrum to mature milk, there is variation in the composition of mother's milk within each nursing period. The foremilk, which accumulates in the alveoli between nursings, has a higher concentration of lactose and whey protein (lactalbumin), while the hindmilk, which is secreted during the nursing period, is higher in fat and casein.[4] There are also differences in composition of breast milk according to the time of day of the nursing period.

Immunological and Antiallergic Factors

Human milk and colostrum have been shown by many recent studies to be rich in defense factors, such as immunoglobulins, lactoferrin, enzymes, macrophages, lymphocytes, and *Lactobacillus bifidus* (a growth enhancer of lactobacilli). "These components promote a 'normal' bacterial colonization of the gastrointestinal tract and also suppress the invasiveness of certain pathogenic microorganisms. They may be of major importance to the newborn's system of defense against infection. However, further studies are needed to verify this view and to fill in some of the gaps in our knowledge."[5]

One known advantage of the immunoglobulin secretory IgA, which is present in human milk, is the protective anti-absorptive effect it has in keeping protein molecules from passing through the intestinal walls. During the first six months of life, foreign proteins are more likely to be absorbed through the intestinal wall than they are in later life, which can lead to allergies. The protein in cow's milk is one of the most common food allergens encountered in infancy. Human milk proteins, on the other hand, are virtually nonallergenic to humans.[6]

Psychological Aspects

The psychological advantages of breast-feeding are not as easily documented, and sometimes it is said that bottle-feeding and breast-feeding are interchangeable for the emotional well-being of mother and child. However, breast-feeding, by establishing a more direct and intimate biologic relationship between infant and mother may very well influence the quality of the mother–child interaction.[3]

Other Aspects

For the baby, breast milk can be safer because it is not subject to incorrect mixing or contamination. The baby does not have to wait to eat—if mother is nearby the milk is always available and at the right temperature. The action of sucking at breast is different from sucking on a bottle, and may help the mouth and jaw to develop better (see Fig 33-6).

For the mother, an early benefit is promotion of uterine involution stimulated by the release of oxytocin when the infant sucks. The mother also has the convenience of not having to prepare bottles or incur the added expense of buying formula. When a woman breast-feeds her infant, she is less likely to conceive again during the first eight to ten months of lactation. As a means of birth control, this, of course, is not as reliable as modern contraceptive measures but can be helpful for those who cannot afford or accept artificial contraception.[6] (See References and Suggested Reading for a more complete discussion of advantages of breast-feeding.)

Choosing to Bottle-Feed

Throughout recorded history, women have sought alternatives to breast-feeding their infants. Although the most popular alternative was the use of a wet-nurse, attempts at artificial feeding were widespread, as can be seen from the remains of spouted feeding pots, artificial teats, and other mechanical feeding devices. Historical writings show that women were often urged to breast-feed their own children, but many ignored these admonitions for various reasons.[7]

Women still give a variety of reasons for choosing artificial feeding. Some feel that breast-feeding is too tiring, confining, or simply distasteful; some may be afraid that it will disfigure their breasts. Others fear that they will fail at breast-feeding, especially if previous attempts to breast-feed a child were unsuccessful.

The mores and pressures of the mother's socioeconomic class and peer group also are important. Bottle-feeding may be the accepted practice in the community or neighborhood; relatives, friends, and others may be either very much for or against breast-feeding. Return to employment for the mother may be a very significant factor.

Certain conditions in both the mother and the

infant also can have a bearing on the decision and outcome. Diseases and infection (*i.e.,* syphilis, tuberculosis, staphylococcal infections, communicable diseases) generally are contraindications for breast-feeding. Similarly, certain infections and anomalies in the infant may make nursing impossible, at least temporarily. Breast infection or painful, cracked, or fissured nipples also may require temporary discontinuation of breast-feeding. Becoming pregnant usually is considered to be an indication for weaning because of the physiological strain that it places on the mother.

Breast-Feeding

If breast-feeding is the method of choice for a new mother, the degree to which she perseveres in this endeavor is often influenced by her care in the hospital. A consistent approach to assisting with breast-feeding is important. A "breast-feeding protocol," as suggested by Dutton, can be developed in a hospital setting to help "standardize teaching and eliminate contradictory guidance."[8]

Recent studies have shown that many breast-feeding mothers perceive nurses as being negative or neutral toward breast-feeding.[9] After returning home, many mothers encountered problems that they felt could have been prevented if they had been given more anticipatory guidance by the nurses in the hospital about possible problems.[10] In light of these findings, it seems safe to say that support from knowledgeable nursing personnel, permissive hospital policies, and anticipatory teaching can do much to make breast-feeding a pleasant and successful experience for mother and infant.

Mechanisms of Lactation

A working knowledge of how the breasts function in the lactation process can help the nurse to guide the new mother. The anatomy of the breasts and the physiology of lactation have been discussed in Chapters 28 and 30. The student is referred to these chapters for a renewal of background understanding of the subject. Figure 33-1 also reviews the anatomical structures of the breast.

Secretion of Milk

Two major mechanisms are involved in lactation. The first of these is the secretion of milk. It is believed, that the hormone prolactin is responsible for the initiation of lactation and that the release of this hormone is enhanced by the sucking of the infant. Milk continues to be secreted by the alveoli or acini cells for as long as the breasts are sufficiently emptied. Frequent emptying of the breasts is very important, especially in the early stages of lactation. Both the production of milk and the quantity produced are dependent on *frequent* and *complete* emptying of the breasts. If the breasts

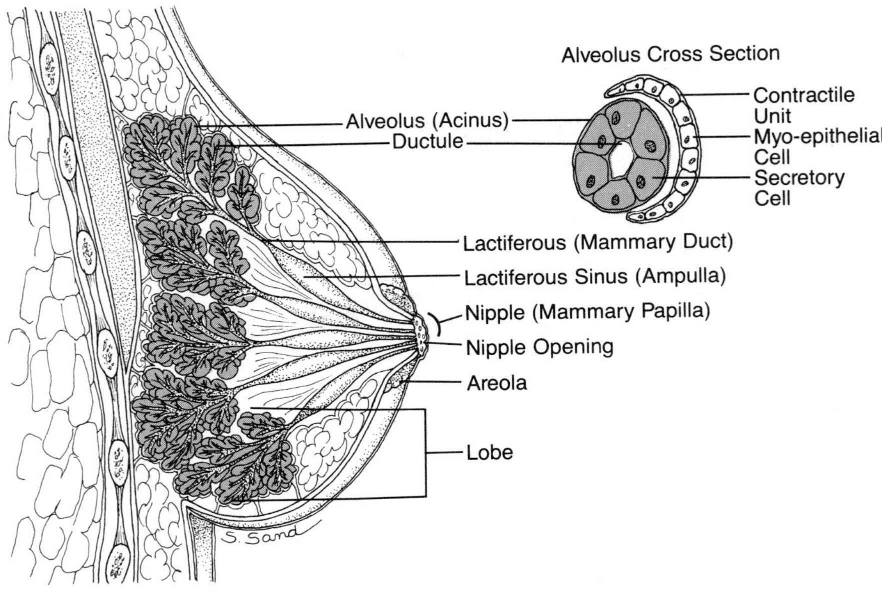

Figure 33-1. Schematic diagram of the breast. (Redrawn from Riordan J, Countryman BA: Basics of breast-feeding, part II: The anatomy and psychophysiology of lactation. JOGN Nurs 9, 4:210, July/August 1980)

are not entirely emptied, and the back pressure in the alveoli is not relieved, milk secretion decreases and eventually stops.

The first stage of milk production begins with the secretion of a yellow-colored fluid called *colostrum* by the lining of the alveoli and ductules. This early milk, or pre-milk, is usually present toward the end of pregnancy and is the infant's food for the first day or two after birth. Colostrum is higher in protein and lower in fat and lactose than milk. It also contains greater amounts of other substances such as sodium chloride and zinc and is rich in antibodies. Besides its nutrient purpose and anti-infective function, it also may act as a laxative in facilitating the passage of meconium.[11] As the prolactin levels continue to increase and the estrogen and progesterone levels drop, newly secreted milk is progressively mixed with the colostrum for a transitional period of 7 to 10 days until the mature milk stage is reached. During this time there is a decrease in the concentration of immunoglobulins and total protein and an increase in lactose, fat, and total calories.[12]

In the early stages of lactation, milk secretion can be stimulated by having the infant nurse from both breasts at each feeding and by increasing the frequency of the feedings. Milk production begins slowly in some mothers, but it can be stimulated by allowing the infant to nurse both breasts every 2 to 3 hours.

Milk-Ejection Reflex

The second mechanism involved in lactation is the milk-ejection or let-down reflex. Initiated by the infant's sucking, oxytocin released from the posterior pituitary stimulates the myoepithelial cells in the alveoli to contract and eject the milk through the ducts into the lactiferous sinuses. This reflex affects the quantity of milk the infant is able to obtain because the milk has to be in the sinuses before it can be removed by the infant's sucking. The quality of milk is also affected because the fat-containing hindmilk is not secreted until the foremilk is removed. Failure of the let-down reflex may be a direct or indirect cause of early termination of breast-feeding in many women (see Possible Consequences of an Inadequate Let-down Reflex).

Possible Consequences of an Inadequate Let-Down Reflex

1. Let-down reflex doesn't occur. (Mother tense, nervous, in pain, and so forth.)
   ↓
2. Milk is not propelled into ducts by contraction of myoepithelial cells.
   ↓
3. Insufficient milk available to infant = hungry baby.
4. Mother afraid she doesn't have enough milk → further inhibits let-down → gives infant formula → less sucking stimulation → decreased milk production.
   ↓
5. Engorgement due to inadequate emptying of breasts → more difficult for infant to suck → may lead to infection from stasis of milk.
   ↓
6. Termination of breast-feeding—reasons given: "I didn't have enough milk." Or, "My breasts were too sore." Or, "My breasts were infected so the doctor told me to stop."

Initiation of Breast-Feeding

Depending on the condition of both mother and infant, breast-feeding may be started shortly after birth, in the delivery or recovery room. The newborn usually is awake and alert for the first hour or so after birth and will often be seen trying to suck on his fist. Taking advantage of this heightened sucking reflex will give an opportunity for a successful initial breast-feeding experience.[10] Of course, if the mother has been heavily medicated or has experienced a difficult delivery, the infant may be sleepy and initial breast-feeding may have to be postponed. The Committee on Fetus and Newborn of the American Academy of Pediatrics recommends that breast-feeding begin as soon as possible after delivery.[13]

Some physicians still prefer to give the baby one or two bottles of plain water or glucose water before allowing breast-feeding to begin. The purpose of this is to help the infant regurgitate any mucus or secretions that may have been swallowed during delivery, although the same function can be served by colostrum. Another reason for using the bottle at this time is to provide an opportunity to observe the infant for any possible congenital anomalies, such as tracheoesophageal fistula. It is also felt that if such a condition exists, water will be safer than colostrum. However, others argue that colostrum, because it is a physiological secretion, is probably just as safe because it would not have the irritating effects of a foreign substance.[14] Those advocating early breast-feeding also point out that an observant nurse would be quick to detect a problem such as tracheoesophageal fistula in the initial breast-feedng sessions and would then obtain help quite readily.

Assistance with Breast-Feeding

It is important to remember that *both* mother and baby must learn how to work as a team during the breast-feeding process. Hence, practice is essential. Even though the mother may have breast-fed before, there is a wide range of nursing behaviors among infants, and the experience of breast-feeding each infant can be somewhat "new." The mother will need to learn how to handle the infant appropriately, how to interpret cues of hunger and satiety, and how to help the infant to grasp the nipple and to withdraw the milk successfully. The infant, in turn, must learn to associate the nipple with food and to coordinate grasping of the nipple with sucking and swallowing in such a way as to get food successfully. No wonder that mother and baby often take a few days to become adept at this process!

An interested and experienced nurse should be immediately available to mothers in their first experiences with their new babies. Maternity nurses in the hospital can play a major role in facilitating the mothers' efforts to breast-feed their babies (Fig. 33-2).

Many of the problems associated with unsuccessful breast-feeding experiences can be prevented or solved through purposeful nursing action. Nurses need to accept the responsibility of helping mothers gain the knowledge and skill necessary to successfully breast-feed their babies.[15]

Preparing the mother *before* the actual breast-feeding experience plays a large part in giving effective care. This includes instructions about hand-washing, sterile technique procedures, and other rituals associated with the feeding of the infant in the hospital. If these tasks have to be carried out after the infant is brought to the mother for feeding, the delay can be frustrating and stress-producing for both mother and baby.

Whenever it is indicated, the mother should be informed about the feeding reflexes of her infant. During the actual nursing period the nurse can reinforce this information (as necessary) and *show* the mother how to elicit these responses. It is essential that the mother be able to evoke these reflexes herself, since she ultimately must assume total responsibility. Too often the nurse takes over these aspects, and the mother does not get sufficient practice to acquire any skill during these first days in the hospital. It is not easy to "stand by" and watch the inexperienced mother trying to breast-feed her baby with-

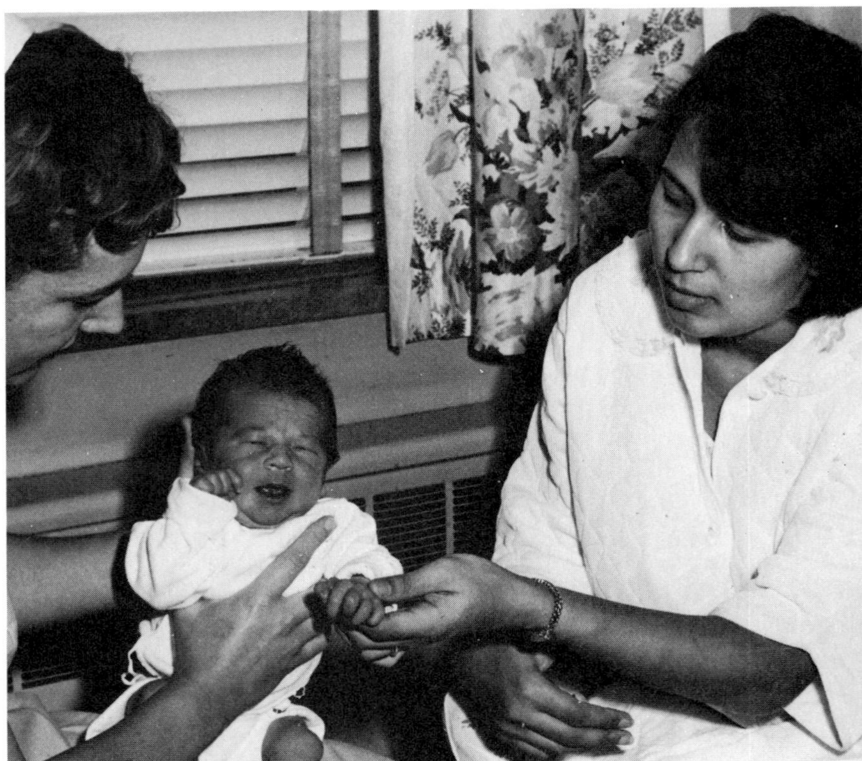

Figure 33-2.
The nurse demonstrates methods of handling the baby prior to feeding.

out offering too much interference. But it is necessary to be careful not to disrupt the learning process.

Whether the first nursing is done in the delivery room, in the recovery room, or in the patient's room later, the nurse who assists the mother should record the type of instruction given and the response of the mother and infant to the experience. This information can help other staff members, working with the mother, to provide needed assistance and consistency.

Positioning

Assisting the mother to experiment with various positions during breast-feeding is another important facet of care. The mother is sometimes asked whether she wants to nurse the baby sitting up or lying down. An inexperienced mother may be unaware of the options and should be given an opportunity to try various positions while help is available. If the mother is shown only one position, she may think there is only one "right" way to do it.

The best positions for any given mother and infant depend on several factors, including the size and shape of the breast, the size of the infant, and the condition of the mother, who may have a sore perineum or tender incisional area from a cesarean section. However, it is a good idea to encourage the mother to avoid using the same position at each feeding. The area of the nipple in line with the infant's nose and chin is subjected to the greatest stress. Varying the nursing positions from one feeding to the next can be helpful because it changes the position of the infant's mouth on the nipple. This allows the breast to empty more completely and prevents the nipples from becoming tender and the ducts from becoming plugged.[16]

To nurse satisfactorily, the infant needs to be held properly by the mother. Although some mothers seem to know how to support a baby at the breast, many are awkward at first and need definite instructions. The following are some helpful teaching points:

1. The mother and baby must be comfortable.
2. The baby should be at the level of the breast so his weight does not pull on the breast.
3. The baby must be able to grasp the nipple and most of the areola. If only the nipple is grasped, the baby will not be able to draw out the milk because the milk sinuses will not be compressed. Possible damage to the nipple may occur along with pain to the mother.

If the mother is lying down (Fig. 33-3), she should be on her side with her arm raised and her head comfortably supported. The baby lies on his side, flat on the bed or supported so that he can grasp the breast easily. Tucking the baby's feet close to the mother's body will help give him room to breathe. If the mother prefers to sit up to nurse, she may be most comfortable in a chair, with a stool to support her feet, if necessary. If she stays in bed, the high Fowler's position is probably best so she can lean over slightly, toward the infant on her lap. It is often helpful to place a pillow under the arm that is supporting the infant to reduce the tension on the muscles (Fig. 33-4) or to place a pillow under the baby to raise him to a sufficient height to reach the breast easily. An alternate position for the baby is facing the breast with his body supported on a pillow along the mother's side and under her arm in the "football hold" (Fig. 33-5). This is especially helpful for the mother who has delivered by cesarean section, or the mother who wants to nurse twins simultaneously.

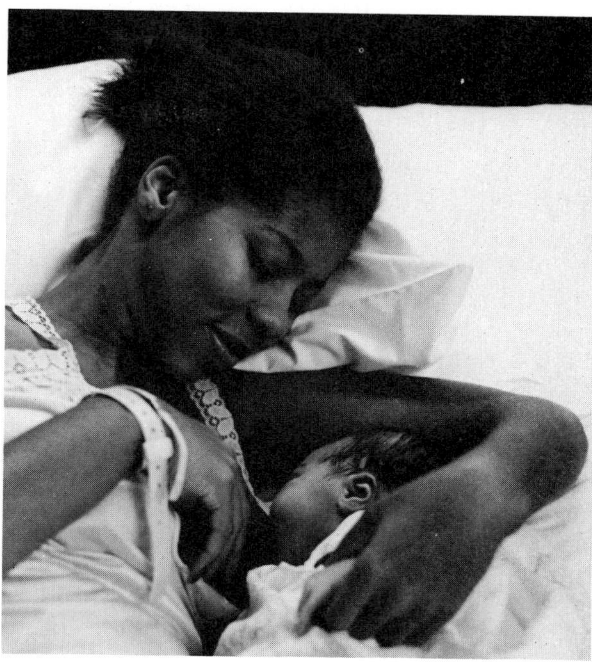

Figure 33-3.
The mother may breast-feed her child while lying down.

The nurse may have to work with the mother a bit to be sure that she is comfortable. Often, in their eagerness to get the baby on the breast, mothers become very tense and assume quite uncomfortable positions (although they assure the nurse they are "comfortable"). Patience and gentle reminding on the part of the nurse encourage these mothers to relax more readily.

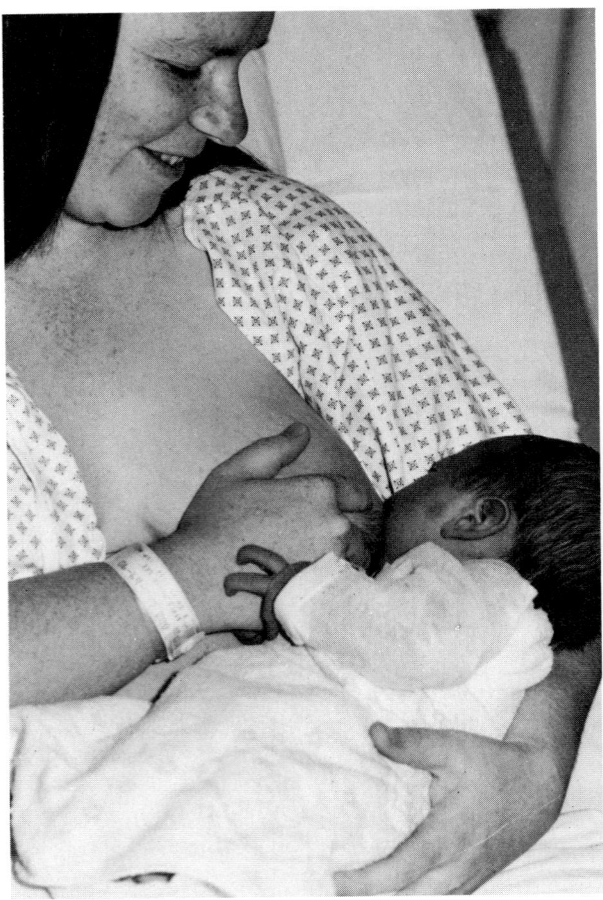

Figure 33-4.
The mother may prefer to assume a sitting position when nursing her infant.

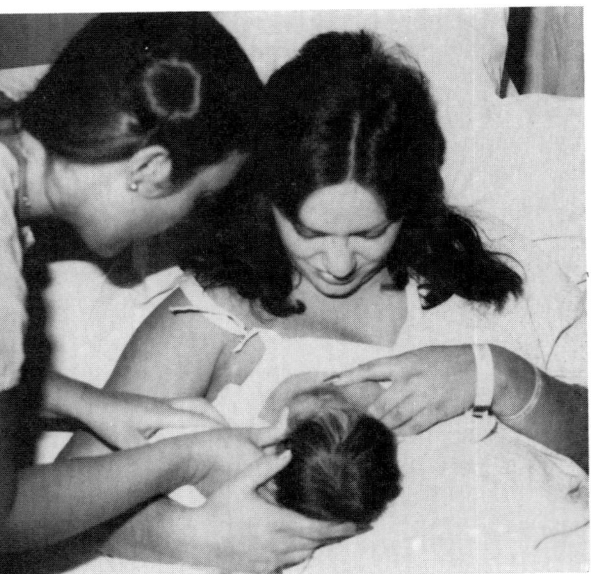

Figure 33-5.
The nurse assists the mother in positioning the infant in the football hold for breast feeding.

Orientation of Infant

After being placed beside the mother, the baby needs to be allowed a little time to become accustomed to the new environment and to hunt for the nipple. The baby should not be forced to nurse immediately, especially if he is hesitant or shows disinclination. If the rooting reflex is well developed (and as he smells the milk), the baby will turn toward the nipple or any object that brushes the cheek. Thus, if the mother or the nurse touches his cheek gently with the nipple, he will turn toward it, open his mouth and grasp it.

The mother can help the baby grasp the nipple by making a V with two fingers of her free hand, placing one finger on the upper edge of the areola and the other on the lower edge, while shaping the breast to better correspond to the shape of the infant's mouth. Sucking usually follows closely thereafter. If the infant seems to have some difficulty in finding and grasping the nipple, although he seems to be eager, the mother or nurse can gently cup a hand around the baby's head and guide him to the nipple.

When the mother assumes the sitting position, the infant's head can be held in the bend of the mother's arm while she guides the infant toward the breast by moving her arm. Care should be taken, however, not to touch his cheek or to force his head, since he will only turn away and resist the pressure. In addition, he may cry, and a crying baby tends not to grasp a nipple successfully even though he may be hungry.

Sucking Behavior of Infant

Babies exhibit a wide variety of sucking behaviors. Some, after finding the nipple, suck vigorously without stopping until they are satisfied. Others may suck vigorously for a time, appear to sleep or to rest, and then resume sucking. Still others mouth the nipple before actually sucking, but eventually nurse well. Others seem rather disinterested in the whole thing and dawdle throughout the nursing period. When the milk comes in, however, a change usually is noted, and even the seemingly disinterested infants begin to nurse more in earnest.

The important point here is that individual differences do exist in infants, apparently from birth; hence care must be taken to allow for these differences. To try to force the infant into a style or speed that is not natural for him will only result in screaming, resistance, and refusal; the nursing period should be adapted to the infant and not the infant to the nursing period.

Mothers, especially, are appreciative of learning about this; often they think there is "a way to nurse" and do not realize that infants have different eating behaviors. Giving mothers anticipatory guidance and instruction in this aspect of nursing a baby is a very important component in nursing care.

If breast-feeding has not begun early and the infant has had experience with a rubber nipple, he may be "nipple confused." The sucking behavior required to obtain milk from the bottle is quite different from that of breast-feeding, described below. The milk from the bottle comes into the infant's mouth with very little effort on his part, and instead of using his tongue to help extract the milk, he has to thrust his tongue forward to control the flow of milk (see Fig. 33-6 F). It is not surprising that many infants have some difficulty in switching from bottle to breast, but with a little time they usually do well. It is helpful for the mother to know about these sucking differences so she doesn't become frustrated.

If the infant is to suck effectively on the breast, he must place the nipple well back in his mouth, close his lips tightly around the areola, and squeeze the nipple against his palate with his tongue. He then can compress the lactiferous sinuses behind the areola and draw the milk into his mouth by sucking. He empties the breast through a combination of compression and suction. As he nurses, he moves his jaws up and down to compress and empty the sinuses; his tongue, as it draws the nipple back against the palate, suctions the milk from the nipple. Swallowing occurs when enough milk has been obtained to induce the reflex. This activity is carried on rhythmically, interspaced with periods of rest, until the infant is satisfied (see Fig. 33-6 A–E).

Sometimes the let-down reflex is so active that the milk literally streams, and the baby not only does not have to suck very hard but may have difficulty in swallowing fast enough to keep up with the stream. Placing the baby in a more upright position sometimes helps to prevent choking in these cases. He may have to nurse a bit, stop, and then continue as he learns to cope with the increased stream.

When assisting the mother, the nurse should be sure that the baby has the nipple on top of his tongue and that enough of the areola is in his mouth to prevent damage to the nipple. If he has a good grasp, his jaws will move up and down regularly, and sucking and swallowing movements can be seen in his cheeks and throat. If his grasp is poor, sucking and swallowing may be infrequent or absent, although his jaws may continue to move. If the breast tissue seems to press against the infant's nose and thus obstruct his breathing, the nurse can instruct the mother to take her forefinger and gently compress the tissue so that the breast no longer impinges on the infant's nose (note the hand positions of mothers in Figs. 33-3, 33-4, and 33-5). Care should be taken not to pull the nipple away from the infant in this maneuver.

Usually, getting the nipple in his mouth and tasting the milk seem to increase the baby's interest and ability to nurse. If the infant does not seem too interested or adept, moistening the nipple by expressing a few drops of colostrum or milk often encourages sucking.

Occasionally, a breast shield may be used to start the infant nursing if for some reason he cannot grasp the nipple. Continued use of this appliance is unwise, since the breasts cannot be emptied because the lacteal sinuses are not compressed during the nursing. The shield can be useful during the first few minutes of nursing to draw the nipples out if they are flattened by engorgement or inversion. Usually, however, even inverted nipples become prominent if the alveolar area is compressed gently by the fingers before nursing; they generally evert more as the infant sucks.

Sometimes a baby will be sleepy and difficult to arouse. If the mother unwraps him, plays with his hands, sings to him, or uses some other type of loving stimulation, it may be enough to awaken him. If it does not, the mother should be reassured that the baby will nurse when he is hungry. The nurse should then make sure that the baby is brought to the mother as soon as he awakens and is not given any feeding in the nursery. If possible, the infant should be left at the mother's bedside, so that she is available when the baby is ready to eat.

Once the infant is sucking well, the mother should be reminded to break the suction before removing him from the breast. Failure to do this can result in pain or trauma to the nipple. To break the suction, a clean little finger can be placed in the corner of the infant's mouth or the infant's chin can be pulled down. Sometimes the mother needs to pull away a little at the same time so the infant does not grasp the nipple again.

The mother may also inquire about bubbling or burping the infant. This may be done when she changes breasts and at the end of the feeding period. If the infant was crying hard before the feeding, she may want to bubble him before beginning. For the infant who has difficulty getting started, it might be better to bubble him only at the end of the feeding. Breast-fed

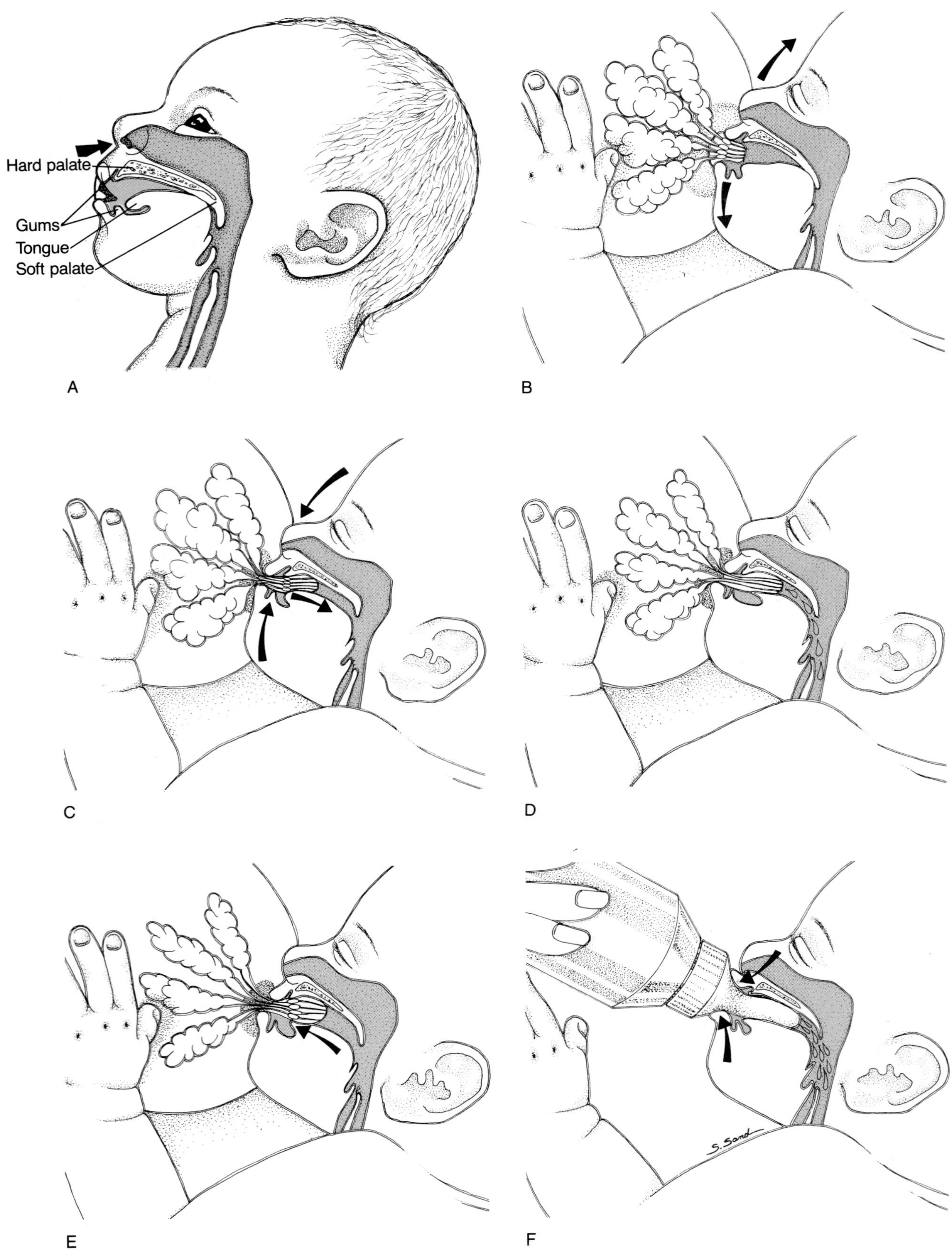
Hard palate
Gums
Tongue
Soft palate
A
B
C
D
E
F
S. Sand

babies tend not to swallow as much air as bottle-fed infants, hence the need for bubbling usually does not present much of a problem.

Giving Support and Supervision

Once the infant has taken the breast without difficulty and has been sucking well for several minutes, the nurse probably does not need to remain in constant attendance at the bedside. The mother needs some opportunity to feel that she can manage on her own. Letting her have reasonable periods of managing breast-feeding by herself will help to instill some confidence. However, she should never be left without adequate instruction and reassurance. The nurse might find something else to do in the room or can place a call-bell within easy reach so that the mother can ring for help if need be. The nurse should make a point of looking in occasionally to observe the progress. The reassurance that the nurse is readily available may be all the encouragement the mother needs.

Since some infants do not nurse well during the first few days, the nurse will want to remind the mother that the first week is a time of learning for both the nursing mother and the child. Many mothers feel that all infants are born knowing how to suck and that if their infant does not latch on immediately, it must be because of something the mother is doing wrong. Some mothers even have a feeling of being rejected, stating, "The baby doesn't like me," or "The baby doesn't want my milk." Actually, taking milk from the breast is more than just a simple act of sucking, and some infants do need help in learning how. If the mother is helped to understand this, she will be less inclined to blame herself and more able to enjoy the nursing experience.

Because hospital stays are so short, there is less time available to provide professional assistance to the new mother. Most women still need support after leaving the hospital. In some cases the father fills this need, but in others another support person is needed. In the past, information and positive feelings about breast-feeding were passed from mother to daughter. However, since breast-feeding has not been a universal practice recently, grandmothers or other relatives may not have breast-feeding experiences to relate. Also, in our mobile society and with the trend toward nuclear families, female family members are not always available to give support to the new mother. To fill this void, nursing mothers' groups have been started across the country. One particularly popular group is La Leche League International, which holds classes about breast-feeding for women either before or after the baby is born. This organization also publishes a book about breast-feeding *(The Womanly Art of Breast Feeding)* along with other pamphlets, including one called "How the Nurse Can Help the Breast-Feeding Mother." In many communities there are 24-hour phone numbers that nursing mothers may call if they are having problems with breast-feeding.

The mother may also be referred to a public health agency if necessary. Some hospitals are now encouraging mothers to call the nursery or obstetric unit if they need support or help with problems. While many mothers are reluctant to call, they welcome the chance to ask questions if the nurse makes the call or a home visit. Some hospitals and some private doctors are hiring nurses to make follow-up visits after the woman leaves the hospital.

Schedule

A self-regulatory or self-demand schedule is the usual accepted practice today, especially for breast-fed babies; that is, the baby is fed when he indicates hunger by crying and body posture. The infant cries when he is hungry because actual contractions in his stomach cause him pain. If he is fed when he cries and is experiencing pain, he learns to associate food with the relief of pain. Thus food and the mother who supplies it become pleasant factors in his life. If, on the other hand, he is made to wait until "time" for feeding, he may not nurse well because he is exhausted from crying or has lost his feeling of hunger. Similarly, if a baby is "sleepy" and not allowed to wake up sufficiently by himself, he also will not nurse well and will soon resent efforts to wake him up.

Figure 33-6.
(A) Normal breathing for a young baby is through the nose; the back of the mouth is closed by contact of tongue and palate. *(B)* Infant opens mouth to receive the breast and the tongue comes forward to grasp nipple and areola. *(C)* Nipple is sucked far back into mouth. The gums close on areola while elevation of the tongue, traveling from front to back, presses nipple against hard palate, squeezing milk out of sinuses. Note how lips curl in around areola, forming an air-tight seal. *(D)* When milk reaches the back of the throat the swallowing reflex is initiated. *(E)* The gums then open, allowing sinuses to refill. The tongue comes forward, and the cycle is repeated. Enough suction is maintained to keep nipple back in the mouth and the infant continues to breathe through the nose, one breath to one or two swallows. *(F)* Rubber nipple is less pliable, reaches farther into mouth and may strike soft palate, interfering with normal tongue action and sometimes causing gagging. Milk comes more freely and tongue is thrust forward against gums to control overflow. Note the lips flaring outward from pressure of widened area of nipple.

Slapping the soles of his feet, spanking his bottom, and the like generally are not effective.

Problems of this type can often be avoided in a rooming-in situation, because with the mother and baby together most of the time, the mother knows when the infant is awake for a feeding. She also has the opportunity to learn to recognize the cry and behavior which indicate that her baby is hungry.

Most breast-fed babies will want to nurse every two to three hours at first. This is helpful in stimulating milk production and in satisfying the infant's sucking needs. The nursing pattern will vary greatly in the early weeks of life. Each time the infant has a growth spurt he will want to nurse more frequently for a few days until the supply catches up with his increased demand. The mother will be encouraged to know that her baby will gradually go longer between feedings and that his eating pattern will become less varied.[17]

Length of Nursing Time

In the early stages of breast-feeding, some authorities suggest that the sucking time be limited and then gradually increased each day as a means of preventing sore nipples. Whitley found that of the women who restricted nursing time, fewer developed sore nipples while in the hospital, but more developed soreness at home.[18] If the time limitation is drastic, such as starting with one minute on each breast at each feeding and increasing by one minute each day, the let-down reflex will not have a chance to function before the baby is removed from the breast. Another disadvantage is that the mother becomes too involved in clock watching to have a pleasant, relaxed time with her baby.

It is best to offer both breasts at each feeding to provide maximum stimulation for the mother and an adequate supply of milk for the infant. If initial sucking time is going to be limited, 5 to 7 minutes on each side for the first day's feedings is probably reasonable. This allows time for the let-down reflex to occur and the ducts to be emptied. The time can then be gradually increased up to 10 to 15 minutes on the first breast and as long as the infant desires on the second. The condition of the mother's nipples should be considered and the time shortened if there are problems.

When the breasts are full and the let-down reflex is functioning well, the baby usually gets most of the milk in the first 5 to 10 minutes of sucking. Therefore, the mother need not worry that the baby is not getting enough milk if she has to limit nursing time for a short period due to nipple soreness. Nursing should begin on the side used last at the previous feeding. A safety pin on the bra strap will help the mother remember which breast to start with.

Not Enough Milk

Many mothers worry that they will not have enough milk. The mother can be assured that the baby is probably getting an adequate amount of milk if he is wetting four to six diapers a day, sleeping fairly well, and gaining weight at a steady rate. The wet diapers may be the best guide, because "colicky" babies cry for reasons other than hunger and usually gain well, and some breast-fed babies are slow weight gainers even when the milk supply is adequate.

If the mother thinks her baby is not getting enough milk, putting the baby to breast more often will usually increase the supply. The concept of supply and demand, that the more milk the baby takes from the breast, the more the mother will produce, is important for the mother to remember. Sometimes women mistakenly think that they can "save" their milk and have more for the next feeding if they give the baby a bottle at one feeding. Getting more rest and increasing fluid and protein intake may also help increase the milk supply.

Some mothers fear that they are losing their milk at the time when engorgement subsides because their breasts go back to a more normal size and feel less full. An explanation that this might happen and that it is just the swelling that has gone down, not the milk supply, would help prevent worry.

If the mother's breasts seem full but the infant does not seem to be getting enough, there could be a problem with the let-down reflex. It may be helpful to the mother to learn how to recognize whether or not the let-down reflex is occurring. Mothers usually feel the let-down as a kind of tingling or drawing sensation in the nipple, followed by a fuller, heavier feeling of the breasts. Since let-down occurs bilaterally, another sign is dripping of milk from one breast while the infant is sucking on the other. Also there is often a change in the infant's sucking as the milk begins to flow more freely and he doesn't have to work as hard.

The let-down reflex can be influenced profoundly by psychic factors and the mother's emotions. If let-down is not occurring, the nurse can help the mother determine and eliminate disturbing factors. The mother may need to lie down, have a warm drink, or discover other ways of relaxing before the feeding time. A relaxed atmosphere, adequate assistance, effective pain relief, and a supportive attitude on the part of the nurse and family are important to the establishment of the let-down reflex.

Sometimes mothers are concerned that their milk isn't "rich enough" because they compare the thin, bluish white color of breast milk with the creamy color of cow's milk. They need to know that human milk is naturally different from cow's milk in many ways, including color. They may be interested in the fact that the milk of each animal species has a characteristic color. For example, buffalo's milk is completely white and kangaroo's milk is pink.[11]

Supplementary or Complementary Feedings

A bottle given instead of a breast-feeding is called a *supplementary feeding,* while one given in addition to the breast-feeding is called *complementary* (Fig. 33-7).

This subject has long been controversial. Some physicians (and mothers) feel that giving the infant any artificial feedings diminishes the success of breast-feeding and is extremely detrimental to establishing and maintaining lactation (see References and Suggested Reading). Others feel that there are legitimate indications for an occasional artificial feeding. A variety of feedings may be used (*i.e.,* plain water, glucose water, dilute formula, full-strength formula). It is sometimes suggested that these be given by spoon or dropper to avoid the use of a rubber nipple.

If the mother is to use supplemental or complementary feedings when she returns home, the nurse will want to be sure that the mother understands how to prepare these feedings, the kind and the amount of feedings, and the indications for their use.

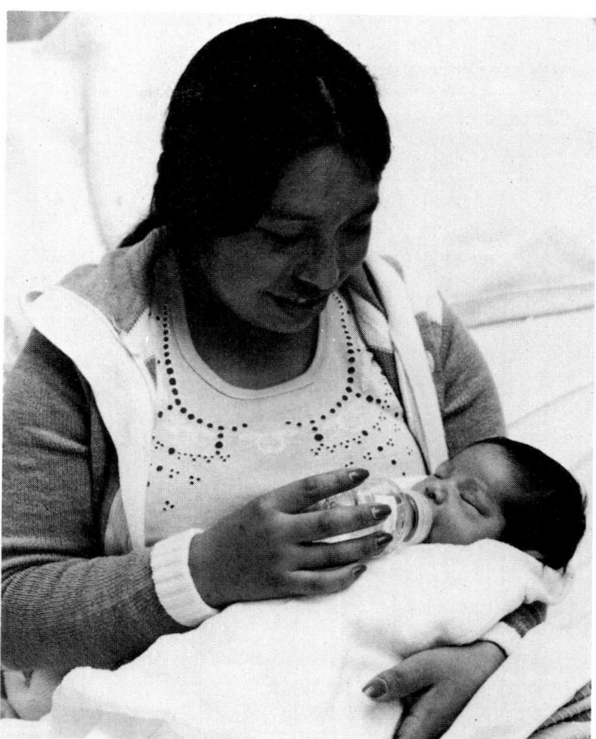

Figure 33-7.
A mother cuddling her infant while giving a complementary bottle of water.

Care of the Nipples

To facilitate breast-feeding, it is important to discuss nipple care with the new mother. Cleanliness is important in breast-feeding, but it is the hands that need washing, not the nipples. There is a natural antisepsis provided in the oils secreted by the nipple and by enzymes in the milk.[16] Washing the breasts with plain water at the time of the daily bath or shower is thought to be enough. The use of soap should be avoided, because it is drying and can lead to cracking. There are many commercial nipple ointments and creams available, but hydrous lanolin has also been found to be soothing to tender nipples. Whatever is used should be safe for mother and baby and not have to be washed off before nursing. The nipples should be dried and the ointment or cream applied lightly so air circulation will not be obstructed. Keeping the nipples dry is another important aspect of their care. Air drying after each nursing period and leaving the bra flaps down for 15 to 30 minutes several times a day is suggested.[16] Also, plastic liners of any kind in the bra should be removed because they hold the moisture in. In case of some milk leakage, especially in the first days after the milk comes in, something absorbent, such as a breast pad or a clean, folded, man's handkerchief, can be helpful to keep the nipple drier and prevent the outer clothing from getting wet. They should, of course, be changed frequently when they get damp.

Common Concerns and Problems of Nursing Mothers

Painful Nipples

Nipple pain is frequently a reason mothers give for discontinuing breast-feeding. Although it may not be possible to prevent or eliminate this problem completely, it can be minimized with good care. Measures to prevent nipple trauma include the following:

1. Make sure most of the areola is in the infant's mouth so that he does not just chew on the nipple.
2. Change nursing positions with each feeding so that different areas of the nipple are subjected to the greatest stress from sucking.
3. Do not allow the breasts to become engorged so that the infant has difficulty grasping the breast.
4. Feed the infant on demand so that he does not become overly hungry, causing him to suck the nipple too vigorously.

Assisting the New Mother with Breast-Feeding

1. Assess knowledge and needs.
2. Provide conducive environment.
   a. Provide privacy.
   b. Assist mother to find comfortable position.
   c. Assist in positioning infant.
3. Teach:
   a. About sucking patterns
   b. Importance of areola in infant's mouth
   c. Ways of waking baby
   d. How to break suction when removing infant from breast
   e. Burping methods
   f. Nipple care
4. Give support and reassurance.

5. Start each feeding on alternate breasts so that both breasts are subjected to the vigorous sucking that occurs at the beginning of the feeding.
6. Limit sucking time as necessary.

The mother should also avoid allowing the infant to suck on empty ducts. Before the let-down reflex is established, she can manually express a few drops of colostrum or milk to fill the ducts prior to allowing the baby to begin nursing.

The mother can probably benefit from some anticipatory guidance about nipple soreness. She needs to know that it is not unusual and is usually self-limiting. The discomfort is often most noticeable as the baby begins to suck but diminishes rapidly as the let-down reflex occurs. The discomfort with the first few sucks can last for several days or weeks and does not mean that there is anything wrong.

It is possible, of course, for the nipples to develop fissures, erosions, or blisters, which can serve as entryways for bacteria and possible infection. If any of these do develop, the nurse should check with the mother to be sure she is carrying out proper nipple care. The nipples may be exposed to a lamp with a 40-watt bulb for 15 to 20 minutes. Grassley and Davis also suggest that an application of cold tea to the nipples can aid healing because of the tannic acid it contains.[19]

If symptoms of mastitis or breast abscess develop, such as localized increased warmth, tenderness, or redness, the physician should be consulted so that treatment can be started immediately. Since these problems usually occur after the woman has left the hospital, she should be given some guidance prior to discharge and instructed to observe her breasts for signs of infection. Antibiotics are usually the treatment of choice. Many physicians now feel that it is best for the woman to continue breast-feeding even when these difficulties develop.[4]

Engorgement

When the milk "comes in," the breasts suddenly become larger, firmer, and more tender. New mothers experience varying degrees of discomfort at this time. Two factors thought to be involved in causing this discomfort are venous and lymphatic congestion and the filling of the alveolar cells with milk. Ideally, the lymphatic and venous engorgement is transitory, and with early and frequent sucking by the infant, the let-down reflex will be established, the alveoli will be periodically emptied, and engorgement will not occur.

In some women, probably at least partly due to delayed emptying, the breasts do become distended or "engorged", sometimes so much so that the skin appears shiny. The tissue surrounding the nipple may also become taut to the extent that it actually retracts the nipple, making it extremely difficult for the baby to grasp the nipple and the areola adequately. The breasts may be reddened and warm to the touch, but engorgement is *not* an inflammatory process, so if fever occurs, some other cause should be suspected. With severe engorgement, the breasts can become very painful, especially when touched or moved, and throbbing pains sometimes extend into the axilla.

Although this condition is transitory and usually disappears in 24 hours to 48 hours, prompt treatment is to be instituted, not only for the mother's comfort but also to prevent the condition from progressing. If engorgement is allowed to become marked, emptying of the breasts (which is the basis of treatment) becomes very difficult because the ducts become occluded by the surrounding congested tissues and the thick and tenacious character of the retained secretions. Secondary lymphatic and venous stasis may occur because the milk cannot be emptied.

Prevention of engorgement is preferable to treatment and is generally possible with good management. Early and regular nursing is considered by many to be the best preventive measure. When the mother and infant are together around the clock as in rooming-in, engorgement tends to occur less often because the baby can nurse in response to the mother's needs as well as his own. If rooming-in is not available, the infant can be taken to the mother as soon as her breasts begin to fill and as often thereafter as is necessary to maintain her comfort.

If engorgement does occur, management is directed toward removing the milk and relieving the discomfort. To assist in moving the milk from the alveoli to the sinuses where the baby can obtain it, Murdaugh and Miller suggest that the breasts be massaged before nursing.[20] This helps to open the lacteal ducts and relieve breast tightness by increasing circulation, thus making the breast softer and the nipple area easier to grasp. The mother can be instructed to place both hands at the upper part of the breast near the clavicle. With continuous downward pressure the fingers move out and around on opposite sides of the breast until they encircle it, then slide smoothly over the tip. Some lubrication, such as lotion, should probably be used for this procedure. When the breasts begin to soften, the infant can be placed at the breast.[20]

The use of an oxytocin nasal spray by the mother before the baby nurses may also facilitate the removal of milk by encouraging the let-down reflex.

Another aid to emptying the breast and further relieving engorgement is alternate massage. To do this, the infant's sucking movements should be observed during nursing. When they become short and choppy instead of long and rhythmic, it indicates that the milk is no longer flowing as freely. Without removing the infant from the breast, the mother can alternately massage different areas of the breast to bring more milk down into the ducts where the infant can remove it by sucking.[20]

Manual expression, use of a breast pump, or use of a nipple shield to help the baby grasp the nipple are other possible recommendations. Some mothers find that the use of hot packs or a hot shower before nursing improves the flow of milk.

For relief of discomfort, ice packs applied between nursing periods may be useful. The use of a bra for good uplift support should be stressed. Analgesics such as aspirin, acetaminophen, or codeine may be needed for pain relief. They should be given in adequate dosage and with appropriate timing so that the mother can be relatively comfortable during nursing.

Expression of Milk

There are some instances in which the mother wishes to breast-feed, but for certain reasons the infant cannot be "put to breast." There are also situations in which the breast-fed infant is not able to empty the breast completely. At such times it becomes necessary to empty the breasts of milk by artificial means. Otherwise, if this condition is allowed to persist for several days, lacteal secretion is inhibited, and the future milk supply may be jeopardized. Before attempting to empty the breast by hand or pump, the mother may find it helpful to use measures to facilitate the let-down reflex, such as taking a warm shower, having a warm drink, or gently massaging the breasts.[16]

Manual Expression. It is helpful if a woman can learn this technique before the baby is born, but it can be taught afterward if necessary. The mother should have the opportunity to try it in the hospital where she can have guided practice under the supervision of the nurse, so that she will be able to do it with more confidence when she returns home.

A sterile glass or wide-mouthed container should be ready before beginning, and if the milk is to be fed to the infant, a sterile bottle and cap also will be needed. It may be desirable first to massage the breast for a few seconds to stimulate the flow of milk, as described in the section on engorgement.

The hands of the person expressing the milk are washed thoroughly with warm water and soap and dried on a clean towel. Since the daily care of the breast is designed to maintain cleanliness, the same cleansing ritual required before putting the baby to breast would be used here.

1. One hand is used to support the breast and to express the milk; the other is used to hold the container that will receive the milk. Although some authorities advocate that the right hand be used to milk the left breast, the decision as to which hand is used should depend on how the mother can accomplish this with the greatest ease.
2. The forefinger is placed below and the thumb above the outer edge of the areola. The first action is gentle but firm pressure toward the chest wall and the second is movement of the finger and thumb toward each other, then drawing forward with a slight milking motion. The forefinger is kept straight so that pressure can be exerted between the middle of this finger and the ball of the thumb. As the finger and thumb are alternately brought together and released, compressing the area of the lactiferous sinuses between them, milk is forced out in a stream (Fig. 33-8). It is of paramount importance to avoid pulling, pinching, or squeezing movements, since these can possibly bruise and damage the breast tissue.
3. The fingers should not slide forward on the areola or the nipple during the milking process. However, the position of the thumb and forefinger should be changed as the sinuses are emptied, moving in a clockwise direction, so that milk can be removed from all the sinuses.

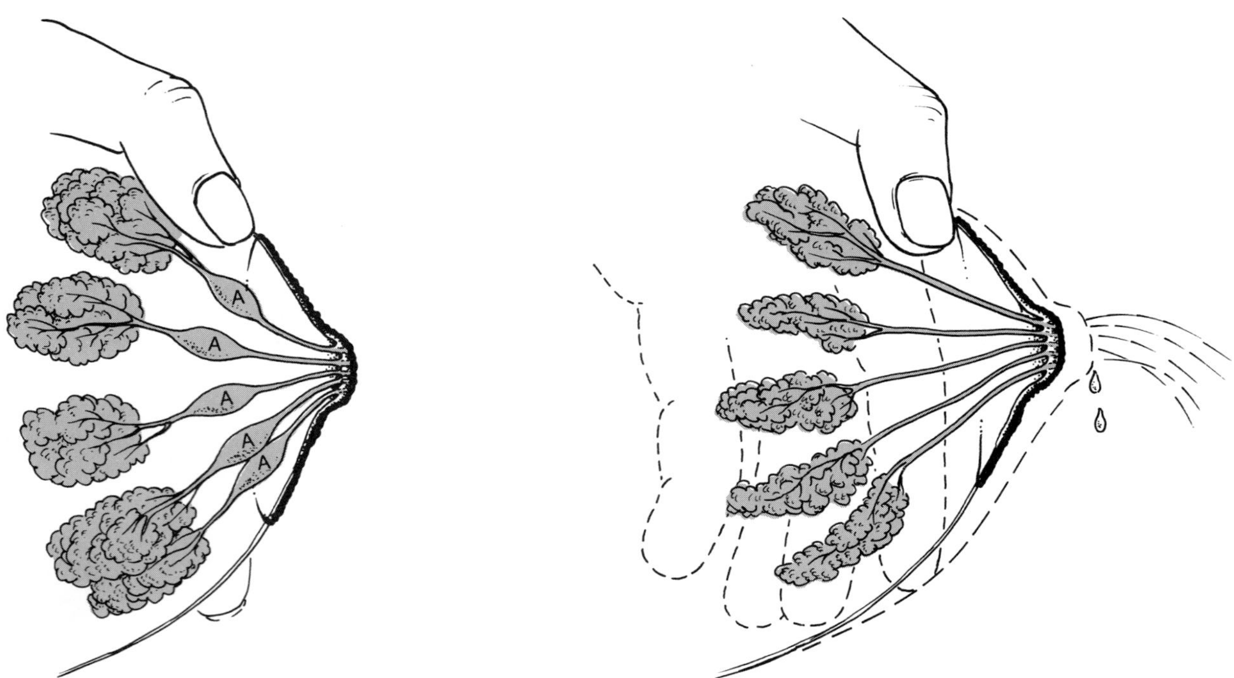

Figure 33-8.
A lateral view of the left breast showing the method of expressing the milk from the breast. The thumb and forefinger are placed on opposite sides of the breast just behind the areola. The lactiferous sinuses (ampulla A) are compressed and milk is forced out, as the thumb and forefinger are brought together. See text for complete explanation.

Many authorities advocate this method of emptying the breast rather than using the breast pump, because the action more nearly simulates the action of the infant's jaws as he nurses. Furthermore, since no mechanical equipment is required, it is a method that can be readily used when necessary after discharge from the hospital.

Electric-Pump Expression. When an electric pump is used, there is always the potential danger of traumatizing the breast tissue. This was particularly true of the older-style electric pumps that were originally designed for other purposes and then modified for use as a breast pump. The more recently introduced electric breast pumps have been specifically designed for pumping the breast and have a physiological sucking action, which decreases the danger of trauma (Fig. 33-9). Mothers using these pumps have found them efficient and easy to use.

Before using any pump, the mother should be given explanations about why it is used, how it works, and how to use it. If this information is not offered, the mother may experience fear and anxiety, which could retard the flow of milk. The nurse should stay with the mother and assist her the first few times until she feels confident to use the pump alone.

It takes approximately 5 minutes to 12 minutes to empty a breast completely, depending on the stage of lactation, but pumping should be stopped as soon as milk ceases to flow. A breast should never be pumped longer than 10 minutes at any one time. If the mother experiences back or chest pain, an indication that the breast is dry, the pumping should be stopped immediately.

The breast milk obtained is measured and the amount recorded. When only one breast is pumped at a time, the record should indicate whether it was the right or the left breast, so that the next time the other breast can be pumped. If the milk is to be fed to the infant, it can be poured into a sterile nursing bottle, labeled with the infant's name and the time and the date, and refrigerated immediately.

The electric breast pump may be used for more than one mother and thus should be washed with soap or detergent each time that it is used. In addition, certain removable parts, such as the breast-pump bottle and cap, the breast funnel, and the rubber connection tubing, must be washed thoroughly, wrapped, and autoclaved immediately after use.

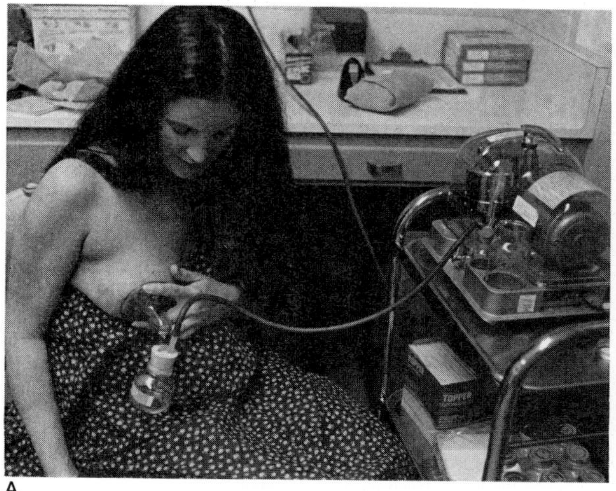

A

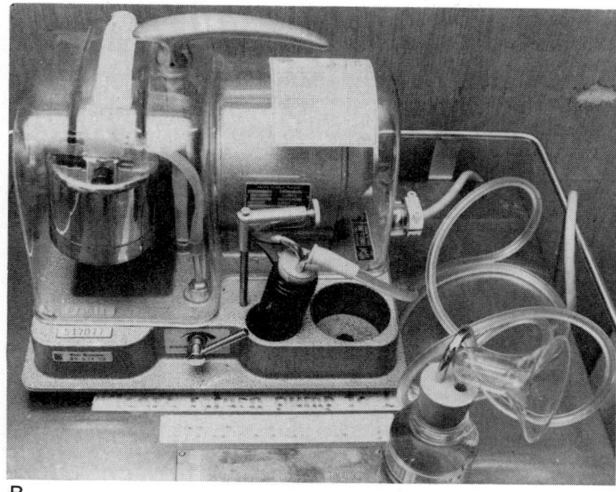

B

Figure 33-9.
Electric breast pump. *(A)* Mother using electric breast pump; *(B)* close-up of electric breast pump.

Hand-Pump Expression. The most common type of manual breast pump is the one that looks a little like a bicycle horn, with a glass cone and a rubber bulb. To minimize pain and nipple damage, which may occur if the hand pump is used improperly, the inside of the cone should first be lubricated with warm water and the bulb compressed half-way before the cone is placed on the breast and the bulb released to create suction. The bulb is alternately compressed and released to extract the milk. This pump is not very effective and the hand action can be tiring for the mother, but it is probably the least expensive.

There are several newer, nonelectric pumps on the market, which, although more expensive, are more efficient and less traumatic to breast tissue. The Kaneson Breast Milking Unit (Fig. 33-10) uses a piston-type action to remove the milk. It is small and portable and has been found to be effective and comfortable to use by many women. The Loyd-B hand pump operates with a trigger action that creates a vacuum that can be controlled by the mother, and the Ora'Lac pump operates by suction from a tube that the mother puts in her mouth.[16]

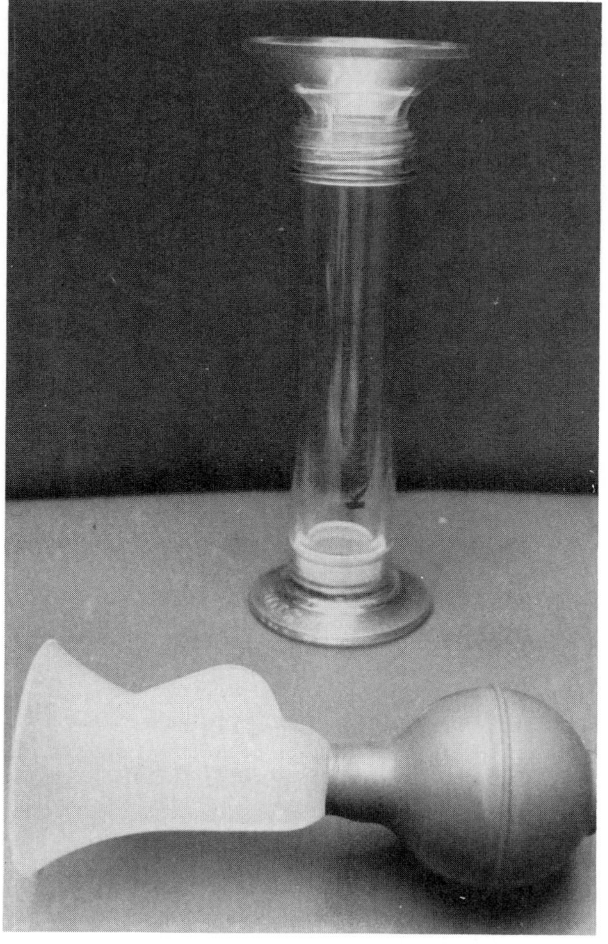

Figure 33-10.
Hand breast pumps. *(A)* Kaneson breast milking unit, *(B)* Bicycle horn pump.

Hygiene of the Nursing Mother

Rest

Rest is one of the most important considerations for the lactating mother. The detrimental effects of fatigue and worry already have been discussed. In the hospital the nurse is able to act as a buffer between the mother and some of these problems. In addition, the mother is relieved of household responsibilities and is able to have meals served to her. When she leaves the hospital, she no longer has this somewhat protected environment. Thus, it is important for the nurse to make sure that the parents understand the importance of rest and that they have made adequate plans to provide for it. If it is at all possible, the mother should have help at home. Her main energies then can be directed to the care of the infant and other family members. Housekeeping chores will have to be simplified and the mother's activity restricted so that she will get sufficient rest. Since her sleep will be broken at night, naps during the day become particularly *essential*—they should not be considered a luxury. Without adequate rest, the milk supply soon will be reduced to a dribble. If heretofore the woman has been very active, she may need special help to realize the importance of naps and rest periods. It is helpful, also, if visitors (including relatives) are restricted at first. They can become fatiguing to the mother, and they may be a source of potential infection to the newborn.

Diet

The daily diet of the lactating mother should be similar to that recommended during pregnancy (see Chap. 20) except that, according to the Food and Nutrition Board of the National Research Council, the need for calories, vitamin A, vitamin C, niacin, riboflavin, and iodine is greater than during pregnancy. It is hoped that the new mother has become more aware of good nutrition during her pregnancy and will be able to incorporate the proper foods into her diet to meet these increased needs. The nurse should discuss the recommendations with her, assess her knowledge, and give instruction as necessary.

If the mother's diet was adequate in pregnancy, additions rather than changes are all that will be necessary. Often nursing mothers, not realizing that their nutritional needs increase even over the needs of pregnancy, go back to their prepregnant diet or limit their intake in the hope of losing weight. Dieting should be discouraged during lactation. Any limitation of maternal nutrient intake during lactation can interfere with quantity of milk produced and, if the limitation is severe, with the composition of the milk.

Individual caloric needs will vary with the body size of the woman and with the quantity of breast milk produced. Since it is difficult to determine exactly how much milk is being produced, a caloric intake of 800 to 1000 calories over that recommended for a nonpregnant woman is usually suggested. The mother's weight is one of the best criteria in determining adequate caloric intake—it should remain stationary. Wide fluctuations will require that the diet be adjusted, most likely in the amount of carbohydrates and fats consumed, assuming that protein intake is adequate.

The value of protein in the diet should be stressed. The efficiency of converting the dietary protein into milk protein is about 75%, so that about three fourths of the extra protein taken in by the lactating woman is secreted in the milk she produces.[21]

Increasing the milk intake to at least 1½ quarts daily will meet the additional protein, thiamin, riboflavin, calcium, phosphorus, and niacin needs. Supplementing the citrus fruit recommendations in pregnancy with generous servings of other fruits and vegetables will meet the vitamin C requirements. To further ensure optimum vitamin and mineral intake, many physicians will prescribe that the vitamin supplement capsules taken during pregnancy be continued.

A high fluid intake also is necessary for milk production. Between 2,500 ml and 3,000 ml is recommended for the mother engaged in usual activity under pleasant environmental conditions. More may be required in hot weather or with physical exertion. This fluid intake should include a good deal of water as well as other beverages. Many mothers find that taking a beverage prior to nursing facilitates the letdown reflex. Concentrated urine or constipation may be indications of inadequate fluid intake.

Mothers have often heard that there are foods, such as chocolate and cabbage, that should be avoided during lactation. Although some babies are bothered by certain things their mothers eat, this is not universally true. Most mothers can eat any nutritious food without causing the baby any distress. If the mother herself is bothered by a particular food, she would be wise to avoid it because it could also have an effect on the baby. Eating large quantities of some foods, such as chocolate, seems to upset many babies, so moderation should be the rule. Also, some babies seem to have more sensitive taste buds and object to certain flavors that come through in the milk.

Drugs

Most drugs ingested by the mother while she is lactating are secreted in the milk, but in varying amounts and with differing effects on the infant. Concentration of the drug in the breast milk depends on several factors, including the concentration in the mother's blood, the lipid solubility of the drug, the degree of ionization, and the composition of the milk. Usually the amount of drug in the milk is small, but the cumulative effect over a 24-hour period may give the infant a fairly large dose. Some drugs seem to have highest concentrations shortly after they are ingested; therefore, taking them after breast-feeding rather than before might help to minimize the infant's exposure.[22] Delayed excretion or inactivation of drugs due to the immaturity of the infant's renal and hepatic functions can be a factor in the concentration of the drug in the infant's body. Decreased renal function in the mother can also lead to increased concentrations of drugs in the milk.

Interpreting the data concerning concentration of drugs in breast milk is hampered by the fragmentary and contradictory nature of the information available. Most drug companies state in their inserts that "Safety in pregnancy and lactation has not been established and the benefits of the drug must be weighed against possible risks." When drugs are prescribed for a nursing mother, she should remind the physician that she is breast-feeding. If she is taking drugs for a chronic condition, she should discuss their possible effects with the physician during pregnancy, before she decides on the method of feeding her infant.

Drugs that have been shown to have adverse effects on some infants should be avoided (Table 33-2). If any of these drugs are given to the mother, the infant should be kept under close observation.

Some nonprescription medications also contain drugs that can be harmful to the infant when passed through the breast milk. Mothers need to be warned to read the label of any medication they are going to take to determine the presence of any potentially dangerous components. The following examples are given by Rothermel.[23] Bromo-Seltzer and some over-the-counter sleeping aids contain bromides, which are contraindicated during lactation. Laxatives containing cascara or senna may cause diarrhea in the infant. Some preparations for migraine headaches contain ergot, which can cause vomiting, diarrhea, a weak pulse, and unstable blood pressure in the nursing infant.

Contaminants in Breast Milk

Ever since investigators first discovered DDT in breast milk in the 1950s, people have been asking if breast milk is still safe for babies. A variety of contaminants are now known to be present in breast milk, including DDT, pesticides, and other chemicals. Pesticides are stored in body fat from whence they are mobilized and enter into milk fat. Toxic chemicals, such as PCB (polychlorinated biphenyls) and PBB (polybrominated biphenyls), have also been detected in human milk. None of these substances have yet been shown to have damaging effects on human infants as a result of ingestion from mother's milk, but newborn rats were shown to have a higher mortality rate when their lactating mothers were heavily dosed with DDT.[24] Lead, another contaminant of human milk, is found in larger amounts in other forms of milk. More research is needed to determine the possible long-term effects of contaminated breast milk. The benefits of breast-feeding still seem to outweigh the possible dangers in most cases. Excessive exposure to contaminants should prompt mothers to have their milk analyzed to aid them in making a decision about the method of feeding. Nurses should join with others in attempts to rid the environment of pollutants as a more permanent solution to the problem.

Weaning

When it comes to initiating breast-feeding, many mothers receive advice and counseling. However, frequently, little is said about how or when they should stop nursing. Although stopping abruptly at a time set by the physician has sometimes been the accepted method of weaning, this can be very uncomfortable and distressing to both mother and baby. Most recent professional advice advocates that the infant be weaned slowly at a time chosen by either mother or infant. The mother should be helped, from the beginning, to feel comfortable with any length of time she chooses, even if it is considerably longer or shorter than usual.

The mother can begin to wean her infant by omitting either the feeding the infant is least interested in or the one that is least convenient for her. Parsons suggests substituting the feeding with another comforting experience that the baby enjoys, such as rocking, singing, or sucking on a pacifier.[25] Anywhere from a week to a month later, when both mother and baby are ready, another feeding may be dropped. This can be continued with periodic omissions until the child is completely off the breast. Additional omissions should be avoided when there are stressful situations in the family, such as illness, traveling, or guests. The child can be weaned to a cup or to a bottle depending on age and sucking needs.

Weaning is as likely to be traumatic to the mother as it is to the baby, especially if nursing has been a satisfying experience. Support from the father or another significant person may help guide her through this difficult time.

Sudden weaning is seldom necessary because the mother can express milk for a short time if she and the baby must be separated because of illness or absence

(Text continued on page 726)

Table 33-2.
Drugs in Breast Milk

Drug or Agent	Contra-indicated	R_X With Caution	No Apparent Harm	Insufficient Information	Comment
Analgesics					
Acetaminophen			x		
Aspirin			x		
Propoxyphene (Darvon)			x		
Anticoagulants					
Ethyl biscoumacetate	x				Bleeding infant
Phenindione	x				Bleeding infant
Heparin			x		No passage into milk
Warfarin Na (Coumadin)			x		
Bishydroxycoumarin (Dicumarol)		x			
Anticonvulsants					
Phenobarbital			x		Low levels in infant
Primadone (Mysoline)			x		? Drowsiness
Carbamazepine				x	Significant infant levels; no reported effects
Diphenylhydantoin (Phenytoin, Dilantin)			x		Low levels in infant, methemoglobin, 1 case
Antihistamines					
Diphenhydramine (Benadryl)			x		Small amounts excreted
Trimeprazine (Temaril)			x		Small amounts excreted
Tripelennamine (Pyribenzamine)			x		Small amounts excreted
Anti-infective Agents					
Aminoglycosides (Kanamycin, (gentamicin)			x		Significant excretion in milk; not absorbed
Anti-infective Agents					
Chloramphenicol	x				Bone marrow depression; gastro-intestinal and behavioral effects
Penicillins			x		Possible sensitization
Sulfonamides		x			Hemolysis, G-6-PD deficiency, bilirubin displacement
Tetracyclines			x		Limited absorption by infant
Nalidixic acid		x			Hemolysis
Nitrofurantoin		x			Possible G-6-PD hemolysis
Metronidazole (Flagyl)		x			Low absorption but potentially toxic

Table 33-2.
Drugs in Breast Milk

Drug or Agent	Contra-indicated	R_x With Caution	No Apparent Harm	Insufficient Information	Comment
Isoniazid		x			High levels in milk, possible toxicity
Pyramethamine	x				Vomiting, marrow suppression, convulsions
Chloraquine			x		Not excreted
Quinine		x			Thrombocytopenia
Anti-inflammatory					
Aspirin			x		
Indomethacin		x			Seizures, 1 case
Phenylbutazone		x			Low levels, ? blood dyscrasia
Gold	x				Found in baby; nephritis, hepatitis, hematologic changes
Steroids				x	Low levels with prednisone and prednisolone
Antineoplastic					
Cyclophosphamide	x				Neutropenia
Methotrexate	x				Very small excretion
Antithyroid					
Radioactive iodine	x				Thyroid suppression
Propylthiouracil	x				Thyroid suppression
Bronchodilators					
Aminophylline			x		Irritability, 1 case
Iodides	x				Thyroid suppression
Sympathomimetics				x	Inhalers probably safe
Cardiovascular Agents					
Digoxin			x		Insignificant levels
Propanolol			x		Insignificant levels
Reserpine	x				Nasal stuffiness, lethargy
Guanethidine (Ismelin)			x		Insignificant levels
Cardiovascular Agents					
Methyldopa (Aldomet)				x	
Cathartics					
Anthroquinones (Cascara, danthron)	x				Diarrhea, cramps
Aloe, senna		x			Safe in moderate dosage
Bulk agents, softeners			x		

(Continued)

Table 33-2.
Drugs in Breast Milk

Drug or Agent	Contra-indicated	Rx With Caution	No Apparent Harm	Insufficient Information	Comment
Contraceptives, Oral*					
Diethylstilbestrol	x				Possible vaginal cancer
Depo-provera		x			May affect lactation
Noresthisterone		x			May affect lactation
Ethinyl estradiol		x			May affect lactation
Diuretics					
Chlorthalidone				x	Low levels, but may accumulate
Thiazides		x			May affect lactation; low levels in milk
Spironolactone			x		Insignificant levels
Ergot Alkaloids					
Bromcriptine	x				Lactation suppressed
Ergot	x				Vomiting, diarrhea, seizures
Ergotamine				x	
Ergonovine	x				Brief postpartum course may be safe
Methylergonovine	x				Brief postpartum course may be safe
Hormones					
Corticosteroids				x	Low levels with short-term prednisone or prednisolone
Sex hormones (see above contraceptives, oral)					
Thyroid (T_3 or T_4)			x		Excreted in milk; may mask hypothyroid infant
Insulin			x		Not absorbed
ACTH			x		Not absorbed
Epinephrine			x		Not absorbed
Narcotics					
Codeine			x		In usual doses
Meperidine (Demerol)				x	
Morphine			x		Low infant levels on usual dosage
Heroin	x				Addiction, withdrawal in infants
Methadone		x			Minimal levels
Psychotherapeutic Drugs					
Lithium	x				High levels in milk
Phenothiazines		x			Drowsiness; chronic effects uncertain
Tricyclic antidepressants				x	Low levels; effects uncertain

*Controversy in literature; long-term effects uncertain; one case of gynecomastia

Table 33-2.
Drugs in Breast Milk

Drug or Agent	Contra-indicated	R_x With Caution	No Apparent Harm	Insufficient Information	Comment
Diazepam (Valium)	x				Lethargy, weight loss, EEG changes
Meprobamate (Equamil)	x				High levels in milk
Chlordiazepoxide (Librium)			x		Low levels in milk
Radiopharmaceuticals					
^{131}I	x				72 hr, no breast-feeding
Technetium (99M Tc)	x				48 hr, no breast-feeding
^{131}I albumin	x				10 days, no breast feeding
Sedatives-hypnotics					
Barbiturates		x			Short-acting, less depressant
Chloral hydrate		x			Drowsiness
Bromides	x				Depression, rash
Diazepam (Valium)	x				Depression, weight loss
Flurazepam				x	Chemically related to diazepam
Nitrazepam				x	
Social-recreational Drugs					
Alcohol			x		Milk levels equal plasma, moderate consumption apparently safe, high levels inhibit lactation
Caffeine			x		Jitteriness with very high intakes
Nicotine			x		Low levels in milk
Marijuana			x		Minimal passage in milk
Miscellaneous					
Atropine		x			May cause constipation or inhibit lactation
Dihydrotachysterol		x			Renal calcification in animals

(Avery GB (ed): Neonatology, 2nd ed, p 1216. Philadelphia, JB Lippincott, 1981)

(Text continued)

for some other reason. If it does become necessary, a good supportive bra and mild analgesics for discomfort will probably be helpful for the mother. Breast-drying medications used during the early puerperium do not stop established lactation.

Artificial Feeding

The mother who chooses to bottle-feed her infant may have as many concerns about feeding as the breast-feeding mother, especially if this is her first child. Depending on what she has heard about the comparison between breast milk and formula, she may feel a little uncertain about her choice and become defensive if questioned. She may also have heard about formulas disagreeing with some infants or causing allergies so that it becomes necessary to switch from one formula to another. By keeping up to date on the latest information about infant nutrition, the nurse can help allay the mother's fears about the adequacy of formulas, instruct her in safe preparation, and give guidance about when to seek medical assistance.

Comparison of Formulas

In today's hospital nursery the infant will probably receive ready-to-feed formula in a disposable bottle. However, since formula in disposable bottles is expensive, one of the other packaging methods will be recommended once the baby is ready to go home (Table 33-3). Formula is available in various sized cans in ready-to-use, concentrated, or powdered form.

Table 33-3.
Types of Formula

Type	Packaging Available	Comments
Ready-to-Feed	Small cans, large cans, bottles	Most convenient; most expensive; should not be diluted
Concentrate	Large or small cans	Less expensive; must be diluted 1:1 with water from safe source
Powder	Large cans	Least expensive; simple to prepare individual bottles with warm water from safe source; sometimes difficult to dissolve

The model usually used in planning a formula is human milk. Companies that manufacture infant formula are continually making adjustments to match new discoveries concerning the composition of human milk (Table 33-4).

To provide adequate nutrition for an infant, a formula must meet the following criteria: it must have an appropriate distribution of calories from protein, fat, and carbohydrate; it must meet the infant's need for water, energy, vitamins, and minerals; and it must be readily digestible. Recommended standards for calories, protein, fat, vitamins, and minerals in formulas have been published by the Committee on Nutrition of the American Academy of Pediatrics.[26]

Cow's milk has more protein, sodium, and calcium and less carbohydrate than human milk, but is about the same in fat, calories, and the ratio of water to solids. The protein in cow's milk is quite different from that in human milk and contains much more casein and less whey protein. The approximate whey/casein ratios are 20:80 in cow's milk and 60:40 in human milk. The increased casein leads to a tougher curd, which is more difficult to digest. Boiling or pasteurizing fresh milk, and using the process employed in making evaporated milk, will soften the curd and make it more digestible. Adding water to the milk also softens the curd and dilutes the composition, bringing it closer to human milk. However, since the dilution lowers the proportion of carbohydrate, corn syrup or dextro-maltose is usually added.

Before commercially prepared formulas became widely available, evaporated milk formulas were most commonly used. They are still less expensive than the commercial formulas and are in use in some areas. Evaporated milk contains adequate amounts of vitamins A, B, and K and is usually fortified with vitamin D, but along with fresh whole milk, it fails to meet current recommendations for vitamin C, vitamin E, and essential fatty acids.

Many ingredients and processes are used in an effort to make commercial formulas meet the recommended nutritional standards and come as close as possible to human milk. Most of the formulas, such as Similac and Enfamil, use a nonfat cow's milk base with added vegetable oil and carbohydrate. Another group, called "humanized" formulas, attempts to duplicate the 60:40 whey/casein ratio by using dialyzed whey. The dialysis removes electrolytes, bringing the formula closer to the lower-electrolyte human milk. An example of this type is SMA.

Some infants are not able to tolerate formulas based on cow's milk. Many formulas have been developed to try to meet the nutritional needs of these infants. Some of these, such as meat-based formulas,

Table 33-4.
Composition of Frequently Used Milks and Formulas

Milk or Formula	Cal/dl	Percentage Composition Pro	Fat	CHO	mmol/dl Na	K	mg/dl Ca	P	Type of Carbohydrate	Type of Protein	Remarks
Human milk	74	1.1	4.5	6.8	0.7	1.3	34	121	Lactose	Human	
Cow's milk	67	3.5	3.7	4.9	2.2	3.5	117	92	Lactose	Cow	
Goat's milk	67	3.2	4.0	4.6	1.5	4.5	129	106	Lactose	Goat	Insufficient folate
Enfamil	67	1.5	3.7	7.0	1.2	1.8	55	56	Lactose	Cow	
Enfamil with Iron	67	1.5	3.7	7.0	1.2	1.8	55	46	Lactose	Cow	
Similac	67	1.6	3.6	7.2	1.1*	2.0*	51	39	Lactose	Cow	
Similac with Iron	67	1.6	3.6	7.2	1.1*	2.0*	51	39	Lactose	Cow	
Similac PM 60/40	67	1.6	3.5	7.6	0.7	1.5	40	20	Lactose	Casein, whey	60/40 lactalbumin; casein
SMA	67	1.5	3.6	7.2	0.6	1.4	44	33	Lactose	Whey from cow, cow	60/40 lactalbumin; casein
Advance	54	2.0	2.7	5.5	1.3	2.2	51	39	Corn syrup, lactose	Cow, soy	16 cal/oz
Isomil	67	2.0	3.6	6.8	1.3	1.8	70	50	Corn syrup, sucrose, corn starch	Soy, methionine	
i-Soyalac	67	2.1	3.8	6.7	1.4	1.9	63	52	Sucrose, tapioca	Soy, methionine	
Nursoy	67	2.3	3.6	6.8	0.9	1.9	64	44	Sucrose	Soy, methionine	
ProSobee	67	2.5	3.4	6.8	1.8	1.9	79	53	Corn syrup solids	Soy, methionine	
Soyalac	69	2.2	3.8	6.6	1.5	2.0	63	52	Dextrose, maltose, sucrose	Soy, methionine	
Meat base	67	2.8	3.3	6.3	0.8	1.0	99	66	Sucrose, tapioca	Beef	High protein, low sodium

*Slightly higher if made from powder
(After Avery GB (ed): Neonatology, 2nd ed. Philadelphia, JB Lippincott, 1981)

may be difficult for the mother to accept since they do not look like milk. Soybean-derived products are commonly used as the protein source in these artificial formulas. Soy protein isolate has a lower biologic value than casein and whey, so slightly larger amounts are needed to meet the infant's nutritional needs.

Sometimes an infant will be given milk other than a formula. In our weight-conscious society it might seem that *nonfat milk* would be a good choice for an infant who was gaining weight too rapidly. Or nonfat dry milk may seem desirable for economic reasons. But nonfat milk is not recommended for infants under one year because it provides an excessive intake of protein with inadequate calories. In order to meet energy requirements and growth needs, body fat is mobilized. The infant may look healthy but have little reserve for illness. Nonfat milk also lacks an adequate content of iron, ascorbic acid, and essential fatty acids. *Low-fat* (2%) milk is midway between nonfat and whole milk in fat content, but probably would not meet all the infant's energy needs.[27]

Commercial milk substitutes such as filled milk or imitation milk are also available. *Filled milks* consist of a combination of true milk solids and a nonmilk fat. They usually have all the nutrients of regular milk but may have more carbohydrate. Depending on which nonmilk fat is used, one or more of the essential fatty acids may be missing along with the fortified vitamins that are usually found in regular milk. Thus they usually are not recommended for infants. *Imitation milk* is available in a few states. Although it may be cheaper than regular milk, it is also nutritionally inferior and should not be given to infants or children as a substitute for milk.[28]

Feeding in the Hospital

Most hospitals have a routine for when the bottle-fed baby will receive the first water feeding and when the formula feedings will start. In some hospitals it is the rule that the first water is given by the nurse in the nursery. Other hospitals are more permissive and allow the mother to give the first water. If this is the case, the nurse should show the mother how to use the bulb syringe because the water often causes the infant to bring up mucus. The nurse should also stay nearby to observe the infant's responses to the water.

The first feeding experiences can be very important for mother and infant. The mother begins to learn how the infant communicates his wants and needs, while the infant, besides learning to coordinate his feeding behaviors, begins to find out how the discomfort from hunger is relieved and who provides the relief. The nurse can help the mother and infant with these tasks by being available during initial feeding periods to observe their behaviors, assess the interaction, and intervene with suggestions or demonstrations as necessary. When intervening, the nurse should be careful not to make the mother feel as though she is incompetent or inadequate.

Before feeding begins, the mother should be helped to get into a comfortable position. She may want to sit up in a chair instead of in the bed. Holding the baby in a semireclining position will allow any air that is swallowed to rise to the top of the infant's stomach where it is more easily expelled. To minimize the amount of air swallowed, the bottle should be tilted enough to keep the nipple filled with milk (Fig. 33-11).

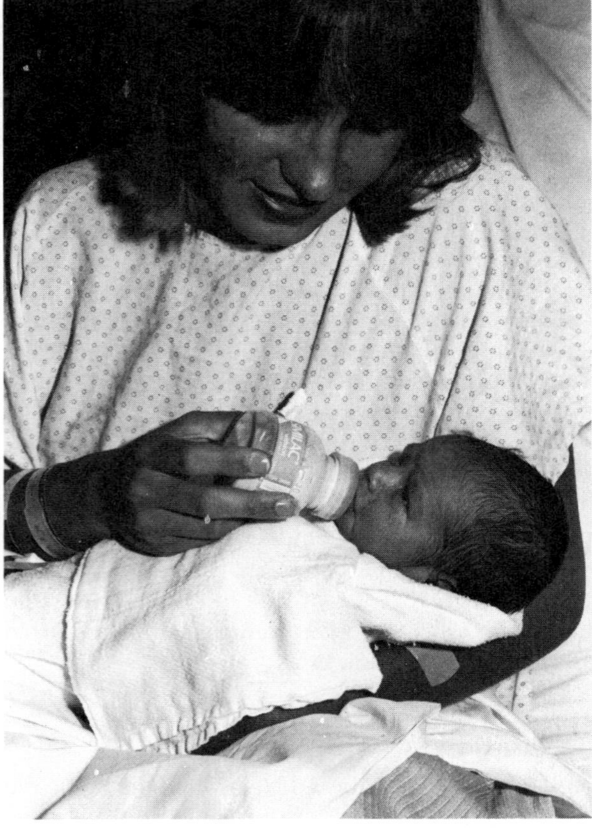

Figure 33-11.
When bottle feeding her infant, the mother tilts the bottle in such a way that the nipple is filled with milk.

The mother may need some help in getting the infant started on the bottle. If the infant does not open his mouth readily, gently stroking the lips with the nipple might help. Some babies elevate their tongue when opening their mouths and an inexperienced mother may not recognize that the nipple is under the tongue. Having the baby open his mouth wide enough so that the tongue can be seen usually helps in placing the nipple in the right position. Also, care should be taken that the nipple is not pushed too far into the mouth where it may cause gagging if it strikes the soft palate.

As the baby sucks, air bubbles rise in the bottle, indicating that the baby is getting milk. If air bubbles do not appear, the nipple should be checked to see if the hole is clogged or too small. If the milk is coming too fast the nipple holes may be too large. Nipple holes can be checked by holding the bottle upside down. The milk should drop freely but not run in a stream. If milk is coming at the right speed a feeding should take 15 to 20 minutes. If it takes much longer the infant may get too tired, but if it is much shorter the infant may not meet his sucking needs.

Babies have many different feeding behaviors, some of which may not correspond to the mother's expectations. Identifying the infant's individual behavior patterns and interpreting the baby's individuality to the mother can help to avert potential problems.[29]

If the mother is concerned that the baby is not taking enough milk, it may help her to know that babies are often sleepy the first few days after birth but that they are born with reserves of fat and water and do not really need many calories until the second or third day.[27] The bottle-fed baby, like the breast-fed baby, should have the opportunity to be on a self-demand schedule. Some babies get hungry more frequently than every 4 hours and some will want to wait longer than that between some feedings.

Before the mother and baby leave the hospital, the mother should be given some anticipatory guidance in how much formula the infant may take and how to prepare it.

According to the Recommended Dietary Allowances established by the Food and Nutrition Board of the National Academy of Sciences in 1973, infants from birth to 5 months need approximately 117 calories/kg (51 calories/lb) each day. From 6 months to a year the need decreases to 108 calories/kg (47 calories/lb).[30] Using this as a guide, the nurse can help the mother calculate the infant's daily caloric needs. Most formula contains 20 calories per ounce, so a 7-pound baby would need about 17½ ounces a day, or a little less than 3 ounces at each of six feedings. As the infant grows, he will increase his consumption. At times of particularly fast growth, he will want to eat more at each feeding or more frequently. Again, the reminder should be given that each baby is an individual and that babies of the same age and weight may have different needs.

Preparation of Formula at Home

Bottles and Nipples

With the wide variety of bottles and nipples available on the market, selection depends on the parents' preference. Some will prefer glass bottles with plastic nipple caps; others will opt for the boilable plastic bottles that are nonbreakable. There are also kits that have a hollow plastic holder in which a disposable plastic bag containing the milk is suspended. Supposedly less air will be swallowed with this method because the bag collapses rather than filling with air when the milk is sucked out. However, the infant can still swallow air around the nipple.

Nipples also come in several shapes and sizes. One supposedly resembles the mother's breast in appearance; another (Nuk) is supposed to elicit sucking responses more like the breast. The number of bottles and nipples needed will depend on the method of preparation. (For examples of bottles and nipples available, see Fig. 33-12).

Methods of Preparation

Strict sterilization procedures for preparing formulas have been considered a must in the past. Some recent studies have shown that formulas that are prepared at home and sterilized are frequently contaminated.[31] Many physicians are no longer insisting that bottles or formulas be sterilized if there is an uncontaminated water source and good refrigeration, and if hands and equipment are cleaned properly, since this clean technique is proving to be as safe as sterilization. There was no higher incidence of illness or infection when infants were fed formula prepared by the clean technique than when infants were fed formula prepared by terminal sterilization.[32]

There are four basic methods of formula preparation (Table 33-5). Points common to all methods of preparation are the following:

1. Hands should be washed well before starting.
2. If canned milk is used, the top of the can should be washed with soap and water using friction and

Figure 33-12.
Types of bottles and nipples. From left to right: a disposable bag and nipple cover; the bottle and nipple that is used with the disposable bag; regular bottle with Nuk nipple; and ready-to-feed bottle with standard nipple.

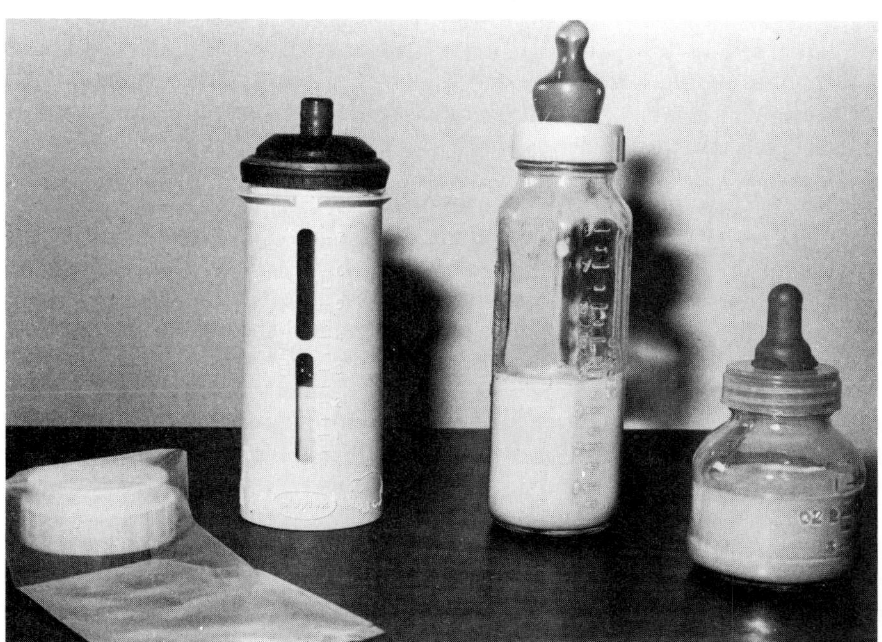

Table 33-5.
Formula Preparation Using Concentrated Formula

One Bottle Method	Clean Method	Aseptic Method	Terminal Sterilization
1. Open can of concentrated formula; pour ½ of total amount desired into bottle. 2. Add equal amount of fresh tap water from safe source. 3. Feed within 30 minutes of preparation. 4. Discard if not used within 1 hour.	1. Same as one bottle method, but prepare day's supply at one time. 2. Refrigerate immediately after preparation.	1. Equipment includes glass or enamel pitcher; measuring cup and spoons, mixing spoons, funnel, can opener, tongs. 2. Sterilize bottles, nipples, nipple caps, and equipment by boiling for 10 minutes in pan or sterilizer half full of water. 3. Mix formula in pitcher. 4. Pour into bottles. 5. Put on nipples and caps. Refrigerate until needed.	1. Prepare as in clean method. 2. Apply nipples and caps loosely. 3. Place in sterilizer with water in bottom and cover with tight-fitting lid. 4. Boil for 25 minutes. 5. Tighten nipple collars. 6. Refrigerate until needed.

For all methods start by washing hands, formula can top, bottles, nipples, and equipment well.
Ready-to-feed and powdered formula can be prepared by any of the above methods.
Ready-to-feed formula needs no water or mixing.
For powdered formula follow directions on can for proportions.

then rinsed thoroughly. Hot water can be poured over the top just before opening.

3. All equipment should be washed thoroughly in warm soapy water. A bottle and nipple brush should be used and water should be squeezed through the nipple to make sure no milk particles or residue remain. Rinse thoroughly so all soap or detergent is gone.
4. Opened cans of formula or milk should be covered with fresh foil or plastic wrap, placed in the refrigerator, and used within 48 hours.

One Bottle Method. This is the method recommended in the pamphlet, *Infant Care,* put out by the Children's Bureau of HEW.[33] According to these recommendations, a concentrated prepared infant formula is poured directly into the bottle once the four steps mentioned above are carried out. One half of the total amount of formula desired is measured according to the markings on the bottle. For example, if 4 ounces of formula is needed, 2 ounces of concentrated formula would be used. Assuming a safe water supply, an equal amount of fresh tap water is added. The formula in the bottle should be fed to the infant within 30 minutes of the time it is made. If it is not used within an hour, it should be discarded.

Clean Method. The major difference between the clean method and the one bottle method is that in the former the whole day's formula is prepared at one time. The bottles should be refrigerated immediately after preparation.

Since some physicians still recommend sterilization and since some people still live under conditions where sterilization is necessary, the aseptic method and terminal sterilization are included in this discussion.

Aseptic Method. In this method, the bottles, nipples, nipple caps, and equipment used in making the formula are sterilized before the formula is prepared. The mother will need a glass or enamel pitcher in which to mix the formula, a measuring cup, measuring spoons, tablespoon (to mix the formula), funnel (depending on the size of the bottle mouth), can opener (if canned milk is used), and some kind of tongs that can be sterilized. The tongs will be used as a forceps to handle the equipment. These items, together with the bottles, caps, and nipples, are placed in a large pan or sterilizer half full of water and boiled vigorously for 10 minutes. The equipment and the bottles, nipples, and so on may be done separately if the sterilizer cannot accommodate such a large load. Care should be taken to place the forceps in such a way that the mother can reach the handles easily after sterilization without burning her hand and contaminating the water when she picks them up. After sterilization the formula is made according to directions. A specific amount of the formula is put into each bottle. The bottles are then nippled, capped, and refrigerated.

Terminal Sterilization. In this method, the formula is prepared under a clean but not aseptic technique. The equipment, bottles, nipples, and nipple caps are washed thoroughly but are not sterilized. The formula is prepared and poured into the bottles, and the nipples and the caps are applied loosely. They then are placed in the sterilizer, covered with a tight-fitting lid, and sterilized by having the water boil rapidly in the bottom of the sterilizer for 25 minutes. In this method, formula, bottles, nipples, and protectors are all sterilized in one operation. Before the formula is refrigerated, the screw collar should be made secure.

Common Concerns in Infant Feeding

There are several topics related to infant feeding that are of concern to the new mother regardless of the method of feeding.

Hunger

The mother may wonder how she can tell if her infant is getting enough to eat. She can be told that most babies when awakened from sleep by hunger "pains" will fuss and cry and make sucking movements with their mouths, but that at first the infant may have difficulty distinguishing between hunger and other discomforts. If the baby awakens a short time after a feeding, the mother should try other comfort measures such as holding, changing the diaper, and bubbling, before assuming he is hungry. Occasionally a baby appears hungry when in reality he is only thirsty and will be satisfied with a small amount of water. If he is obviously hungry and crying, refuses water with apparent disgust, and when a feeding is offered seizes the nipple ravenously and nurses with great vigor, he may need to eat more frequently for a while if he is breast-fed or be offered more in his bottle at each feeding if he is bottle-fed.

Bubbling (Burping)

After 5 minutes or so, or in the middle and at the end of each feeding, the infant should be held in an upright position and his back *gently* patted or stroked (Fig. 33-13). Pounding the baby on the back vigorously is neither effective for bubbling him nor conducive to his well-being. The change in position (from semi-reclining to upright) is an important factor in eliciting a bubble. Often holding the infant upright and pressing him against the breast is all that is necessary.

Assisting the New Mother with Bottle-Feeding

1. Assess knowledge and needs.
2. Assist in finding comfortable position for mother and infant. Stress importance of holding infant for feeding.
3. Teach techniques of feeding:
   a. Feeding reflexes
   b. Placement and positioning of bottle in infant's mouth
   c. Angle to hold bottle to keep nipple full
   d. Burping method
4. Teach about formula preparation:
   a. Types of formula available.
   b. Methods of preparation.
5. Give support and reassurance.

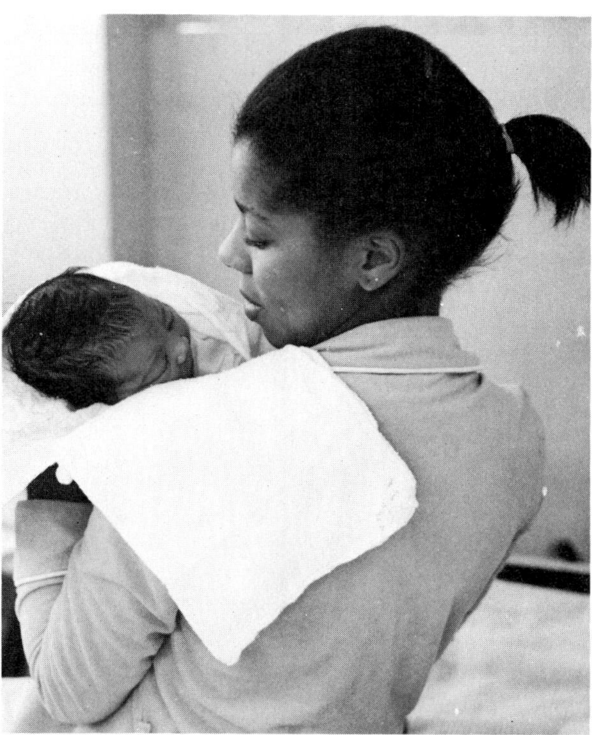

Figure 33-13.
One method of bubbling or burping an infant is to place him in an upright position over the shoulder where he can be pressed against the breast.

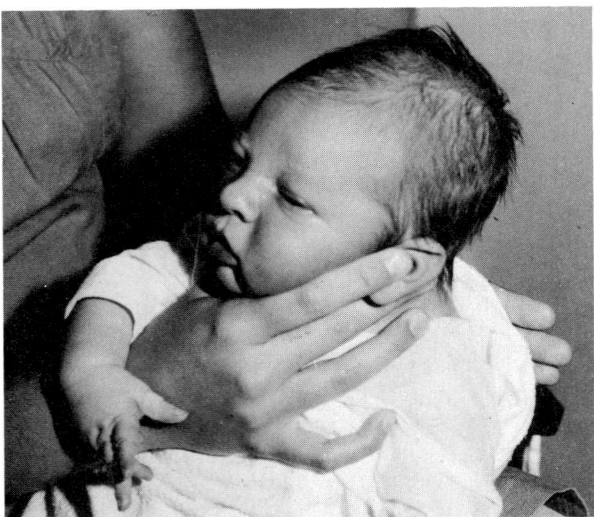

Figure 33-14.
When bubbling the infant in the nursery, the nurse sits the infant up in her lap, with his chest resting on her hand and his chin supported by her thumb and index finger.

An alternate position is for the mother to sit the infant up on her lap, with his chest resting on her hand and his chin supported by her thumb and index finger, while she pats him with her other hand. A third position is to place the infant prone over her knees with the knee nearest the head elevated slightly. The last two positions are sometimes preferred by nurses in the newborn nursery because they keep the infant away from the nurse's face and hair (Figs. 33-14 and 33-15).

Because the new infant's gastrointestinal tract is labile, milk may be eructated with the gas bubbles. A diaper is usually kept in front of the infant while he is being bubbled, in case this occurs (Fig. 33-13). If there is doubt about whether or not the infant has brought up all the air when he is placed in his crib, putting him on his right side or in a prone position will help bring up the air and also prevent the infant from choking on any milk that might be regurgitated with the air.

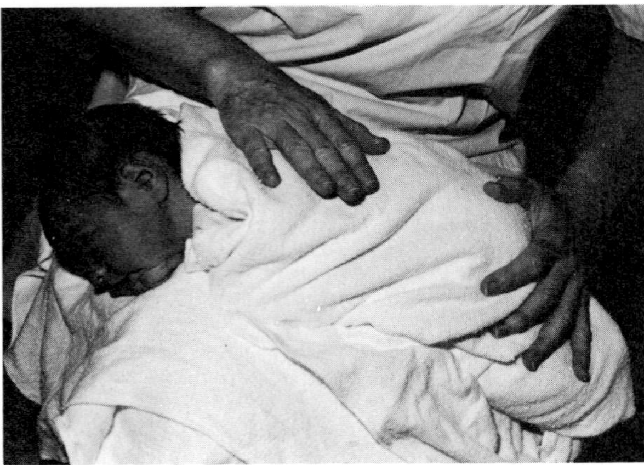

Figure 33-15.
For an alternate method of bubbling, the infant is placed over the knees while his back is gently rubbed.

Regurgitation

Regurgitation, which is merely an overflow and often occurs after nursing, should not be confused with vomiting, which may occur at any time, is accompanied by other symptoms, and usually involves a more complete emptying of the stomach. This regurgitation is the means of relieving the distended stomach and usually indicates that the baby either has taken too much food or has taken it too rapidly.

Hiccups

Some mothers need reassurance that hiccups are not unusual for infants and really do not seem to bother them. If the mother is disturbed, she can try giving the infant a few sips of water, but the hiccups go away by themselves without treatment.

Constipation

This is almost nonexistent in breast-fed babies and uncommon in those fed commercially prepared formulas, but mothers frequently express concern about possible constipation. Many parents believe that an infant is constipated if he misses having a bowel movement one day. The nurse can explain that it is quality not frequency of the stool that indicates the presence of constipation. An infant is considered to be constipated when the stools are hard, formed, and difficult to pass.

Nutritional Considerations During the First Year

Diets for infants are sometimes based on temporary scientific fashions or local customs. Long-term effects of infant diets are not known. Standards for formulas and baby foods are based on infant growth, but it is not known whether a diet that is optimum for growth in infancy will offer freedom from allergy, obesity, arterial disease, or cancer later in adult life.

During the first year of life the infant's growth exceeds that of any future period. In the first four months he usually doubles his birth weight and may triple it by one year. Watching the infant grow is pleasing to the parents, and they often see the chubbiness of the infant as evidence of good health and their good parenting. This attitude can lead to overfeeding.

The infant's caloric needs per unit of body weight are relatively constant during the first year. This is because as he becomes more physically active from the fourth month on, his rate of growth is slowing down, and energy is relocated from growth to activity.

Introduction of Solid Foods

The time for adding solid foods is an area where recommendations in the literature and actual practice often differ markedly. Although an adequate amount of all essential nutrients can be provided during the first six months without the addition of solids, many babies in the United States are receiving solid foods before they are a month old.[34] This early feeding often occurs because the parents request it, thinking it will help the baby sleep through the night or considering it a sign that he is more advanced than infants who are "only taking milk."

There are many reasons suggested for delaying the introduction of solids until the infant is 4 to 6 months old. First, the baby is not developmentally ready to deal with nonliquid foods until about the end of the third month, and his tongue will usually push them out of the mouth. Also, the large protein molecules from the foods may pass through the mucosa of the infant's immature gastrointestinal tract and become antigens, sensitizing the infant and causing allergic reactions. After 6 months the gastrointestinal system is more mature and the infant's antibody production has reached a more desirable level. In the breast-fed infant, early introduction of solids may interfere with the desire for breast milk, decreasing the infant's sucking and subsequently decreasing the milk supply. Other drawbacks to early feeding of solids are the potential for not supplying the infant's nutritional needs, the relatively high cost of the food, and the possibility of overfeeding.

Infantile obesity has become a growing concern in recent years because of its possible relation to adult obesity. Growth during infancy is mostly due to cell hyperplasia (tissue growth involving increases in the number of cells). It is felt that the obese infant will have more fat cells than normal throughout life and therefore be more prone to continuing obesity.[35]

Some suggestions for avoiding infant obesity are as follows:

1. Help parents use factors other than weight gain to evaluate their role as parents.
2. Help mothers discover the infant's satiety behavior and avoid encouraging the infant to get down the last drop or bite.
3. Encourage practices that promote more physical activities in infants.
4. Avoid early introduction of solids.

Nutritional Supplements

Vitamins

Woodruff states that since both breast milk and prepared formulas contain adequate vitamins for normal infants, routine supplementation should be abandoned.[27] However, some sources still recommend a vitamin D supplement for breast-fed babies. If the infant is on a formula made of fresh or evaporated cow's milk, a vitamin C supplement might be necessary.

Iron

Iron-deficiency anemia is currently the most common specific nutritional deficiency encountered. Infants and children between the ages of 6 and 30 months, especially those from lower socioeconomic groups, are particularly vulnerable. Breast-fed infants rarely have iron-deficiency anemia and it is now recommended that formulas be fortified with iron at a level of 10 mg to 12 mg per liter. Infant cereal has been fortified with iron for a long time, but the form of iron used was recently found to be poorly absorbed and has now been changed to a more absorbable form in most cereals.

These sources of iron would probably be adequate, but they may not continue to be available to the infant as he grows older. By the age of 6 months many infants are switched to fresh cow's milk. This causes two problems. First, cow's milk is low in iron. Second, there is increasing evidence that drinking fresh cow's milk during infancy is associated with occult blood loss from the intestine, resulting in iron-deficiency anemia. The latter is less likely if the milk is boiled. Prepared formulas fortified with iron are recommended for the nonbreast-fed baby for the first 12 months of life.[27]

References

1. Neumann CC, Jelliffe DB: Foreword. Symposium on Nutrition in Pediatrics. Pediatr Clin North Am 24, 1:1, February, 1977

2. Smith C, Nelson N: The Physiology of the Newborn Infant. Springfield, IL, Charles C Thomas, 1979

3. Jelliffe DB, Jelliffe EFP: Current concepts in nutrition, Breast is best; Modern meanings. N Engl J Med 912–915, October 27, 1977

4. Nichols BL, Nichols VN: The biologic basis of lactation. Compre Ther 4, 10:63–70, October 1978

5. Grams KE: Breast feeding: A means of imparting immunity? MCN 3, 6:340–344, November/December, 1978

6. Gunther M: The value of breast feeding. In Early Nutrition and Later Development. Chicago, Year Book Medical Publishers, 1976

7. Gerard A: Please Breast-feed Your Baby, Chap. 7. New York, Hawthorn Books, 1970

8. Dutton MA: A breastfeeding protocol. JOGN 8, 3:151–155, May/June 1979

9. Lawson B: Perception of degrees of support for the breast-feeding mother. BFJ 3:2, Summer, 1976

10. Johnson NW: Breast feeding at one hour of age. MCN 121:12–16, January/February, 1976

11. Jelliffe DB, Jelliffe EFP: Human Milk in the Modern World, p. 30. Oxford, Oxford University Press, 1978

12. Lawrence RA: Breastfeeding—A Guide for the Medical Profession, p. 47. St. Louis, CV Mosby, 1980

13. Committee on Fetus and Newborn: Hospital Care of Newborn Infants, 6th ed, p. 73. Chicago, American Academy of Pediatrics, 1977

14. Countryman BA: Hospital care of the breastfed newborn. Am J Nurs 71:2365–2367, December, 1971

15. Iffrig SM: Nursing care and success in breast feeding. Nurs Clin North Am 3:353, June, 1968

16. Nichols MG: Effective help for the nursing mother. JOGN 7, 2:22–30, March/April, 1978

17. Haire D, Haire J: The nurse's contribution to successful breast-feeding; and The medical value of breast-feeding. Implementing Family Centered Maternity Care with a Central Nursery, New Jersey, ICEA

18. Whitley N: Preparation for breastfeeding. JOGN 7, 3:44–48, May/June, 1978

19. Grassley J, Davis K: Common concerns of mothers who breastfeed. MCN 3, 6:347–351, November/December, 1978

20. Murdaugh Sr A, Miller LE: Helping the breast-feeding mother. Am J Nurs 72:1420–1423, August, 1972

21. MacKeith R, Wood C: Infant Feeding and Feeding Difficulties. Edinburgh, Churchill Livingstone, 1977

22. Horning MG et al: Identification and quantification of drugs and drug metabolites in human breast milk using GC-MS-COM methods. In Modern Problems in Paediatrics—Milk and Lactation 15:73–79, Basel, S. Korger, 1975

23. Rothermel BS, Faber MM: Drugs in breastmilk—A consumer's guide. BFJ 2, 3:76–88, Summer, 1975

24. Doucette JS: Is breast feeding still safe for babies? MCN 3, 6:345–346, November/December, 1978

25. Parsons LJ: Weaning from the breast. JOGN 7, 3:12–15, May/June, 1978

26. American Academy of Pediatrics, Committee on Nutrition: Commentary on breast feeding and infant formulas, including proposed standards for formulas. Pediatrics 57:278–285, February, 1976

27. Woodruff C: The science of infant nutrition and the art of infant feeding. JAMA 240, 7:657–661, August 18, 1978

28. Brown MS, Murphy MA: Ambulatory Pediatrics for Nurses. New York, McGraw-Hill, 1975

29. Scahill MC: Helping the mother solve problems with feeding her infant. JOGN 4, 2:51–54, March/April, 1975

30. Slattery J: Nutrition for the normal healthy infant. MCN 2, 2:105–112, March/April, 1977

31. Kendall V, Kusakcroglu: A study of preparation of infant formulas. Am J Dis Child 122:215, 1971

32. Hargrove T, Hargrove C: Formula preparation and infant illness. Clin Pediatr 13:1057, 1974

33. Children's Bureau, U.S. Department of Health, Education, and Welfare: Infant Care, p. 11. Washington, D.C., U.S. Government Printing Office, 1973

34. Anderson TA, Fomon S: Beikost. In Infant Nutrition, 2nd ed. Philadelphia, WB Saunders, 1974

35. Parham E: The effect of early feeding on the development of obesity. JOGN 3, 3:58–61, May/June, 1975

Suggested Reading

Arafat I et al: Maternal Practice and Attitudes Toward Breast-feeding. JOGN 10, 2:91–95, March/April, 1981

Avery GB, Fletcher AB: Nutrition. In Avery GB (ed): Neonatology, 2nd ed. Philadelphia, JB Lippincott, 1981

Broome ME: Breast-feeding and the working mother. JOGN 10, 3:201–202, May/June, 1981

Cadwell K: Improving nipple graspability for success at breast-feeding. JOGN 10, 4:277–279, July/August, 1981

Foman SJ (ed): Infant Nutrition. Philadelphia, WB Saunders, 1974

Giacoia GP, Catz CS: Drugs and pollutants in breast milk. Clin Perinatol 6, 1:181–196, March, 1979

Hambraeus L: Proprietary milk vs human breast milk in infant feeding. Pediatr Clin North Am 24, 1:17–35, February, 1977

Jelliffe DB, Jelliffe EFP: Human Milk in the Modern World. New York, Oxford University Press, 1978

Lawrence RA: Breast-Feeding: A Guide for the Medical Profession. St Louis, CV Mosby, 1980

Lawrence RA (ed): Counseling the Mother on Breast-Feeding. Report of the Eleventh Ross Roundtable on Critical Approaches to Common Pediatric Problems. Columbus, Ohio, Ross Laboratories, 1980

L'Esperance CM: Pain or pleasure: The dilemma of early breast-feeding. BFJ 7, 1:21–26, Spring, 1980

Markesbery BA, Wong WM: Watching baby's diet: A professional and parental guide. MCN 4, 3:177–180, May/June, 1979

Riordan J, Countryman BA: Basics of breast-feeding. Parts I and II. JOGN 9, 4:207–213, July/August, 1980; Parts III and IV, JOGN 9, 5:273–283, September/October, 1980; Parts V and VI, JOGN 9, 6:357–366, November/December, 1980

Waletzky LR (ed): Symposium on Human Lactation. Rockville, MD, U.S. Department of Health, Education and Welfare, Bureau of Community Health Services, 1976

Worthington-Roberts B et al: Nutrition in Pregnancy and Lactation, 2nd ed, Chaps. 7 and 8. St. Louis, CV Mosby, 1981

Study Aids for Unit VI:
Postpartal Assessment and Management of the New Family

Conference Material

1. Discuss in detail the mechanisms by which lactation occurs, including hormonal preparation of the breasts, neurohormonal control of milk secretion and ejection, effects of noxious stimuli, and approaches to the suppression of lactation. What implications for nursing care can be found by understanding the physiology of this delicate mechanism?

2. Describe the patterns of return of menstruation and ovulation in nonlactating and lactating women. Include in your discussion anovulatory versus ovulatory menses, the influence of breast-feeding upon both ovulation and menstruation, and the risk of pregnancy with unprotected intercourse. How would you counsel a postpartum patient who was (a) not breast-feeding, and (b) breast-feeding, about what to expect regarding first menstruation and return of fertility?

3. A mother experienced a sudden postpartum hemorrhage after delivery and the infant had to be taken to the nursery immediately after birth. What assessments and interventions might you plan to aid in reinstituting the bonding process?

4. Rita R. delivered her second baby 3 days ago and is to be discharged home this afternoon. Mother and infant are healthy and have adapted well to each other during their hospital stay. Rita is breast-feeding and her milk just began to come in today. Her husband, who will take her home later, has been able to take 1 week off from work. Their chid at home is 2½ years of age. You have set aside 30 minutes to counsel Rita about the first few weeks at home. What topics will you include in this discussion, and what key points will you make concerning each? How did you set priorities for these topics?

5. Elizabeth S. is an 18-year-old primipara who underwent a long but normal labor and delivery. She and her 20-year-old husband are fascinated with their new son, although neither have experience caring for children. On her second postpartum day, Elizabeth experiences severe discomfort from her large mediolateral episiotomy, to the point of not wanting to care for the baby. What measures will you initate to promote her comfort? What will be the primary focus of your nursing care plans for the remainder of her hospital stay?

6. What approach would you use to help a mother who was undecided about whether or not to breast-feed her infant?

7. A mother tells the nurse that she wants to breast-feed her infant for 6 months to 8 months because she knows she can not become pregnant as long as she is nursing. What information should the nurse include in her reply?

8. A mother who is bottle-feeding tells the nurse she does not know anything about preparing formula so she thinks she will buy "ready-to-feed" formula that comes in bottles. What do you think about this plan? How can the nurse help her in choosing the type of formula to use and the method of preparation?

Study Aids for Unit VI:
Postpartal Assessment and Management of the New Family

Multiple Choice

Read through the entire question and place your answer on the line to the right.

1. The principles found to be involved in bonding are

A. There is a species-specific response between the parents and infant when the infant is first given to them.
B. The attachment process is structured around monotropy.
C. The infant must give some signal with eye or body movements to the parents.
D. Individuals who witness the birth process become strongly attached to the infant.
E. There is no particular sensitive period after the birth.
F. It is difficult for parents to attach to an infant while mourning the loss or expected loss of another person.
G. Some early events may have a long-lasting effect on the raising and caretaking of the infant.

Select the number corresponding to the correct letter or letters.

1. All but A
2. All but B
3. All but D
4. All but E
5. All of the above ____

2. Engrossment refers to

A. The infant becoming interested in moving objects and smiling faces
B. The parents' interest in their infant
C. The behavior noted in fathers when they are interacting with their infants
D. The behavior noted in mothers when they are interacting with their infants

Select the number corresponding to the correct letter or letters.

1. A only
2. B only
3. C only
4. C and D
5. A and B
6. All but A ____

3. Research indicates that fathers who attend the birthing process

A. Feel a significant strengthening of the marital bond
B. Exhibit much more loving behavior to their mates
C. Exhibit significantly more attachment behavior to their infants
D. Have significantly more desire to have more children

Select the number corresponding to the correct letter or letters.

1. A only
2. C only
3. A and B
4. A and C
5. All of the above ____

4. Rubin's description of the tasks of mothering includes
A. Determining her relationship with her child
B. Identifying the child
C. Redefining her relationship with her husband
D. Guiding and restructuring the family constellation

Select the number corresponding to the correct letter or letters.
1. A only
2. B only
3. D only
4. All but D
5. All but C
6. All but A _____

5. To keep the nipples in good condition for breast-feeding, which of the following should be included in their daily care?
A. Wash with plain water once a day.
B. Air dry after each nursing period.
C. Wash with mild antiseptic solution prior to each feeding period.
D. Cover the nipples with clean plastic squares to avoid contamination.
E. If nipple is sore, discontinue breast-feeding until tenderness subsides.

Select the number corresponding to the correct letters.
1. A and B
2. A, C, and D
3. B, D, and E
4. All of the above _____

6. The young mother asks how she will know when her baby is hungry. Which of the following responses would be most appropriate for the nurse to give?
A. "All crying indicates hunger."
B. "Feed the baby whenever he is awake."
C. "He will cry, fret, and suck on anything in contact with his lips."
D. "Offer him water first; if he refuses the water, feed him." _____

7. How does the composition of mother's milk compare with cow's milk?
A. Human milk contains more whey protein.
B. Human milk contains more casein.
C. Human milk forms a tougher curd.
D. Human milk contains more carbohydrates.
E. Human milk contains less sodium.

Select the number corresponding to the correct letters.
1. A and C
2. A, D, and E
3. B, C, and D
4. All of the above _____

8. Which of the following is true of the let-down reflex?
   A. It occurs unilaterally.
   B. It is under voluntary control.
   C. It is usually felt by the mother as a tingling or drawing sensation in the nipple.
   D. It is not affected by external stimuli. ____

9. What is the principle underlying the concept of demand feedings for the newborn infant?
   A. Maintaining a regular 4-hour schedule to establish eating habits
   B. Feeding the infant every 2 hours to 3 hours to stimulate digestion
   C. Fitting individual feedings to individual needs
   D. Permissive feeding schedule causes less conflict with the mother's household activities
   E. More frequent feedings assure an adequate nutritional intake ____

Discussion

10. What are the physiological processes that affect involution of the uterus?

11. When is involution completed for the following organs and tissues: uterus, cervix, vagina, ureters, and fallopian tubes?

12. Describe the progression of the lochia after delivery.

13. What differences are commonly found between nulliparous and multiparous cervices?

14. Muscular-fascial relaxation of the vagina after birth may cause what clinical conditions?

15. Why is the early postpartum period the time of greatest risk of heart failure in women with heart disease?

16. What physiological changes and processes are responsible for the marked postpartal diuresis?

17. What is the average time after delivery of first menstruation in nonlactating and lactating women?

18. Why is constipation a frequent problem in the early postpartum period?

19. How much weight is generally lost after delivery, and what are the sources of this loss?

20. The removal of the inhibitory effect of which two hormones, in the presence of continued secretion of which other hormone, are keys to the initiation of lactation?

21. What is the cause of postpartal afterpains?

22. Why is it important for mother, father, and newborn to spend some time together privately during the first hour after birth?

23. What is included in the postdelivery observations?

24. Describe the procedure for checking the condition of the uterine fundus in the postdelivery period.

25. What is the danger of a boggy uterus?

26. What signs alert the nurse to postpartum hemorrhage?

27. Why is early ambulation after delivery important for promoting maternal health?

28. What advice is the postpartum mother given regarding showers and baths?

29. How can the nurse determine that the patient is adequately emptying her bladder?

30. What measures are useful in alleviating postpartal constipation?

31. What instructions are included in teaching the patient perineal care?

32. How may the nurse identify possible thrombophlebitis?

33. What is the recommended breast care for both lactating and nonlactating mothers?

34. What recommendations are given regarding exercises?

35. How is the postpartum mother counseled about contraception before her discharge from the hospital?

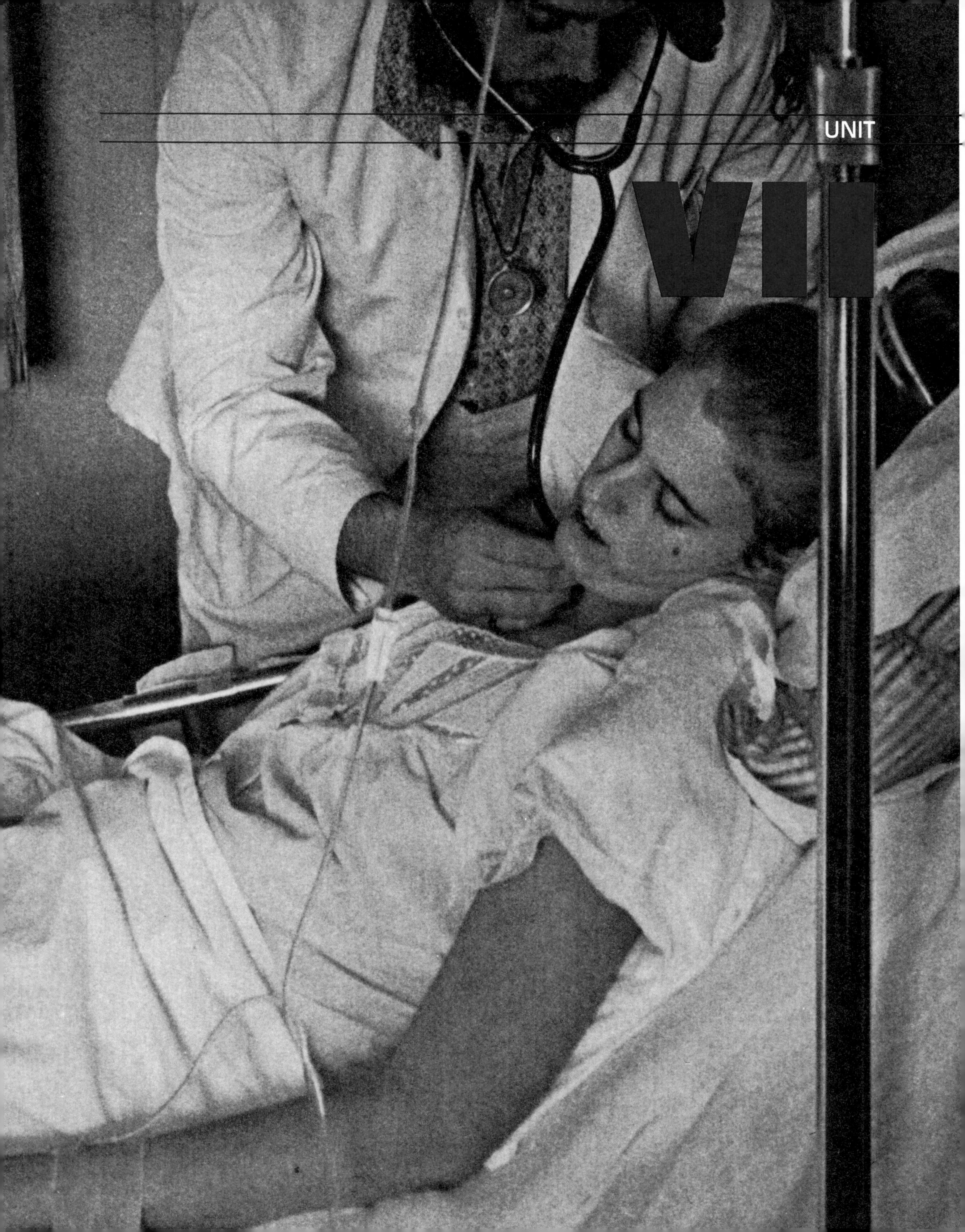

UNIT VII

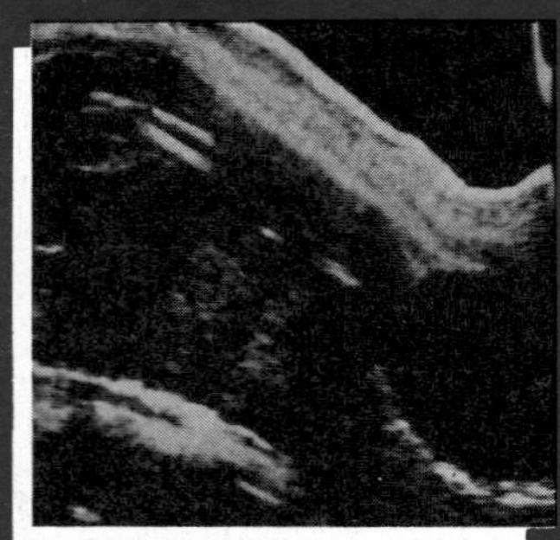

34 Complications of Pregnancy

Hemorrhagic Complications of Early Pregnancy

Hyperemesis Gravidarum

Hemorrhagic Complications of Late Pregnancy

The Hypertensive Disorders of Pregnancy

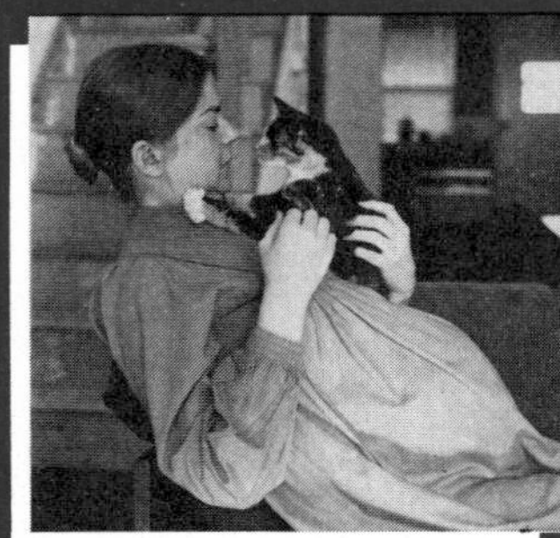

35 Concurrent Diseases in Pregnancy

Hematologic Disorders

Heart Disease

Diabetes Mellitus

Disturbances in Thyroid Function

Renal Disease

Infectious Diseases

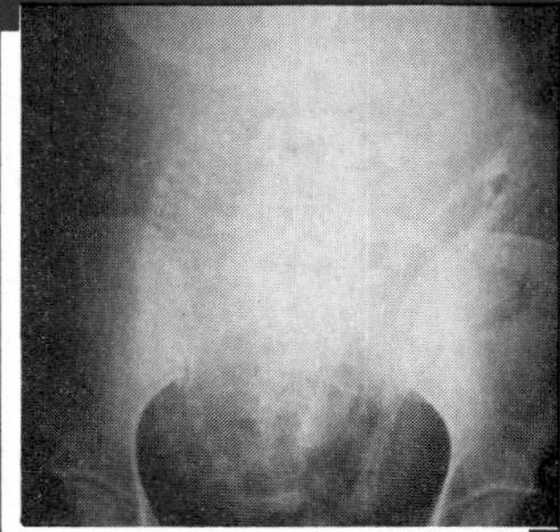

36 Complications of Labor

Dystocia due to Abnormalities of Labor Mechanics

Hemorrhagic Complications

Prolapse of Umbilical Cord

Amniotic Fluid Embolism

Multiple Pregnancy

Assessment and Management of Maternal Disorders

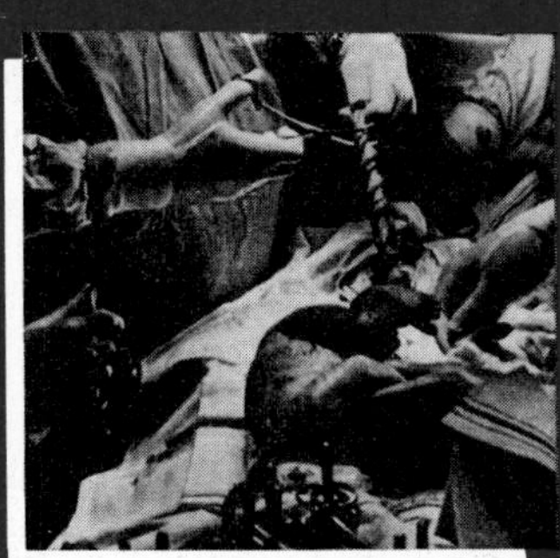

37 Operative Obstetrics

Repair of Lacerations

Forceps

Vacuum Extraction

Version

Cesarean Section

Destructive Operations

Induction of Labor

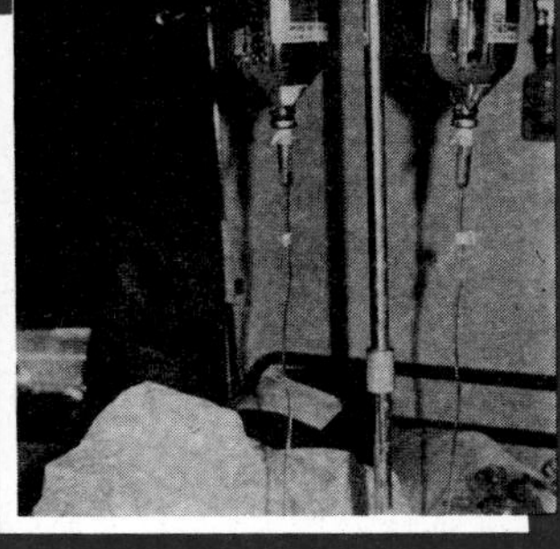

38 Postpartal Complications

Postpartum Infections of the Genital Tract

Pulmonary Embolism

Subinvolution of the Uterus

Vulvar Hematomas

Mastitis

Urinary Tract Infection

Other Complications

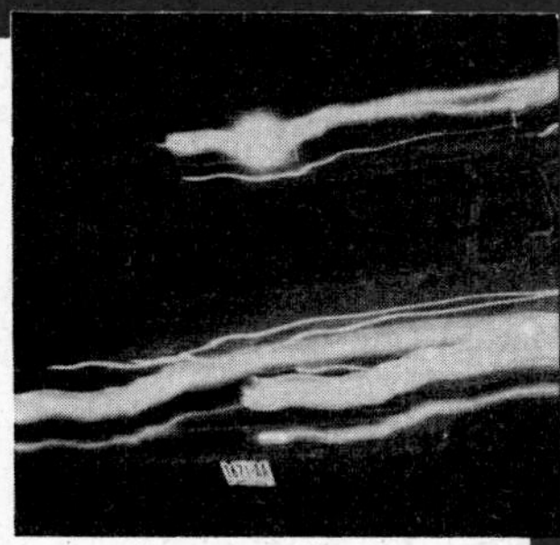

39 Emergencies in Maternity Practice

Precipitate and Emergency Deliveries

Continuing Care for Mother and Infant

Large Scale Disasters

Commonalities of Disaster Situations

Nuclear Disaster

Organization of Disaster Nursing Services in the Hospital

Disaster Protection for Mothers and Infants

Psychological Reactions in Emergency Situations

Reactions of Nurses to Disaster Situations

CHAPTER

34

CHAPTER 34

Complications of Pregnancy

From a biological point of view childbearing is considered to be a normal process. Nevertheless, the borderline between health and illness is less distinct in this time because of the numerous physiological changes that occur during the course of pregnancy. The importance of early and continued health supervision during pregnancy for the total well-being of the mother and her infant is paramount, for such preventive care makes possible the early detection of warning signals of potential pathologic conditions. Serious problems can be averted or controlled by prompt treatment.

Certain "common complaints" are experienced by most expectant mothers to some degree. These are the so-called minor discomforts of pregnancy, which in themselves are not serious but detract from the mother's feeling of well-being. Since these discomforts are usually related to physiological changes occurring within the mother's body and are not in themselves pathologic, they have been included in the chapter on antepartal care (see Chap. 21).

Certain complications of pregnancy may seriously jeopardize the health of both the mother and her unborn infant. Although dramatic progress has been made in reducing maternal and perinatal morbidity and mortality, some problems remain unsolved. Despite expanding social programs, a great many underprivileged women receive inadequate or no prenatal care. These women, in contrast to those with optimal care, have an increased rate of complications, morbidity, and mortality, both maternal and perinatal.

Pregnancy-related maternal disorders are divided into two broad categories—complications related to the pregnancy itself and not seen at other times, and diseases which are not pregnancy-related but occur coincidentally. The latter may arise in the nonpregnant patient as well, but when they occur during pregnancy they may complicate the pregnancy and influence its course or may be aggravated by the pregnancy. Such conditions are considered in Chapter 35.

There are only a few major complications that result from pregnancy, but these may present serious health hazards. These complications, which will be considered here, include the following: (1) hemorrhagic conditions of early pregnancy (abortion, ectopic pregnancy, and hydatidiform mole), (2) hyperemesis gravidarum, (3) hemorrhagic complications of placental origin in late pregnancy (placenta previa and abruptio placentae), and (4) hypertensive disorders of pregnancy, formerly called *toxemia* (preeclampsia and eclampsia).

Hemorrhagic Complications of Early Pregnancy

The causes of bleeding in pregnancy are usually considered in relation to the stage of gestation in which they are most likely to cause complications. Frequent causes of bleeding during the first half of pregnancy are abortion, ectopic pregnancy, and hydatidiform mole. Although hydatidiform mole is a less common cause (it occurs once in about 2000 pregnancies), it is nevertheless important, because uterine bleeding is its outstanding symptom. The two most common causes of hemorrhage in the latter half of pregnancy are placenta previa and abruptio placentae.

Abortion

Definitions

Abortion is the termination of pregnancy at any time before the fetus has attained a stage of viability, that is, before it is capable of extrauterine existence. The term *miscarriage* is commonly used by lay persons to denote an abortion that has occurred spontaneously rather than one which has been induced. Since *abortion* is the accepted medical term for either, this point should be clarified in discussions with patients to avoid confusion or misinterpretation. In medical parlance the word miscarriage is rarely employed.

It is customary to use the weight of the fetus as an important criterion in abortion. Modern advances in the management and care of preterm infants have made it possible for smaller and smaller infants to survive, so fetuses weighing only 800 g to 900 g (1 lb, 13 oz–2 lb) may live. For this reason many authorities now maintain that fetal weight of 1000 g or less but more than 500 g is classified as *immature,* and that fetal weight of 500 g (about 20 weeks of gestation) or less constitutes an *abortion.* In many states a birth certificate is prepared for any pregnancy terminating beyond the twentieth week of gestation or when the fetus weighs 500 g or more. It is obvious, therefore, that how the termination of pregnancy is classified in different hospitals depends wholly on the interpretation to which they subscribe.

A preterm infant is one born after the stage of viability has been reached but before it has the same chance for survival as a full-term infant. By general consensus, an infant that weighs 2500 g or less at birth is termed *preterm;* one that weighs 2501 g (5½ lb) or more is regarded as *full term.*

It is important to remember that preterm labor does not refer to abortion. *Preterm labor* is the termination of pregnancy after the fetus is viable but before it has attained full term. Although the cause of many preterm labors cannot be explained, the condition can be brought on by maternal diseases such as chronic hypertensive vascular disease, abruptio placentae, placenta previa, untreated syphilis, congenital uterine anomalies or a mechanical defect in the cervix.

Types of Abortions

The term abortion includes many varieties of termination of pregnancy prior to viability but may be subdivided into two main groups—spontaneous and induced.

Spontaneous abortion is one in which the process starts of its own accord through natural causes. *Induced abortion* is one which is artificially induced whether for therapeutic or other reasons. Induced abortion has been considered in Chapter 14.

Threatened Abortion. An abortion is regarded as threatened if vaginal bleeding or spotting occurs in early pregnancy. This may or may not be associated with mild cramps. The cervix is closed. The process has presumably started but may abate.

Inevitable Abortion. Inevitable abortion is so called because the process has gone so far that termination of the pregnancy cannot be prevented. Bleeding is copious, and the pains are more severe. The membranes may or may not have ruptured, and the cervical canal is dilating.

Incomplete Abortion. An incomplete abortion is one in which part of the products of conception has been passed, but part (usually the placenta) is retained in the uterus. Bleeding usually persists until the retained products of conception have been passed.

Complete Abortion. Complete abortion is the expulsion of all the products of conception.

Missed Abortion. In a missed abortion the fetus dies in the uterus but is retained. The term is generally restricted to cases in which two months or more elapse between fetal death and expulsion. During this period the fetus undergoes marked degenerative changes. Of these, maceration, or general softening, is the most common. Occasionally it dries up into a leatherlike structure (mummification), and very rarely it is converted into stony material (lithopedion formation). Symptoms, except for amenorrhea, are usually lacking, but occasionally such patients complain of malaise, headache, and anorexia. Hypofibrinogenemia, a hemorrhagic complication, may result.

Habitual Abortion. This term indicates a condition in which spontaneous abortion occurs in successive pregnancies (three or more). This is a most distressing condition, some women having six or eight spontaneous abortions.

Criminal Abortion. Criminal, or perhaps better stated, extra-hospital (or extra-clinic) abortion is the termination of pregnancy outside of appropriate medical facilities, generally by nonphysician abortionists, regardless of the validity of the indication. The frequency of such abortions is not precisely known but has dropped precipitously in the United States following the Supreme Court decision of 1973. In years past, estimates ranged from 200,000 to 1,200,000 per year in the United States. In most urban areas, abortions were responsible for the majority of maternal deaths, with estimates of 800 to 5000 abortion deaths per year.

Attempts at producing abortion are generally made by the ingestion of drugs such as quinine or castor oil, which usually do nothing or, if taken in sufficient quantities to produce an abortion, place the woman in serious jeopardy.

Another common approach involves the placement of a foreign body, such as a urethral catheter, into the uterus with or without the instillation of toxic substances. Severe infection, often with shock and renal failure, is a common consequence of such crude efforts at pregnancy termination. Patients so affected surely are some of the most critically ill that the nurse may ever have to care for and, unfortunately, they sometimes succumb in spite of the best efforts of all concerned.

Manifestations and Causes

Clinical Picture. About 75% of all spontaneous abortions occur during the second and the third months of pregnancy, that is, before the twelfth week. The condition is very common; it is estimated that about one pregnancy in every ten terminates in spontaneous abortion. Almost invariably the first symptom is bleeding due to the separation of the fertilized ovum from its uterine attachment. The bleeding is often slight at the beginning and may persist for days before uterine cramps occur; or the bleeding may be followed at once by cramps. Occasionally the bleeding is torrential, leaving the patient in shock. The uterine contractions bring about softening and dilatation of the cervix and either complete or incomplete expulsion of the products of conception.

Causes. What causes all these spontaneous abortions that are so tragic and shattering to so many women? If the evidence is reviewed with some perspective and with full fairness to all concerned, it is the inevitable conclusion that most of these abortions, far from being tragedies, are blessings in disguise, for they are Nature's beneficent way of extinguishing imperfect embryos. Indeed, careful microscopic study of the material passed in these cases shows that the most common cause of spontaneous abortion is an inherent defect in the products of conception. This defect may express itself in an abnormal embryo, an abnormal *trophoblast* or both abnormalities.

In early abortions, 80% are associated with some defect of the embryo or trophoblast that is either incompatible with life or would result in a grossly deformed child. The incidence of abnormalities after the second month is somewhat lower but not less than 50%. Whether the germ plasm of the spermatozoon or the ovum is at fault in these cases, it is usually difficult, if not impossible, to determine.

Abortions of this sort are obviously not preventable and, although they are often bitterly disappointing to the parents, they do serve a useful purpose.

Spontaneous abortions may result from causes other than defects in the products of conception. Severe acute infections, such as pneumonia, pyelitis and typhoid fever, often lead to abortion. Occasionally, abnormalities of the generative tract, such as a congenitally short cervix or uterine malformations, produce the accident. Abortion is common in women whose mothers were treated with diethylstilbestrol (DES) during pregnancy. Retroposition of the uterus rarely causes abortion, as was formerly believed. Many women tend to explain abortion as a result of an injury or excessive activity. Women exhibit the greatest variation in this respect. In some the pregnancy may go blithely on despite falls from second-story windows and automobile accidents severe enough to fracture the pelvis. In others a trivial fall, anxiety, or overfatigue may appear to be related to abortion, but there is obviously no way to determine a cause-effect relationship.

Management

The severity of the symptoms manifested in threatened abortion determines the treatment prescribed. If the patient is having only slight vaginal bleeding or even spotting, without pain, she should be advised to stay in bed and eat a light well-balanced diet. If she appears to be apprehensive, a mild sedative may be given. Some physicians do not restrict activity, based on the concept that the uterus is well insulated from outside influences.

Uniformly the patient should be advised to save all perineal pads, as well as all tissue and clots passed, for inspection. In cases where bed rest has been prescribed, if the bleeding disappears within 48 hours, the woman may get out of bed but should limit her activities for the next several days. Coitus should be avoided for 2 weeks following the last evidence of bleeding.

In cases in which pain accompanies the vaginal bleeding, the prognosis for saving the pregnancy is poor. Usually bleeding is observed first, and a few hours, sometimes days later, uterine contractions ensue. When the pain and the bleeding increase, the patient should be hospitalized, if this has not already been done.

If the abortion is incomplete, ordinarily efforts are made to aid the uterus in emptying its contents. Oxytocin may be administered, but if this is ineffectual, surgical removal of the retained products of conception should be done promptly. Active bleeding may make this urgently necessary. Many times the tissue lies loose in the cervical canal and can simply be lifted out with ovum forceps; otherwise, curettage of the uterine cavity must be done. The instruments commonly used in completing an incomplete abortion are shown in Figures 34-1 and 34-2. The suction curet may also be used.

If evidence of infection is present (*e.g.,* fever, foul discharge, or suspicious history of criminal abortion), evacuation of the uterus should be delayed only long enough to obtain appropriate studies (especially smears and cultures) and to initiate antibiotic therapy. Such prompt and aggressive management of the patient with an infected abortion effectively reduces the incidence of more serious complications such as septic shock, thrombophlebitis, and renal failure, and reduces morbidity and hospital stay as well.

Nurse's Responsibilities in Abortion Cases

Bleeding in the first half of pregnancy, no matter how slight, always must be considered as threatened abortion. The patient must be put to bed and the physician notified. An episode of this nature is indeed distressing to the expectant mother, many times alarming. The nurse should bear in mind that although it is important to give emotional support, the patient should never be reassured that "everything will be all right," because in fact the patient may lose this pregnancy.

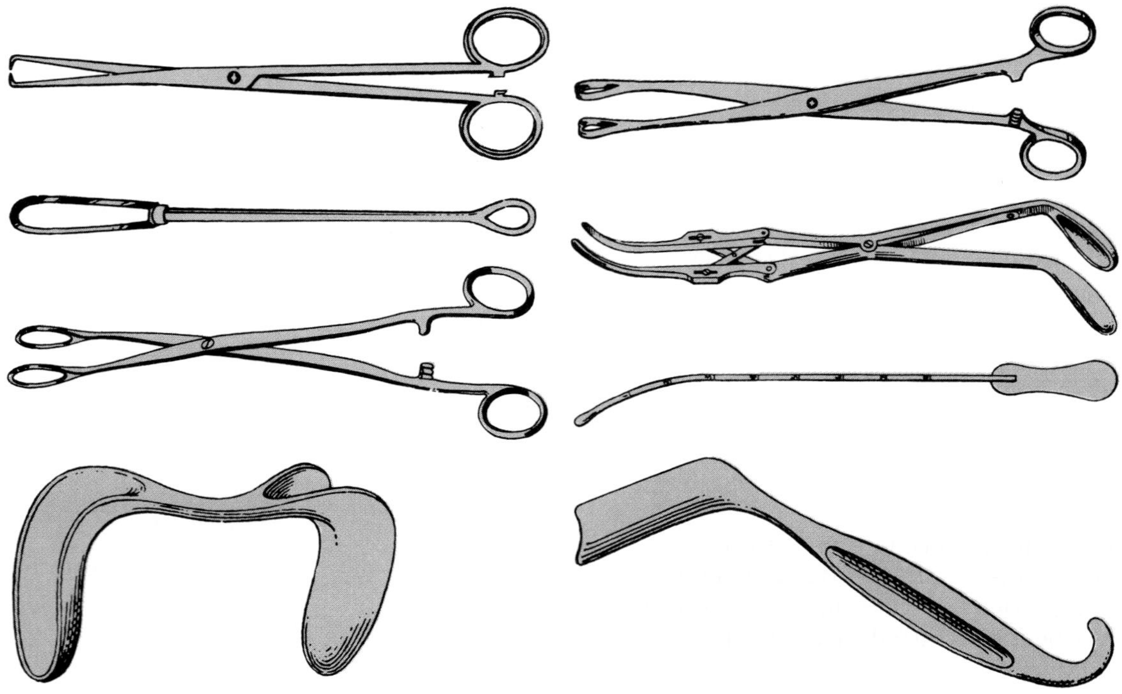

Figure 34-1.
(Left, top to bottom) Bullet forceps used in grasping the lips of the cervix. Sims's sharp curet, a scraper or spoonlike instrument for removing matter from the walls of the uterus. Sponge holder. Sims's speculum for inserting into the vaginal canal so as to expose the cervix to view. *(Right, top to bottom)* Placental forceps with heart-shaped jaws. Modified Goodell–Ellinger dilator used for enlarging the canal of the cervix. Uterine sound. Schroeder vaginal retractor for drawing back the vulvar or vaginal walls during an operation.

Perineal pads and all tissue and blood clots passed by the patient should be saved to determine the amount of bleeding. When tissue has been passed, it is useful to examine the products of conception to ascertain whether or not the abortion is complete.

If bleeding is so copious as to be alarming, elevate the foot of the bed (shock position) while awaiting the physician. If surgical completion of the abortion is to be carried out, the same aseptic regimen is carried out as for delivery.

Incompetent Cervical Os

A mechanical defect in the cervix, known as incompetent cervical os, has gained recognition as a cause of late habitual abortion or preterm labor. When repeated termination of pregnancy in the second trimester is due to an anatomical factor such as this, surgical treatment may make it possible to save the fetus.

Shirodkar Technique

One type of treatment used to prevent relaxation and dilatation of the cervix when it is incompetent is the modified Shirodkar technique. In this, the vaginal mucous membrane is elevated and a narrow strip of some material such as Mersilene is carried around the internal os of the cervix and tied. Then the vaginal mucosa is restored to its original position and sutured. The procedure may be done between pregnancies, if the diagnosis is clearly established, or during pregnancy. When done during pregnancy, it is usually elected to wait until the early part of the second trimester (12 weeks–14 weeks) to avoid the possibility of having to remove the suture if a spontaneous first trimester abortion occurs.

Postoperatively, the main concerns are rupture of the membranes and uterine contractions. If the membranes rupture, the suture must be removed and the uterus emptied because of the risk of infection. If contractions ensue, the patient should be placed at bed rest immediately, and a pharmacologic agent such as ritodrine hydrochloride may be given in an effort to control the contractions. Attempts to control contractions should not be persistent if they are not effective promptly, since there is a risk of uterine rupture.

Decisions regarding the type of delivery a patient is to have are generally based on the position of the suture when the patient reaches term or when labor begins. If the suture is in good position, with the cervical closure maintained, cesarean section may be elected to preserve the suture for future pregnancies. If the suture has loosened or rolled down on the cervix, it is not adequate for subsequent pregnancies. In that case, it is removed when labor begins and vaginal delivery is permitted.

McDonald Technique

Another more simple procedure used to treat the incompetent cervix is the McDonald technique. This involves placing a nonabsorbable suture, such as No. 1 nylon, around the cervix high on the cervical mucosa. The McDonald procedure is usually carried out during pregnancy when premature dilatation of the cervix is detected or electively in the fourth month. The suture is easily removed near term to allow spontaneous delivery.

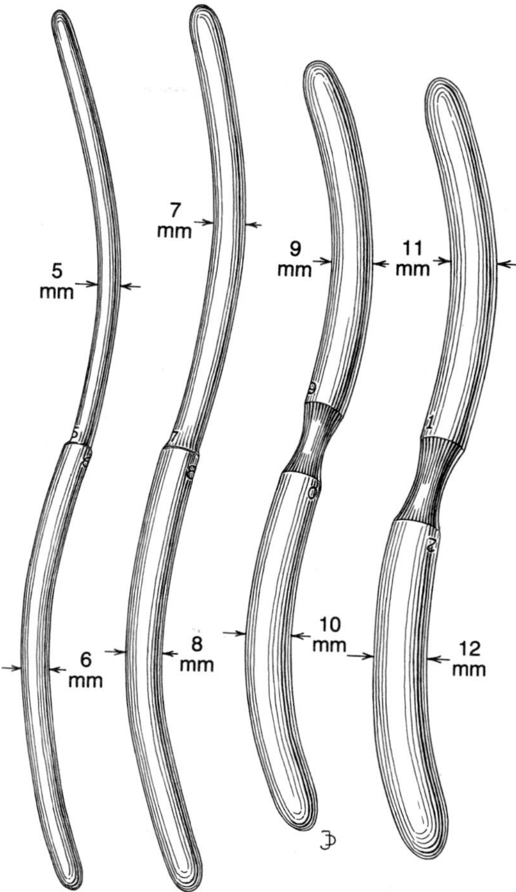

Figure 34-2.
Hegar dilators of graduated diameters from 5 mm to 12 mm. Larger sizes are also used (Mattingly, RF: Telinde's Operative Gynecology, 5th ed. Philadelphia, JB Lippincott, 1977)

Ectopic Pregnancy

An ectopic pregnancy is any gestation located outside the uterine cavity. The majority of ectopic pregnancies are tubal gestations. Other types, which make up about 5% of all ectopic pregnancies, are interstitial (in the interstitial portion of the tube), cornual (in a rudimentary horn of a uterus), cervical, abdominal, and ovarian gestations.

About once in every 300 pregnancies the fertilized ovum, instead of traversing the length of the fallopian tube to reach the uterine cavity, becomes implanted within the wall of the fallopian tube. This condition is known as "ectopic pregnancy" (literally, a pregnancy which is out of place) or as "tubal pregnancy" or "extrauterine pregnancy" (Fig. 34-3). Since the wall of the tube is not sufficiently elastic to allow the fertilized ovum to grow and develop there, rupture of the tubal wall is the inevitable result. Rupture most frequently occurs into the tubal lumen with the passage of the products of conception, together with much blood, out the fimbriated end of the tube and into the peritoneal cavity—so-called tubal abortion. Or rupture may occur through the peritoneal surface of the tube directly into the peritoneal cavity; and, again, there is an outpouring of blood into the abdomen from vessels at the site of rupture. In either case, rupture usually occurs within the first 12 weeks.

Occasionally an ectopic pregnancy may develop in that portion of the tube which passes through the uterine wall, a type known as "interstitial pregnancy." In very rare instances, the products of conception, after rupturing through the tubal wall, may become implanted on the peritoneum and develop to full term in the peritoneal cavity. This extraordinary occurrence is known as "abdominal pregnancy." Surprisingly, living infants have been delivered in such cases by means of abdominal incision.

Tubal ectopic pregnancy may be caused by any condition which narrows the tube or brings about some constriction within it. Under such circumstances the tubal lumen is large enough to allow

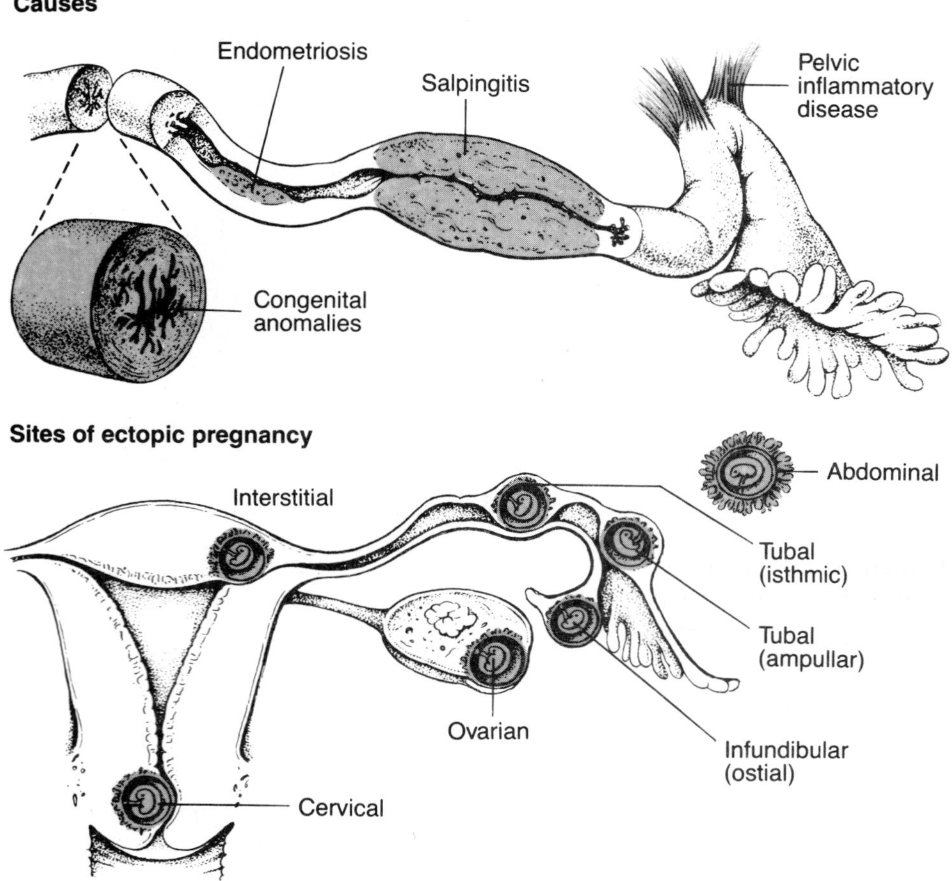

Figure 34-3.
Causes and sites of ectopic pregnancy.

spermatozoa to ascend the tube but not big enough to permit the downward passage of the fertilized ovum (see Fig. 34-3). Among the conditions which may produce such a narrowing of the fallopian tube are previous inflammatory processes involving the tubal mucosa and producing partial agglutination of opposing surfaces, such as gonorrheal salpingitis; previous inflammatory processes of the external peritoneal surfaces of the tube, causing kinking, such as puerperal and postabortal infections; endometriosis of the tubal wall and lumen; and developmental defects resulting in a segmental narrowing of the tubes.

Manifestations

In cases of ectopic gestation the woman exhibits the usual early symptoms of pregnancy and, as a rule, regards herself as being normally pregnant. After missing one or two periods, however, she suddenly experiences knifelike pain, often of extreme severity, in one of the lower quadrants. This is usually associated with slight vaginal bleeding, commonly referred to as "spotting." Depending on the amount of blood that has escaped into the peritoneal cavity, she may or may not undergo a fainting attack and show symptoms of shock.

Ectopic pregnancy is a grave complication of pregnancy and is a significant cause of maternal death. Moreover, if a woman has had one ectopic pregnancy, she is more likely to have another in a subsequent pregnancy.

Management

In the vast majority of cases the tube has already ruptured and the fetus is dead when the patient is first seen by the physician. It is the rupture that produces the acute clinical picture. The treatment is to remove the tube and replace blood as necessary. Occasionally the ovary must be removed with the tube. Under certain circumstances in which subsequent fertility must be maintained, the tube may be preserved by removing the products of conception from the tube, either through a linear incision (salpingostomy) or by milking the conceptus out of the tubal lumen by external pressure applied with the fingers. This approach is applicable if the contralateral tube is badly diseased or has been previously removed and it is the patient's wish to preserve fertility.

Nursing Intervention

During the transportation of such a patient to the hospital or in the interval when the patient is awaiting operation, the nurse can be of immeasurable assistance in combating the shock that is frequently present. An intravenous infusion should be maintained so that blood or plasma expanders can be administered as needed and the patient's vital signs should be monitored and recorded.

Hydatidiform Mole

Hydatidiform mole is a benign neoplasm of the chorion in which the chorionic villi degenerate and become transparent vesicles containing clear, viscid fluid. The vesicles have a grapelike appearance and are arranged in clusters involving all or part of the decidual lining of the uterus (Fig. 34-4). Although there is usually no embryo present, occasionally there may be a fetus and only part of the placenta involved. Hydatidiform mole is rather an uncommon condition, occurring about once in every 2000 pregnancies.

The pregnancy appears to be normal at first, although in about 50% of cases the uterus enlarges more rapidly than a normal pregnancy, and is larger than expected for the duration of pregnancy by dates. Then bleeding, a usual symptom varying from spotting to heavy bleeding, occurs, so that one might suspect threatened or inevitable abortion. If the patient does not abort, the uterus enlarges rapidly, and profuse hemorrhage may occur, at which time these vesicles may be evident in the vaginal discharge. Vomiting in rather severe form may appear early. Preeclampsia, a complication that does not usually occur until the later months of pregnancy, may appear early in the second trimester. When diagnosis of hydatidiform mole is suspected, it may be confirmed by sonographic examination (Fig. 34-5).

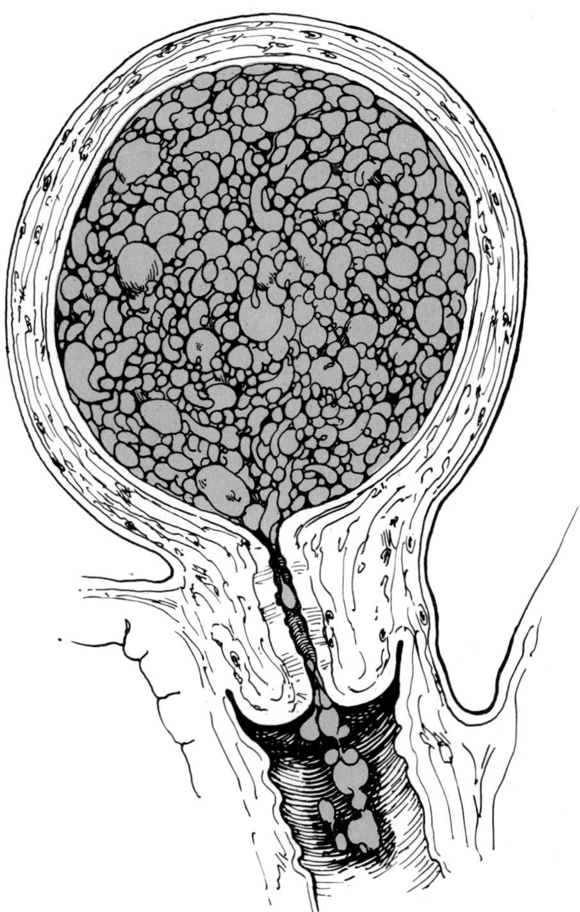

Figure 34-4.
Hydatidiform mole.

Management

The treatment consists of emptying the uterus. The approach used for evacuating the uterine contents varies, depending on the size of the uterus at the time molar pregnancy is diagnosed. If the uterus is less than the size of a ten-week gestation, dilatation of the cervix, followed by suction curettage, is the usual procedure. This must be carried out with great care to avoid injury to the uterine wall, which is weakened and spongy due to the growth of the mole. If uterine size is larger, labor is stimulated with a continuous oxytocin infusion. After a portion of the uterine contents have been expelled, curettage is carried out to evacuate uterine contents completely.

The tissue obtained must be carefully evaluated by the pathologist, because, while a mole is a benign process, choriocarcinoma, an extremely malignant tumor, sometimes complicates the picture. For this reason also, follow-up care is very important in cases of molar pregnancy.

Hyperemesis Gravidarum

A mild degree of nausea and vomiting, morning sickness, is the most common complaint of women in the first trimester of pregnancy. This manifestation is considered in the realm of a minor discomfort rather than a complication, and it usually responds to measures

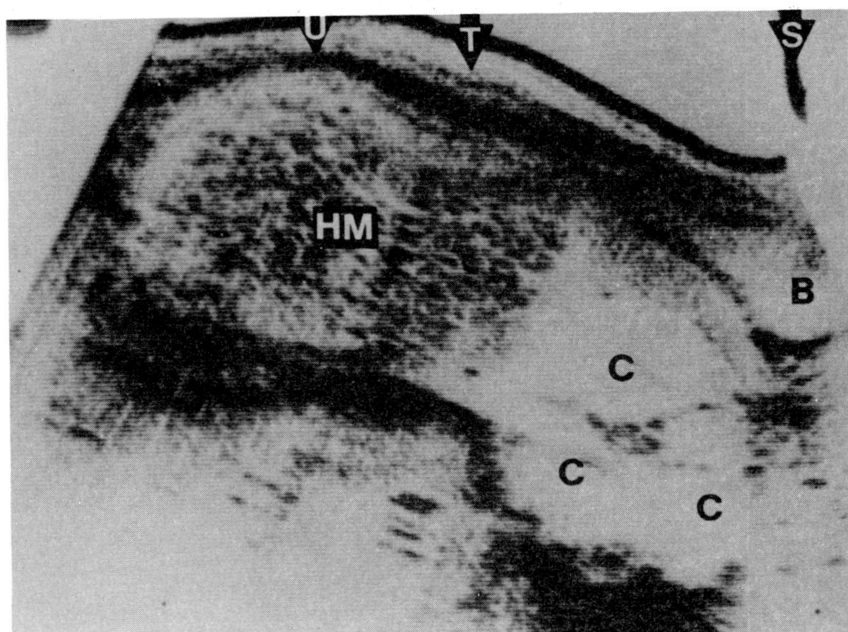

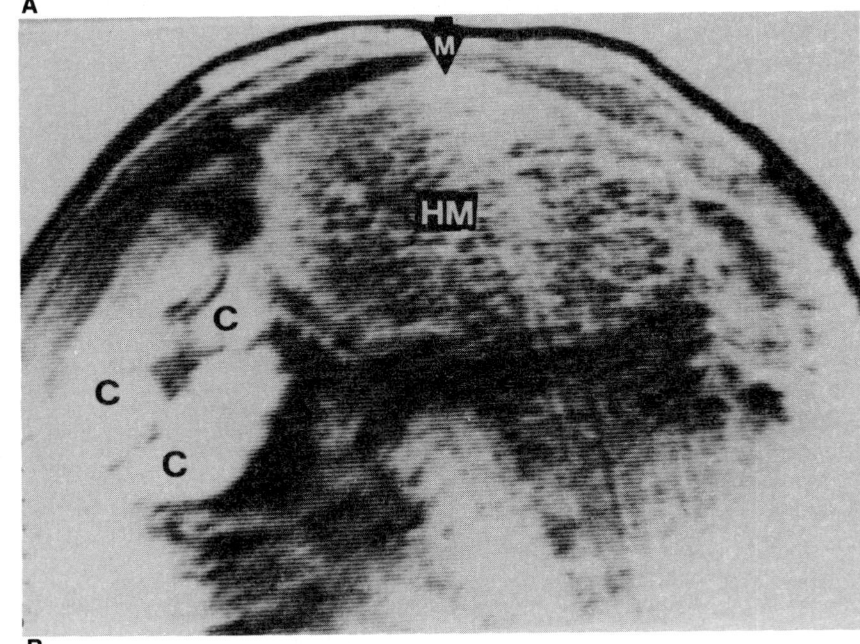

Figure 34-5.
T, point at which transverse scan is obtained. Hydatidiform mole with theca-lutein cysts in a gravida, at 20 weeks' gestation, presenting with nausea and vomiting. *A.* Longitudinal midline scan shows a complex multilocular cyst *(C)* in the cul-de-sac displacing the lower aspect of the uterus to the left side. The upper portion of the uterus is filled with echoes consistent with a hydatidiform mole (HM). *B.* Transverse scan at T shows the echo pattern of hydatidiform mole and the cystic structure *(C)* (theca-lutein cysts) on the right side. (Sabbagha RE [ed.]: Diagnostic Ultrasound Applied to Obstetrics and Gynecology, Hagerstown, MD, Harper & Row, 1980. Courtesy of Carlos Reynes, M.D., Loyola Hospital, Maywood, Illinois)

discussed in Chapter 21. It is uncommon today for this mild form of nausea and vomiting to progress to such a serious extent that it produces systemic effects (*i.e.,* marked loss of weight and acetonuria), but when it becomes thus exaggerated, the condition is *hyperemesis gravidarum,* sometimes called pernicious vomiting.

Because even the gravest case of hyperemesis starts originally as a simple form of nausea, all cases of nausea and vomiting should be treated with proper understanding and judgment, and none should be regarded casually. When simple remedies do not prove to be effective, and symptoms of hyperemesis appear to be imminent, the patient should be hospitalized for more intensive treatment. Appropriate measures should be taken to rule out other disease such as cholecystitis, hepatitis, peptic ulcer, and gastroenteritis. At the present time grave cases of hyperemesis gravidarum are rare, and recovery of those who are admitted to the hospital is usually rapid.

Causes and Manifestations

Cause. It is currently recognized that during pregnancy there are certain organic processes that are basic to all cases of vomiting, regardless of whether the symptoms are mild or severe. The endocrine and metabolic changes of normal gestation, fragments of chorionic villi entering the maternal circulation and the diminished motility of the stomach might well give rise to clinical symptoms.

It has long been thought that hyperemesis gravidarum is in large measure a *neurosis.* The term "neurosis," it will be recalled, is employed very loosely to designate a large array of conditions in which symptoms occur without demonstrable pathologic explanation, the symptoms being due, it is thought, to a disturbance of the patient's psyche. As many examples show (quite apart from pregnancy), nausea is often psychic in origin. For instance, a repellent sight, an obnoxious odor, or the mere recollection of such a sight or odor may give rise to nausea and even vomiting. Our general use of the adjective "nauseating" to describe a repulsive object is further acknowledgment that an upset mind may produce an upset stomach.

Clinical Picture. The clinical picture of the patient suffering from pernicious vomiting varies in relation to the severity and the duration of the condition. In any event, the condition begins with a typical picture of morning sickness. The patient experiences a feeling of nausea which may be most pronounced on arising in the morning but may occur at other times of the day. With the majority of these patients this pattern persists for a few weeks and then suddenly ceases.

A small number of patients who have "morning sickness" develop persistent vomiting which lasts for 4 weeks to 8 weeks or longer. These patients vomit several times a day and may be unable to retain any liquid or solid foods, with the result that marked symptoms of dehydration and starvation occur. *Dehydration* is pronounced, as evidence by a diminished output of urine and a dryness of the skin.

Starvation, which is regularly present, manifests itself in a number of ways. Weight loss may vary from 5 lb to as much as 20 lb or 30 lb. This is tantamount to saying that the digestion and the absorption of carbohydrates and other nutrients have been so inadequate that the body has been forced to burn its reserve stores of fat in order to maintain body heat and energy. When fat is burned without carbohydrates being present, the process of combustion does not go on to completion. Consequently, certain incompletely burned products of fat metabolism make their appearance in the blood and the urine. The presence of acetone and diacetic acid in the urine in hyperemesis is common. In severe cases considerable changes associated with starvation and dehydration become evident in the blood chemistry. There is a definite increase in the nonprotein nitrogen, uric acid, and urea, a moderate decrease in the chlorides and little alteration in the carbon dioxide combining power. Then, too, vitamin starvation is regularly present, and in extreme cases, when marked vitamin B deficiency exists, polyneuritis occasionally develops and disturbances of the peripheral nerves result.

The severe type of vomiting may occur in either acute or chronic form. With prompt, persistent, and intelligent therapy, the prognosis of hyperemesis is excellent.

Management and Nursing Care

The principles underlying the treatment of hyperemesis gravidarum are as follows: (1) rule out other underlying causes of nausea and vomiting, principally hepatitis, by appropriate diagnostic measures; (2) combat the dehydration by liberal administration of parenteral fluids; (3) combat the starvation by administration of glucose intravenously and thiamine chloride subcutaneously and, if necessary, by feeding a high-caloric, high-vitamin fluid diet through a nasal tube; (4) combat the emotional component with sedatives, supportive measures, and an understanding attitude.

Hospitalization is essential because isolation from relatives, change of atmosphere, and better facilities for intravenous medication confer unusual benefits in this condition.

The success of the treatment depends largely on the tact, the understanding, and the attitude of the nurse. Although optimism must be the keynote of the nurse's approach to the patient, this must be coupled with a plainly avowed determination to conquer the complication. Most of these patients are in psychological conflict because of family, financial or social difficulties, and many are averse to the whole idea of pregnancy. If one can only get to the root of these difficulties in a tactful, empathic way, and help the patient to become reconciled to becoming a mother, a great deal will have been accomplished.

The nurse must exercise great care in preparing and serving trays for patients suffering from hyperemesis. The portions should be extremely small and attractively arranged. Cold liquids such as ginger ale or lemonade must be ice-cold; and hot foods, such as soups, cocoa, and tea, must be steaming hot because lukewarm liquids may be nauseating. It is best not to discuss food with the patient, even when serving the tray, but simply to assume that she will enjoy it and talk about other matters. At all times keep the emesis basin out of view, since the sight of it may start vomiting. Likewise, the smell of food may be nauseating; accordingly, the patient's room should be kept well aired and should be as far from the food preparation area as possible.

Even the most severe cases of hyperemesis usually respond favorably to the treatment described if patience and persistence are exercised.

Hemorrhagic Complications of Late Pregnancy

Placenta Previa

Although abortion is the most frequent cause of bleeding early in pregnancy, the most common cause during the later months is placenta previa. In this condition the placenta is attached to the lower uterine segment (instead of high up in the uterus as usual) and either wholly or in part covers the region of the cervix. There are three types, differentiated according to the degree to which the condition is present (Figs. 34-6 and 34-7)—*total placenta previa* occurs when the placenta completely covers the internal os; *partial placenta previa* occurs when the placenta partially covers the internal os; and *low implantation of placenta* occurs when the placenta encroaches on the region of internal os, so that it can be palpated by the physician on digital exploration about the cervix but does not extend beyond the margin of the internal os.

Painless vaginal bleeding during the second half of pregnancy is the main symptom of placenta previa. Indeed, a diagnosis of placenta previa should be seriously considered and ruled out whenever there is painless bleeding in the last trimester.

The bleeding usually occurs after the seventh month. It may begin as mere "spotting," or it may start with profuse hemorrhage. The patient may awaken in the middle of the night to find herself in a pool of blood. The bleeding is caused by separation of the placenta as the result of changes which take place in the lower uterine segment during the later months. This separation opens up the underlying blood sinuses of the uterus from which the bleeding occurs.

Fortunately, placenta previa is not a very common condition, occurring about once in every 200 deliveries. It occurs much more frequently in multiparae than in primigravidae. Placenta previa must always be regarded as a grave complication of pregnancy. Until recent years it was associated with a maternal mortality of approximately 10%. Modern methods of management, plus the more liberal use of blood transfusion, have reduced this figure considerably. The fetus may be compromised not only because the placental separation interferes with the infant's oxygen supply, but also because many of the babies are very premature when delivery must necessarily take place.

Diagnosis and Management

The presence of a placenta previa causes two main problems for the mother—bleeding and obstruction of the birth canal. For the baby, the most significant concern is prematurity. These problems provide the guides to treatment.

Conservative Management. Conservative management is in order when the fetus is premature (by weight or dates) and the bleeding is not excessive. The natural history of placenta previa is such that uncontrolled bleeding is not likely to occur with the first episode. There may be, in fact, several episodes of bleeding, starting early in the third trimester, before there is sufficient bleeding to force the obstetrician to intervene and terminate the pregnancy. Under such circumstances, bed rest and observation often result in cessation of the bleeding and provide valuable days for the maturation of the fetus.

It is important that the obstetrician rule out other causes of bleeding under these circumstances. A speculum examination of the vagina is generally done to rule out other sources of bleeding such as cervicitis and cervical polyps. The examiner does *not,* however, insert a finger through the cervix under these circumstances, since such a maneuver might well precipitate bleeding and therefore the delivery of a premature infant.

Cervical manipulation must be postponed, if a course of expectancy appears reasonable, to allow additional time for fetal maturation. In any case, a more complete examination should never be carried out unless all preparations have been made for immediate cesarean birth. Other techniques of placental localization are useful in confirming the diagnosis. Such measures as isotope scans, amniography and soft tissue abdominal x-rays have been used with varying degrees of success. These have been largely supplanted by sonography (Fig. 34-8). Placental localization by ultrasound "B" scanning offers 95% accuracy and should be used when available. When the placenta is found to be normally located and thus a diagnosis of placenta previa is not substantiated, the physician may elect, in the absence of bleeding, to

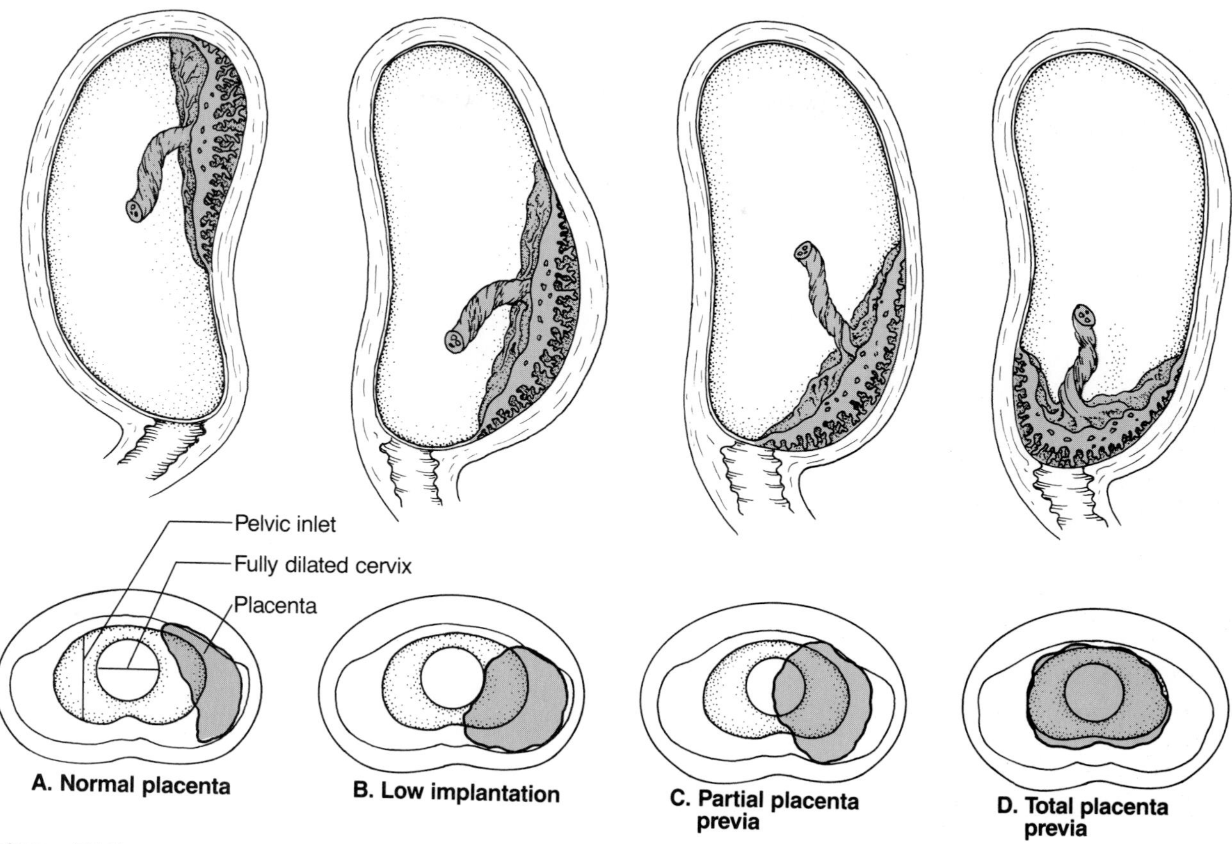

Figure 34-6.
Placenta previa. *(A)* Normal placenta, *(B)* low implantation, *(C)* partial placenta previa, *(D)* total placenta previa. (Redrawn from Benson RC: Handbook of Obstetrics and Gynecology, 6th ed. Los Altos, CA, Lange Medical Publications, 1977)

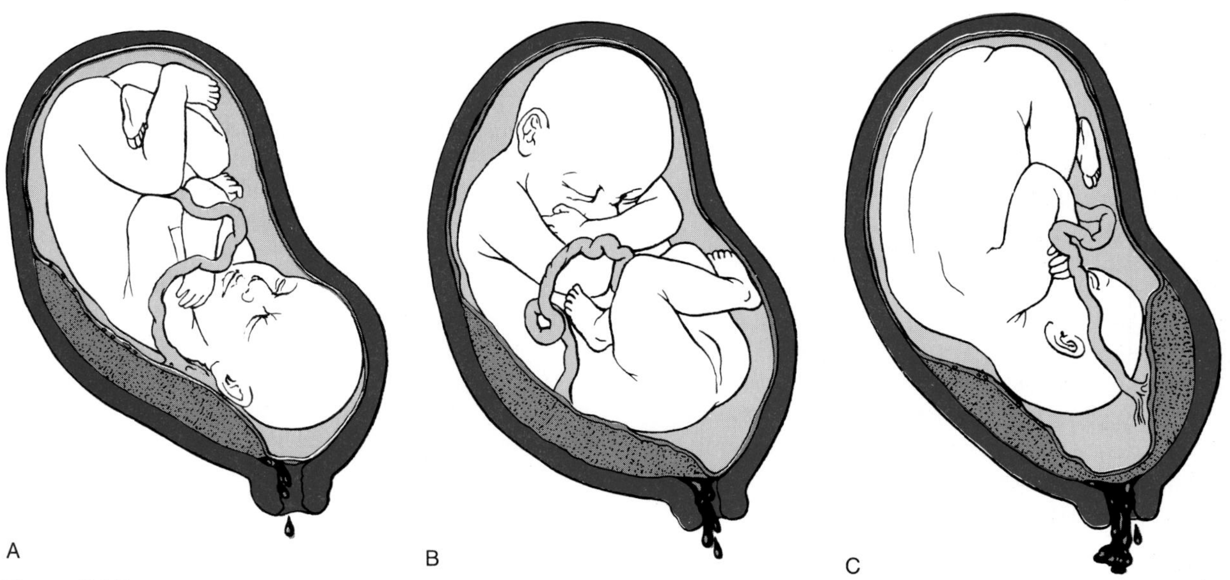

Figure 34-7.
Placenta previa. *(A)* Low implantation. *(B)* Partial placenta previa. *(C)* Central (total) placenta previa.

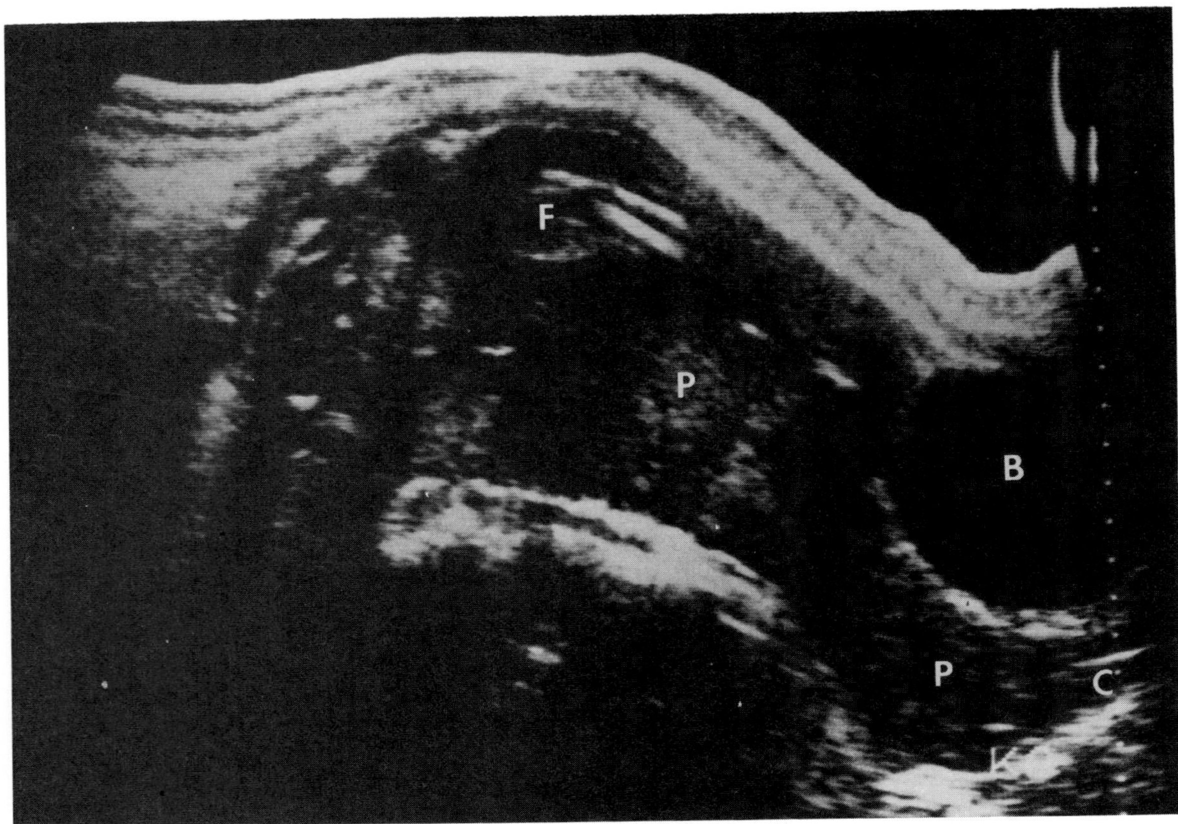

Figure 34-8.
Ultrasonogram of 25 weeks' gestation, showing placenta previa. The placenta *(P)* is located on the posterior wall of the lower uterine segment and extends anteriorly to cover the cervix *(C)*. Bladder *(B)* is outlined in front. Fetal echoes *(F)* are seen in the upper part of the uterus.

discharge the mother from the hospital with the admonition that she is to report promptly at the first sign of recurrence of bleeding.

When the diagnosis is confirmed, in general, the patient should remain hospitalized at bed rest. Further bleeding must be carefully observed and recorded, and all perineal pads must be saved to allow a reasonable assessment of the amount of additional blood loss. The fetal heart tones should be monitored at frequent intervals until the bleeding has subsided completely, and the uterus should be palpated periodically to detect contractions suggesting onset of labor. Any increase in uterine activity or bleeding should be reported promptly.

Active Management. An active approach is indicated if the fetus is at term by size and dates, if labor has begun, or if bleeding is sufficient to threaten the mother. Then, the patient is taken to the operating room where a "double setup" examination is usually performed. This means that everything is prepared for an immediate cesarean birth, should the examination confirm the diagnosis. This precaution is necessary, since digital examination of the cervix might precipitate increased bleeding.

In all instances of total and partial placenta previa, and in most instances of low implantation of the placenta, cesarean birth is the approach of choice for delivery. In an occasional case of low implantation, especially if the baby is small and the cervix is already partially dilated, the obstetrician may elect to rupture the membranes in the hope that the presenting part may enter the pelvis and control the bleeding by compressing the area of placenta that has separated. If this does occur, vaginal delivery may sometimes be accomplished. By and large cesarean section is the procedure of choice as it is generally associated with a better fetal survival.

Nursing Intervention. Bleeding, shock, and infection are the main dangers. Before the arrival of the physician, the nurse should keep a careful watch on the amount of bleeding and the pulse rate and watch for signs of oncoming shock (pallor, increased pulse rate, cold extremities, and so on). Should the bleeding be profuse, elevation of the foot of the bed and application of external heat may forestall shock. In determining the amount of bleeding, the patient should be instructed to report if she feels any fluid escaping from the vulva. The nurse, in turn, should inspect the pad or bed frequently for hemorrhage.

Abruptio Placentae

Abruptio placentae (meaning that the placenta is torn from its bed) is a complication of the last half of pregnancy, in which a normally located placenta undergoes separation from its uterine attachment. The condition is frequently called "premature separation of the normally implanted placenta;" other synonymous terms such as *accidental hemorrhage* (meaning that it takes place unexpectedly) and *ablatio placentae* (ablatio means a carrying away) are sometimes used. Bleeding may be apparent, in which case it is called *external hemorrhage,* or concealed, in which case it is called *concealed hemorrhage.* If a separation occurs at the margin, the blood is apt to lift the membranes and trickle down to the cervical os and thus escape externally. If the placenta begins to separate centrally, a huge amount of blood may be stored behind the placenta before any of it becomes evident (Fig. 34-9). Ultrasonography is often helpful in establishing the diagnosis (Fig. 34-10). Although the precise cause of the condition is unknown, it is frequently encountered in association with cases of hypertensive disorder of pregnancy (toxemia).

Premature separation of the normally implanted placenta is characterized not only by bleeding beneath the placenta but also by pain. The pain is produced by the accumulation of blood behind the placenta, with subsequent distention of the uterus. The uterus also enlarges in size as the result of the accumulated blood and becomes distinctly tender and exceedingly firm. Because of the almost woody hardness of the uterine wall, fetal parts may be difficult to palpate. Shock is often out of proportion to blood loss, as manifested by a rapid pulse, dyspnea, yawning, restlessness, pallor, syncope, and cold, clammy perspiration.

Management

Treatment is dependent upon the condition of the fetus and the mother at the time the diagnosis is made. If the fetus is alive, prompt delivery is in order and should be by cesarean birth, unless vaginal delivery can be accomplished promptly. If the fetus has already succumbed, this is usually an indication of an extensive placental separation. The complications of abruptio placentae to be described subsequently are all time-related and occur with greater frequency with more extensive separation. Therefore, although a vaginal delivery is desirable with a dead baby, one should not persist for too long.

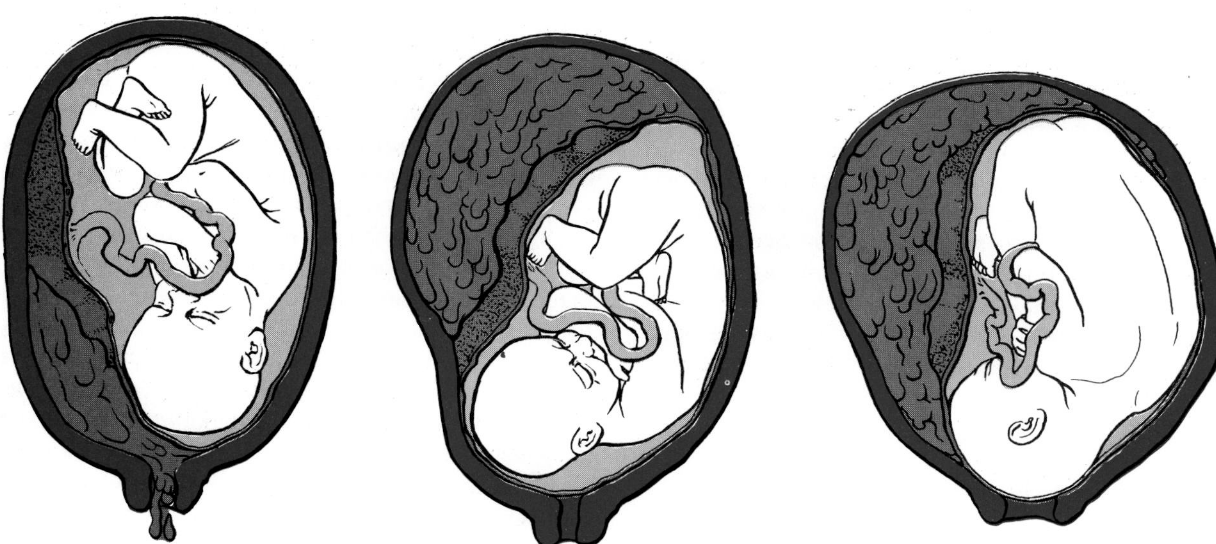

Figure 34-9.
Abruptio placentae at various separation sites.

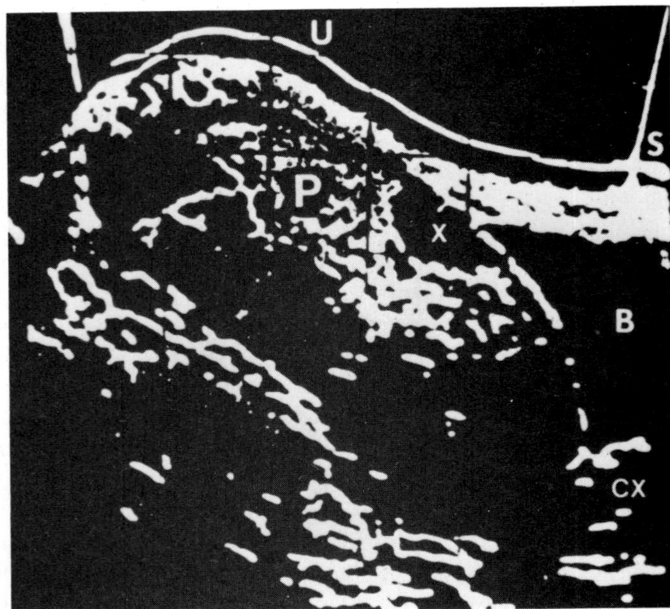

Figure 34-10.
Ultrasonography of placental abruption at 27 weeks. The clear space, *X*, represents a retroplacental blood clot between the placental basal plate and the uterine wall. (Sabbagha RE (ed): Diagnostic Ultrasound Applied to Obstetrics and Gynecology. Hagerstown, MD, Harper & Row, 1980)

Further Complications

Hemorrhagic shock is a common complication and demands vigorous treatment with blood replacement and control of the bleeding by emptying the uterus in the most expeditious manner. Occasionally, with a severe abruption, a coagulation defect, *hypofibrinogenemia,* develops. This complication is also seen with other entities such as amniotic fluid embolus, prolonged retention of a dead fetus, and septic abortion. It is brought about by the entry into the circulation of thromboplastin from the uterus and placenta, which causes small fibrin clots in the capillaries and consumes fibrinogen, leaving the patient with nonclotting blood. Treatment involves the use of blood and fibrinogen replacement and termination of the pregnancy. Also, in severe abruptions, when coagulation is impaired, there is extensive bleeding into the uterine muscle, producing the so-called Couvelaire uterus. Such a uterus occasionally does not contract well after delivery, causing further bleeding and even necessitating hysterectomy. Finally, *renal failure* may result, either on the basis of acute tubular necrosis or bilateral cortical necrosis. In the latter case, the outlook is grave.

Mistaken Diagnosis of Hemorrhage

A false alarm concerning hemorrhage is sometimes due to a normal "show" at the beginning of labor. It simply means that dilatation of the cervix has begun, causing slight bleeding. No treatment is required. However, the nurse should reassure the patient and watch to determine whether or not the bleeding which is present is more than the normal show.

The Hypertensive Disorders of Pregnancy

A condition that is characterized by hypertension and is peculiar to pregnancy is sometimes encountered during gestation or early in the puerperium. Until recently, *toxemia* was the term used to describe this syndrome, which is characterized by one or more of the following signs: hypertension, edema, proteinuria, and in severe cases, convulsions and coma. The term "toxemia of pregnancy" was coined when it was believed that the condition was caused by toxins derived from the products of conception circulating in the blood. Because this theory is no longer tenable, the term toxemia has fallen into disfavor, although it is still used in common parlance. The terms *preeclampsia* and *eclampsia* are used to describe pregnancy–induced or aggravated hypertension, usually associated with edema or proteinuria. Preeclampsia and eclampsia represent one and the same process, but the term *eclampsia* is used when the patient's clinical course has advanced to generalized convulsions or coma. The hypertensive disorders of pregnancy include other conditions associated with hypertension, which present concomitantly with pregnancy but have not arisen *de novo* as a result of pregnancy. They are included because their clinical course may be aggravated by the pregnancy, and the patient may develop a superimposed preeclampsia or eclampsia.

Hypertensive disorders of pregnancy are a very common complication, being seen in 6% or 7% of all gravidae. They rank among the three major complications (hemorrhage and puerperal infection being the other two) responsible for the vast majority of maternal deaths and account for some 250 maternal deaths in the United States each year. As a cause of fetal death they are even more important. It can be estimated conservatively that at least 25,000 stillbirths and neonatal deaths occur each year in the United States from hypertensive diseases of pregnancy, and those newborns who survive may suffer impairments that affect the quality of their lives. The great majority of perinatal deaths are related to prematurity.

The huge toll of maternal and infant lives taken by hypertensive disorders of pregnancy is in large measure preventable. Proper antepartal supervision, particularly the early detection of signs and symptoms of incipient preeclampsia, and appropriate treatment arrest many cases and so ameliorate others that the outcome for baby and mother is usually satisfactory. Nurses are often the first to encounter the early signs and symptoms, not only in the hospital's outpatient department, but also on home visits, and their detection is of utmost importance so that treatment can be instituted at the earliest possible moment.

Classification

A number of classifications have been proposed to categorize the various forms of hypertensive disorders of pregnancy. Because of changing concepts and the complexity of these conditions, a standard and uniformly acceptable classification has not yet been devised. One which has recently been proposed by Welt and Crenshaw (see Suggested Reading) is reproduced here in modified form for purposes of discussion and clarification.

- I. *Pregnancy-associated hypertensive diseases*
  - A. Preeclampsia and eclampsia
  - B. Gestational hypertension
  - C. Superimposed preeclampsia and eclampsia
- II. *Concurrent hypertension and pregnancy*
- III. *Hypertensive diathesis*

The term *pregnancy-associated hypertensive diseases* covers those specific conditions that develop as a direct result of pregnancy. *Preeclampsia* is characterized by hypertension with edema or proteinuria or both. When the preeclampsic patient develops convulsions or coma, unrelated to other cerebral conditions, the term *eclampsia* is used. If hypertension develops without edema or proteinuria during pregnancy, or in the first ten postpartum days, it is described as *gestational hypertension.* The term *superimposed preeclampsia and eclampsia* is used when the patient who already has underlying hypertensive vascular or renal disease develops preeclampsia and eclampsia, which is heralded by a significant rise in blood pressure with edema or proteinuria.

The term *concurrent hypertension and pregnancy* is used when the two separate conditions, pregnancy and hypertensive disease, are present in the same patient at the same time, but a causal relationship is not evident. *Hypertensive diathesis* refers to a predisposition to hypertension as a result of physiological stress. The hypertension may be manifest in pregnancy for the first time as preeclampsia, eclampsia, or gestational hypertension.

This classification is designed to cover all of the contingencies associated with hypertensive disorders in pregnancy. No doubt, as these various conditions are better understood, new classifications will be proposed. For purposes of discussion, it is useful to consider hypertensive disorders in pregnancy in two broad categories—those disorders that occur only in pregnancy, namely preeclampsia and eclampsia and hypertensive disorders not confined to pregnancy but which may exist during pregnancy and may be complicated by superimposed preeclampsia or eclampsia. The latter include essential hypertension and various forms of renal disease.

Preeclampsia

Preeclampsia is characterized by elevation in blood pressure, proteinuria, or edema in a gravida after the twentieth week of pregnancy who previously has been normal in these respects. It is a forerunner or prodromal stage of eclampsia; in other words, unless the preeclamptic process is checked by treatment or by delivery it is likely that eclampsia (*e.g.,* convulsions or coma) will ensue. The rise in blood pressure may occur suddenly, or it may be gradual and insidious.

The criteria for hypertension which are applied include the following:

1. a systolic blood pressure of 140 mm Hg or more, or an elevation of 30 mm Hg or more above the previously observed levels;
2. a diastolic pressure of 90 mm Hg or more or an

elevation of 15 mm Hg or more above that previously observed;
3. observation of the abnormal blood pressure on two occasions or more at least 6 hours apart, as a single reading may be misleading.

The earliest warning signal of preeclampsia is *sudden development of hypertension.* Accordingly, the importance of frequent and regular blood pressure readings during pregnancy cannot be emphasized too strongly. The absolute blood pressure level is probably of less significance than the relationship it bears to previous determinations and the time in gestation when these determinations were recorded. The normal patient often exhibits a lower than normal blood pressure in the midtrimester of pregnancy, and hence a baseline reading in midpregnancy may be misleading. For example, a pressure of 120/80 may actually indicate hypertension in a patient whose midpregnancy pressure has been running in the 100/70 range.

The next most constant sign of preeclampsia is *sudden excessive weight gain.* If cases of preeclampsia are studied from the viewpoint of fluid intake and output, it is at once apparent that these sudden gains in weight are due entirely to an accumulation of water in the tissues. Such weight gains represent occult edema and almost always precede the visible face and finger edema that is so characteristic of the advanced stages of the disease. From what has been said, it is apparent that scales are essential equipment for good antepartal care. Weight gain of 1 lb a week or so may be regarded as normal. Sudden gains of more than 2 lb a week should be viewed with suspicion; gains of more than 3 lb a week, with alarm. Weight increases of the latter magnitude call for more frequent blood pressure determinations, and if these latter are also abnormal, hospitalization may be indicated. In investigating suspected edema, it is important to ask the patient if her wedding ring is becoming tight, since finger and facial edema is a more valuable sign of preeclampsia than is swelling of the ankles. In the facies of a patient with outspoken preeclampsia, the eyelids are swollen, and, associated with the edema, marked coarseness of the features develops (Fig. 34-11).

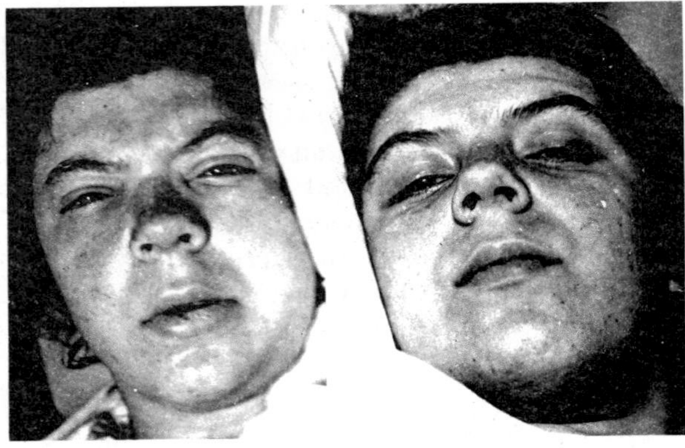

Figure 34-11.
(Left) Facies in preeclampsia. Note edema of eyelids and facial skin and general coarsing of features. *(Right)*) Same patient ten days after delivery.

The sudden appearance of *protein in the urine,* with or without other findings, should always be regarded as a sign of preeclampsia. A complete urinalysis, including a microscopic examination, helps to exclude infection as a cause of proteinuria. Usually it develops later than the hypertension and the gain in weight and for this very reason must be regarded as a serious omen when superimposed on these other two findings.

But the very essence of preeclampsia is the lightninglike fulminance with which it strikes. Although the above physical signs of preeclampsia usually allow ample time to institute preventive treatment, it sometimes happens that these derangements develop between visits to the office or the clinic, even if they are only a week apart. For this reason it is imperative that all expectant mothers be informed, both orally and by some form of printed slip or booklet, about certain danger signals which they themselves may recognize.

The following symptoms demand immediate report to the physician:

1. Severe, continuous headache
2. Swelling of the face or the fingers
3. Dimness or blurring of vision
4. Persistent vomiting
5. Decrease in the amount of urine excreted
6. Epigastric pain (a late symptom)

It should be emphasized that the three early and important signs of preeclampsia, namely, hypertension, weight gain, and proteinuria, are changes of which the patient is usually unaware. All three may be present in substantial degree, and yet she may feel quite well. Only by regular and careful antepartal examination can these warning signs be detected. By the time the preeclamptic patient has developed symptoms and signs which she herself can detect, such as headache, blurred vision, and puffiness of the eyelids and the fingers, she is usually in an advanced stage of the disease, and much valuable time has been lost.

Headache is rarely observed in the milder cases but is encountered with increasing frequency in the most severe grades. In general, patients who develop eclampsia often have a severe headache as a forerunner of the first convulsion. The visual disturbances range from a slight blurring of vision to various degrees of temporary blindness. Although convulsions are less likely to occur in cases of mild preeclampsia, the possibility cannot be entirely eliminated. Patients with severe preeclampsia should always be considered as being on the verge of having a convulsion.

Management

Prophylaxis is most important in the prevention and control of preeclampsia. Because in its early stages preeclampsia rarely gives rise to signs or symptoms that the patient herself will notice, the early detection of this disease demands meticulous antepartal supervision. Rapid weight gain or an upward trend in blood pressure, although still in the "normal" range, is a danger signal. Every pregnant woman should be examined every week during the last month of pregnancy and every two weeks during the two previous months. Finger edema is a frequent forerunner of preeclampsia, which may precede the hypertension by several weeks and is a valuable warning sign.

Ambulatory Patient

When the patient's symptoms are mild (*i.e.*, there is minor elevation of blood pressure with minimal or no signs of edema and proteinuria), treatment may be instituted at home in the hope that symptoms will abate. During this period the patient should be examined at least twice a week, and she should be given a strict regimen to follow, as well as careful instructions about symptoms to report promptly, such as the following:

1. The patient's activities should be restricted, and she should understand that bed rest during the greater part of the day is most desirable.
2. Sedative drugs may be prescribed to encourage rest and relaxation.
3. The diet should be well balanced. It should contain ample protein, particularly lean meat, fish, and eggs.

Although in the past some have suggested that sodium restriction and routine therapy with thiazide diuretics would prevent preeclampsia, in a group of high-risk patients it has now been clearly established that this is not true. The value of diuretic therapy has been questioned because it has been shown to decrease both placental and renal clearance.

Hospital Patient

In the event that the patient's condition does not respond promptly to restricted activity at home, she should be hospitalized without delay. Hospitalization becomes mandatory if proteinuria appears. A systematic method of study, such as the one that follows, should be instituted upon admission to the hospital.

1. A general physical examination and history should be obtained promptly, followed by constant vigilance for the development of such symptoms as headache, visual disturbances, and edema of the fingers and the eyelids.
2. Body weight should be obtained on admission and daily thereafter.
3. Blood pressure readings should be taken every 4 hours except between midnight and morning, unless the midnight blood pressure has risen.
4. Daily fluid intake and output records should be kept, and urine specimens should be sent to the laboratory daily for analysis for protein and casts.
5. Retinal examination is always included as part of the admission physical examination and is done every 2 days to 3 days thereafter, depending on the findings.
6. Once the patient is admitted to the hospital, complete bed rest is essential.

Magnesium Sulfate. When severe preeclampsia develops, immediate and intensive therapy is imperative. Sedation is of major importance to forestall convulsions. The dosage of drugs employed should be regulated so that they produce drowsiness and sleep, from which the patient can be easily awakened, and also suppress the hyperactive reflexes of the patient. Magnesium sulfate is most often used as a sedative and an anticonvulsant under these circumstances. In addition to being an excellent anticonvulsant, magnesium causes vasodilatation and, therefore, is also effective in lowering blood pressure.

For rapid action, an IV dose of 20 ml to 40 ml of a 10% solution (2 g–4 g) is used. Very often the drug is given intramuscularly in doses of 10 ml to 20 ml of a 50% solution (5 g–10 g). The dose is divided, half given into each buttock, and often 1 ml to 2 ml of 1% procaine is added to the injection to minimize discomfort.

A repeat dose of magnesium sulfate should not be given unless the reflexes and respiratory rate have been checked, since it depresses both. The antidote is calcium, and an ampul of calcium gluconate should always be readily available when magnesium is being administered.

For nursing protocol for the administration of magnesium sulfate see the chart on Nursing Protocol for Administration of Magnesium Sulfate.

Other Sedatives. Barbiturates have long been used, the dose being larger (60 mg–120 mg every 4 hr–6 hr) than for mild cases, and they are administered parenterally. The possibility has been raised, however, of adverse effects such as depletion of fetal coagulation factors or delay of fetal lung maturation. Furthermore, if the patient is in labor, barbiturates should be avoided because of their depressant effect on the fetus. Although many use morphine in the management of severe preeclampsia, it would seem best reserved for the patient who has the added stimulus of pain (*i.e.,* labor). Minimizing this stimulus certainly reduces the likelihood of a seizure.

Another drug which is an effective anticonvulsant is diazepam (Valium) in 5- to 10-mg doses intramuscularly or, if the situation warrants, intravenously.

Diazepam is usually reserved for severe cases and is discussed further in the management of eclampsia.

Antihypertensive Drugs. Agents that reduce peripheral blood pressure find occasional use in the treatment of the patient with extreme degrees of hypertension. Opinions differ as to their general effectiveness, largely because they are known to decrease placental perfusion and hence may have an untoward effect on the fetus. Nevertheless, they are sometimes prescribed in cases of severe preeclampsia and eclampsia when the diastolic blood pressure exceeds 100 mm Hg. They are used as a temporary measure to reduce blood pressure and thus decrease the possibility of a cerebrovascular accident. They have also been found to improve kidney function and are associated with some improvement in cardiac output. The most widely used antihypertensive agent at present is hydralazine (Apresoline). This is given intravenously in a dilute solution by slow drip. The use of these agents has not been shown in careful studies to improve either fetal or maternal survival, and their long-term use in preeclampsia is generally not recommended.

Delivery. The treatments which have been discussed are useful only as temporary measures. The only definitive cure for preeclampsia is delivery. Careful medical judgment must be exercised in deciding how long a pregnancy should be continued when preeclampsia has supervened. This is a particularly difficult decision when the preeclampsia has developed early in the last trimester, as a premature infant may not survive extrauterine life. Monitoring fetal well-being with serial serum or urinary estriol levels may be of considerable value. If the estriol levels remain stable, continued expectancy with concomitant treatment is appropriate to allow further *in utero* maturation. In some circumstances evaluation of placental function with a weekly NST or oxytocin challenge test (OCT) is recommended (see Chap. 40). If the OCT is positive, the pregnancy should not be allowed to continue.

Despite all efforts, the condition may persist to a marked degree, and in that event induction of labor may become necessary for the welfare of mother and infant. In some instances, especially when preeclampsia is severe and fulminating and conditions for induction of labor are not favorable, cesarean section may be the procedure of choice.

Postpartum

The signs and symptoms of preeclampsia usually abate rapidly after delivery, but the danger of convulsions does not pass until 48 hours have elapsed postpartum. Therefore, continuation of sedation throughout this interval is indicated. In the majority of cases the elevated blood pressure as well as the other derangements have returned to normal within 10 days or 2 weeks. In about 30% of cases, however, the hypertension shows a tendency either to persist indefinitely or to recur in subsequent pregnancies. For this reason prolonged follow-up of these patients is highly important.

Nursing Management

The nurse's responsibility in the detection and care of cases of preeclampsia is manifold. Since this complication of pregnancy is common and may occur antepartally, intrapartally, or postpartally, it is important for the nurse to observe all maternity patients closely for the first indication of early symptoms, and to report any evidence pointing to an aggravation of the process. The early symptoms and the manifestations related to more severe preeclampsia, such as persistent headache, blurred vision, spots or flashes of light before the eyes, epigastric pain, vomiting, torpor, or muscular twitchings, are all vastly important. Data collected in relation to these symptoms, in addition to an accurate record of weight gain, fluid intake and elimination, diet and attitudes, and behavior, when accurately recorded, can be of great assistance in planning the course of therapy.

In setting the therapeutic atmosphere, the nurse should see that the environment is as comfortable and pleasant as possible. The patient should be in a single room, free from noise, strong lights, and the presence of unnecessary equipment which might frighten her. The nurse must protect the patient from needless traffic into the room; otherwise, the coming and going of personnel to the bedside may be so constant that it could interfere with the efficacy of the treatment being carried out. Every effort should be exerted to relieve the patient's anxiety, which sometimes is brought about by apprehension regarding her illness

Nursing Protocol for Administration of Magnesium Sulfate*

Preparation of the $MgSO_4$

1. IM dose
   $MgSO_4$ 10 g or 5 g
   a. 10 g of $MgSO_4$ in 20 ml of a 50% solution.
   b. Divide into 2 doses, 10 ml in 2 syringes.
   c. Add .5 ml of Lidocaine to each 10 ml of $MgSO_4$ in the syringe.
2. IV dose
   $MgSO_4$ 2 g to 4 g, IV stat by soluset.
   a. 2 g to 4 g of $MgSO_4$ in 20 ml to 40 ml of a 10% solution.
   b. Add ordered grams of $MgSO_4$ to soluset, fill to 100 ml with IV fluid.
   c. Infuse medication over a 10-minute period.

   $MgSO_4$ 1 g, IV by IMED
   a. 1 g of $MgSO_4$ in 2 ml.
   b. Add 10 g of $MgSO_4$ in 20 ml to a 500 ml of D_5/u.
   c. Infuse medication at 50 ml/hr by IMED to give $MgSO_4$ 1 g/hr.

Nursing Assessment of Patient Receiving Magnesium Sulfate

1. Detection of the signs of magnesium intoxication
   a. Early signs mother may experience and you recognize are as follows:
      1. Hot all over
      2. Flushing
      3. Thirsty
      4. Sweating
      5. Depression of reflexes
      6. Hypotension
      7. Flaccidity
   b. Later signs of hypermagnesemia are as follows:
      1. CNS depression
      2. Respiratory paralysis
      3. Circulatory collapse
2. Deep tendon reflexes should be checked hourly if the patient is receiving continuous IV infusion or before each dose of intermittent therapy is administered. Disappearance of the patellar reflex is one of the most important clinical signs to detect increasing hypermagnesemia. However, if the patient has received regional anesthesia (epidural) you will have to test the biceps or radial reflex.
3. CNS depression is at first characterized by anxiety. This changes to drowsiness, lethargy, slight slurring of speech, ataxic gait, and a tendency to fall sideward while standing erect. Constantly evaluate patient's orientation to person, place, and time.
4. Intake and output of the patient are monitored carefully. Specific gravity should be obtained. Urine should be observed for color and volume. The volume should be 30 ml or more/hour; if not, the next dose of $MgSO_4$ should be withheld.
5. If the patient is receiving an IV infusion, BP and TPR should be evaluated at least every 15 minutes to 30 minutes. For patient on intermittent therapy of $MgSO_4$, a BP and TPR should be taken before and after each administration.
6. Do not administer $MgSO_4$ if the patient respirations are less than 12 to 14 per minute or there is a drop in pulse rate, blood pressure, or FHR or any other sign of fetal distress.
7. a. Complaints the patient may have are headache, malaise, nausea, and vomiting. The nurse must assess whether these signs are due to progression of toxemia or drug therapy.
   b. Another complaint that the mother may have if she is receiving $MgSO_4$ intramuscularly is pain at the site of the injection.
8. Calcium gluconate (10% solution) is kept at the patient's bedside.
   a. This is the antidote for magnesium intoxication (usually reverses respiratory depression and heart block). The dosage should be 5 mEq to 10 mEq (10 ml–20 ml) given intravenously over a 3-minute period.

(Continued)

Nursing Protocol for Administration of Magnesium Sulfate*

Testing Deep Tendon Reflexes

1. As outlined above, deep tendon reflexes should be tested hourly.
   a. Absence of or decrease in the patellar reflex indicates that a toxic blood level (7 mg/liter–10 mg/liter of Mg) has been reached.
   b. The reflexes that are tested besides the patellar reflex (knee jerk) are the biceps and radial reflexes. These reflexes are tested by striking the tendon and watching for contraction of the appropriate muscle. The muscle need not contract forcefully enough to move the limb but must simply contract.
   c. These reflexes are difficult to elicit when the patient is tense, so relaxation is important for proper testing.
   d. Reflexes are compared from one side of the corresponding side and expressed with an arbitrary scale.
      0 = Reflex absent
      +1 = Reflex hypoactive
      +2 = Normal reflex
      +3 = Reflex hyperactive
      +4 = Clonus
2. In testing a muscle reflex, it is actually the tendon that is stimulated; the reflex is involuntary. A sensory impulse is initiated when a stimulus is applied to the tendon and in return a motor response is elicited.
   a. When testing reflexes on a patient who has recently received an epidural or spinal anesthesia, motor responses will be diminished. An accurate response will not be elicited if the knee jerk is used. The biceps or radial reflex will have to be used.
3. Knee jerk reflex or patellar tendon reflex
   a. The knee should be positioned halfway between the longest and shortest positions.
   b. Support is given under the knee with the foot off the bed (45° angle).
   c. Patellar tendon is struck (tapped) just below the patella and the quadriceps muscle group should be observed for contraction (slight movement). The lower leg should extend in response.
4. Biceps reflex
   a. The forearm should be resting on the patient's trunk.
   b. Place your thumb firmly on the patient's biceps tendon (antecubital space) and strike the thumbnail briskly with reflex hammer.
   c. The biceps muscle will respond by slight movement. The lower arm should flex in response.
5. Radial reflex
   a. The patient's hand and forearm should be resting on the patient's trunk. Place a finger over the tendon and gently tap your finger with the reflex hammer.
   b. The brachioradial tendon is located on the lateral surface of the lower end of the radius. It is often difficult to feel this tendon. If the tendon cannot be felt, tap the lateral surface of the lower end of the radius. The brachioradial muscle will respond by a slight movement. The response consists of the hand jerking.
6. For relaxation
   a. If the patient is having difficulty relaxing, two techniques can be tried.
      1. Testing the knee jerk—have patient lock her fingers together and pull in the opposite directions (monkey grip). This technique will help the patient relax her leg by having her concentrate on a physical activity.
      2. Testing the biceps or radial reflexes—have the patient bite down hard. This technique will help patient relax her arm by having her concentrate on doing something else.
   b. If it is necessary to try either of these techniques while testing the reflexes, it is likely that the reflexes are slightly depressed.
   c. *Clonus* is the sudden stretching of a hypertonic muscle, producing reflex contraction. If the stretch is maintained during subsequent relaxation, further reflex contraction occurs and this may continue almost indefinitely, unless the stretch stimulus is released. It is demonstrated by dorsiflexion of the foot or by sharply moving the patella downwards, but it may be present at any joint. Clonus represents an increase in reflex excitability and may be present in a very tense patient.

*Used at the Hospital of the University of Pennsylvania.

or may be due to concern for the welfare of her family at home.

Regardless of the severity of the preeclampsia, certain responsibilities are carried out by the nurse. Medications ordered must be administered promptly, the prescribed diet should be supervised, a careful record of intake and elimination need to be kept, blood pressure readings and basal weights need to be taken, specimens need to be collected and labeled accurately, and observations of slight symptoms or change in condition should be reported immediately, both orally and on the patient's record.

Since rest is a major consideration in the care of this patient, the nurse should plan a schedule of activities so that the patient is disturbed as little as possible. Medications, treatments, and nursing procedures should be administered at the same time as far as the physician's orders will permit, but always with the thought in mind that only as much as will not overtire the patient should be planned for any one time. When any treatment is ordered, the procedure is best carried out after sedation has been administered. Before heavy sedation is initiated, any removable dentures or eyeglasses should be stored in a secure place. If the patient is not in labor, the nurse must be alert to watch for signs of labor, particularly after sedation has been given. Any time an intravenous fluid is administered, if the rate at which the fluid is to flow has not been specified, it should be given slowly.

The nurse should see that the equipment necessary for the safe and efficient care of the patient is immediately available and in good working order. A padded mouth gag should always be ready for use at the bedside to prevent the patient from biting her tongue if a convulsion develops. Trays for catheterization equipment and for the administration of special medications constitute part of the necessary equipment. Since water retention plays such a large role in the disease, and urinary output is likely to be diminished, an indwelling bladder catheter may be ordered to ensure accuracy in obtaining output from the kidneys. Since the urinary output must be watched carefully, it is imperative to see that the retention catheter is draining properly at all times. In severe cases suction apparatus should be readily available for aspirating mucus, as well as equipment for administering oxygen, should symptoms such as cyanosis or depressed respiration indicate the need.

Eclampsia

Clinical Picture

As indicated, the development of eclampsia is almost always preceded by the signs and symptoms of preeclampsia. A preeclamptic patient, who may have been conversing with you a moment before, is seen to roll her eyes to one side and stare fixedly into space. Immediately, twitching of the facial muscles ensues. This is the *stage of invasion* of the convulsion and lasts only a few seconds.

The whole body then becomes rigid in a generalized muscular contraction; the face is distorted, the eyes protrude, the arms are flexed, the hands are clenched, and the legs are inverted. Since all the muscles of the body are now in a state of tonic contraction, this phase may be regarded as the *stage of contraction;* it lasts 15 seconds or 20 seconds.

Suddenly the jaws begin to open and close violently, and forthwith the eyelids also. The other facial muscles and then all the muscles of the body alternately contract and relax in rapid succession. The muscular movements are so forceful that the patient may throw herself out of bed, and almost invariably, unless protected, the tongue is bitten by the violent jaw action. Foam, which is often blood tinged, exudes from the mouth; the face is congested and purple, and the eyes are bloodshot. Few pictures which the nurse is called upon to witness are so horrible. This phase in which the muscles alternately contract and relax is called the *stage of convulsion;* it may last a minute or so. Gradually the muscular movements become milder and farther apart, and finally the patient lies motionless.

Throughout the seizure the diaphragm has been fixed, with respiration halted. Still no breathing occurs. For a few seconds the woman appears to be dying from respiratory arrest, but just when this outcome seems almost inevitable, she takes a long, deep, stertorous inhalation, and breathing is resumed. Then coma ensues. The patient does not remember anything about the convulsion or, in all probability, events immediately before and afterward.

The coma may last from a few minutes to several hours, and the patient may then become conscious, or the coma may be succeeded by another convulsion. The convulsions may recur during coma, they may recur only after an interval of consciousness, or they may never recur at all. In the average case, from five to ten convulsions occur at longer or shorter intervals, but as many as 20 are not uncommon. Convulsions may start before the onset of labor (antepartum), during labor (intrapartum), or anytime within the first 48 hours after delivery (postpartum). About a fifth of the cases develop postpartally.

Upon physical examination, the findings of eclampsia are similar to those in preeclampsia, but exaggerated. Thus, the systolic blood pressure usually ranges around 180 mm Hg and sometimes exceeds 200 mm Hg. Proteinuria is frequently extreme, from 10 g per liter to 20 g per liter. Edema may be marked but sometimes is absent. Oliguria, or diminution of urinary excretion, is common and may progress to complete anuria. Fever is present in about half the cases.

In favorable cases the convulsions cease, the coma lessens, and urinary output increases. However, it sometimes requires 1 day or 2 days for clear consciousness to be regained. During this period eclamptic patients are often in an obstreperous, resistant mood and may be exceedingly difficult to manage. A few develop actual psychoses. In unfavorable cases the coma deepens, urinary excretion diminishes, the pulse becomes more rapid, the temperature rises, and edema of the lungs develops. The last is a serious symptom and usually is interpreted as a sign of cardiovascular failure. Edema of the lungs is readily recognizable by the noisy, gurgling respiration and by the large quantity of frothy mucus which exudes from the mouth and the nose. Toward the end, convulsions cease altogether, and the final picture is one of vascular collapse, with falling blood pressure and overwhelming edema of the lungs.

Like preeclampsia, eclampsia is a disease of young primigravidae, with the majority of cases occurring in first pregnancies. It is more likely to occur as full term approaches and is rarely seen prior to the last 3 months. Eclampsia is particularly likely to develop in twin gestations, the likelihood being about four times that in single pregnancies.

Prognosis

Eclampsia is one of the gravest complications of pregnancy; the maternal mortality in different localities and in different hospitals ranges from 5% to 15%. The outlook for the baby is particularly grave, as the fetal mortality is about 20%. Although it is difficult in a given case to forecast the outcome, the following are unfavorable signs: oliguria, prolonged coma, a sustained pulse rate over 120, temperature over 39.5C (103°F), more than ten convulsions, 10 or more g of protein per liter in the urine, systolic blood pressure of more than 200, and edema of lungs. If none of these signs is present, the outlook for recovery is good; if two or more are present, the prognosis is definitely serious.

Even though the patient survives, she may not escape unscathed from the attack but sometimes continues to have high blood pressure indefinitely. This applies to both preeclampsia and eclampsia. Even though the patient survives, unrecognized hypertension may result in continued high blood pressure. It is even more important to note that a still larger percentage of these women (about 50% of preeclamptics and 30% of eclamptics) again develop hypertensive toxemia in any subsequent pregnancies. This is known as "recurrent" or "repeat" toxemia. These facts make it plain that careful, prolonged follow-up of those mothers who have suffered from preeclampsia or eclampsia is imperative. Moreover, the prognosis for future pregnancies must be guarded, although, as the figures indicate, such patients stand at least an even chance of going through subsequent pregnancies satisfactorily.

Principles of Management

Because the cause of eclampsia is not known, there can be no "specific" therapy, and treatment must necessarily be empirical, which means use of those therapeutic measures which have yielded the best results in other cases. Empirical treatment is thus based on experience. Because the experience of different physicians and different hospitals varies considerably, the type of therapy employed from clinic to clinic differs somewhat in respect to the drugs used and in other details. However, the general principles followed are almost identical everywhere. These are enumerated as follows:

1. *Prevention.* Let it be emphasized again that eclampsia is largely (but not entirely) a preventable disease. Vigilant antepartal care and the early detection and treatment of preeclampsia does more to reduce deaths from eclampsia than the most intensive treatment after convulsions have started.
2. *Termination of Pregnancy.* Although the precise cause of preeclampsia and eclampsia is not known, it is quite clear that since they occur in pregnancy, the one sure "cure" is to render the patient nonpregnant. In almost all instances of eclampsia, efforts to effect delivery should be undertaken as soon as the patient is stabilized. This involves control of seizures as well as hyperreflexia by using adequate doses of anticonvulsants and initiating diuresis. It is often helpful to monitor central venous pressure in addition to urinary output in an attempt to optimize fluid balance.

   Efforts to accomplish delivery before the patient is stabilized may result in increased maternal morbidity and mortality. The method of delivery should be by the most expeditious route. Prolonged attempts at induction in the face of an unripe cervix are not indicated; however, the possibility of vaginal delivery should not be discounted even at early gestational age since, for unexplained reasons, the cervix often quickly becomes favorable for induction. Occasionally the obstetrician is faced with the dilemma of an eclamptic with an immature fetus. Although it is tempting to try to prolong the pregnancy in the interest of bringing about greater fetal maturity, such attempts are generally unsuccessful, with impaired placental function and failure of the fetus to prosper.

3. *Sedation.* The purpose of administering sedative drugs is to depress the activity of the brain cells and thereby stop convulsions. The drugs most commonly employed are described below:

Magnesium Sulfate. This drug is an excellent central nervous system depressant, and therefore an anticonvulsant and also a smooth muscle relaxant that causes dilatation of peripheral blood vessels and thereby reduces blood pressure. For these reasons it is probably the most common drug used in eclamptic patients. The routes of administration, doses, and precautions have already been discussed. The drug is most often given intravenously, at least initially, because the situation with the eclamptic patient is so urgent.

Diazepam (Valium). Intravenous diazepam is widely used for seizure control. Generally 40 mg is diluted in 500 ml of 5% dextrose in water, and this is administered at a rate of 30 drops per minute. Diazepam can cause neonatal depression if more than 30 mg are used within 15 hours to 20 hours before delivery. For this reason, magnesium sulfate remains the sedative drug of choice.

4. *Protection of Patient from Self-Injury.* The eclamptic patient must never be left alone for a second. When in the throes of a convulsion, she may crash her head against a bedpost or throw herself onto the floor, or she may bite her tongue violently. To prevent the latter injury, some device should be kept within easy reach which can be inserted between the jaws at the very onset of a convulsion. A piece of heavy rubber tubing, a rolled towel or a padded clothespin is often employed. The nurse must take care in inserting it not to injure the patient (*e.g.,* lips, gums, teeth) and not to allow her own fingers to be bitten.

   Eclamptic patients must never be given fluids by mouth unless thoroughly conscious. Failure to adhere to this rule may result in aspiration of the fluid and consequent pneumonia.

5. *Protection of Patient from Extraneous Stimuli.* A loud noise, a bright light, a jarring of the bed, a draft—indeed, the slightest irritation—may be enough to precipitate a convulsion.

Nurse's Responsibilities in Eclampsia

The nurse's responsibilities in the management of a patient with eclampsia are serious. Some of them have already been mentioned in the discussion of treatment. Although eclampsia usually is regarded as the climax to a mounting preeclampsia that has been present, the nurse must remember that it is occasionally observed as a fulminating case in an apparently normal woman who may develop severe symptoms in the span of 24 hours. In the event that eclampsia occurs, the highest quality of nursing care is necessary. The attack may come on at any time, even when the patient is sleeping.

During the seizure it is necessary to protect the patient from self-injury. Never leave the patient for an instant unless someone is actually at the bedside to relieve you. Gentle restraint should be used to guide the patient's movements whenever necessary to prevent her from throwing herself against the head of the bed or out of it. The padded mouth gag should be inserted between the upper and lower teeth at the onset of a convulsion to prevent the tongue from being bitten.

Regardless of the fact that the nurse is exceedingly "busy" with the patient during a seizure, careful and complete observations of the duration and the character of each convulsion, the depth and duration of coma, the quality and the rate of pulse and respiration and the degree of cyanosis are important. A record should be kept so that this information can be used in treating the patient.

During the coma which follows, care must be taken to see that the patient does not aspirate. It is understood, of course, that one never gives an eclamptic patient fluids by mouth unless it is certain she is fully conscious. The position of the patient in bed should be such that it promotes drainage of secretions and the maintenance of a clear airway. It may be necessary to raise the foot of the bed of the comatose patient a few inches to promote drainage of secretions from the respiratory passage. When this measure must be resorted to, it is particularly important to watch for signs of pulmonary edema, which would be aggravated by this position. The head of the bed may need to be elevated to relieve dyspnea.

The patient should be protected from extraneous stimuli. Light in the room should be eliminated except for a small lamp, so shaded that none of the light falls on the patient. Although the room should be darkened, the light should be sufficient to permit observations of changes in condition, such as cyanosis or twitchings. A flashlight, directed well away from the patient's face, may be used during catheterization and during examinations. Sudden noises, such as the slamming of a door or the clatter of a tray as it is placed on a table, and jarring of the bed must be avoided, because they are often sufficient stimuli to send the patient into convulsions. Only absolutely necessary conversation should be carried on in the room, and this should be in the lowest tones possible.

The fetal heart tones should be checked as often as time permits. Also, the nurse must watch for signs of labor. In eclampsia this may proceed with few external signs, and occasionally such a patient gives birth beneath the sheets before anyone knows that the process is under way. Be suspicious when the patient grunts or groans or moves about at regular intervals, every 5 minutes or so. If this occurs, feel the consistency of the uterus, watch for "show" and bulging and report your observations to the physician. Convulsions that occur during labor may speed up this process, and more rapid preparation for delivery should be made. During the delivery, the same atmosphere of quiet should be maintained, and glaring lights should be kept away from the patient's face.

Throughout the care of the eclamptic patient a careful account of fluid intake and output should be recorded, along with all the other observations and pertinent data. And, since further complications of pregnancy may occur in eclampsia, the patient should be observed for signs and symptoms of cerebral hemorrhage, abruptio placentae, pulmonary edema and cardiac failure.

Concurrent Hypertension and Pregnancy

As the name implies, this is a process in which high blood pressure is present before pregnancy. Difficulty is encountered in establishing such a diagnosis, because many women are not seen between pregnancies and blood pressures are, therefore, not recorded. Also, there is normally a decrease in blood pressure during the second trimester that could mask a preexisting hypertension if the patient does not report for care until the fourth or fifth month of gestation. The diagnosis is justified if hypertension is detected prior to the 24th week of gestation. Most often patients with chronic hypertension are multiparae and commonly over the age of 30.

At least 75% of such patients are able to complete their pregnancies successfully, with no significant change in the status of their hypertension. Fifteen percent develop superimposed preeclampsia, an occurrence which carries an ominous fetal prognosis (20% mortality), and even an increase in maternal mortality.

The treatment, then, for the majority of pregnant patients with chronic hypertension is no different from treatment for the nonpregnant patient. The pregnancy is allowed to run its normal course under such circumstances, unless the pregnancy aggravates the already existing hypertension. When the gravida with this chronic process develops a further elevation of blood pressure, significant proteinuria, or edema, the condition is called *superimposed preeclampsia.*

In the case of superimposed preeclampsia, after 24 hours to 48 hours of intensive medical therapy, pregnancy termination is generally indicated. Even though the fetus may be preterm, its chances for survival under these circumstances are generally better outside the uterus.

In a small number of patients the hypertension will be so severe, with evidence of kidney involvement, severe retinal changes, or cardiac involvement, that therapeutic abortion might be considered if the patient comes to medical attention in the first trimester. It is also important to consider the advisability of postpartum tubal ligation in this group of patients who are generally older, with established families, and for whom additional pregnancies may represent a serious health hazard. This, of course, can only be a recommendation; the final decision rests with the patient.

Suggested Reading

Cavanagh D, O'Connor TCF: Eclamptogenic toxemia. In Cavanagh D, Woods RF, O'Connor TCF (eds): Obstetric Emergencies, 2nd ed, pp 105–132. Hagerstown, Md., Harper & Row, 1978

Gant NF, Worley RJ, Cunningham FG, Whalley PJ: Clinical management of pregnancy induced hypertension. Clin Obstet Gynecol 21:397, June, 1978

Welt SI, Grenshaw MC Jr: Concurrent hypertension and pregnancy. Clin Obstet Gynecol 21:619, September 1978

Wingate MB, Iffy L, Kelly JV, Birnbaum S: Diseases specific to pregnancy. In Romney SL, Gray MJ, Little AB, Merell JA et al (eds): Gynecology and Obstetrics, The Health Care of Women, 2nd ed. pp 718–776. New York, McGraw–Hill, 1980

Woods RF, Cavanagh D: Hemorrhage in early pregnancy. In Cavanagh D, Woods RF, O'Connor TCF, (eds): Obstetric Emergencies, 2nd ed, pp 133–176. Hagerstown, Md., Harper & Row, 1978

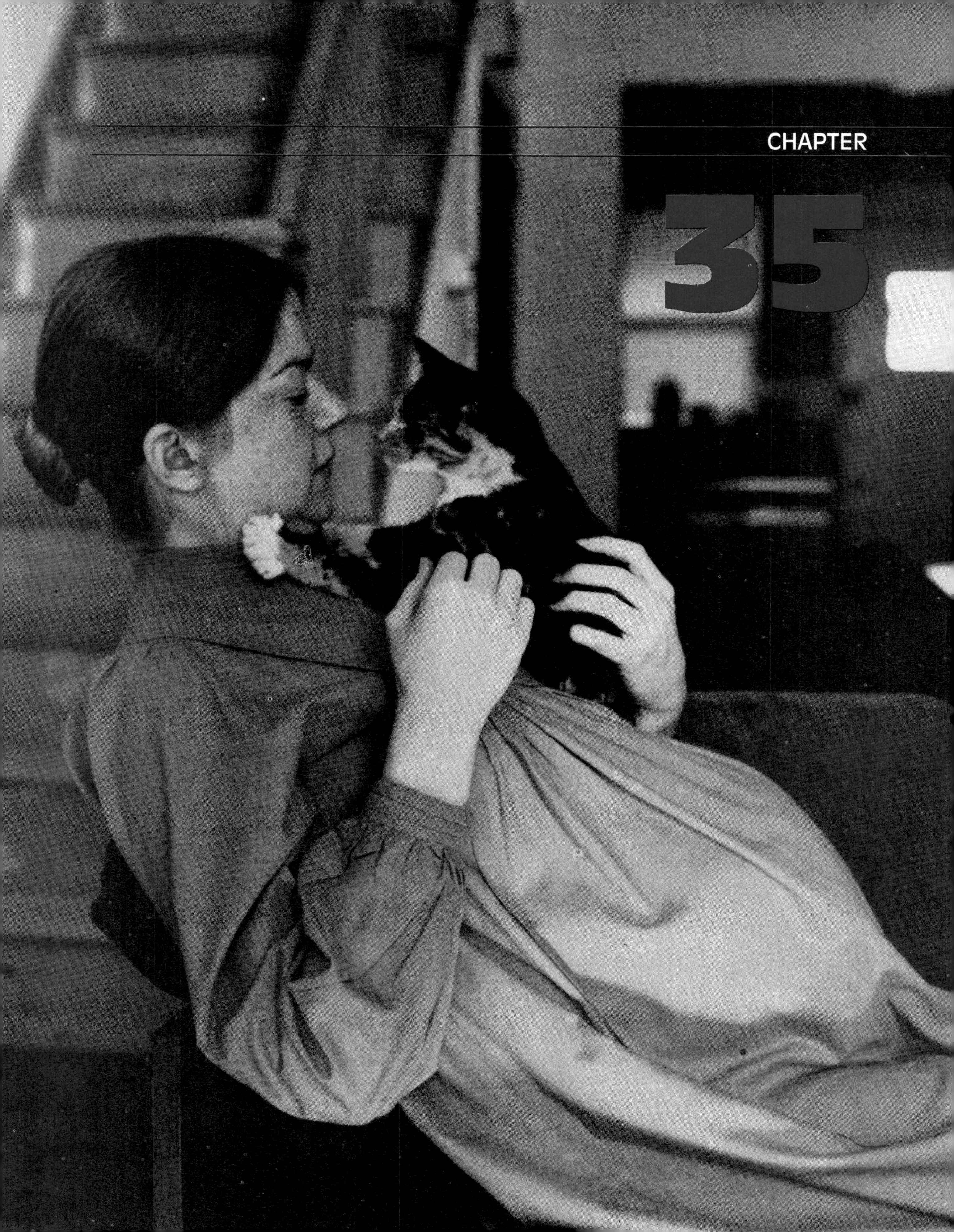

CHAPTER 35

CHAPTER 35

Concurrent Diseases in Pregnancy

It has been said wisely that the pregnant woman can have any disease which her nonpregnant counterpart can have, except for infertility. One must be aware that many disease states are modified by the physiological changes of pregnancy. Pregnancy may alter the classic clinical picture of a disease state and, indeed, some of the normal physiological changes of pregnancy mimic disease. Therapeutic approaches must be altered in some cases, especially with regard to possible effects on the fetus. For most coincidental diseases, the effects of pregnancy on the disease and of the disease on pregnancy are negligible and do not influence the management of either. Some diseases, however, have profound fetal effects, as discussed in Chapter 39, others have a predominantly maternal effect; and some, such as diabetes, affect both. The more common diseases in the latter two categories are discussed in this chapter.

Hematologic Disorders

Iron Deficiency Anemia

Iron deficiency anemia is the most common hematologic disorder in pregnancy. Because of the expanded blood volume there is an element of hemodilution with a resultant fall in hemoglobin concentration unless the need is met by augmented hematopoiesis. There is, in addition, the fetal requirement for iron to contend with. Since many women have depleted iron stores as a result of regular menstrual blood loss, these added demands often result in the total depletion of storage iron and the development of overt anemia. The socioeconomically deprived patient with poor general nutrition is more susceptible to this condition.

In most patients with mild to moderate anemia, the signs and symptoms are few and often indistinguishable from the normal symptoms of pregnancy. Such patients are detected by frequent antepartum hemoglobin or hematocrit determinations. Severely anemic patients are symptomatic and in the most severe cases can even develop heart failure as a result of the anemia.

Treatment for mild to moderate cases consists of iron-rich diet and an oral iron compound such as ferrous sulfate or gluconate. Similar recommendations hold for the nonanemic gravida as prophylaxis. It has been estimated that the pregnant patient requires 3 mg of iron per day to 5 mg of iron per day to supply the needs of mother and fetus, with demands for iron increasing in the last 5 months of pregnancy to as much as 3 mg per day to 7.5 mg per day. Thus, oral iron supplementary therapy is recommended throughout pregnancy, but especially in the latter half. 200 mg of ferrous sulfate three times a day or 320 mg of ferrous gluconate three times a day satisfies this need. Injectable iron therapy is rarely required because absorption is generally not a limiting factor. More often a failure to respond to oral iron therapy is the result of failure to take the medication (iron tends to produce gastrointestinal symptoms) or a concurrent folic acid deficiency.

Folic Acid Deficiency

Folic acid deficiency can produce severe anemia of the megaloblastic type in pregnancy. Megaloblastic anemia is much less common than iron deficiency anemia, occurring in less than 3% of gravidae. In its full-blown form there is also a reduction in white cells and platelets and is usually associated with glossitis and a sore tongue.

Treatment consists of oral folic acid and diet. Prevention is achieved by the inclusion of folic acid in prenatal vitamin–mineral supplements.

Hemoglobinopathies

Hemoglobinopathies present special problems in pregnancy. The most commonly encountered of the hemoglobinopathies are sickle-cell anemia and sickle cell hemoglobin C disease. These are inherited diseases that are seen principally in the black population and are invariably associated with an increased maternal morbidity and mortality, perinatal mortality, and abortion.

Sickle-cell anemia occurs when the gene for the production of S hemoglobin is inherited from both parents. When S hemoglobin is transmitted from one but not the other, the individual does not exhibit frank anemia but has *sickle-cell trait.* Pregnant patients with sickle-cell trait have a predisposition to urinary tract infections but are otherwise normal. About 1 in 12 black individuals has sickle-cell trait.

The theoretical incidence of sickle-cell anemia is about 1 in 500. Its actual occurrence in pregnancy, however, is only one third as high, probably because many affected individuals do not survive to childbearing age. The anemia is exacerbated during pregnancy, and life-threatening hemolytic crises can occur. About one half of the pregnancies end in spontaneous abortion, neonatal death, or stillbirth. Patients with sickle-cell anemia require the most meticulous of prenatal care. Multiple transfusions are sometimes used to suppress the patient's bone marrow from forming abnormal cells while at the same time permitting her to exist on transfused cells during the period of risk. Throughout pregnancy, diet should be supplemented with folic acid because of the rapid turnover of red blood cells.

Sickle-cell hemoglobin C disease occurs when the gene for the production of hemoglobin C is inherited along with that for hemoglobin S. It is much less common and certainly less serious in the nonpregnant state. During pregnancy and the puerperium, however, mortality and morbidity are greatly increased, with a maternal mortality reported in some series as high as 2%. In contrast to sickle-cell anemia disease, the perinatal mortality is increased only slightly.

In managing hemoglobinopathies, detailed counseling is called for. One must consider not only the impact of pregnancy in precipitating crises but also the genetic implications and the fact that patients with sickle-cell anemia have a limited life expectancy. Patients with sickle-cell anemia might well wish to consider limiting childbearing or even avoiding pregnancy completely.

■■■

Heart Disease

Rheumatic heart disease has for some time been the most common type of heart disease seen in pregnancy. Recognition of the role of streptococcal infection and its appropriate therapy has reduced the frequency of rheumatic fever and its cardiac consequences and congenital heart disease is now relatively more commonly encountered in pregnancy. Another dimension has been added by cardiac surgeons. Surgically treated patients, even some with valve replacements, now often proceed through pregnancy uneventfully.

The diagnosis of heart disease during pregnancy is made somewhat more difficult by the physiological changes that occur. In normal pregnancy functional systolic heart murmurs are rather common. Upward displacement of the diaphragm and heart by the enlarging uterus moves the apex of the heart laterally. This may create a false impression of cardiac enlargement. Progesterone stimulates the respiratory center, accentuating breathing effort which is reminiscent of the dyspnea sometimes seen in heart disease. Edema of the lower extremities that is commonly encountered in normal pregnancy is also a sign of cardiac failure. These normal changes must be considered when the cardiac status of the pregnant patient is evaluated. The most useful criteria in establishing a diagnosis of heart disease in pregnancy include a diastolic, presystolic, or continuous heart murmur; unequivocal cardiac enlargement; a harsh systolic murmur associated with a thrill; or a significant cardiac arrhythmia.

Changes in the circulatory system in pregnancy must also be considered. During the course of pregnancy, there is a decrease in vascular resistance and blood pressure and an increase in blood volume. Cardiac output increases during the first trimester and continues to be elevated throughout the remainder of pregnancy. Since venous return to the heart is retarded by pressure of the enlarged uterus when a pregnant woman is in the supine position, cardiac output is decreased, increasing when the patient is moved to the lateral recumbent position. Because of the increased body mass in pregnancy, cardiac output in response to exercise is, of course, greater as pregnancy progresses. The first stage of labor is associated with a modest increase in cardiac output, and there is an appreciable change associated with the expulsive efforts of the second stage.

Management

For most types of heart disease, the major threat imposed by pregnancy is that the increasing blood volume will precipitate congestive heart failure. With appropriate therapy and restriction of activities, however, most patients can tolerate that stress and carry a pregnancy to a successful conclusion. The exception might be that individual falling into functional class IV (symptomatic at rest) in the first trimester, especially if she does not have a surgically correctable lesion. It is now the very rare cardiac patient who should be considered for therapeutic abortion on medical grounds.

Appropriate therapy demands close cooperation between the obstetrician and cardiologist, with the nurse playing a major role by coordinating information for the patient as well as providing day-to-day patient supervision. Treatment is governed to a considerable extent by the functional capacity of the patient, and rest is one of the most important ingredients, with bedrest being necessary in some advanced cases. Digitalis, diuretics, and salt restriction may all be required, depending upon the severity. In the case of valvular lesions, penicillin prophylaxis is recommended during labor and at delivery to prevent bacterial endocarditis, to which patients with valvular lesions are susceptible.

As for all patients with heart disease, any respiratory infection can be devastating, and consequently, patients should avoid any predisposing situation and report even a sore throat or cold to the nurse or physician. The patient with heart disease who develops a cough should be examined forthwith, as coughing is one of the early symptoms of pulmonary congestion and cardiac failure.

Because the onset of heart failure may be insidious, it behooves the nurse to be alert to the signs and symptoms of this problem. These might include inability to carry on normal activities, increased dyspnea on exertion, and paroxysmal nocturnal dyspnea, tachycardia, palpitations, and cough, especially if blood or rusty sputum is evident.

Very special problems are presented by the patients with valve prostheses, since they require anticoagulant therapy. Sodium warfarin (Coumadin) and related drugs are contraindicated because they cross the placenta; this requires changing such patients to heparin therapy for the duration of pregnancy.

Diabetes Mellitus

Diabetes mellitus illustrates the interplay between the altered physiology of pregnancy and the pathophysiology of disease. In contrast to the majority of disease states which do not alter or are not affected by pregnancy, there is a significant change in the course of diabetes when pregnancy supervenes, and diabetes has a profound effect on the course of pregnancy as well as on the fetus. In addition to participating in the regular medical and prenatal care of the diabetic gravida, the nurse can serve a very important counseling role. Care is a team effort and must involve cooperation among obstetrician, internist, pediatrician, nurse, and nutritionist.

Diabetes can have a deleterious effect on pregnancy in the following ways: (1) infection, especially urinary tract infection is more common and more serious; (2) the fetus is often larger (macrosomia), which increases the possibility of a difficult vaginal delivery and postpartum hemorrhage; (3) there is a fourfold overall greater incidence of preeclampsia or eclampsia, with an increase even when there is no associated preexisting vascular disease; (4) there is an increased incidence of hydramnios, and if this is coupled with fetal macrosomia, it can cause cardiopulmonary symptoms; (5) the fetus and newborn can also be affected adversely in several ways (see Chap. 44).

In recent years, the number of pregnant diabetics has increased, partly because with modern management, diabetics are now able to conceive and maintain pregnancies, and partly because there is presently an increased recognition of the milder forms of gestational diabetes.

Pregnancy Alterations in Insulin and Carbohydrate Metabolism

During the course of pregnancy, the placenta produces HPL, which is an insulin antagonist and exerts a powerful effect on insulin action. The estrogen and progesterone produced by the placenta also influence insulin, albeit to a lesser degree. The effect of these placental products on insulin increases the maternal requirement for insulin during the course of pregnancy. In other words, more insulin must be produced in order to make up for the antagonistic effect of these hormones. The placenta also produces placental insulinase, an enzyme which accelerates the degradation of insulin, and this also increases insulin requirements.

During the course of normal pregnancy, there is a lower fasting blood sugar level. There is, however, no difference between the pregnant and nonpregnant intravenous glucose tolerance test, and the degree of induced hyperglycemia is the same during the course of this test in the pregnant and nonpregnant states. When the oral glucose tolerance test is used, the hyperglycemia persists somewhat longer in pregnancy because of slower and more prolonged absorption of glucose from the gastrointestinal tract.

Diagnosis

During the course of normal pregnancy, glucose may appear in the urine with blood sugars as low as 100 mg% because of a lowered renal threshold to glucose excretion. Although the presence of glucose in the urine does not necessarily indicate high glucose blood levels, any patient exhibiting glucosuria should be suspected of having diabetes, and the diagnosis should be established or ruled out by evaluation of glucose blood levels. A fasting blood glucose of over 130 mg% is almost invariably associated with diabetes. However, if a woman has already been identified as being diabetic prior to pregnancy, diagnostic glucose tolerance tests are not required.

Diabetes may become manifest during pregnancy only to regress completely following delivery. In these circumstances, the condition is referred to as gestational diabetes. It should be suspected on the basis of the following:

1. Previous large babies
2. Family history of diabetes
3. Glucosuria
4. Obesity
5. Unexplained pregnancy wastage

In these patients the appropriate screening test is a 2-hour postprandial blood sugar. Fasting blood sugars are not adequate since the fasting sugar is normally reduced in the first trimester. When a normal value is obtained initially, the patient should be screened for diabetes again in the second and third trimesters. Abnormal values indicate the need for a full glucose tolerance test.

A special diagnostic problem occurs when a patient is not suspected of being diabetic until after delivery, as might be the case if she has delivered an unusually large baby or an unexplained stillborn. Since the diabetogenic effects of pregnancy disappear quickly following delivery, a normal glucose tolerance test 48 hours to 72 hours postpartum is not necessarily reassuring. The so-called steroid enforced glucose tolerance test in which cortisone is administered prior to the testing may bring out the abnormality.

Classification

The most universally used classification of diabetes is that by White, which is as follows:

Class A—glucose tolerance test diabetes

Class B—onset: over age 20
duration: 0 years to 9 years
vascular disease: 0

Class C—onset: 10 years to 19 years
duration: 10–19 years
vascular disease: 0

Class D—onset: under age 40
duration: 20+ years
vascular disease: calcification in legs, retinitis

Class F—patients with nephritis

Class R—proliferative retinopathy

Although this classification has some pitfalls in that duration of disease and vascular disease are not always absolutely parallel, in general perinatal wastage can be related to the class. Wastage is invariably greater in those patients with vascular disease (Classes D, F, and R), and less in Classes A, B, and C. It should also be noted that mothers with significant vascular involvement have small rather than large-for-date babies.

Management

Careful medical management of the pregnant diabetic is the key to a successful outcome. The initial evaluation should include examination of the optic fundi for detection of vascular disease, and also urine analysis and culture to detect asymptomatic bacilluria, a precursor to overt pyelonephritis, to which the diabetic is especially prone.

Diet

Diet is of paramount importance, and the nurse must be prepared to assist the patient in this area. The caloric requirement for the normal-weight patient is approximately 2200 calories with 1 g of protein per kg of body weight to 1.5 g of protein per kg of body weight. In the case of many gestational diabetics who are overweight, total calories must be reduced to control blood sugar. It is difficult to go below 1500 calories and still maintain adequate protein intake and a palatable formulation. Standard diabetic diets tend to lack the protein needed in pregnancy. Occasionally one needs to increase carbohydrate and total calories because of the patient's activities, or in some cases of juvenile diabetes, the large amount of glucose lost in the urine. Food costs and ethnic dietary habits must also be considered when making such recommendations.

Preeclampsia and hydramnios both occur relatively frequently in diabetic pregnant patients. These serious complications should be kept in mind and watched for throughout the entire course of prenatal care.

Insulin

Although diet alone may control many gestational diabetics, if the two-hour postprandial sugar exceeds 150 mg% to 160 mg%, despite the diet, insulin therapy is indicated. Although occasionally used, the oral hypoglycemics are not cleared for use in pregnancy. Progressive insulin resistance is characteristic of pregnancy and it is not unusual for insulin requirements to increase as much as fourfold. This commonly necessitates the use of evening as well as morning doses of insulin to achieve good control. Although in the majority of patients, insulin requirements increase as pregnancy progresses; about 35% require the same dose or less. This variability highlights further the importance of meticulous management of insulin needs during the prenatal course.

Obstetrical Considerations

Obstetrical management involves evaluating fetal well-being and determining the timing and method of delivery. Since the major target of diabetes is the small blood vessels, it is not surprising that the placenta may also be involved, and therefore, placental insufficiency and even fetal death may occur. This result is far less common in gestational diabetics than in prepregnancy diabetics and is the basis for the common practice of delivering diabetic patients 3 weeks to 4 weeks prior to the expected date of confinement. This is not, however, always necessary if one can identify the fetus at risk by another type of technique, such as serial 24-hour urinary estriol determinations (see Chap. 39).

In those patients with no evidence of fetal compromise and who are otherwise stable (good diabetic control, absence of preeclampsia, and no significant hydramnios), pregnancy may be allowed to go to term, with careful surveillance. The method of delivery is a matter of obstetrical judgment at the time. Early deliveries are carried out more often by cesarean birth because the cervix is not prepared for induction, and even at term there is an increased need for section because of the mechanical problems created by the fetal macrosoma.

During vaginal deliveries fetal size may cause problems in the form of shoulder dystocia.

Newborns of diabetic mothers show a high incidence of congenital anomalies. It is reported as high as 8%. They also display a greater incidence of respiratory distress syndrome and neonatal hyperbilirubinemia.

The problems of the diabetic offspring are discussed in detail in Chapter 42. However, it is important to realize that even under the best of circumstances the perinatal mortality is two to three times that in the nondiabetic, and pregnancy is a very major undertaking for the diabetic and her family.

Disturbances in Thyroid Function

Hyperthyroidism is probably the second most significant endocrinopathy in pregnancy, second only to diabetes mellitus. Although a woman with uncontrolled hyperthyroidism is likely to be anovulatory and thus unable to conceive, many with milder disease do conceive, and in some cases the hyperthyroidism is first diagnosed during pregnancy. If the condition is not detected and treated properly, spontaneous abortion and premature labor are common. Diagnosis may be somewhat of a problem in milder cases since some thyroid enlargement and confusing hyperdynamic symptoms occur in normal pregnancy. Laboratory studies may also be confusing since there is increased protein binding of thyroid hormone in pregnancy resulting in higher values for studies such as the protein bound iodine and total T_4, with lower T_3 uptake. Multiple studies and newer methods, however, can overcome the confusion.

Once-popular surgical treatment (subtotal thyroidectomy) has been replaced by medical approaches, except in special cases (*e.g.,* reaction to the antithyroid drugs, unusually large dosage requirements). The problem with medical therapy is that the antithyroid drugs do cross the placenta and if doses are excessive the fetal thyroid can be suppressed, leading to fetal goiter or even cretinism. This is best avoided if the level of control is maintained at slightly hyperthyroid levels.

Patients with exophthalmic goiter produce a long-acting thyroid stimulator (LATS), which is a gamma-g globulin. This does cross the placenta and if present can cause hyperthyroidism in the newborn.

Hypothyroidism and parathyroid disorders are reported in pregnancy, but they are rare. Adrenal, pituitary, and ovarian disorders generally result in infertility.

Renal Disease

Almost all forms of acute and chronic renal disease have been reported in association with pregnancy. Not infrequently, specific diagnosis is difficult during pregnancy because proteinuria and hypertension may mimic preeclampsia and also because definitive studies such as renal biopsy and intravenous urography are relatively contraindicated. Chronic renal disease, especially if accompanied by hypertension, may be associated with fetal growth retardation and increased perinatal mortality.

The most common renal problem in pregnancy is urinary tract infection. Anatomical changes as well as hormonal effects cause narrowing of the lower ureter with dilatation of the upper ureter and renal pelvis. These changes result in delayed emptying and an increased risk of infection. The risk increases as pregnancy progresses and continues into the puerperium.

Symptoms include chills, fever, frequency, dysuria, and pain in the kidney area. Severity may vary from extremely mild to extremely toxic, with nausea, vomiting, and abnormal distention. Uterine irritability is an important complication of pyelonephritis. It is wise to look for urinary tract infection in any patient with premature labor.

In order to treat the patient adequately, a carefully collected midstream clean catch urine specimen must be obtained. To assure an adequate specimen the nurse should instruct the patient as to the proper method of collecting the sample. An examination of the urinary sediment as well as a culture and antibiotic sensitivity studies should be carried out. In addition to the selection of an appropriate antibiotic, it is imperative that a good fluid intake be maintained, parenterally if necessary. Antimicrobial therapy should be continued for 7 days to 10 days even if the response is good, and the urine should be recultured once therapy is stopped. Recurrences are common, causing some authorities to recommend long-term suppressive antimicrobial therapy.

Asymptomatic bacteriuria in pregnancy is significant because of its high association with subsequent pyelonephritis and consequently should be treated. Association with other obstetrical problems such as prematurity has been suggested, but it is likely that these are simply coincidental findings in a group of high-risk patients.

Infectious Diseases

Although most infectious diseases have no established specific ill effects on mother or baby, there are those that produce profound effects. Diseases with particular fetal effects are discussed in Chapter 42.

The Common Cold

Susceptibility to acute upper respiratory infections is apparently slightly greater during pregnancy. The common cold often precedes more serious conditions affecting the upper respiratory tract. Therefore, the pregnant woman should make every effort to avoid contacts with these infections.

Influenza

Although the pregnant woman is not more likely to contract influenza, she is more prone to the development of complicating pneumonia, especially if she is in the third trimester during which time the diaphragm is elevated and respiration is compromised.

The development of pneumonia represents a serious threat to the gravida. In the face of an epidemic involving a specific strain of influenza virus, immunization with a killed or attenuated virus vaccine is indicated. Nonspecific polyvalent vaccines are probably ineffectual.

Measles

Ill effects are not commonly noted in pregnancy, but pregnant women who contract measles are said to be more likely to have premature labor. No other definite effects are reported, although eruptions have been noted on infants at birth.

Typhoid Fever

Typhoid fever, which is now relatively rare in the United States, may cause serious complications in pregnancy, resulting in abortion, prematurity, and infant mortality. Immunization is not contraindicated during pregnancy, and antityphoid vaccine should be administered when necessary.

Tuberculosis

The average case of tuberculosis in itself has only a slight effect on the course of pregnancy, since it rarely predisposes to abortion, premature labor, or even stillbirth. Fortunately, the disease is seldom acquired congenitally, although a small number of authentic cases have been reported in which, in addition to a tuberculous condition of the placenta, tubercle bacilli were found in the cord blood, together with tuberculous lesions in the baby.

Medical opinions differ, but the consensus is that pregnancy does not exert an adverse effect on tuberculosis when properly managed. It is generally agreed, however, that only a patient in an arrested state should consider becoming pregnant. Pregnancy is undertaken with some risk, for although a tuberculous lesion may remain latent for an indefinite time, provided that the natural resistance is not overtaxed, it must be noted that pregnancy is one of the factors responsible for overtaxing the resistance sufficiently to convert a latent, inactive lesion into an active one. Maintenance of proper nutrition does much to prevent activity in a latent focus.

Treatment with modern antituberculosis drugs, streptomycin, isoniazid (INH), and para-aminosalicylic acid (PAS), has completely altered management in general, as well as during pregnancy. New advanced cases are rare and a majority of patients are managed as outpatients. No deleterious effects of these agents on the mother or the fetus have been reported.

Labor and delivery are conducted in a normal fashion, avoiding inhalation anesthesia, and mother and baby are separated if disease is active. Breastfeeding is unwise even when the disease is inactive. Some authorities recommend INH therapy in the third trimester and puerperium for the inactive patient who has had active disease within 2 years of pregnancy.

Poliomyelitis

This disease generally does not complicate pregnancy or delivery, except in the very unusual cases in which respiratory paralysis develops; in these rare cases cesarean birth has given satisfactory results. Fortunately, as a result of immunization, the disease has virtually disappeared.

Viral Hepatitis

The hepatitis viruses (hepatitis A and B) are the most common causes of liver disease in pregnancy. Anorexia, nausea, and vomiting are the most characteristic symptoms of hepatitis. Since 75% of affected patients do not exhibit clinical jaundice, the diagnosis may be missed or delayed in patients exhibiting the nausea and vomiting characteristic of pregnancy, or cases may be misdiagnosed as hyperemesis gravidarum. In contrast to the latter, in hepatitis the liver is characteristically enlarged and tender and bilirubin levels rise as high as 25 mg%. When nausea and vomiting persist unabated in pregnancy, hepatitis should be considered and ruled out.

Hepatitis is associated with an increased incidence of abortion, premature labor and stillbirth. Maternal mortality from viral hepatitis varies, and has been reported at from 1% to 17%. Its course is substantially influenced by the nutritional status of the patient, and hence maternal mortality is higher in the less developed regions of the world. Prompt diagnosis and treatment with bedrest, good nutrition, and intravenous therapy generally result in a favorable maternal outcome.

The fetus may acquire the virus *in utero* or during delivery, and the newborn may develop active hepatitis or a carrier state. Prompt treatment of the newborn with hyperimmune gammaglobulin has been recommended. Since hepatitis B surface antigen has been detected in breast milk, and since the virus is present in maternal serum and could be transmitted from excoriations around the nipple, breast-feeding should be avoided.

Syphilis

In the past the major hazard of syphilis in pregnancy was the occurrence of intrauterine infection and late abortion or stillbirth. Congenital syphilis has now been reduced nearly to the point of elimination. The antenatal blood test for syphilis is required by law and, except for the instances in which prenatal care is nonexistent, maternal syphilis should be detected and adequately treated, thereby protecting the fetus.

Syphilis can occur at any stage during pregnancy. The primary and secondary stages are usually apparent because of their lesions. In latent syphilis, the diagnosis is based upon a positive serology; the most difficult problem occurs when the serology is repeatedly positive and the patient denies a history. Biological false positives do occur in a number of circumstances, but, fortunately, new, more specific tests are now available that can be used in the questionable case.

Treatment is indicated in the following circumstances:

1. When a diagnosis of early syphilis is made, regardless of stage
2. When late symptomatic syphilis is discovered
3. When latent syphilis is diagnosed by repeated positive serologic tests and the patient's history corroborates the diagnosis, and when there has been either inadequate or no treatment
4. When the diagnosis is made by repeated positive tests, even though the history does not confirm, and when either the more specific tests are not available or there is not time for adequate therapy. Retreatment in subsequent pregnancies is necessary if there is any doubt about the adequacy of previous therapy

The treatment consists of a course of penicillin or a suitable substitute if penicillin allergy exists. Both mother and baby should be carefully followed by serologic tests postpartum. It is important to know that even the unaffected baby will have a positive test because the mother's test is positive; however, the titer in the baby will be lower than that of the mother and will become negative within 3 months.

Gonorrhea

Gonorrhea is of special concern in maternity care because of the consequences to the mother at the time of labor and during the puerperium, as well as the risk of permanent injury to the baby's eyes at the time of birth.

The disease is caused by *Neisseria gonorrhoeae,* an organism which may attack the mucous membrane but most commonly affects the mucosa of the lower genital tract. The endocervical glands and urethra are common foci, but for complete detection, the anus and oropharynx should be cultured.

Gonorrhea is spread by sexual contact and in the

majority of women remains asymptomatic except for a nonspecific vaginal discharge. This is particularly the case in pregnancy, in which the normal route of spread through the endometrial cavity to the tubes is occluded by the pregnancy. The rate of asymptomatic carriers in pregnancy is reported to be as high as 5% to 10% in many clinics.

Although gonorrhea causes few problems for the patient during pregnancy, it can produce serious puerperal infection if present in the cervix at the time of delivery. Routine gonorrhea cultures are recommended during pregnancy. Gram-stained smears are suggestive but not conclusive in women.

The treatment of asymptomatic gonorrhea involves a single injection of 4.8 million units of aqueous procaine penicillin intramuscularly, preceded by 1 g of probenecid to produce the high level of penicillin needed to eradicate the increasingly resistant gonococcus. Cure should be proven by reculture, although reinfection is possible and should be watched for. Sexual partners should be evaluated and treated appropriately.

The organism can infect the infant's eyes at birth, and if prophylactic treatment of the eyes is not adequate, blindness may result.

Genital Herpes

Two types of herpes viruses that are immunologically and clinically distinct may involve the genital tract. Type I herpes hominis is mainly associated with nongenital lesions, but may also involve the genital tract. Type II herpes hominis is almost entirely genital and is sexually transmitted.

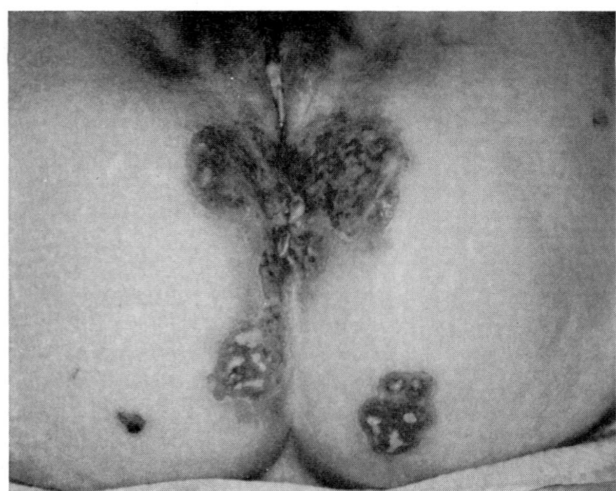

Figure 35-1.
Herpes genitalis lesions are characterized by painful vesicles in the vulva and perineal areas.

Between 1% and 2% of pregnancies are complicated by herpes virus infection. The lesions are characterized by painful vesicles in the vulva and perineal areas that commonly rupture and become secondarily infected (Fig. 35-1). The cervix and vagina may also be involved, but these lesions are asymptomatic and may persist for several months. Cytologic smears reveal large multinucleate cells with eosinophilic inclusion bodies, and unsuspected herpes is frequently diagnosed as an incidental finding by Papanicolaou smear.

The maternal infection is only rarely transmitted transplacentally to the fetus, but when this occurs, severe fetal abnormalities may result (see Chap. 36). The fetus can, however, be infected following rupture of the membranes or during the course of delivery. Detection of active herpes infections prior to delivery is most important, as congenital and neonatal herpes is often lethal, and ocular and CNS damage occurs in nearly half of the survivors. See Chapter 42 for further discussion.

Since there is at present no effective treatment for genital herpes, cesarean birth is recommended to avoid exposure to the lower genital tract when viral cultures are positive.

Suggested Reading

Burrow GW: The thyroid gland and reproduction. In Yen S, Jaffe RB (eds): Reproductive Endocrinology, pp 373–387. Philadelphia, WB Saunders, 1978

Cohen AW, Gabbe SG: Intrapartum management of the diabetic patient. Clin Perinatol 8:165, 1981

Gabbe SG: Diabetes in pregnancy: Clinical controversies. Clin Obstet Gynecol 21:443, 1978

Gabbe SG, Hagerman DD: Clinical application of estriol analysis. Clin Obstet Gynecol 21:353, 1978

Marchant DJ: Urinary tract infections in pregnancy. Clin Obstet Gynecol 21:921, 1978

Rovinsky JJ: Diseases complicating pregnancy. In Romney SL, Gray MJ, Little AB et al (eds): Gynecology and Obstetrics, The Health Care of Women, pp 777–866. New York, McGraw-Hill, 1975

Sever JL: Viral infections in pregnancy. Clin Obstet Gynecol 21:477, 1978

Tejanic N, Klein SW, Kaplan M: Subclinical herpes simplex genitalis infections in the perinatal period. Am J Obstet Gynecol 135:547, 1979

Ueland K: Cardiovascular diseases complicating pregnancy. Clin Obstet Gynecol 21:429, 1978

CHAPTER

36

CHAPTER 36

Complications of Labor

A complicated labor requires sensitive and astute nursing care, for it represents a period of great stress for the laboring woman, her partner, nurses and physicians. The principles of nursing care during normal labor (see Chap. 24) also apply when the labor is complicated, with certain modifications depending upon the nature of the problems. The nurse's ability to use clinical judgment is crucial, as the nursing diagnoses and care deriving from such judgments may be of life-saving significance for both the mother and the infant. Assessment skills including observation, interviewing, and physical examination provide important data on the nature and extent of the problem. Reporting, recording, and professional intercommunication promote accurate decision making and implementation of appropriate treatment. Physical and emotional supportive measures assist the mother and father to understand and cope with the unusual events in the labor experience, which is often prolonged and painful.

Dystocia Due to Abnormalities of Labor Mechanics

Dystocia, or difficult labor, can result from abnormalities in the machinery of labor. When there is cessation or delay of progress in the labor process due to such abnormalities, it is termed dystocia and may be due to the following four distinct abnormalities which may occur singly or in combination:

1. The uterine forces are not sufficiently strong or appropriately coordinated to effect cervical dilatation and effacement.
2. Forces generated by the voluntary muscles during the second stage of labor are inadequate to overcome the resistance of the bony pelvis and maternal soft parts.
3. There is faulty presentation or abnormal development of the fetus of such a character as to prevent entrance into or passage through the birth canal.
4. There are variations in the size and shape of the bony pelvis which create an obstacle to the entrance or descent of the fetus.

Frequently two or more of these conditions occur together. For instance, faulty fetal presentation and a contracted maternal pelvis are associated with uterine dysfunction.[1]

To further understand the nature of these problems, the process of labor can be thought of as divided into three components, each of which must be normal for progress to be made and birth to occur. These components may be described as the *forces* of labor, the *passenger,* and the *passage.* The *forces,* including uterine contractions with the addition of maternal "bearing down" during the second stage, must be of adequate strength with coordination of muscle activity. These forces propel an irregular object, the infant or *passenger,* through the birth canal or *passage.* The *passenger* must be of appropriate size and shape, and able to undergo the necessary maneuvers to pass through the different dimensions of the birth canal. The *passage* must also be of normal size and configuration, not presenting any undue obstacles to the descent, rotations, and expulsion of the baby.

Thus, when nature tries to propel the fetus through the birth canal and fails to do so, there can be problems in the forces—uterine dysfunction (inertia), the position of the infant, or the size of the infant and the birth canal.

Uterine Dysfunction

Definition

When the stages of labor are described diagrammatically by plotting elapsed labor time on the abscissa and cervical dilatation on the ordinate of a graph, an S-shaped curve results (Fig. 36-1). The first stage of labor is divided into a latent and an active phase. Normally, the *latent phase* is a period of some effacement and slow dilatation of the cervix, lasting perhaps an average of 8½ hours in a nullipara. About a 4 cm dilatation is accomplished in this stage.[2,3,4] The *active phase,* or clinically apparent labor, is briefer and consists, according to Friedman, of an acceleration phase, a phase of maximum slope, and a deceleration phase, before full dilatation is accomplished. This phase of labor lasts approximately 3½ hours to 4 hours in the primigravid patient.[2] Hendricks and his associates describe slightly different curves in normal labor (Fig. 36-2). They found in normal active labor that there is a rather constant active acceleration phase without the *deceleration* described by Friedman. Also, these investigators found that cervical dilatation progressed at about the same rate in both nulliparae and multiparae after 4 cm dilatation was reached.[5] Despite these divergent points of view, any significant

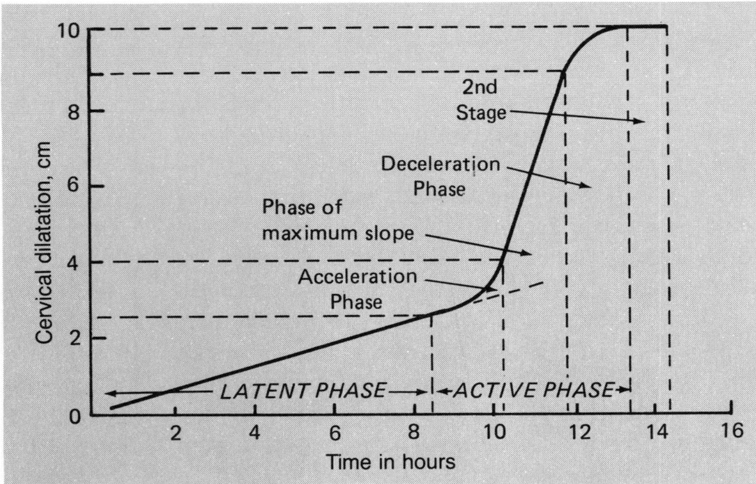

Figure 36-1.
A composite Friedman labor curve based on 500 nulliparas. (Friedman E: Primigravid labor. Obstet Gynecol 6:569)

prolongation of any of the phases described by Friedman or any significant variation from the curves presented by Hendricks and associates constitutes uterine dysfunction.[2]

Etiological Factors

When there is failure to progress despite the presence of uterine contractions, one of the first factors to consider is whether or not the patient is actually in labor. It is not unusual for a woman in late pregnancy to experience Braxton–Hicks contractions that are so strong and regular that they can easily be mistaken for true labor. Progressive cervical changes must be present to signify true labor, as effective contractions gradually accomplish effacement and dilatation. Appearance of bloody show assists in the diagnosis of labor, particularly when it accompanies cervical changes. Without these other signs to confirm labor, uncomfortable uterine contractions signify false labor. For the diagnosis of dystocia, cervical changes must have occurred and progressed, only to have continued progression in effacement and dilatation slowed or halted at some point.

The chief factors associated with uterine dysfunction are injudicious use of analgesia (*i.e.*, excessive or too early administration of the drugs), minor degrees of pelvic contraction, and fetal malposition of even a small degree, such as a slight extension of the head as seen in some occiput posterior positions. Similarly, postmaturity and a large infant have been found to be significantly related to dysfunctional labor. These conditions may occur singly or in combination in cases of dysfunction.

Other factors that are associated with this condi-

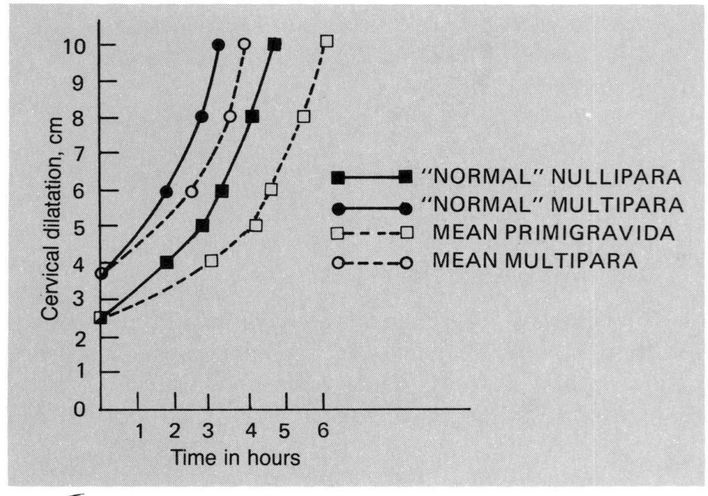

Figure 36-2.
Cervical dilatation in normal nulliparous and multiparous women after the onset of true labor. (Hendricks, Brenner, Kraus: Am J Obstet Gynecol 106:1065, 1970)

tion include overdistention of the uterus, grand multiparity, excessive cervical rigidity, and maternal age. The latter group of factors has been shown to play some etiological role although not such an important one as was once believed. In over 50% of the cases, the cause is often unknown. Considering the possible role of cortical steroids in the initiation of labor, and their relation to stress states, the effects of emotional factors in dystocia cannot be overlooked when no other cause is apparent. More research at the cellular level will have to be done to obtain increased definitive knowledge concerning the etiological factors in this condition.

Complications

The complications of uterine dysfunction are unfortunate for both mother and infant. Fetal injury and death are the most serious outcomes of this disorder. For the mother, exhaustion and dehydration may occur if labor is allowed to become too prolonged. Elevation of the maternal temperature and pulse are the clinical signs that herald the onset of secondary complications. Acetonuria is another sign of exhaustion and dehydration. These symptoms are to be reported immediately. Generally, in patients having dysfunctional labor, supportive intravenous therapy and electrolyte replacement are instituted before this syndrome occurs.

Intrauterine infection is another common maternal complication in these types of labor; broad-spectrum antibiotics are the usual choice of treatment. It is particularly important not to allow intrauterine infection to occur, because it contributes heavily to the increased perinatal mortality even though the mother is placed on antibiotics.

Dysfunctional labor appears to have some long-term consequences. Research has indicated that difficult labors and deliveries may have a deleterious effect on future childbearing.[6] Apparently, the more difficult the labor and delivery, the less inclination there is to have future children. In addition, the fear and anxiety that are engendered by a complicated childbirth become a special concern of the perinatal team if these patients do have subsequent children.

Fortunately, there have been several significant advances in the treatment of uterine dysfunction in the past decade. First, it is now realized that undue prolongation of labor contributes to perinatal mortality and morbidity. Second, the judicious use of dilute intravenous oxytocin in the treatment of some types of uterine dysfunction has been introduced. Third, cesarean sections are used more frequently to effect delivery in place of the difficult midforceps delivery when oxytocin fails or is inappropriate for use.[1]

Types of Uterine Dysfunction

Several groups of investigators have contributed to our understanding of the problem of uterine dysfunction. Larks described the stimulus of a contraction as starting in one cornu, followed several milliseconds later in the other cornu, with the contraction waves then joining and sweeping down over the fundus and the upper segment, thus pulling up the isthmus and cervix.[7] Caldeyro–Barcia and associates in Montevideo furthered the work of Reynolds by determining that the pressure of a contraction necessary to dilate the cervix is at least 15 mm Hg.[1,8] Finally, Hendricks and his coworkers found that a normal uterine contraction may exert as much as 60 mm Hg.[1] Thus, contractions have come to be described in terms of Montevideo units, which are the product of contraction intensity and frequency per 10 minutes. Optimal results are achieved in labor with a frequency of about 22 contractions per hour together with 50 mm Hg to 60 mm Hg amniotic pressures (140 Montevideo units to 180 Montevideo units).[9]

Uterine dysfunction has been classified according to two types—*hypertonic* and *hypotonic*. In the former there is incoordinate uterine action; in the latter there is coordinate activity but the intensity is not strong enough (less than 15 mm Hg) to produce dilatation.

Hypertonic Dysfunction

Hypertonic dysfunction generally comes at the onset of labor. The gradient of the contraction is distorted, perhaps by contraction of the midsegment with more force than the fundus or perhaps by complete asynchronism of the electrical impulses originating in each cornu. There is constant tension in the muscle but the contractions are of poor quality.

Friedman has a somewhat different classification of dysfunction which uses length of the phases of labor rather than the quality of the contractions. However, his *prolonged latent phase* occurs during the onset and first part of labor and hence is associated with hypertonic dysfunction. By definition, the latent phase is prolonged if it lasts longer than 20 hours in the primigravida and 14 hours in the multigravida. In practice, however, the diagnosis should be suspected and treatment instituted many hours before these time intervals have elapsed. Treatment is the same as for hypertonic dysfunction.[2]

Although the contractions in this type of dysfunction are ineffectual in accomplishing dilatation, they are extremely painful and have been described as "colicky."

It is particularly important to help mothers with this type of labor to distinguish between the anticipation of pain and the actual pain (see Chap. 24), for as labor wears on and no progress is made, the mother's strength and ability to cope with the contractions diminish, and hence the pain seems to be intensified. The anxiety and fear which are generated can easily lead to panic, which is detrimental to resumption of a successful labor course.

It is of paramount importance for the nurse to be able to accurately evaluate the intensity of labor contractions without relying exclusively on the electric monitor. At the height of an efficient uterine contraction it is impossible to indent the uterine wall with one's fingertips, and during a fairly good contraction it may be possible to cause some slight indentation, but if the uterine wall can be indented easily at the height of a contraction, it is a poor one. In evaluating the intensity of a labor contraction, reliance should be placed on tactile examination and data from the electronic monitor and not on the amount of "complaining" done by the patient about her pain.

Management. Treatment for this type of dysfunctional labor generally consists of rest and fluids. When medication is indicated to produce the needed rest and relaxation, an injection of 10 mg to 15 mg of morphine may be prescribed because it usually stops the abnormal contractions. In addition, a 0.1-g to a 0.2-g dose of a short-acting barbiturate may be administered. Intravenous fluids are used to maintain hydration and electrolyte balance, and in most instances normal labor resumes when the patient awakens. Certain tocolytic agents such as ritodrine and slabutamol have been used in other countries with some stated success. However, their use in this country to date has not been widespread.

Oxytocin is contraindicated in treating this type of dysfunction. With the uterus in a constant state of increased muscle tone, oxytocin presents the danger of causing an even greater resting tension, which might interfere with fetal oxygenation. Moreover, it does not correct the uncoordinated action of the two segments, which underlies this problem.

Occasionally the contractions remain uncoordinated and ineffective even after the patient has had a good rest. In these cases, cesarean section is employed if the fetal heart rate becomes abnormal.[1] Thus, the nurse needs to be particularly attentive to the mother's progress.

Complications. Fetal distress tends to appear quite early in labor when there is hypertonic dysfunction. Fetal heart rate must be carefully monitored, and other signs of distress, such as meconium-stained amniotic fluid, must be noted. Occasionally in cases of hypertonic dysfunction, membranes will have been ruptured 24 hours or more without effective labor. In this situation, bacteria are likely to ascend into the uterus and give rise to infection. This is *intrapartal infection* and is a serious complication. It is signaled by a rise in temperature, often in association with a chill.

Because of the danger of intrapartal infection, it is customary to take temperatures every 2 hours in patients whose labors have lasted more than 24 hours or who have ruptured membranes. Even an elevation of half a degree should be reported to the physician at once. Intrapartal infection is much more likely to occur if the membranes have been ruptured for a long time. As previously stated, treatment is usually in the form of antibiotics. Cesarean section is resorted to if fetal distress occurs and in the case of prolonged rupture and before fetal stress is apparent.

Hypotonic Dysfunction

After the onset of true labor, contractions in hypotonic dysfunction decrease in strength and the tone of the uterine muscles is less than usual. Minimum uterine tension during the resting stage is about 8 mm Hg to 12 mm Hg in the normally functioning uterus, while normal labor contractions reach an intrauterine pressure of 50 mm Hg to 60 mm Hg at acme. These values are reduced in hypotonic dysfunction, and contractions are not strong enough to affect dilatation. Contractions may become farther apart and irregular.

Dysfunction often is nature's protection against pelvic contraction and abnormal fetal position, and it signifies the need for careful assessment for these factors. Thorough vaginal examination to determine position of the presenting part, dimensions of the pelvis, and state of the cervix are usually done by the obstetrician. The cervix is at least 3 cm dilated if the diagnosis of hypotonic dysfunction in the active phase of labor is correct. X-ray pelvimetry is often done for accurate measurement of the pelvis and to confirm abnormal fetal position or abnormalities of development.

This condition usually occurs in the accelerated or active phase, or even during the second stage of labor; the contractions become infrequent and of poor quality, and the uterus is easily indentable at the acme of a contraction. Table 36-1 compares hypertonic dysfunction to hypotonic dysfunction.

Friedman describes two types of dysfunction that can occur at this time. *Active phase dysfunction* is recognized by a maximum slope phase of less than 1.2 cm of dilatation per hour in the primigravid patient or less than 1.5 cm in the multigravida (Fig. 36-3). The majority of these patients, with supportive fluids, reassurance, and *minimum* sedation go on to dilate fully, although more slowly than is optimal. However, about 10% develop the most serious dysfunction, *secondary arrest dysfunction*. This occurs when there is no cervical dilatation for 2 or more hours in the active phase of labor. Cephalopelvic disproportion is suspected in these cases.[2]

Treatment. Early and accurate diagnosis of hypotonic dysfunction is a major factor in reducing fetal death and injury. If a marked degree of disproportion exists or if there is an uncorrectable malposition, then cesarean section is employed to effect delivery. If these conditions are not present, stimulation of labor is generally the treatment of choice rather than "watchful waiting" for more effective labor to resume spontaneously. The main reason for this is the increased perinatal loss and injury that accompany unduly prolonged first or second stages of labor.

If membranes are intact, initial treatment may include artificial rupture. This procedure alone may stimulate effective labor contractions.

Oxytocin augmentation, however, is usually resorted to when strong, regular contractions with progressive effacement and dilatation or fetal descent fail to occur, or if membranes are already ruptured. Ten units of oxytocin are mixed with 1000 ml of 5% glucose in a balanced salt solution or water for controlled intravenous drip. Initially, the infusion is begun at a flow of 2 mU of oxytocin per minute. This amount does not initiate tetanic contractions in true hypotonic dysfunction unless there is hypersensitivity to the drug. Contractions and fetal heart rate are carefully evaluated, and if no problems develop, the infusion can be gradually increased up to 20 mU of oxytocin. Flows above this rate are rarely necessary, for if effective contractions are not initiated by this dosage of oxytocin, greater amounts are also unlikely to do so and present serious dangers to both the baby and the mother.

Table 36-1.
Criteria for Differentiating Dysfunctional Labor

Criteria	Hypertonic	Hypotonic
Phase of labor	Latent	Active
Symptoms	Painful	Painless
Fetal distress	Early	Late
Medication		
Oxytocin	Unfavorable reaction	Favorable reaction
Sedation	Helpful	Little value

(Modified from Pritchard JA, McDonald PC: Williams Obstetrics, 16th ed. New York, Appleton-Century-Crofts, 1980, p 660)

A constant infusion pump is often used to administer oxytocin, as this method enhances the precision of dosage. The older *Harvard pump* or the newer *Ivac peristaltic pump* are two types commonly used. The oxytocin solution, which is in a separate bottle, flows into a syringe mounted on the pump, which delivers an exact amount of solution depending on the drip rate set. This solution can be piggybacked into a plain glucose infusion, if the two-bottle set-up is used. Although the pump method allows more precise regulation of the oxytocin flow than simply adjusting clamps attached to the intravenous tubing, both approaches require constant and careful monitoring. Clamps can slip and the pump can malfunction. The dangers of an excessive dosage of oxytocin include uterine tetany with resultant fetal hypoxia or rupture of the uterus with fetal anoxia and maternal hemorrhage and shock.

Oxytocin stimulation is contraindicated in cases of fetal-pelvic disproportion, overdistension of the uterus, and great parity (para 5 and over). Signs of fetal distress must be carefully watched for, and the infusion must be immediately slowed or stopped if these occur. Use of external or internal monitors is manda-

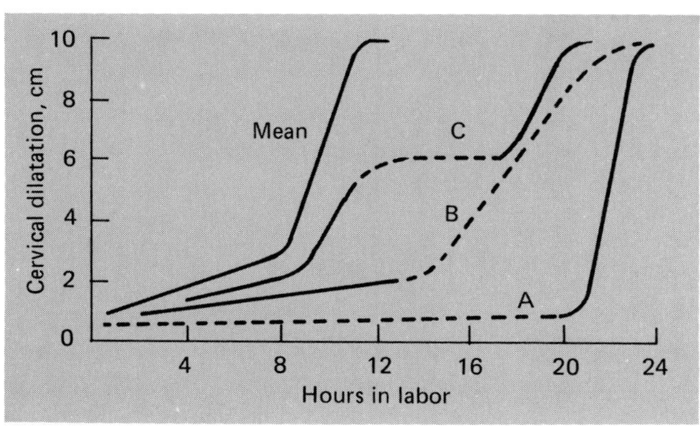

Figure 36-3.
The major labor aberrations shown in comparison with the mean cervical dilatation time curve for nulliparae. A = prolonged latent phase, B = protracted active phase dilatation, and C = secondary arrest of dilatation. (Friedman E: Greenhill Obstetrics, 13th ed. Philadelphia, WB Saunders)

tory when oxytocin stimulation of labor is employed. With internal monitoring, the strength of contractions as well as continual rate of the fetal heart may be constantly evaluated.

Formerly, intramuscular or buccal oxytocin has been used to augment labor. However, these methods do not allow accurate control of blood levels, either to accomplish effective contractions or to avoid the dangers of excessive dosage. Most recently the use of buccal oxytocin has been disapproved by the Food and Drug Administration.

The use of the powerful uterotonic agents, prostaglandins F_2 and E_2, have not been approved by the Food and Drug Administration for use in induction and augmentation of labor in this country. Because these drugs are so powerful, even the carefully monitored intravenous infusion can cause untoward problems. They have been used in other countries with some reputed success, especially for softening an unfavorable cervix in women who were to have induced labor.[1]

Complications. Untreated hypotonic uterine dysfunction exposes the mother to the dangers of exhaustion, dehydration, and intrapartum infection. Signs of fetal distress often do not appear until intrapartum infection has developed. While treatment of intrauterine infections with antibiotics offers protection to the mother, this is of little value to the fetus. Nursing observations include assessment of the mother for signs of infection, as previously discussed.

Nursing Care

In addition to observing and reporting the maternal and fetal conditions as noted above, nursing care includes offering explanations to the parents and providing emotional support.

Psychosocial Support. Labors of this type are extremely discouraging for the mother and the father. The diagnostic procedures as well as the therapy take a certain amount of time, and carrying out these measures requires patience and waiting on the part of everyone concerned.

It is essential that the couple know and understand this fact. The physician and the nurse need to spend sufficient time with the parents to explain what is happening in depth and in terms that are appropriate for them. It is very possible that repeated reinforcement of the explanations, progress, and so on will be needed. Feedback from the parents should be encouraged, so that their level of understanding and acceptance can be ascertained. The normal tension and anxiety found in any labor certainly is intensified, and it is important that it not be compounded by fantasy or misunderstanding.

Since dysfunctional labor is so variable, it is often impossible (and unwise) to give the parents any definite reassurances as to when effective labor will commence. Yet, some kind of boundaries must be placed on when this ineffective phase will end and progress will begin, so that the mother will have some goal to look forward to and to work for. Therefore, it is important to reassure the patient, reminding her that her case is not unique (patients think after many hours that theirs is the longest labor in obstetrical history), that certain specific measures are known and can be taken to help effective labor to begin, and that competent medical and nursing care will be given throughout labor.

An explanation of the plan for treatment enables the parents to anticipate more realistically what is in store and therefore reassures them that certain definite measures are available and are being employed.

Comfort Measures. In addition, all the comfort measures that promote relaxation should be used. Sponge baths, various positioning, soothing backrubs, clean, dry linen, quiet conversation, reading or other diversionary activities, as well as a quiet restful environment are all appropriate. However, isolating the patient in a dark room on the premise that she needs sleep or rest only contributes to her fear unless she is actually sleeping, and then frequent observations are needed to see when she awakens. Human contact is one of the most important items of "treatment" in cases of complicated labor and should never be neglected. The presence of the same person, nurse, or physician, is very helpful for the reasons already mentioned in Chapter 24. Coaching the mother in breathing patterns and relaxation techniques also conserves her strength.

The physician may want the patient to have fluids by mouth, or may order intravenous infusions to maintain hydration and electrolyte balance. A total of 2000 ml or more of intravenous fluid may be given in 24 hours.

Oxytocin Monitoring. If oxytocin stimulation of labor is used, the patient must have someone in attendance at all times during the infusion. Uterine contractions and fetal heart tones are to be monitored continuously. Maternal blood pressure and pulse are checked every half hour. As the physician specifies the dosage, the nurse (or other attendant) ascertains that the infusion is running at the prescribed drops per minute and reports any maternal or fetal aberrations immediately. Many institutions have an "Oxytocin

NC Nursing Care: Priorities for Patients with Dysfunctional Labor*

Assessment	Intervention	Evaluation
Monitor level of fatigue and ability to cope with pain	Stay with patient or have partner stay continually; help patient relax between contractions; record and report behavior Assist as needed with effleurage, concentration, or distraction for pain management; reassure, explain labor progress, and support as indicated; provide quiet environment	Patient works with contraction Exhaustion avoided Panic and discouragement alleviated
Determine hydration level	Monitor intravenous fluids for infiltration Check condition of lips and skin for dryness	Dehydration avoided
Bladder hygiene	Encourage patient to void frequently; catheterize as necessary	Bladder distention avoided
Vital signs	TPR and BP of 2° or more frequently as indicated	Secondary infection avoided or alleviated
Monitor oxytocin or antibiotics if necessary	Record all contractions and FHR; report as necessary; give and record administration of antibiotics if indicated	Labor progress Tetanic contractions avoided, fetal distress avoided

*In addition to nursing care for normal labor, with these priorities to be considered uppermost.

Record" or a "Pitocin Sheet" that provides space for recording times, amount and frequency of the oxytocin given, fetal heart tones, maternal blood pressure and pulse, frequency, intensity and length of contractions, and other relevant comments. This type of sheet gives an easily accessible record of the patient's progress during the infusion.

Recording and reporting the physiological signs and symptoms cannot be stressed enough during these infusions. However, supportive care is also to be maintained. Adequate explanation and reassurance can be given, and since the nurse will be with the mother continuously, this time can be used to establish a relationship of rapport. While the infusion stimulates contractions, and therefore discomfort, the mother and her partner often look upon this treatment optimistically, for it marks the end of a desultory, ineffective period in labor and brings with it promise of termination of a difficult time. This positive attitude can be especially reinforced if the nurse provides explanation and assurance. See Chapter 37 for further details in monitoring these impressions.

Persistent Occiput Posterior Positions

The fetal head usually enters the pelvis inlet transversely and therefore must transverse an arc of 90° in the process of internal rotation to the direct occiput anterior position (see Fig. 7-3).

In about a quarter of all labors, however, the head enters the pelvis with the occiput directed diagonally posterior, that is, in either the R.O.P. or the L.O.P. position. Under these circumstances the head must rotate through an arc of 135° in the process of internal rotation.

With good contractions, adequate flexion, and a baby of average size, the great majority of these cases of occiput posterior position undergo spontaneous rotation through the 135° arc as soon as the head reaches the pelvic floor. This is a normal mechanism of labor. It must be remembered, however, that labor is usually prolonged, and the mother has a great deal of discomfort in her back as the baby's head impinges against the sacrum in the course of rotating.

Nursing intervention is aimed at relieving the back pain as much as possible. Sacral pressure, backrubs, and frequent change of position from side to side can be helpful, and they should be employed to the degree that seems to be well tolerated by the patient.

In a minority of cases, however (perhaps 10% or less) these favorable circumstances do not exist, and rotation may be incomplete or may not take place at all. If rotation is incomplete, the head becomes arrested in the transverse position, a condition known as *transverse arrest*. If anterior rotation does not take place at all, the occiput usually rotates to the direct occiput posterior position, a condition known as *persistent occiput posterior*. Both transverse arrest and persistent occiput posterior position represent deviations from the normal mechanisms of labor. It is thought that narrowing of the mid pelvis plays a role in the etiology.

Some controversy persists in the management of persistent occiput posterior. When labor progresses, although first and second stages tend to be prolonged in primigravidas, management is the same as for occiput anterior positions and results in no increased risk to the fetus. Premature operative intervention, particularly if the station is high, seems contraindicated. Forceps rotation on the perineum is appropriate to reduce lacerations if this can be easily accomplished.[1]

Sometimes the mechanical problem associated with abnormal uterine action is an abnormal position of the presenting head. Hence, these conditions of posterior or transverse arrest of the occiput appear to have, in some cases, an adverse effect on uterine behavior. Here the malposition is the cause rather than the effect of uterine inefficiency. This conclusion can be verified by the following findings. (1) When the fetal head is rotated or rotates spontaneously, uterine action improves. (2) Oxytocin therapy for dysfunction associated with an occipitoposterior position does not cause the infant's head to rotate.

It should be remembered that the uterus of the multigravid patient usually reacts to mechanical obstruction by becoming more active and ultimately rupturing itself. On the other hand, when the primigravid uterus encounters resistance it nearly always responds by inertia or incoordinate behavior. It is imperative, then, that the obstetrician rules out mechanical obstruction before deciding that labor is prolonged due to idiopathic faulty uterine action. Since disproportion may be slight and therefore easily overlooked, only the most careful observation and study can disclose the important association between faulty uterine action and smallness of the pelvis or large size of the baby. The nurse can make an important contribution in this diagnosis by her continuous and critical observations of the character and frequency of the contractions, the amount of the mother's discomfort, her vital signs and general condition, and the fetal heart rate.

Breech Presentations

The breech is the presenting part in 3% to 4% of singleton deliveries and is more common when the baby is premature or there is multiple gestation. The reasons for breech presentations are not always apparent, although associated factors include great parity, twinning, hydramnios, hydrocephalus, placenta previa and implantation of the placenta in the cornual fundal regions of the uterus. Recent studies indicate no positive correlation between breech presentation and contracted pelvis.[11]

Possible Complications. There is no significantly increased danger for the life of the mother in breech presentations, although there is increased incidence of lacerations of the birth canal, episiotomy extensions, cesarean sections, and postpartum infections. Labor is not prolonged, contrary to previous belief.[1]

For the infant, however, there is considerably increased risk of both death and injury in comparison to vertex presentations. Uncorrected perinatal loss is about 12% in the United States, and when corrected for congenital anomalies and maternal disease, fetal loss is still three times higher in single breech than in vertex. Traumatic morbidity is 12 times higher, including fractures, dislocations, and peripheral nerve injuries.[11] Although pulmonary morbidity (*e.g.*, pneumonitis, atelectasis, or respiratory distress syndrome) occurs with similar frequency in both breech and vertex, brain damage from asphyxia resulting in neurologic abnormalities at one year is increased in breech infants.[12]

The major cause of perinatal death is trauma sustained in delivery. Tentorial tears and subsequent intracranial hemorrhage are twice as common in breech presentations as they are in cephalic presentations. The symptoms and nursing care associated with these conditions are discussed in Chapter 43. Lesions of the spinal cord and extrusion of the medulla into the foramen magnum also account for a large portion of deaths. In footling presentations (Fig. 36-4C), prolapse of the umbilical cord is common. Even in the most skilled hands, and considering only full-term infants, about 1 breech infant in 15 succumbs as the result of delivery.

Unrecognized fetopelvic disproportion is the primary cause in the increase in perinatal mortality and

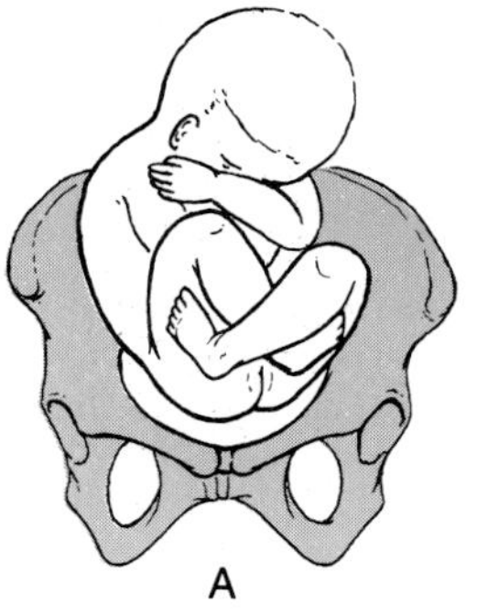

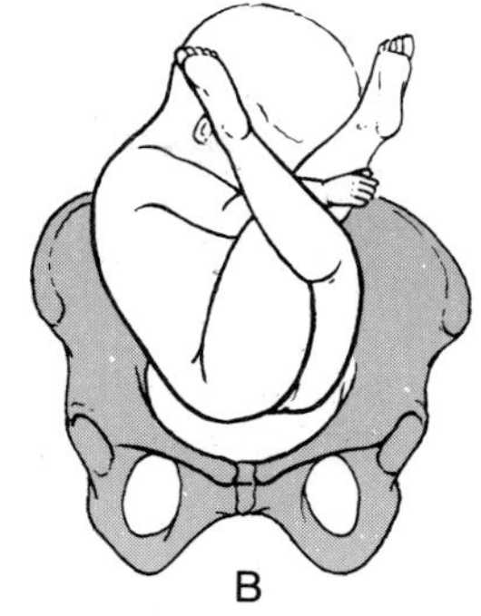

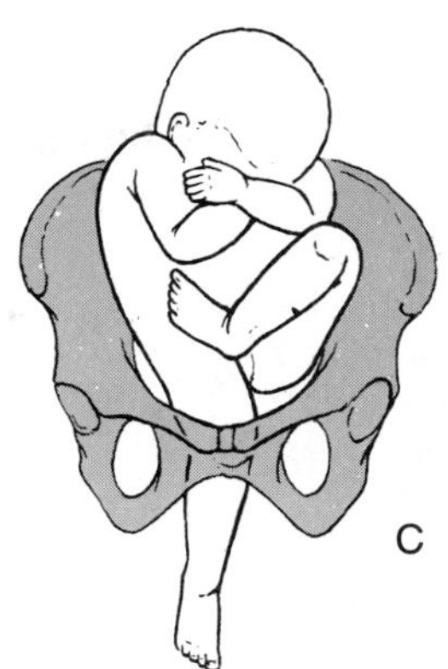

Figure 36-4.
Breech presentation may be *(A)* complete breech, *(B)* frank breech, and *(C)* an incomplete or footling breech.

morbidity in breech deliveries. Recommendations for medical management to reduce these complications include accurate sonographic and x-ray pelvimetry, at least mean normal pelvic measurements and fetal size to permit trial labor, constant monitoring of fetal heart rate for signs of asphyxia, and cesarean section for estimated fetal size of above 8.5 lb, minimal fetopelvic disproportion, failure to progress in labor, and signs of fetal distress.[11]

Classification. Breech presentations are classified as follows:

Complete—the buttocks present with the feet and legs flexed on the thighs and the thighs flexed on the abdomen (Fig. 36-4A)

Frank—the buttocks present with the hips flexed and the legs extended against the abdomen and chest (Fig. 36-4B); this is the most common type of breech presentation

Incomplete—one or both feet or the knees extend below the buttocks (Fig. 36-4C); this type of presentation is also known as a single or double footling breech (Fig. 36-5)

Compound—the buttocks present together with another part such as a hand

Mechanism of Labor in Breech Delivery

If the powers, passage, and passenger are of adequate capacity and functioning properly, delivery in a breech presentation progresses at about the same rate as in vertex presentations. Descent is slower initially in the case of a breech but among patients with similar parity, dilatation and effacement are approximately the same for breech and vertex presentations. Whether spontaneous or assisted, the delivery of the fetus is most efficiently accomplished when the largest planes of the fetus descend into the largest planes of the pelvis. The mechanism of delivery is as follows:

1. *Descent* of the breech basilic diameter through the pelvic inlet usually occurs in the oblique plane with the fetal anterior hip leading (Fig. 36-6A).
2. *Internal rotation* toward the AP plane of the pelvis occurs as pelvic muscle resistance is met and the posterior hip then descends as *lateral flexion* of the fetal back occurs (Fig. 36-6B and C).
3. *Delivery* and *external rotation* of the hips to the lateral back-up position occur as the bisacromial

(Text continued on page 794)

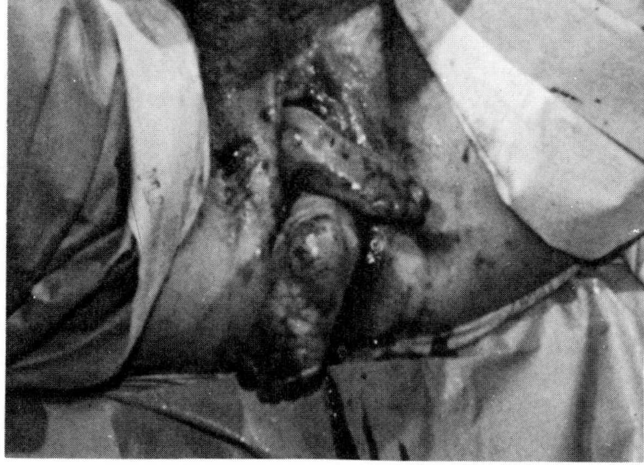

Figure 36-5.
Double footling breech. (From the film Human Birth, published by JB Lippincott, Philadelphia)

Figure 36-6.
(A) Engagement, RSA. The bitrochanteric diameter has passed through the inlet of the maternal pelvis (side view). *(B)* Internal rotation of the breech, RSA to RST. With further descent, the anterior hip of the fetus meets the resistance of the pelvic floor of the mother and rotates 45° so that the bitrochanteric diameter of the fetus lies in the anteroposterior diameter of the maternal pelvic (side view). *(C)* Birth of the buttocks by lateral flexion. Birth of the posterior buttock over the perineum (side view). *(D)* Birth of the anterior buttock under the pubic arch (side view). *(E)* Birth of the baby up to the umbilicus. Loop of cord is being brought down. *(F)* Engagement of the shoulders. The bisacromial diameter is in the right oblique diameter of the maternal pelvis (perineal view). *(G)* Delivery of the anterior shoulder under the pubic arch (side view). *(H)* Delivery of the posterior shoulder over the perineum (side view) *(I)* Mauriceau-Smellie-Veit maneuver (with an assistant). The occiput is directly under the symphysis pubis. The assistant applies suprapubic pressure (side view). *(J)* Delivery of the head is attempted after the hairline is visible at the introitus (perineal view). *(K)* Mauriceau-Smellie-Veit maneuver continuing. Delivery of the head by flexion upward over the perineum with continuous suprapubic pressure (side view).

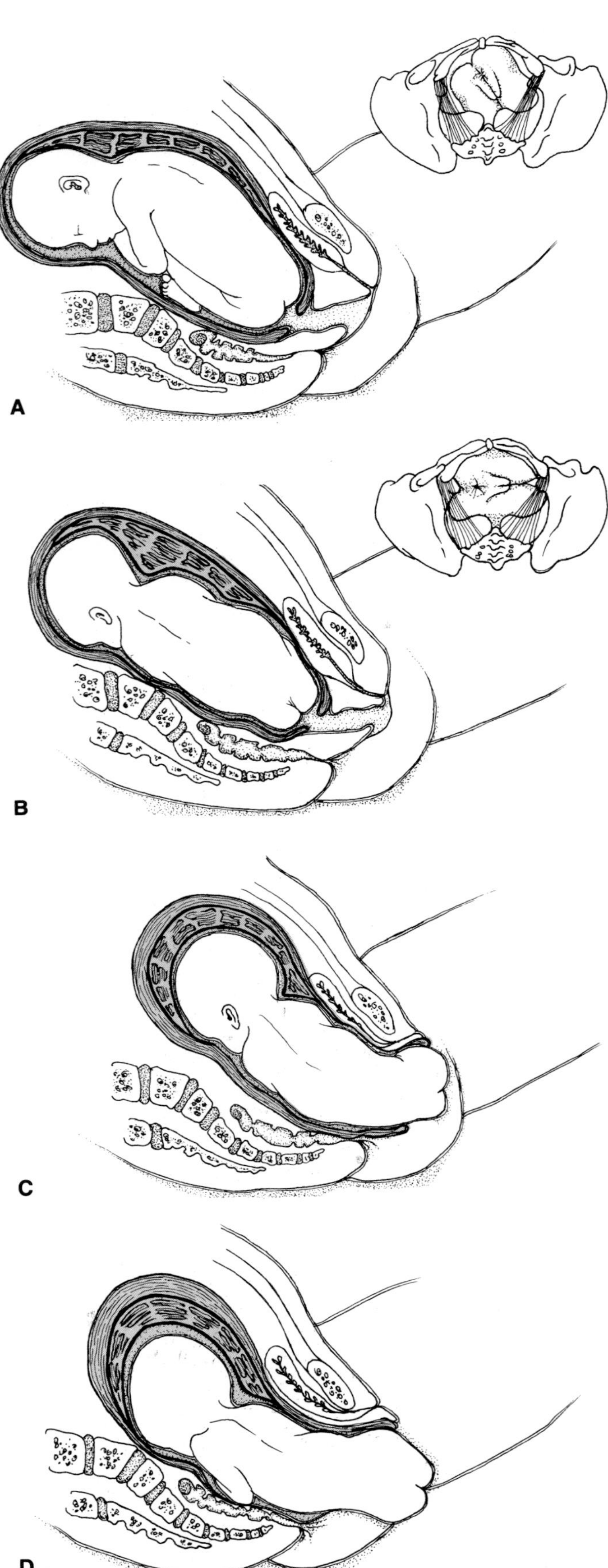

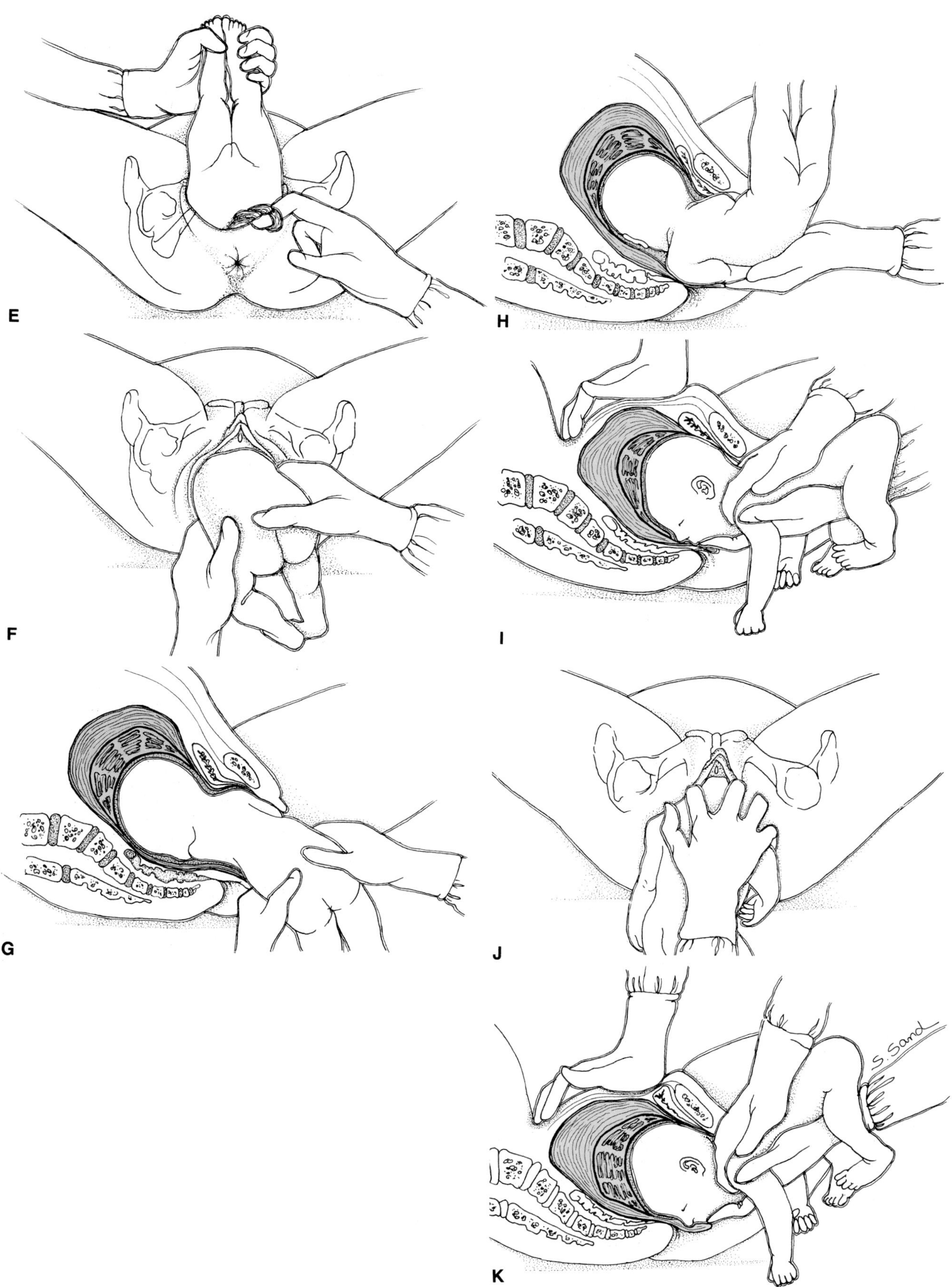
E
F
G
H
I
J
K
S. Sand

(Text continued)

plane of the shoulders enter the pelvis in the oblique maternal plane (Fig. 36-6D).

4. The descending shoulders are delivered after the arms in the AP plane (Fig. 36-6G). The anterior shoulder descends to behind the symphysis and the posterior shoulder descends into the hollow of the sacrum with resultant *lateral flexion* (Fig. 36-6G). In a spontaneous delivery, the posterior shoulder and arm may be delivered next, which allows the body to drop posteriorly and the anterior shoulder to be delivered from behind the symphysis. Next, the flexed head descends, internally rotates to the AP plane (Fig. 36-6I) and is delivered by flexion (Fig. 36-6J, K). The obstetrician may assist this by slightly extending the infant's body to allow easier flexion of the head.[13]

Delivery

There is becoming more of a consensus that cesarean section should be used liberally, especially if there is dysfunctional labor, prematurity, or small pelvis[12] because the perinatal mortality and morbidity is so high in this kind of presentation. In those instances when delivery is attempted vaginally, especially in the primigravida, it is often necessary for the physician to perform a partial or complete breech extraction.

Selection of a Delivery Method. Occasionally there is no choice of delivery method if the patient arrives in the labor suite when delivery is imminent. Thus, physicians need to be skilled in atraumatic vaginal delivery techniques. Cesarean section is used for such conditions as acute fetal distress, abruptio placentae, placenta previa, cord prolapse, dysfunctional labor, and those conditions directly related to the breech presentation.[13]

Vaginal Delivery. Several scoring systems are used to evaluate the feasibility of vaginal delivery in breech presentations. The Zatuchni–Andros system and its modifications are used extensively (Table 36-2). These systems give an estimate of whether the shoulders and head can traverse the pelvis without undue delay when the fetus is maintained in the most advantageous position. Some investigators have reported the effectiveness of low scores in predicting infants at risk for mortality and morbidity, prolonged labor, and eventual cesarean section. A score of three or less justifies a section. A score of four requires further observation and subsequent evaluation. A score of five will hopefully result in a successful vaginal delivery. Unfortunately, serious fetal morbidity, mortality, and low Apgar scores are found with vaginal delivery of patients with high Zatuchni–Andros scores in whom cephalopelvic disproportion (CPD) is not a problem. Moreover, dysfunctional labor and resuscitation of the infant frequently accompany vaginal delivery. Thus, in many tertiary care centers, breech presentation is an indication for cesarean section in term or near term primigravidae and in multiparae with a fetus estimated at 7½ lb when labor is desultory or when complications are apparent.[1,13,14]

Breech delivery has been classified according to the amount of professional assistance that is required to effect delivery.

A *spontaneous breech delivery* is one in which the mother essentially delivers herself in a more or less emergency situation (*i.e.,* en route to the hospital) or is found in the labor room with her infant delivered. This latter case indicates sheer neglect on the part of the staff. This type of delivery is often found with premature labor.

An *assisted breech delivery* requires minimal intervention from the physician. The mother may be a multipara in strong labor who has made optimal progress. Her infant may be smaller than average.

Partial breech extraction requires the assistance of the physician with delivery of the shoulders and head (Fig. 36-7).

The following steps are usually performed:

1. The cord is extracted to prevent compression as soon as the umbilicus appears, after the feet and legs have been delivered. If there is a short cord or nuchal cord, it is doubly clamped and cut.
2. After delivery of the cord, a deep *mediolateral* episiotomy is done to prevent tearing and to minimize perineal resistance. A midline episiotomy is contraindicated in a breech extraction because of the danger of extension into surrounding structures.
3. The infant's trunk is wrapped in a towel to provide warmth and prevent slippage when traction is applied. Traction together with slight rotation results in the bisacromial diameter of the infant coming into the AP plane of the maternal pelvis. The posterior shoulder can then be delivered by inserting two fingers into the vagina and elevating the fetus upward toward the mother's inguinal area. The posterior shoulder then rests on the perineum, the arm and hand are delivered, and the anterior arm can be extracted with the fingers. If the infant has an arm extended above the head, it can be passed downward across the chest by passing two fingers over the shoulder. Rough traction on the arm is to be avoided because neurologic damage can result.
4. The aftercoming head may be delivered by application of the Piper forceps (see Chap. 34) or

Table 36-2.
Zatuchni–Andros Prognostic Index*

	Points		
	0	1	2
Parity	Primigravida	Multipara	
Gestational age	39 weeks or more	38 weeks	37 weeks or less
Estimated fetal weight	8 lb (3630 g)	7 lb–7 15/16 lb (3629 g–3176 g)	< 7 lb (3173 g)
Previous breech†	0	1	2 or more
Dilation‡	2 cm	3 cm	4 cm or more
Station‡	−3 or higher	−2	−1 or lower

*Zatuchni GI, Andros GJ: Prognostic index for vaginal delivery in breech presentation. Am J Obstet Gynecol 98:854, 1967
†Greater than 2500 g
‡Determined by vaginal examination on admission

by the Mauriceau–Smellie–Veit or the Bracht maneuvers.

a. In the Mauriceau–Smellie–Veit maneuver, the fetus is placed astride the physician's left arm. Two fingers of the left hand are placed firmly over the mandible to flex the head. The right hand is placed over the back, with the fingers over the shoulders to guide the shoulders and head. The torso is elevated slowly with flexion of the head maintained by the maxillary pressure. Suprapubic pressure is applied by an assistant during these maneuvers to aid the descent of the head into the pelvis and eventually with the suprapubic and maxillary pressure, the occiput is delivered (Fig. 36-8).[13]
b. In the Bracht maneuver, the back is gently arched toward the mother's abdomen when the scapulas are seen. The arms then tend to deliver spontaneously. Suprapubic pressure is applied to assist descent of the head into the pelvis and the suspended body continues to be brought *slowly* to the mother's abdomen. The face and occiput should then deliver spontaneously. This maneuver requires no intravaginal invasion or traction and hence is often preferred. However, if the infant is not in the right position or tries to breathe before the head is delivered, or the mother cannot work with the operators, this is not the maneuver of choice.

A *complete breech extraction* also may be called "decomposing" or "breaking up" a breech or a total breech extraction. As the name implies, the small parts are rearranged so that labor resumes and progress can be made. Decomposition may be effected in a frank breech by bringing the legs down for traction by means of *Pinard's* maneuver. Here the physician's hand is inserted into the vagina and the thigh is abducted, which causes the knee to flex. The foot is grasped and delivered. Traction is applied downward and if the buttocks descend, delivery can proceed as previously described. If the breech does not descend, the other foot may be extracted.[13] We would make the point again that cesarean section is by far the method of choice over assisted breech deliveries.

Anesthesia. Many physicians prefer local or pudendal anesthesia because it does not interfere with labor and allows the mother to participate actively. Epidural anesthesia is also preferred for the same reasons and also because it permits comfortable intravaginal manipulation and extraction. Some physicians prefer a general anesthetic such as halothane if the breech must be decomposed, since these agents inhibit uterine contractions and intravaginal manipulation is easier. Both conduction and general anesthesia have been used successfully for cesarean section.

Nursing Care

The nurse should be extremely meticulous in her monitoring of the mother. This means not just relying on electronic equipment, but also frequent physical checks, comfort measures, and explanations to the parents.

In breech presentation the infant often passes meconium from the rectum during the course of labor, and after the membranes are ruptured, and the liquor amnii has escaped, the nurse may find the black, tar-colored material coming from the patient's vagina. She needs to ascertain that the presentation is, in fact, a breech, for if such a phenomenon occurred in a vertex presentation, it would be an indication of probable fetal distress.

Explanation and appropriate reassurance are important for mothers who have breech presenta-

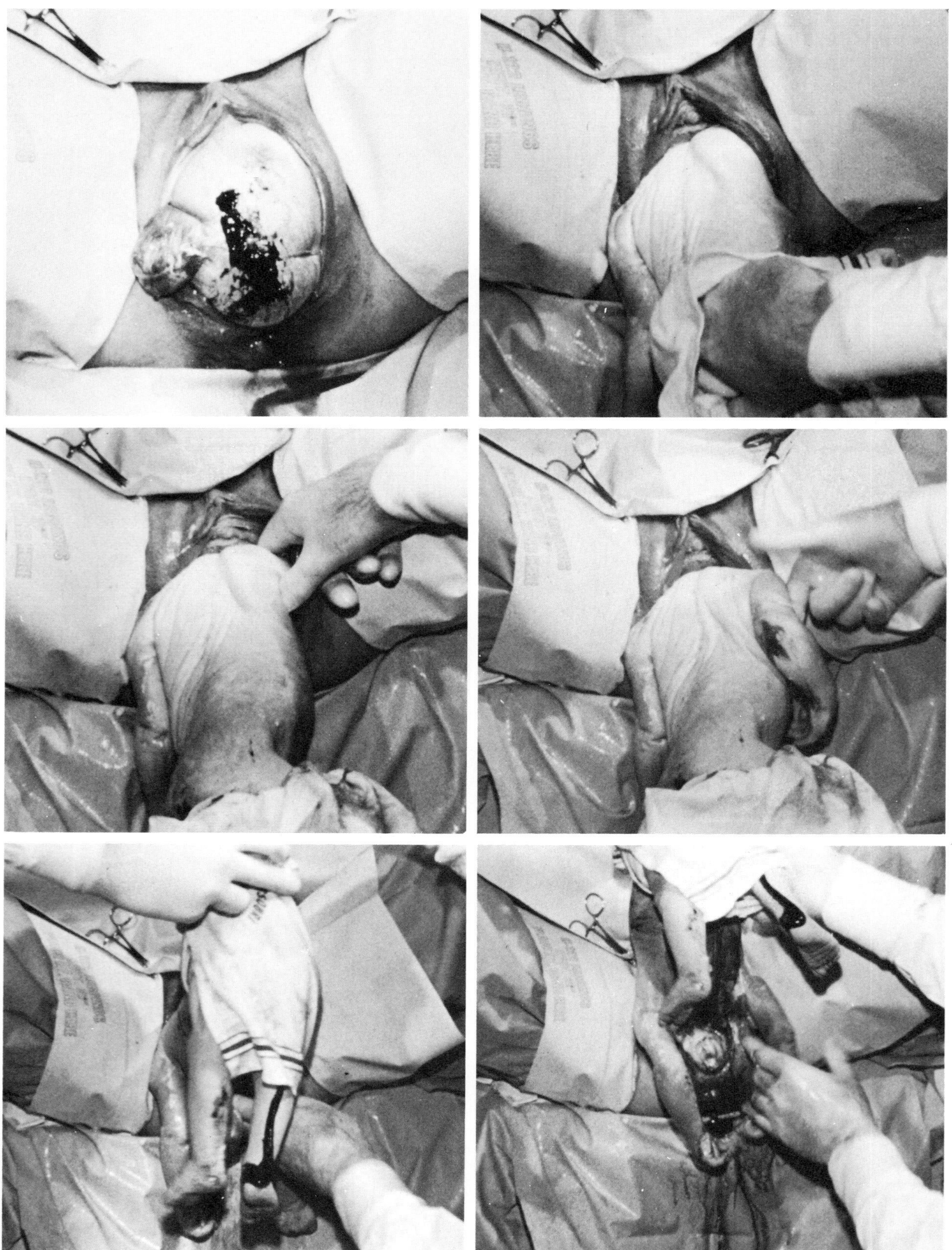

Figure 36-7.
Partial breech extraction. (From the film, Human Birth, published by JB Lippincott, Philadelphia)

tions, as they are for any patient having an abnormal presentation or complicated labor of any type. Many patients are steeped in old wives' folklore of the fearfulness of a breech birth and become exceedingly anxious and terrified as soon as they find out (or overhear) that theirs is this type of presentation; the same is often true of their partners, and the anxiety and fear that are communicated between them can impede the patient's working effectively with her labor. With modern obstetrical techniques and knowledge, labor need not be prolonged or exceptionally painful, and cesarean section is a safer viable alternative to vaginal delivery.

Shoulder, Face, and Brow Presentations

In shoulder presentations the infant lies crosswise in the uterus instead of longitudinally. This complication occurs about once in every 300 cases and is seen most often in multiparae. Frequently an arm prolapses into the vagina, making the problem of delivery even more difficult.

Shoulder presentation is a serious complication, with an increased maternal mortality rate and an extremely high perinatal mortality with vaginal delivery—about 30% for term infants. External version in late pregnancy or early labor is occasionally successful, especially in multiparae, in converting the shoulder to a longitudinal lie. Internal podalic version and extraction is a very hazardous procedure (see Chap. 37), the second most common cause of rupture of the uterus, and associated with high perinatal mortality. Its use is hardly justified, except in carefully selected cases. Virtually all transverse presentations should be delivered by cesarean section, which reduces perinatal mortality to about 4%.

Face presentations are seen in about one out of 600 patients. Factors that favor extension of the head and prevent flexion are implicated in these presentations, a contracted pelvis being paramount among these. These infants may deliver spontaneously if labor is effective and the pelvis is adequate. The face comes through the vulva with the chin anterior. However, if there is indication that the pelvis is contracted or that there is fetal distress, cesarean section is employed for delivery. As edema of the scalp is common in vertex presentations, facial edema is often present to the extent that the landmarks resemble a breech presentation. The edema and purplish discoloration disappear within a few days but the infant's appearance gives the parents a great deal of concern. The nurse can be very helpful in reassuring the parents that the condition is temporary and will resolve without sequelae.

Brow presentations are somewhat more rare than the other malpresentations. They are impossible to deliver as long as the brow presentation persists since the largest diameter of the fetal head, the occipitomental, presents. They are, however, an unstable presentation, and often spontaneously convert to an occiput or face presentation. The same etiological factors that underlie a face presentation pertain here. The principles of treatment are the same as for face presentations. If the labor is progressing and it is not unduly vigorous and there is no fetal distress in the closely monitored infant, no intervention is necessary. If labor does become tumultuous or, more likely, desultory, then prompt cesarean section is indicated.[1]

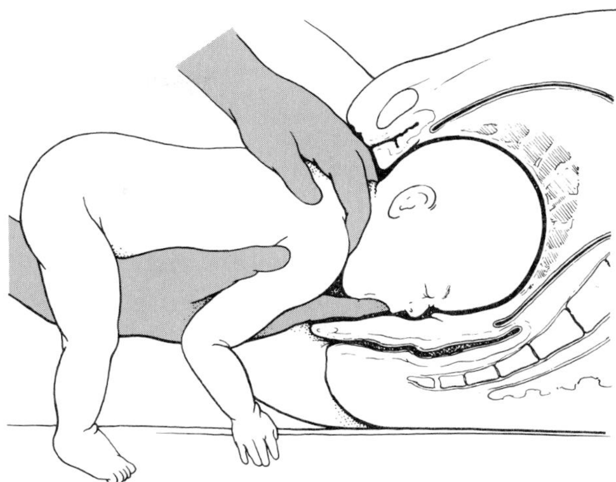

Figure 36-8.
Mauriceau-Smellie-Veit maneuver for extracting head in breech delivery.

Cephalopelvic Disproportion

Contracted Pelvis

Disproportion between the size of the infant and that of the birth canal, commonly spoken of as cephalopelvic disproportion, is caused most frequently by contracted pelvis. The pelvis may be contracted at the inlet, the midpelvis, or the outlet. In the case of inlet contraction, the anteroposterior diameter of the inlet is shortened to 10 cm or less, or the greatest transverse diameter is 12 cm or less. The sacrum is broader and less concave from side to side, thinner from behind forward, and shorter from above downward.

Inlet contraction is most often due to rickets, a fact indicating how much good may be accomplished by the prevention of rickets in infants and children through an adequate intake of vitamin D. Contracted pelvis due to rickets has been found to be more common among black people than among white people.

In midpelvic contraction, the distance between the ischial spines is diminished; it is often found in conjunction with outlet contraction. In outlet contraction, the angle formed by the pubic rami is narrow, and the ischial tuberosities are close together; it thus resembles a male pelvis insofar as the outlet is concerned. This type of pelvic contraction occurs with equal frequency in white people and black people, but its cause is not known. It is not only likely to hinder the egress of the infant at the outlet but also may be responsible for deep lacerations because the narrow pubic rami tend to push the infant's head posteriorly in the direction of the rectum.

One purpose of antepartal care is to detect pelvic contraction during pregnancy, so that long before labor begins, some intelligent decision can be reached about how best to deliver the infant. Of course, in a case of extreme pelvic contraction, cesarean section is obligatory. But all gradients of contracted pelvis are encountered, and, depending on the size of the infant and other factors, many patients with moderate degrees of the condition can be delivered vaginally with care.

In doubtful cases, the physician may give the patient a "trial labor," that is, 4 hours to 6 hours of labor to ascertain whether or not with adequate contractions the head will pass through the pelvis. For these patients labor may be even more anxiety provoking than usual (depending in part on the extent and the depth of supportive antepartal counseling), and if cesarean section is the ultimate outcome, there may be a great deal of disappointment and perhaps even a feeling of failure. The warm empathic attitude of the nurse is particularly needed with these patients. Frequent reports on the progress of labor should not be overlooked when the progress is favorable; if it is not, then explanation and anticipatory guidance regarding cesarean section may be given. The perinatal team does the patient a disservice in avoiding the subject if progress is not made in labor.

Oversized Baby

Excessive size of the infant (4000 g or more) may be a cause of serious dystocia, especially when the fetus weighs over 4500 g (10 lb). About 1 infant in 138 falls into this class. The trauma associated with the passage of such huge infants through the birth canal causes a decided increase in fetal mortality; this has been estimated as 13% (almost 1 in 7), in contrast with the usual death rate of 4% for normal-size infants. Uterine dysfunction is frequent in labors with excessive-size infants because the head becomes not only larger but harder and less malleable with increasing weight. Even though these infants are born alive, they often do poorly in the first few days because of a variety of conditions.

Excessive size of the fetus is usually due to maternal diabetes, large size of one or both parents, or multiparity. Postmaturity due to prolonged gestation is thought to be a cause of excessive-size infants in some instances. Tremendously large infants weighing over 13 lb are extremely rare, and almost all are born dead. Most oversized babies are boys. Although studies have shown a relationship between maternal diet and growth and survival of the fetus, it is doubtful that strict regulation of diet during pregnancy can significantly reduce excessive growth of the infant. However, large women who are heavy may tend to have larger babies.

Shoulder Dystocia. One serious complication of an oversized infant is shoulder dystocia. After the head has passed through the pelvic canal, the infant's unusually large shoulders may arrest at either the pelvic brim or the outlet. The incidence of shoulder dystocia is 1.7% in infants over 4000 g, with mortality of about 16%. The time between delivery of the head and delivery of the body must be short to ensure an uncompromised fetus. A large mediolateral episiotomy and adequate anesthesia are mandatory. The infant's nose and mouth are cleared. Then, without using force, the physician sweeps the posterior arm across the chest and delivers it. The shoulder girdle is then rotated into one of the oblique pelvis diameters (Fig. 36-9). At this time the anterior shoulder can usually be delivered. Care must be taken not to apply vigorous traction on the head or neck or to excessively rotate the body. Occasionally deliberate fracture of the clavicle is necessary to save the infant's life.[1]

Hydrocephalus

Hydrocephalus, or an excessive accumulation of cerebrospinal fluid in the ventricles of the brain with consequent enlargement of the cranium, is encountered in approximately 1 fetus in 2000 and accounts for some 12% of all malformations at birth. Associated defects are common, spina bifida being present in about one third of the cases. Varying degrees of cranial enlargement are produced, and frequently the circumference of the head exceeds 50 cm, sometimes reaching 80 cm. The amount of fluid present is usually between 500 ml and 1500 ml, but as much as 5 liters has been reported. Since the distended cranium is too large to fit into the pelvic inlet, breech presentations are exceedingly common, being observed in about one third of such cases.

Whatever the presentation, gross disproportion

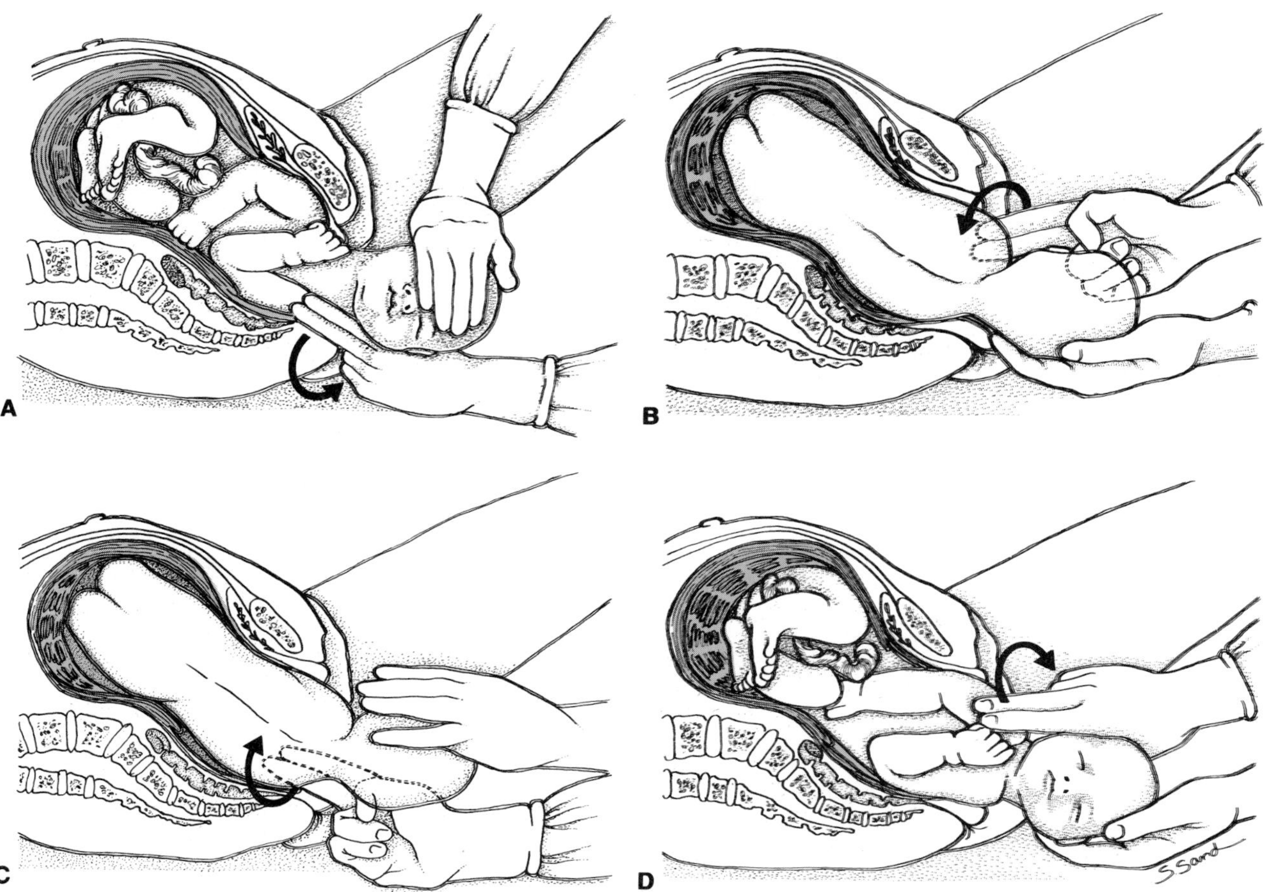

Figure 36-9.
Maneuvers to relieve shoulder dystocia. *(A)* First phase beginning. The posterior shoulder is rotated 180°. *(B)* First phase is completed. Former anterior shoulder is now posterior, and former posterior shoulder is now anterior. There will be an attempt to deliver the shoulders normally at this time. If the attempt fails, the physician proceeds to the second phase. *(C)* Second phase beginning. The newly posterior shoulder is rotated 180°. *(D)* Second phase is completed. Original anterior shoulder is now anterior once again, and the original posterior shoulder is now posterior once again. The remainder of the delivery is performed in the usual way.

between the size of the head and that of the pelvis is the rule, and serious dystocia is the usual consequence (Fig. 36-10). This is a tragic and serious complication of labor, with diagnosis based on sonography and x-ray film.

The obstetrician finds it necessary, as a rule, to puncture the cranial vault and aspirate as much of the cerebrospinal fluid as may be necessary to permit delivery. When aspiration is necessary, fetal mortality is as high as 70% (this percentage includes very mild forms of the disease).

Births of this type are a terrible tragedy for all concerned; the mother must undergo a difficult labor at great risk to herself, the father suffers with her, the fetus may expire, and the physician and the nurse must cope with a grave crisis with a poor prognosis. It is often difficult to describe the emotional climate at this time; perhaps it is impossible if one has not experienced a similar loss or disappointment. A state of emotional shock prevails, in which disbelief, noncomprehension and, sometimes, denial prevail. This is a situation in which the nurse is called on to exercise nursing skill to the utmost, not only during labor but after the delivery, and particularly if there is an obvious abnormality, or if a fetal demise occurs. The components of care that are useful in helping the parents in such a crisis are discussed fully in Chapter 43.

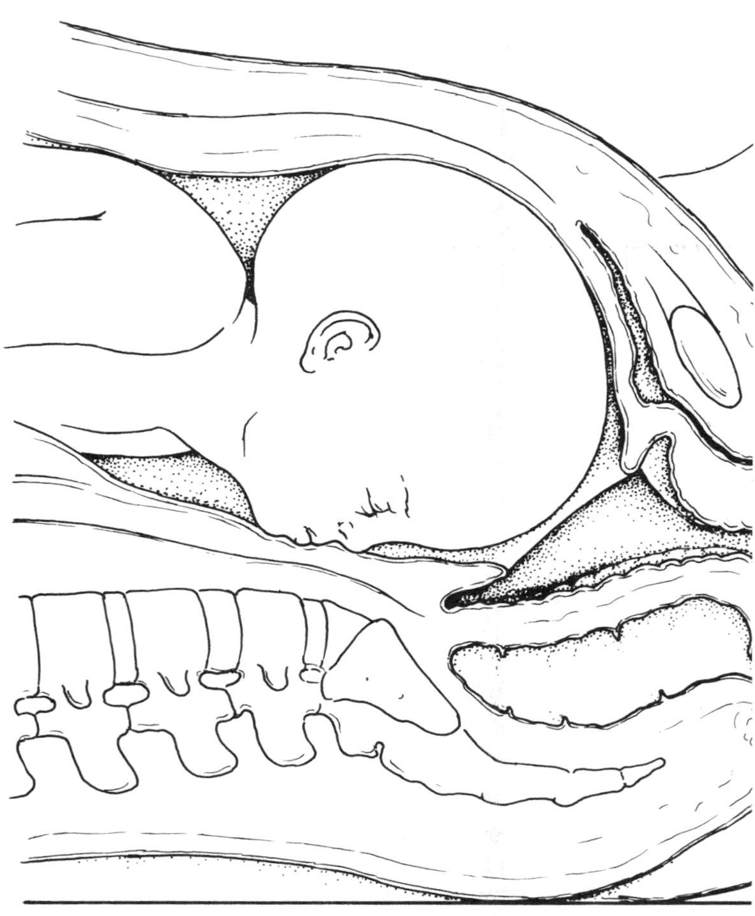

Figure 36-10.
Severe dystocia from hydrocephalus, cephalic presentation. Note the disparity between the small size of the face compared to the rest of the cranium.

Hemorrhagic Complications

Hemorrhage is probably a more important cause of maternal death in the United States than statistics indicate, because national vital statistics are based only on the *immediate* cause of death. The death of a woman who hemorrhaged after labor, contracted postpartum infection, and died would be classified as due to infection, although hemorrhage was the real underlying cause. The major causes of hemorrhage associated with childbearing are placentae previa and abruptio (see Chap. 34) and uterine atony.

Postpartum Hemorrhage

Hemorrhage during the postpartum period is the most common cause of serious blood loss associated with pregnancy, and it causes about one fourth of all maternal deaths from hemorrhagic complications. The debilitation and lowered resistance that often accompany it are related to postpartum infections, another leading cause of maternal death. To a large extent, death from postpartum hemorrhage is preventable if the condition is diagnosed early and treated aggressively.

Definition and Incidence

Postpartum hemorrhage is commonly defined as loss of more than 500 ml of blood during the first 24 hours after giving birth. However, ordinary blood loss following vaginal delivery frequently is more than 500 ml by accurate measurement. Most obstetricians estimate the amount of bleeding at delivery, and studies show that estimated blood loss is usually only about one half of actual loss. Therefore, an *estimated* blood loss over 500 ml serves to alert the nurse and physician that the patient has bled excessively and is in danger of postpartum hemorrhage.

Bleeding of this degree occurs once in every 20 or 30 cases despite the most skilled care. Hemorrhages of 1000 ml and over are encountered once in about every 75 cases, whereas blood losses of even 1500 ml and 2000 ml are encountered less frequently. Postpartum hemorrhage is a fairly common complication of

NC Nursing Care: Priorities in Abnormal Presentations

Assessment	Intervention	Evaluation
Meticulous attention to the status of the mother and infant	Remain with patient Check electronic monitor frequently for signs of uterine contractions and fetal distress	Labor progress; fetus uncompromised
Comfort measures	Frequent backrubs, linen change, oral hygiene as tolerated. Sacral pressure as appropriate in back labor	Patient relatively comfortable
Orientation to continuing labor	Reassurance and explanation as indicated	Discouragement/panic alleviated
Determine hydration level	Monitor IV if present. Check skin and lips for dryness	Dehydration avoided
Bladder hygiene	Encourage frequent voiding. Catheterize as necessary	Bladder undistended

labor. Moreover, it is one with which the nurse must be intimately familiar, as nurses are expected to assume an important role in the prevention and treatment of the condition.

Causes

In order of frequency, the three immediate causes of postpartum hemorrhage are as follows: uterine atony; lacerations of the perineum, the vagina, and the cervix; and retained placental fragments.

Clotting defects, uterine tumors and infections as well as obstetrical accidents such as inversion of the uterus, can also be classified as causes, but they are less common and are of a more indirect nature.

Uterine Atony. Uterine atony is by far the most common cause of postpartum hemorrhage. The uterus contains huge blood vessels within the interstices of its muscle fibers, and those at the placental site are open and gaping. It is essential that the muscle fibers contract down tightly on these arteries and veins if bleeding is to be controlled. They must *stay* contracted down, because relaxation for only a few seconds gives rise to sudden, profuse hemorrhage. They must stay *tightly* contracted down, because continuous, slight relaxation gives rise to continuous oozing of blood, one of the most treacherous forms of postpartum hemorrhage.

In a study of 56 maternal deaths from pregnancy-related hemorrhage over a 9-year period in California, 19 were due to uterine atony. The majority of these women died within 4 hours of delivery, possibly before the seriousness of their bleeding was recognized. Generally, these patients were older multiparae with spontaneous term deliveries; most of their deaths were avoidable had the hemorrhage been diagnosed earlier and adequate blood and fibrinogen replacement been instituted in time. Most of their babies survived.[1]

Lacerations. Lacerations of the perineum, the vagina and the cervix are naturally more common after operative delivery. Tears of the cervix are particularly likely to cause serious hemorrhage. Bright red arterial bleeding in the presence of a hard, firmly contracted uterus (no uterine atony) suggests hemorrhage from a cervical laceration. The physician establishes the diagnosis by actual inspection of the cervix (retractors are necessary) and, after locating the source of bleeding, repairs the laceration.

Perineal and vaginal tears also contribute to postpartal blood loss. In addition, perineal tears may do great damage in destroying the integrity of the perineum and in weakening the supports of the uterus, the bladder, and the rectum. Unless these lacerations are repaired properly, the resultant weakness, as the years go by, may cause prolapse of the uterus, cystocele (a pouching downward of the bladder), or rectocele (a pouching forward of the rectum). These conditions, which originate from perineal lacerations at childbirth, give rise to many discomforts and often necessitate operative treatment.

Lacerations of the birth canal sometimes occur during the process of normal delivery and may be unavoidable even in the most skilled hands.

Retained Placental Fragments. Small, partially separated fragments of placenta may cause postpartum hemorrhage by interfering with proper uterine contraction (Fig. 36-11). Careful inspection of the placenta to determine whether a piece is missing should be routinely carried out at delivery. If a portion is missing, exploration of the uterus is indicated to remove the placental fragment. In the case of continued postpartum bleeding, retention of placental fragments is generally ruled out by manual exploration. However, this is rarely a cause of immediate postpartum hemorrhage, and is more commonly implicated in late hemorrhage in which profuse bleeding occurs suddenly a week or more after delivery.

Predisposing Factors

There are certain factors which predispose to postpartum hemorrhage, so that to a certain extent it may be anticipated in advance. Among these, one of the most important is the size of the infant. With a 9-pound infant, the chances of postpartum hemorrhage are five times as great as they are with a 5-pound infant. Excessive bleeding is twice as common in twin pregnancy. Hydramnios (excessive amount of amniotic fluid) is another predisposing factor. It has been shown, however, that with the careful use of oxytocin in the placental stage and special care to achieve effective contraction in this stage, the incidence of hemorrhage due to overdistention can be reduced considerably.

Operative delivery with deep general anesthesia, prolonged labor with maternal exhaustion, and mismanagement of the third stage of labor greatly increase the likelihood of this complication. Other conditions in which postpartum hemorrhage is extremely frequent are high parity and premature separation of the placenta.

It should be noted also that a small woman withstands blood loss less well than a woman of average size or larger. An average-sized, relatively healthy mother can lose up to 1% of her blood volume without immediate crises. It is not difficult to relate body weight to blood volume since 1 ml of blood equals 1 g. Therefore, if a woman loses 1% of her body weight through blood loss, she is considered to have a hemorrhage.[9]

Hemorrhage and Shock

During any stage of pregnancy, hemorrhage poses a severe threat to the mother. This is especially true of postpartal hemorrhage because the shock that accompanies the blood loss is often out of proportion to the amount lost.

Pathophysiology of Shock. When hemorrhaging occurs, the body activates certain compensatory mechanisms. The adrenals release catecholamines which cause the arterioles and venules of the skin, liver, gastrointestinal tract, lungs, and kidneys to constrict. This diverts blood to the brain and heart. When shock persists, cellular oxygenation continues to be reduced, which results in accumulation of lactic acid and consequent acidosis. Serum acidosis in turn causes arteriole vasodilatation, but venule vasoconstriction persists. Thus, a downward spiral is established in which the decreased perfusion, increased tissue acidosis and anoxia, edema, and blood pooling further decrease perfusion of the tissues. Eventually, cellular death occurs and the patient dies.[16]

Clinical Picture. Excessive bleeding may occur prior to the birth of the placenta, but it is seen more commonly thereafter. Although it is occasionally torrential in character, the most common type is a continuous trickle—minute by minute. These small constant trickles are not alarming in appearance; consequently, no one may become concerned and no action may be taken.

Such hemorrhages are particularly treacherous for this reason. The condition and size of the patient determines the amount of blood loss that can be tolerated, with exhaustion from prolonged labor or antecedent anemia or chronic disease reducing the ability of the body to compensate. When hemorrhage has been profuse enough, the pulse becomes rapid and thready, the skin becomes pallid and clammy; and chills and disturbed vision occur. As shock deepens air hunger develops, with restlessness and sweating; then unconsciousness and death may follow. The pulse and blood pressure may not change significantly until large amounts of blood have been lost; then the vascular mechanism fails and shock ensues. Vascular collapse may lead to death when intravenous infusion cannot be maintained for blood replacement. Cardiac arrest may also occur at this point.

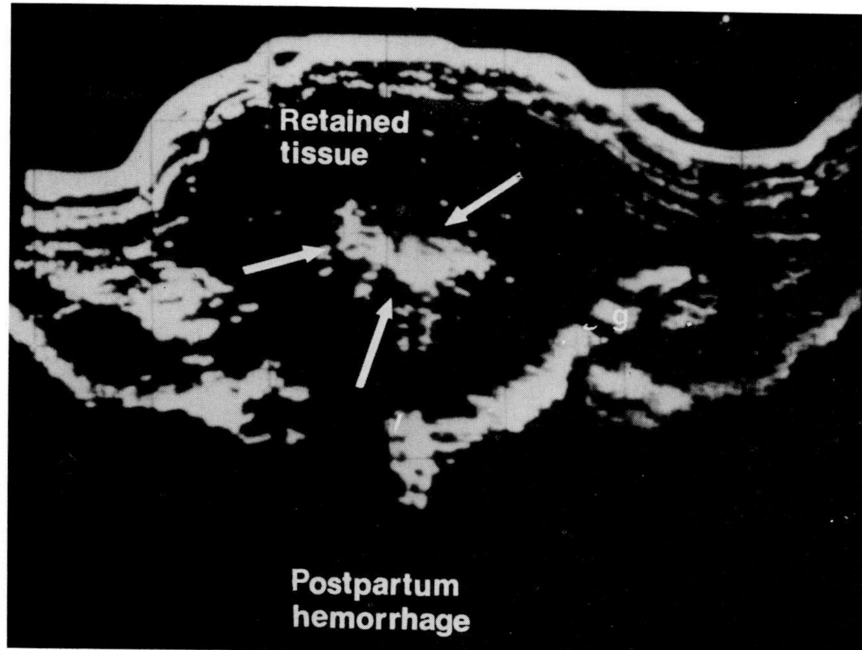

Figure 36-11.
Postpartum hemorrhage. Retained tissue demonstrated on sonogram. This requires surgical evacuation. (Cavanagh D, Woods RE, O'Connor TCF, Knuppel RA: Obstetric Emergencies, 3rd ed. Philadelphia, Harper & Row, 1982)

Treatment

If one suspects that a woman may be hemorrhaging, it is important that the nurse remain with her constantly. The fundus should be checked immediately. The physician needs to be notified, and the emergency equipment must be easily accessible, including intravenous fluid packs, tubing and large bore (#18) needles, oxygen equipment, retention catheter, suction, blood pressure, and central venous pressure apparatus. Signs of shock are to be monitored through the appropriate vital signs, skin, urinary output, and level of consciousness (Fig. 36-12 and Table 36-3).

The physician ascertains the reason for the hemorrhage. If it is the result of vaginal or uterine injuries or retained placental fragments, the patient is returned to the delivery room for repair or uterine evacuation. However, it is far more likely that uterine atony is to blame and the nurse plays a key role in managing this condition.

Massaging the Fundus. The uterus should be grasped immediately and massaged gently but firmly. The lower uterine segment is supported with the edge of the hand a little above the mother's symphysis, while the fundus is massaged with the other hand (Fig. 36-13). Thus, the uterus is cupped between the two hands and is supported as it is massaged. Massage is to be continued until the uterus assumes a woody hardness; if the slightest relaxation occurs, the massage must be reinstituted. In many cases the uterus stays contracted most of the time but occasionally it relaxes; it is therefore obligatory to keep a hand on the fundus constantly for a full hour after bleeding has subsided. When the uterus is well contracted, care should be taken to *avoid overmassage,* because such practice contributes to muscle fatigue, which in turn further encourages uterine relaxation and excessive bleeding.

It must be remembered that relaxation sometimes occurs two or more hours after delivery; in these cases the uterus may balloon with blood, with very little escaping externally. Accordingly, the consistency, size, and height of the uterus should be checked frequently until several hours have elapsed. Ordinarily, the height of the fundus after delivery is about at the level of the umbilicus. If the uterus becomes distended with blood, or if the bladder becomes full and presses upward against the uterus, causing it to rise in the abdomen, then the fundus can be palpated several centimeters above the umbilicus. The nurse must make absolutely certain that the uterus is in fact being massaged, and not a roll of abdominal fat or a distended bladder. When properly contracted, the uterus should feel like a small-to-large hard apple.

Frequently, a big, boggy, relaxed uterus is difficult to outline through the abdominal wall, and it may be necessary to push the hand well posteriorly toward

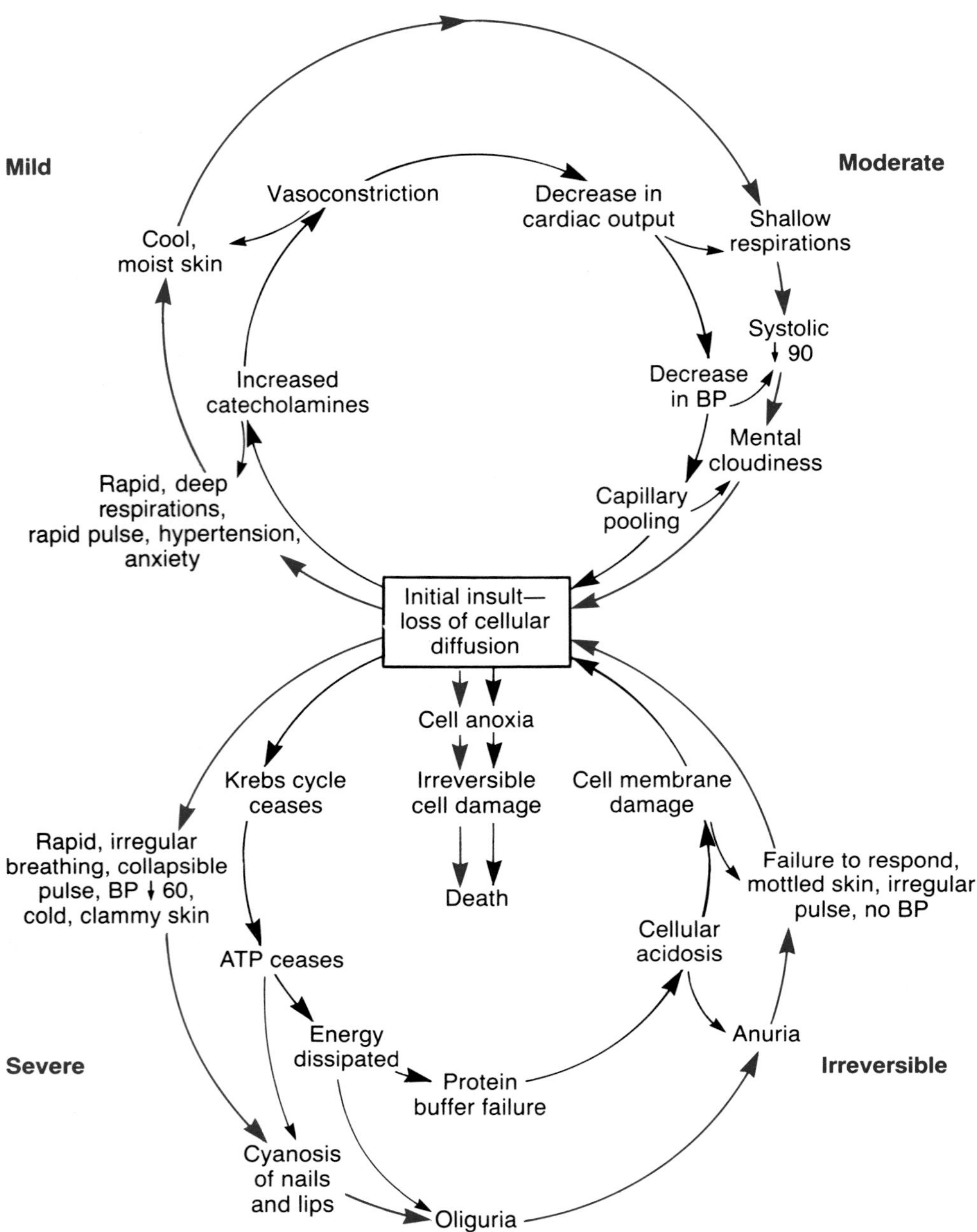

Figure 36-12.
Diagram of physiological alterations in shock in relation to symptoms. (Royce JA: Shock: Emergency nursing implications. Nurs Clin North Am 8:377, 1973)

the region of the sacral promontory to reach it. The very fact that the uterus is hard to identify usually means that it is relaxed.

Allaying Anxiety. The frequent massage and deep palpation are often painful to the mother; at best, they are disturbing, since they come at a time when she wants nothing more than to rest and sleep after her great effort. If she is awake and alert, then the continued attention and scrutiny may increase her anxiety. It must be remembered that apprehension is a natural concomitant of hemorrhage and shock. Quick and efficient nursing observations and appropriate explanation and reassurance help allay the concerns of both the mother and her partner.

This aspect of nursing care may be difficult to implement. If the mother or the father expresses concern and questions the activity by asking "What's

Table 36-3.
Symptoms of Shock

	Mild	Moderate	Severe	Irreversible
Respirations	Rapid, deep	Rapid, becoming shallow	Rapid, shallow, may be irregular	Irregular, or barely perceptible
Pulse	Rapid, tone normal	Rapid, tone may be normal but is becoming weaker	Very rapid, easily collapsible, may be irregular	Irregular apical pulse
Blood pressure	Normal or hypertensive	60 mm Hg–90 mm Hg systolic	Below 60 mm Hg systolic	None palpable
Skin	Cool and pale	Cool, pale, moist, knees cyanotic	Cold, clammy, cyanosis of lips and fingernails	Cold, clammy, cyanotic
Urine output	No change	Decreasing to 10 ml/hr–22 ml/hr (adult)	Oliguric (less than 10 ml) to anuria	Anuric
Level of consciousness	Alert, oriented, diffuse anxiety	Oriented, mental cloudiness or increasing restlessness	Lethargy, reacts to noxious stimuli, comatose	Does not respond to noxious stimuli
CVP	May be normal	3 cm H_2O	0 cm H_2O–3 cm H_2O	

(Royce JA: Shock: Emergency nursing implications. Nurs Clin North Am 8:377, 1973; Wagner MM: Clinical Nursing Specialist, University of Iowa Hospitals and Clinics.)

wrong?", then the nurse can simply say, "The uterus has a tendency to relax, and must be massaged so that it will contract down as it should." Usually, such a statement suffices. This indicates the reason for the continued activity without associating hemorrhage and its fearsome consequences with the actions of the attendants. If the mother drifts off to sleep between the nurse's observations, then the nurse can gently rouse her by speaking her name before commencing massage, so that the mother is not awakened abruptly to the painful sensation of someone squeezing her abdomen.

Other Aspects of Care. Vital signs must be checked every 5 minutes to 15 minutes, and any variation, however slight, is to be reported immediately. Skin condition, level of consciousness, and urinary output are also monitored.

One way that the nurse can keep a more accurate account of the blood loss is by keeping a perineal pad count. A record is kept of the number of pads saturated, how fully they are saturated, and the time it took for the saturation to occur. Thus, the nurse's notes might read: "Two pads ¾ saturated in 20 minutes." This type of report is more helpful to the physician than a more general, vague statement like, "Saturating perineal pads quickly."

If the bleeding occurs prior to delivery of the placenta, the physician may find it necessary to extract the placenta manually. (A change of gloves as well as gown may be called for to ensure strict asepsis, since the uterine cavity is to be invaded.) Oxytocics will invariably be requested. Ergonovine or oxytocin, or both, are administered intramuscularly. One or the other of these may be given intravenously.

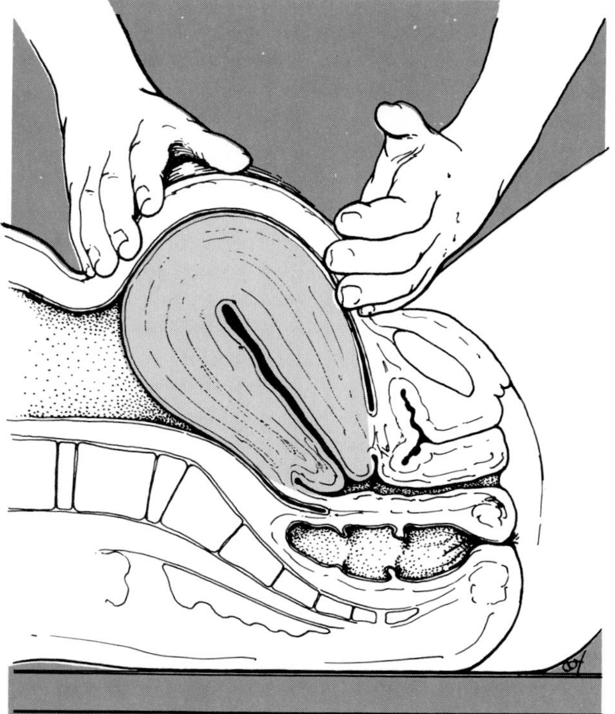

Figure 36-13.
Massaging the uterus.

It is necessary that there be *fluid replacement* for serious hemorrhage to combat hypovolemia. Pritchard recommends two general guidelines. First, lactated Ringer's solution and whole blood are given in amount and proportion to maintain a urine flow of at least 30 ml per hour and preferably 60 ml per hour (1 ml per minute). In addition, the hematocrit is maintained at 30% or slightly higher. Second, if initial vigorous fluid replacement therapy does not maintain or restore the urine flow, then the CVP is monitored, and fluids are adjusted accordingly.

Central Venous Pressure. *CVP readings* measure the contractility of the heart and the adequacy of the blood volume. The normal range is between 6 mm H_2O and 12 mm H_2O. Falling values indicate hypovolemia and rising values indicate impaired contractility. To institute this type of monitoring, a catheter is inserted into the subclavian vein, between the clavicle and first rib (Fig. 36-14). The data obtained provide a more precise estimate of the amount of fluid replacement necessary to combat shock.[9]

Since *blood transfusion* plays an important role in preventing serious shock, the blood groups of *all* maternity patients should be known before labor, and crossmatched blood should be available for those in whom hemorrhage is anticipated or appears imminent. Seeing that the bloodtyping is carried out, ordering and calling for the cross match, and making sure that the blood is sent to the unit are usually responsibilities of the nurse. Time is of the essence for these patients; therefore, the nurse must preplan and establish priorities with rapidity.

If oxytocin therapy fails to stop the bleeding, the physician probably will carry out bimanual compression of the uterus. This provides the most efficient means of compressing the site of bleeding. Packing the uterus with gauze, a procedure once considered valuable to promote hemostasis in such cases, is seldom used today. It is considered by many authorities

Figure 36-14.
(A) Insertion of CVP catheter into subclavian vein. *(B)* Plastic catheter and central venous pressure setup in place. (Modified from Malinak et al: Am J Obst Gynecol 92:447, 1965)

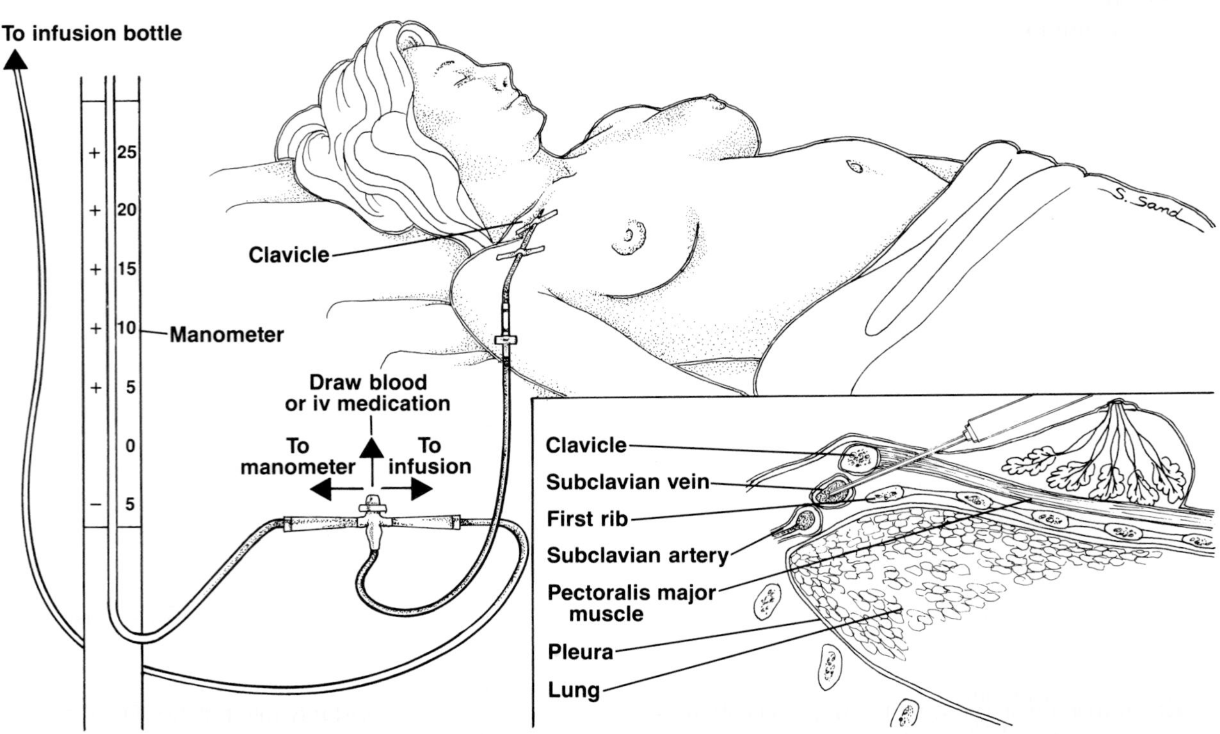

(*e.g.,* Hellman, Cosgrove, Leff, and Berkeley) to be inadequate and conducive to infection. If shock threatens, the right hip is elevated, external heat is applied, and preparations for blood transfusion and fluid replacement are made. An airway may be inserted.

In the handling of a case of postpartum hemorrhage, the nurse often assumes the important tasks of massaging the uterus, giving oxytocics, helping with the infusions, and caring for the infant. The nurse must be prepared to act quickly and efficiently if the lives of these mothers are to be saved.

If postpartal hemorrhage occurs after the physician has left, the nurse gently grasps the uterus at once and presses out as much blood as possible by gentle but vigorous massage, and notifies the physician immediately. If massage fails to stop the bleeding, the physician usually does not object if the nurse gives the patient an intramuscular injection of ergonovine or oxytocin. If possible, this arrangement should be understood beforehand.

Late Postpartum Hemorrhage

Occasionally, postpartum hemorrhage may occur later than the first day following delivery. These late postpartum hemorrhages may take place any time between the second day and sixth week and are usually sudden in onset and may be so massive as to produce shock. Fortunately, late postpartum hemorrhage is uncommon, occurring perhaps once in 1000 cases.

While this condition is relatively uncommon, it is most dangerous because the mother is usually alone at home, and without professional attendance. Thus, if the hemorrhage is massive, she may be in immediate danger. Even if the bleeding is not great, there is still considerable difficulty getting medical assistance, and all of this can produce a great deal of anxiety and fatigue.

Arrangements must be made for the care of the infant even if the mother is to be seen only for a short while in the emergency room. Partners must be contacted, transportation arranged, and often myriads of other details worked through so that the mother can receive medical attention. This is why it is so important that the mother know where she can readily contact her physician should she need him in an emergency. Moreover, it becomes clearer why the mother should have someone who is readily available and responsible to help her for the first weeks of the puerperium.

Factors that most often cause these late hemorrhages are retention of placental fragments, recurrent bleeding from lacerations or episiotomy and subinvolution of the placental site. The latter condition is especially interesting because, as yet, the pathogenesis is unknown. The regeneration of the placental site takes longer than the rest of the uterus. It is accomplished in about 6 weeks as compared with about 21 days for the rest of the endometrium. The regeneration of the placental site begins from the remains of the epithelial glands; if these are not viable, then regeneration must occur from the spread of the surrounding epithelial tissue in the rest of the uterus. Until the site is firmly epithelialized, sloughing of clots may cause bleeding. Certain factors have been found to be associated with clot sloughing and hemorrhage; among them are low grade fever, a history of abortion or uterine bleeding during pregnancy, hormonal influences, and the lack of breast-feeding. Often, however, none of these factors are found to be present, and the reason for the subinvolution remains a mystery. The physician will probably want to examine the patient and then carry out instrumental dilatation of the cervix, at which time any placental fragments that are present will be removed with a curet or ovum forceps, and any lacerations or incisions will be repaired.

Use of ultrasonic scanning of the uterus to detect the presence of retained products of conception, thus avoiding unnecessary curettage, has been suggested.[17]

If the mother must return to the hospital, this undoubtedly upsets the beginning relationship with the newborn to some degree. If the mother is nursing her infant and it is within a 2-week period after delivery, the physician often can arrange to have the mother room-in with her infant for the short one- or two-day hospital stay. If the mother is bottle-feeding, then relatives, husband, or "mother's helpers" can help in the interim until the mother's return. The nurse should remember that much of the mother's apparent anxiety or desire to return home as quickly as possible arises from these often abrupt and temporary arrangements that she has had to make. Understanding and counseling the mother to help her get adequate rest upon her return home is one of the helpful measures that the nurse can offer.

Rupture of the Uterus

Rupture of the uterus is fortunately a rare complication, occurring about once in every 2000 pregnancies. It constitutes one of the gravest accidents in obstetrics, however, since the mortality rate for the infant is 50% to 75% and virtually all untreated mothers succumb to hypovolemia from hemorrhage or, less often, to infection. In this condition, the uterus simply bursts because the strain placed upon its musculature is more than it can withstand. Uterine rupture may occur in pregnancy but is far more frequent in labor.[1]

While the incidence has not changed to any degree in the last several decades, the etiology has changed, and the outcome has improved significantly. Today, the most common cause is attributed to rupture of the scar from a previous cesarean section. So great is this condition indited that the dictum "once a cesarean, always a cesarean" continues to be valid in the opinion of many clinicians.[20] The second most common etiological agent is felt to be injudicious stimulation of labor with oxytocin. Other contributing factors include previous surgery involving the myometrium, prolonged or obstructed labor, certain faulty positions or fetal abnormalities, multiparity, excessive fetal size, and traumatic delivery, such as version and extraction, or injudicious use of forceps.[9]

When rupture occurs, the patient complains of a severe, sudden, lacerating pain during a strong labor contraction. The rupture may be complete or incomplete; pain and abdominal tenderness are usually present in both cases. If there is complete rupture, regular contractions cease because the torn muscle can no longer contract. There is an outpouring of blood into the abdominal cavity and sometimes into the vagina. The uterus may be palpated abdominally as a hard mass lying alongside the fetus. The patient soon exhibits signs of shock.

If the rupture is incomplete, the contractions may continue, and the signs of shock may be delayed, since the blood loss is slower. As soon as the diagnosis of rupture of the uterus is made, rapid preparations for an abdominal operation should ensue as hysterectomy is the usual treatment. In addition, antibiotics are administered to combat infection, and blood transfusions and fluids are given to replace blood loss and to alleviate shock.

Since this accident gravely compromises the lives of both the infant and the mother, prevention, early diagnosis, prompt treatment, blood transfusions, and antibiotics are essential components in improving the prognosis.

The nursing care is essentially that for any complicated delivery and postpartum hemorrhage and shock. Whenever possible it is advisable to have the nurse who has been attending the mother during labor remain with her until the anesthetic for the cesarean section is given. This provides some measure of continuity of care and help in reassurance and comfort of the parents.

Inversion of Uterus

Inversion of the uterus is a highly fatal accident of labor in which, after the birth of the infant, the uterus turns inside out. Shock is profound, and hemorrhage may occur, which if not treated quickly will cause the death of the mother.

There are two common causes of this accident, both of which are preventable, (1) pulling on the umbilical cord and (2) trying to express the placenta when the uterus is relaxed. In the former case, the traction on the attached placenta simply pulls the uterus inside out, while in the latter, the hand pushes the relaxed muscular sac inside out. Thus, umbilical cord should never have strenuous traction applied nor should the uterus be pushed downward unless it is firmly contracted.

It is imperative that several steps in treatment be taken promptly and simultaneously. (1) Two intravenous infusions systems are instituted, one with lactated Ringer's solution and one with whole blood. These are given promptly to refill the intravascular compartment and support cardiac output. (2) An anesthesiologist gives a general anesthetic, usually halothane, to relax the uterus. The placenta is left in place until the infusions are operational and uterine relaxation has been accomplished. If the placenta is removed prematurely, hemorrhage is increased. Attempts are then made to replace the uterus in the vagina by placing the palm of the hand on the center of the fundus with the fingers extended to identify the cervical margins. The fundus is then pushed up through the cervix. When the uterus is returned to its normal shape, anesthesia is discontinued and oxytocin is begun to help the uterus remain contracted. Bimanual compression also aids in this. The uterus is then monitored transvaginally until normal tone is assured.

If the uterus cannot be placed from below because of a constriction ring, a laparatomy is performed so that the uterus can be pulled up simultaneously from above and pushed up from below. The constriction ring may be incised. A traction suture in the fundus aids in repositioning. Treatment continues as previously described. Subsequent inversion is unlikely.[1]

Disorders of Placental Attachment

Other important causes of bleeding associated with pregnancy and labor are placenta previa and abruptio placentae. These have been discussed previously as complications of pregnancy in Chapter 34. However, at times the first signs of these problems occur during

NC **Nursing Care: Priorities in Postpartum Hemorrhagic Complication**

Assessment	Intervention	Evaluation
Status of fundus	Hold fundus; massage gently until firm (not continuously); express clots as needed	Bleeding controlled
Amount of flow	Pad count (amount saturated in amount of time)	
Vital signs TPR, BP	Check q 5 min–15 min Record and report	Profound shock avoided
Skin	Provide warmth with clean, dry, warm blankets	
Urine output	Record, report accurately; maintain @ 30 ml/hr–60 ml/hr	
Level of consciousness	Check frequently; speak to patient to ascertain if she is oriented; reassure couple as indicated	
Monitor intravenous/oxytocin	Check frequently to be sure needle is in place, uterus contracted	Uterus contracts and patient hydrated
Monitor CVP if necessary	Maintain approximately 6 mm H_2O–12 mm H_2O; record and report as indicated	Blood volume more precisely ascertained
Type and cross match blood	Order if indicated; follow through with lab	In readiness if continued hemorrhage

labor, and the nurse in the delivery suite must be familiar with their diagnosis and management.

The cardinal sign of *placenta previa* is painless, bright red vaginal bleeding. If partial separation occurs after the onset of labor, contractions may confuse the situation; identification depends upon accurately assessing the extent of vaginal bleeding. Overt hemorrhage with huge blood loss is not difficult to diagnose, but it requires fine judgment to decide when bloody vaginal discharge ceases to be heavy "show" and becomes potential hemorrhage. It is wise to report any vaginal bleeding which the nurse believes is excessive to the physician and to refrain from digital examination of these patients.

Abruptio placentae can be a true obstetrical emergency if the area of separation is extensive. The signs that alert the delivery room nurse to this complication include a hypertonic uterus that does not relax well between contractions, an area of extreme sensitivity when the uterus is palpated, sudden sharp and persistent uterine pain, and symptoms and signs of shock which seem greater than the observable blood loss would indicate. An extremely hard, boardlike uterus that cannot be indented and does not relax indicates a severe degree of placental separation and bleeding.

Marginal sinus rupture was formerly treated as a separate clinical entity, but now is felt to be a mild type of abruptio placentae in which slight separation occurs at the edge of the placenta. The marginal sinus is located under the edge of the placenta, and is one of the large maternal sinuses bathing the placental villi. If the placenta separates at a point along its margin, this maternal sinus is disrupted and bleeding occurs. There is usually no increased pain or uterine tension, and the amount of vaginal bleeding may vary considerably. If the area of separation is small, as it usually is in marginal sinus rupture, there is no danger of hypoxia to the fetus and generally no changes in fetal heart rate. When there is excessive vaginal bleeding during labor, and placentae previa and abruptio have been ruled out, the most probable cause is a small marginal separation of the placenta.[19] Nursing care is the same as for other hemorrhage conditions.

Prolapse of Umbilical Cord

In the course of labor, the cord prolapses in front of the presenting part about once in every 400 cases. It is a grave complication for the fetus, since the cord is then compressed between the presenting part and the

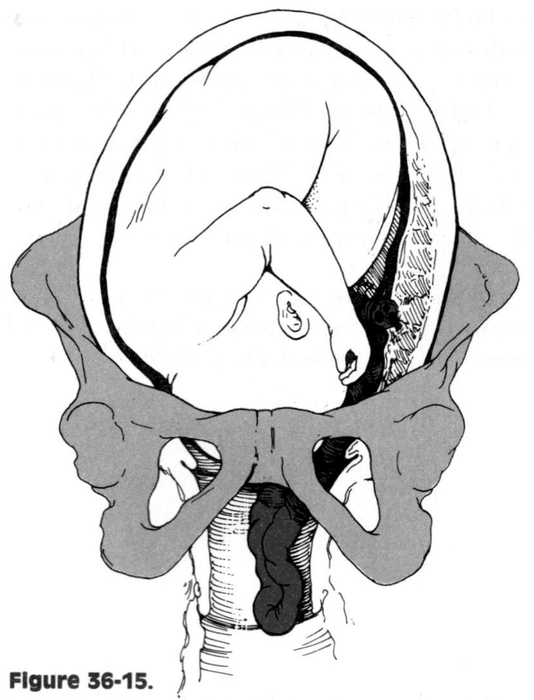

Figure 36-15.
Prolapse of the cord. As the head comes down, the compression of the cord between the fetal skull and the pelvic brim will shut off its circulation completely.

bony pelvis, and the fetal circulation is shut off (Fig. 36-15). Any factor which prevents proper adaptation of the presenting part to the maternal pelvis predisposes to prolapse of the cord. The accident occurs more commonly in shoulder and footling breech presentations, and less often with frank breeches and multiple pregnancy. In cephalic presentations, it rarely occurs unless there is pelvic contraction or excessive development of the fetus. There is an increased incidence with prematurity, probably because the small fetus is poorly fitted to the pelvic inlet.

Prolapse frequently occurs following rupture of the membranes when the head, the breech, or the shoulder is not sufficiently down in the pelvis to prevent the cord from being washed past it in the sudden gush of amniotic fluid. After the membranes rupture, the cord comes down, and it may be either a concealed or an apparent prolapse. In the latter instance, the diagnosis is made when the cord is seen; but when the cord is not visible, the correct diagnosis is made when the patient is examined and the cord is felt or examination of the fetal heart reveals distress due to pressure on the cord. This is why it *must* be a routine practice to listen to and to record the fetal heart sounds immediately after the membranes rupture and again in about 5 minutes to 10 minutes. When fetal heart rate is monitored internally, a characteristic slowing of the fetal heart with onset early during the contraction and persistence of bradycardia beyond the end of contraction are suggestive of cord compression.

The immediate treatment of cord prolapse is to minimize the pressure of the presenting part upon the cord and the resultant impaired umbilical circulation. The head of the bed or table should be lowered, or the patient should be placed in a knee-chest position to raise the level of the hips above the shoulders and allow the presenting part to gravitate away from the pelvi (Fig. 36-16). Additionally, the presenting part may be pushed upward by pressure from a sterile gloved hand in the vagina.

The physician and other staff must be notified at once so emergency procedures can be instituted. No attempt should be made to reposition the cord, and

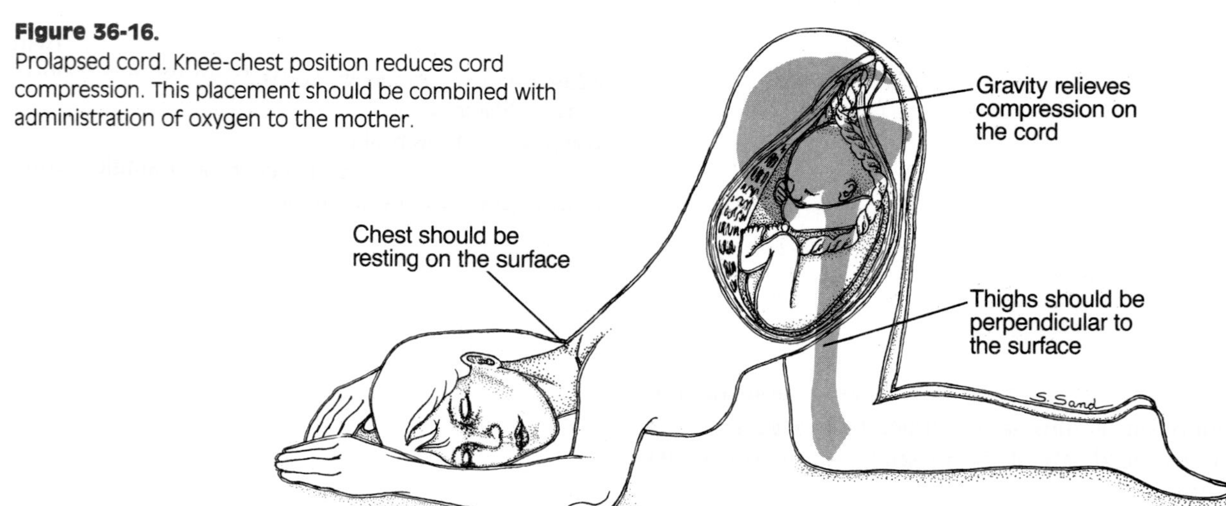

Figure 36-16.
Prolapsed cord. Knee-chest position reduces cord compression. This placement should be combined with administration of oxygen to the mother.

with a live baby near term, the goal of therapy is to effect delivery as soon as possible. If dilatation is incomplete, immediate cesarean section yields the best results for fetal salvage. In occasional carefully selected cases, prolapsed cord in vertex presentations with nearly complete dilatation can be delivered with minimal trauma to mother and infant using vacuum extraction.

Perinatal mortality with cord prolapse, which is usually about 26%, can be reduced to 5% to 10% when delivery is accomplished within one half hour after diagnosis. More frequent vaginal examinations, checking fetal heart after rupture of membranes, and active rapid treatment combine to reduce mortality.

This particular complication is not painful for the mother; however, it can be very frightening, for many patients realize it can result in their infant's death. Also whether they realize the grave implications or not, the various frantic positions and quickened responses of the attendants give them an indication that all is not well. Therefore, again, the calmness, warmth, and efficiency of the nurse can do much to reassure the patient that all possible measures are being taken to bring the situation under control.

It goes without saying that these patients never should be left unattended, and their partners, if they are present, should be treated with consideration. It is difficult, when any crises occur, to deal with the relatives of the patient with appropriate thoughtfulness, since most of the energy is directed toward meeting the pressing (and often life-saving) demands of the situation. However, it must be remembered that the patient and her family are considered as a unit, and a few moments usually can be found to provide essential information.

Amniotic Fluid Embolism

At any time after the membranes have ruptured there is a possibility that amniotic fluid may enter the gaping venous sinuses of the placental site as well as the veins in the cervix, be drawn into the general circulation, and in this way reach the pulmonary capillaries. Since the amniotic fluid invariably contains small particles of matter, such as vernix caseosa, lanugo, and sometimes meconium, multiple tiny emboli may reach the lungs in this manner and cause occlusion of the pulmonary capillaries. This complication, amniotic fluid embolism, is almost invariably fatal and, as a rule, causes the death of the mother within one or two hours. Fortunately, this tragic condition is rare, occurring only once in many thousand labors.

The clinical characteristics of the condition are sudden dyspnea, cyanosis, pulmonary edema, profound shock, and uterine relaxation with hemorrhage. A highly important feature of amniotic fluid embolism is a diminution in the fibrinogen content of the blood, or hypofibrinogenemia. The mechanism is similar to, if not identical with, that which occurs in abruptio placentae and missed abortion, as described in Chapter 34.

The treatment consists of oxygen therapy, blood transfusion and the intravenous administration of fibrinogen, but, as indicated, this is usually futile.

Multiple Pregnancy

When two or more embryos develop in the uterus at the same time, the condition is known as multiple pregnancy. Multiple pregnancies account for about 2% to 3% of all viable births. The frequency of identical (monozygotic or one-egg) twins is apparently relatively constant throughout the world at about 1 set in every 250 pregnancies. Moreover, their appearance is largely independent of race, heredity, maternal age, parity, infertility drugs, and environmental factors. On the other hand, fraternal (dizygotic, two-egg) twins are influenced by these factors. Their incidence in the white race is about 1 set in 95 and in the black race 1 set in 78. Twinning among orientals is less common. Women who were themselves a dizygotic twin tend to have more multiple pregnancies. Similarly, increased age, parity, endogenous gonadotropin, and taking infertility drugs also increases the probability of multiple pregnancy.[20]

Types of Twins

Multiple fetuses result from two basic processes. Twin fetuses more commonly result from the fertilization of two different ova. This type of twin is known as dizygotic, or fraternal twin. About one third as often, twins arise from the fertilization of a single ovum, monozygotic or identical twin. Either or both processes may be at work in the production of larger numbers of fetuses in one birth. Quadruplets, for instance, may arise from one to four ova.[1] An interesting feature of twinning is that although dizygotic twins are not in the strict sense true twins because they result from the union of two separate ova and sperm, if they are of the same sex, they often resemble each other more closely than a pair of monozygotic twins. The process of the division of one fertilized zygote into two does not always result in an equal sharing of the protoplasm; thus, the growth of monozygotic twins is often dramatically discordant.[1]

Basically, two types of placentae exist in twins, those with monochorial (one chorion) and those with dichorial (two chorions) membranes (Fig. 36-17). Also, the placentae may be fused, separate, or a single disk, and there may be one or two amnions. However, each fetus usually has its own umbilical cord. The possible combinations thus include the following:

1. Monozygotic (identical)
   a. Diamniotic dichorionic (two amnions, two chorions), 30%
   b. Diamniotic monochorionic (two amnions, one chorion), common
   c. Monoamniotic monochorionic (one amnion, one chorion), very rare
2. Dizygotic (fraternal or nonidentical)
   a. Diamniotic dichorionic (two amnions, two chorions)

Examination of the fetal membranes is used to assist in diagnosing the zygosity of twins but is not always accurate. Only monozygotic twins can have a single chorion, which establishes identical twinning. Two chorions are always present in dizygotic twins, but are also the placentation of about 30% of monozygotic twins. If the sexes are different, the twins are obviously fraternal; but if twins are the same sex and dichorionic, the diagnosis is uncertain.[1,20] The usual twin placentations are shown in Figure 36-18. In the United States, 33% of twins are identical.

Diagnosis

Twins are suspected whenever uterine size is greater than ordinarily expected for any point in pregnancy. In addition, the palpation of three or four large parts in the uterus, the appearance of two fetal heart tones of differing frequency, and the history of twins "running in the family" all serve to alert the obstetrician and nurse to the possibility of a multiple pregnancy. Sonography can confirm the diagnosis.

Twins are likely to be born about 2 weeks before the calculated date of delivery. Even though pregnancy goes to full term, twins are usually smaller than single infants by nearly 1 lb. There is greater perinatal risk for twins than singletons which persists into the first year of life. Hence, early diagnosis and monitoring antepartally are necessary.

Pathophysiology of Multiple Pregnancy

Several high-risk conditions are associated with multiple pregnancy. These include premature delivery (50%), hemorrhage (20%), hypertensive disorders, preeclampsia and eclampsia (25%), abnormal presen-

Figure 36-17.
Twin pregnancy *(A)* Fraternal twins with two placentas, two amnions, and two chorions. *(B)* Identical twins with one placenta, one chorion, and two amnions.

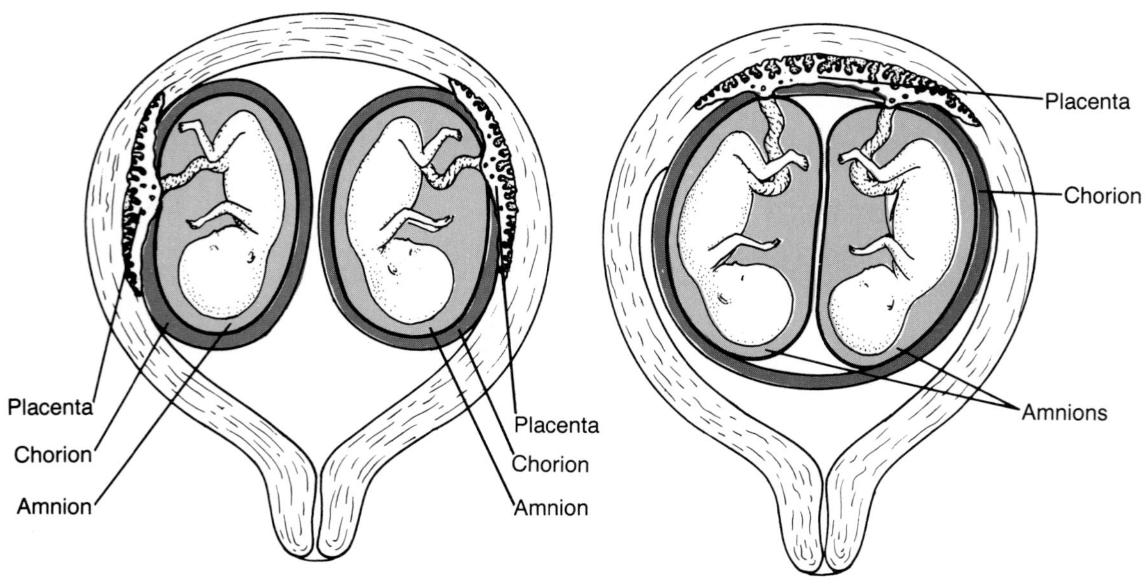

tation and position (10%), hydramnios (7%) and uterine dysfunction (10%). Cord compression and entanglement, intrauterine growth retardation, and operative delivery also contribute to morbidity and mortality. In addition, monozygotic twins are less hardy than dizygotic twins. Weight differences are more pronounced, and they have a higher incidence of congenital anomalies and neonatal mortality.

Some of these problems may be due to the monochorionic placenta which is thought to be less competent than the dichorionic variety. The problems center on placental vascular disorders.

The most serious of these is the shunting of blood due to vascular anastomosis which results in a twin-to-twin transfusion syndrome (intrauterine parabiosis). The anastomosis may be artery-to-artery, artery-to-vein, or vein-to-vein. An artery-to-vein anastomosis is the most serious and accounts for the disparity in size and appearance seen in these supposedly identical infants. The *donor* twin is pallid, anemic, dehydrated, growth retarded, and hypovolemic. Hydrops and cardiac decompensation may be present as well as polyhydramnios. In contrast, the *recipient* twin appears healthy, large by contrast, and ruddy. However, this appearance is due to edema, plethora, and hypertension. Kernicterus, ascites, glomerular-tubal hypertrophy, enlarged heart and liver, or congenital heart anomalies may be accompaniments. Fetal polyuria and hydramnios may also be present. These infants are at great risk for death in the first 24 hours of life.[1,21]

Figure 36-18.
Single- and double-ovum twin differences. *(A and B)* Double-ovum twins. There are two chorions. *(B)* The two placentas have fused. *(C)* Single-ovum twins. There is only one chorion and one placenta.

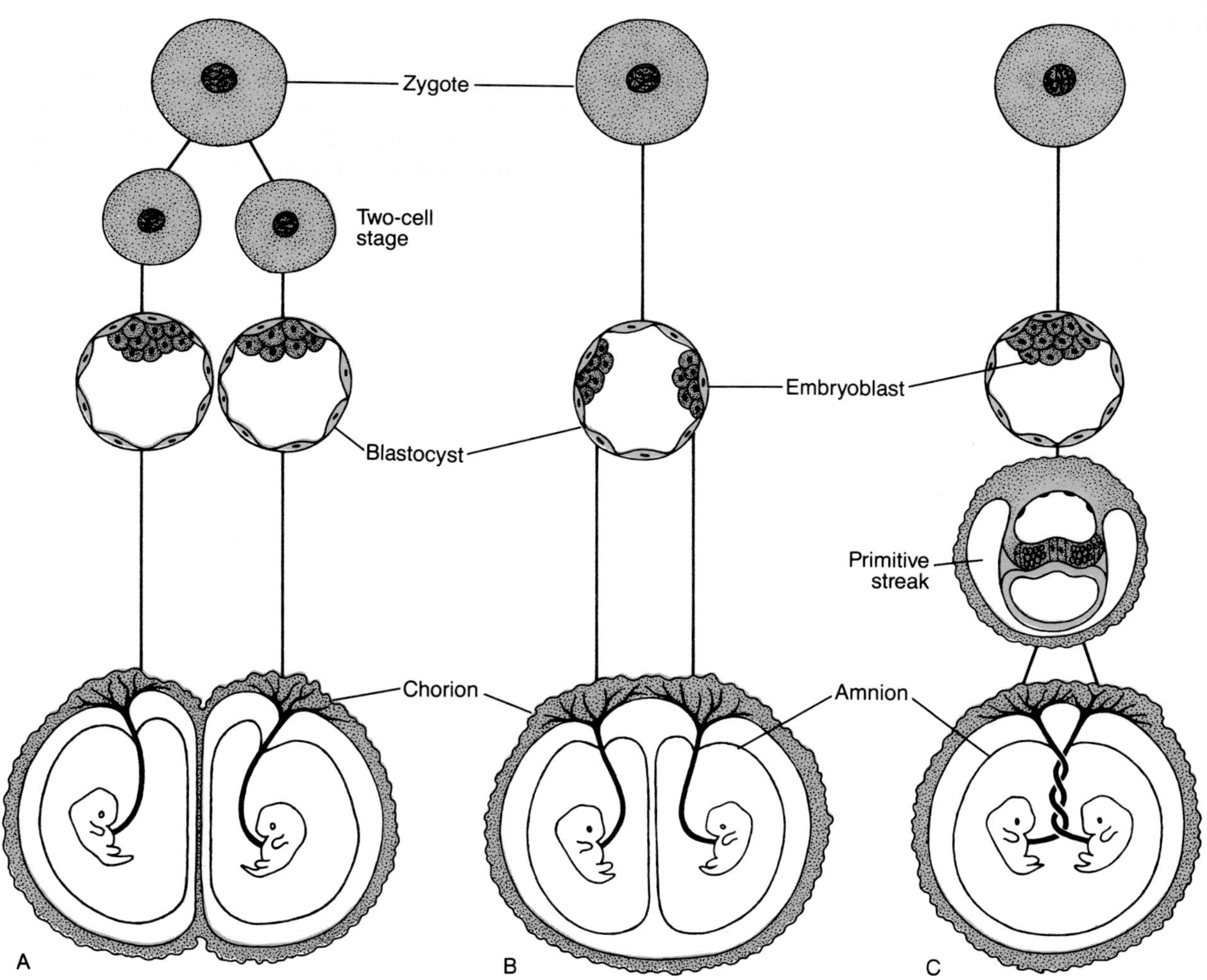

Management of Multiple Pregnancy

Because of the antepartal and perinatal risk, the mother needs to be monitored carefully during the antepartum period. She is asked to see the obstetrician more frequently, at least every 2 weeks in the second trimester and at least weekly in the third trimester if there are no complications. Diet is regulated to allow for adequate weight gain. An increase of 300 Kcal or more per day in energy sources in the diet is not too much. Protein intake is supervised, and iron, folic acid, and vitamin supplements are increased. Rest periods on the side may be prescribed although the efficacy of complete bed rest even in the last trimester for higher socioeconomic status patients seems equivocal.[1] Pritchard and associates, however, have found that patients who are socioeconomically deprived seem to benefit from hospitalization with some ambulation privileges during the last trimester. In their opinion there are better outcomes in the incidence of premature labor and preeclapsia and a generally lowered perinatal mortality.[1]

The latter weeks of a twin pregnancy are likely to be associated with heaviness of the lower abdomen, back pains, and swelling of the feet and the ankles. Abdominal distention makes sleeping difficult, and therefore the physician may prescribe a hypnotic. A well-fitting maternity girdle makes daytime more comfortable. Because of the excessive abdominal size, the patient may find that frequent small feedings are more suitable than the usual three larger meals a day. The nurse can be very helpful in giving the mother anticipatory guidance regarding these matters during the antepartal period.

Travel is curtailed because labor may begin at any time without warning, and delivery in strange surroundings may be hazardous.

A spontaneous delivery is particularly desired in instances of twins, since this type of delivery results in less blood loss and maternal morbidity and a greater likelihood of healthy, undamaged infants.

Delivery

The patient is requested to come to the hospital at the first sign of labor. If she is found to be in labor, she is kept in the labor and delivery area. If labor cannot be confirmed, she may be kept in the emergency admitting room until a definitive diagnosis is made.

When labor has been established, several steps are taken to insure a successful outcome for the dyad. First, the mother is attended at all times by a qualified perinatal team member. Here the nurse can be invaluable. Fetal heart rates must be monitored continuously and maternal vital signs recorded. A combination of external and internal fetal monitoring after the membranes have ruptured proves satisfactory. A liter of crossmatched blood or its equivalent is to be available and in the area. In addition, an intravenous infusion system capable of delivering the blood is to be instituted. Lactated Ringer's solution alternated with a 5% dextrose solution at 60 ml per hour to 120 ml per hour has been found to be satisfactory in the absence of hemorrhage or metabolic disturbance during labor.[1]

It is recommended that two obstetricians be available and scrubbed for the delivery and an anesthesiologist be in attendance, especially for the contingency of a cesarean section. Moreover, *two* individuals who are skilled in resuscitation are needed for *each* fetus at the time of delivery.

A local or pudendal block is preferred to minimize the effect of anesthetic on the infants. However, a combination of thiopental, nitrous oxide plux oxygen, and succinylcholine given in timed, appropriate doses has been found to be effective when cesarean section is indicated. The general anesthetic, halothane, may be used when operative intervention is needed.[1]

The first twin is delivered either by vertex or assisted breech delivery. If the first infant is transverse, an external version is used to bring about a deliverable presentation.

If the twins are monozygotic, the first infant's cord must be clamped to prevent the second twin from bleeding through it. The cords should be labeled. The position of the second twin is ascertained and it is brought into position by a combination of vaginal and abdominal manipulation. If there is a second sac, it is carefully ruptured to allow a slow loss of fluid and to guard against cord prolapse. A spontaneous or a prophylactic forceps vertex delivery is preferred. If the breech presents, then the physician may have to assist in the extraction. If descent does not come about, then a version and extraction may be required. These require astute management on the part of both the obstetrician and the anesthesiologist.[1]

After delivery of the second twin, 1 ml oxytocin is given intravenously. The uterus is not massaged until after the placenta(s) separate, then massage is continued until the uterus remains hard and contracted (15 min–30 min); 1 ml of ergonovine is given after the placenta(s) separate if the mother's condition does not contraindicate it.

As with any delivery, the nurse has the responsibility of supportive care for the patient as well as assisting the physician in whatever activities are indicated. Since these infants are apt to be small, oxygen or resuscitative measures may be necessary. The care is similar to that for the premature baby (see Chap. 42).

Any supplies or equipment that may be needed (*e.g.*, resuscitator, oxygen apparatus, *etc.*) should be procured early in the delivery and kept in readiness (but out of the patient's sight, if possible). Maternal vital signs as well as the fetal heart rate should be checked frequently.

Postpartum

When there is a twin birth, there is frequently a decided psychological and economic (albeit somewhat delayed) shock to the parents even though the twins were expected. Emotionally, one additional child may be desired and acceptable; two may impose a burden, particularly if this pregnancy was to be "the last." The parents may wonder if they can manage the care of two newborn infants simultaneously. Problems may be compounded in feeding, especially if the mother wants to nurse her infant. In addition, two of everything must be provided, instead of one, and this additional cost may put a strain on the budget. In terms of long-range planning, the present housing may be inadequate, especially if the children are of different sexes and eventually will require separate rooms. The cost entailed in additional construction or new housing is considerable. None of these problems is insurmountable, but resolution takes time and effort.

Recent data suggest that there may be special problems with identification and attachment to twins as well as with the twins' separation-individuation process. Sometimes parents just do not see their infants as separate individuals and tend to treat the children as "the same," hence the children fail to see themselves as individuals with separate identities.[22,23] Sater suggests that maternal behaviors which will affect the separation-individuation process fall into two categories—childrearing practices and attitudinal communication. In childrearing practices, if the mother behaves in ways that definitely and clearly show that she regards each infant as separate, she is making appropriate progress. She may, for instance, dress each child differently, have nonrhyming names and address each separately, not in the "you" plural. If, in her attitudinal communications, she conveys that she does expect differences, she can be thought of as giving appropriate communication.[23] The student is referred to the Suggested Reading for further exploration of this topic.

Some parents need an understanding and emphatic person to help them over the initial adjustment period. In some cases they may need the help of a social worker or a public health nurse to plan for the unexpected new baby. Many parents seem to adjust nicely through being able to ventilate their concerns. If the twins are undiagnosed, that is, not discovered until labor, then these problems are compounded.

The parents also benefit from any assistance or advice that helps them simplify their household schedule. The mother needs to have adequate rest and additional help, if it can be afforded. Household chores and responsibilities need to be as simple and flexible as possible. If at all possible, the father should be an active participant in the home and child care responsibilities.

If the babies must remain in the hospital, there may be problems in bonding and sibling rivalry. The parents may need help in working out a schedule of visiting the infants that allows the mother to recover her strength and yet provides some communication with the infants. Anticipatory guidance of the other children can be helpful in preventing intense sibling rivalry. All of these contingencies require astute discharge planning on the part of the physician and the nursing staff.

References

1. Pritchard JA, McDonald PC: Williams Obstetrics, 16th ed, Chapter 26. New York, Appleton–Century–Crofts, 1980
2. Friedman EA: Labor, Evaluation and Management. New York, Appleton–Century–Crofts, 1978
3. Niswander KR: Obstetric and Gynecologic Disorders. Flushing, Medical Examination, 1975
4. Niswander KR: Obstetrics, 2nd ed, Chapter 11. Boston, Little, Brown 1981
5. Hendricks, CH et al: The normal cervical dilatation patterns in late pregnancy and labor. Am J Obstet Gynecol 106:1065, 1970
6. Steer CM: Effect of type of delivery on future childbearing. Am J Obstet Gynecol 60:395, 1950 170–175
7. Larks SD: Electrohysterography. Springfield, Il, Charles C Thomas, 1960
8. Caldeyro-Barcia R et al: A better understanding of uterine contractility through simultaneous recording with an internal and seven channel external method. Surg Obstet Gynecol 91:641, 1950
9. Douglas RG, Stromme WB: Operative Obstetrics, 3rd ed. New York, Appleton–Century–Crofts, 1976
10. Phillips RD, Freeman M: The management of the persistent occiput posterior position. Am J Obstet Gynecol 43:171, February 1974
11. Rovinsky JJ et al: Management of breech presentation at term. Am J Obstet Gynecol 115:497–513, February 15, 1973
12. Benson WL et al: Management delivery in the primigravida. Am J Obstet Gynecol 40:417–428, 1972
13. Brenner WE: Breech presentation. In Makowski EL (ed): Clinical Obstetrics and Gynecology. New York, Harper & Row, 21:2 June 1978, 511:31

14. Brenner WE et al: The characteristics and perils of breech presentation. Am J Obstet Gynecol 118:700, 1974

15. Hammond H: Death from obstetric hemorrhage. Calif Med 117:16–20, August 1972

16. Royce JA: Shock, emergency nursing implications. Nurs Clin North Am 8:377, 1973

17. Malvern J et al: Ultrasonic scanning of the puerperal uterus following secondary postpartum hemorrhage. J Obstet Gynecol Br Comm 80:320–324, April 1973

18. Klein T, O'Leary JH: Rupture of the gravid uterus. J Reprod Med, 6:43–47, May 1971

19. Robello Y: Placenta previa, placenta abruptio. Paper read at the National Symposium of Perinatal Nursing, San Francisco, June 7–10, 1978

20. Benirschke K, Chung KK: Multiple pregnancy, Part 1. N Eng J Med 288:1276–1284, June 14, 1973

21. Newman HH: The Physiology of Twinning. Chicago, Chicago Press, 1923

22. Gromada K: Maternal–infants attachment: The first step toward individualizing twins. MCN 6:129–134, March/April 1981

23. Sater J: Appraising and promoting a sense of self in twins. MCN 4:218–220, July/August, 1979

Suggested Reading

Bowes WA Jr: Breech delivery: Evaluation of the method of delivery on perinatal results and maternal morbidity. Am J Obstet Gynecol 965–973, December 1, 1979

Dickerson PS: Early postpartum separation and maternal attachment to twins. JOGN Nurs 10:120–123, March/April 1981

Foley KL: Caring for parents of newborn twins. MCN 4:221–226, July/August 1979

Gromada K: Maternal–infants attachment: The first step toward individualizing twins. MCN 6:129–134, March/April 1981

Hart G: Maternal attitudes in prepared and unprepared cesarean deliveries. JOGN Nurs 9:243–245, July/August 1980

Komaromy B, Lampe L: The value of bedrest in twin pregnancies. Int J Gynecol Obstet 15:262–266, 1977

CHAPTER

37

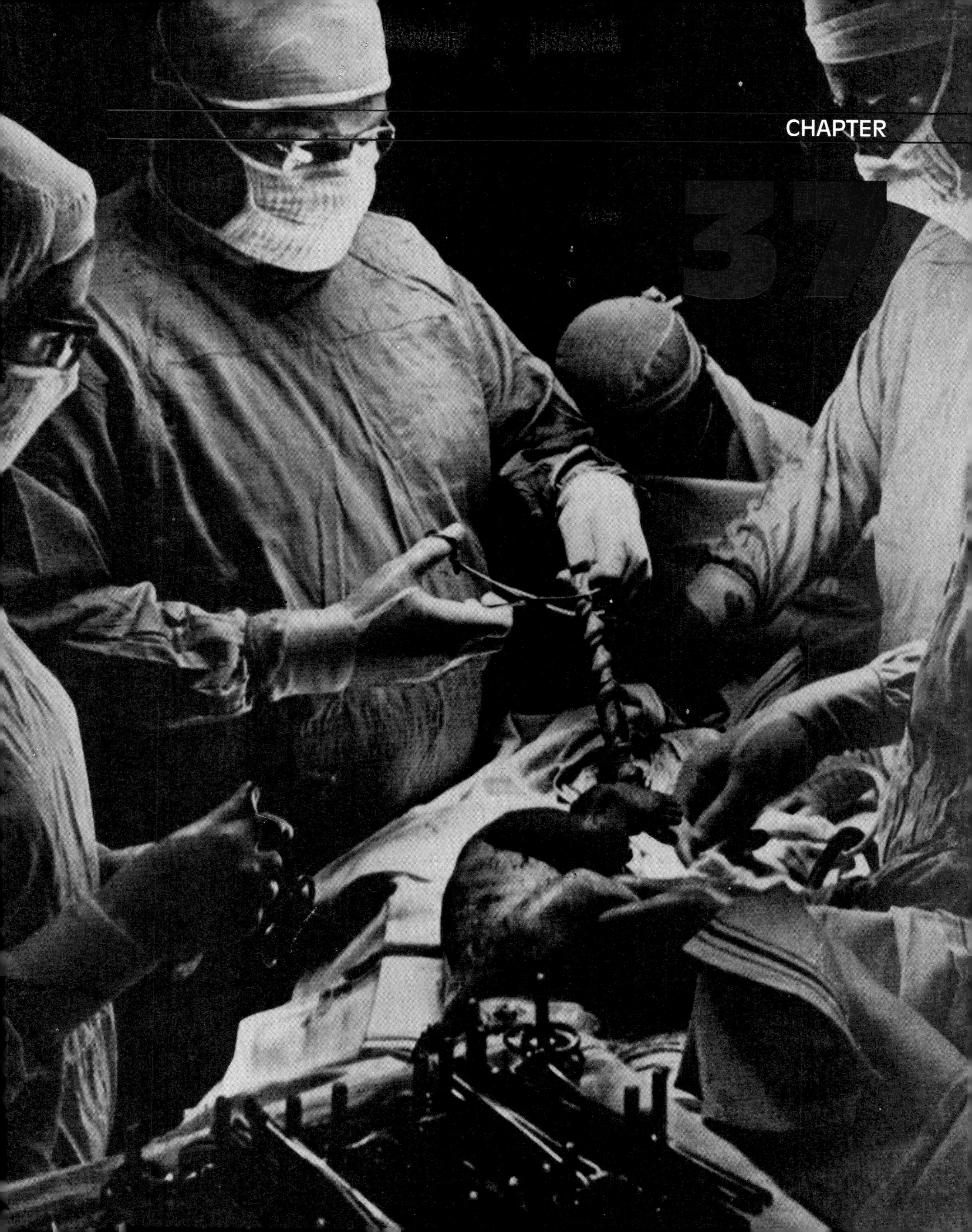

CHAPTER 37

Operative Obstetrics

A number of special procedures that the physician may use to assist the mother in labor and delivery come under the heading of operative obstetrics. These include repair of lacerations, the application of forceps or vacuum extractor, destructive operations on the fetus, version, cesarean birth, and induction of labor.

Repair of Lacerations

Except for clamping and cutting the umbilical cord, episiotomy is the most common operative procedure performed in obstetrics. In view of the fact that this incision of the perineum, made to facilitate delivery, is employed almost routinely in primigravidae, the procedure has been discussed in the section on the conduct of normal labor (see Chap. 24).

Lacerations of the perineum and the vagina that occur in the process of delivery have also been discussed previously, because some tears are unavoidable, even in the most skilled hands. The suturing of spontaneous perineal lacerations is similar to that employed for the repair of an episiotomy incision, but may be more difficult because such tears often are irregular in shape with ragged, bruised edges.

Forceps

Some of the common types of obstetrical forceps are illustrated in Figure 37-1. The instrument consists of two steel parts that cross each other like a pair of scissors and lock at the intersection. The lock may be of a sliding type, as in the first three types shown, or a screw type, as in the Tarnier instrument.

Each part consists of a handle, a lock, a shank, and a blade; the blade is the curved portion designed for application to the sides of the fetal head. The blades of most forceps (the Tucker–McLean is an exception) have a large opening or window (fenestrum) to give a better grip on the head, and usually consist of two curves—a cephalic curve, which conforms to the shape of the head, and a pelvic curve, to follow the curve of the birth canal. Axis-traction forceps, such as the Tarnier, have a mechanism attached below that permits the pulling to be done more directly in the axis of the birth canal. An axis-traction handle is also available for use on standard forceps.

The two blades of the forceps are designated as right and left. The left blade is the one which is introduced into the vagina on the patient's left side; the right blade goes in on the right side. If the nurse anticipates assisting the obstetrician, it is helpful to articulate and disarticulate the forceps to be able to know which blade is which.

Reasons for Forceps Delivery

It may become necessary to deliver the baby by forceps for the mother's welfare (maternal indications), or because of conditions associated with the baby's condition (fetal indications). Maternal indications include inability of the mother to push after full dilatation of the cervix because of conduction anesthesia, exhaustion, heart disease, or any condition affecting the mother that is likely to be improved by delivery.

The chief fetal indications for forceps delivery are fetal distress, as suggested by a slow, irregular fetal heart and, in general, conditions which would potentially cause fetal distress, such as placental abruption or prolapsed umbilical cord.

Many obstetricians, however, deem it desirable to deliver almost all primigravidae with forceps electively, in the belief that the operation spares the mother many minutes of bearing-down efforts and relieves pressure on the baby's head. This is usually referred to as "elective forceps."

Forceps delivery is never attempted unless the cervix is completely dilated and the vertex is engaged (*i.e.,* the greatest biparietal diameter of the fetal head is at, or has already traversed, the pelvic inlet). Usually, but not always, when engagement has occurred, the vertex is at or below the ischial spines.

Types of Forceps Deliveries

In the vast majority of instances today, the forceps delivery is carried out at a time when the fetal head is on the perineal floor (visible or almost so) and internal rotation may have already occurred, so that the fetal head lies in a direct anteroposterior position. This is called *low forceps,* or "outlet forceps." When the head is higher in the pelvis but engaged and its greatest diameter has passed the inlet, the operation is called *midforceps.* If the head has not yet engaged, the procedure is known as *high forceps.* High-forceps delivery is an exceedingly difficult and dangerous operation for both mother and baby and is rarely done. Increasingly, cesarean birth is preferred to a potentially difficult midforceps delivery.

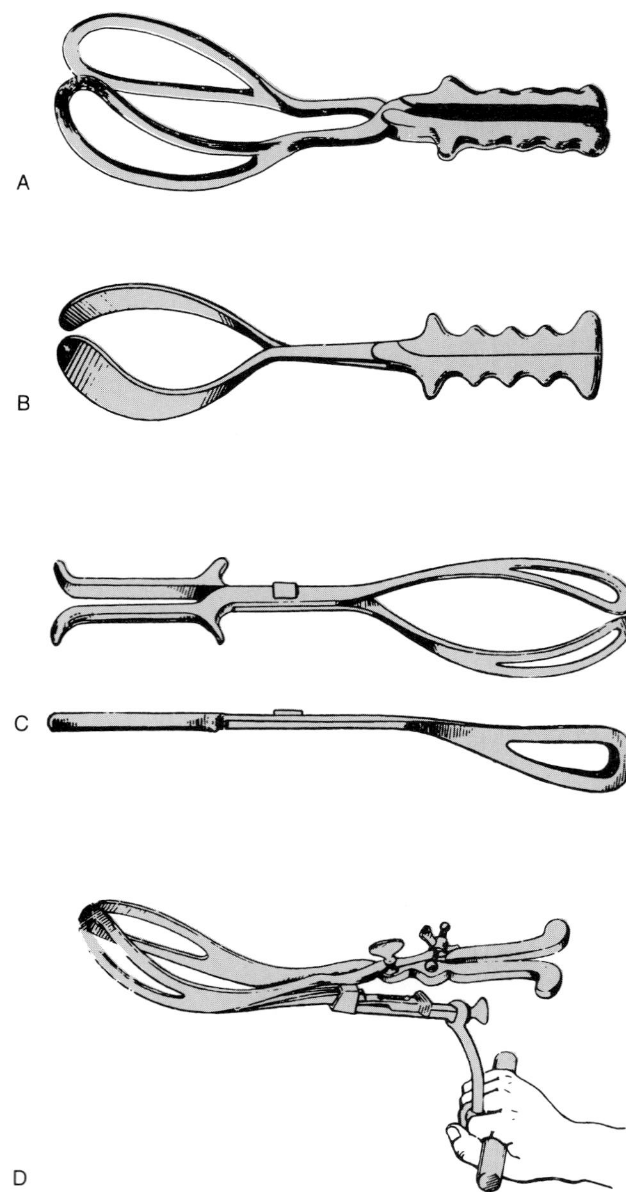

Figure 37-1.
Types of forceps. *(A)* Simpson forceps; *(B)* Tucker-McLean forceps; *(C, top)* Kielland forceps, front view; *(C, bottom)* side view; *(D)* Tarnier axis-traction forceps.

After a decision is made to use forceps, the obstetrician selects the type of instrument to be used. Several pairs of the generally approved forceps, each encased in suitable wrappings, are autoclaved and kept in the delivery room for immediate use. The other instruments needed for a forceps delivery are the same as those required for a spontaneous delivery.

Procedure

Anesthesia is recommended, but in low-forceps deliveries it may be light, and in most institutions this type of operation is performed successfully under pudendal block anesthesia. The patient is placed in the lithotomy position and prepared and draped in the usual fashion. For a midforceps delivery the bladder should be emptied by catheterization.

After checking the exact position of the fetal head by vaginal examination, the physician introduces two or more fingers of one hand into the left side of the vagina; these fingers guide the left blade into place and at the same time protect the maternal soft parts (vagina and cervix) from injury. The other hand is used to introduce the left blade of the forceps into the left side of the vagina, gently insinuating it between the baby's head and the fingers of the hand (Fig. 37-2). The same procedure is carried out on the right side, and then the blades are articulated. Traction is not continuous but intermittent (Fig. 37-3), and between traction, the blades are partially disarticulated in order to release pressure on the fetal head. Episiotomy is routine nowadays in these cases.

Piper Forceps for Breech Delivery

The Piper forceps have been designed to assist in the delivery of the after-coming head in breech presentations (Fig. 37-4). They are applied after the shoulders have been delivered and the head has been brought into the pelvis by gentle traction combined with suprapubic pressure. Suspension of the body and arms with a towel facilitates application of the blades. The left blade is introduced in an upward direction along the fetal head on the left side, and the right blade is then applied in a similar fashion. The forceps are locked in place, and their position on the head is confirmed by palpation. An episiotomy is made and, as traction is applied, the chin, mouth, and nose emerge over the perineum. The Piper forceps are often used electively as a substitute for the Mauriceau–Smellie–Veit maneuver, or when the Mauriceau–Smellie–Veit maneuver for delivery of the fetal head has failed (see Chap. 36).

■■■

Vacuum Extraction

Occasionally, an instrument known as the vacuum extractor is used in place of the forceps. The vacuum extractor consists of a metal cup that is applied to the fetal head and tightly affixed there by creating a vac-

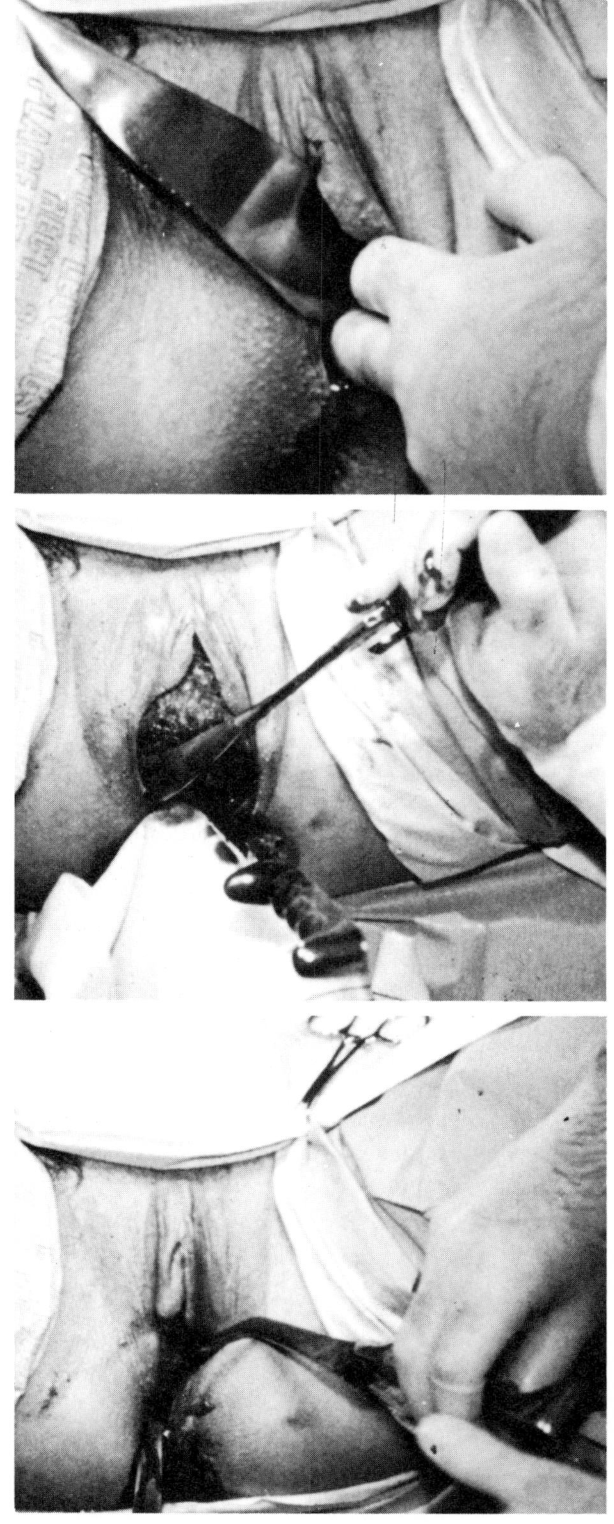

Figure 37-2.
Insertion of the two blades of the forceps. (From the film, Human Birth, published by JB Lippincott, Philadelphia)

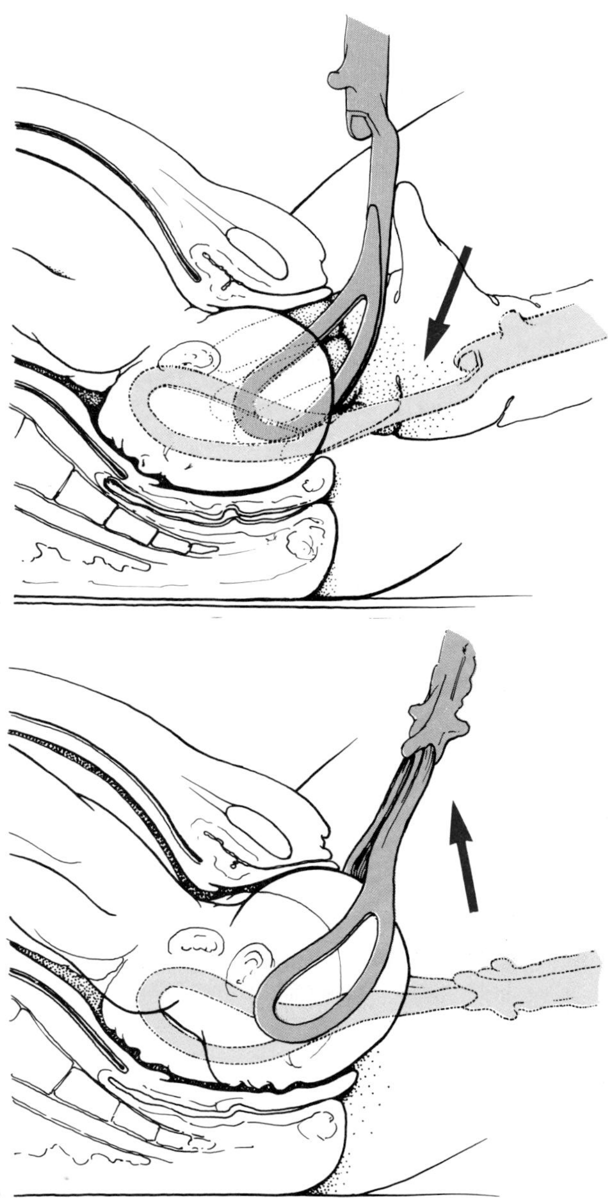

Figure 37-3.
(A) Insertion of forceps blade and *(B)* applied forceps and direction of traction.

uum in the cup through withdrawal of the air by a pump (Fig. 37-5). Cups are supplied in various sizes. The largest cup that can be applied with ease is selected for use. Vacuum is built up slowly, and the suction creates an artificial caput within the cup, providing a firm attachment to the fetal scalp. Traction can then be exerted by means of a short chain attached to the cup, with a handle at its far end.

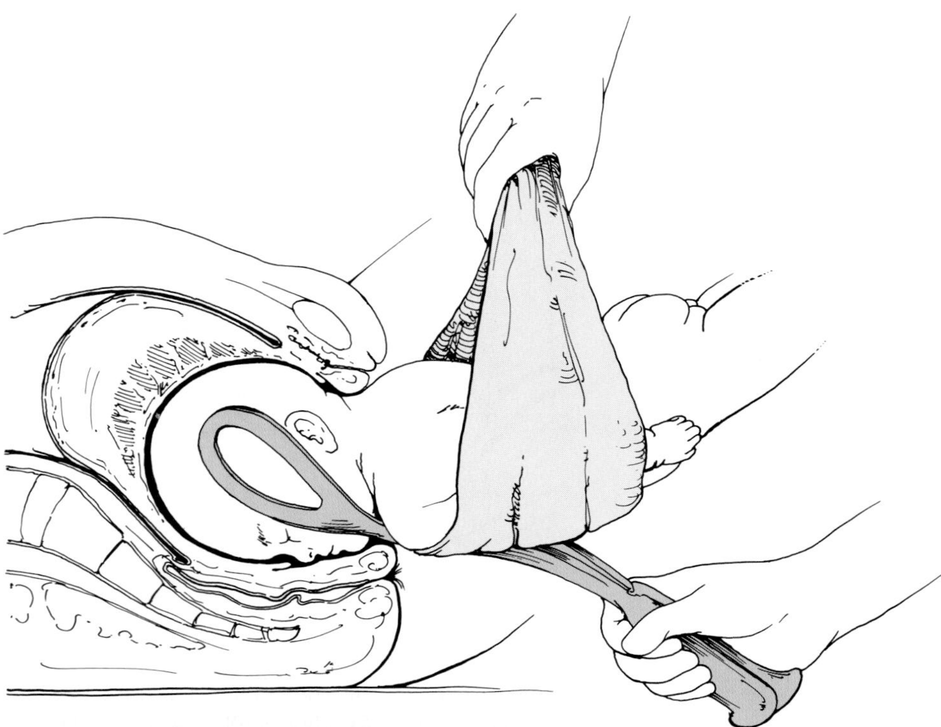

Figure 37-4.
Use of Piper forceps in breech delivery.

Version

Version consists of turning the baby in the uterus from an undesirable position to a desirable position. There are two types of version—external and internal.

External Version

This is an operation designed to change a breech presentation into a vertex presentation by external manipulation of the fetus through the abdominal and the uterine walls. It is attempted in the hope of averting the difficulties of a subsequent breech delivery. Obstetricians find the procedure most successful when done about a month before full term; it often fails, however, either because it proves to be impossible to turn the fetus around, or because the fetus returns to its original position within a few hours. Some obstetricians disapprove of it altogether.

Internal Version

Internal version is sometimes called internal podalic version, which is a maneuver designed to change whatever presentation may exist by converting it into a breech presentation (see Fig. 37-6).

When cervical dilatation is complete, the whole hand of the operator is introduced high into the uterus, one or both feet are grasped and pulled downward in the direction of the birth canal. With the external hand, the obstetrician may expedite the turning by pushing the head upward. The version is followed by breech extraction.

Internal version is most useful in cases of multiple pregnancy in which the birth of the second twin is delayed or when the second twin is in a transverse lie. It is now almost never used in other circumstances.

Cesarean Section

Cesarean section is the removal of the fetus from the uterus through an incision made in the abdominal wall and the uterus.

The main indications for cesarean section fall into the following five groups:

1. Disproportion between the size of the fetus and that of the bony birth canal—that is, contracted pelvis, tumor blocking birth canal and so on
2. In certain cases in which the patient has had a previous cesarean section, myomectomy, or uter-

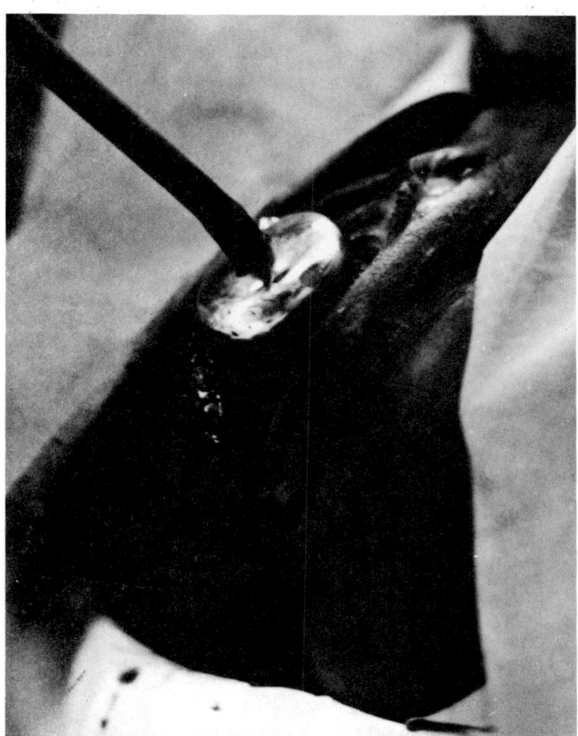

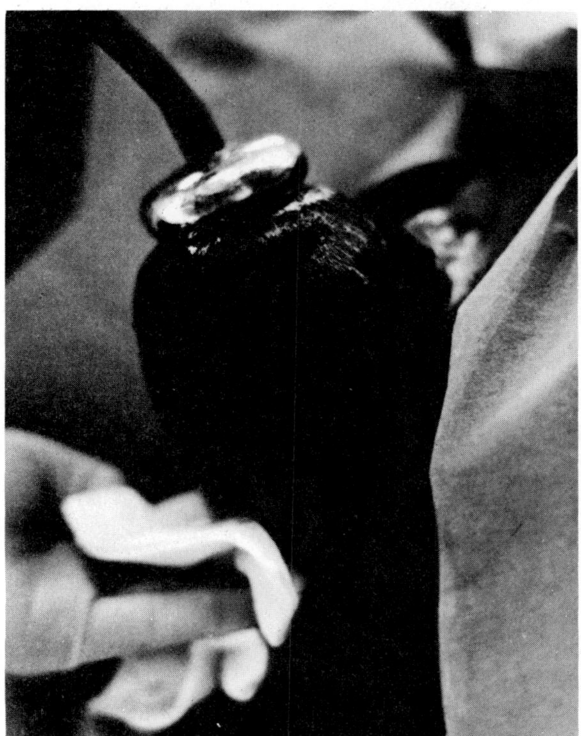

Figure 37-5.
Application of the vacuum extractor and delivery of the fetal head.

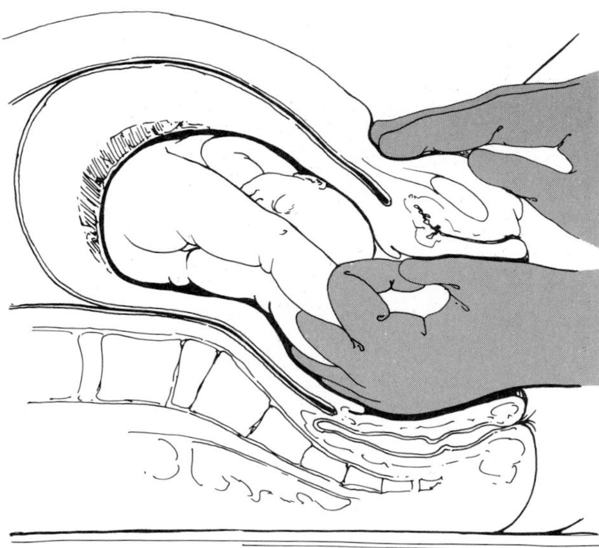

Figure 37-6.
Internal podalic version.

ine reconstruction, the operation is done because of the fear that the uterus will rupture in labor
3. Certain cases of severe preeclampsia or eclampsia
4. Certain cases of placenta previa and premature separation of the normally implanted placenta
5. Actual or pending fetal distress
6. Malpresentation (breech or transverse)

When a cesarean section is done prior to the onset of labor, as the result of a prearranged plan, it is called *elective* cesarean section (as with elective low forceps, the obstetrician is not forced to perform the operation immediately, but elects to do it as the best procedure for mother and baby).

Prematurity is the most common fetal complication of elective cesarean section, occurring because the duration of gestation is misjudged. This can now be avoided by evaluating fetal maturity preoperatively through determination of amniotic fluid L/S (lecithin-sphingomyelin) ratio (see Chap. 39).

The incidence of cesarean section has increased dramatically in the past several years. In the state of California, for example, the cesarean section rate increased from 4.8% in 1960, to 12.7% in 1975. In some larger referral centers, where the incidence of complicated obstetrical cases is high, the section rate is now as high as 22%. This substantial increase has engendered a great deal of controversy, and the necessity for the large numbers of operative deliveries has come under public scrutiny. By and large, the increase in the incidence of cesarean section is attributable to fetal indications. Fetal monitoring has permitted earlier diagnosis of fetal distress, and mod-

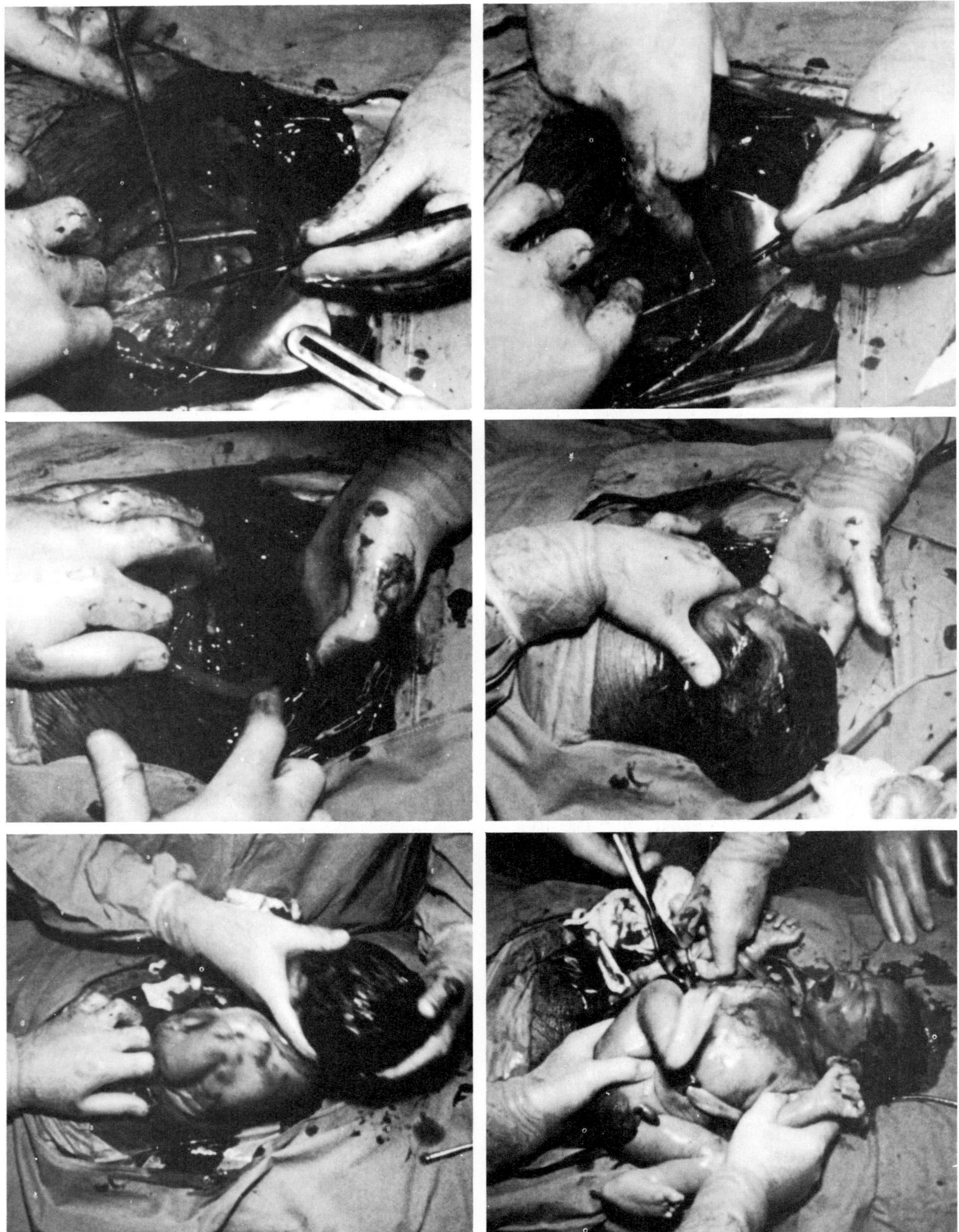

Figure 37-7.
Cesarean section. (From the film, Human Birth, published by JB Lippincott, Philadelphia)

ern methods for assessment of fetal well-being during the course of pregnancy also provide a basis for early delivery. In the latter circumstances, cesarean section is a justifiable substitute for prolonged and difficult medical induction. Cesarean section is a less traumatic substitute for some previously preferred operative procedures, such as difficult midforceps and vaginal breech delivery in the primagravida or patient in preterm labor to avoid trauma to the aftercoming head. Those who support this trend point to a markedly reduced perinatal mortality or morbidity. This does not mean, however, that the decision to carry out a cesarean section can be taken lightly. Maternal morbidity is still more frequent and more severe than with vaginal delivery. For this reason, cesarean section should not be performed unless there is obstetrically sound justification.

Main Types of Cesarean Section

Although there are four types of cesarean section, the lower segment section is usually the operation of choice. In this operation, the uterus is entered through an incision in the lower segment. Other types of cesarean section include the classical cesarean section, in which the incision is made directly into the wall of the body of the uterus; the extraperitoneal cesarean section, in which the operation is arranged anatomically, such that the incision is made into the uterus without entering the peritoneal cavity; and cesarean section–hysterectomy, which involves a cesarean section of any variety followed by removal of the uterus.

The Low-Segment Cesarean Section

This procedure is usually the operation of choice for a number of important reasons. Since the incision is made in the lower segment of the uterus, which is its thinnest portion, there is minimal blood loss, and the incision is easy to repair. The lower segment is also the area of least uterine activity, and thus the possibility of rupture of the scar in a subsequent pregnancy is lessened. Since the incision can be properly peritonealized, the operation is associated with a lower incidence of postoperative infection.

The initial incision (the abdominal cavity having been opened) is made transversely across the uterine peritoneum, where it is attached loosely just above the bladder. The lower peritoneal flap and the bladder are now dissected from the uterus, and the uterine muscle is incised either vertically or transversely. The membranes are ruptured, and the baby is delivered (Fig. 37-7). After the placenta has been extracted (Fig. 37-8) and the uterine incision sutured, the lower flap is imbricated over the uterine incision. This two-flap arrangement seals off the uterine incision and is believed to prevent the egress of infectious lochia into the peritoneal cavity.

Classic Cesarean Section

A vertical incision is made directly into the wall of the body of the uterus; the baby and the placenta are extracted, and the incision is closed by three layers of absorbable sutures. Thus, this approach requires traversing the full thickness of the uterine corpus. It is still recommended in certain circumstances. It is particularly useful when the bladder and lower segment

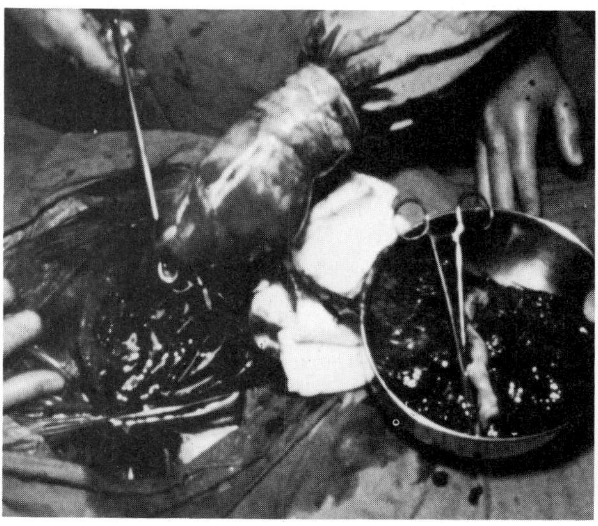

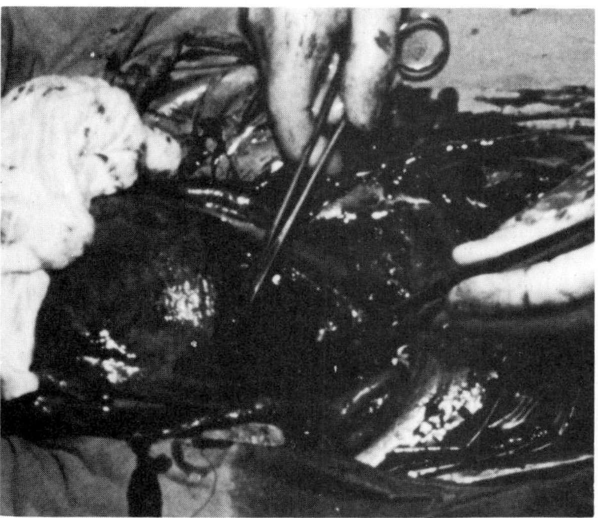

Figure 37-8.
Extracting the placenta in cesarean section. (From the film, Human Birth, published by JB Lippincott, Philadelphia)

are involved in extension adhesions resulting from a previous cesarean section, and occasionally is selected when the fetus is in a transverse lie or when there is an anterior placenta previa.

Extraperitoneal Cesarean Section

By appropriate dissection of the tissues around the bladder, access to the lower uterine segment is secured without entering the peritoneal cavity. The baby is delivered through an incision in the lower uterine segment. Since the entire operation is done outside the peritoneal cavity, neither spill of infected amniotic fluid nor subsequent seepage of pus from the uterus can reach the peritoneal surfaces. This approach was used extensively in the preantibiotic era, but is rarely employed today.

Cesarean Section—Hysterectomy

Cesarean section–hysterectomy is also known as Porro's operation. This operation comprises cesarean section followed by removal of the uterus. It may be necessary in certain cases of *premature separation of the placenta,* in patients with multiple *fibroid tumors of the uterus,* and in some circumstances is done electively for sterilization purposes.

Preparation

Preparations for cesarean sections are similar to those for any other abdominal operation, except that in these cases it includes preparations for the care of the infant. An elective cesarean section allows ample time for a physical examination, routine laboratory studies, typing and crossmatching blood, and other customary procedures. However, if there is an emergency, or if labor has started, then such preparations must be made with expediency. In any event, the usual hospital procedure should be followed.

Nursing Management

Preoperative Preparation

When the patient is admitted for an elective cesarean section, nursing care that is routine for any waiting mother (*e.g.,* checking fetal heart tones and being alert to prodromal signs of labor) is employed. A short time before the operation the abdomen is shaved, beginning at the level of the xiphoid cartilage and extending out to the far sides and down to the pubic area. A retention catheter is inserted to ensure that the bladder remains empty during the operation and attached to a constant drainage system. One should make certain that the catheter is draining properly before the procedure.

Atropine is usually the preoperative medication ordered. The use of narcotic drugs prior to delivery is avoided because of their depressant effect on the infant, but these medications should be readily available. Oxytocic drugs (*e.g.,* oxytocin and ergonovine) should be ready in the operating room so that they can be administered promptly on the verbal order of the obstetrician when the infant is born.

Preparation for Infant

In addition to the preparation of the operating room for the surgical procedure, preparation for the care of the infant must be accomplished. There must be a warm crib and equipment for the resuscitation of the infant. An infant resuscitator, equipped with heat, suction, oxygen (open mask and positive pressure), and an adjustable frame to permit the proper positioning of the infant is most useful. A competent person should be present at cesarean section to give the infant initial care and to resuscitate if necessary. This person may be an experienced nurse, but in many hospitals today it is customary to have a pediatrician at hand to take over the care of the infant as soon as it is born and thus free the obstetrician to devote full attention to the mother.

Postoperative Management

Usually postoperative care is the same as that following any abdominal surgery. It is important to remember that the patient who has had a cesarean section has had both an abdominal operation and a delivery.

Assessing for Hemorrhage

As with any delivery, the patient must be watched for hemorrhage by frequently inspecting the perineal pad and checking the fundus. If the abdominal dressings are bulky, it may be difficult to palpate the fundus to see if the uterus is well contracted, but if the dressings are not massive and do not extend above the level of the umbilicus, the nurse may feel the consistency of the fundus. Oxytocics may be ordered to keep the uterus contracted and to control bleeding. The vital signs should be checked regularly until they have stabilized, and if there is any indication of shock or hemorrhage, it should be reported promptly. Although there may be no visible signs of external hemorrhage, one would suspect internal hemorrhage if the pulse rate becomes accelerated, the respiration increases in rate, or the blood pressure falls, bearing in mind, of course, that the drop in blood pressure could be due to the effects of some types of anesthetic drugs.

Input and Output

If the retention catheter is to remain in place until the following morning, it should remain attached to "constant drainage" and should be watched to see that it drains freely. Intravenous fluids are usually administered during the first 24 hours, although small amounts of fluids may be given by mouth after nausea has subsided. A record of the mother's intake and elimination is kept for the first several days or until the need is no longer indicated.

Comfort and Respiratory Function

Analgesic drugs should be used to keep the mother comfortable and encourage her to rest. Her position in bed during the early postoperative hours may be dictated by the type of anesthesia that she received. She should be encouraged to turn from side to side every hour. Deep breathing and coughing should also be encouraged to promote good ventilation. Today most mothers who deliver by cesarean section are allowed early ambulation. It is felt that this contributes considerably to maintaining good bladder and intestinal function.

Psychosocial Considerations

Nursing management of the patient must also include additional emotional support. The parturient finds herself in a situation when at a very special time in her life she must face the additional burden of an abdominal operative procedure. The anxiety level can be reduced considerably if she is prepared for the procedures which will be carried out in interest of her physical well-being. The role of the nurse is critical in this regard and is discussed in detail in Chapter 44. When the cesarean section can be carried out under epidural anesthesia (Chap. 27), the adjustment is much easier, and any anxiety over fetal outcome is alleviated immediately when she can be awake to hear the baby's first cry and receive immediate assurance that all has gone well. The mother also has the satisfaction of being able to see her newborn shortly after delivery. In many centers, arrangements can be made to have the father present at the delivery to provide added support (see Chap. 27). Under other circumstances, the father should be permitted to visit as soon as it is feasible. The mother will be anxious to see her infant, too, and it should be brought to her as soon as she is able to see it. The nurse should remain with the mother while she has her infant with her. Communication is the key, and the role of the nurse in keeping the patient and family informed both before and after the operative delivery is most important.

General Postpartum Care

The general care of the mother is similar to that given any postoperative or postpartal patient. Daily breast care and perineal care are carried out per routine. The mother may have the afterpains, engorgement of the breasts, and the emotional reactions which often accompany a normal delivery.

Nursing Management Following Cesarean Section

Assessing for Hemorrhage

1. Inspect perineal pads frequently.
2. Palpate fundus to see if uterus is contracted.
3. Administer oxytocin if prescribed, to contract uterus and control bleeding.
4. Check vital signs regularly until stabilized. Signs of internal hemorrhage are accelerated pulse rate, increased rate of respiration, and fall in blood pressure (due in some cases to effects of anesthesia).

Monitoring Intake and Output

1. Check to see that retention catheter (if left in place) is draining freely.
2. Attend to IV therapy, which is usually given during first 24 hours postoperatively.
3. Record intake and output for several days postop or as indicated.

Assuring Adequate Respiratory Function

1. Encourage deep breathing and coughing.
2. Encourage mother to turn from side to side every hour.

Attending to Comfort Measures

1. Give analgesic medication as prescribed.
2. Position as indicated by the type of anesthesia.

Providing General Postoperative Care

1. Give daily breast care and perineal care.
2. Relieve breast engorgement and afterpains.

Destructive Operations

Destructive operations (designed for the most part to reduce the size of the baby's head and thus to expedite delivery) are rarely done in modern obstetrics. Even in large maternity hospitals many years may pass without a single destructive operation. This salutary state of affairs is attributable in part to the widespread extension of prenatal care, in part to better management of women in labor, and in part to the availability of cesarean section, which makes it safe to effect abdominal delivery even in neglected cases. In the event that a destructive operation is necessary, the obstetrician chooses the necessary instruments.

Induction of Labor

Induction of labor means the artificial initiation of labor after the period of viability. Induction of labor is indicated when continuation of pregnancy would affect maternal health or when there are conditions in the mother that would affect fetal well-being. Complications of pregnancy that may require induction include hypertensive disease of pregnancy, diabetes, hemolytic disease, and postmaturity (see Chap. 34, Complications of Pregnancy).

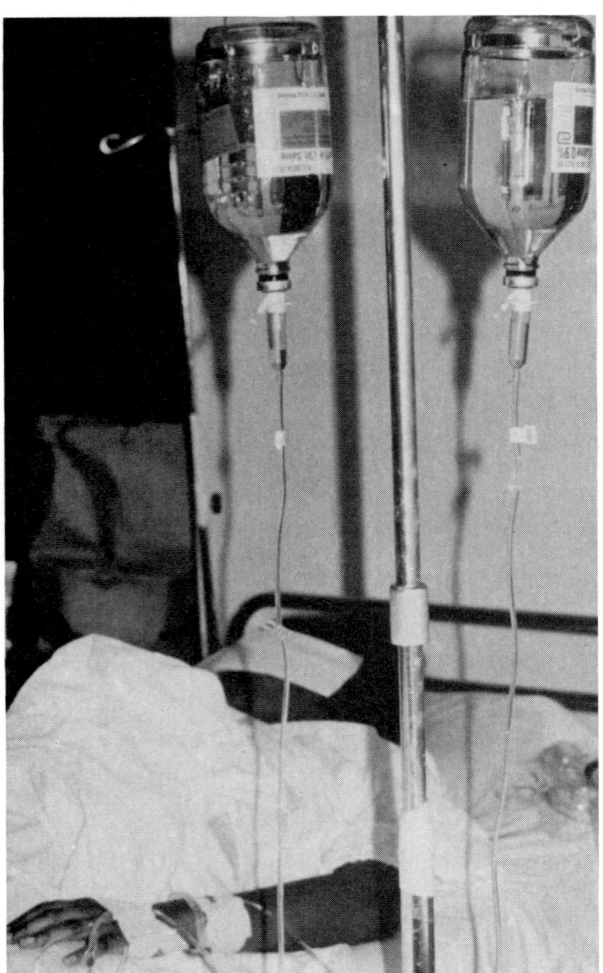

Figure 37-9.
Administration of pit drip with piggyback technique.

Since it was believed that the intestinal peristalsis produced by a cathartic is somehow transferred to the uterus, with the consequent initiation of uterine contractions, castor oil has long been employed to induce labor. It was often followed by the administration of a hot soapsuds enema. While this is a harmless approach, it is at the very least uncomfortable and it usually fails.

Oxytocin Induction

An efficient and safe method for the induction of labor is the administration of oxytocin by intravenous drip. The properties of this oxytocic agent and its use in the third stage of labor have already been discussed in Chapter 24.

Rate of Administration

Since oxytocin has dangerous potentialities when administered to a pregnant woman, the dosage used is always extremely small. Administration by intravenous drip assures a uniform, although infinitesimal, concentration of the agent in the bloodstream. The amount of oxytocin being administered can be readily controlled and is governed by the response of the uterus. Oxytocin has also been administered intramuscularly, but this approach is no longer recommended. Because the response of a given patient is not predictable, there is no way to select an appropriate intramuscular dose.

For the intravenous administration of oxytocin, the physician usually asks for a flask containing 500 ml of 5% glucose or balanced salt solution to which the indicated quantity of oxytocin is added. The intravenous equipment is set up as usual so that the number of drops flowing per minute can be closely observed in the observation tube. This is extremely important, and the physician specifies the precise number of drops per minute. Initially, the drip should be run very slowly—4 drops per minute to 5 drops per minute. The rate of administration should be increased gradually thereafter, always being governed by the response of the patient. To avoid a sudden infusion of oxytocin during placement of the intravenous, a piggyback system is usually recommended (Fig. 37-9). After an infusion of 5% D + W is running, the solution containing the pitocin is introduced for a second intravenous setup by placing the needle into the rubber adaptor of the infusion already in place. The amount of pitocin delivered can then be regulated—increased, decreased, or discontinued—without interfering with the continuity of the IV delivery system. Oxytocin administration can also be very accurately controlled with the use of a constant infusion pump.

Protocol for Oxytocin (Pitocin) Induction and Augmentation*

Physician Responsibility

1. The physician evaluates the patient and determines if patient is to be started on intravenous oxytocin.
2. The physician obtains at least a 10-minute baseline monitor strip of uterine contractions and fetal heart rate, using an external system if membranes are intact.
3. The physician writes on patient's order sheet that oxytocin is to be started at 0.2 mU/minute or at a level to be determined by the physician and may progress to 10 mU/minute by using the increments listed below. The oxytocin infusion may be increased every 15 minutes to 20 minutes.

Table 1

Oxytocin infusion starts at	0.2 mU/minute
and increases to	0.4 mU/minute
	1 mU/minute
	2 mU/minute
	4 mU/minute
	8 mU/minute
hold at	10 mU/minute

4. The physician evaluates the patient when the dosage of oxytocin reaches 10 mU/minute. If continuation is needed, the physician writes on patient's order sheet that the oxytocin infusion be increased every 15 minutes to 20 minutes until a dose of 20 mU/minute is reached. The following dose schedule should be used:

Table 2

Oxytocin infusion continues at	12 mU/minute
	16 mU/minute
hold at	20 mU/minute

5. The resident physician consults with the Chief Resident when oxytocin infusion has reached 20 mU/minute.
6. The physician must be present on the Labor and Delivery Floor while oxytocin is being infused. (At least one physician is present at all times.)
7. The physician frequently observes the patient's progress, at least hourly or more often if indicated.

Nursing Responsibilities

1. Prepare the oxytocin solution as follows:
   a. 5 U of oxytocin are added to 250 ml of normal saline, 0.9% solution. This yields a solution with a concentration of 20 mU of oxytocin/ml to be used with Harvard Pump.

   OR

   b. Add 2.5 U of pitocin to 500 ml of normal saline, 0.9% solution. This yields a solution with a concentration of 5 mU of oxytocin/ml to be used with IMED or constant infusion (2620 Harvard) Pump.
2. Take infusion pump to bedside.
3. Assemble infusion pump with oxytocin solution.
4. Set infusion pump to correspond to the oxytocin dosage which was ordered.
5. Start oxytocin infusion (secondary line) by inserting needle into the connector most proximal to the primary line. Be sure to keep primary line running at a slow rate.
6. Turn on oxytocin infusion pump at set rate.
7. Observe contraction pattern and fetal heart rate on the monitor. If no abnormalities are noted in 15 minutes to 20 minutes, increase the oxytocin infusion according to Table 1 so that the uterine contractions are observed every 2 minutes to 3 minutes and last approximately 60 seconds.
8. Once a regular contraction pattern is established, hold the oxytocin infusion at that rate or decrease the infusion rate and determine if a regular contraction pattern will still be sustained.
9. If at any time a question arises as to the possibility of hyperstimulation (less than 2 minutes between contractions or contractions lasting longer than 60 seconds) or an abnormal fetal heart rate pattern, the nurse immediately does the following:
   a. Turns off oxytocin infusion.
   b. Turns patient on left side.
   c. Starts oxygen by mask at 6 liters/minute to 8 liters/minute.
   d. Notifies physician.

(Continued)

Protocol for Oxytocin (Pitocin) Induction and Augmentation*

10. Notify the physician if the contraction pattern slows and labor is not well established.
11. Check the oxytocin infusion bottle as to the amount being absorbed and the rate of infusion, at least every ½ hour.
12. Remember that all patients receiving intravenous oxytocin must be continuously observed by a qualified member of the nursing staff who is under the direct supervision of a registered nurse.
13. Continuously assess the patient's progress both physically and emotionally as well as by the monitor tracings. Remember that the patient, and not the monitor, is being treated.
14. Notify the physician when 10 mU/minute of oxytocin is reached so that an evaluation of the patient may be made by the physician.
15. Carry out the written prescription for oxytocin infusion, if it is to be continued to 20 mU/minute, according to Table 2.
16. Take vital signs and fetal heart rate every 15 minutes and record these on the intrapartum flow sheet as well as on the monitor strip.
17. Record the characteristics of the contraction pattern every 15 minutes on the intrapartum flow sheet. These observations include palpation of the intensity of the uterine contraction and their frequency at least every ½ hour.

Note. If in doubt at any time about the response of the patient or fetus to oxytocin, turn the oxytocin infusion off and notify the physician immediately.

Chart Notations

Intrapartum Flow Sheet

1. Dosage of oxytocin, the name, and amount of the solution
2. Rate of the flow of oxytocin increased, held, or decreased
3. Contraction pattern every 15 minutes
4. Vital signs and fetal heart rate every 15 minutes
5. Vaginal exams and results done by the physician
6. Adjustment to the monitor

Nurse's Record

1. Intake
   a. Oral
   b. Intravenous
2. Output
   a. Urine
   b. Vomitus
   c. Other
3. 8-hour summary of intake and output
4. Vaginal exams and results done by the physician
5. Treatments
6. Nursing care
   a. Physical
   b. Emotional
   c. Teaching

Monitor Tracings

1. Dosage of oxytocin and time started
2. Time and the dosage of oxytocin when increased, held, or decreased
3. Vital signs every 15 minutes and the time
4. Exams and procedures by physician and the time
5. Any movement or changes to the patient or monitor that may interfere with recording of the tracing

*Hospital of the University of Pennsylvania, Department of Nursing, Department of Obstetrics and Gynecology

Precautions

The administration of oxytocin to a gravida carries certain hazards, and it is obligatory for her safety and for the baby's safety that a physician or a nurse be in constant bedside attendance to make certain that the number of drops flowing per minute does not change and to watch for the following untoward effects.

1. The observer must check the rate of flow of the oxytocin solution at frequent intervals to make certain that it remains constant.
2. The duration and the intensity of each uterine contraction must be watched closely and recorded.
3. Any contraction lasting over 90 seconds indicates that the quantity of solution is too great, and the rate of flow should either be decreased or temporarily discontinued altogether.
4. Furthermore, the fetal heart rate should be counted and recorded. In many hospitals continuous electronic fetal monitoring is used routinely when oxytocin is administered.
5. The fetal heart tones should return to their normal rate and rhythm within 15 seconds or so after the termination of a contraction. Any persistence of fetal bradycardia is an indication for discontinuation of the oxytocin drip.
6. If any abnormality in the uterine contractions or the fetal heart tones is observed, the solution should be turned off *immediately* and the findings reported to the physician. The major advantage of the oxytocin drip is that it may be discontinued immediately in the event that untoward effects should be observed—an obvious safety factor.

Some obstetrical units have found it helpful to use a protocol for oxytocin induction or augmentation of labor. See pages 829 and 830 for an example.

Artificial Rupture of the Membranes

Amniotomy, or artificial rupture of the membranes, is a common method of enhancing labor. Amniotomy has also been used to induce labor. When the patient is near term and the cervix is favorable, it is almost always followed by labor within a few hours.

The membranes serve as a barrier against bacterial invasion. For this reason, once this barrier has been eliminated by amniotomy, delivery should be accomplished expeditiously. Many obstetricians now feel that the primary use of amniotomy for labor induction is tantamount to burning one's bridges and that the procedure should be delayed until after the initiation of good contractions with intravenous oxytocin.

Amniotomy is accomplished after placing the patient in the lithotomy position and carrying out antiseptic preparation of the vulva. The first two fingers of one hand are inserted into the cervix until the membranes are encountered. A long hook, similar to one blade of a disarticulated vulsellum tenaculum, or an Allis clamp, is inserted into the vagina, and the membranes are simply hooked and torn by the tip of the sharp instrument. As much fluid as possible is allowed to drain. The quality of the fluid should be noted. Normally, it is watery and clear.

Fetal heart tones should be checked immediately after amniotomy; extra care should be exercised, as there is an increased possibility of cord prolapse.

Suggested Reading

Boyd ST, Mahon P: The Family-Centered Cesarean Delivery. MCN 5:May/June 1980

Prichard JA, Macdonald PC: Williams Obstetrics, 6th ed. New York, Appleton–Century–Crofts, 1980

Shearer E: NIH Consensus Development Task Force on Cesarean Childbirth: The process and the result. Birth and the Family Journal, 8:1, Spring 1981

Willson SR, Carrington ER: Obstetrics and Gynecology, 6th ed. St. Louis, CV Mosby, 1979

CHAPTER 38

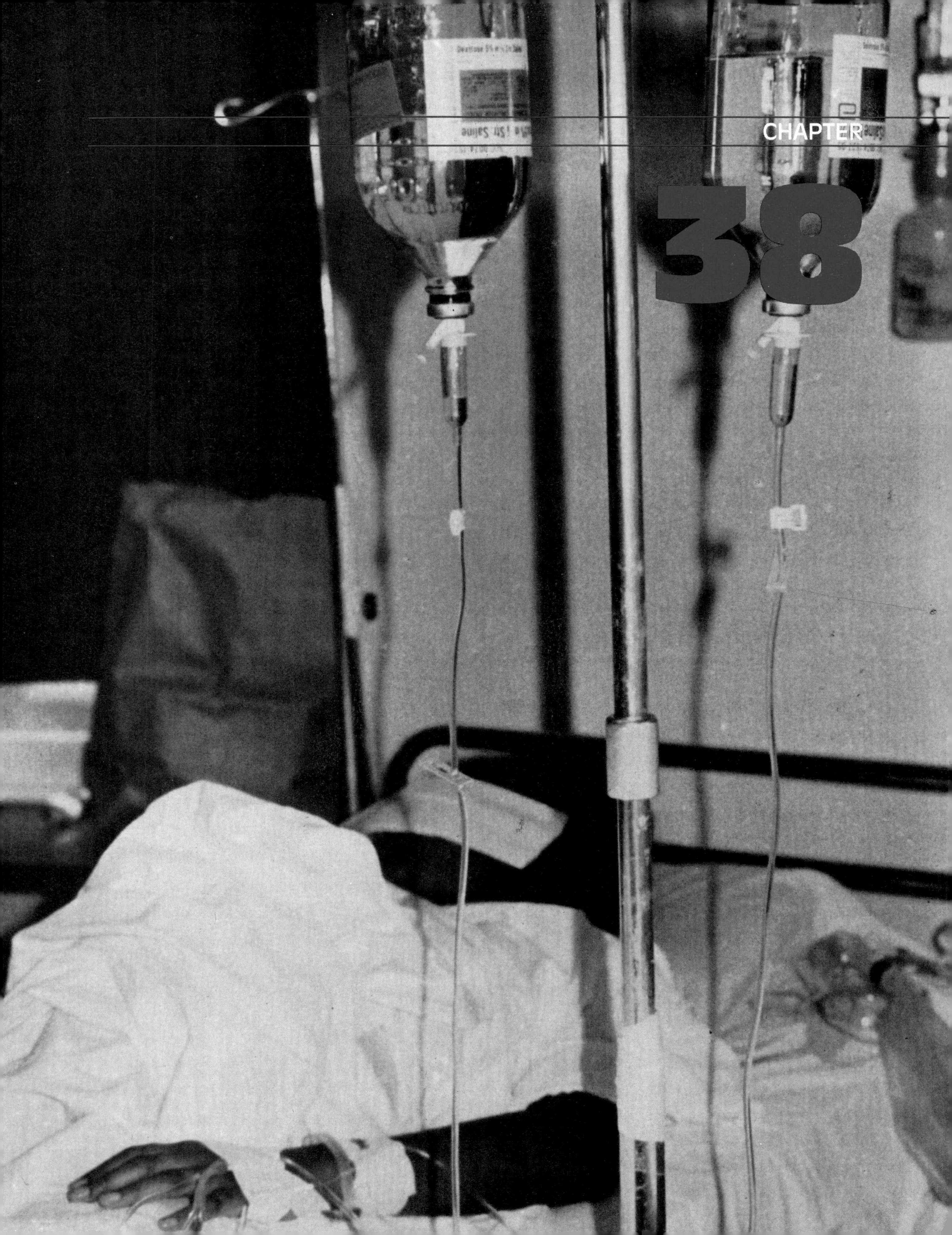

CHAPTER 38

Postpartal Complications

The postpartal period is a time of increased physiological stress, as well as a phase of major psychological transition. During this time the woman's body is more vulnerable because of the energy depletion and fatigue of late pregnancy and labor, the tissue trauma of delivery, and the blood loss and propensity for anemia which frequently occur. Most women recover from the stresses of pregnancy and childbirth without significant complications. When postpartal complications do occur, the most common are *infection* involving the genital tract, urinary system, and breasts; *hemorrhage,* immediate or delayed; *embolic clotting disorders;* and *uterine subinvolution.* The potentially critical nature of many postpartal complications, the associated pain and procedures, medications, frequent need to be isolated or removed from the maternity unit, and emotionally disruptive effects of the physiological malfunction can interfere with the maternal–infant bonding process. Nursing care must minimize physical separation of mother and infant and encourage attachment through such means as frequent discussions about the baby's behavior and characteristics, pictures of the baby, visits to the nursery observation window; or, when the complication is noninfectious, assisting and supporting the mother in holding and caring for her infant as much as her condition allows. Prompt diagnosis and treatment of postpartal complications to reduce their dysfunctional effects is also important.

Common Postpartal Complications

- Genital tract infections
  - Infection of episiotomy or lacerations
  - Endometritis
  - Parametritis (pelvic cellulitis)
  - Pelvic abscess
  - Peritonitis
  - Salpingitis
- Pelvic or femoral thrombophlebitis
- Cesarean section wound infection
- Pulmonary embolism
- Subinvolution of the uterus
- Vulvar hematomas
- Mastitis, breast abscess
- Urinary tract infection
  - Cystitis
  - Pyelonephritis

Postpartum Infections of the Genital Tract

When inflammatory processes develop in the birth canal postpartally, as a result of bacterial invasion of these highly vulnerable areas, the condition is known as puerperal infection. It is really a postpartal wound infection of the birth canal, usually of the endometrium. As is true of other wound infections, the condition often remains localized but may extend along various pathways to produce diverse clinical pictures. Febrile reactions of more or less severity are the rule, and the outcome varies according to the portal of entry, the type, the number and the virulence of the invading organisms, the reaction of the tissues and the general resistance of the patient. Puerperal infection is one of the most common causes of death in childbearing.

Febrile morbidity in the postpartum period is defined as a temperature elevation of 38°C (100.4°F) or more occurring after the first 24 hours postpartum on two or more occasions that are not within the same 24 hours.[1] Low-grade temperature elevations postpartally are not uncommon and have been attributed to such factors as dehydration, infusion of fetal protein, breast engorgement, and respiratory infection. However, the endometrial cavity is the site of significant anaerobic bacterial growth in the immediate postpartal period, and probably most women with temperature elevations in the first 24 hours do have genital tract infections. When delivery has occurred vaginally, the spontaneous clearance of necrotic decidua and blood from the uterine cavity is adequate to remove bacteria in most cases. The transient temperature elevation seen in the first 24 hours after delivery represents this process. When the delivery has been by cesarean section, there is a much higher risk of postpartum infection, with the risk of death 26 times greater than from vaginal delivery.[2] The incidence of postpartum infection has been reported as 5.9% to 7.2%.[3] Figures 38-1 and 38-2 show febrile patterns of transient temperature elevation in the first 24 hours and clinically significant postpartum infection.

Causative Factors

The most common organisms causing postpartum infections are anaerobic nonhemolytic streptococci, coliform bacteria, bacteroides, and staphylococci. There is reduced incidence of beta-hemolytic streptococcal infection due to improvements in obstetrical

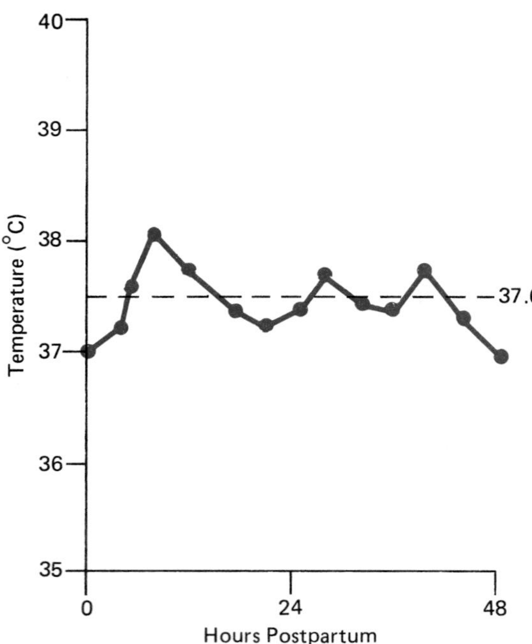

Figure 38-1.
The pattern of resolving postpartum fever (single spike) following spontaneous vaginal delivery. (Filker R, Monif GRG: The significance of temperature during the first 24 hours postpartum. Obstet Gynecol, 53, 3:358–361, 1979)

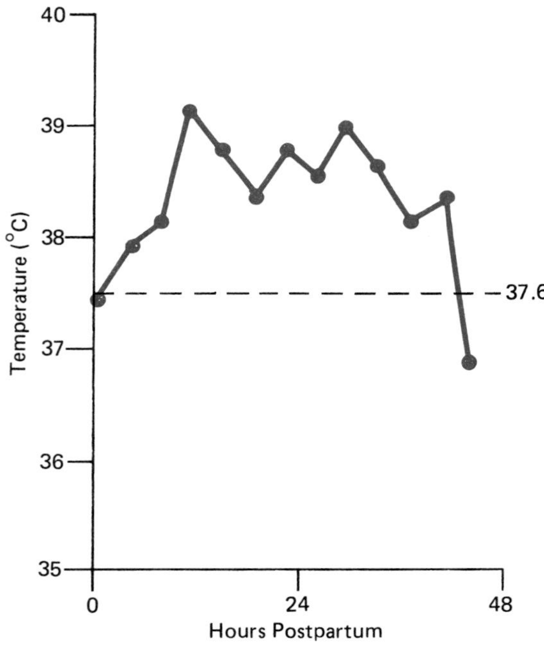

Figure 38-2.
The pattern of fever (>38.4 C) in the first 24 hours postpartum following either spontaneous vaginal delivery or cesarean section. (Filker R, Monif GRG: The significance of temperature during the first 24 hours postpartum. Obstet Gynecol, 53, 3:358–361, 1979)

care and aseptic technique. Multiple bacterial pathogens are present in the cervix and lower uterine segment during pregnancy and for a short time after delivery. Generally, such organisms harbored in the female genital tract do not cause infections, but the trauma of birth and alteration of immunologic function and resistance caused by fatigue and stress make the postpartal woman more susceptible. Hemorrhage and anemia also predispose to postpartal infection.

Endogenous infections are caused by bacteria in the genital tract that enter and colonize wounds in the perineum, vagina, cervix, or endometrium at the site of placental attachment. Existing infections in other organs or septicemia may also be a cause. Exogenous infections are caused by introduction of organisms into the genital tract. Nurses, physicians and other personnel are the most frequent source of exogenous (nosocomial) infections.

Although attending personnel wear gloves, the hands and the instruments used may become contaminated by pathogenic bacteria as the result of droplet infection from the nasopharynx or improper sterilization. Even in modern obstetrics, this is a very common mode of infection, and unless the utmost vigilance is used in masking all attendants in the delivery room (both nose and mouth) and in excluding all persons suffering or recovering from an upper respiratory infection, it is a constant source of danger.

Although a less common means of transfer today than a few decades ago, careless physicians and nurses have been known to carry bacteria to the parturient from countless extraneous contacts—from other cases of puerperal infection, from suppurative postoperative wounds, from cases of sloughing carcinoma, from patients with scarlet fever, from infants with impetigo neonatorum, and from umbilical infections of the newborn. The physician and nurse, themselves, may have an infection such as an infected hangnail or furuncle.

Coitus late in pregnancy may introduce extraneous organisms to the birth canal or carry upward bacteria already present on the vulva or in the lower vagina. However, there is little risk unless the membranes are ruptured, in which case coitus should be avoided.

During the second stage of labor, the chances of fecal matter being transferred to the vagina are great, another source of introducing coliform bacteria.

In addition to traumatic labor and postpartal hemorrhage, other factors are prolonged labor, prolonged rupture of the membranes, retention of placental tissue, and retained blood clots.

Pathophysiology

Uterine-peritoneal puerperal infection is most commonly a result of colonization of these tissues by bacteria present in the cervix or vagina. Cervicovaginal organisms enter the uterine cavity during labor, which explains the high correlation between duration of labor and postpartum endometritis. Although in most cases the organisms enter the amniotic fluid when the membranes are ruptured, the presence of organisms within amniotic fluid with intact membranes has recently been demonstrated. Amniotic fluid colonization during labor (with intact membranes) may be a common occurrence, but without clinically significant infection resulting. Amniotic fluid has an antibacterial effect, related to a polypeptide linked with zinc and other lysozyme and immunoglobulin systems.[3]

The upper endometrial cavity is probably sterile in most women without postpartal infection. However, it is known that the postpartum cervix and vagina contain numerous potentially pathogenic bacteria, and these increase during the postpartal period. The lower uterus is probably colonized by such bacteria, but at some point colonization ceases and the uterine cavity becomes sterile. The exact location in the cavity at which colonization ceases is unknown, but is presumed to be close to the cervical-endometrial junction.

When large numbers of virulent bacteria enter the uterine cavity during labor (by mechanisms such as discussed in the preceding section), they can attach to the uterine decidua following delivery and cause endometritis. In some cases, the bacteria gain entrance into the large venous vascular channels to produce parametritis, or bacteria enter the fallopian tubes to cause salpingitis. It is often difficult to accurately identify the causative organism in such infections because of the lack of sensitivity and specificity in sampling and diagnostic techniques. For example, transcervical sampling of the uterine cavity almost always is contaminated by cervical organisms, blood cultures may identify only one organism in a mixed infection, and fundal aspiration is infrequently done because of difficulty in obtaining the sample and being certain that it is from the uterine cavity.

Types of Genital Tract Infection

Genital tract (puerperal) infection can be divided into two main types—*local lesion processes* and *extensions of the original lesion process.* When a lesion of the vulva, the perineum, the vagina, the cervix, or the endometrium becomes infected, the infection may remain localized in these wounds. However, the original inflammatory process may extend along the veins (the most common way) and cause thrombophlebitis and pyemia, or through the lymph vessels to cause peritonitis and pelvic cellulitis.

Lesions of the Perineum, the Vulva, and the Vagina

These lesions are highly vulnerable areas for bacterial invasion in the early puerperium. The most common is a localized infection of a repaired perineal laceration or episiotomy wound.

The usual symptoms are elevation of temperature, pain and sensation of heat in the affected area, and burning on urination. The area involved becomes red and edematous, and there is profuse seropurulent discharge. If a wound of the vulva becomes infected, the entire vulva may become edematous and ulcerated. Infections involving the perineum, the vulva, and the vagina cause the patient considerable discomfort and alarm.

These local inflammatory processes seldom cause severe physical reactions, provided that good drainage is established and the patient's temperature remains below 38.4°C (101°F). To promote good drainage, all stitches may be removed to lay open the surface. Because the drainage itself is a source of irritation and contamination, the wound must be kept clean and the perineal pads changed frequently. Care must be exercised in cleansing the wound to see that none of the solution runs into the vagina.

Treatments by such means as sitz baths or the perineal heat lamp are generally used for the relief of pain. Antibiotics are prescribed to combat the infection. If drainage is impaired, the patient not only has more pain but also may have a chill, followed by a sudden elevation of temperature.

Endometritis

This is a localized infection of the lining membrane of the uterus. Bacteria invade the lesion, usually the placental site, and may spread to involve the entire endometrium (Fig. 38-3).

When endometritis develops, it is usually manifest about 48 hours to 72 hours after delivery. In the milder forms the patient may have no complaints or symptoms other than a rise in temperature to about 38.4°C (101°F) which persists for several days and then subsides. On the other hand, the more virulent infections are often ushered in by chills and high fever, with a comparable rise in pulse rate (Fig. 38-4). In the majority of severe cases the patient experiences a chilly sensation or actual chills at the onset and often complains of malaise, loss of appetite, headache, backache, and general discomfort.

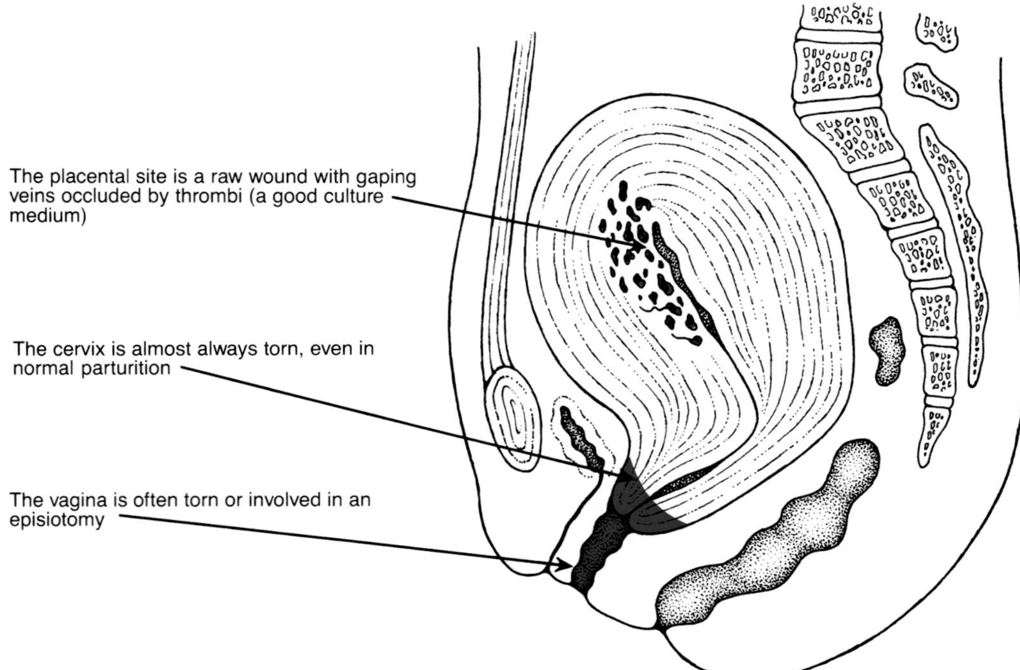

Figure 38-3.
Sites of common postpartal infection.

It is not unusual for the patient to have severe and prolonged afterpains. The uterus is usually large and is extremely tender when palpated abdominally. The lochial discharge may be decreased in amount and distinguished from normal lochia by its red brown appearance and foul odor. In some cases, particularly those caused by the hemolytic streptococcus, the lochia may be odorless.

If the infection remains localized in the endometrium, it is usually over in about a week or 10 days. But when extension of the infection occurs to cause peritonitis, pelvic thrombophlebitis, or cellulitis, the

Figure 38-4.
Febrile pattern in endometritis. The four classical signs of postpartal endometritis are temperature elevation 101°F (38.4°C), increase in pulse rate (100–120), delayed involution with fundal height not decreasing, and lochia remaining red with foul odor. *R* = red, *B* = brown.

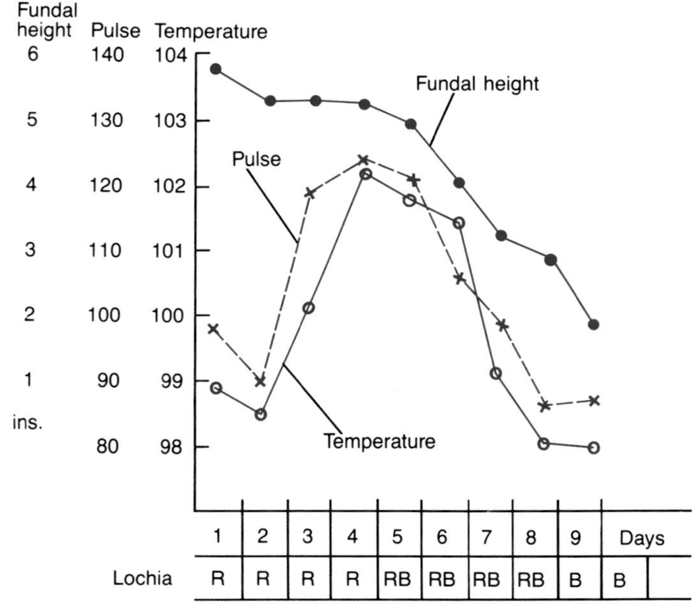

Table 38-1.
Antibiotic Activity Against Common Endometrial Infections

	Penicillin	Penicillin & Aminoglycoside	Ampicillin	Cephalosporin	Aminoglycoside & Clindamycin	Penicillin & Chloramphenicol
Aerobic organism						
Streptococci	+	+	+	+	+	+
Enterococci	−	+	+	−	−	±
E coli	±	+	±	+	+	+
Gardnerella vaginalis	+	+	+	+	+	+
S aureus	−	+	−	+	+	±
Anaerobic organism						
Peptostreptococci	+	+	+	+	+	+
Peptococci	+	+	+	+	+	+
Bacteroides sp.	+	+	+	+	+	+
B fragilis or *B bivius*	−	−	−	−	+	+

+ = 95% of organisms susceptible; ± = greater than 50% of organisms susceptible; − = less than 50% of organisms susceptible
(Eschenbach DA, Wager GP: Puerperal infections. Clin Obstet Gynecol 23, 4:1020)

disease may persist for many weeks, often with dramatic temperature curves and repeated chills.

Treatment depends on the severity of the condition. Mild cases with temperature under 100°F and no chills are best handled by simple measures. Fowler's position facilitates lochial drainage. Ergonovine four times daily for 2 days promotes uterine tone, and forced fluids provide additional support. The lochia is cultured and the patient is treated with the appropriate antibiotic (Table 38-1). Isolation is desirable to protect other patients and to afford the mother greater rest. In this group it is unnecessary to discontinue breast-feeding.

In severe cases, breast-feeding is discontinued not only because it exhausts the mother but also because it is usually futile in the presence of high fever.

Pelvic Cellulitis, or Parametritis

Pelvic cellulitis is an infection that extends along the lymphatics to reach the loose connective tissue surrounding the uterus. It may follow an infected cervical laceration, endometritis, or pelvic thrombophlebitis. The patient has a persistent fever and marked pain and tenderness over the affected area. The problem is usually unilateral but may involve both sides of the abdomen. As the process develops, the swelling becomes very hard and finally either undergoes resolution or results in the formation of a pelvic abscess. If the latter occurs, as the abscess comes to a point, the skin above becomes red, edematous, and tender. Recovery is usually prompt after the abscess is opened (Figs. 38-5 and 38-6).

Parametritis usually occurs later than endometritis, during the second postpartal week. Fever and malaise are the typical presentation, and lochia usually remains red and is heavy. There is less pain than might be expected. This condition is treated with antibiotics.

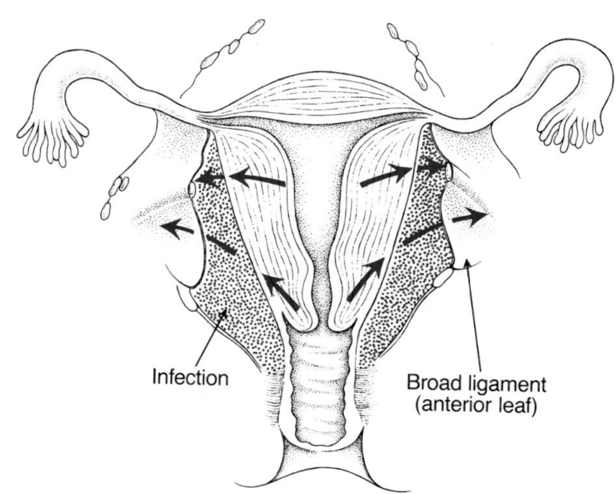

Figure 38-5.
Parametritis or pelvic cellulitis. Infection may spread from the uterus, a cervical laceration, or thrombophlebitis into the loose connective tissue. It may extend retroperitoneally in any direction, commonly between leaves of the broad ligament, and around the vagina or rectum. Pelvic examination reveals a large, hard mass representing a pelvic abscess in some instances.

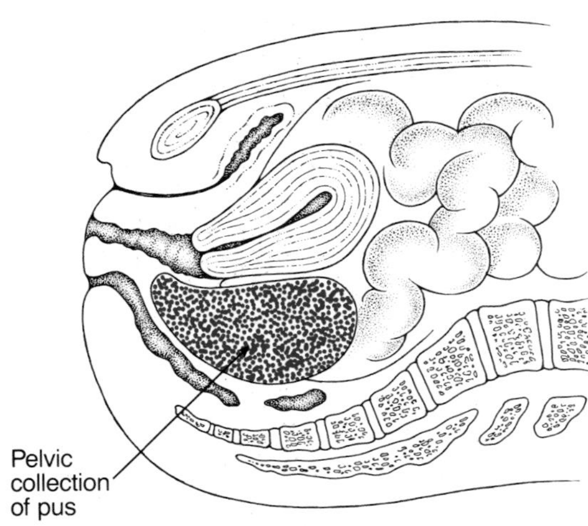

Figure 38-6.
Pelvic abscess.

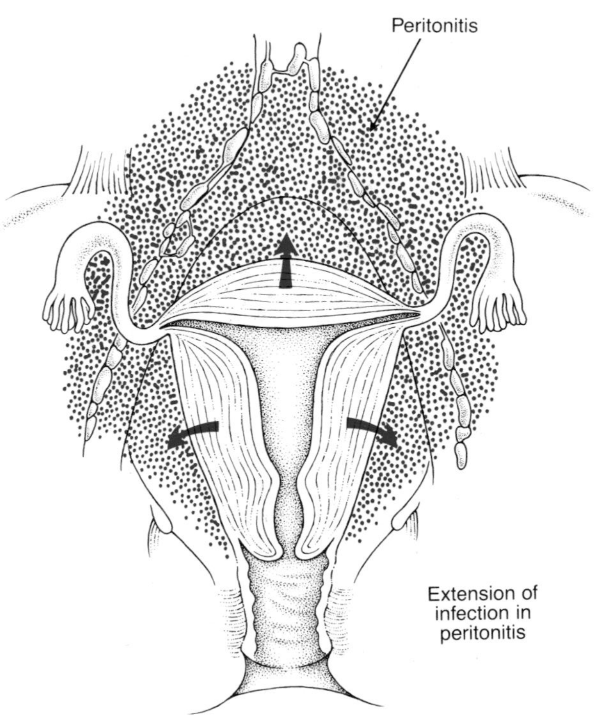

Figure 38-7.
Postpartal peritonitis. The pelvic peritoneum may become involved in an infection in the same ways as the parametrium. Generalized peritonitis may occur with development of paralytic ileus. Although uncommon, peritonitis can be severe and life threatening.

Peritonitis

Peritonitis is an infection, either generalized or local, of the peritoneum. Usually the infection reaches the peritoneum from the endometrium by traveling through the lymphatic vessels, but peritonitis may result also from the extension of thrombophlebitis or parametritis (Fig. 38-7).

The clinical course of pelvic peritonitis resembles that of surgical peritonitis. The patient has a high fever, rapid pulse and, in general, has the appearance of being profoundly ill. She is usually restless and sleepless and has constant and severe abdominal pain. Hiccups, nausea and vomiting, which is sometimes fecal and projectile, may be present.

Antimicrobial therapy is given to combat the infection, while analgesic drugs are prescribed for discomfort and mild sedative drugs to relieve the restlessness and apprehension. If there is intestinal involvement, oral feedings are withheld until normal intestinal function is restored; meanwhile, fluids are administered intravenously. Blood transfusions and oxygen therapy may be indicated for supportive treatment. A record of intake and output must be kept.

Salpingitis

Acute salpingitis is infection of the fallopian tubes following childbirth. Bacterial ascent from the uterine cavity or by venous route can cause salpingitis. The symptoms resemble peritonitis and the two are difficult to distinguish diagnostically. High fever, rapid pulse, nausea and vomiting, abdominal pain, and rigidity are common findings. Although usually bilateral, unilateral salpingitis may be impossible to distinguish from appendicitis when it occurs on the right side. An exploratory laparotomy or laparoscopy may be necessary to establish the correct diagnosis.

Treatment is with antibiotics, analgesics, and sedatives as with peritonitis. Tubal patency and subsequent fertility is always a concern with salpingitis (Fig. 38-8).

Thrombophlebitis

This is an infection of the vascular endothelium with clot formation attached to the vessel wall. It may be of two types—pelvic thrombophlebitis, an inflammatory process involving the ovarian and the uterine veins, or femoral thrombophlebitis, in which the femoral, the popliteal, or the saphenous vein is involved (Fig. 38-9). Early ambulation may be a factor in preventing this complication.

Femoral Thrombophlebitis. This condition presents a special group of signs and symptoms. It is a disease of the puerperium characterized by pain, fever, and swelling in the affected leg. These symptoms are due to the formation of a clot in the veins of the leg itself, which interferes with the return circulation of the blood. When this condition develops, it usually appears about 10 days after labor, although it may manifest itself as late as the twentieth day. As in all acute febrile diseases occurring after labor, the secretion of milk may cease.

The disease is ushered in with malaise, chilliness, and fever, which are soon followed by stiffness and pain in the affected part. If it is in the leg, the pain may begin in the groin or the hip and extend downward, or it may commence in the calf of the leg and extend upward. In about 24 hours the leg begins to swell, and although the pain then lessens slightly, it is always present and may be severe enough to prevent sleep. The skin over the swollen area is shiny white in color.

The acute symptoms last from a few days to a week, after which the pain gradually subsides, and the patient slowly improves.

The disease lasts 4 weeks to 6 weeks. The affected leg is slow to return to its normal size and may remain permanently enlarged and troublesome.

The prognosis is usually favorable. However, in some of the very severe cases, abscesses may form and the disease may become critical and produce fatality. Since the clot tends to be attached to the vessel wall somewhat loosely, there is a tendency for the clot to dislodge and produce a pulmonary embolism which is also fatal in the majority of cases.

Treatment of femoral thrombophlebitis consists of rest, elevation of the affected leg, and analgesics as indicated for pain. Anticoagulants, such as heparin and dicumarol, may be prescribed to prevent further formation of thrombi. Antimicrobial drugs may be used in cases where more generalized infection is known or suspected. A "cradle" is used to keep the pressure of the bedclothes off the affected part. Heat or icebags may be used along the course of the affected vessels.

Surgical treatment may be indicated in some severe or nonresponding cases and consists of incision of the affected vessel, removal of the clot, and repair of the vessel. Ligation of the major vessels is sometimes resorted to as a preventive measure for pulmonary embolism.

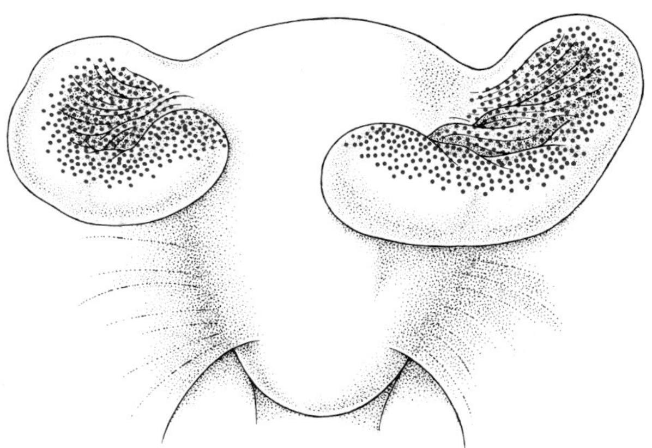

Figure 38-8.
Postpartal salpingitis. Infection of the fallopian tubes leads to hyperemia, edema, and purulent discharge into the tubal lumina. The tubes are enlarged, swollen, and tender. Tubal abscesses may occur, creating tender adnexal masses.

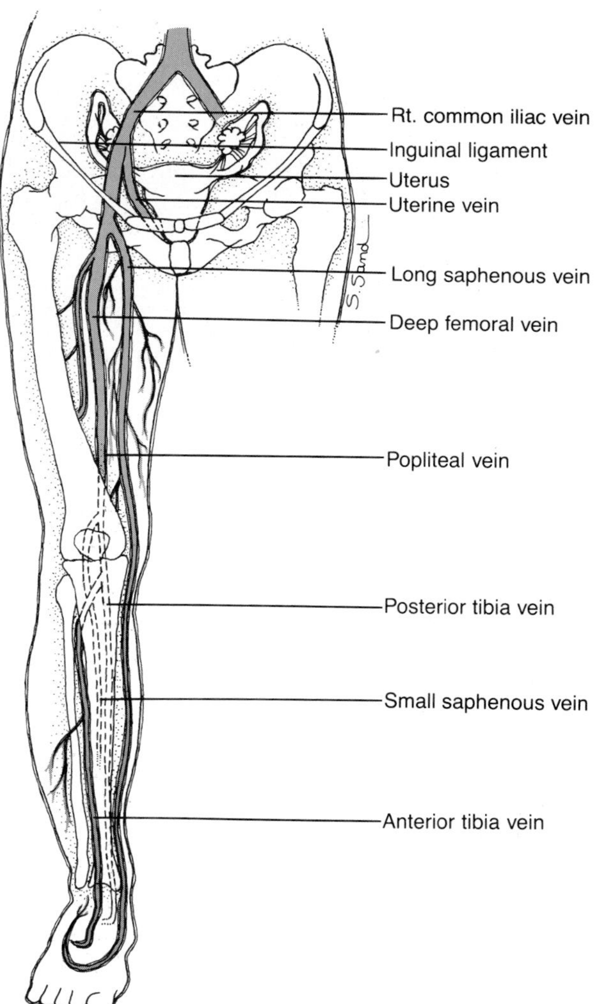

Figure 38-9.
Sites of postpartal thrombophlebitis. Pelvic thrombophlebitis involves the uterine and ovarian veins. Femoral thrombophlebitis involves the femoral, popliteal, and the long saphenous veins. When the small saphenous vein is involved, the term is phlebothrombosis, because the thrombis is caused more by stasis than infection, although deep calf thrombi do become infected.

Under no circumstances should anyone rub or massage the affected part. The leg should be handled with the utmost care when one is changing dressings, applying a bandage, making the bed, or giving a bath.

Pelvic Thrombophlebitis. This is a severe complication in the puerperium. The onset usually occurs about the second week following delivery with severe repeated chills and dramatic swings in temperature. The infection is usually caused by anaerobic streptococci, and although it is difficult to obtain a positive blood culture, bacteria are present in the bloodstream during chills. Antimicrobial therapy is used and is effective in treating most strains of this organism; as long as the chills and the fever persist, blood transfusions may be given. Heparin and dicumarol may be prescribed to prevent the formation of more thrombi. A further problem is likely to arise with metastatic pulmonary complications, such as lung abscesses or pneumonia.

These patients are often depressed, discouraged, and feel physically unwell. Breast-feeding may have been interrupted and the significant emotional and physiological changes following childbirth may be compounded by the illness.

Astute nursing care at this time is particularly essential. Accurate observing, recording, and reporting, and paying particular attention to details of the physical care aspects are extremely important in helping to resolve the disorder and to prevent further complications. Supportive care to help the mother (and family) work through the depression and discouragement is another crucial aspect of care. The principles outlined in the discussion of grief are appropriate here (see Chap. 42).

Signs and Symptoms

It is very important that the nurse recognizes and reports early signs and symptoms of postpartal genital tract infection so that proper treatment may be instituted without delay. When such puerperal infection develops, one of the first symptoms usually seen is a rise in temperature. Although temperature elevations in the puerperium may be caused by upper respiratory infections, urinary tract infections and the like, the majority are due to genital tract infection.

The symptoms may vary, depending on the location and the extent of the infectious process, the type and the virulence of the invading organisms, and the general resistance of the patient. The affected area is usually painful, reddened and edematous, and the source of profuse discharge. The patient may complain of malaise, headache, and general discomfort. As mentioned above, the temperature is elevated, and in the more severe infections, chills and fever may occur.

In its typical form each of the clinical types of puerperal infection presents a very characteristic set of signs and symptoms, although occasionally one form of the disease is combined with another. The distinctions between these different types of infections are important because the clinical course, the treatment, and the prognosis depend on the particular form of infection (Table 38-2).

The nurse can maintain particular alertness for symptoms and signs of puerperal infection in providing care for women with increased risk factors. The risk factors that increase the probability of developing postpartum uterine and pelvic infections fall into three major categories—factors related to general risk of infection, factors related to events during labor, and factors related to operative procedures. Table 38-3 lists these risk factors by each category.

Women are at increased risk for thrombophlebitis during the postpartal period if they cannot ambulate soon after delivery, and if they have a previous history of embolic disorders.

Management

The use of antimicrobial therapy provides highly effective treatment and has vastly improved the prognosis of puerperal infection. Antibiotic drugs are effective in combating most of these infections, but, nevertheless, the management and the care of patients with puerperal infections are highly important and demand the utmost skill. Penicillin is effective against the hemolytic streptococcus, the clostridium bacillus, and certain staphylococcus. Since penicillin is not effective against the colon bacillus and certain strains of staphylococci, a broad-spectrum antibiotic such as ampicillin, tetracycline, or cephalosporin may be prescribed for infections caused by these organisms. Many types of antimicrobials are available, some specifically for the gram positive or gram negative organisms and the penicillin resistant organisms (see Table 38-1). The selection and dosage of these drugs depend upon the severity of the disease and the type of offending organism. Sensitivity series are often done to help determine the appropriate antibiotic. Uterine cultures are taken to gain information about the organism; in severe cases blood cultures may be taken, but if they are to be of real diagnostic value, they must be taken at the time of the chill. The infected lesions are treated the same as those of any surgical wound. Drainage must be established, and since this discharge is of a highly infectious nature, care must be taken to see that it is not spread and that all contaminated pads and dressings are wrapped and burned.

Table 38-2.
Types of Postpartum Genital Tract Infections

Type of Infection	Etiology	Signs and Symptoms	Treatment
Perineal and vulvar lesions	Bacterial invasion of episiotomy, laceration, traumatized tissue	Fever, localized pain Edema, erythema, seropurulent discharge from lesion	Antibiotics Removal of stitches and promotion of drainage, sitz baths, perineal heat lamp, analgesics
Endometritis	Bacterial invasion of placental site or entire endometrium	Fever about 38.4°C or 101°F, chills, rapid pulse Malaise, headache, backache, loss of appetite, cramps Relaxed, tender uterus with foul-smelling discharge, dark or profuse lochia	Antibiotics, ergonovine Fowler's position to promote drainage, hydration
Pelvic cellulitis or parametritis	Bacterial invasion via lymphatics to tissue surrounding uterus (often following endometritis)	Fever, chills Pain and tenderness of lower abdomen, edema Signs of endometritis may be present also	Antibiotics Hydration, blood transfusion for dropping hemoglobin Bedrest, analgesics
Femoral thrombophlebitis	Infection of thrombi and vascular endothelium	Fever, chills, malaise Stiffness, pain, swelling of affected area	Rest, elevation of leg, heat or ice to leg Anticoagulants, antibiotics, analgesics
Pelvic thrombophlebitis	Infection of thrombi and pelvic veins	Severe repeated chills and dramatic temperature swings	Anticoagulants, antibiotics, blood transfusion, bedrest
Peritonitis	Spread of infection to peritoneum, local or generalized	High fever, rapid pulse Severe abdominal pain Vomiting, restlessness Distention	Antibiotics, analgesics, sedatives Bedrest, hydration, blood transfusion, oxygen, IV infusions

Table 38-3.
Risk Factors for Developing Postpartal Infections

Related to General Infection Risk	Related to Labor Events	Related to Operative Risk Factors
Anemia Poor nutrition Lack of prenatal care Obesity Low socioeconomic status Sexual intercourse after rupture of membranes	Prolonged rupture of membranes Chorioamnionitis Intrauterine fetal monitoring Number of exams during labor	Cesarean section General anesthesia Urgency of operation Breaks in operative technique Manual placental removal Hemorrhage Forceps delivery Episiotomy Lacerations

(Eschenbach DA, Wager GP: Puerperal infections. Clin Obstet Gynecol 23, 4:1004, 1980)

Nursing Intervention. The curative treatment is antibiotic therapy, but good nursing care is also essential. The patient should be kept as comfortable and quiet as possible, for sleep and rest are important. Conserving the patient's strength in every way, along with giving her nourishing food and appropriate amounts of fluids, helps to increase her powers of resistance. The head of the bed should be kept elevated to promote drainage and to keep the patient comfortable.

Care must be exercised to prevent the spread of the infection from one patient to another. Isolation of infected patients from others is desirable in order to protect the healthy maternity patients. Ideally, the patient with puerperal infection should be away from the maternity divisions. If it is impossible to arrange for such complete segregation, the nurse must consider every patient with puerperal infection as "in isolation" and follow scrupulous technique accordingly.

Regardless of the situation, the nurse who is caring for a patient with puerperal infection (or any infection, for that matter) should not attend other maternity patients. The hands of all attendants need special attention and should be scrubbed thoroughly after caring for a mother who has an infection. In certain cases strict isolation technique, with special gowns, masks, and rubber gloves, is essential. Clean isolation gowns, masks, and gloves should be available for all persons who attend the isolated patient, and after being used should be left in the room and disposed of in special hampers or containers. This apparel should not be worn outside the patient's room. Nurses who care for these patients must be fully acquainted with principles of good isolation technique.

Genital Tract Infection Following Cesarean Section

The incidence of genital tract infection is significantly increased when delivery is by cesarean section. This is frequently related to several factors, such as duration of ruptured membranes, number of vaginal examinations, length of labor, various complications, and the need for invasive procedures. However, the operative trauma itself increases infectious morbidity, generally caused by a mixed anaerobic/aerobic infection by organisms present in the genital tract at the time of labor and delivery. Surgical trauma, with devitalization of tissue and collection of blood and serum in the myometrium or endometrium, which have become infected with organisms that have ascended from the lower genital tract to the amniotic fluid, plays a key role in the development of postpartal endometritis, myometritis, incisional wound abscesses, and pelvic abscesses.[4]

Treatment is by antimicrobial therapy and drainage of abscesses; the antibiotics commonly used include penicillin, tetracycline, kanamycin, and clindamycin. The organisms most frequently causing infections following cesarean section are anaerobic streptococci, aerobic streptococci, Bacteroides species, *E coli,* and less often Clostridium species and staphylococci. A particularly strong relationship has been found between membranes ruptured for longer than 6 hours and postcesarean section infection (myometritis).[4]

Wound Infections

The incidence of wound infection following cesarean section is between 6% and 11%. Risk factors for development of wound infections include obesity, diabetes, number of vaginal examinations, length of time in the hospital prior to delivery, emergency cesarean section, duration of operation, use of electrocautery, and placement of wound drains. The bacteria causing wound infections usually originate from the patient's own flora, either bacteria from the skin or coliforms or anaerobes from the uterine cavity. However, some particularly virulent infections are due to hospital-acquired organisms.

The initial signs of wound infection usually begin on or after the second postoperative day, with unexplained temperature elevation often occurring before other physical findings. Pain, induration, and erythema of the incision are the classical signs and symptoms. Areas of fluctuance often develop, and these, as well as abscesses, need to be drained. Treatment also consists of debridement of necrotic tissue and packing the wound to keep it open and draining several times daily with saline sponges, as well as antibiotics. Suggested preventive measures include wound irrigation with topical antimicrobials instead of saline during surgery, prophylactic systemic antibiotics, and delayed primary closure in cases complicated by obesity or established infection.

The complications of abdominal wound infection may be most serious. Synergistic bacterial gangrene widens the wound and must be treated by wide surgical excision and systemic antibiotics. Necrotizing fasciitis may be difficult to diagnose initially, requires debridement of the entire necrotic area, and has high mortality rates. Wound dehiscence has mortality rates as high as 35%, with predisposing factors including obesity, ileus with vomiting and coughing, intestinal obstruction, fluid and electrolyte imbalance or hypoproteinemia, and wound infection. This surgical emergency needs immediate exploration of the wound, debridement, and secondary fascial closure with retention sutures. Postoperatively, nasogastric decompression and systemic antibiotics are usually needed.[3]

Prevention of Infection

The prevention of infection throughout the maternity cycle is an important factor in the maintenance of health and the prevention of disease. During pregnancy, complete blood counts or hematocrit and hemoglobin tests are done routinely and iron is prescribed as necessary, not only for the immediate value but also because anemia predisposes to puerperal infection. Health teaching is emphasized at this time, particularly in regard to diet, rest, exercise, and general hygiene. The patient is advised to avoid possible sources of infection, especially upper respiratory infections.

During labor care should be exercised to limit bacteria from extraneous sources. In the hospital, cleanliness and good housekeeping are imperative, but, nevertheless, individual care technique reduces the chance of contamination from other patients. Each patient should have her own equipment, which includes her own bedpan. This bedpan should be cleansed after each use and sterilized once a day. Careful hand washing on the part of all personnel after contacts with each patient helps to prevent the transfer of infection from one patient to another.

The strictest rules should be enforced for surgical cleanliness during labor and delivery. No one with an infection of the skin or the respiratory tract should work in the maternity department. The nasopharynx of attendants is the most common exogenous source of contamination of the birth canal. Regular nasopharyngeal cultures of maternity personnel are often required. To be effective, masks worn during delivery must cover the nose and the mouth and be clean and dry; thus, they must be changed frequently and should not hang around the neck when not in use.

During the puerperium the same precautions should be carried out. For many days following the delivery, the surface of the birth canal is a vulnerable area for pathogenic bacteria. The birth canal is well protected against the invasion of extraneous bacteria by the closed vulva, unless this barrier is invaded. Patients, therefore, are to be taught the principles of perineal hygiene and how to care for themselves

Prevention of Postpartal Infection

- Well-balanced diet, good nutrition before and during pregnancy
- Prompt recognition and treatment of anemia
- Early and regular prenatal care
- Healthful activities during pregnancy (*e.g.,* adequate rest, exercise, general hygiene, maintaining normal weight)
- Accurate diagnosis and early treatment of urinary tract infections during pregnancy
- Infection control and monitoring in the hospital
- Conscientious aseptic technique by hospital personnel
- Regular nasopharyngeal cultures of maternity personnel
- Minimization of pelvic examinations during labor
- Avoidance of early rupture of membranes
- Intrauterine fetal monitoring only when absolutely necessary
- Prevention of Cesarean section
- Avoidance of general anesthesia
- Avoidance of manual removal of placenta
- Prevention of hemorrhage
- Minimization of delivery trauma (*e.g.,* forceps, episiotomy, lacerations)

without using the fingers to separate the labia, because this permits the cleansing solution to enter the vagina.

Pulmonary Embolism

Pulmonary embolism is usually due to the detachment of a small part of a thrombus, which is washed along in the blood current until it becomes lodged in the right side of the heart. In many cases the thrombus originates in a uterine or a pelvic vein, although its origin may be in some other vessel. When the embolus occludes the pulmonary artery, it obstructs the passage of blood into the lungs, either wholly or in part, and the patient may die of asphyxia within a few minutes. If the clot is small, the initial episode may not be fatal, although repeated attacks may prove so. The condition may follow infection, thrombosis, severe hemorrhage, or shock; and it may occur any time during the puerperium, especially after sudden exertion.

Manifestations

The symptoms of pulmonary embolism are sudden intense pain in the chest; severe dyspnea; unusual apprehension; syncope; feeble, irregular, or imperceptible pulse; pallor in some cases, cyanosis in others; and eventually air hunger. Death may occur at any time from within a few minutes to a few hours, according to the amount or degree of obstruction to the pulmonary circulation. If the patient survives for a few hours, it is likely that she may recover.

Management

The treatment consists, first of all, in preventing the accident by careful attention to all details of surgical asepsis and to the proper management of labor and delivery. Following delivery, early ambulation may be an additional prophylactic measure, since circulatory stasis is undoubtedly a causative factor. In some instances it is almost impossible to prevent a fatal attack, because the patient may be recovering without elevation of temperature and without complications and yet, on the seventh or tenth day, she suddenly cries out, and passes into coma and shock due to cor pulmonale.

When embolism occurs, rapid emergency measures to combat anoxia and shock must be carried out promptly. Oxygen is administered without delay, and anticoagulants are given. Morphine or Demerol may be given to help relieve the patient's apprehension and pain. Dicumarol and heparin therapy is continued to prevent recurrent emboli, for as long as 6 weeks to 6 months, depending on clinical response. During hospitalization the patient must be kept warm, quiet, comfortable, and as free from worry as possible. She may be given a light, nourishing diet during early convalescence.

Subinvolution of the Uterus

Subinvolution is the term used to describe the condition that exists when normal involution of the puerperal uterus is retarded. The causes contributing to this condition may be lack of tone in the uterine musculature, imperfect exfoliation of the decidua, retained placental tissue and membranes, endometritis, and presence of uterine fibroids.

Subinvolution is characterized by a large and flabby uterus, lochial discharge prolonged beyond the usual period, sometimes with profuse bleeding, backache, and dragging sensation in the pelvis.

Treatment is aimed at correcting the cause of subinvolution. Oxytocic medication, such as methylergonovine maleate (Methergine) or ergonovine, may be administered to maintain uterine tone and prevent the accumulation of clots in the uterine cavity. Curettage is employed to remove any retained placental tissues or secundines. Endometritis requires antimicrobial therapy.

Early ambulation is believed to have decreased the incidence of subinvolution. And, since it is recognized that breast-feeding stimulates uterine contractions, the fact that the mother is *not* breast-feeding plus the fact that she is usually taking a lactogenic suppressing drug, may be influencing factors when subinvolution occurs.

Vulvar Hematomas

Blood may escape into the connective tissue beneath the skin covering the external genitalia or beneath the vaginal mucosa to form vulvar and vaginal hematomas, respectively. The condition occurs about once in every 500 to 1000 deliveries.

Vulvar hematomas manifest themselves by severe perineal pain and the sudden appearance of a tense, fluctuant, and sensitive tumor of varying size covered by discolored skin. When the mass develops in the vagina, it may temporarily escape detection, but the pain and the patient's inability to void should alert the nurse to this complication.

Since these symptoms may also be indicative of other types of complications, a careful examination of the perineum and an accurate report of its condition is important. The new parturient has great difficulty in localizing any pain that she may have. Therefore, the nurse usually has to explore with the mother the nature and location of her discomfort, gradually moving from general statements to more specific and more accurate ones. A vaginal examination which confirms the diagnosis is usually performed.

Small hematomas are usually treated supportively and allowed to resolve of their own accord. However, if the pain is severe or the tumor enlarges, incision and evacuation of the blood, with ligation of bleeding points, is required. Large genital hematomas nearly always result in a blood loss that is more than the clinical estimate. Hypovolemia and anemia should be prevented by blood replacement as necessary.

Vulvar or vaginal hematomas may become infected, particularly those that must be opened and drained. Therefore, attention must be given to prevention of contamination both through careful aseptic technique of attendants and by teaching the patient perineal and bowel hygiene. Dressings or perineal pads must be changed frequently and early signs of infection such as foul-smelling discharge or temperature elevation reported at once. Broad-spectrum antibiotics may be instituted.

Mastitis

Mastitis, or inflammation of the breast, may vary from a "simple" inflammation of the tissues around the nipple to a suppurative process that results in abscess formation in the glandular tissue. Mastitis is always the result of an infection, usually caused by *S aureus* or hemolytic streptococcus organisms. The disease in most instances is preceded by fissures or erosions of the nipple or the areola, which provide a portal of entry to the subcutaneous lymphatics, although under conducive conditions organisms present in the lactiferous ducts can invade the tissues and cause mastitis.

Manifestations

Puerperal mastitis may occur any time during lactation but usually occurs about the third or fourth week of the puerperium. There is usually marked engorgement of the breast preceding mastitis, although engorgement per se does not cause the infection. When the infection occurs, the patient complains of acute pain and tenderness in the breast and often experiences general malaise, a chilly sensation or, in fact, may have a chill followed by a marked rise of temperature (40.5°C or 105°F) and an increased pulse rate. On inspection the breast appears hard and reddened. The obstetrician should be notified at once and treatment instituted promptly before the infection becomes localized as an abscess (Figs. 38-10 and 38-11).

Management

For the most part, puerperal mastitis is preventable by prophylactic measures. An important measure is initiated when the expectant mother learns about breast hygiene and begins to take special care of her breasts during the latter months of pregnancy (see Chap. 21).

After delivery, appropriate breast care continues to help prevent the development of lesions, but if they do occur, proper treatment must be given promptly. Any time the mother complains of sore, tender nipples, they should be inspected immediately. At this time there may be no break in the surface, but if the condition is neglected, the nipple may become raw and cracked. The alert nurse often can detect even a very small crack in the surface of the nipple if it is inspected carefully. Once a break in the skin occurs, the chances of infection mount, because pathogenic

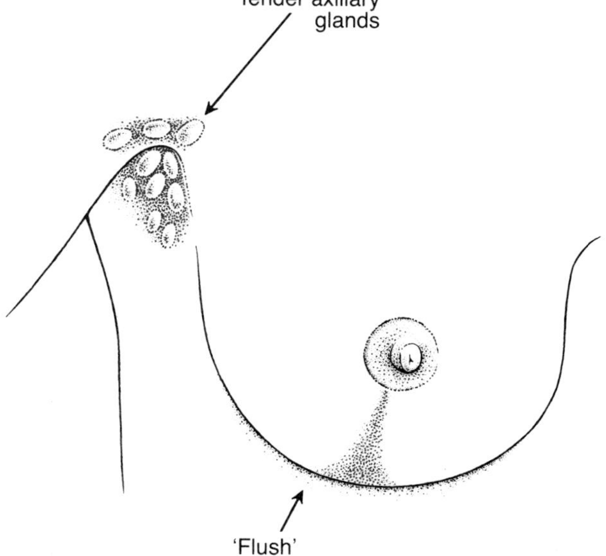

Figure 38-10.
Early mastitis. Fever is followed by a painful area on the breast and a "flush" which is red and tender but not fluctuant or swollen.

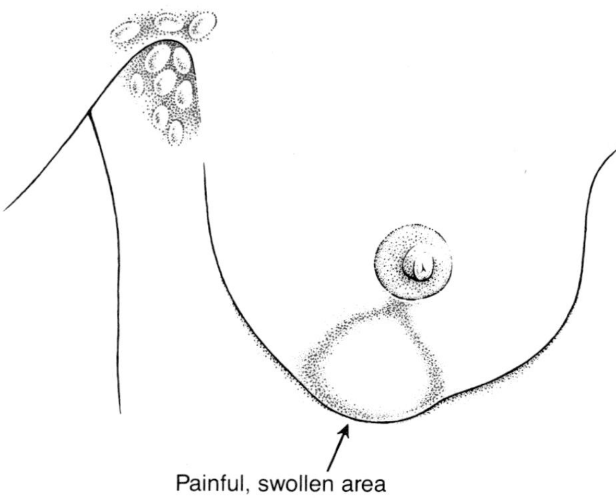

Figure 38-11.
Overt inflammation in mastitis. A swollen, painful, red to brawny area develops. The purulent drainage gradually localizes into an abscess; when fluctuant, it must be incised and drained.

organisms are frequently brought to the breast by the hands or may reach the breast from the patient's nightgown or bedclothes.

With early treatment by antibiotics, the inflammatory process may be brought under control before suppuration occurs. A broad-spectrum antibiotic is effective in treating acute puerperal mastitis if the therapy is started promptly, and often symptoms subside within 24 hours to 48 hours. The breasts should be well supported with a firm breast binder or well fitted brassiere. While the breasts are very painful, small side pillows used for support may give the mother some measure of comfort. Icecaps may be applied over the affected part, but if in time it becomes apparent that suppuration is inevitable, heat applications may be ordered to hasten the localization of the abscess. It is usually advised that breast-feeding be discontinued immediately in cases of mastitis.

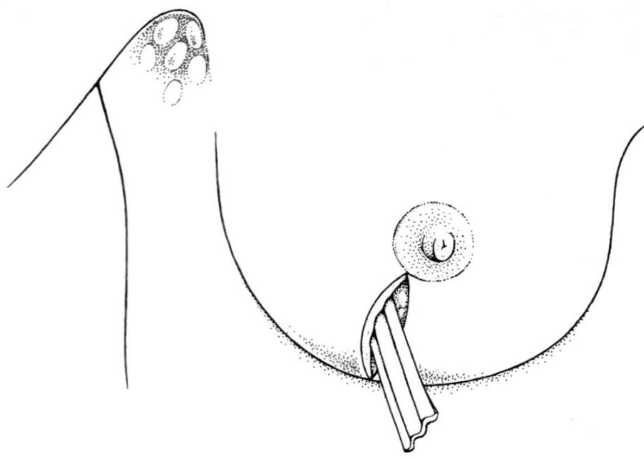

Figure 38-12.
Drainage of breast abscess. A radial incision is made in the breast, to avoid injuring the lactiferous ducts, that extends from near the areolar margin toward the periphery. All pus pockets must be broken down and evacuated. A gauze drain is left in for about 3 days. The wound is closed when clean. Antibiotic therapy is given.

If the treatment described above is unsuccessful, measures have to be taken to remove the pus when abscess formation occurs. In some cases it may be preferable to aspirate the pus rather than resort to incision and drainage. When incision and drainage are done, the incision is made radially, extending from near the areolar margin toward the periphery of the gland, in order to avoid injury to the lactiferous ducts. After the pus is evacuated, a gauze drain is inserted (Fig. 38-12). Following the operation the care of the patient is essentially the same as for a surgical patient. Complete recovery is usually prompt.

Another possible route for transmission of organisms to the mother's breasts is from the nasopharynx of her infant, who has become colonized by staphylococci in the hospital nursery. There need be no break in continuity of the skin of the breast or nipple. Once these organisms are introduced into the mother's breast, milk provides a superb culture medium for them. Efforts to prevent puerperal mastitis cannot be limited to the care of the mother's breasts but must extend to the hospital nursery, where the infant may acquire this penicillin-resistant strain. In the nursery such equipment as soap-solution containers, cribs, mattresses, blankets, and linens, as well as floors, can harbor the organisms. Some methods to help control the spread of infection at its source include careful nursery aseptic technique on the part of all personnel, measures to prevent the spread of organisms from infant to infant, such as proper spacing of cribs, and the exclusion of carriers from the maternity divisions as soon as they are identified.

It should be remembered that in maternity hospitals the nasopharynx of newborn infants tends to become readily infected with *S aureus,* and, moreover, the infection may persist for some weeks after the infant leaves the hospital. Where intensive studies have been carried out and puerperal mastitis or breast abscess appeared after discharge from the hospital, the cultures of the mothers' nares on admission to the hospital did not show evidence of the resistant strain of the organism. In these cases the infants were the source of infection, because the offending organism was cultured from the nose, the throat, and the skin of the infants.

When such infections occur, in either the mother or the infant, the nurse, in her care of the mother, should emphasize health teaching, not only concerning hygienic measures for the prevention of skin infections but also the urgency for prompt treatment of any member of the family if carbuncles, boils, burns, or other skin lesions develop.

Urinary Tract Infection

Postpartum urinary retention is a common occurrence due to increased bladder capacity, decreased tonus, and decreased perception of the urge to void due to perineal trauma. If the patient is unable to fully empty the bladder, the urine which is retained serves as a culture medium for bacterial growth, often leading to cystitis or pyelonephritis. Urinary tract infections occur in about 5% of postpartum patients and are usually caused by coliform bacteria. This incidence increases to 15% in women who receive intrapartal catheterization.[3]

The increased circulatory volume of the mother that was necessary for the growth and development of the fetus during pregnancy diminishes rapidly after delivery. The two main avenues for the diminution of the circulating blood volume are the skin and the kidneys. Consequently, the newly delivered mother perspires copiously and excretes large quantities of urine within 24 hours to 48 hours of delivery. As much as *500 ml to 1000 ml* may be voided at *each* urination; that is, as we know, two to three times what is usual in the nonparturient. The nurse should be particularly careful of bladder hygiene at this time because of the increase in urinary production and the danger of overdistention. Thus, one should not wait for any designated time to elapse to indicate when the bladder should be emptied; rather, the nurse should observe for evidence indicating the degree of bladder distention, because the bladder may fill in a relatively short span of time. If the patient is unable to void, catheterization is needed.

Retention of urine due to the inability to void is more frequently seen after operative delivery. It often lasts 5 days or 6 days but may persist longer. The main cause is probably edema of the trigone muscle, which may be so pronounced that it obstructs the urethra. Very temporary urinary retention may be due to the effects of analgesia and anesthesia received in labor.

As already stressed, the nurse should make every effort to have the patient void within 6 hours after delivery (see Chap. 28). If the patient has not done so within 8 hours, or depending upon the degree of distention, catheterization is necessary.

Because of the trauma of labor or operative delivery, the bladder usually is not as sensitive to distention as it was prior to pregnancy and delivery. Overdistention and incomplete emptying may occur; thus, the problem of residual urine frequently results. Repeated catheterization may be necessary for several days although in these persistent cases an indwelling catheter needs to be inserted to provide constant drainage.

When the mother continues to void small amounts of urine at frequent intervals, the nurse may suspect that these voidings are merely an overflow of a distended bladder and that there is residual urine there. Catheterization for residual urine, to be completely accurate, must be done within 5 minutes after the patient voids. If 60 ml or more of urine still remains in the bladder after the patient has voided, it is usually considered that the voiding has been incomplete. It is not uncommon for the catheterization to yield 800 ml or more of residual urine. Large amounts of urine (from 60 ml–1500 ml, as shown by catheterization) may remain in the bladder, even though the patient may feel she has completely emptied the bladder when she voided. The condition is due primarily to lack of tone in the bladder wall and is more likely to occur when the mother's bladder has been allowed to become overdistended during labor. A distended bladder requires prompt attention because of the resultant trauma; moreover, it may be a predisposing cause of postpartal hemorrhage.

In many cases of residual urine the patient is without symptoms other than frequent, scanty urination, but in others there may also be suprapubic or perineal discomfort. The treatment of this condition is usually confined to catheterization after each voiding until the residual urine becomes less than 30 ml; in severe cases constant drainage by means of an indwelling catheter may be employed.

Cystitis

The normal bladder is very resistant to infection, but when stagnant urine remains in a traumatized bladder, and infectious organisms are present, there is danger of cystitis. When cystitis occurs, the patient often has a low-grade fever, frequent and painful urination, and marked tenderness and discomfort over the area of the bladder. A catheterized specimen of urine for microscopic examination is collected, and if pus cells are present in association with residual urine, the diagnosis of cystitis is confirmed. Since it is important in the presence of bladder infection to avoid accumulations of stagnant urine in the bladder, an indwelling bladder catheter may be inserted. In addition, antimicrobial agents are prescribed, and fluids should be forced.

If the infection spreads and involves the ureters and kidneys, the patient has a high fever and chills and a good deal of pain over the affected kidney(s). Diagnosis and treatment for pyelonephritis are essentially the same as for cystitis.

Collection of Urine Specimens

It is the nurse's responsibility to obtain the urine specimens which are used for the microscopic examinations and, occasionally, for cultures. The technique of catheterization already has been discussed in Chapter 30.

However, it may be preferable to avoid catheterization, especially if the mother is having no particular difficulties in voiding. This procedure only enhances the possibility of promoting more infection. Therefore a "clean catch" specimen may be indicated. Different terminology for this procedure exists in various parts of the country, but the procedure is essentially the same. It consists of the collection of a "clean" urine specimen that is uncontaminated by lochia.

One method for this type of collection is as follows:

1. The patient is requested not to void for at least 2 hours and to drink as much fluid as she can in the meantime.
2. Then she is taken to the bathroom (or placed in a sitting position on a bedpan if she cannot ambulate) and the vulva and introitus are cleansed.
3. A large sterile cotton ball is placed over the introitus.
4. The mother is then requested to void a little urine forcefully into the toilet or bedpan, but *not to empty her bladder.*
5. Next, a sterile urine specimen bottle or sterile basin is placed under the stream and a specimen of urine is caught. It is sent to the laboratory for examination.

This method yields very good results with respect to uncontaminated specimens, if done carefully under the continued supervision of the nurse. It avoids the possibility of introducing bacteria into the bladder at the time of catheterization.

Management

Diagnosis of urinary tract infection is confirmed by urine culture. Sensitivity studies are usually performed to identify the appropriate antibiotic for the causative organism. Medication is usually administered orally, except in acute febrile pyelonephritis in which intravenous antibiotics are often used. Symptoms are usually relieved within 24 hours to 48 hours, and treatment is continued for 10 days to 2 weeks. Repeat urine cultures are performed following the course of therapy to be certain the urine is free of organisms.

When indwelling catheters are necessary because of inability to void and residual urine which persists, it has been found that patients with catheters in place for longer than 4 days have a significantly higher incidence of bacteriuria than those whose catheters are removed before this time. Almost all such infections are caused by *E coli.* Therefore, it is recommended that patients with indwelling catheters for longer than 24 hours be treated with suppressive antimicrobial therapy, usually with such antimicrobial drugs as nitrofurantoin, sulfamethoxazole, or ampicillin.[5]

Other Complications

Sheehan's Syndrome

This uncommon complication, also called postpartum anterior pituitary necrosis, occurs in about 15% of women who survive severe hypovolemic shock associated with postpartum hemorrhage. There is loss of function of the pituitary gland, resulting in deficiency in thyroid, adrenocortical, and ovarian functions. Symptoms include failure of lactation, decreased breast size, loss of pubic and axillary hair, genital atrophy, and myxedema in severe cases. Most women never menstruate again, although in less severe cases, there may be occasional ovulation and scanty menses.

Treatment consists of hormone replacement, usually thyroid, cortisone, and estrogen. A high protein diet with ample carbohydrates is prescribed to counteract the typical cachexia. The prognosis depends on the degree of pituitary deficiency, and infertility is usual. Reasonable health can often be maintained with proper hormone replacement, but premature aging frequently results.

Chiari–Frommel Syndrome

This rare condition is characterized by prolonged lactation (galactorrhea) which can occur following normal delivery, whether or not the mother is breast-

Nursing Care: Postpartal Complications

Assessment	Intervention	Evaluation
Physiological assessment		
Vital signs Patterns of temperature elevation Condition of perineum and uterus Character of lochia Tenderness and pain Condition of legs Condition of breasts Status of bladder and voiding	Record and report signs and symptoms Administer medications and treatments Monitor vital signs Monitor fluids and hydration Collect specimens	Vital signs remain stable Afebrile Able to void completely No symptoms of pain, dysuria, malaise, loss of appetite Uterus and lochia normal for stage of involution Breasts normal
Physical comfort		
Rest and sleep Appetite, nutrition, and hydration Pain or discomfort	Provide physical care to promote comfort (*e.g.*, bath, backrub, clean and dry linens, positioning) Enhance fluid and food intake (relaxed atmosphere, preferences) Carry out treatments promptly and efficiently (*e.g.*, sitz baths, medications, dressings)	Able to rest and sleep well Intake of fluids and food adequate Reports relief of pain and discomfort
Psychosocial assessment		
Relation to infant Response to complication Response of partner	Encourage maximum mother–infant contact, provide continuous information on infant Explain and discuss complication, expected course and treatment Involve partner in education about complication, relating to infant, understanding mother's emotional needs, providing support Respond to needs for support and encouragement, working through grief and fear	Assumes as much caretaking of infant as condition permits Maintains interest in infant Understands treatment and expected course of complication Partner understands above, is able to provide support Able to express grief and fear

feeding. There is profuse leakage of fluid from the breasts, with headaches, hearing or visual loss, and genital atrophy. The cause is often unknown, but it may be due to pituitary tumor or prolonged phenothiazine therapy. Gonadotropin and urinary estrogen excretion are reduced or absent. There is no effective treatment, although clomiphene citrate may induce ovulation and menstruation, and abnormal lactation can be suppressed by 2-bromocriptine. Estrogen therapy or oral contraceptives may also control galactorrhea, but symptoms usually recur following discontinuation of medication.

Postpartum Vulvar Edema

An unusual syndrome that is frequently fatal, involves massive perineal edema. In the instances reported, following normal pregnancy, labor, and delivery, in which local or regional anesthesia and episiotomy were used, unilateral perineal edema and induration developed beginning about the second postpartum day. This progressed to generalized vulvar, vaginal, perineal, and gluteal edema and induration. Over 2 days or 3 days, the edema gradually spread to the other side and into the inner pelvis. Fever and marked leukocytosis also occurred, and in those patients who died, there was also vascular collapse. No definite etiology has been found, and while infections were present in some cases, this was not always true. Treatment consisted of various antibiotics, local heat, heparin, steroids and crystalloids, but none was particularly effective. Early recognition of asymmetric vulvar edema, associated with low-grade fever and an elevated white blood count, is recommended as possibly preventing maternal death by aggressive treatment with antibiotics and steroids.[6]

References

1. Benson RC: Current Obstetric and Gynecologic Diagnosis and Treatment, p 764. Los Altos, CA, Lange Medical Publishers, 1978

2. Filker R, Monif GRG: The significance of temperature during the first 24 hours postpartum. Obstet Gynecol 53, 3:358–361, March 1979

3. Eschenbach DA, Wager GP: Puerperal Infections. Clin Obstet Gynecol 23, 4:1003–1037, December 1980

4. Gilstrap LC, Cunningham FG: The bacterial pathogenesis of infection following cesarean section. Obstet Gynecol 53, 5:545–549, May 1979

5. Harris RE: Postpartum urinary retention: Role of antimicrobial therapy. Amer J Obstet Gynecol 133, 2:174–175, January 15, 1979

6. Ewing TL, Smale LE, Elliott FA: Maternal deaths associated with postpartum vulvar edema. Amer J Obstet Gynecol 134, 2:173–179, May 15, 1979

CHAPTER 39

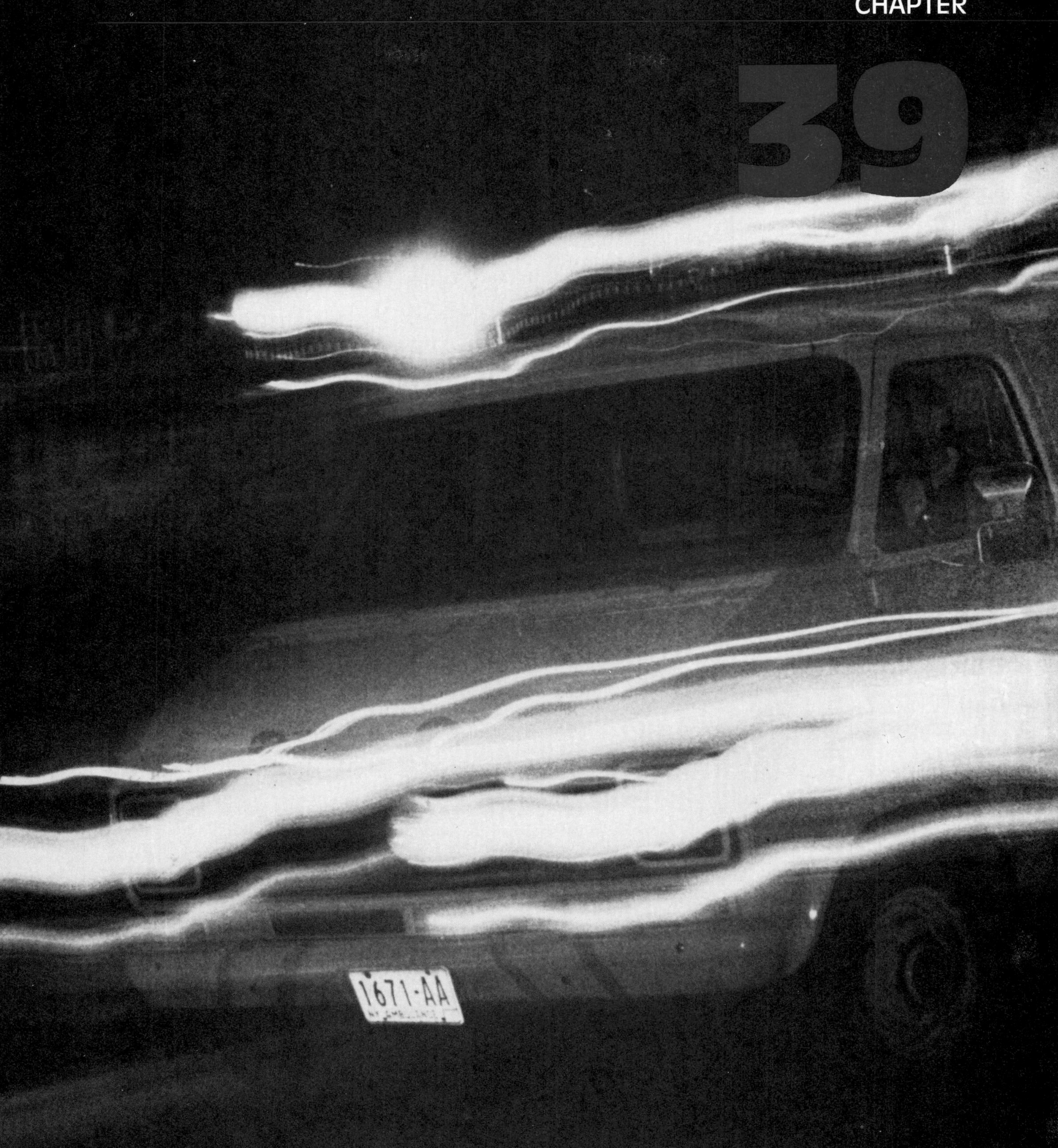

CHAPTER 39

Emergencies in Maternity Practice

Precipitate and Emergency Deliveries

In the course of labor one occasionally encounters the so-called *precipitate* delivery, a rapid spontaneous delivery of less than 3 hours from onset of labor to birth. The infant is generally born without benefit of asepsis. These deliveries tend to occur in certain multiparous women, particularly if the soft parts of the pelvis offer little resistance or if the contractions are unusually strong and forceful. A precipitate delivery can also occur if the mother does not experience the usual discomforting sensations during labor and thus has inadequate warning that the delivery is approaching.

This type of delivery is to be avoided because the mother may suffer lacerations of the tissues as the result of tumultuous labor. Similarly, the infant is endangered because, in its rapid progress through the birth canal, it may suffer cerebral trauma or the umbilical cord may be torn in the process of delivery. Moreover, if the mother is unattended, the infant may be in jeopardy from lack of care during the first few minutes of life.

At other times the labor may not be precipitate, but the laboring woman is far from a hospital or labor is brought on unexpectedly by an unforeseen emergency. Her only attendant may be a member of the family or a nurse. Figure 39-1 illustrates common circumstances that often surround emergency deliveries.

Thus, for those nurses who practice in the area of maternity nursing, a basic working knowledge for providing a safe birth without benefit of the usual institutional supports is crucial. The following review is not meant to minimize the knowledge, skill, and extensive preparation for a fully qualified birth attendant; however, in the absence of such an attendant, a knowledgeable maternity nurse can help to ensure a safe birth and an emotionally satisfying experience for those involved.

It should be stressed that the nurse's composure and ability to convey calm is one of the cornerstones in a successful delivery. Whenever possible, the mother should be told what to anticipate and what she can do to cooperate effectively. Teamwork with the mother is essential and can be accomplished if confidence is instilled by competence in both the physical and emotional aspects of care. If the father is present, he can help care for the mother and infant in whatever capacity seems most appropriate and in accord with his ability. He might be involved directly in some aspect of the delivery or he might help best by taking care of the other children or by calling the physician. If it seems more desirable that he be away from the immediate vicinity, then the reasons for his leaving should be understood by all. He is not to be dismissed summarily from the situation.

General Considerations for Delivery

The Location for Delivery

If the mother is laboring on a delivery table, it is wise *not to break* the table because it takes practice to handle the infant over a dropped table while accomplishing the following three critical objectives:

- Holding the baby close to the introitus to prevent tension and pulling on the cord
- Holding the baby's head down to promote drainage of secretions
- Holding the infant at or above the level of the introitus to prevent transfusion of the baby by gravity flow[1]

If the mother is laboring in a bed or stretcher, there are certain advantages and disadvantages to these conveyances. First, they are generally more comfortable to the mother. Secondly, if the mother remains on them, there is no danger of the infant being born while the mother is being moved to the delivery table. The infant's head cannot be controlled if the actual birth occurs while the mother is in transfer. However, there are certain disadvantages. There

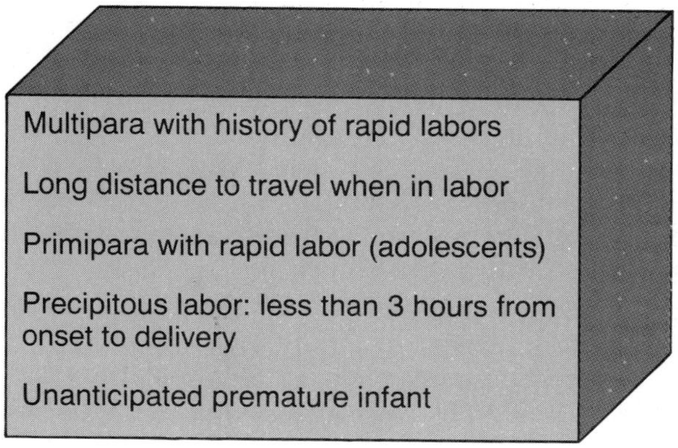

Multipara with history of rapid labors

Long distance to travel when in labor

Primipara with rapid labor (adolescents)

Precipitous labor: less than 3 hours from onset to delivery

Unanticipated premature infant

Figure 39-1.
Common circumstances surrounding emergency deliveries.

may not be sufficient space to deliver the shoulders, especially if the stretcher is narrow and the nurse is inexperienced. Also, the perineum may not be readily visible and it may be difficult to keep the infant's nose and mouth free from the blood and amniotic pool, especially when it comes time for suctioning the infant.

These disadvantages can be overcome by placing an upside down padded bedpan (or similar object) under the mother's hips. This gives about five extra inches of space between the perineum and the bed. If there is no bedpan or similar object available, the nurse can ask the mother to raise her hips by placing her feet firmly on the bed. If this is not feasible, then one or two persons can raise her buttocks a few inches off the bed until the necessary procedures are performed.[1]

Positioning the Mother

The mother's head needs to be elevated about 45° by any means available. If the mother is flat during delivery her vena cava and aorta are compressed and the uteroplacental blood flow is compromised in the supine position. This is likely to result in a hypoxic baby, and in an emergency situation the nurse wants to avoid this circumstance at all costs.

Elevating the head also helps the mother to maintain eye contact with her attendants. This can help allay any fears she might have and help her to see and hear instructions.

Many authorities recommend the lateral Sims position for emergency deliveries because it places the least strain on the perineum and affords the best possible visualization of the birth. It also allows for necessary space for delivering the shoulders.[1,2]

Maintaining Clean Technique

Sterility and asepsis are not priorities since surgery, vaginal intrusion, or the use of instruments is not involved in these deliveries. One must remember that normally the vagina has a high bacterial count and few women have sterile uterine cavities during the postpartum period. Moreover, it is repeated vaginal examinations and cross contamination that are the primary causes of puerperal infection. The infant also does not need to be in a sterile environment after birth.

Hence, the priorities for clean technique are as follows: (1) cleansing the attendant's hands, (2) cleansing the mother's skin, (3) putting on gloves if they are available, (4) placing clean or sterile drapes on the mother if they are available, and (5) preventing fecal contamination of the birth canal and baby.[2]

Priorities in Clean Technique

1. Cleanse attendant's hands
2. Cleanse mother's perineum and thighs
3. Attendant puts on gloves if available
4. Drape mother if drapes available
5. Prevent fecal contamination of birth canal and baby

Protecting the Perineum

It is important that the nurse not perform an episiotomy unless she is legally and professionally qualified to do so. The nurse's greatest contribution is assisting a slow birth of the infant's head (Fig. 39-2). Again, massaging and supporting the perineum may be helpful, but for the inexperienced attendant there are other steps that take priority.[1]

The Delivery

Delivery of the Head

As the head distends the perineum at the acme of a contraction, gentle, even pressure is exerted against the head to control its progress and thereby to prevent undue stretching of the perineum. This kind of *control* applied during each contraction prevents the head from suddenly pushing through the vulva and causing subsequent complications. *The head must never be held back.* The mother should be encouraged to blow through the contraction to deter bearing-down efforts on her part, particularly as the head, which is supported by the nurse, is being delivered. Preferably, the head is delivered between contractions. It is important to remember not to put the fingers into the vagina since this increases the chance of infection. As the head extends upwards, the mouth and nose are wiped gently to remove mucus and fluid.

Rupture of the Membranes

If the membranes have not ruptured previously, they may remain intact until they appear as a smooth, glistening object at the vulva. If they protrude, they may rupture with the next contraction. But if the membranes have not ruptured before the head is delivered, they must be broken and removed immediately (by nipping them at the nape of the infant's neck) to prevent aspiration of fluid when the infant takes its first breath.

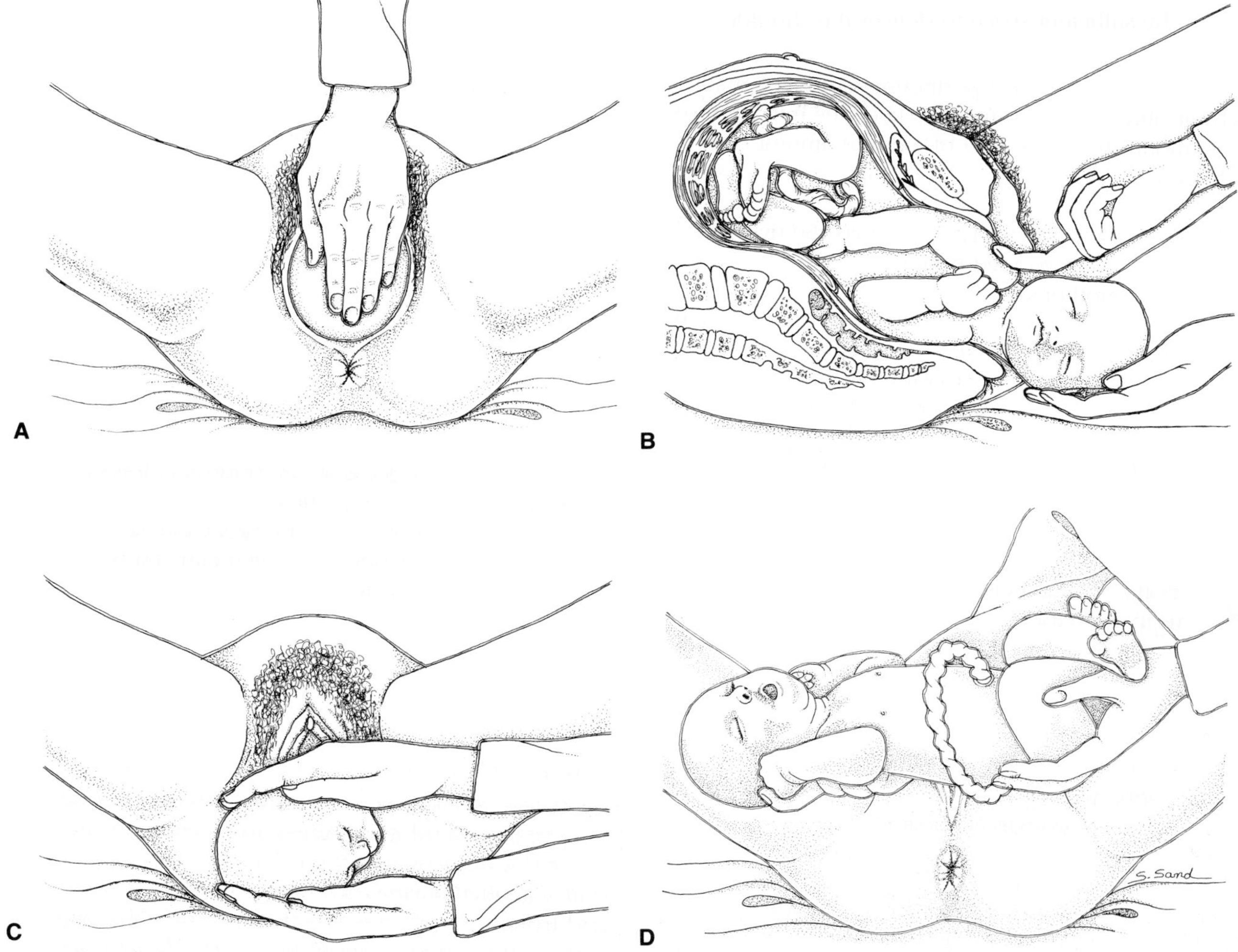

Figure 39-2.
Assisting an emergency birth. *(A)* Apply gentle, even pressure with the flat of your hand, fingers and thumb close together, on the emerging head to slow the baby's progress and protect the mother's perineum. *(B)* While gently supporting the head, during restitution and external rotation, feel around the neck for the umbilical cord, pulling gently to slacken it if necessary. *(C)* Placing palms over baby's ears, apply gentle traction downward until the anterior shoulder appears fully at the introitus; then upward to lift out the other shoulder. *(D)* As the body emerges, slide your hand down the baby's back, cradling the buttocks in one hand, the head and the upper back in the other. Hold the head lower than the trunk.

Precautions Concerning the Cord

As soon as the head is delivered, the nurse should feel for a loop or loops of cord around the neck and, if any is found, gently slip it over the baby's head, if this can be done easily or pull on it gently to slacken it. If the cord is coiled too tightly to permit this, it must be doubly clamped and cut (between the clamps) before the rest of the body is delivered. One or more loops of cord around the fetal neck occur in about a quarter of all deliveries.

Delivery of the Infant's Body

After external rotation of the head, which is usually spontaneous, there is no occasion for haste in the delivery of the body. Gentle downward pressure with the hands on either side of the head, over the ears, may be exerted to direct the anterior shoulder under the symphysis pubis, then reversed upward in order to deliver the posterior shoulder over the perineum. The *posterior* shoulder should be controlled by the nurse's hand. When the axilla of the *anterior* shoulder is seen, the hand is slid along the posterior shoulder to hold the upper arm close to the infant's body to prevent its flapping with delivery and tearing the mother's perineum. The infant's body now follows easily and quickly and should be supported as it is born.

As the body emerges, the nurse can slide her hand down the baby's back, cradling the buttocks in one hand and the head and back in the other. The head is always held lower than the trunk. The infant can then be placed on the mother's abdomen and steadied until she can hold him. She should be helped to keep the head lower than the rest of the body.

Immediate Care of the Infant

After the baby is born the nurse clears the airway of any blood or mucus, holding the infant at the level of the introitus. A bulb syringe is useful for suctioning, but cleansing the *face* with the hand or soft towel can be done if there is no syringe. The mouth or nose should never be invaded with a towel or gauze. Gentle stimulation by rubbing the back as the infant is dried is also helpful to stimulate crying and respiration after the airway is clear. Care should be taken to see that it is clear, since the child only aspirates material into the lungs if encouraged to cry with an occluded airway.

The infant must be kept warm. This is most easily done by having the mother, who should assume a semisitting position, hold the baby skin-to-skin. The pair can then be covered by warmed, dry blankets or several layers of whatever cloth is available. The baby's head should be covered. The mother's body serves as a reliable heat source, and the layers of cloth prevent heat loss through evaporation.[1]

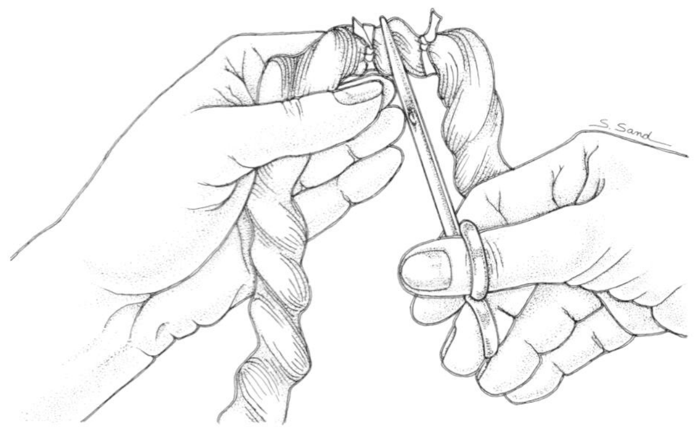

Figure 39-3.
Placement of tapes and scissors for cutting the cord. To prevent the possibility of neonatal tetanus, it is important to use sterile materials.

If necessary, the airway can continue to be cleared and the Apgar can be done. After the airway is cleared, the mother is encouraged to put the baby to breast. Even if the infant only nuzzles or licks rather than sucks, oxytocin is released from the mother's pituitary, which stimulates uterine contractions and aids in the separation of the placenta and prevention of hemorrhage.

Care of the Cord

There is some disagreement in the literature, but most neonatologists advise against encouraging placental transfusions by milking the cord or waiting for the pulsations to cease before clamping the cord. Placental transfusions can lead to hyperviscosity and significant problems for the infant. Thus, most experts recommend clamping the cord at about 1 minute of age.[3,4]

The rate of placental transfusion is dependent on several factors—time, gravity, and constriction of the umbilical vessels. The entire volume of placental blood can be transfused in as little as 3 minutes, depending on the level of the infant in relation to the introitus. Minimal transfusion takes place when the baby is at the level of the mother's breast when she is semirecumbent. Significant and rapid transfusion takes place if the infant is at the level of the introitus or below. Effective constriction of the umbilical arteries occurs by about 45 seconds to 60 seconds. The umbilical vein remains patent somewhat longer.[1]

The nurse needs to remember that only sterile equipment is to be used to clamp and cut the cord. Materials can be boiled in water if no sterile packs are available and can include a Kelly clamp, an umbilical clamp, or tape or boiled shoelaces. If the cord is clamped with unsterile materials, neonatal tetanus can result, which is a highly fatal but preventable condition.[1] Fig. 39-3 illustrates placement of tapes and scissors for cutting the cord. Double loops of tape or laces need to be placed around the cord and secured with at least two square knots. The cord should then be observed frequently for any bleeding.

Delivery of the Placenta

It is important to *wait* for the placenta to separate before attempting to deliver it. More harm is done by injudicious "assistance" than by letting nature take its course. When the signs of placental separation are apparent (see Chap. 24), the mother usually feels another urge to push, have a contraction, or feel pressure in her vagina. The nurse can then lift the placenta from the vagina by holding onto the umbilical cord. Uterine inversion can be guarded against by placing the flat of one hand gently but firmly on the lower abdomen just above the symphysis pubis. Force is not to be used and the placenta can be guided along the curve of Carus (the curved angle from the cervix to the introitus that forms almost the lower fourth of a circle). If the umbilical cord is held near the introitus, it is less likely to break or tear than if held further back.[1]

The membranes may trail behind the placenta and can be teased out with a gentle up, down, and out motion. When all material is delivered, the uterus can be massaged gently to maintain firmness and to help the uterine vessels constrict down. Vigorous or continuous massage is to be avoided to prevent muscle fatigue or prolapse or inversion of the uterus (see Chap. 24).

Continuing Care for Mother and Infant

When the infant is breathing satisfactorily, he can remain skin-to-skin with the mother and the pair is covered with warmed dry, clean covers if they are available. It is important to be sure the infant's head is covered because that is his largest body area and heat dissipates very readily with no covering. Later, if clean clothes are available for the infant, he can be dressed after the vernix and birth secretions are *wiped* away. There is no need under emergency conditions to attempt to bathe the infant. The infant can also be allowed to nurse at will.

As stated earlier, it is important that the nurse proceed slowly and carefully through the delivery. Her reaction to the situation provides a role model to the mother and family. If she remains poised and unfaltering, those whom she is attending are more likely to do likewise.

Large-Scale Disasters

When any large-scale emergency arises, it is usually sudden and calls for immediate action, whether it is caused by earthquake, hurricane, flood, fire, or war. In the event of such a catastrophe, babies are likely to be born rapidly, and many woman may abort. When organized rescue work is hampered, it may fall to those who are in the immediate area to manage as best they can. The nurses in the area need to be able to assist with measures for the safety and the welfare of maternity patients and their newborn infants.

All nurses who have completed the basic course in maternity nursing are familiar with antepartal care, the conduct of labor, and the immediate care of the newborn infant, but their preparation has been carried out, for the most part, in an organized environment, such as a hospital, where supplies, equipment, and medical direction are available. It requires considerable imagination on the part of the nurse to conceive of an emergency situation in which she might be required to work without the availability of these facilities. Yet in any large-scale disaster, whole communities may be isolated and left to their own resources when telephone and radio communications are wrecked; roads may become impassable if they are inundated by water and blocked by debris, and an area may be without safe water, means of power and light, and medical supplies.

Commonalities of Disaster Situations

It has been established that all disaster emergencies have certain similarities and differ only in scope, intensity, and effect.[5] It has also been demonstrated that there are usually two kinds of people remaining, those who *need* help and those who *are able* to help. It is safe to assume that in any extreme, large-scale emergency, the medical-health requirements of the surviving population leads to an unprecedented need for hospital space (improvised if necessary) and for skilled professionals to care for the ill and injured and to keep the well well.

In extreme disaster conditions nursing care is usually administered on an austere basis, but still, whenever possible, in accordance with established medical principles designed to save life, prevent the spread of disease, alleviate suffering, and promote recovery. If the emergency is dire but confined to an area, the resources and manpower of the unaffected regions can be brought to bear upon the situation, thus allowing all health care to proceed along the above lines. In the case of a thermonuclear holocaust involving a whole nation, survival will depend on self- and buddy-help, with only life-sustaining care provided by the necessarily limited resources that must be conserved for a prolonged period.

Every responsible practitioner will want to familiarize herself with basic emergency and disaster nursing techniques (see Suggested Reading). It is important to remember, however, that the required knowledge and skills for nursing under these conditions are essentially the same as those required in daily patient care; *only the priorities change.* Thus, treatment will be based on available personnel, drugs, supplies, and equipment.

Nuclear Disaster

This type of catastrophe is given particular attention because of all the disaster situations, it is without a doubt the most severe. The medical and health problems that arise from it require special physical facilities and particular attention with respect to modification of priorities.

The early 1950s brought a threat of actual thermonuclear war. In subsequent decades, concern turned from actual bombing and the consequent Hiroshima-type devastation to concern about fallout from possible radioactive accidents from the nuclear power plants being built around the country. Now with the advent of the neutron bomb, which kills populations by radiation, but does less damage to property, there is again heightened concern for the effects from both bombing and radiation fallout.[6,7] For more indepth discussion of the devastation at Hiroshima and the problems of the present-day survivor, as well as the reactions of the inhabitants of the Three Mile Island nuclear accident, the student is referred to the articles by Wert, and McClelland and Isler in the Suggested Reading.

Fallout Shelters

As previously stated, the advent of the nuclear age and the continuing development of nuclear weaponry brought with it not only the possibility of war, but also the risk of nuclear accidents and the hazards of radioactive fallout. To meet these contingencies, the United States Government enacted the Federal Civil Defense Act in 1950; each state followed with similar legislation soon after. Thus, Civil Defense has come to represent government in emergency and its guiding principle is that disaster preparedness is a responsibility of each citizen, assisted by the local, state, and federal government. Original civil defense planning provided for mass casualty care which used emergency medical facilities that could be mobilized in a short time. With the threat of fallout, however, concepts changed and attention turned to providing shelter against radiation for as many persons as possible. These "fallout" shelters were marked and stocked with emergency equipment by the federal government. Supplies included survival biscuits, water, sanitation kits, and basic medical supplies sufficient to provide for total capacity of the shelter and to last 14 days. Each community was responsible for providing any additional supplies it could to make living more comfortable.[8]

These shelters received scant attention in the 1970s, and it is unclear at this time how they might be used, if at all. If, however, it appears that the threat of nuclear disaster is real, they will no doubt be reactivated for service.

The ABGs of radiation

Radioactivity—The process of spontaneous disintegration of an atom's nucleus, resulting in the emission of radiation in the form of alpha, beta, and gamma rays. Alpha rays are positively charged and beta rays are negatively charged. Gamma rays, more penetrating than either of the others, are emitted in electromagnetic radiation (like x-rays), and in nuclear accidents.

X-ray—A form of energy produced when high-speed electrons collide abruptly with an object.

Roentgen—A unit of x-ray exposure in air.

Rad—The standard unit of "radiation absorbed dose." (Equivalent to the rem for gamma rays and electrons.)

Millirad—One thousandth of a rad.

Rem (Roentgen equivalent man)—A unit of measurement of the biological effectiveness of a given radiation dose. (Equivalent to the rad for gamma rays and electrons).

Average exposure (in rems) in one year—Estimated to be about 100 millirems to 200 millirems, from sources including the sun, cosmic rays, television sets, and diagnostic x-rays. One chest x-ray, depending on the equipment and technique used, yields 30 millirems to 60 millirems exposure.

Permissible levels of exposure (as established by the National Council on Radiation Protection and Measurement)

General population—500 millirems per year

Nuclear plant workers—up to 5000 millirems (5 rems) per year

Hospital personnel working with radionuclides—3000 millirems (3 rems) per 13 weeks. Maximum permissible lifetime rem exposure, however, is determined by using the formula 5(N-18), where N is the age of the individual. For example, a 30-year-old nurse could receive 5(30-18) rems—a total of 60 rems—during her lifetime, including the average number of rems received from nonwork related sources. The radiation safety officer in each hospital's nuclear medicine department should keep records of each employee's exposure, to insure that the maximum permissible limit is not exceeded.

(Isler C: Could you cope with a nuclear accident? RN June 1979)

"In the event of radiation exposure . . ."

The following protocol for handling victims of radiation contamination and poisoning is based on the emergency plan of New York's Mount Sinai Hospital. It is the responsibility of the senior Emergency Department staff member on duty, on receipt of notification of the momentary arrival of a case involving radiation exposure or contamination, to do the following:

1. **Notify the responsible staff physician or radiation safety officer** (trained health physicist or trained technician from the Nuclear Medicine or X-ray Department). When the responsible person is not on duty, the administrator should be notifed so he can contact the responsible person.

2. **Obtain an appropriate survey meter** from the Radiation Safety Office; if the office is closed, Security has keys to it. When a meter is removed from the office, a note must be left indicating who has it and where it can be found. If no survey meter can be procured in the hospital, notify the administrator or radiation safety officer, so that equipment can be obtained from the Police Department.

When the Patient Arrives at the Hospital

3. **Check the patient for contamination** while he is on the stretcher (preferably as the stretcher is being removed from the ambulance), and perform a survey of his clothing and the ambulance, before undertaking any other activity or bringing the patient inside the hospital.

4. **If clothing is contaminated, place in a special container marked "Radioactive—Do Not Discard."** Handle contaminated patient and objects as in surgical procedures, using gown, gloves, cap, mask, *etc.*

5. **Notify the hospital administrator** so he may seek expert professional consultation for technical management of the case.

6. **Prepare a separate examining room or outside hallway** immediately adjacent to the entrance to the Emergency Department. Cover the floor—in an area adequate for the stretcher-cart, disposal hampers, and working space—with absorbent paper. Mark and close off this area. If dust is involved, be prepared to shut off air circulation system to prevent spread of contamination.

When the Patient is Brought into the Examination Treatment Area

7. **If seriously injured,** give emergency lifesaving assistance immediately.

8. **If possible external contamination is involved** save all clothing, bedding from ambulance, blood, urine, stool, vomitus, and other objects (*e.g.,* jewelry, belt buckles, dental plates). Label with patient's name, body location, time, and date. Save in containers marked "Radioactive—Do Not Discard."

9. **Begin decontamination,** if medical status permits, with cleansing and scrubbing of the areas highest in contamination first. If an extremity alone is involved, clothing may serve as an effective barrier; the affected limb should still be scrubbed. Initial cleansing should be done with soap and hot water. If the body as a whole is involved or if clothing is generally permeated, showering and scrubbing is necessary. Pay special attention to hair, body orifices, and body folds. Remeasure with survey meter and record measurement after each washing or showering.

10. **If a wound is involved, prepare and cover it with self-adhering disposable surgical drape.** Cleanse neighboring skin surfaces. Seal off cleansed areas with self-adhering disposable surgical drapes. Remove wound covering and irrigate wound with sterile water, catching the irrigating fluid in a basin or can to be marked as above. Each step in the decontamination process should be preceded and followed by monitoring and recording of the location and extent of contamination.

11. **Save physicians', nurses', and attendants' scrub or protective clothing** as described for patients. Staff must follow the same monitoring and decontamination procedures as the patients.

12. **If confronted with a grossly contaminated wound** (dirt particles and crushed tissue), the physician in attendance should be prepared to do a preliminary simple wet debridement. Further measurements may necessitate use of sophisticated wound counting detection instruments supplied by the consultant, who advises further definitive debridement when necessary.

Standing Orders

When the accident has occurred at a plant, university, or medical unit that regularly works with nuclear material, the health physicist or supervisor, a co-worker, or the patient should be able to inform the rescue squad of the nature of the accident, type of radiation exposure or radioactive contamination involved, and possible body areas that may be affected.

Isler C: Could you cope with a nuclear accident? RN June 1979

The Packaged Disaster Hospital

These hospitals are units stored at various sites throughout the country. They contain sufficient supplies to set up an emergency disaster hospital and keep it in operation for 30 days. There is an admitting and sorting area (triage), operating rooms, wards, an x-ray, a laboratory, a pharmacy, and a central supply. In addition, each hospital has its own generators, water pump, and storage tank. The hospitals belong to the federal government and are loaned to various states for use primarily in nuclear emergency. Community medical-health and government leaders are responsible for the storage of the hospital unit, and unless otherwise arranged, are also responsible for preparing its use.

Packaged disaster hospitals are used in major emergencies to augment existing hospital facilities or to establish independent hospital facilities. It is planned that in the case of a nuclear catastrophe, these units will be in the forefront when the stage of postshelter rehabilitation is begun. There is no way to predict the conditions under which this type of hospital will be used. However, any disaster of the magnitude requiring its activation is bound to make severe demands on the staff. Hours will be long and staff and supplies short. The basic objective of an emergency unit of this type is to assist in meeting the health needs of the surviving population. The actual situation may vary from *early activation* with a large number of traumatic injury casualties to *delayed activation* with less injuries but more illness. These units must conserve their resources and so casualties will undergo triage by a physician and appropriate ancillary personnel who will establish priorities for patient care and the possible methods of treatment.

While each packaged unit has its own basic supplies, the continued use as well as the general functioning of the unit depends on services originating in the community. These would include such things as ambulance and transportation services, communication facilities, decontamination capabilities, refuse and body waste disposal, mortuary services, and food and laundry facilities. The organization and activation of these units will depend on full cooperation and coordination with other hospitals and community services within the area.[8]

Additional Support Facilities

In the immediate thermonuclear postdisaster period, nurses will also be needed in a variety of other places. One of these is the Field Aid Points which are simple fixed or temporary facilities where the sick and injured are taken to receive initial treatment. They serve as a collecting area where patients can be held until transportation to a Principal First Aid Station or hospital can be provided. It is in these reception areas (and also in the Principal First Aid Stations) that the majority of pregnant women and infants will be cared for if there is time for evacuation. These areas may be located anywhere that is commensurate with existing conditions—homes, stores, or even street corners. The Principal First Aid Stations also may be fixed or temporary, but treatment is administered under the direction of professional doctors, nurses, and allied personnel. These stations are usually located in shelter areas, schools, churches and other substantial buildings if they are available. These units will administer to the surviving population as well as the immediate casualties.

Mass Care Centers are planned for refugees who are homeless or unable to return to their residence. Workers who are engaged in rehabilitation activities will also be allowed to share these facilities. Recuperation centers will be located on college campuses, motels, or homes where simple convalescent bed and ambulatory care can be readily available without requiring the services of a full-time nursing staff. Thus, in all disasters, nurses find themselves with a dual responsibility of citizen and skilled professional. We must not only be prepared to contribute to the community's disaster preparedness, but we must also enhance our own survival chances through knowledge and preparedness.[8]

Organization of Disaster Nursing Services in the Hospital

As we know, more conventional disasters strike with little if any warning, and a hospital's emergency department must be prepared to face almost any situation. Definitions of disaster vary. Some disaster authorities define a major accident as having occurred when there are 50 or more living casualties. From a hospital's point of view, a disaster or emergency occurs when, with no warning, more casualties of varying severity arrive than the hospital is prepared or staffed to handle at that particular time.

With all the attendant noise, confusions, horror, and tragedy of a disaster, there is no time to begin planning the management of mass casualties. Thus, planning must have been carried out beforehand and be in readiness.

The following paragraphs provide an outline of one suggested plan that has proven successful.

The Alert

When such facilities are available, the emergency or accident service usually has the responsibility of alerting the rest of the hospital; the message can be conveyed to the hospital telephone operator by some person designated as the alerting or casualty officer. Hospitals that do not have specific emergency room facilities per se can set aside some room that might serve this purpose. If the physical plant is such that this is impossible, these hospitals might act as "overflow" facilities for those casualties who are not so badly injured.

When the various wards of the hospital are alerted, the following information about the disaster needs to be given: the type of disaster, where and when it took place, the number of casualties involved, and the nature of the injuries. The hospital's preparation for multiple injury cases from a plane crash, for instance, differs from that required for a large number of burned patients or casualties suffering from smoke inhalation or exposure to cold.

The Phased Response

The casualty officer (person designated to give the alert) is responsible for deciding the level of response initially required by the hospital to cope with the disaster. For instance, a Phase 1 response might be designed to cope with an internal disaster affecting the hospital itself, such as fire, explosion, or bomb threat. A Phase 2 response might cope with a small number of casualties involving just the emergency room facilities. Finally, a Phase 3 response alerts and mobilizes the entire hospital to deal with a classic disaster.[5]

The Disaster Chest

Once a disaster has been declared, the nurse or other member of the staff in charge (and there should be a special person so designated) goes to the "disaster chest," which is easily identifiable and contains all the necessary documents and equipment for organizing the emergency service. Some item of identification, an armband, badge, and the like, must be available for the disaster officer to wear. This is also appropriate for any of her deputies, as many bottlenecks and disorganization are created by not being able to identify appropriate personnel in charge of activities. In addition to the identifying material, each box ought to contain a number of "action" cards which incorporate written information, advice, and instruction for members of the nursing staff. Standard 5″ × 8″ cards can be used for basic instructions; for more complicated diagrams, larger cards may be necessary. These instructions need to be clear, short, and unambiguous.[5]

Basic Contents of a Disaster Chest

- Applicator sticks
- Armbands (medical)
- Baking soda
- Bandages (adhesive, gauze roller, head, muslin roller, triangular)
- Basins (emesis)
- Bedpans
- Blankets (disposable, fireproof, and waterproof)
- Cotton (absorbent)
- Cups (paper)
- Dressings (tubular gauze, 4 × 4s and other sizes)
- Eyepads (adult and child sizes)
- Instrument sets (4 hemostats, 1 tissue forceps, 1 scissors)
- Matches (safety)
- Muslin (uncut)
- Paper toweling
- Pencils (indelible, red and white skin-marking)
- Pitchers (2-quart)
- Safety pins
- Salt (table)
- Sanitary pads, binders, or belts
- Scissors
- Soaps (hand, tincture of green soap)
- Splints (basswood)
- Swabs (alcohol)
- Tags (medical)
- Tape (adhesive)
- Tongue depressors
- Tourniquets
- Twine

The contents of the disaster chest are described above.[9] These chests and their contents are also suitable for transfer to the scene of a disaster (with suitable action cards) if it is advisable to give emergency treatment at the scene. Hospital and civil disaster officials caution against including drugs, particularly narcotics, in the disaster chest, even when it is to be used exclusively in the hospital, because they are subject to theft and deterioration. Arrangements can be made to assure that local physicians, hospitals, police, and ambulance and rescue teams provide drugs at the disaster scene if the chest is to be transported there.

Triage or Casualty Sorting

The process of casualty sorting in the saving of lives bears repeating here. The aim of this endeavor is to identify those casualties whose lives can be saved by the early application of medical skills and resuscitation procedures and to concentrate available medical and nursing resources on these people. An experienced physician is appointed as triage officer and as each casualty is brought in, he is rapidly assessed and assigned one of the following priorities: Priority 1—these individuals can easily die and may need blood transfusions, plasma infusions for burns, or surgery soon to close cavity wounds. Laboring women, especially if wounded, are assigned to this category and the delivery as well as treatment of injuries is given first priority. Priority 2—these casualties are unlikely to die immediately or soon from the injuries sustained. Pregnant women who are not in labor may be given this priority unless they are wounded or some complication is anticipated. Priority 3—these persons are obviously dying from the injuries sustained.

It has been suggested that Priority 2 patients be given first aid, and then be left in the care of first aiders until more help can be given. After Priority 1 casualties have been attended to and when resources permit, attention can then be redirected to Priority 2 casualties. Those who are dying need to be offered comfort and compassion by auxiliary personnel but not by medical and nursing personnel, whose efforts need to be directed toward saving the lives of those who can be helped.[10]

Primary Treatment Areas

Several kinds of facilities are needed; they may have to be improvised. The *resuscitation rooms* must be close to the ambulance entrance and suitably equipped so that hemorrhage can be controlled, airways established by tracheostomy if necessary, and fractures supported and stabilized. Once the patient has been resuscitated he can be reassessed and moved to another treatment area as quickly as possible.

In the *urgent treatment area,* wounds are covered, splints are applied, shock is treated, and patients are prepared for later care. Operation priorities are made before the patients leave this area. In the *nonurgent treatment area,* which may include the *ambulatory casualty area,* patients are received for care of minor wounds, burns, and simple fractures. Special provision is made for those with minimal or no injuries who are suffering from the effects of emotional shock. If a woman is near term or is having any cramping, she may be held in the ambulatory area until further assessment can be made.

It is recommended that two registered nurses staff each of these areas, one of whom has some experience with disaster nursing. In addition, two nurses need to help the triage officer, while the casualty officer supervises the total operation. Nursing auxiliary personnel or volunteers can escort patients to other parts of the hospital.[5,10]

Some communities have instituted a mobile Disaster Nurse Corps whose members go to the scene of a disaster and carry out most of the procedures described above. Working with physicians and other paramedical personnel, they are able to render lifesaving care to many victims whose injuries would have been compounded by improper handling.[10]

Disaster Protection for Mothers and Infants

Insuring the lives and health of pregnant women and their newborn during national or extensive local disasters requires planning that is predicated on the belief that detailed plans and preparations prior to these events are essential and imperative.

In planning for the safeguarding of mothers and newborn infants prior to a disaster, certain assumptions can be made and specific factors considered. Pregnant women will be subject to all of the risks and injuries to which men and nonpregnant women will be exposed. Their general care needs to be in accordance with provisions made for the population at large However, their obstetrical care does require additional planning and facilities, for it should be separate from hospital and emergency facilities for casualties if possible. Two lives are at stake, lives of particular importance to the future of the country. The need for care of the pregnant woman is predictable, since sooner or later she must inevitably be delivered, and in the process will need medical attention to a greater or lesser extent. In the vast majority of instances, probably in 90% of all cases, the birth process, whether it results in a viable infant or abortion, will be essentially uncomplicated. The most formidable complications to be encountered with any frequency will be hemorrhage, obstructed or prolonged labor, infection, and mild and severe toxemias of pregnancy and miscellaneous medical and surgical conditions accompanying pregnancy.

It is estimated that at any given time approximately 2% of the total population will consist of women in various stages of pregnancy. In applying this prevalence rate to a given geographic area, allowance must be made for the character of the area because the rate will, of course, be affected by the presence of large industrial plants and offices employing large numbers of males.

If the foregoing concepts are accepted and remain valid in disaster planning, what then should be the planning for minimal essential care for mothers and newborn infants in disaster situations? To the extent that it is possible, the facilities that are normally available for pregnant women during the antepartal, delivery, and postpartal periods should be available.

However, we have learned from experience that in the event of large-scale catastrophes, such as tornados, hurricanes, floods, or bombings, these facilities may not be functioning. Therefore, adequate preparation for the care of mothers and babies during a disaster, particularly a large-scale one, requires that thought be given and plans be made for the training of families for their own protection and survival. This is especially true for the pregnant woman and her family. Thus, a large percentage of the population needs to be trained to carry out minimal essentials of care (buddy system) to save the lives of other people.

As we have said, it can be assumed that in any major disaster, physicians, nurses, and other specially trained professional personnel will be almost completely absorbed in the task of caring for casualties; normal women in labor at such times will have to rely largely on nonprofessional personnel for their needs. Just who will these nonprofessional people be? They will have to be other women who have received instruction in the procedures described. In other words, each community should contain a corps of laywomen who understand the basic concepts contained in this brief review and have been given at least minimal training in providing this type of care. Preparation for disaster is a family affair. Every citizen and every family need to have the information necessary to protect the individual, the family, and the community well in advance of a disaster or an enemy attack. Those responsible for planning and implementing disaster plans have the unique responsibility for making this information available to individuals in communities in a way that they can understand and accept.

The only hope we have for the saving of lives of mothers and newborn infants depends on the family's ability to carry out the plans made with and for them.

Hence, every expectant mother needs to know her physician's expectation of the kind of delivery she will have, so that if she needs any special facilities, she will be able to go where these are available. She needs to understand the care she and her baby will need during delivery and immediately afterward.

There are differences of opinion about how much information pregnant women should have about their own condition and the conduct and outcome of the delivery. It is assumed that in the event of large-scale disasters, women will have to carry much of the responsibility for their own safety. Therefore, adequate information about what to do, where to go, and what constitutes essential equipment will be comforting to them rather than alarming.

Essential Equipment

Essential equipment is quite minimal and is available to almost every woman in her own home. A package should be made up and kept accessible with other emergency supplies if the area is disaster prone. Contents include a clean sheet, towels, washcloth, and soap; blankets, clothing, a nipple and a bottle for the baby; a pair of blunt scissors; two pieces of clean linen tape, 6 in long and ¼ in wide, separately wrapped from the other articles; and a package of powdered milk for the mother. A 72-hour supply of bottled drinking water is also imperative. A can of powdered infant formula is also good insurance in the event that the establishment of lactation is delayed.

Emergency Obstetrical Equipment for Pregnant Women

- Clean sheet
- Clean towels, washcloth, soap
- Blankets
- Clothing
- Bottle and nipple for infant
- Blunt scissors
- Two pieces of clean linen tape (6 in long, ¼ in wide) or white shoe laces, separately wrapped
- Package of powdered milk for mother
- Can of powdered infant formula in case lactation is delayed

Meeting the Pregnant Disaster Victim's Needs

Those who are giving care to pregnant women need to understand that the pregnant woman's normal dependent needs may be greatly enhanced by separation from and concern for her husband and family and by increased fear for herself and her baby. Understanding in meeting this exaggerated need for mothering and providing a warm accepting environment increases the confidence of the pregnant woman in her ability to have her baby and comforts her and relieves some of her fear and apprehension. Every effort needs to be made to have someone with the patient throughout labor. The emotional support which patients in labor (who have had some preparation) derive from each other should be used.

Preparations for Impending Labor and Delivery

There are certain preparations for impending labor or abortion that can be made in the immediate period of evacuation. As quickly as possible after a shelter, Field Aid Point or First Aid Station is occupied, all pregnant women should be registered and the expected date of birth recorded. As we stated previously, the nurse may be the only health professional on the scene; in that event she may want to delegate this activity to someone who appears able to carry it through *accurately.* The pregnant women of special concern are those who are in labor or expecting at any time, those who are expecting within a week or two, and those who have had difficulty with previous confinements or who have reason to expect difficulty by reason of disease or abnormalities. *They should be apprised of these facts by their physicians.*

The nurse can assign someone to assist the laboring mother. In all probability, the nurse will be too occupied with other activities to assist herself if she is the only health professional. The attendant is to be informed of the expected date of birth and any information that the mother may have learned during her prenatal care. In addition, the nurse will need to instruct the attendant in the course of labor and the activities necessary at the time of birth. A delivery area can be selected away from the general living or gathering area if space permits. It should be prepared with respect to quiet, warmth or coolness, cleanliness, available supplies, and equipment. The mother will need a clean surface to lie on for the actual delivery. Clean plastic material or paper can be used for padding the actual delivery bed. The mother will need clean towels or a clean garment or sheet. A warmer covering such as a sweater, jacket, or blanket is also desirable. Hopefully, she will have brought these articles for the baby with her. The infant's crib can be improvised from a carton and lined with any suitable material (*e.g.,* paper or a blanket) available. It goes without saying that the mother's confidence may be temporarily shattered, but her courage may not be. If the nurse can convey that although conditions may be very austere, labor and delivery can progress normally, she will do much toward helping the mother mobilize her resources to proceed through labor. The nurse will instruct the mother or attendant to report the first evidence of the onset of labor. This will usually give enough time to make the immediate preparations for delivery.

Essentials of care during labor and delivery do not differ significantly from those described early in the chapter.

Continuing Care

Mother and newborn baby can be considered an inseparable unit. If a mother cannot take care of her baby, full-time mothering care must be provided to enhance the baby's chances of survival and to promote his well-being. Irregularities in breathing, mucus in air passages, weak sucking reflex, skin irritation, and unstable temperature-regulating mechanism point to the importance of constant observation and an environment adapted to meet the needs of the individual infant.

Breast-feeding is preferable. The infant may be put to breast immediately after birth and as necessary thereafter until the milk supply is established. Once the milk supply is sufficient to satisfy the baby, feedings are given as often as necessary to meet the need. Artificial feedings may be necessary in instances in which the mother is unable to nurse. Formula may be prepared from powdered infant formula or dried skim milk immediately prior to feeding, as there will be no refrigeration facilities. If a bottle and nipple are unavailable, the baby can suck on a teaspoon placed on his lower lip, or milk can be dropped on the inside of the cheek with a medicine dropper. The formula does not have to be heated. Disposable diapers are preferred, but sheets substitute nicely. Of course, any absorbent material can be used if these are not available.

The newborn is particularly susceptible to infection. Anyone with any evidence of infection, such as rash, diarrhea, or upper respiratory infection, should not give infant care.

When the infant is found to be premature and in need of special care, or to have congenital malformations, the emergency facilities that have been developed for such conditions can be used.

When the mother and infant are to be discharged from the place where care has been given during labor and delivery, it is important for arrangements to be made with the family and others for the mother to be relieved of responsibilities, except the care of her baby and herself, if possible. The mother, the family, and the attendant should know where and whom to call if she or the baby have any conditions or symptoms that need medical care.

To increase the number of people with some training in the care of pregnant women and newborn infants, existing educational programs need to be expanded. These include mother and baby care classes, such as those given by the Red Cross and other health agencies, parent education groups, home nursing classes, first-aid training, classes for baby sitters and junior and senior high school students, and midwifery training programs. Planning for training and the achievement of the training of persons who carry this responsibility in a disaster are not easy.

During a disaster, it is assumed that it will be the responsibility of nurses and certified nurse–midwives to carry on an intensive program of on-the-job training of whoever is available to help and to supervise the care of mothers and babies.[11,12]

Psychological Reactions in Emergency Situations

It has been found that in disaster, human behavior, like human behavior in other life situations, falls into fairly predictable patterns. Since the nurse's role is so vital in the event of disaster, she will need to have knowledge of these reactions because coping with large numbers of persons suffering massive emotional shock will become every bit as important as rendering help for physical trauma and illness. Moreover, it will help the nurse to better understand her own responses to the catastrophe.

Periods of a Disaster

For purposes of our analysis, disaster can be said to have various periods. These may include a prodromal or warning period, an impact period, an immediate-reaction period, and finally, a delayed-response period. During these segments there are characteristic modes of behavior that people may exhibit.

In the *prodromal or warning period* certain persons tend to demonstrate disorganized or destructive behavior. They mill around, disobey instructions, break things, or lash out at anyone getting in their way. Others, however, are able to function in the face of even grave personal danger incredibly effectively; still others become immobilized and, for all practical purposes, helpless.

Some of the above individuals may respond to the warning signals as if catastrophe had already occurred and demonstrate a penchant for ineffective action. These persons fall into two general groups. The first are those who have been through a similar experience before in which they were helpless and have developed a subsequent fear or helpless response to disaster or its warnings. The second group is those who always become helpless in any dangerous or frightening situation. These persons often present a difficult problem for helping personnel because if left to themselves, they often precipitate wild panic in others due to their own panicky behavior. They need to be taken aside and given definite tasks to do, no matter how simple. Clear, brief instructions, and frequent reassurance help these people to regain control of their emotions.[13]

At the *impact period,* almost everyone will experience many frightening feelings, no matter how adequate the training or drilling; thus, there will be at least some period of confusion. This is especially true in the case of an emergency in which there is no warning, such as a dam breaking, a sudden explosion, or an electrical storm. Many respond with physical signs and symptoms. They may exhibit shortness of breath, rapid pulse, and respiration, trembling, sweating and so on. Adequate anticipatory training and drilling have been found to shorten the period of this uncontrolled activity, thus reducing the confusion period.

The *immediate reaction period* after impact is most crucial. Noneffective behavior at this point exacts a heavy toll in terms of the lives and well-being of the survivors. On the other hand, effective action will save lives, diminish disability, reduce abnormal behavior, and decrease the confusion immeasurably. It is imperative that normal behavior be resumed as quickly as possible, not only for each individual's personal safety but also to assure help for those unable to act because of an injury.

Immediately following impact, especially in a disaster of any magnitude, almost all persons will be unable to think, move, or express concern, although given a reasonable length of time, most will make a tremendous effort to adjust. Some will manage this more quickly than others, and they will have to help their slower brethren in their adjustments. Help will usually be available from the relatively uninjured since professionals are often not available, as we have stressed. Thus, it is wise for the less able to team with those who appear more able; the buddy system is more effective and often invaluable.[13]

The *delayed response period* begins when the immediate danger has passed. Groups often unite for mutual protection and it is at this period that the less acutely affected psychological casualties can be salvaged. It is important to remember that minimal attention may be all that is needed, but it *must be given* and *given early* in this period. Those afflicted are often highly suggestible and will follow almost any advice or take cues for action from the behavior of others. This can be a double-edged sword, for while they respond well to instructions and reassurances, they also tend to become infected easily with anxiety and panic, and will, in turn, precipitate panic reactions in others if they are not carefully watched. It is important at this time for all to realize that the menace has passed; thus, verbal reinforcement and reiteration are important. Valuable information can also be conveyed by signs and facial expressions to aid individuals in achieving some measure of security.[13]

Types of Behavior

We have spoken of the different periods in a disaster and of some of the general behavior that might be exhibited. It is important at this point to expand on the various types of behavior that can be demonstrated in response to danger or threat in general.

Normal Reactions

Apparent calmness, at least for a time, is a normal reaction during disaster. More usually seen, however, are physical or body manifestations such as sweating, trembling, weakness, or rapid pulse. Included here also are nausea, vomiting, and diarrhea of a temporary nature. Confusion, crying, and immobilization of a short duration are not uncommon and can still be classified as "normal." The ability and the length of time required to collect oneself with or without help seem to be the most likely criteria for classification in the "normal" category.[13]

Abnormal Reactions

When the above reactions become prolonged or incapacitating, the individual condition is thought of as more serious. "Conversion hysteria" can occur in which the person unconsciously converts his massive fear into a belief that some part of his body has ceased to function. And in fact, the organ does not function in spite of the fact that no organic damage can be demonstrated. These people cannot be treated as malingerers or "fakers." Since the disability is at the level of the unconscious, the person is as truly disabled as if he had had physical injury to the limb or organ. Nausea and vomiting arising from emotional origins are also seen in prolonged and incapacitating cases. Difficulty arises in diagnosis because these symptoms are indicative of radiation sickness also. Moreover, the person may interpret his symptoms as due to radiation exposure. Problems of isolation and decontamination multiply. These cases tax both the diagnostic astuteness and the emotional reserve of those dealing with them.

Panic and Depression

Somewhere between the normal reactions and the gross abnormal reactions fall panic and depressed and overactive responses. Panic is not expressed as frequently as one might expect, but its danger lies in its contagiousness. It can spread and cause a mass headlong flight of a crowd. Persons in the grip of this phenomenon often crush and trample one another as they are driven by a compulsion to flee. Purposeless uncontrolled motor behavior is indicative of a panic stage; it is evidenced by such behavior as uncontrolled weeping and running around. Sheer horror, such as the sight of maimed family, or the belief that avenues of escape are being blocked are the two most frequent precipitating conditions. Helping to move indviduals and a crowd away from the presenting danger *in an orderly fashion* is the best preventive for this phenomenon.

Depressed reactions are characterized by a general slowing down of motor and mental processes. Persons sit and stare; they seem numb and confused. They do not respond when spoken to or if they do, it is with monosyllables. These individuals cannot initiate action even to escape threat. Fortunately, they can be salvaged if help can be given to get them moving before too long a period. Other victims respond with a flurry of overactive responses. They will chatter ceaselessly about inappropriate topics, they run back and forth and are avid rumor spreaders. If given a task, they are soon off doing something else, although to their minds, they have completed it to perfection. An unreal confidence in their abilities is their hallmark. This causes them to assume more responsibility than they can possibly discharge and to become very intolerant of other ideas or plans. They are especially troublesome to those who are demonstrating effective leadership.[13]

Principles of Behavior for Helping in Disasters

It is not possible to present a blueprint for dealing with these situations and behavior. There are some principles of behavior that the nurse can use and which can be easily conveyed to those who will help her. First of all, she should try to accept *each person's right to his own feelings.* A quick appraisal of one's own feelings at this time makes one realize how difficult it is to make a conscious choice of one's deeper feelings. An ability to make a conscious choice depends upon what we do about our feelings to relieve the tensions they create within us. Nothing is gained by trying to deny the existence of the distressed feelings in ourselves or others, simply because they appear different from what we would ordinarily expect or experience in everyday life. If we can help someone to take appropriate action, the distressed feelings may change, either quickly or gradually. Each person brings to the disaster a varied experiential background that contributes greatly to his coping with the effects of the disaster. Letting a person know that you understand *how he feels at the moment* will be the first step toward helping him. As with any patient, pity will overwhelm him; if the nurse can convey by gesture or short conversation that she is trying to see the events through his eyes, she will be helping him to find constructive outlets for his feelings and thereby aid him in rehabilitation.[13]

A second principle involves *accepting a person's limitations.* If a person is obviously physically shattered, one does not expect him to carry on as usual. Yet, when the nurse finds herself tired, frustrated, and trying to maintain her own emotional equilibrium, she is apt to resent enormously the vague "unseen" disabilities of others. This is, perhaps an understatement, for the feeling of irritability will be enhanced because others will seem to have "pulled themselves together" considering the circumstances. Again, these patients need understanding and patience, not resentment, because they too are laboring under a great load.

A third principle involves the *ability to accurately and quickly assess the capabilities of others.* A very upset person can easily cause the nurse to forget that he can be of real assistance; therefore, it is wise to be on the lookout for skills and other assets that might be revived and used. The nurse can begin to help the patient reorganize his world by inquiring into what has happened to him and letting him reply in his own way. Allowing him to talk of his experiences, without letting him ramble on or become more upset, will greatly relieve some of his feelings of despair and helplessness. The nurse can briefly explore his concern about his family and friends, giving him an honest estimate regarding the possibility of his reestablishing contact with his dear ones. If he is too depressed to talk freely, she can talk to him about what may have happened to him and to them. This may increase his confidence in the nurse to the point where he can make conversation. Brief questions regarding his occupation will give clues to his interests and basic capabilities. The nurse can then draw conclusions as to how he can best be used. While this may sound exploitive, keeping someone gainfully occupied is a genuine therapeutic coup. Treating someone as a potentially valued member of the disaster team will increase his effectiveness immeasurably.[13]

Finally, the last but perhaps the most important principle—try to *accept your own limitations in the relief role.* We have stressed the responsibility of the nurse's role to herself and others, perhaps to the detriment of the real limitations in herself that the nurse will encounter. There will be much that the nurse will want to do in a disaster; some things, however, will be beyond her strength and skill. Thus, the nurse will need to establish a set of priorities, not only with respect to what she must do for patient care but what she must undertake in the realm of responsibility generally. The first priority is to whatever emergency job that she has been assigned or has volunteered for. In practice this job may well be more than full time; therefore, the nurse must select those activities that will be worth trying and those that would be a waste of time. While she will be pushing herself to the limits of her capacity, it is imperative that she not extend herself beyond those limits because she may become as ill as those whom she treats. If pushing herself beyond endurance is a personality characteristic, then it is wise that she acknowledge it early and pace herself accordingly. A reasonable candid self-appraisal is an important prerequisite for anyone attempting psychological first aid. If one is to deal effectively with others, then one's own concerns must be dealt with *first and promptly.* If they are, the nurse will be less likely to become bogged down when she is trying to aid others. No matter how thorough the nurse's training has been, it is important that she recognize that she will not be immune to all personal disturbance if her community is torn apart by a terrible tragedy. Her first psychological job then is to look to her own defense. If she understands herself reasonably well, she may justifiably hope to endure and control her own anxieties in the midst of a community-wide disaster and render excellent assistance to those who need her.[13]

Principles of Behavior for Helping in Disasters

1. Accept each person's right to his own feelings.
2. Accept the person's limitations.
3. Assess others' capabilities quickly and accurately.
4. Accept your own limitations.

Reactions of Nurses to Disaster Situations

Research has indicated that while nurses may experience a great deal of anxiety and stress in a disaster while ministering to patients, this does not apparently interfere with effective performance.[14,15] Causes of greatest stress for the nurse appear to be the excessive physical demands made on her and concern for her own safety. Next most stressful is concern about supplies, either because supplies are inadequate or because they cannot be replenished. Other concerns include worry about one's own family, disorganization, and concern for those who have lost their home and all their possessions.

Excerpts from the following interviews with nurses who have encountered disasters are instructive.

Physical Demands

We had to walk up several flights of stairs, back and forth, up and down, for anything we needed (no elevators because of power loss). We carried water up the stairs. We helped carry trays up. The hardest thing was having to move all the patients into the halls. It was hard physical work because we had all the windows shut and there was no air conditioning and it was very hot.

Evacuating the patients from the top floors was the hardest. We could not use the elevator, just had to carry them down the stairs, two and three flights.[15]

Concern for Safety

I think, trying to safeguard the patients during the worst part of the hurricane, when it just looked like the walls were going to come down. I heard that all the windows had blown in and I tried so desperately to get over there. Some men forced open the hall door so I could go down the stairwell and I was kind of sorry after I got in the stairwell, because I was in there by myself and I have never felt such pressure in my life. I felt as though my ears would burst.

I was worried and concerned because I had a patient on a Stryker frame that I couldn't take down the stairs. Finally, the engineers took her down the elevator by hand-pulling the ropes. It seemed like it took 30 minutes just to come down from the sixth floor to the third floor.

Safety of the patients and myself. I was really frightened. Of course, I tried to control my feelings. I couldn't let the patients see that I was frightened and really think I would have been more frightened if I had not had so much to do. In trying to see to the patients' care and trying to keep them calm and protected from the flying debris, the flying gravel, rocks, and glass, and protect them from the slamming doors, I just didn't have time to be as afraid as I possibly should have been because it was real, real bad.[15]

Other Concerns

I didn't know what was happening to my family; that was the most stressful thing. I didn't know until three o'clock the next day, except I knew they weren't dead because there weren't that many people killed. I felt like they weren't.

I was mainly concerned about the children. So many were hurt by broken glass.

I think what really got me most was the people with large families that had small children. Small children that didn't even have a place to lie down or rest, and not a change of clothes, and no food. One lady with six or eight children came in and I asked her what I could do for her. She said, "Oh, I'm not too concerned about myself right now; I am more concerned about my children, and if I could just get a bottle of water for my children and for my baby."[15]

These quotes illustrate that the nurse is, indeed, human and vulnerable. As we have said previously, however, if she understands herself reasonably well, she will be able to cope when a disaster occurs and render excellent assistance to those who are in need of her services.

References

1. Jennings B: Emergency delivery and how to attend to one safely. MCN 4:148–153, May/June 1979

2. Fowler S, Butler–Manuel R: Modern Obstetrics for Student Medicine, p 360. Chicago, Year Book Medical Publishers, 1974

3. Yao AC, Lind S: Cord clamping time—influence on the newborn. Birth Family Journal 4:98–101, Fall 1977

4. Kraybill E: Needs of the term infant. In Avery G (ed): Neonatology, p 57. Philadelphia, JB Lippincott 1975

5. Hirst W, Savage P: Disaster planning. Nursing Times 70:186–189, February 1974

6. McClelland M: Hiroshima—the effect of the atom bomb. Nurse Mirror pp 19–22, September 1, 1977

7. Wert BS: Stress due to nuclear accident: A survey of an employee population. Occupational Nursing 2:16–24, September 1979

8. Eicherly EE: Nursing in thermonuclear disaster. Nurs Clin North Am 2:325–335, June 1967

9. Zanotelli P: Civil disasters? These nurses are ready. RN 34:50–52, September 1971

10. Zanotelli P: Major disasters and plans to deal with them. Nursing Mirror 130:40–41, June 28, 1974

11. Felter SE et al.: Bulletin of Maternal Welfare, 49:9–15, 1957

12. Isler C: Could you cope with a nuclear accident? RN pp 67–77, June 1979

13. Isler C: The psychology of disaster. Nurs Clin North Am 2:349–368, June 1967

14. Rayner J: How do nurses behave in disaster? Nurs Outlook 6:572–576, October 1956

15. Laub J: Psychological reactions of nurses in disaster. Nurs Res 22:343–347, July/August 1973

Suggested Reading

Antonetti M: Staff training for fire emergencies. Journal of American Health Care Association 1:49–50, July 1975

Blakely J: The Care of Radiation Casualties. London, William Heinemann Medical Books, 1968

Ede L, et al: Emergency care and the nurse. Nursing Care 6:23–27, September 1973

Eicherly EE: Nursing in thermonuclear disaster. Nurs Clin North Am 2:325–335, June 1967

Emergency Health Programs. Journal South Carolina Med. Assoc. 65:23–24, January 1969

Isler C: Could you cope with a nuclear accident? RN pp 67–77, June 1979

McClelland M: Hiroshima—the effects of the atom bomb. Nursing Mirror pp 19–22, September 2, 1977

Melber R: The nurse's role in obstetrical emergencies in the hospital setting. Nurs Clin North Am 2:261–269, June 1967

Psychology of Disaster. Nurs Clin North Am 2:349–358, June 1967

Rosenblum EH, Jones AL: What would you do in a disaster? Nursing 76 pp 72–73, September 1976

Wert BJ: Stress due to nuclear accident: A survey of an employee population. Occupational Health Nursing pp 16–24, September 1979

Study Aids for Unit VII:
Assessment and Management of Maternal Disorders

Conference Material

1. A mother, Para 2, is admitted to the hospital at 42 weeks' gestation for induction of labor. Her membranes have been artificially ruptured and intravenous oxytocin has been started. Discuss the nursing care of this mother from this time until she is in active labor.

2. What specific nursing care would you give to a mother who sustained a third-degree perineal laceration as the result of a maximal breech delivery?

3. A 38-year-old gravida 5 had an uneventful pregnancy until the last trimester, when she developed preeclampsia. Now, at term, she is admitted to the hospital because of suspected abruptio placentae and, after consultation, is to have an emergency cesarean section. Discuss the nursing care of this mother from time of admission until she is taken to the operating room for surgery.

4. A primigravida, who has 3-year-old adopted twins, is delivered by low cervical cesarean section because of pelvic injuries received in an auto accident 6 years earlier. Discuss the nursing care of this mother following cesarean section.

5. J.W. is a 25-year-old multipara whose labor was prolonged with early rupture of membranes. There were no complications of delivery. On her second postpartum day, her temperature spiked to 39°C with a pulse rate of 118. She also reported increased afterpains and headache. On examination, you note fundal tenderness and a foul odor to the lochia, which is decreased and red–brown in color. After the physician's examination, the diagnosis of endometritis is established, cultures are taken, and antibiotic therapy is begun. J.W. is breast-feeding her infant and planning to leave the hospital early tomorrow. How will you counsel her regarding (a) the infectious process and treatment, (b) breast-feeding, and (c) hospital discharge? What physical care activities will be added to the care plan as part of the management of her endometritis?

6. Three common infectious processes during the postpartum period are mastitis, urinary tract infection, and thrombophlebitis. For each of these conditions, discuss the following:
   A. Measures that may be taken prenatally, intrapartally, and postpartally to prevent their development
   B. The mechanisms by which these infections develop
   C. Their clinical manifestations (signs and symptoms)
   D. Their medical management and delegated nursing functions
   E. The nursing care plan which you would institute, including the areas of patient education, maternal–infant bonding, postpartal psychological processes, infant care and feeding, discharge planning, and follow-up care after hospitalization.

7. You are caring for a mother having her fourth child who is in very active labor. Suddenly, the membranes rupture, and she begins to bear down. As you observe the perineum, you see the infant's head crowning. Since you are alone with this mother at the time, what will you do?

8. Your community has been devastated by a sudden tornado. What types of behavior would you expect from some of the survivors? What interventions would you plan to help them?

9. How would you go about finding out what preparations your community has taken for disaster protection?

Multiple Choice

Read through the entire question and place your answer on the line to the right.

1. Which of the following signs and symptoms should the nurse anticipate when a pregnant patient has a history of heart disease?
   A. Dyspnea
   B. Slow pulse rate
   C. Decrease in blood pressure
   D. Hemorrhage

   Select the number corresponding to the correct letter or letters.
   1. A only
   2. B only
   3. A, C, and D
   4. All of the above ____

2. Which of the following factors influence the answer which you have given in Question No. 1?
   A. Increased need for oxygen intake
   B. Increase blood volume
   C. Toxic damage to the heart
   D. Failure of kidneys to excrete

   Select the number corresponding to the correct letters.
   1. A and B
   2. A and C
   3. B, C, and D
   4. All of the above ____

3. Which of the following signs and symptoms would the patient with a ruptured fallopian tube manifest?
   A. Hegar's sign
   B. Intense pain
   C. Profound shock
   D. Irregular fetal heart tones
   E. Vaginal bleeding

(Continued)

Multiple Choice
(continued)

Select the number corresponding to the correct letters.
1. A and B
2. A, C, and D
3. B, C, and E
4. B, D, and E ____

4. In the management of hypertensive disorders of pregnancy, which of the following symptoms during labor should be reported to the physician promptly?
A. Regular uterine contractions
B. Epigastric pain
C. Dimness of vision
D. Headache
E. Decrease in urinary excretion

Select the number corresponding to the correct letters.
1. A, C, and D
2. A, C, and E
3. B, C, and D
4. B, C, D, and E ____

5. Which of the following are causes of bleeding in the first trimester of pregnancy?
A. Abortion
B. Abruptio placentae
C. Placenta previa
D. Ectopic pregnancy

Select the number corresponding to the correct letters.
1. A and B
2. A and D
3. A, B, and C
4. B, C, and D ____

6. Which of the following are common causes of bleeding in the third trimester of pregnancy?
A. Menstruation
B. Abortion
C. Abruptio placentae
D. Placenta previa
E. Ectopic pregnancy

Select the number corresponding to the correct letters.
1. A and B
2. A, B, and C
3. C and D
4. A, D, and C ____

7. By what criterion or criteria is an incomplete abortion distinguished from a threatened abortion?
   A. Dilatation of the cervix
   B. Bleeding
   C. Passage of placental tissue
   D. Pain

   Select the number corresponding to the correct letter or letters.
   1. A only
   2. A and B
   3. C only
   4. A, C, and D ____

8. A patient in the third trimester of pregnancy reports to the nurse by phone that she has experienced vaginal bleeding. This is unassociated with pain and she feels otherwise well. She should be advised
   A. To report to the hospital immediately for evaluation
   B. To go to bed and call again if bleeding persists
   C. That this is commonly seen just prior to labor and not to worry
   D. To report this to the physician at the time of the next prenatal visit ____

9. The patient described above continues to bleed vaginally. The most serious condition which must be ruled out is
   A. Placental abruption
   B. Bloody show
   C. Chronic cervicitis
   D. Placenta previa ____

10. The warning signals of preeclampsia that should be watched for during the course of routine prenatal care include
   A. Sudden excessive weight gain (greater than 2 lb/week–3 lb/week)
   B. Generalized skin rash
   C. An elevation of blood pressure greater than 14 mm Hg in diastolic pressure over previously observed levels
   D. An elevation of more than 30 mm Hg in systolic pressure above previously observed levels

   Select the number corresponding to the correct letters.
   1. A, B, and C
   2. A, C, and D
   3. A and D
   4. B and C ____

(Continued)

Multiple Choice
(continued)

11. Match the statements below with the hemoglobinopathy they most accurately describe.
A. No increased fetal morbidity or maternal morbidity, but an increased incidence of urinary tract infection in pregnancy ____
B. Only slight increased perinatal mortality but greatly increased maternal morbidity and mortality ____
C. 50% of pregnancies end in spontaneous abortion, neonatal death, or stillbirth ____

1. Sickle cell trait
2. Sickle cell hemoglobin C disease
3. Sickle cell anemia

12. Diabetes may have a deleterious effect in pregnancy in the following ways:
A. Increased fetal size with a greater risk of difficult vaginal delivery
B. A 4-fold increase in the incidence of preeclampsia
C. An increased incidence of hydramnios
D. Increased incidence of urinary tract infection

Select the number corresponding to the correct letters.
1. A and B
2. A and C
3. A, B, and C
4. All of the above ____

13. Match the following statements with the condition listed below.
A. Potentially lethal infection of the newborn which may occur during delivery ____
B. Eyes may be affected at birth and unless promptly treated, blindness may result ____
C. Characterized by anorexia, nausea, vomiting, and elevated serum bilirubin levels ____

1. Gonorrhea
2. Herpes genitalis
3. Viral hepatitis

14. Breech presentations
A. Should never be delivered vaginally
B. Cause a considerable increased risk of mortality and morbidity for the infant
C. Cause an increased risk of morbidity for the mother
D. Generally result in prolonged labor
E. Always require cesarean section

Select the number corresponding to the correct letters.
1. All of the above
2. A, B, and C
3. C, D, and E
4. B, C
5. C, D ____

15. The three most frequent causes of postpartum hemorrhage are
A. Retained placental fragments
B. Full bladder
C. Uterine atony
D. Lacerations of the perineum, cervix, and vagina
E. Clotting defects
F. Uterine infections

Select the number corresponding to the correct letters.
1. A, B, and C
2. A, C, and D
3. B, C, and D
4. C, E, and F
5. B, C, and F ____

16. What is the effect of tetanic contractions on the pregnant uterus?
A. Descent and rotation are hastened.
B. Ruptured uterus is a great risk.
C. Fetal head may be compressed and ruptured.
D. Uterine inertia may follow.
E. Perineal lacerations may occur.

Select the number corresponding to the correct letter or letters.
1. A only
2. B only
3. A, C, and D
4. B, C, and E ____

17. A patient in the first stage of labor develops hypertonic dysfunctional labor. Which of the following are important in the treatment of this condition?
A. Pitocin
B. Sedation
C. Fluids
D. Bed rest
E. Ambulation

Select the number corresponding to the correct letters.
1. A, B, and D
2. A, C, and E
3. B, C, and D
4. B, C, and E ____

(Continued)

Multiple Choice (continued)

18. Which of the following principles should be observed in the use of intravenous oxytocin to stimulate labor?
   A. The condition of the fetus must be satisfactory.
   B. It should be used only in cases of primary uterine inertia.
   C. It should not be given to a multipara who has had five or more full-term pregnancies.
   D. It should be used in cases of borderline pelvis.
   E. A responsible person should be in constant attendance while the mother is receiving intravenous oxytocin.

   Select the number corresponding to the correct letters.
   1. A and B
   2. A, C, and E
   3. B, D, and E
   4. All of the above ____

19. What specific treatment should be included in the care given a mother who has had a repair of a third-degree laceration of the perineum?
   A. Give daily routine perineal care.
   B. Begin stool softeners early.
   C. Omit enemas until the fifth postpartal day.
   D. Limit activities in regard to early ambulation.
   E. Encourage the mother not to sit erect until wound has healed.

   Select the number corresponding to the correct letter or letters.
   1. A only
   2. A and B
   3. A, C, and D
   4. All of the above ____

20. After a cesarean section, which of the following symptoms might indicate that the patient is having excessive bleeding?
   A. Accelerated pulse and respiration and drop in blood pressure
   B. Pain and tenderness in operative area
   C. Abdominal distention
   D. Sanguineous drainage from the abdominal wound and the vagina
   E. Apprehension and restlessness

   Select the number corresponding to the correct letters.
   1. A and B
   2. A, C, and D
   3. A, D, and E
   4. All of the above ____

21. In caring for a mother who has been delivered by cesarean section, which of the following are usually employed to keep the uterus contracted and control bleeding?
   A. Oxytocic drugs
   B. Vigorous massage of the fundus if it becomes relaxed

C. Icebag to the operative area
D. Pressure dressings and tight abdominal binder
E. Keep the patient flat in bed for the first 6 hours postoperatively

Select the number corresponding to the correct letter or letters.
1. A only
2. A, C, and D
3. B, C, and E
4. All of the above ____

22. Which of the following structures are involved when an episiotomy is performed?
A. The vaginal mucosa
B. The levator ani muscle
C. The glans clitoris
D. The cardinal ligament
E. The fourchette

Select the number corresponding to the correct letter or letters.
1. A only
2. A and B
3. A, B, and E
4. All of the above ____

23. Obstetrical forceps are frequently used to facilitate delivery. In which of the following conditions could it be indicated to deliver the infant by forceps?
A. The cervix fails to dilate completely
B. The mother has heart disease
C. The mother has a contracted pelvis
D. Prolapse of the umbilical cord
E. Passage of meconium-stained amniotic fluid in vertex presentation at full dilatation

Select the number corresponding to the correct letters.
1. A and B
2. B, D, and E
3. C and E
4. All of the above ____

Discussion

24. What are four common causes of postpartal uterine and peritoneal infections?

25. By what routes do bacteria usually colonize these tissues?

26. List the four classical signs of endometritis.

27. How does peritonitis differ from parametritis?

28. List the signs and symptoms of femoral thrombophlebitis.

(Continued)

Discussion (continued)

29. What are five risk factors that increase the probability of developing postpartal infection?

30. Describe measures that are generally used in treatment of postpartal infections (medical and nursing).

31. What are four factors that increase the risk of wound infection after cesarean section?

32. List five measures that can contribute to preventing postpartal infections.

33. What are the signs and symptoms of pulmonary embolism?

34. What is the treatment of puerperal mastitis?

35. What are four measures to prevent mastitis?

36. What is the relationship between overdistention of the bladder, retention of urine, the postpartum period, and urinary infection?

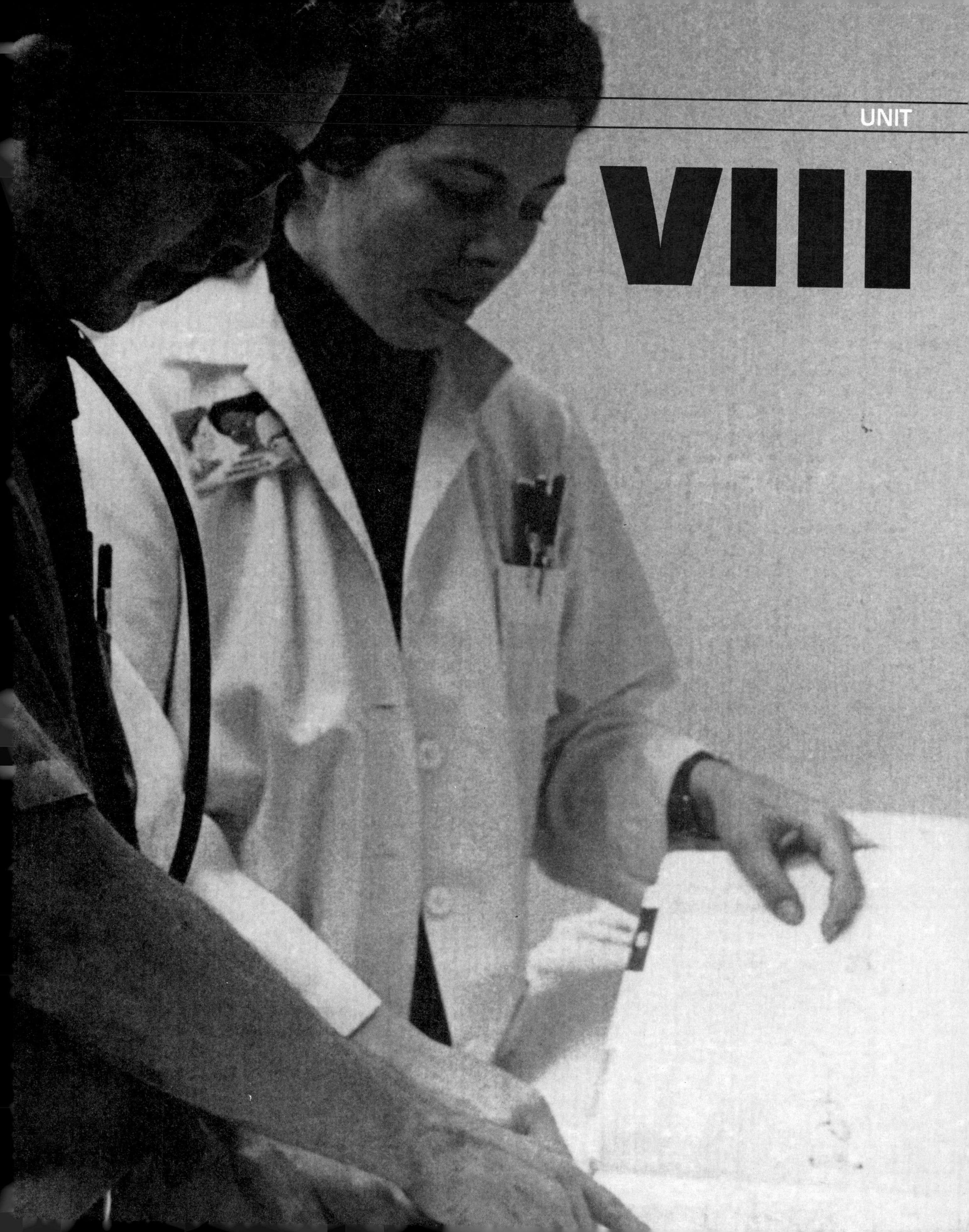
UNIT
VIII

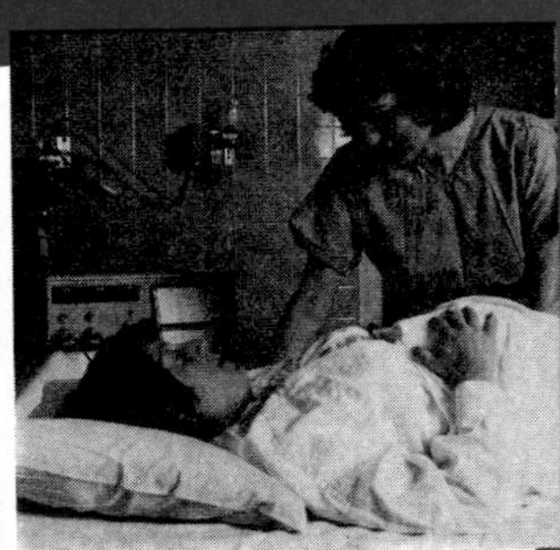

41 Electronic Fetal Monitoring and Fetal Intensive Care

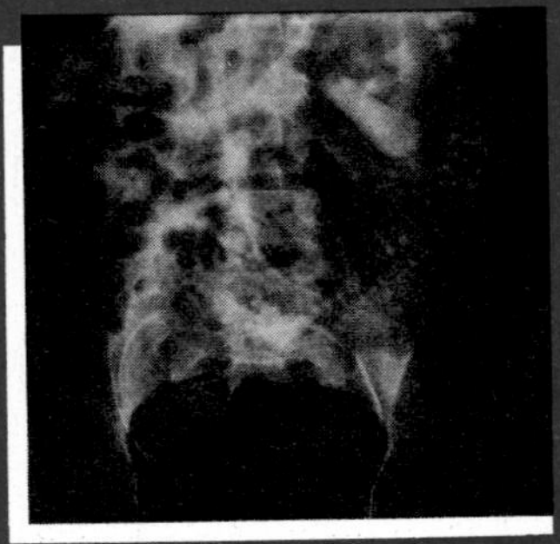

40 Fetal Diagnosis and Treatment

UNIT VIII

Assessment and Management of Perinatal Disorders

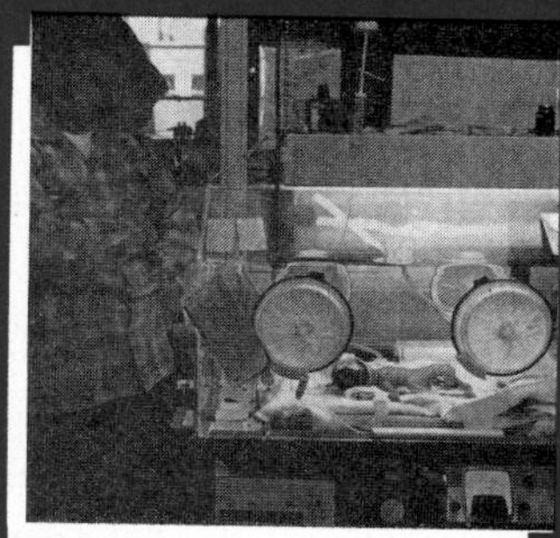

42 The High-Risk Infant: Disorders of Gestational Age and Birth Weight

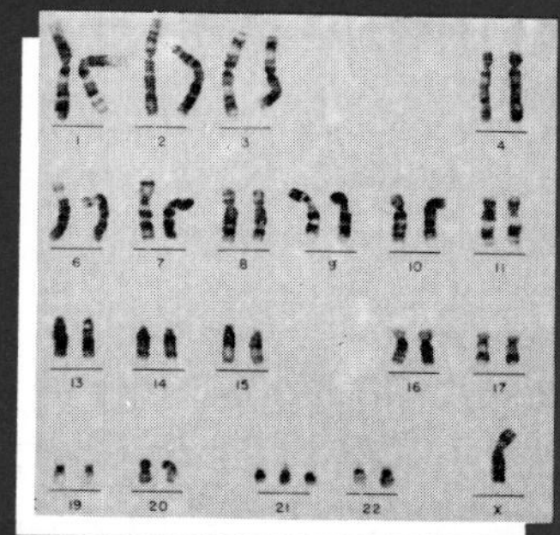

43 The High-Risk Infant: Developmental Disorders

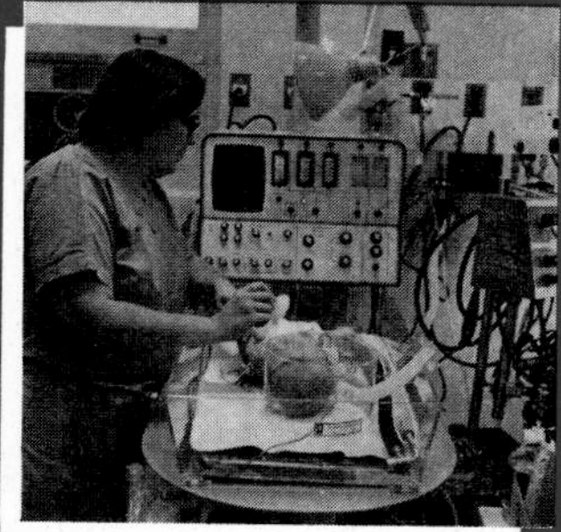

44 The High-Risk Infant: Acquired Disorders

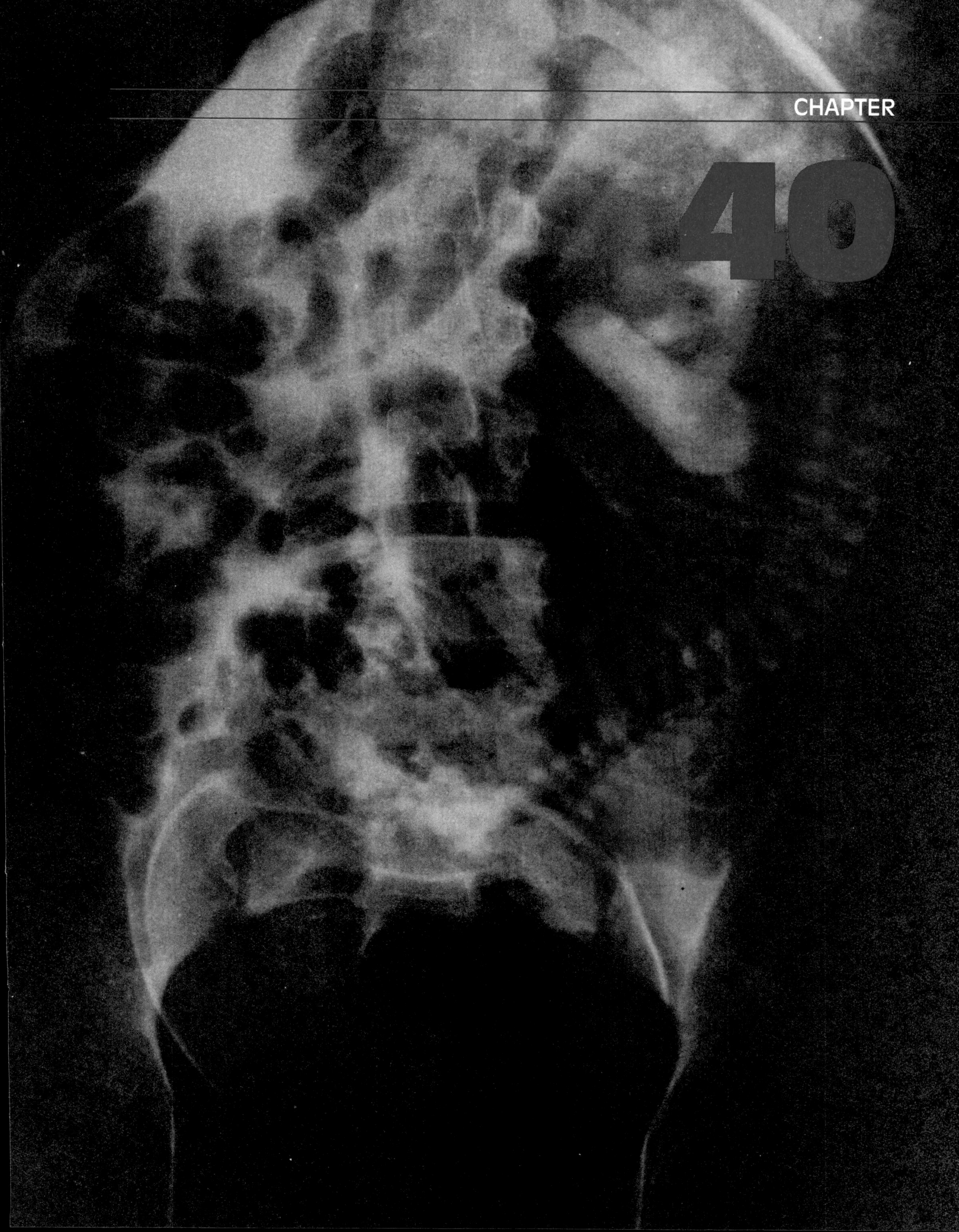

CHAPTER

40

CHAPTER 40

Fetal Diagnosis and Treatment

Prior to the middle of the twentieth century the fetus was generally regarded as a passive participant in the entire reproductive process. Fetal evaluation was limited to gross observation of growth and auscultation of the fetal heart. X-ray films were used to assess fetal position and major bony abnormalities, but these methods clearly fell short of precisely determining fetal age and well-being. In the last few decades, however, a series of rapidly evolving developments have opened the way to increasingly accurate approaches. These developments include safer use of amniocentesis, which has allowed greater access to amniotic fluid, along with cytogenetic, biochemical, cytologic, and biophysical assessment of the fluid, B-mode and real-time ultrasound techniques, and electronic and biochemical fetal monitoring.

In addition to these technical advances, which permit evaluation of the fetus, there have been advances in understanding that permit significant, albeit limited, treatment of the fetus beyond simply converting the fetus to a newborn. The proliferation of this technology has been accompanied by a parallel proliferation in professional and supportive personnel in the broad area of perinatology. Subspecialties have evolved for both maternal and fetal medical specialists and neonatologists. Obstetrical anesthesia has emerged as a growing and well-defined area of study. Training programs have been developed for perinatal nurse clinicians and the concept of the perinatal team has been well established. Such a team includes the obstetrician, neonatologist, anesthesiologist, nurse specialist, nutritionists, social worker, and other supporting consultants.

Regionalization of Perinatal Care

Facilities are a concern because it is impractical for every hospital regardless of size and population served to have all the personnel and equipment necessary to deliver the most sophisticated levels of care. The concept of regionalization or centralization of perinatal care, in which three levels of care can be identified, has evolved. As previously stated, the basic level of care would provide for the management of only normal maternity patients and newborns. Mothers or newborns with complications would have to be transferred to level 2 or level 3 institutions. Level 2 care would be provided in institutions with a significant maternity practice. These institutions should have the equipment and personnel to handle all but the most sophisticated and unusual problems. These facilities should provide care for some premature infants as well as most high-risk mothers. Level 3 institutions providing the most specialized types of care for unusual problems would serve larger populations.

Implicit in this concept is the identification of the high-risk mother or newborn and the transfer of that patient as required to a hospital with the appropriate level of care. Scoring systems and computerized and problem-oriented record systems have been developed to aid in identifying these patients. The key is early recognition of problems by the health-care provider in order that transport may be carried out at the earliest and most optimal time. Whenever possible, infant transport is best accomplished *in utero* rather than after birth, when the newborn is already in a compromised state. There is considerable evidence that the outcome is far superior when intensive neonatal care begins at the moment of delivery. This is not always possible because occasionally high-risk babies are born to low-risk mothers, and even when the mother at risk is identified, delivery before transfer can be accomplished may be inevitable. Despite the obvious value of this concept of regionalization and mother and infant transport, there are significant problems relating to the social and emotional aspects of patient care. Separation of patients from their families, familiar surroundings, and physicians can create tremendous anxiety and require special sensitivity on the part of all involved in their care.

In the general area of fetal diagnosis, two broad areas of concern are the determination of fetal age or maturity and the evaluation of fetal well-being. In the latter category are included assessment in early pregnancy for congenital disorders, later evaluation of well-being in pregnancy complications, and, finally, intrapartum monitoring by electronic or biochemical means. Genetic diagnosis and intrapartum monitoring are covered in Chapters 16 and 41, respectively.

Determination of Fetal Age

Although it is customary to use Naegele's rule to determine the period of gestation and estimated date of confinement from the first day of the last menstrual period, this method is fraught with error for various reasons. These include failure to remember exact dates, irregular cycles, bleeding in the first trimester, and late registration for prenatal care. In the case of an uncomplicated pregnancy, not knowing the exact length of gestation may not represent a serious problem. However, in the high-risk patient for whom timing of the delivery is critical, the information is vital. Thus, the degree to which the determination should be pursued depends upon the clinical situation.

Means for Determining Fetal Age

Physical Measurements

Estimation of uterine size by pelvic examination in the first trimester is a helpful indicator of gestational growth, whereas determination of uterine size in the second trimester is less valid. Measuring the fundal height above the pelvic symphysis at each visit can give useful information about growth or lack of growth, but not about the exact period of gestation. Estimation of fetal weight is notoriously inaccurate, with the greatest error at the higher and lower weights.

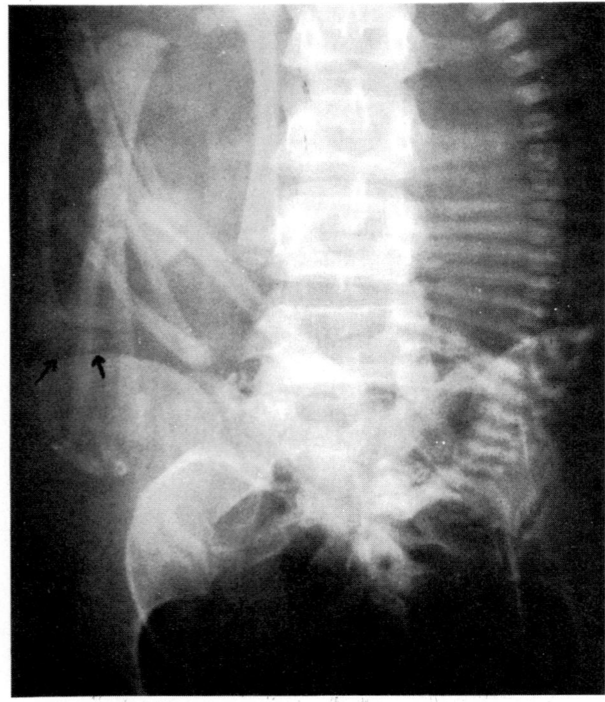

Figure 40-1.
Abdominal roentgenogram showing a fetus with calcification of both the distal femoral and proximal tibial epiphyses *(arrows).*

Radiographic Studies

Radiographic studies can be helpful in determining maturity. If both the distal femoral and proximal tibial epiphyses are calcified, one can be assured of a mature fetus (Fig. 40-1). However, if the epiphyses are not calcified one cannot assume immaturity, since there is considerable variation based on sex, race, and fetal weight, along with technical problems related to the position of the fetal knee relative to the maternal skeleton. Because of these inaccuracies, as well as concerns about radiation and the fetus, radiographs are no longer a preferred approach for the purpose of determining fetal age.

Ultrasound

Diagnostic ultrasound is now widely used in obstetrics for a variety of purposes, including early diagnosis of pregnancy, confirmation of fetal viability, placental localization, confirmation of fetal death, and estimation of fetal age. The most useful techniques are the B-mode scan with or without gray scale, and the real-time scan. The B scan provides a visual cross-sectional picture that allows identification of the size, shape, and location of structures. Real time utilizes a generator that produces multiple pulses and echoes. Since these are activated in sequence, they detect movement, including vessel pulsations, cardiac action, and breathing. The diagnosis of early pregnancy and estimation of the period of gestation can be made by either technique, but real time offers the advantage of documenting viability as well, since cardiac activity as well as fetal movement can be seen by that technique from early on (uniformly by 8 weeks).

The most common approach to the determination of gestational age is to measure the biparietal diameter of the fetal head. This is especially useful if done during the linear phase of growth of the fetal head between 20 and 30 weeks and is further enhanced by making two measurements, 3 to 4 weeks apart, which will not only better fix the gestational age, but also confirm a normal rate of growth.

Fetal head growth generally proceeds at a normal rate despite late pregnancy problems that might retard overall fetal growth. This occurs because the brain is spared under such circumstances and brain growth is the major determinant of head size. To detect this type of growth retardation with head sparing, additional measurements must be made, including the thoracic diameters, crown–rump lengths, or calculations of the total intrauterine volume. It must be emphasized that, although it is commonly done, a single measurement of the biparietal diameter late in the third trimester is of very little value in establishing the period of gestation.

Concerning the safety of diagnostic ultrasound, there is no available evidence to suggest any harmful fetal effects. This is not to say, however, that it should be used without restraint. Indeed, for some practitioners, ultrasound has become routine for all pregnancies, an approach that may not be justifiable at this time.

Endocrine Studies

Of all the assays available, estriol (or total estrogens) and human placental lactogen (HPL)—also known as human chorionic somatomammotropin (HCS)—are the most commonly used. Both have normal curves that rise progressively during pregnancy. Serum and 24-hour urine samples are assayed. The range of normal is wide, however, making these techniques less valid in determining fetal age than fetal well-being. It is possible for a given value to be in the normal range for both 35 and 40 weeks and, therefore, the age differentiation cannot be made.

Amniotic Fluid Studies

Transabdominal amniocentesis has become a standard technique in modern obstetrical practice (see Fig. 16-8). It must not be regarded as a totally innocuous procedure and should be undertaken only on the basis of well-founded indications. Potential complications include fetal bleeding, placental disruption, Rh sensitization, and fetal puncture. The frequency of these complications is poorly recorded and is greatly influenced by such factors as the experience of the person carrying out the procedure and the use of ultrasound to localize the placenta. The incidence of complications is probably in the 1% range. Given a sample of amniotic fluid, the following determinations are useful in evaluating fetal age.

Gross Appearance. The presence of large amounts of vernix caseosa generally indicates maturity. Meconium is often present in the significantly postdate pregnancy. Neither, however, is sufficiently consistent for precise age estimation because the meconium may be present as a sign of fetal distress in the less than mature pregnancy.

Cytology. The cells in amniotic fluid come from the fetus and the membranes. The bulk of fetal cells are desquamated squamous cells from the skin. Cells from the respiratory, urinary, and gastrointestinal tracts are also present. If amniotic fluid is mixed with a vital stain for fat (Nile blue sulfate) and a smear is made, a varying number of the squamous cells take up the stain and appear orange on the smear. These cells normally first appear at 34 to 35 weeks of gestation and increase in number as term is approached. Generally 15% to 20% indicates a mature fetus, while at term the presence of 50% fat-containing cells and free-fat droplets is the rule. This technique has the distinct advantage of being easily done and the information can be immediately available.

Creatinine. The concentration of creatinine in amniotic fluid gradually rises as the fetus' kidneys mature, increasing their ability to excrete creatinine, and also as the fetus' muscle mass increases, which causes an increase in creatine to creatinine metabolism. Values of 2 mg per 100 ml are indicative of fetal maturity.

Bilirubin. Although the determination of bilirubin in amniotic fluid by spectrophotometry has its greatest application in evaluating the fetus in Rh sensitization, it can also be applied in evaluating the age of the fetus in nonsensitized patients. Because of the maturation of the fetal liver and the placenta, the concentration of bilirubin in amniotic fluid is progressively decreased toward term and disappears at about 37 to 38 weeks, strongly suggesting fetal maturity. This evaluation is not sufficiently valid to be used as the sole standard but does complement the other assays.

Osmolality. Although amniotic fluid in early pregnancy is isotonic with maternal plasma, as pregnancy progresses the fluid becomes more hypotonic, presumably because of the increasing contribution of fetal urine. Values of 250 mOsm per liter per kilogram or less are generally associated with maturity, but variation is considerable.

Phospholipids. The most important and germane studies of fetal maturity have evolved through extensive investigation of fetal pulmonary fluids and the genesis of respiratory distress syndrome. Because there are respiratory movements *in utero,* the composition of amniotic fluid does reflect the content of pulmonary fluids. Consequently, several techniques measuring surfactant activity in amniotic fluid have been devised to determine fetal pulmonary maturity.

Surfactant is synthesized by the type II cells in the lung and although present in small quantities from midpregnancy, the mature pathway for surfactant synthesis (choline incorporation) is activated at 35 weeks in the normal pregnancy. In certain stressful circumstances such as preeclampsia, class D and F diabetes, and premature rupture of the membranes, the process is accelerated. In others, such as class A, B, and C diabetes, it may be delayed. As will be discussed subsequently, the administration of corticosteroids may, under certain conditions, accelerate pulmonary maturity.

There are several techniques for measuring this activity, including the "Shake" test, L/S ratio, and Felma measurement. The Shake test determines the stability of foam on the surface of mixtures of ethyl alcohol and various dilutions of amniotic fluid (Fig. 40-2); maturity is indicated when the foam is stable in the presence of a 2:1 dilution.

The most widely used technique is the lecithin/sphingomyelin (L/S) ratio. Since the concentration of sphingomyelin remains relatively constant, a rising L/S ratio indicates increasing surfactant production (lecithin is a major constituent of surfactant). The separation of lecithin and sphingomyelin is achieved by thin-layer chromatography. The ratio is determined either by visual inspection or by densitometry. Pulmonary maturity is established when the L/S ratio exceeds 2:1.

With another technique, the fetal lung maturity (Felma) apparatus measures total concentrations of amniotic fluid phospholipid by an electro-optical approach. This equipment is somewhat expensive, but if the method is validated by further studies its reproducibility may make it a desirable technique. More recent studies of specific phospholipids in amniotic fluid, phosphatidylglycerol (PG), and phosphatidylinositol (PI) have proved to be valuable in borderline cases and especially in patients with class A, B, and C diabetes where pulmonary maturity is often delayed to 37 weeks or later. When PG and PI are both present maturity seems assured.

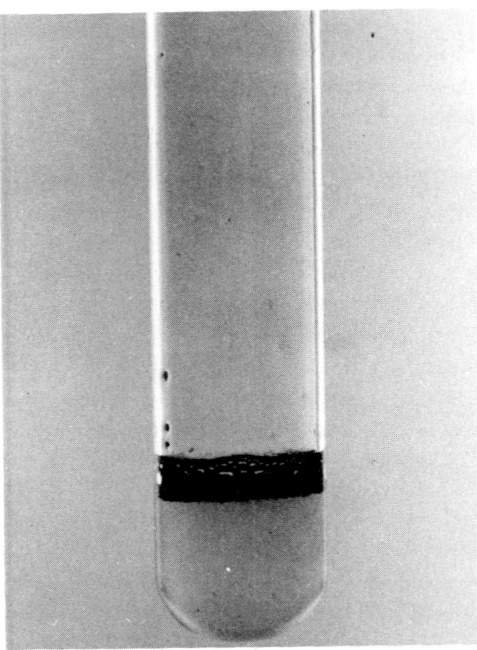

Figure 40-2.
Shake test. Note bubbles on the surface maintained by surfactant in the amniotic fluid.

Evaluation of Fetal Well-Being

There are a number of circumstances in obstetrical practice in which the fetus might be in jeopardy, and it is therefore desirable to evaluate the fetal status. Such instances range from the first trimester patient with a threatened abortion, with whom there is the need to determine the viability of the pregnancy, to mid-trimester pregnancy studies to determine congenital disorders (see Chap. 16). In the third trimester, serial evaluations are necessary in chronic disorders such as diabetes and hypertension as well as in more acute problems such as preeclampsia and the postdate pregnancy. At the present time the application of sophisticated tests to determine fetal well-being is limited to patients with a determined fetal risk, while normal pregnancies are evaluated largely by clinical means. It is entirely possible that some or all of these techniques may soon be routinely applied as a form of antenatal screening.

Antepartal Fetal Evaluation

The action to be taken by the obstetrician when the fetus at risk is in fact in jeopardy is limited and determined by the period of gestation. If in the first trimester it is determined that the pregnancy is nonviable, the uterus can be evacuated. This is basically an all-or-none evaluation, and qualitative assessment of the first trimester pregnancy is not currently possible. As one deals with the midtrimester and a previable fetus, evaluation of well-being is of little moment because there is generally no recourse if serious fetal problems are uncovered, given the fact that delivery is unacceptable. There are some exceptions to this in which therapy can be directed toward the fetus while allowing the pregnancy to continue. The classic example of this situation is intrauterine transfusion in the severely affected fetus with Rh hemolytic disease. In the vast majority of cases, however, these evaluations are done in the third trimester and the choice is between delivery of a potentially viable premature infant or prolongation of intrauterine life with the risk of fetal death. When the indications of *in utero* jeopardy are severe, the decision to deliver often results in the birth of a seriously ill newborn and a potential neonatal death. More commonly, however, the studies are reassuring and permit prolongation of the pregnancy.

Early Pregnancy Evaluation—Threatened Abortion

A common problem in the first trimester is evaluating the significance of bleeding and deciding whether a pregnancy is viable and should be allowed to continue despite the persistent symptoms. Standard immunologic pregnancy tests may remain positive for some time following the point at which viability is lost. The more specific beta subunit assay is particularly reassuring if its values are appropriate for the gestational period. B-mode ultrasound scans can define a gestational sac as early as 5 weeks following the last menstrual period. The integrity of the sac and its appropriate dimensions are reassuring up to 10 weeks. The fetus is generally visible with the sac by 8 weeks, and fetal activity and heartbeat can be discerned by 10 weeks with real-time equipment. These techniques have considerably more precision in assessing progress than clinical examinations evaluating uterine growth. They can therefore provide reassurance in a situation involving considerable anxiety and offer a definitive answer in situations of nonviability, thereby permitting uterine evacuation.

Late Pregnancy Evaluation

Estrogens

Estrogen levels in maternal serum and urine rise progressively during the course of normal pregnancy, following a sigmoid curve as seen in Figure 40-3. Although estrone and estradiol also increase during pregnancy, it is estriol that is the predominant estrogen, increasing 1000-fold and accounting for 90% of the total estrogen. This makes it feasible in the case of 24-hour urinary determinations to measure either estriol or total estrogens. Even more important in the clinical application of estriol measurements for problem pregnancies is the fact that at least 90% of the estrogen precursors are produced by the fetal zone of the fetal adrenal cortex, largely as sulfates of dehydroepiandrosterone (DHEAS) and 16αOH DHEAS. Much of the DHEAS is converted to 16αOH DHEAS by the fetal liver. The conversion of these androgen precursors to estriol is a function of the placenta by processes involving the splitting off of the sulfate and conjugation. Finally, estriol is excreted by the maternal kidney mostly in the conjugated form. Thus it becomes clear that, in order for there to be a normal quantity of estriol in a 24-hour urine specimen, the several parts of the cycle must be intact, including the live healthy fetus with intact adrenals producing normal amounts of androgen precursors, a normally functioning placenta capable of making the conversion to estriol, and healthy maternal liver and kidneys competent to conjugate and then excrete the estriol. Consequently, estriol values that are normal for the gestational age are quite reassuring. Most commonly, measurements are made in 24-hour urine collections. Although there may be some day-to-day variation, a fall of more than 30% to 40% must be considered significant and the impression of fetal jeopardy pursued. Serial measurements must be done, and the frequency of determination is dependent upon the seriousness and the stability of the clinical situation. In a hospitalized unstable diabetic, daily estriols may be needed, while less frequent studies are sufficient in a less critical situation.

Because urinary estriols require a 24-hour collection, with the possibility that it may be incomplete as well as inconvenient for the patient, and because this, in effect, brings about a lag in the assessment process, a number of alternatives have been suggested. Simultaneous measurement of urinary creatinine can provide a constant which then enables the clinician to use shorter collection periods, of 4 or 8 hours, for example, and still get meaningful information by calculating the estriol/creatinine ratio. It should also be noted that there are a number of factors that can interfere with urinary estriol determinations. Obviously, in the presence of impaired maternal renal function, the test loses its validity and cannot be used to assess the fetal status. Maternal administration of ampicillin, Mandelamine, and corticosteroids all interfere with the measurement, as does a large quantity of glucose in the urine. The latter can be dealt with by diluting the specimen for the assay.

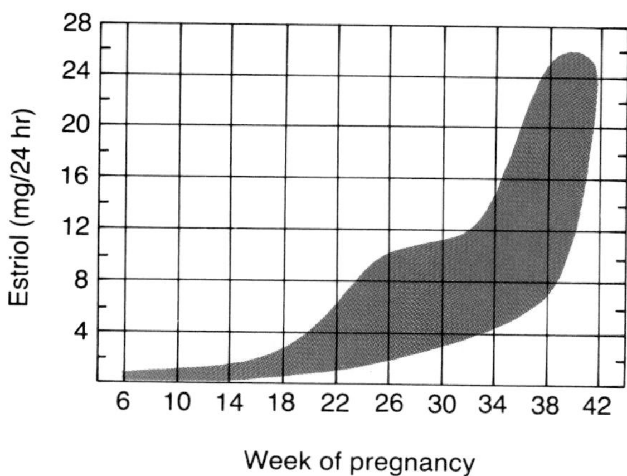

Figure 40-3.
Pattern of urinary estriol excretion in normal pregnancy.

Because of these problems, a number of workers have turned to the use of plasma estriol measurements. The normal curve is similarly shaped to that for urinary measurements, although the quantities are measured in micrograms rather than milligrams. The use of plasma values does not eliminate all problems because levels vary during the day. Therefore, samples must be obtained at the same time each day for proper comparison. Abnormal renal function can result in false elevations of plasma levels. Furthermore, this technique is somewhat more difficult than urinary assays. The methodology has been improved, however, by the use of radioimmunoassay, and currently this technique, applied to unconjugated estriol, is gaining in favor.

Estetrol (15αhydroxyestriol) measurements have been proposed by some as a better means of fetal evaluation. This estrogen is derived from placental estradiol and estrone with the final synthesis taking place in the fetal liver. Both serum and urinary assays have been suggested, but the current consensus, after an initial surge of enthusiasm, is that estetrol measurements offer no advantage over estriol.

Progesterone

This steroid hormone is produced by the placenta in progressively increasing quantities during pregnancy. It can be measured as serum progesterone or urinary pregnanediol, but has little value in evaluating fetal well-being, since progesterone does not require fetal precursors and can, in fact, persist in significant quantities even after an intrauterine fetal death has occurred.

Human Chorionic Gonadotropin (HCG)

This hormone, produced by the trophoblast, normally peaks in early pregnancy and falls off to relatively low levels in the second and third trimesters. It is the basis for most pregnancy tests, as well as for the follow-up of hydatid moles and choriocarcinoma, but is of limited value in problem pregnancies. An exception occurs in the case of severely affected erythroblastotic infants. Because of placental hypertrophy, HCG values may be quite high; however, by the time these values are reached, the fetus is usually beyond saving.

Human Placental Lactogen (HPL)

Also known as human chorionic somatomammotropin, HPL is synthesized by the syncytiotrophoblast of the placenta in progressively increasing quantities throughout pregnancy. HPL shows an incomplete immunologic cross reaction with human pituitary growth hormone. The value of this assay in monitoring fetal well-being has been a rather controversial subject, and one can probably conclude that HPL is a valuable adjunct but should not be regarded as the sole end point for testing fetal jeopardy. It is generally concluded that those clinical situations in which fetal compromise is the direct result of impaired placental function will be heralded by falling HPL values approaching a danger zone (below 4 mg/ml after 30 weeks of gestation). Thus, HPL assay is most useful with hypertension disorders of pregnancy, placental insufficiency with fetal growth retardation, and especially postdate pregnancies. Because placental function is not impaired in such conditions as class A and B diabetes without hypertension, congenital malformation, and hemolytic disease, the study has no predictive value for such patients.

Maternal Blood Enzyme Measurement

A number of enzymes increase in concentration in maternal serum during pregnancy, including heat-stable alkaline phosphatase (HSAP), diamine oxidase (DAO) and oxytocinase.

Heat-Stable Alkaline Phosphatase (HSAP).

This isoenzyme of alkaline phosphatase originates in the placenta and rises in concentration progressively throughout pregnancy. A sudden rapid rise in late pregnancy seems to indicate placental damage and potential fetal death. In some studies this has been shown to take place prior to a drop in estriol. As with HPL, most feel this easy-to-do study is a good adjunct but not an end in itself.

Plasma Diamine Oxidase (DAO). This enzyme is probably produced by retroplacental decidua, perhaps to protect the pregnant woman against histamine produced by the fetus. It rises at a rapid linear rate in early pregnancy, but, unfortunately, it tends to plateau in the third trimester, making it less useful for fetal evaluation.

Oxytocinase. Cystine aminopeptidase enzyme (oxytocinase) inactivates oxytocin during pregnancy and is synthesized by the placenta. As with HPL and HSAP, it seems to be a rather pure indicator of placental function, does not reflect distress, which is primarily fetal, and is therefore useful as an adjunct but not for primary evaluation of well-being.

Physiological Studies

Because it is not feasible to measure directly the critical respiratory and nutritional function of the placenta, a number of indirect approaches have been developed. Two of these studies, the oxytocin challenge test and the nonstress test, are discussed in Chapter 41. Fetal movements and especially a change in the pattern of fetal movement are felt to be indicators of well-being. Some have suggested that patients be instructed to count the number of fetal movements in a given time period each day and record the information. Even without this formal quantifying of fetal movement, when a patient reports a reduction in fetal movements, it must be evaluated further, especially if there is an underlying reason to suspect fetal jeopardy.

With the advent of real-time ultrasound, which enables one to observe fetal activity, it is possible to observe cardiac activity and respiratory movements. The latter, it has been suggested, is a good index of fetal well-being; however, the approach has not yet achieved practical clinical application, especially since long periods of observation may be needed for proper information.

Amniotic Fluid Studies

Most amniotic fluid studies are directed toward the determination of fetal maturity or genetic diagnosis, which is discussed in Chapter 16. A major exception is the measurement of bilirubin in amniotic fluid as a means of judging the severity of hemolytic disease.

When chorioamnionitis is suspected, but the diagnosis is not clear, examination of amniotic fluid for the presence of polymorphonuclear leukocytes and Gram-stained bacteria may be helpful. Although there are some conflicting reports concerning the importance of the white blood cells, the presence of bacteria is clearly significant.

The presence of meconium in amniotic fluid is an indication that there may have been an episode of fetal stress at some time prior to the observation, but not necessarily as an ongoing situation. Indeed, the presence of meconium does not indicate a fetus in distress unless there are other indicators, such as a significant alteration in the fetal heart rate. The mechanism of passage of meconium is presumably hyperperistalsis secondary to the hypoxic insult. In most cases, the observation of meconium-stained fluid is made intrapartum after rupture of the membranes, although transabdominal amniocentesis or transvaginal amnioscopy may also be used. The latter procedure is limited to late pregnancy when the cervix is open enough to admit the lighted speculum. An advantage is that the procedure can be done repeatedly to monitor well-being in certain cases, such as the postdate pregnancy. Disadvantages of the technique are that fluid samples cannot be obtained for analysis and that occasionally the membranes may be inadvertently ruptured.

Specific Fetal Problems

Acute fetal distress is covered in Chapter 41 in relation to intrapartum fetal monitoring, although many of the chronic fetal problems that are discussed here can produce acute distress as well. In addition, some of these problems, such as preeclampsia, have significant maternal implications that are covered elsewhere.

Hemolytic Disease—Rh Factor

Hemolytic disease is one of the complications of pregnancy in which there may be devastating fetal effects with virtually no maternal risk. Although the fetal pathology of severe hemolytic disease had been described before the turn of the century, the exact nature of the problem was not known until after the discovery of the Rh factor in 1940. The disease is most unusual in that within 30 years the cause, treatment, and methods for prevention have been worked out. Most of the attention has been focused on the Rh factor as a cause, but the ABO blood groups may also cause a form of hemolytic disease, as do other lesser blood groups.

The incidence of hemolytic disease is related to the occurrence of blood groups. In the Caucasian population, 15% are Rh-negative. In blacks, orientals and American Indians this figure is only 5%. The frequency of Rh hemolytic disease is therefore much less in these groups. Approximately 13% of American marriages have the setup for Rh problems (Rh-negative wife, Rh-positive husband), and 22% have the combinations for ABO disease. Ninety-eight percent of all hemolytic disease is related to either Rh or ABO incompatibilities. Fetal involvement with hemolytic disease formerly occurred with a frequency of approximately 1 in 100 deliveries; however, this incidence has been markedly reduced by the introduction of prevention by Rh immunoglobulin.

Anti-D Globulin

The ability to prevent Rh sensitization has been an established fact since Rh (anti-D) globulin became commercially available in 1969. This substance, which was initially obtained from the plasma of sensitized women, is now obtained by deliberately sensitizing Rh-negative male volunteers. It prevents sensitization by clearing the fetal cells from the material circulating and perhaps also by depressing the patient's immune response. A single dose (300 μg) is capable of clearing up to 15 ml of fetal erythrocytes. Lower doses (50 μg) have been made available for use in situations where only small fetomaternal transfusions are likely, such as first trimester abortion and ectopic pregnancy.

Candidates for Rh immunoglobulin are unsensitized Rh-negative patients who (1) have delivered Rh-positive babies, (2) have had untypable pregnancies such as stillborns, ectopic pregnancies, or spontaneous or induced abortions, or (3) received ABO-compatible Rh-positive blood. It is of no value in the patient who is already sensitized, and although the recommendation is that it should be administered within 3 days of delivery this should not preclude administration at a later time if for some reason the 72-hour deadline has been missed.

Although many failures to prevent sensitization are due to failure to administer Rh immunoglobulin or inadequacy of the dose to cover the size of the fetomaternal bleed, there is a small risk (1% to 2%) of sensitization even when proper technique is followed. The inadequate dose problem can be dealt with by doing appropriate follow-up studies 48 hours after the anti-D globulin. This involves doing either a Kleihauer Betke smear to demonstrate that fetal cells are no longer present, or, even more simply, an indirect Coombs' test to show that there is excess antibody present. If the indirect Coombs' test is negative at 48 hours, an additional dose of immunoglobulin should be given. The remainder of the failures are probably related to fetomaternal bleeding episodes that occurred long enough prior to delivery that the postpartum administration of anti-D globulin will not protect. Several projects are underway to reduce this problem by evaluating the administration of immunoglobulin antepartum in the third trimester either routinely or when there are predisposing occurrences such as third trimester bleeding.

With all of these developments, Rh hemolytic disease is becoming increasingly uncommon, but there does seem to be an irreducible group of patients who are sensitized for the reasons mentioned above. Because the problem is becoming more rare, it is important that the care of the severely sensitized patient be delegated to a perinatal center.

Pathophysiology

The pathogenesis of Rh hemolytic disease is based on the fact that, even though the maternal and fetal circulations are normally completely separated, breaks in this barrier permit the entry of fetal red cells into the maternal circulation during the second and third trimesters and at delivery in up to 50% of pregnancies. Such breaks also occur with abortions beyond 6 to 8 weeks of pregnancy. If these cells are Rh-positive (*e.g.,* containing the Rh+ or D antigen), the mother may react to this mismatched "minitransfusion" by forming protective antibodies. Since the formation of antibodies takes time, and since the unsensitized woman probably does not react until after she delivers, there is rarely a problem in the first pregnancy unless the patient has received a mismatched transfusion in the past. Antibodies formed as the result of the first exposure persist for life. When the woman becomes pregnant again, and the fetus is Rh-positive, she will respond with rapid antibody formation as soon as she is exposed to Rh-positive cells. Thus, once antibodies have been formed, all subsequent pregnancies with Rh-positive infants will be a problem.

There are two types of Rh antibodies. The larger type (gamma M, or 19S) does not cross the placenta as readily as the smaller (gamma g, or 7S). In the case of ABO disease where the mother who lacks the antigen has the antibody (*e.g.,* type O has neither A nor B antigen, but has both anti-A and anti-B antibodies, type A has A antigen and anti-B antibody, and so on), these naturally occurring antibodies are the large 19S variety. Also, because these antibodies require a break in the placental barrier to get into the fetal circulation, and because this is most likely to occur at the time of delivery of the placenta, ABO disease is almost always milder than Rh disease, and rarely is the child stillborn or severely affected at birth. In addition, because the AB antigens are present in all body cells, this tends to absorb excess antibody and reduce the effect on the red cells. However, in Rh disease, there are both 19S and 7S antibodies (the result of sensitization). The 7S antibodies cross readily into the fetal circulation by a facilitated transport mechanism and are responsible for the destruction of the fetal red blood cells. This produces anemia, and if it is severe enough, heart failure results in an edematous hydropic infant, and possibly a stillbirth.

While the fetus is *in utero,* the mother is able to remove the breakdown products of the red cells (bilirubin) and handle them in her own liver; thus, the baby is not born jaundiced. However, once separated from the mother, the newborn must handle the continuing breakdown of red cells, and its liver, especially in prematures, lacks the necessary enzymes to do this efficiently. The affected newborn rapidly develops jaundice and, if untreated, brain damage may result from the deposition of the bile pigments in vital areas of the brain (kernicterus). This is the most severe form of pathology, but it is not only possible but likely that an Rh-negative woman may have one, two, or even more pregnancies without significant difficulty.

Genetic Determination

The inheritance of Rh blood type follows the simple dominant recessive rules, with Rh+ being a dominant. Each person receives two genes (one from each parent) to determine Rh blood type. It is necessary to

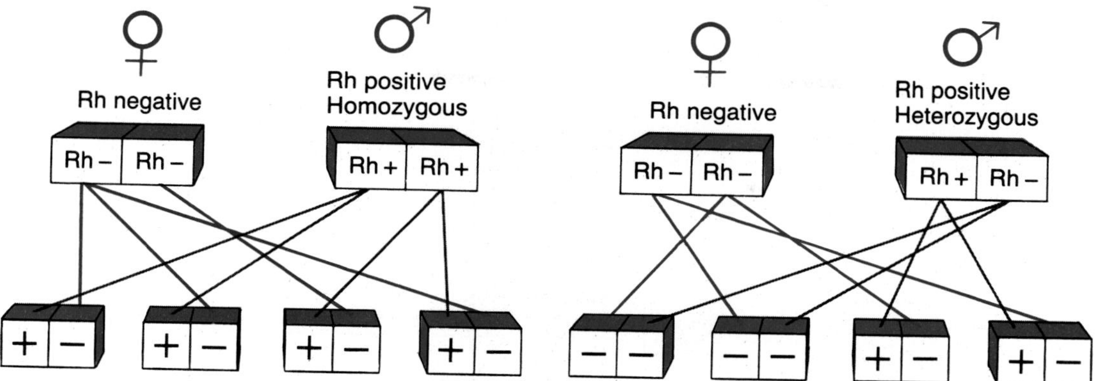

Figure 40-4.
Inheritance patterns for the Rh factor.

receive two Rh-negative genes to be negative, whereas one can be Rh-positive with one Rh-positive and one Rh-negative gene (heterozygous) or two Rh-positive genes (homozygous). Thus, if the husband is heterozygous, there is a 50–50 chance of having an Rh-negative, unaffected child (Fig. 40-4). If the father is homozygous, all offspring will be Rh-positive and subject to hemolytic disease.

In the ABO system, a person may have genes for A, B, AB, or no antigens. Thus, the contribution to the offspring may be A or B or none. For example, type O individuals receive neither A nor B from the parents; a type A individual may receive an A gene from each (AA) or an A from one and none from the other (AO). The same is true for the type B individual (BB or BO). The AB individual receives an A from one parent and a B from the other.

All pregnant patients should have a blood group determination, at least with the first pregnancy. If adequate records are available, this need not be repeated with subsequent pregnancies. If the patient is Rh-negative or type O (the most common maternal type for ABO disease), the husband's blood should also be typed. If he is Rh-positive, a genotype may be done to determine whether he is homozygous or heterozygous. Also, the Rh-negative woman's blood should be examined for the presence of antibodies to the Rh factor (D). This is accomplished by the indirect Coombs' test and is reported in dilutions (*e.g.*, positive 1:2, 1:4, 1:8, and so on). If the initial screening or titer is negative (*i.e.*, shows no antibodies), this should be repeated at approximately 30 and 36 weeks of pregnancy. If both of those titers are negative, it is safe to assume that there will be no significant problem and to permit the pregnancy to run its normal course. If the titer is positive, it becomes necessary to decide how seriously the fetus is affected (*i.e.*, how anemic it is). Because it is not possible to approach the fetus directly and do a hemoglobin or hematocrit, less direct means must be used. In the past, the physician merely repeated the antibody titer, watching for a rise, and combining with this the patient's past history, arrived at a plan of management.

Bilirubin Levels in Fetal Diagnosis

It has now been well established that the severity of the hemolytic anemia in the fetus can best be determined by the quantity of *bilirubin* in the amniotic fluid (*i.e.*, the higher the bilirubin level, the lower the fetal hemoglobin). Thus, amniocentesis with analysis of the bilirubin in the fluid is the best basis for making therapeutic decisions in the sensitized patient. Because the quantity of bilirubin is small in the mildly sensitized or unsensitized patient, standard techniques for measuring bilirubin cannot be used, and therefore a spectrophotometric approach is used. Bilirubin produces an optical density peak at 450 and it is the height of this peak (or the ΔOD_{450}) that is used to evaluate fetal involvement (Fig. 40-5). Amniocentesis is used to evaluate the fetus in all patients with significant sensitization. In most laboratories, a significant antibody titer below which fetal morbidity is unlikely can be determined. Although this varies from institution to institution, titers above 1:8 to 1:16 are generally considered significant. Amniocentesis is usually instituted at 24 to 25 weeks, since intrauterine transfusion is impractical before that, although in instances with previous early stillbirths, the procedure may be instituted as early as 20 weeks. The frequency of repeated amniocentesis is determined by the level of the ΔOD_{450}, weekly taps being indicated if values are high.

The common method for evaluating the ΔOD_{450} is the Liley chart illustrated in Figure 40-5. Values in the lower zone for the particular gestation indicate a mildly or even unaffected fetus, whereas those in the

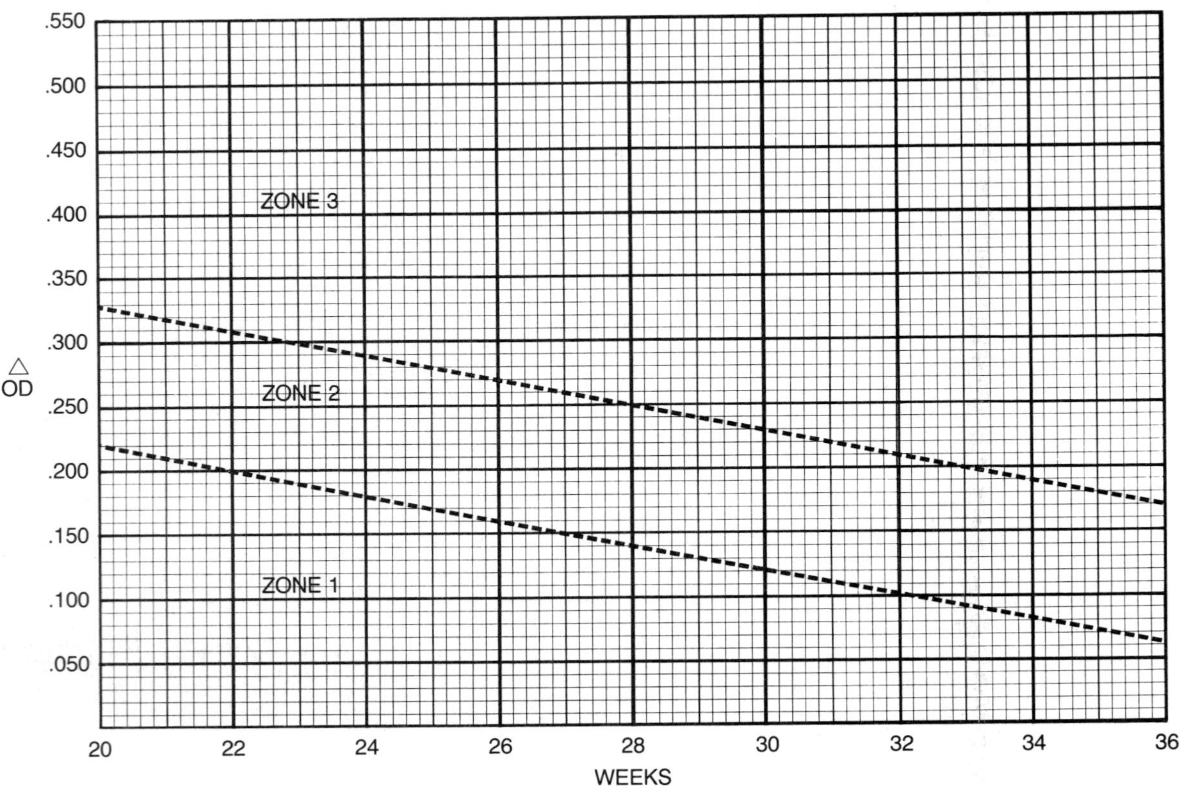

Figure 40-5.
Modified Liley graph for relating ΔOD_{450} to weeks of gestation in determining severity of hemolytic disease. (Management of Erythroblastosis [Technical Bulletin, No. 17]. ACOG, Chicago, July 1972)

middle zone indicate an affected fetus, but one not in immediate danger of death. Values in the upper zone suggest the fetus will not survive 10 to 14 days without intervention. Management decisions are not based on single values but rather on the trend. If the ΔOD_{450} remains in the lower zone, no interference is indicated and the pregnancy can be allowed to proceed to term. If the values remain in the middle zone, the fetus is best delivered as soon as there is evidence of maturity, especially of the lung, by using the L/S ratio. Upper zone values indicate immediate intervention by delivery if beyond 33 to 34 weeks or by intrauterine transfusion if before that gestational age.

This dramatic procedure was first described in 1963 by Liley and involves the instillation of Rh-negative red cells into the peritoneal cavity of the fetus under fluoroscope or more recently by using ultrasound control. The fetus is able to absorb these intact cells. If the procedure is repeated successfully every 10 to 14 days until the point of maturity (approximately 34–35 weeks), a stillbirth may be avoided. Only 40% to 50% of treated fetuses can be saved because the procedure is rather gross, especially in the smaller fetus, and often the fetus is very sick when the procedure is initiated. Of course, these results are far better than no survivors, which could be anticipated without the procedure.

Treatment of Newborn

The pediatric management of the newborn involves the use of exchange transfusion to correct anemia and to reduce the bilirubin concentration, thus obviating the brain damage of kernicterus. Exchange transfusion is often supplemented by the administration of albumin to provide more binding sites for bilirubin and the use of light or phototherapy, which controls the rate of increase of bilirubin by converting it to other apparently innocuous pigments. The management of the newborn may be enhanced by the administration of drugs such as phenobarbital to the mother prenatally. This drug in relatively small doses can induce in the fetus the synthesis of enzymes necessary to conjugate bilirubin and thereby make the newborn better able to deal with the jaundice.

Diabetes Mellitus

The total problem of diabetes and pregnancy is considered in Chapter 34. However, it is important to recognize the specific impact of the disease on the fetus, which is best indicated by the increase in perinatal mortality. Despite the fact that there have been marked improvements in perinatal mortality in general and in diabetic pregnancy specifically, the overall perinatal mortality in diabetic pregnancies is approximately three times that in the nondiabetic. The rate is a direct function of the severity (White classification) of the diabetes, with the rate for the class A diabetic being only slightly above that for the general population while the class F/R diabetic may have not more than a 50–50 chance of having a surviving infant. It has long been known that if all diabetic pregnancies were allowed to go to term, there would be a small but significant number of stillbirths based on the impact of diabetes on the blood vessels of the uterus and placenta, producing premature aging. In order to avoid these stillbirths, routine early delivery became the pattern of management. This unfortunately resulted in an increase in neonatal deaths because of the propensity of diabetic offspring to respiratory distress syndrome. Current improved survival is related to selective early delivery and antepartum testing for fetal pulmonary maturity.

The increased susceptibility of the diabetic offspring to the respiratory distress syndrome is felt to be at least sevenfold and is related to a delay in the onset of surfactant production by the type II cells in the lung. This occurs in class A, B, and C diabetics, whereas in class D and F diabetics, in whom vascular disease predominates, pulmonary maturity is accelerated. In addition to pulmonary problems, there are several metabolic problems that are increased in the infant of a diabetic mother. Because glucose crosses the placenta readily by supple diffusion, the fetal glucose level reflects the level in the mother. Insulin, on the other hand, does not cross, and consequently the fetus must deal with its hyperglycemia by hypertrophy of pancreatic islet cells and the production of insulin. The combination of high levels of insulin and glucose along with the growth-hormonelike substance HPL is responsible for the increased size of fetuses in class A, B, and C diabetic pregnancies. The magnitude of the increase in fetal size is related inversely to the adequacy of maternal blood sugar control. Macrosomia increases the likelihood of mechanical problems and fetal injury at delivery and is in part responsible for a high cesarean section rate among diabetics. This same mechanism (fetal hyperinsulinism) is responsible for neonatal hypoglycemia when the maternal source of glucose is eliminated after delivery. These babies are also more prone to hyperbilirubinemia and hypocalcemia.

Another major problem of the diabetic newborn is birth defects. Congenital malformations are increased three times in babies born to diabetic women, and lethal defects are six times as likely. Although many kinds of defects are observed, skeletal defects involving the caudal portion of the skeleton (caudal regression) and ventricular septal defects are the most characteristic.

Finally, there is the question of development of diabetes in the child. The genetics of diabetes is not well understood, and there may be several mechanisms involved. The suggestion that the disease is inherited as an autosomal recessive is refuted by the facts that the concordance rate is not nearly 100% in identical twins and that diabetic matings do not always result in diabetic children. There is also with diabetes the question of expression, which means that a person who has the genetic determinants for diabetes may not express the disease unless confronted with stresses such as pregnancy, obesity, or infection. The best advice to be given the diabetic patient concerning these considerations is that there is an increased chance that the child may develop diabetes and that the magnitude of this increase is related to the amount of diabetes present in the pedigrees of both father and mother.

It is quite apparent then that the overall outlook for the diabetic woman producing a healthy, normal infant is restricted more severely in long-standing severe diabetes, and therefore the cost in dollars, time, and emotional investment is high. Ideally, the diabetic and her family should be apprised of this information prior to undertaking a pregnancy so that the decision can be a well-considered one.

Prolonged Pregnancy

The average duration of pregnancy is 280 days from the first day of the last menstrual period, or 267 days from the time of conception if the menstrual cycle is of average length. Only 5% of women deliver on the actual due date, although most deliver within 10 days to 14 days in either direction from the date. Since the placenta has a normal life span equal to the duration of pregnancy, one may be justifiably concerned that if the due date is exceeded by more than 2 weeks, the aging placenta may no longer be able to support the fetus adequately. Fortunately, in most instances the placenta is capable of such support. In fact, in a great number of patients who are postdates, the date has been miscalculated or based on faulty memory. In addition to those postmature pregnancies in which there is placental insufficiency, there is another group of late pregnancies in which the placenta functions well and the fetus becomes oversized, creating potential mechanical problems in labor and delivery.

If the circumstances including the status of the cervix, the size and position of the baby, and the size of the maternal pelvis are all favorable, induction of labor should be carried out when a pregnancy exceeds the due date by 10 days to 14 days. If there is any question about the dates, efforts should be made to verify the gestational age by techniques already discussed. It is important to recognize, however, that a single determination in late pregnancy has a rather significant inherent error. This is especially true of ultrasound measurements of the biparietal diameter, since linear growth stops after 30 weeks. When a pregnancy is 10 to 14 days postdate and conditions are not favorable for induction of labor, the well-being of the fetus must be established in order to permit the continuation of the pregnancy. Urinary or serum estriols may be used, and this clinical circumstance is one of few in which HPL determinations seem helpful. The frequency of these studies is critical. Because the adequacy of placental function is not necessarily static under such circumstances, these studies can provide only limited assurance and must be repeated two or three times weekly.

The oxytocin challenge test (OCT) and nonstress test, described in Chapter 41, are also valuable in evaluating the postdate pregnancy. Because of the possibility of a rapid progressive decline in placental function, the OCT cannot provide the usually accepted promise of seven days of well-being for the fetus.

In addition to establishing maturity in the case of uncertain gestational age, the examination of amniotic fluid for meconium may be helpful in such cases. Clear fluid is reassuring although it does not rule out fetal jeopardy. Meconium staining and scant fluid both suggest an affected fetus, and, although not sufficient alone to indicate aggressive action, they are confirmatory in the presence of other signs of fetal compromise. Aspiratory and severe pulmonary consequences for the newborn always exist when meconium is present. However, prevention is a dilemma. Even prompt delivery by cesarean section does not necessarily obviate aspiration, since respiratory movements can occur *in utero*.

The affected postmature (sometimes called dysmature) newborn has a typical appearance. It is long for its weight, which makes it appear to have lost weight. The finger- and toenails are long and stained with meconium, as are the cord and membranes. These infants are especially prone to distress during labor and to respiratory problems in the neonatal period.

On the surface, it would seem simple to determine the due date and the probability that the pregnancy has gone beyond that point, but there are a number of pitfalls. Many patients do not record or cannot recall when they had their last period. Others have long cycles, with ovulation and conception occurring later than the fourteenth day. This is especially true in patients discontinuing oral contraceptive therapy, in whom the first ovulation may not occur until 4 weeks to 6 weeks after the last withdrawal flow. One must assess these factors carefully before overtreating a patient for supposed postmaturity.

Preeclampsia–Eclampsia

Although the manifestations of preeclampsia (hypertension, edema, and proteinuria) and eclampsia (convulsions in addition) are primarily maternal (see Chap. 34), the fetal impact cannot be ignored. Progressive placental insufficiency is an inherent part of the syndrome, and intrauterine fetal growth is frequently retarded prior to the development of maternal manifestations. With the appearance of clinically evident preeclampsia, placental function continues to decline and fetal death may result if the pregnancy is allowed to continue. Occasionally, a patient with moderate or severe preeclampsia may appear to respond so favorably to therapy that there is the temptation to allow the pregnancy to continue to permit further fetal maturity. Such a decision is fraught with risk of failure to the fetus to prosper and the possibility of a stillbirth. In most cases it is unwise. Should such a course be considered, amniocentesis for detection of pulmonary maturity (L/S ratio) should be done first because pulmonary maturity is often markedly accelerated in such circumstances. To attempt to prolong a pregnancy in the face of significant preeclampsia is not appropriate if the fetal lungs are already mature. If the L/S ratio is at immature levels, and a conservative course is to be followed, fetal well-being must be carefully assessed. This is not a simple matter since urinary estriol excretion may be reduced by impaired renal function, whereas serum levels may be falsely elevated. Interpretation of OCTs and nonstress tests is also difficult in the immature fetus.

The perinatal wastage in preeclampsia is largely a function of the stage of pregnancy at which the process develops and therefore the degree of maturity of the infant delivered. If preeclampsia does not develop until after the thirty-sixth week of gestation, the perinatal loss should be quite low. Perinatal mortality is high when convulsions (eclampsia) occur. Recent reviews indicate a rate of approximately 20%.

Chronic Hypertension

Approximately 75% of women with benign essential hypertension go through pregnancy with no problems, either maternal or fetal. Unfortunately, some 15% develop preeclampsia. When this happens, the fetal prognosis is very poor, especially if preeclampsia occurs at a time when the fetus is significantly premature (at the end of the second trimester, for example). The perinatal mortality rate in this group is approximately 20%.

In the case of the hypertensive mother without superimposed preeclampsia, the fetal risk is not great, but it is greater than that for women with normal blood pressure. Because of this, it is recommended that fetal evaluation be initiated for all hypertensive patients in the third trimester to identify the occasional benign hypertensive patient whose fetus is in jeopardy and for whom preterm delivery is indicated. There is, in addition, an increased frequency of abruptio placentae in these hypertensive patients, with the added perinatal wastage characteristic of that problem.

TORCH Infections Affecting the Fetus

There is an increasing number of infections with recognized detrimental effects upon the fetus. These may be direct effects on fetus or indirect effects by precipitating abortion or premature labor. The term TORCH (T–toxoplasmosis, O–other, R–rubella, C–cytomegalovirus, H–herpes) has been applied to these infections. Although it does account for the majority of significant perinatal infections there are many others, some of which are listed in Figure 40-6.

Toxoplasmosis

This disease is caused by the protozoan organism *Toxoplasma gondii,* which is contracted from oocytes in cat feces or by eating uncooked meat. Only cats that

Figure 40-6.
Arrows indicate probable routes of fetomaternal infection. (Evans ME, Glass L: Perinatal Medicine, Hagerstown, Harper & Row, 1976)

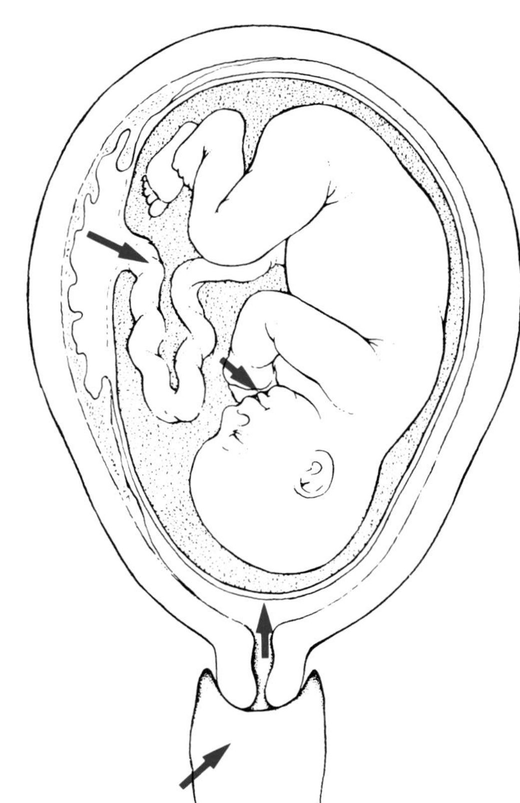

are unconfined and eat infected rodents are a hazard. When primary infection, which is generally asymptomatic, occurs just before or during early pregnancy, congenital infection may result. This can lead to the birth of a child who is mentally and physically retarded with chorioretinitis and microcephaly. Approximately 10% to 15% of these babies die, and most of the survivors are severely compromised. If the disease is recognized clinically or by seroconversion in early pregnancy, abortion is recommended. If abortion is not accepted or the infection occurs later in pregnancy, treatment with triple sulfa may reduce the fetal impact.

Others

Many infections, such as syphilis and varicella, can be included in this category. But group B beta hemolytic streptococcus is most deserving of mention. This organism is not a major pathogen in the mother, but when it causes early neonatal sepsis, it produces a fulminant pneumonia with a very high mortality (greater than 40%). The organism is sexually transmitted and is carried asymptomatically in the cervix and vagina in a significant number (over 20%) of pregnant women. The infection is thought to be contracted by contact during the birth process and is especially likely to occur when predisposing factors such as prematurity, prolonged labor, and premature rupture of the membranes exist. The rate of newborn colonization is high; however, the attack (infection) rate is low (1% to 2% of colonized babies become infected). Screening of all gravidae and treatment of carriers had been recommended, but the practicality of the approach is open to serious question.

A second clinical picture, the late onset, occurs after seven to ten days, with a picture of meningitis; the source is not necessarily the cervix or vagina or even the mother. Mortality in late onset infection is considerably less.

Rubella

Although most concerns are for infection in the first trimester, serious problems are known to occur when the infection happens as late as the fifth month of gestation, and later infections may be responsible for more subtle problems. Infections in the first trimester may result in abortion in more than 33% of cases. Congenital rubella (*i.e.,* the expanded rubella syndrome) may be difficult to differentiate clinically from the other TORCH infections, although cultures of the virus or specific IgM measurements are diagnostic. It is especially important to recognize that these babies are highly infectious, as are the placentas, and contact with nonimmune pregnant personnel should be avoided.

When the pregnant woman is exposed to rubella, she should have immediate serologic testing for rubella antibody. If this indicates immunity she is protected (85% to 90% of adults in the United States are immune). If she is not immune she should be carefully followed for development of clinical rubella or development of antibodies. If either of these developments occur, abortion should be recommended in view of the high rate of fetal involvement. Gamma globulin is not recommended in rubella exposure unless abortion is unacceptable, and then it is important for the patient to realize that, although the disease may be modified, fetal effects are not necessarily obviated.

Immunization against rubella is recommended for all susceptible women in the child-bearing age group, but special care must be taken to avoid immunizing the pregnant woman. Although the exact risk is not known, the vaccine virus is known to have access to the fetus. One convenient time for rubella vaccination is the immediate postpartum period, because pregnancy is unlikely then, and breast-feeding is not a contraindication in rubella vaccination.

Cytomegalovirus

This is the most common of the congenital infections. Approximately two thirds of adult women have antibodies to the virus and the virus can be cultured from the cervix or urine of 3% to 5% of pregnant women. Most adult infections are asymptomatic although this organism is a special problem among immunosuppressed patients—in transplant units, for example—and therefore a special hazard to nurses working in such areas. Congenital infection occurs in about 1% of births with approximately 10% of infected newborns exhibiting permanent damage. The severe form of congenital infection produces a clinical picture not dissimilar to other TORCH infections. The diagnosis can be established by viral culture or serology. There is no specific therapy unless the diagnosis can be established sufficiently early to provide an abortion option.

Herpes Simplex

There are two strains of this virus: type I, which is primarily responsible for oral lesions, and type II for genital lesions. These distinctions are not absolute but hold in the majority of cases. Type II herpes infection can be sexually transmitted and is discussed further in Chapters 35 and 43. Antibodies to the herpesvirus, although specific to types I and II, are cross protective so that a prior type I infection will prevent viremia with a first infection of type II and cause it to behave clinically as a recurrent, rather than primary, infection. Primary genital herpesvirus infections are characterized by multiple lesions, systemic symptoms, and prolonged viral shedding. Once the primary infection has occurred, the virus is sequestered in the dorsal nerve route. There tends to be a series of recurrences at irregular intervals over a period of the next 2 to 3 years.

Two problems are evident in pregnancy. Congenital infection, which is extremely rare, can occur when a primary infection (absent antibodies, viremia) occurs in pregnancy. Like other TORCH infections, the impact is greatest when this occurs in early pregnancy and the result is similar (*i.e.,* mental retardation, microcephaly, cerebral calcification, chorioretinitis). The more common concern is neonatal infection, which is contracted during delivery by exposure to the virus in genital lesions or in the asymptomatic carrier state. Disease in the newborn may be localized or systemic. The prognosis is good in newborns in whom the disease remains localized, but 50% progress to systemic diseases, with a mortality of 90%.

Treatment consists of avoiding the contact by cesarean section if lesions or positive cultures persist at term. Section should be carried out prior to rupture of the membranes or within 4 hours. Long delays after rupture of the membranes are accompanied by a high risk of neonatal infection. Chemotherapy of the infected newborn is under study. The drugs used are toxic but treatment is justified by the high mortality of the disease.

Infections due to Premature Rupture of Membranes

Intrauterine infection as a result of premature rupture of the membranes is probably the most common infectious threat to the fetus. It is well recognized that the frequency of such infection parallels the length of time from the rupture of the membranes to the onset of labor. Infection of the fetus occurs by way of the amniotic fluid to the fetal tracheobronchial tree, as well as from the membranes and placenta through the cord vessels, producing fetal sepsis. The organisms most commonly involved are anaerobic streptococci and gram-negative bacilli.

Since it is difficult to achieve therapeutic levels of antibiotics in the amniotic fluid once the patient becomes febrile, the treatment is delivery either by induction or cesarean section. More important, however, is the prevention of infection. This is accomplished by delivery (most often by induction, but by cesarean section if necessary) of any patient with premature rupture of the membranes whose fetus is larger than 1500 to 1800 g. This weight range is selected because in most clinics the survival data for babies of that size are such that the risk of delivery and prematurity appears to be less than the risk of intrauterine infection. Recent data have suggested, however, that with premature rupture of the membranes, the fetal lung may mature within 24 to 48 hours and therefore a delay may be indicated. This effect has yet to be clearly established in maturing the fetal lung.

Fetal Growth Retardation

Fetal growth retardation is one term applied to the clinical syndrome in which the fetus fails to prosper *in utero.* The terms dysmaturity, placental insufficiency, small-for-date babies, uteroplacental insufficiency, and stunted fetus have also been applied. The syndrome may occur with maternal diseases such as diabetes with severe vascular involvement, chronic renal disease, and chronic hypertension with renal involvement. Intrauterine infection with rubella, toxoplasmosis, and cytomegalovirus are causes. The most severe growth retardation is produced by multiple congenital malformations. In some cases the syndrome may be idiopathic and recurrent. In general, the earlier in gestation that retardation is apparent, the poorer the outlook.

At birth these babies appear to have lost subcutaneous fat, their skin is often wrinkled, and the finger- and toenails are long. The amniotic fluid, cord, and nails are heavily stained with meconium. The stillbirth rate is high, and the frequency of respiratory problems in the newborn is increased. The most significant management problem from the obstetrical viewpoint is differentiating (antepartally) the growth-retarded fetus from a premature fetus of appropriate size. After delivery, this differentiation is less difficult and can be based on weight (particularly weight gain patterns), certain developmental criteria such as ear cartilage development and plantar skin creases, and behavior patterns.

The question of erroneous menstrual dates often arises and this necessitates the use of the method described under fetal diagnosis. Once the diagnosis is suspected, some search for an etiology is indicated. Heroic approaches to the fetus are certainly not indicated if a diagnosis of congenital rubella or cytomegalovirus infection has been established. However, this may not be simple to do if, on the other hand, the diagnosis is not ominous. The fetus must be evaluated and followed with an index of well-being (such as urinary estriol). Delivery must be timed appropriately. In the presence of uteroplacental insufficiency, fetal tolerance to labor may be reduced and the need for cesarean section increased. After birth, newborns with late pregnancy growth retardation and without infection or malformation tend to thrive and rapidly catch up in size with their peers. Those newborns with early pregnancy growth retardation have reduced cell numbers as well as reduced cell size and tend to remain small.

Disproportionate Twin Development

Twins with disparity in size may be accounted for by the possibility of a connection between the placental circulations. This is especially true in single-ovum twins. When this happens in early pregnancy and one heart pumps more strongly than the other, there may be monopolization of a larger area of the placenta by one twin and thus a disparity in size. Such twins are not only greatly different in size at birth, but the smaller one is often anemic and may require transfusion. The larger twin may be hypervolemic and require a phlebotomy to prevent heart failure and jaundice. This type of placental anastomosis, when it occurs in double-ovum twins, accounts for those rare situations known as "chimerism," in which an individual may have two populations of cells, as evidenced by blood groups or sex chromatin. The other important clinical significance of disparity in twin sizes is that difficulties may be encountered in delivery if the smaller of the twins is delivered first through a cervix that is not completely dilated.

Fetal Treatment

The art of fetal treatment is at this time far less developed than fetal diagnosis. The most common approach to the fetus by the obstetrician is to select an appropriate time for delivery, convert the fetus to a newborn, and thus allow active treatment by the neonatologist. Perhaps the most important approach to the fetus is to provide appropriate support throughout the pregnancy. This includes adequate prenatal diet, as well as glucose and oxygen during labor, especially if there is fetal distress.

Treatment in the case of a positive prenatal diagnosis of congenital disease is generally limited to therapeutic abortion. However, in some instances of metabolic errors, maternal dietary modification may be effective in protecting the fetus with an enzyme defect.

Many drugs administered to the mother cross the placenta into the fetal circulation. Transplacental passage is generally a function of the molecular size of the drug. Substances with molecular weights less than 500 cross readily by simple diffusion. Although most often there is concern regarding the deleterious effects of drugs on the fetus, in some instances one can achieve a desirable therapeutic effect. In the case of the sensitized Rh-negative patient, it is possible with certain drugs to induce the fetal liver to produce the enzymes required for bilirubin conjugation. This allows the newborn to cope better with the jaundice and reduces the need for exchange transfusion. The most effective drug is phenobarbital in small doses (15 mg, four times daily) for 1 or 2 weeks prior to delivery.

Another example of fetal drug therapy is the administration of glucocorticoids to the mother to induce the production of surfactant by the type II cells of the fetal lung and thereby reduce the risk of respiratory distress syndrome. The evidence is that if this is done between 26 to 28 and 32 to 34 weeks of gestation, and if delivery can be delayed for 24 to 48 hours, there will be a significant reduction in RDS. The effect appears to be transient, as the frequency of respiratory distress increases when delivery is delayed for more than 7 days following treatment. The effectiveness of this approach is still under investigation. Those who do not favor its use point out that the long-term effects on the child of exposure to glucocorticoids *in utero* are not known, and that glucocorticoids may increase the risk of *in utero* infection. This treatment is still under review.

Intrauterine fetal transfusion in Rh disease is the most publicized form of treatment. Hopefully, the use of Rh immune globulin prophylaxis will ultimately eliminate the need for this rather crude procedure.

The future undoubtedly holds many advances in this area—from the prenatal correction of congenital defects to the unscrambling of genetic mishaps. There may well be treatments of maladies that are presently unknown in this rapidly developing area of fetal medicine.

Suggested Reading

Bolognese RL, Schwarz RH, Schneider J (eds): Perinatal Medicine Management of the Fetus and Neonate, 2nd ed. Baltimore, Williams & Wilkins, 1982

Cohen AR (ed): Emergencies in Obstetrics and Gynecology. New York, Churchill Livingstone, 1981

Depp R: Postmaturity. In Queenan JT (ed): Management of the High Risk Pregnancy. Oradell, NJ, Medical Economics Book Division, 1980

Freeman RK, Garite TJ: Fetal Heart Monitoring. Baltimore, Williams & Wilkins, 1981

Gant NF, Worley RJ: Hypertension in Pregnancy: Concepts & Management. New York, Appleton–Century–Crofts, 1980

Hobbins JC, Winsberg F: Ultrasonography in Obstetrics and Gynecology. Baltimore, Williams & Wilkins, 1977

Scott JR (guest ed): Isoimmunization in pregnancy. Clin Obstet Gynecol 25; 241–456, 1982

Seeds AE (guest ed): Diabetes in pregnancy. Clin Obstet Gynecol 24; 1–324, 1981

Sever JL, Larsen JW, Grossman JH (eds): Handbook of Perinatal Infections. Boston, Little, Brown & Co, 1979

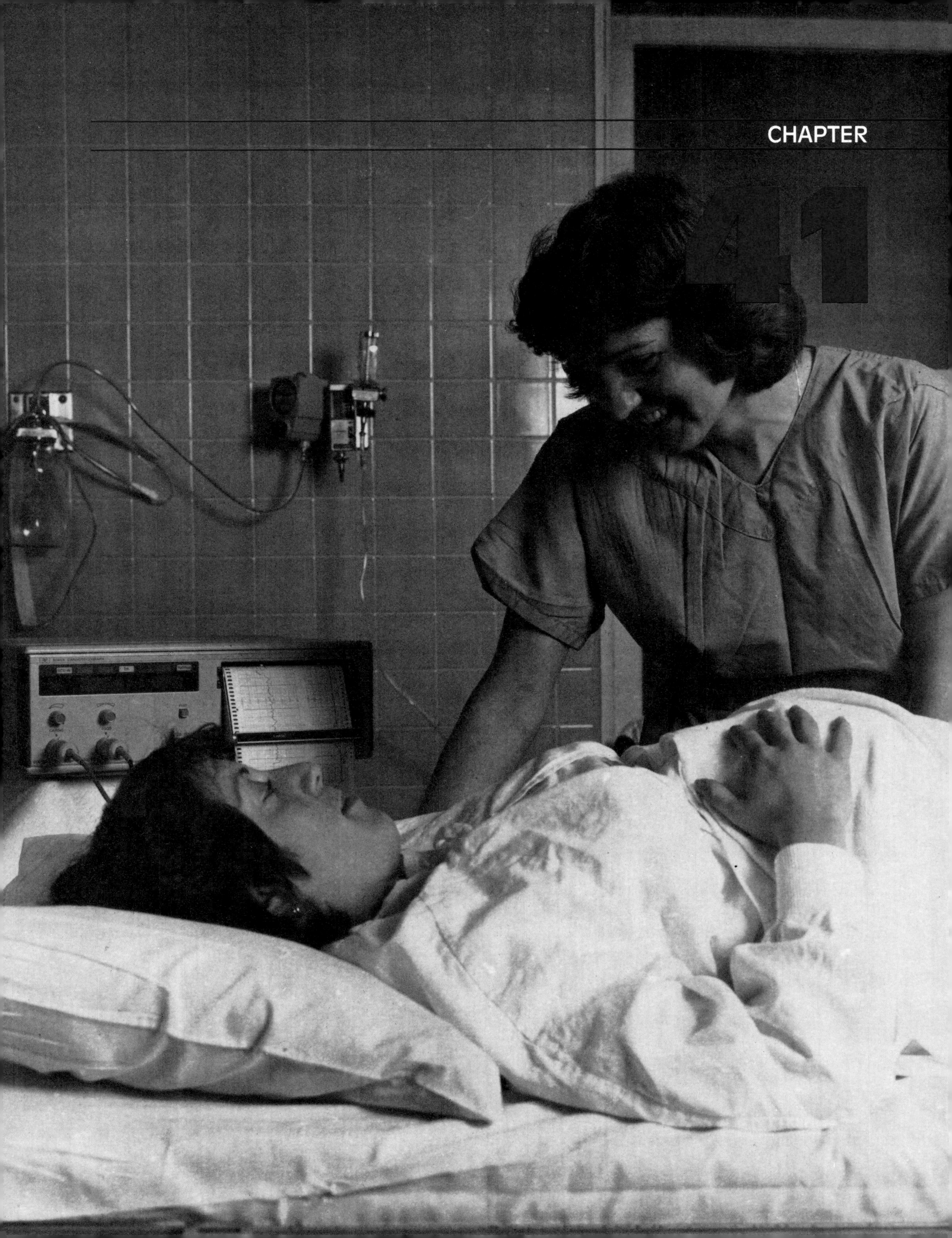

CHAPTER

41

CHAPTER 41

Electronic Fetal Monitoring and Fetal Intensive Care

The fetus, as a "patient," has always been relatively inaccessible to the nurse and the physician. For many years, the forces of labor and the well-being of the fetus could only be evaluated by palpation of the maternal abdomen and by periodic sampling of the fetal heart rate (FHR) through auscultation. A greater understanding of fetal cardiorespiratory physiology and methods to measure certain maternal and fetal functions have developed over the past two decades. Among these methods, continuous electronic monitoring of FHR and uterine activity (UA) have had the widest clinical application. Experience with this instrumentation has resulted in an improved understanding and clinical interpretation of intrapartum events.

The Pros and Cons of Fetal Monitoring

Several studies suggest that the majority of intrapartum fetal deaths should be avoidable when the FHR is monitored continuously. It is also generally considered that continuous fetal monitoring enables early detection of intrapartum fetal hypoxia (distress) and, when accompanied by appropriate therapy, results in lower neonatal morbidity and mortality, as well as improved neurologic development following birth. Most obstetricians believe that continuous fetal monitoring offers substantial benefit in this regard. Clinical studies of its value, however, have produced conflicting results, especially in relation to its use during normal labor. Although the observation of normal fetal monitoring data is predictive of a good fetal outcome, the interpretation of abnormal patterns has been fraught with difficulty and with considerable false-positive diagnosis (*i.e.,* an apparently abnormal finding when the fetus is well). All of this has led the medical community, governmental agencies, and the consumer to question the value of fetal monitoring. It is apparent that valid "cost-benefit" and "risk-benefit" analyses will require more data from long-term prospective studies.

Because methods of fetal monitoring are at times applied internally, several potential risks to the mother and the fetus have been suggested. Complications such as uterine perforations or neonatal scalp infections are uncommon and rarely require therapy. The relationship of internal fetal monitoring to maternal infectious morbidity, although a concern, has generally not proved to be as important as other contributing factors, such as prolonged rupture of membranes and an excessive number of vaginal examinations. Concerns regarding the contributions of electronic fetal monitoring to the increasing rate of cesarean sections have been raised repeatedly. Although this is difficult to evaluate, a number of investigators have suggested that the effect is not substantial. In fact, some have claimed that experience with appropriate use of monitoring can reduce the frequency of cesarean sections that are performed for fetal distress.

In spite of these controversies, the use of electronic fetal monitoring has become commonplace. Because not every high-risk fetus can be identified prior to labor, some physicians advocate electronic monitoring of all patients during labor. However, uncertainty of the benefit in normal pregnancy and limited availability of equipment frequently result in selective monitoring of high-risk patients and those receiving oxytocics or conduction anesthetics. Fetal monitoring has also been extended to the evaluation of the high-risk fetus prior to labor. This form of periodic evaluation, either nonstress testing (NST) or contraction stress testing (CST), is being used effectively to assess fetal well-being in a large variety of pregnancy complications.

With the development of monitoring, the role of the nurse during labor has expanded to caring for the fetus as well as for the mother. As with other diagnostic procedures, it is the nurse's responsibility to inform the patient about the purpose and the procedure of the monitoring and to screen and interpret the data initially. In many institutions, nursing guidelines have been established concerning the application of fetal monitors, the interpretation of data, and the institution of remedial change when abnormalities are detected. Thus, to use the fetal monitor, the nurse must be familiar with the equipment, have an understanding of the fundamental principles involved, and have access to updated information concerning interpretation and management of the data.

Methods of Monitoring

Many different types and models of fetal monitors are available. It is critically important that the nurse be thoroughly familiar with the particular model to be used, including its capabilities, limitations, and method of recording. See Tips for Buyers and Definitions.

Tips for Buyers

Many brands of monitoring equipment are marketed. When one is considering the purchase of a monitoring system, the following information may be helpful:

The system should be designed to monitor externally and internally.

An ultrasonic transducer should have a wide beam, so that the fetal heart rate signal is not easily lost.

The tachometer should measure each fetal heartbeat instead of taking an average of several beats.

The chart speed should be the standard 3 cm per minute.

An engineer should evaluate all components of the system.

The manufacturer should be able to supply all needed accessories, such as ultrasonic jelly, catheters, and so forth.

The system should be portable. Some companies sell monitoring carts with drawers to store accessories.

There should be a warranty.

Servicing should be readily available.

The company should permit a trial period before final purchase, and most companies will agree to this.

Definitions

1. Amplitude of contraction—Pressure exerted by uterus during a contraction; measured from baseline to peak.
2. Amplitude of fetal heart rate—Difference in beats per minute between baseline and the minimum or maximum count.
3. FHR baseline—Modal rate that prevails apart from the periodic accelerations and decelerations occurring with uterine contractions.
4. Periodic fluctuations and changes—Change in fetal heart rate from a baseline rate
   Acceleration—Transient increases lasting less than 10 min.
   Deceleration—Transient decreases lasting less than 10 min.
   A. Tachycardia—Fetal heart rate of more than 160 beats per minute persisting 10 min. to 15 min.
      Mild—160 to 179
      Marked—180 or more
   B. Bradycardia—Fetal heart rate of less than 120 beats per minute persisting 10 min. to 15 min.
      Mild—100 to 119
      Marked—less than 100
5. Abnormal FHR patterns
   A. Uniform patterns of deceleration
      a. Early deceleration (type I Dip). Onset, nadir, and recovery of the FHR coincides with the onset, peak, and end of the contraction. Attributed to compression of fetal head.
      b. Late deceleration (type II Dip). Onset of slowing occurs as contraction intensity peaks. Nadir in FHR reached well after peak, recovery of FHR reached after contraction ended. Attributed to uteroplacental insufficiency.
   B. Nonuniform patterns of deceleration: variable deceleration—FHR decreases begin at no fixed time in relation to contraction; no pattern in wave forms and often nonrepetitive. Classified as mild, moderate, severe, or minimal, average, marked. Attributed to cord compression.
   C. Combined (mixed) patterns of deceleration patterns combining two or more patterns described above.
   D. Sinusoidal pattern
      A repetitive undulation of the baseline resembling a "sine wave." Persistent patterns indicative of fetal hypoxia or severe anemia; unusual, although considered ominous.
6. Reactive baseline—Fetal heart rate normally fluctuating more than 15 beats per minute from baseline.
7. Recovery time—Seconds from end of contraction until fetal heart rate returns to baseline.
8. Lag time—Time between peak of uterine contraction and lowest count of fetal heart deceleration.
9. Variability—Beat to beat variation of the resting fetal heart rate. Normal variability is greater than 5 beats per minute. Diminished variability is less than 5 beats per minute or flat. In the absence of explainable causes, diminished variability is considered ominous and potentially indicative of hypoxia.

The Record

Fetal monitors are equipped to provide a continuous recording of FHR and UA. This information is recorded on perforated paper that folds "accordion style" (Fig. 41-1). The UA is generally recorded on the lower channel. The recording paper provides a vertical scale for measuring the intrauterine pressure, usually in millimeters of mercury (mm Hg). Most monitors are equipped with a zeroing and calibration device to ensure that the record accurately reflects the true intrauterine pressure. The FHR in beats per minute is displayed on the upper channel. Some monitors are also equipped with a digital display of the FHR and a small oscilloscope screen for viewing the fetal electrocardiogram (FECG).

The paper speed is usually set at 3 cm per minute. Divisions on the horizontal scale provide a measurement of the time elapsed and are useful as markers to correlate events on both channels. Numbering on the individual sheets of the record provides a reference for rapid calculation of elapsed time for longer intervals as well as for charting. For example, the nurse's record might reflect the following:

11:30 P.M. Panel #17474—Continuous external fetal monitoring initiated using ultrasound. FHR baseline 136–144 bpm. Uterine contractions every 3 minutes. Jane Doe.

11:50 P.M. Panel #17479—Dilation 6 cm. Effacement complete Station +1. Artificial rupture of membranes. Fluid clear. Internal monitor applied. Jane Doe.

12:30 A.M. Panel #17489—FHR baseline 132–140, variability moderate. UA–baseline 10 mm Hg. Contractions q 2 min, 50 mm Hg. Periodic change—occasional mild variable decelerations to 120 bpm with contractions, duration 30 sec, prompt recovery to baseline. Jane Doe.

Because the data obtained become a part of the patient's permanent record, it is important that a systematic method of identification be used at the beginning and end of each fetal monitor tracing. A sample format for identification is shown in Figure 41-2. In addition, it has become common practice to record the clock-time and important clinical data, such as vital signs, vaginal exams, rupture of membranes, medications (dose and route of administration), and patient activity, directly on the monitor record. This information is important for interpreting the record and is invaluable when reviewed retrospectively for teaching purposes. Monitor tracings as well as nursing notes should be signed by the nurse who is making the observations.

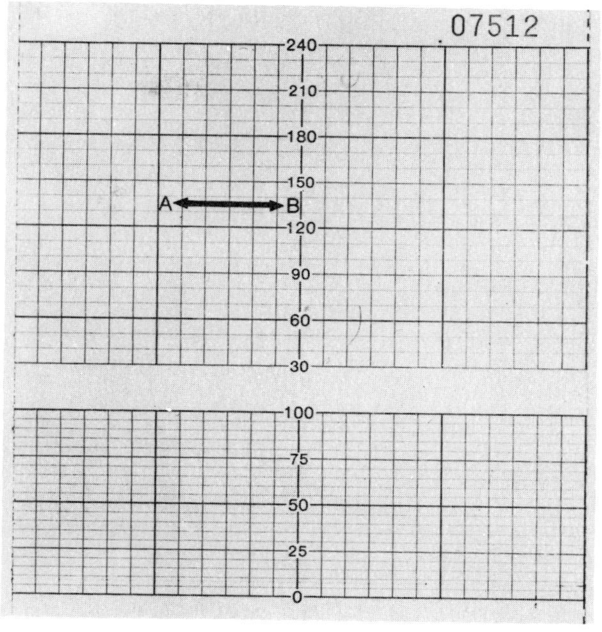

Figure 41-1.
Recording paper for fetal monitor. Note FHR bpm recorded on upper channel, UA mm Hg recorded on lower channel, and panel number at top of sheet. Distance from A to B equals one minute when paper speed is 3 cm/min.

Uterine Activity (UA)

UA may be monitored by either external or internal methods. External monitoring provides a recording of the frequency and duration of uterine contractions (UC), while internal monitoring provides an accurate measurement of intrauterine pressure for assessing both baseline tone and the intensity of the contractions.

The use of an internal pressure catheter permits the most accurate assessment of UA, both quantitatively and temporally. Thus, the internal method is particularly useful in evaluating patients receiving oxytocic drugs or in instances when the temporal relationship of changes in FHR to UC is unclear. Nevertheless, the majority of labors that are monitored can be adequately assessed by the external method. The method used, and any change of method, should be noted directly on the fetal monitoring record as well as in the nursing record.

External Pressure Monitoring

UA is monitored by a pressure transducer called a *tokodynamometer.* A transducer converts one form of energy to another; this transducer converts pressure to electrical signals. The tokodynamometer is a flat

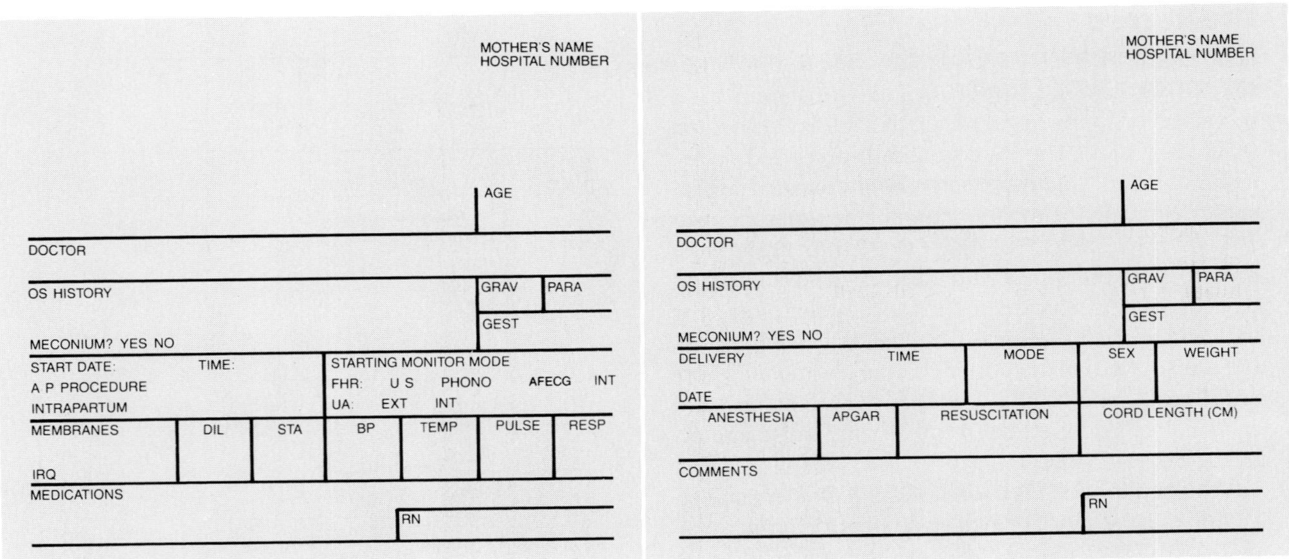

MOTHER'S NAME
HOSPITAL NUMBER
AGE
DOCTOR
OS HISTORY
GRAV PARA
GEST
MECONIUM? YES NO
START DATE: TIME:
STARTING MONITOR MODE
A P PROCEDURE
FHR: U S PHONO AFECG INT
INTRAPARTUM
UA: EXT INT
MEMBRANES DIL STA BP TEMP PULSE RESP
IRQ
MEDICATIONS
RN

MOTHER'S NAME
HOSPITAL NUMBER
AGE
DOCTOR
OS HISTORY
GRAV PARA
GEST
MECONIUM? YES NO
DELIVERY TIME MODE SEX WEIGHT
DATE
ANESTHESIA APGAR RESUSCITATION CORD LENGTH (CM)
COMMENTS
RN

Figure 41-2.
Label on left provides identification and clinical information for interpretation of tracing and is applied when monitoring is initiated. Label on right provides identification and clinical information for correlation of monitor data with neonatal condition.

disk with either a protruding or a flush plunger. It is secured to the mother's abdomen with an elastic belt. As the uterus contracts, the abdominal wall rises and presses against the transducer. The subsequent movement of the plunger is converted into an electrical signal and is recorded on the paper, giving a continuous record of the frequency and duration of contractions.

Correct placement of the tokodynamometer is necessary if interpretable data are to be gathered. The transducer is placed over the area where the greatest displacement of the uterus occurs during a contraction (*i.e.,* the uterine fundus). Displacement of the abdominal wall by the uterus may not be adequate to record UC in a patient with a small uterus (*i.e.,* marked prematurity) or in one who is extremely overweight. Movement of the maternal abdominal wall caused by respirations, coughing, or position changes may be reflected on the fetal monitoring record. Any such interfering factors should be noted as such. It may not be possible to obtain consistent data with this method from patients who are extremely restless. Occasionally, patients who do not have anesthesia find that the firm elastic straps become uncomfortable or interfere with breathing techniques and effleurage. When this occurs, repositioning the tokodynamometer and straps may be useful. If this is not effective, internal pressure monitoring should be considered.

Internal Method

A soft plastic catheter filled with sterile water is passed into the uterus beyond the presenting fetal part by means of a firmer plastic introducer (Fig. 41-3). This, of course, requires that the cervix be partially dilated. Although a catheter or balloon may be placed extra-amniotically, for clinical use, the placement is intra-amniotic and requires that the membranes be previously ruptured. The catheter is connected to a pressure transducer (strain gauge). The intrauterine pressure is transmitted from the amniotic fluid through the sterile water in the catheter to the pressure transducer. Changes in the intrauterine pressure that occur with contractions, the Valsalva maneuver, or coughing and so on are recorded on the monitor.

Because of the invasive nature of the method, the vulva should be cleansed with an antiseptic, and sterile towels should be used to drape the patient and maintain the sterility of the catheter. The catheter is filled with sterile water prior to insertion so that air will not be introduced into the uterus. The catheter tip is protected from contamination during insertion by the plastic introducer. Before the catheter is connected, the transducer should be placed at a height that approximates that of the catheter tip (the xiphisternal junction) and zeroed to atmospheric pressure. If the level of the catheter tip is above the transducer, a false elevated pressure recording results. If the catheter tip is below the transducer, a false low or negative pressure may be recorded. Calibration should be performed periodically on the record to ensure accurate measurement of UA. Function of the catheter can be tested by having the patient cough. This will cause a sudden sharp positive deflection on the recording.

The internal pressure catheter provides a means of sampling amniotic fluid for meconium or bacteria during labor if this becomes clinically useful. If the catheter becomes plugged by vernix, meconium, or blood, intrauterine pressure will not be transmitted to the transducer. Flushing with small amounts of sterile water usually corrects the problem. When this fails, the catheter should be withdrawn slightly and repositioned. The portion of the catheter in the vagina or outside the patient should not be advanced into the uterus. Not only may this result in bacterial contamination, but it is generally ineffective because the flexibility of the catheter will cause it to coil alongside the presenting fetal part. Perforation of the uterus and injury to the placenta should be considered when excessive vaginal bleeding occurs after placement of the catheter and when UC fail to be recorded.

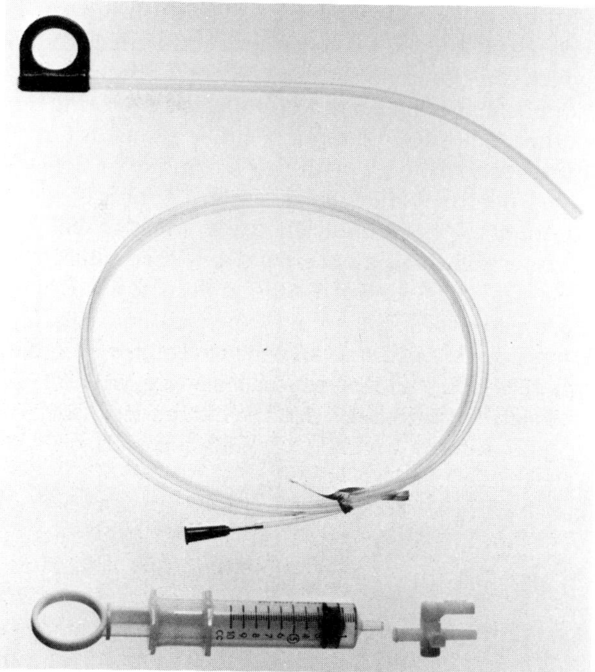

Figure 41-3.
Equipment for internal pressure monitoring—plastic introducer, catheter, stopcock, and syringe.

Fetal Heart Rate (FHR)

Prior to the development of fetal monitoring, evaluation of FHR was restricted to periodic auscultation during the interval between contractions. FHR changes occurring with the contractions or during the first 30 seconds following the contraction were usually not detected. The ability to diagnose fetal distress was limited to sustained and extreme variation in FHR, such as severe bradycardia. With auscultation, the evaluation of periodic changes, that is, those occurring over short time intervals (decelerations or accelerations), was somewhat subjective, especially when they occurred at a rate that was within the normal range.

With continuous FHR monitoring, the time interval between two successive heart beats is calculated at a rate and is recorded graphically. For example, a lapse of 375 milliseconds between beats would constitute a rate of 160 beats per minute. In order for this calculation to be made, the fetal signal obtained with a transducer is amplified and then counted by a cardiotachometer. This is converted to a rate between successive beats and recorded continuously during, and in the interval between, contractions.

External Method

Several methods for monitoring the fetal heart rate through the maternal abdomen are available.

Phonocardiography utilizes a transducer, which is essentially a microphone. With this technique, the heart sounds of the fetus constitute the signal. Extraneous sounds or "noise" from within the uterus, maternal abdomen, or abdominal wall may also be detected as a signal. Thus electronic filtering is required.

Fetal Electrocardiogram (FECG) is a method for obtaining the electrical signal of the fetal heart from the maternal abdominal wall. When the abdominal wall FECG is used as the signal, the larger maternal ECG complex is censored or edited out by the machine. When the maternal signal coincides with the fetal signal, the machine may edit the maternal signal and insert a fetal beat automatically. This is known as *compensation.* Monitoring of the FECG through the maternal abdominal wall will result in clinically useful tracings in only a portion of cases in which it is attempted.

The Doppler or *ultrasound method* is the most commonly used method of external monitoring. With this technique, high-frequency sound waves are transmitted from a crystal and are reflected from the moving fetal heart to a receiving crystal. The difference in frequencies of the transmitted and the reflected sound waves constitutes the signal, which can be amplified for counting by the cardiotachometer and is also heard as an audible signal from the machine. Filtering is needed for other intra-abdominal motion, which constitutes noise. More recently, a bidirectional doppler has been employed in fetal monitoring that permits selection of motion either toward or away from the transducer. With this technique, whichever constitutes the better signal is selected for recording. In order to obtain clinically useful tracings with the doppler, "averaging" over two or three successive beats is performed. Some machines are also equipped with logic circuitry such that rates above a certain level (*e.g.,* 180) will be halved on the recorder, whereas rates below a preset level (*e.g.,* 90) will be doubled. Variations in equipment function such as this illustrate the importance of being familiar with the particular equipment in use.

When the doppler transducer is used, the transducer is applied to an area that is directly over the fetal heart. This site is selected by auscultation and by palpating the fetus. By trial and error, the position from which the sharpest (not necessarily the loudest) audible fetal signal can be heard is determined before securing the transducer with an elastic belt. Periodic changes of fetal or maternal position may require readjustment of the transducer to maintain high-quality data.

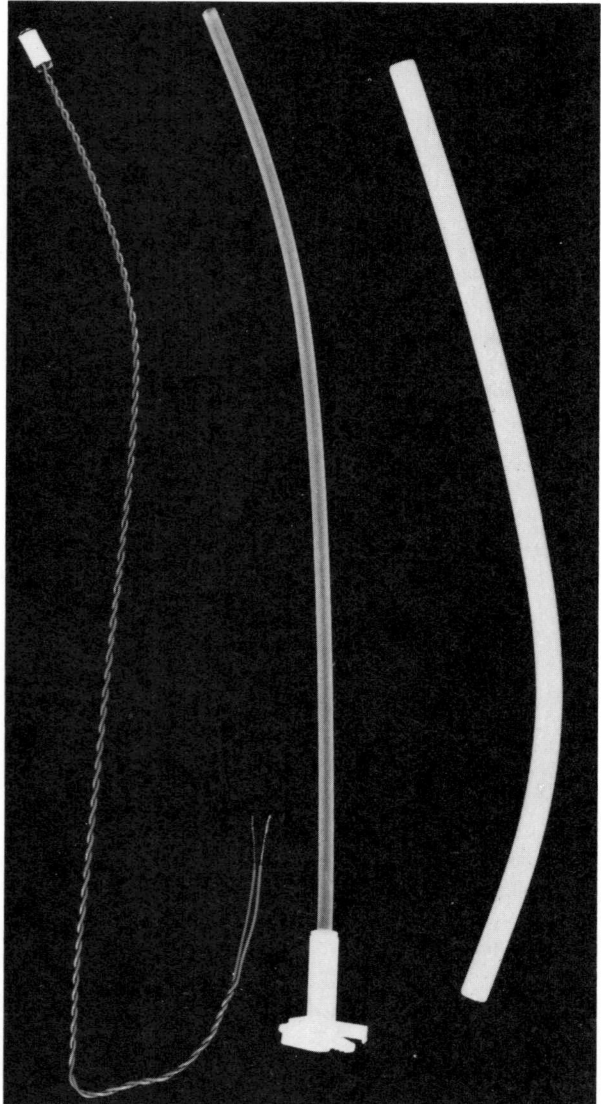

Figure 41-4.
Scalp electrode and introducer for fetal heart monitoring.

Internal Method

Direct FECG is the most widely used method of FHR monitoring during labor. The transducer is a small electrode that is attached to the skin of the presenting part of the fetus, usually the scalp. This small, silver silver-chloride electrode is commonly referred to as a *clip* because the first electrodes available were attached by two prongs to the fetal scalp. At present, the most commonly used electrode is a small spiral wire that is advanced into the fetal skin by clockwise rotation while gentle pressure is applied (Fig. 41-4). Application of the electrode requires that the membranes be ruptured and that the cervix be dilated 1 cm to 2 cm or more. The presenting part must be known and fixed in the pelvis so that the gentle pressure required will not displace the fetus.

The FECG serves as the fetal signal for counting. On occasion, the maternal signal obtained by this method may produce an artifactual tracing; for example, the maternal ECG may be conducted through a dead fetus. Editing of the direct FECG may result in failure to detect fetal cardiac arrhythmias. With direct FECG there is no need for averaging and the true beat-to-beat variation in FHR can be evaluated. Spiral electrodes are easily removed before or after delivery by counterclockwise rotation of the attached wires.

Application of the Fetal Monitor

The decision to apply the fetal monitor should be based on local policy and the consent of the patient. In some institutions, fetal monitoring is applied in all cases. In most programs, the responsibility for selection of patients to be monitored rests with the physician and with the nurse. The nurse's role in selection of patients to be monitored is particularly important when the number of patients who are in labor exceeds the number of available monitors, and priorities for monitoring must be established. In general, the decision to monitor is made on the basis of one of three primary indications:

1. Antepartum risk factors—these include maternal complications such as diabetes and hypertension, or fetal problems such as intrauterine growth retardation
2. Intrapartum risk factors—such as third trimester bleeding, passage of meconium, or abnormalities of FHR by auscultation
3. Other obstetrical factors—for example, to evaluate abnormal labor or the effects of drugs, such as oxytocics.

After the decision has been made to monitor a patient, the method of monitoring is selected. This is contingent upon four factors: (1) status of the cervix and membranes, (2) the indication for monitoring, (3) patient acceptance, and (4) availability. When the membranes are intact or the cervix is not dilated, external methods of monitoring must be used. If adequate data cannot be obtained with the available external systems, or if the belts for the transducers are unacceptable to the patient, internal monitoring should be considered. In cases where the most accurate data are required, for example, true beat-to-beat variation, temporal relationship of decelerations to contractions, or true intrauterine pressures, then internal monitoring must be used.

The application of external devices for fetal monitoring is performed by the nurse. Insertion of intrauterine catheters or attachment of scalp electrodes is frequently performed by the obstetrician, but nurses trained in these techniques routinely perform this function in some institutions. Prior to initiating monitoring, the nurse should explain the basic concepts of monitoring and the equipment to the patient. Ideally, patients should be educated about fetal monitoring during the antepartum period. Most patients readily consent to the use of monitoring when they believe that it might be of value to their fetus. The major drawback for the mother is often the need to restrict physical activity in order to maintain a consistently useful tracing. This problem, as well as interference with effleurage, can be circumvented somewhat by using internal methods. Newer telemetry techniques (*i.e.,* monitoring from a distance) that may become clinically available in the near future reduce these restrictions on patient activity.

Due to most patients' wishes to observe the monitor tracing (Fig. 41-5), the equipment should be placed so that it is within view of the patient, the father, and the nurse. Couples often find that observing the onset and decrement (downslope) of the contractions is useful in applying breathing techniques. This is particularly true for the father. The reassurance obtained from observing or listening to the fetal heart beat during labor is often a secondary benefit to the couple. For this reason it is generally inadvisable to discontinue fetal monitoring once it has been initiated unless there is no further indication to continue and the couple wish to have the monitor disconnected.

It is important that the nurse explain the normal variation in FHR and the functions of the equipment

Figure 41-5.
Patient with external fetal monitor applied. Note that the monitor function can be observed by the patient.

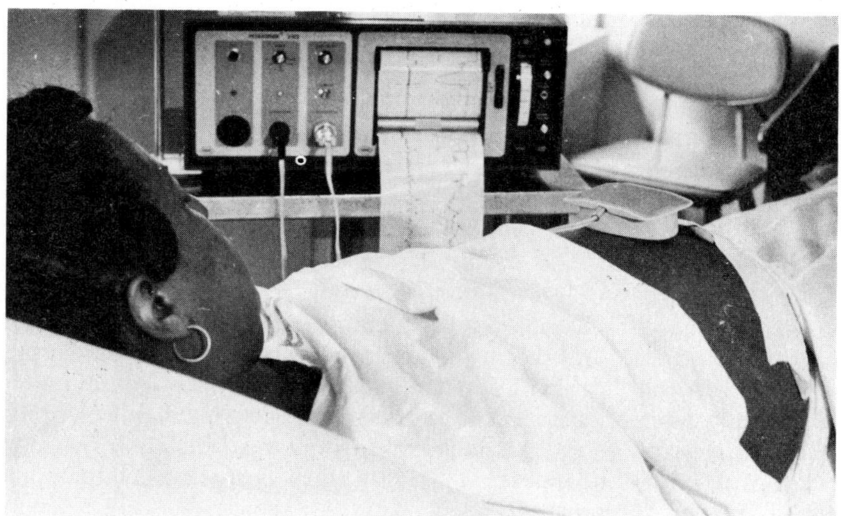

so that patients will not become alarmed by them. When ominous patterns develop, the nurse initiates remedial action in a calm and systematic manner and summons help. Leaving the bedside for more than a moment at such a time may cause undue panic in the patient and can be a decidedly negative feature of monitoring. Providing reassurance by orderly action is a much unrecognized benefit of protocols for remedial measures that have been established in most institutions.

Interpretation of Data

To properly interpret the data obtained from electronic fetal monitoring, a systematic approach should be used to examine the tracings and correlate them with clinical events. The interpretation of monitor tracings can be learned from annotated atlases of monitor tracings (see Selected Reading) and clinical experience. In order to provide teaching in this area, many institutions have periodic in-service programs and, more important, conferences in which tracings are reviewed by members of the team caring for the patients.

Evaluation of Uterine Activity or Uterine Contractions

External Methods

Only the frequency and duration of UC may be determined with external monitoring. The onset of the contraction is determined by the upswing of the pen and is followed by the *increment.* The peak of the contraction or highest level recorded is called the *acme.* The progressive relaxation of the uterus following the acme is referred to as the *decrement.* When the baseline is reached, the contraction is completed. The total duration of the contraction and the interval from the onset of one contraction to the onset of the next contraction may be calculated when the paper speed is known (3 cm/min). Maternal respiratory movement may be noted as fine "saw-tooth" deflections confirmed by comparing the rate with that observed clinically. Coughing, sneezing, and so on appear as large spiking deflections. Bearing-down efforts, or "pushing," cause multiple sharp spikes superimposed on the contractions. Changes of position cause sudden sharp changes of the baseline.

Internal Method

Intrauterine pressure can be calculated (following proper zeroing and calibration) when internal monitoring is used. Baseline tone is measured as the height of the baseline during the interval between contractions and is usually in a range of 5 mm Hg to 15 mm Hg.

Excessive baseline tone may indicate any of the following:

1. Misplacement of the pressure transducer in relationship to the catheter tip
2. Excessive oxytocin administration
3. Abruptio placentae
4. Hypertonic uterine dysfunction

The contraction amplitude may range from 30 mm Hg to 60 mm Hg or more. Although contraction amplitudes of less than 25 mm Hg to 30 mm Hg may occur in normal active-phase labor, they are most frequently associated with early labor or hypotonic uterine dysfunction.

Hypertonic labor occurs when UC amplitudes exceed normal, the frequency between onset of contractions is less than 2 minutes, or the resting interval between contractions is less than 1 minute. Coalescence of UC or a contraction of 2 minutes' or greater duration constitutes a tetanic contraction. Hypertonic labor or uterine tetany is observed with administration of an excessive amount of oxytocic drugs, abruptio placentae, or hypertonic uterine dysfunction. When internal pressure monitoring is applied, the geometric area beneath the contraction can be calculated. This is most easily performed by an on-line computer (*i.e.,* one attached directly to the monitor). Calculation of UA units or total work of the uterus by this method has proven useful for clinical studies of the forces of labor.

Evaluation of the Fetal Heart Rate

FHR Baseline

During very early fetal development, cardiac activity is initiated by the intrinsic rhythmicity of the myocardial cells. Soon after, the sinoatrial node (SA node) assumes the function of initiating the impulses, which are transmitted throughout the conduction system of the heart, resulting in the mechanical events known as the heart beat.

Tachycardia and Bradycardia

The FHR decreases slightly as pregnancy advances and normally ranges between 120 and 160 beats per minute (bpm). Elevation of the FHR baseline to 160 bpm or above is referred to as *tachycardia.* Rates between 161 bpm and 180 bpm are classified as *mild tachycardia* and those greater than 180 bpm as *marked tachycardia.* Rates below 120 bpm are referred to as *bradycardia.* Those between 100 bpm and 119 bpm are classified as *mild bradycardia* and those less than 100 bpm as *marked bradycardia.* Either fetal tachycardia or bradycardia may be related to fetal hypoxia (low oxygen content of the fetal blood or inadequate delivery of oxygen to the fetal tissues). Fetal tachycardia may be an early warning sign of fetal hypoxia, whereas fetal bradycardia occurs somewhat later in the sequence of events. Abnormalities in baseline FHR may also be due to arrhythmias (abnormal discharge or transmission of impulses through the conduction system of the heart). These are usually benign and transient, but may at times be associated with congenital heart defects or heart failure. Fetal tachycardia may also be associated with maternal fever. Because core temperature (internal body temperature) rises earlier and is higher than that measured either orally or rectally, fetal tachycardia may precede maternal fever by a short time. Likewise, fetal bradycardia may be associated with maternal hypothermia, but this is an unusual event clinically. Abnormal FHRs, either tachycardia or bradycardia, may also be caused by drugs administered to the mother.

Beat-to-Beat Variation

As fetal development advances, the autonomic nervous system assumes an increasingly important role in modulating FHR. Discharge of sympathetic nerves causes an increase in rate, whereas discharge of parasympathetic nerves causes a slowing of the heart rate. The normal continuous opposition of these two stimuli results in the beat-to-beat variation noted in the heart rate of the normal fetus. It is reflected by the fine irregularity seen on the normal FHR tracing (Fig. 41-6).

It is important to note that true beat-to-beat variation can be assessed only by direct fetal electrography (*i.e.,* internal monitoring using the spiral electrode). In the past, variability of the FHR baseline was often overlooked as an indicator of fetal status. However, recently it has assumed increasing clinical importance. When beat-to-beat variation is normal (*i.e.,* >5 bpm) it is thought to indicate an intact nervous system with normal regulatory influence over the FHR.

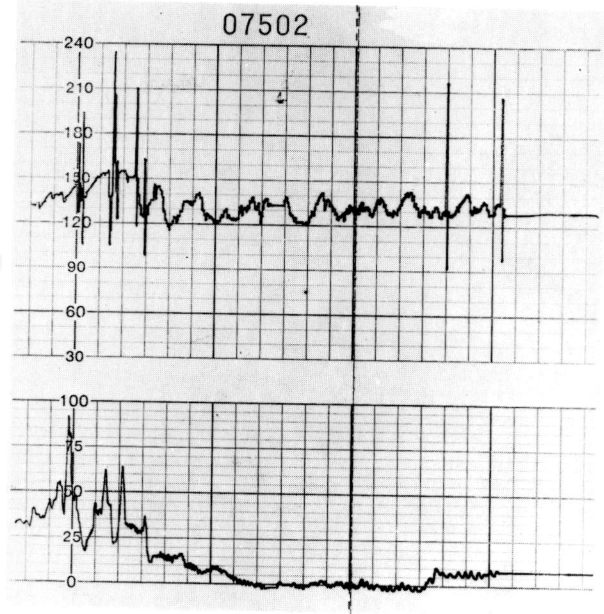

Figure 41-6.
Fetal heart rate tracing. Note fine irregularity or beat-to-beat variability.

Diminished FHR variability (<5 bpm) or a flat FHR baseline in the absence of explainable causes is considered ominous and potentially indicative of hypoxia (Fig. 41-7).

Nowhere in FHR monitoring is the influence of drugs more obvious than in the assessment of FHR variability. It has become increasingly apparent that a large proportion of drugs administered to the mother will cause diminished or absent FHR-variability. For this reason, it is often useful to evaluate FHR-variability by internal monitoring before these drugs are administered.

Periodic Changes

While *in utero,* the fetus is equipped with cardiovascular reflexes that may cause periodic or transient changes in the FHR from its normal baseline. Some of these responses (*e.g.,* accelerations with fetal movement) are indicative of normal fetal status, whereas others (*e.g.,* variable deceleration with cord compression) are designed to compensate for alterations in cardiovascular dynamics. It is these periodic changes that require careful evaluation for the diagnosis of fetal stress or distress.

Accelerations

Transient increases of the FHR (>15 bpm for >15 sec) have been noted during labor since fetal monitoring

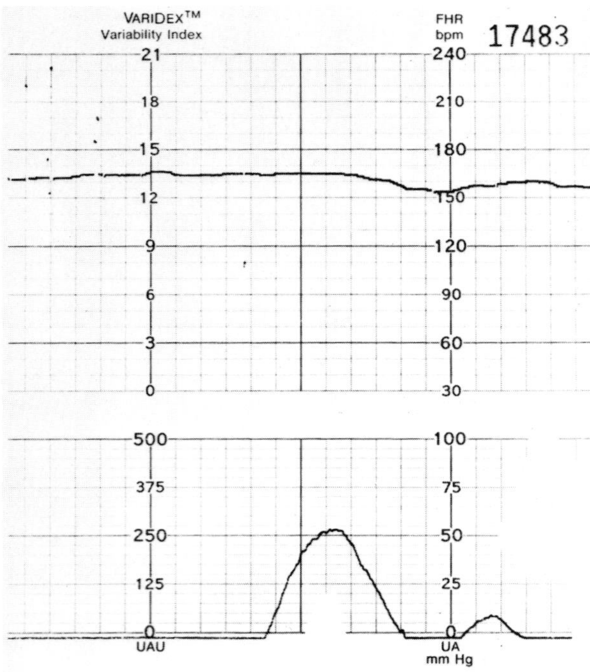

Figure 41-7.
Fetal heart rate tracing with absent beat-to-beat variability. Note subtle late deceleration.

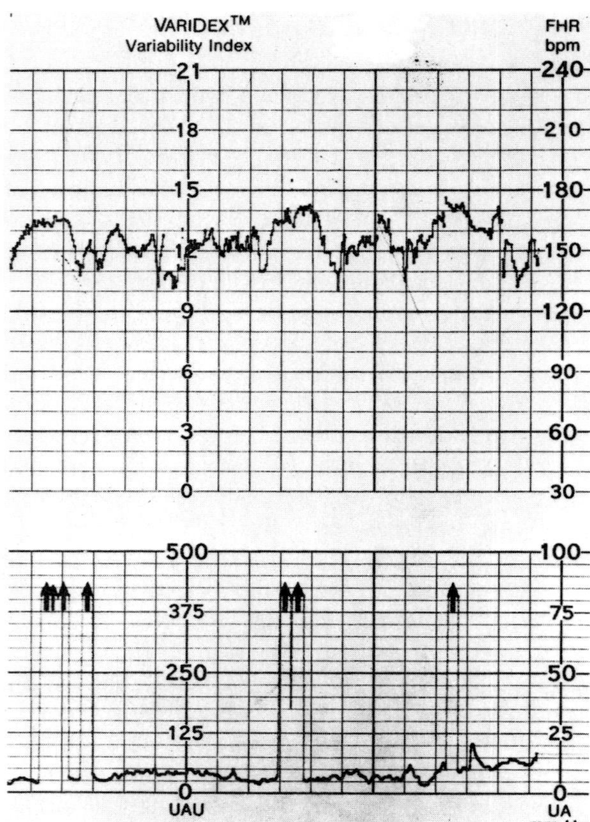

Figure 41-8.
Transient accelerations of fetal heart rate noted during NST. (Arrows) were made by patient to indicate when fetal movements were perceived.

was first used (Fig. 41-8). They are at times associated with contractions but often are unrelated to UA. The outcome of fetuses demonstrating this change has been uniformly good. It is believed that the increased FHR is due to transient discharges of the sympathetic nervous system. It has also been suggested that accelerations associated with contractions might be caused by partial compression of the cord, resulting in diminished venous return to the heart followed by a transient increase of the FHR. More recently, the observation that accelerations are associated with fetal movement in the healthy fetus has led to the development of the nonstress test (NST) for antepartum evaluation of the high-risk fetus.

Early Decelerations (Type I Dips)

Transient slowing of the FHR in a pattern that is almost a mirror image of the contractions is known as an *early deceleration* (sometimes called a *type I dip*). The occurrence of these decelerations is believed to be related to the fetal head compression associated with the contraction, resulting in a parasympathetic discharge mediated by the vagus nerve. Parasympathetic stimulation results in slowing of the FHR. This pattern represents a normal response of the fetus to this stimulus and is associated with a uniformly good outcome.

Characteristically, these decelerations have a wave form that coincides with and resembles an inverted UC (Fig. 41-9). They are uniform in shape, of short duration, and of low amplitude. The FHR at the *nadir* (lowest point) of the deceleration is usually 100 bpm or greater. When slower FHRs are observed with contractions, the decelerations are usually of the variable type (see below). Early decelerations do not respond to oxygen administered to the mother or to position change. They may be abolished when atropine is administered. However, because of the benign nature of this pattern, remedial action is not necessary.

Late Decelerations (Type II Dips)

Like the term *early decelerations,* the designation *late decelerations* indicates a uniform shape and a consistent relationship of the deceleration to contractions. As opposed to early decelerations, the onset of the late deceleration, its nadir, and its recovery do not coincide with the onset, amplitude, and recovery of the UC

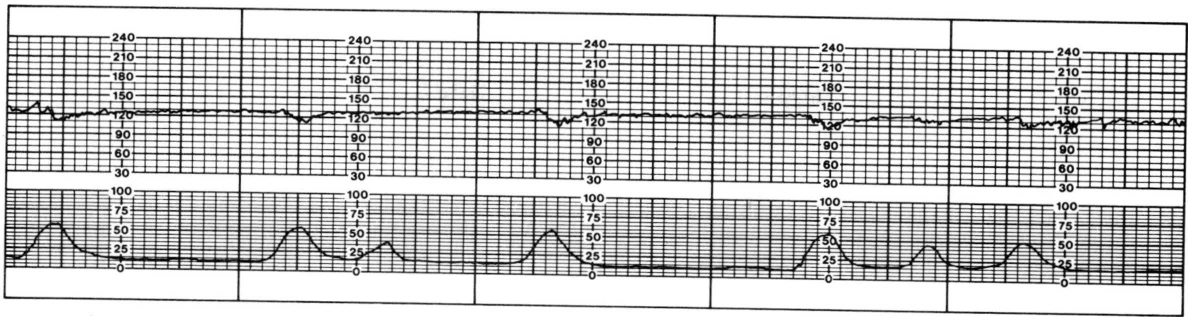

Figure 41-9.
Early deceleration. The FHR baseline is the normal range, with diminished variability. Uterine activity is normal with oxytocin augmentation. Early deceleration patterns are evident, approximating a mirror image of the uterine pressure curve. The nadir of the early deceleration occurs at the same time as the peak of the uterine contraction. (Parer JT, Puttler OL, Jr, Freeman RK: In Freeman RK: [ed]: A Clinical Approach to Fetal Monitoring, San Leandro, CA, Berkeley Bio-Engineering, Inc., 1974)

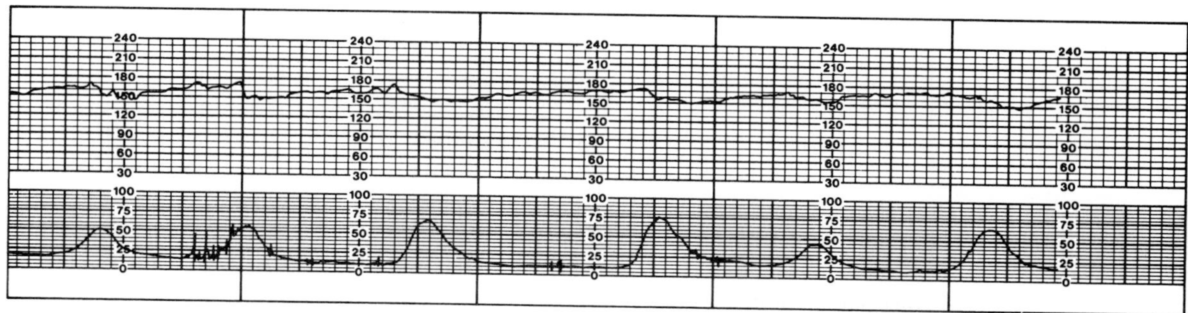

Figure 41-10.
Moderate late deceleration. There is a mild fetal tachycardia, ranging between 160 and 170 beats per minute, with decreased variability. Uterine activity is normal. The nadir of late deceleration occurs when the uterine contraction is nearly over. A scalp capillary blood sample had been taken just prior to the first portion of this panel, and mild fetal acidosis was demonstrated, with scalp blood *p*H 7.21. (Parer JT, Puttler OL, Jr, Freeman RK: In Freeman RK [ed]: A Clinical Approach to Fetal Monitoring, San Leandro, CA, Berkeley Bio-Engineering, Inc., 1974)

but rather are delayed (Fig. 41-10). In contrast to variable decelerations, late decelerations may be quite subtle, entirely within the normal FHR range, and yet ominous. A classification of late decelerations is also given in Table 41-1.

Late decelerations are thought to reflect the effects of direct hypoxia on the fetal myocardium and cardiac conduction system. The hypoxia results from the reduced oxygen exchange by the placenta due to diminished intervillous blood flow that occurs with the UC. A direct and specific relationship between hypoxia and late decelerations has been demonstrated experimentally in monkeys. Hypoxia causing late decelerations may be elicited when less oxygen is delivered to the uterus (*e.g.*, with maternal hypoxia or hypotension), when abnormally strong UC occur, or when relative placental insufficiency exists.

Transient late decelerations associated with maternal hypotension of uterine hypertonus that responds to remedial action are thought to signal fetal stress. Removing or correcting the stress often results in fetal recovery. On the other hand, a pattern of consistent and persistent late decelerations that do not respond to remedial measures suggests fetal distress and is

Table 41-1.
Principles of Grading Variable and Late Decelerations

Criteria of grading	Mild	Moderate	Severe
Variable deceleration			
Level to which FHR drops and duration of deceleration	<30 sec duration irrespective of level >80 bpm irrespective of duration 70–80 bpm <60 sec	<70 bpm >30<60 sec 70–80 bpm >60 sec	<70 bpm >60 sec
Late deceleration			
Amplitude of drop in FHR	<15 bpm	15–45 bpm	>45 bpm

often associated with hypoxia, acidosis, and low Apgar scores at birth. This latter group of findings, of course, indicates prompt delivery.

Variable Decelerations (Type III Dips)

This type of periodic deceleration is the most commonly observed FHR change during labor. The nomenclature of this pattern is based on the fact that the relationships of these decelerations to the contractions and, more importantly, the wave form are both variable (Fig. 41-11). It is believed that these decelerations represent a reflex response to umbilical cord compression. They are often observed in association with UC, a situation in which cord compression is more likely to occur.

Responsibility for the slowing of the FHR in variable decelerations has been attributed to a rise in systemic arterial pressure resulting from cord occlusion. This rise in pressure triggers the baroreceptor (intra-arterial pressure receptor) reflex, activating a vagal impulse that causes slowing of the FHR. More recently, it has been suggested that these decelerations may also be elicited by sudden hypoxia and the triggering of the aortic chemoreceptor response, which also results in vagal discharge. Thus, sudden hypoxia in addition to increased arterial pressure may be important in the pathogenesis of variable decelerations.

Variable decelerations may be classified as mild, moderate, or severe (Table 41-1). Because there is a correlation between the severity of variable decelerations and fetal condition, it is important that the nurse evaluate the frequency, depth, and duration of these decelerations. In addition, other indicators of hypoxia on the FHR tracing, such as abnormally low or high baseline FHR and decreased variability, should be examined. When variable decelerations are noted, remedial action should be initiated. Repetitive moderate or severe variable decelerations, especially those associated with ominous baseline change, that are not

Figure 41-11.
Severe variable deceleration. There is a mild fetal tachycardia with normal baseline variability. Uterine activity is normal. The deceleration is corrected by changing the patient's position. Subsequent deceleration patterns are much less severe. (Parer JT, Puttler OL, Jr, Freeman RK: In Freeman K (ed): A Clinical Approach to Fetal Monitoring. San Leandro, CA, Berkeley Bio-Engineering, Inc., 1974)

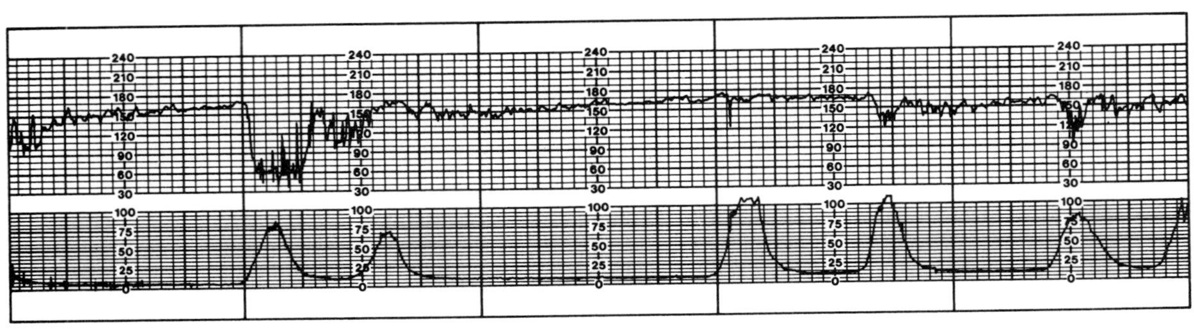

alleviated by remedial measures, may indicate that a sample of fetal scalp blood should be obtained or that a prompt delivery should be carried out.

Sinusoidal Pattern

An unusual abnormality in FHR in which there is a repetitive undulation of the baseline resembling a "sine wave" has been called a *sinusoidal pattern* (Fig. 41-12). Occasionally, tracings of a normal fetus appear to have a transient sinusoidal pattern. This has not been correlated with any particular fetal abnormality. On occasion, a persistent sinusoidal pattern is indicative of fetal hypoxia or severe fetal anemia. The latter is most frequently observed in fetuses suffering from hydrops fetalis due to Rhesus isoimmunization, but has also been seen with fetal anemia due to blood loss.

The pathophysiology of the development of a sinusoidal pattern is not understood. It has been hypothesized that this pattern may reflect an absence of central nervous system control over the FHR due to severe hypoxia. Because of the poor outcome in anemic fetuses when this pattern has been observed, the finding is considered ominous.

Remedial Measures for Fetal Stress or Distress

Fetal hypoxia may result from one or several factors that impair delivery of oxygen to the fetus. As previously discussed, alterations of FHR baseline (tachycardia, bradycardia, or diminished variability) or periodic decelerations (moderate or severe variable, or late decelerations) may indicate fetal hypoxia. When mixed patterns of decelerations (*i.e.,* early and variable, early and late, or variable and late) are observed, the more ominous deceleration should be taken as the indication for action. When abnormal periodic patterns are associated with ominous baseline changes, the fetal situation should be considered more urgent.

The following etiologic factors should be considered and evaluated rapidly when fetal hypoxia is suspected: (1) impaired maternal oxygen delivery; (2) impaired placental oxygen exchange; and (3) impaired fetal circulation or oxygen-carrying capacity.

Impaired Maternal Oxygen Delivery

This situation may result from a number of maternal disorders. Maternal pulmonary dysfunction, associated with an acute severe asthmatic attack, amniotic fluid embolism, thromboembolism, *grand mal* seizure, or general anesthesia, may result in maternal hypoxia that subsequently causes fetal hypoxia. Impaired delivery of normally oxygenated maternal blood to the uterus may occur from abnormalities of cardiac function (pump failure) or decreased peripheral vascular blood flow. The latter is most often associated with hypotension and is the most frequent cause of fetal hypoxia in this category. Hypotension may be related to maternal blood loss or shock, compression of the vena cava by the gravid uterus when the patient is supine, or autonomic blockade associated with conduction anesthesia.

When maternal oxygen uptake or delivery of oxygen to the uterus is impaired, take remedial measures. Oxygen should be administered by mask and the

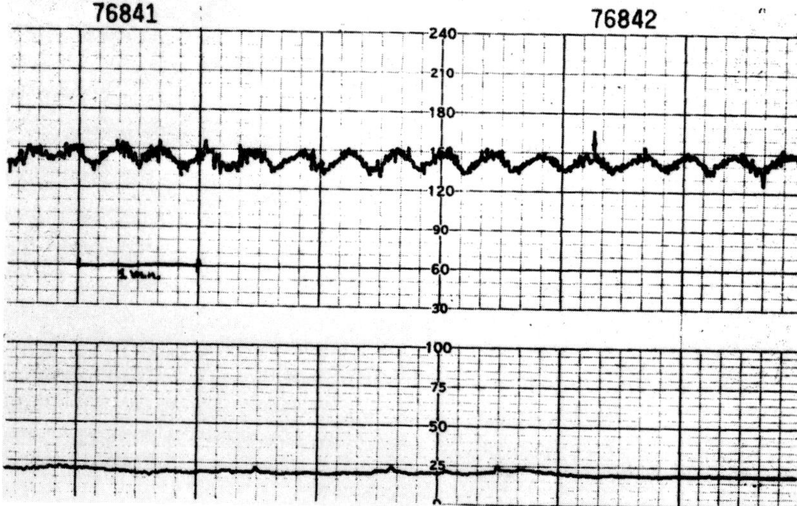

Figure 41-12.
Fetal heart rate tracing demonstrating sinusoidal pattern prior to labor. Fetus was severely anemic owing to Rhesus isoimmunization.

mother turned to the left lateral recumbent position. This position diminishes occlusion of the inferior vena cava by the uterus, thus promoting venous return to the heart and improved cardiovascular function. Then, if necessary, initiate pharmacologic correction of the respiratory or cardiovascular disorder.

Impaired Placental Exchange of Oxygen

The cause of this problem may be placental insufficiency (*e.g.,* associated with intrauterine growth retardation or postmaturity) or excessively strong UC. Such contractions result in transient interruption of blood flow in the intervillous space and thus diminish oxygen exchange. When this occurs, administration of oxytocic drugs should be discontinued if they are being used. Improving maternal oxygenation and oxygen delivery by administration of oxygen and use of the left lateral position are also helpful.

Impaired Fetal Circulation or Oxygen Transport

Cord compression is the usual cause of this problem. In this situation, prolapse of the cord should be determined rapidly by perineal inspection and vaginal examination. This complication requires prompt delivery, usually by cesarean section. When there is evidence of cord compression, the previously mentioned measures should be initiated (*i.e.,* maternal oxygen administration, left lateral position, and discontinuation of oxytocics). Positions other than left lateral (*e.g.,* right lateral or knee-chest) may also be useful in alleviating variable decelerations and should be tried when the pattern does not respond to the initial remedial measures. Fetal oxygen transport to the tissues may also be impaired when there is severe fetal anemia, as is seen in Rhesus isoimmunization associated with a sinusoidal pattern.

When fetal hypoxia is suspected on the basis of monitoring data, a single etiologic factor is often not identifiable. The combination of administering oxygen to the mother, discontinuing oxytocics, and changing the mother's position (left lateral position first) should be instituted simultaneously. Other remedial measures, such as administering tocolytics (UC inhibitors) or fetal alkali (sodium bicarbonate), are considered investigative. When nonremedial fetal distress occurs, the physician may further evaluate the fetus by obtaining a sample of fetal scalp blood or may proceed to prompt delivery.

Other Intrapartum Methods of Fetal Evaluation

A number of other techniques for intrapartum fetal evaluation are under investigation in the laboratory or have reached the stage of clinical trials. These include percutaneous monitoring of oxygen tension, continuous scalp *p*H measurement, electroencephalography, and observation of fetal movements, particularly respirations, using real-time ultrasound.

*p*H of Fetal Blood Scalp Samples

At present, periodic measurement of *p*H of fetal scalp blood has proven to be clinically useful for the diagnosis of fetal distress. For this measurement, a small volume of fetal blood may be obtained by puncturing the fetal scalp and collecting the blood samples in fine glass capillary tubes. As with other invasive techniques, the membranes must be ruptured, the cervix must be dilated 3 cm to 4 cm, and the fetal presenting part must be fixed in the pelvis in order to perform the procedure safely. Although samples of fetal scalp blood may be obtained with the patient in bed, it is easier to carry out this procedure if the mother is in the lithotomy position in a delivery room. Transport of the patient to the delivery room also has the secondary benefit of saving valuable time if immediate delivery becomes necessary.

A plastic or metal truncated cone known as an *amnioscope* is used to visualize the presenting part of the fetus during fetal blood sampling (Fig. 41-13). The term *amnioscope* was first applied because the instrument was initially designed for visualizing the fetal membranes and amniotic fluid through the partially dilated cervix. Because of the invasive nature of the procedure, sterile technique is used throughout. The amnioscope is inserted into the vagina and the dilated cervix. A light source is then attached to the amnioscope. The fetal scalp is cleansed with an antiseptic solution and dried with sterile cotton balls. A light film of petrolatum jelly or silicone spray is applied to the scalp. This causes droplets of fetal blood to bead, making it easier to collect the blood samples in the capillary tubes. A small metal blade attached to a long handle is used to puncture the skin. The narrow detachable blades are mounted in plastic to control the depth to which the skin is penetrated. A single brisk motion is used to penetrate the skin in a manner similar to that suggested for "sticking" the finger to draw blood. The beaded drops of fetal blood are then collected in the long, heparinized capillary tubes. A fine metal bead or short wire is added to the capillary tube prior to sealing it with wax. A magnet passed along the outside of the tube moves the metal wire and stirs the sample to prevent clotting. Exposing the sample to atmospheric air can cause an exchange of oxygen and carbon dioxide, which will alter the hydrogen ion concentration. Placing the capillary tube on ice will retard cellular respiration, which could also result in a change in *p*H.

After an adequate sample of scalp blood is obtained, the physician applies firm pressure to the puncture site for several minutes to retard bleeding. At the conclusion of the procedure, the puncture site is inspected for hemostasis. Repeated scalp blood sampling may be safely performed if necessary. The risks of the procedure include continued bleeding from the puncture site, ecchymosis, hematoma, and infection.

Following scalp blood sampling, the nurse should observe the patient for excessive vaginal bleeding that may be fetal in origin. In addition, sustained fetal tachycardia may be observed on the monitor tracing when fetal blood loss occurs either externally or into the scalp tissues (hematoma).

The partial pressure of oxygen and carbon dioxide as well as bicarbonate ion concentration can be measured on these samples. The *p*H, however, has proven to be the simplest, rapidest, and most clinically useful measurement that can be performed on a small sample of blood. The *p*H of the fetal scalp blood normally ranges between 7.25 and 7.35 during labor. This correlates well with the acid–base status of the blood in the umbilical vessels. A mild progressive decline of *p*H within the normal range has been noted with contractions and as labor progresses. When the fetus becomes hypoxic, anaerobic glycolysis occurs, resulting in an excess production of organic acids (lactic acid) and an increase in hydrogen ion concentration. The increased hydrogen ion concentration is measured as a decrease in *p*H (acidosis). Thus the development of acidosis reflects the effects of hypoxia on cellular metabolism, or respiration.

Clinical studies have demonstrated a correlation between the *p*H of fetal scalp blood and abnormalities in FHR as well as Apgar scores. As a result of these observations, the measurement of the *p*H of fetal scalp blood has become an increasingly important method for diagnosing fetal distress. This measurement helps when the interpretation of fetal monitoring data is unclear and reduces the chances of false-positive diagnoses of fetal distress using fetal monitoring. Traditionally, a scalp blood *p*H of 7.20 or less is considered to be indicative of fetal acidosis or fetal distress.

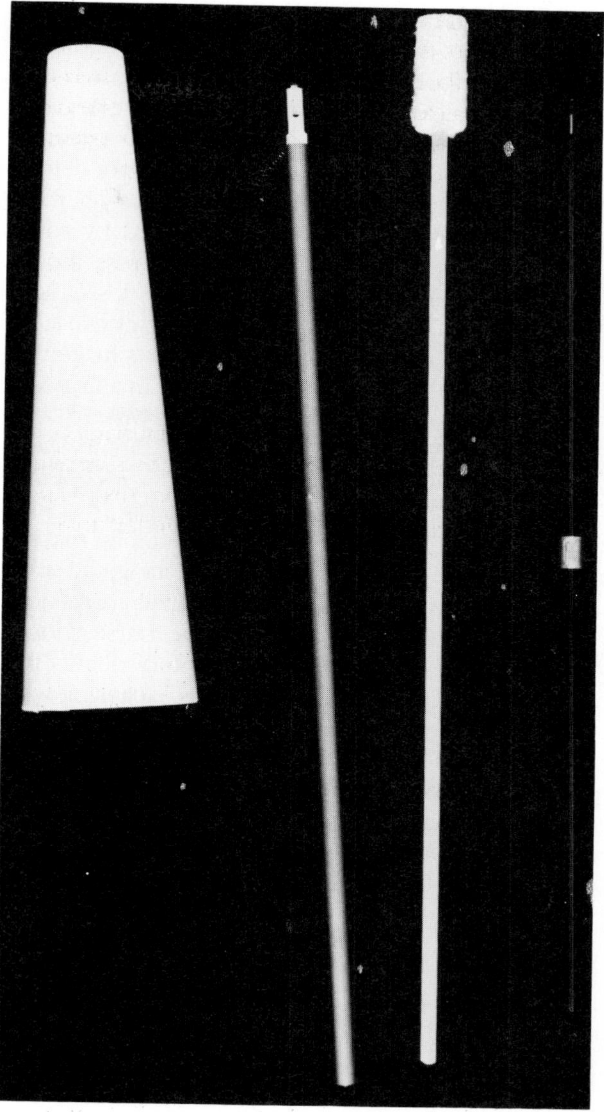

Figure 41-13.
Scalp sampling equipment includes plastic amnioscope, scalpel, cotton sponge, and heparinized capillary tube.

As with other antepartum or intrapartum methods of fetal evaluation, measurement of scalp blood *p*H may produce false-positive results (*i.e.,* normal values when the fetus is hypoxic). Abnormal maternal acid–base status (*e.g.,* abnormal values when the fetus is well) or false-negative results (*e.g.,* maternal acidosis) may be transmitted passively to the fetus through the placenta and account for a portion of the false-positive cases. For this reason, obtaining a simultaneous blood sample from the mother to determine the *p*H of her blood is of value in interpreting the fetal *p*H and will reduce the frequency of false-positive results. Events that occur following fetal blood sampling, but before delivery (*e.g.*, continued cord compression), may account for many of the false-negative results observed. Because these problems occur in only a small proportion of cases, they do not detract substantially from the clinical value of fetal *p*H measurement. In fact, it has been suggested by some physicians that the diagnosis of fetal distress should *always* be based on the finding of fetal acidosis. However, rapid fetal deterioration, inability to obtain samples, or suspicion of false-negative results make this test impractical as an absolute criterion in all cases.

Following delivery of an infant in whom fetal blood sampling has been performed, umbilical venous and arterial blood samples should be obtained from a doubly clamped segment of cord. Measurement of blood gases and *p*H on these samples make it easier to correlate the fetal monitor tracing, the scalp blood *p*H measurements, and the neonatal condition.

When assessing the newborn, the nurse should closely inspect the scalp of the infant to identify the puncture site(s). In many institutions, cleansing with an antiseptic solution and applying an antibiotic ointment are routine. Personnel in the nursery should be notified of the number and the status of scalp puncture sites at the time the infant is transferred to the nursery. In this way, any complications resulting from the procedure can be detected immediately and treated.

Antepartum Fetal Heart Rate Monitoring

Periodic (usually weekly) electronic fetal monitoring during the third trimester has become a common method for evaluating the fetus in a high-risk pregnancy. As with many other forms of fetal evaluation, a normal result is highly accurate in indicating fetal well-being. On the other hand, false-positive results occur with a relatively high frequency. This has required that two or more different tests of fetal well-being be carried out before premature delivery or other remedial measures are instituted.

The observation of changes in FHR associated with spontaneous or evoked fetal movement has become known as the *nonstress test* (NST). Evaluation of FHR in the presence of spontaneous or oxytocin-induced contractions is termed the *contraction stress test* (CST) or *oxytocin challenge test* (OCT). CST was widely applied clinically prior to the more recent development of the NST. The ease of performing the NST and its apparent reliability as a screening tool have greatly reduced the number of CSTs performed. An example of a clinical protocol for applying these tests is given in The Contraction Stress Test and The Nonstress Test charts.

Contraction Stress Testing

The CST requires administration of oxytocin by intravenous infusion. For this reason, it is performed in an in-patient area of a hospital, usually a labor room. Continuous external fetal monitoring is applied, and oxytocin is administered in increasing dosages until UC occur. The occurrence of repeated late decelerations with contractions is classified as a positive or abnormal test. The lack of late decelerations with each of three contractions during a 10-minute interval is classified as a negative result or a passed test.

Other terms used for classification of tests include *unsatisfactory, suspicious,* or *equivocal.* Unsatisfactory tests occur when interpretable tracings cannot be obtained, or the criterion of three contractions in a 10-minute interval is not met. Unsatisfactory tests are repeated within a short time interval (usually 24 hours). It has been suggested by some researchers that the interpretation of the test should be based on a 10-minute testing segment known as a "testing window." The classification of *equivocal* and elimination of the term *suspicious tests* (occasional decelerations) has been proposed in conjunction with the concept of a 10-minute testing window. Equivocal tests are those in which nonrepetitive late decelerations are observed (*i.e.*, no positive or negative testing window) or in which decelerations are associated with maternal hypotension or uterine hyperstimulation. Since external methods of pressure monitoring are used, uterine hyperstimulation cannot be defined on the basis of true intrauterine pressure (mm Hg) but rather is defined on the basis of the frequency of contractions (greater than three contractions in 10 minutes) or a tetanic contraction. It is suggested that equivocal tests be repeated in 24 hours. In some areas of the country, the CST is interpreted without the use of the testing window. If the test shows any late decelerations, it is considered equivocal and is repeated within 24 hours.

Early investigators found that positive CSTs were associated with a relatively high frequency of poor outcome, such as intrauterine fetal death, fetal distress, or poor condition of the infant at birth. A normal CST gave a high degree of confidence for continued fetal survival *in utero* during an arbitrarily set limit of 1 week. Further experience has confirmed this observation. Instances of fetal death within 1 week of a negative CST are very infrequent. When this has occurred, the fetal deaths have often been attributed to factors other than the primary indication for testing (*e.g.*, abruptio placentae or fetal malformation). Some have suggested performing CSTs more frequently when there is deterioration of the maternal condition (*e.g.*, increasing severity of pregnancy-induced hypertension) or in certain very high-risk disorders (*e.g.*, diabetes with vascular disease).

Clinical studies in which patients were induced to labor and electronically monitored following positive CST have demonstrated a high false-positive rate (25%–40%), that is, late decelerations did not recur in labor. Because of this experience, it has been suggested that more than one test of fetal well-being should be carried out before a *preterm* delivery for fetal compromise is indicated. Clearly the greatest benefit of the CST lies in the reassurance that allows continuation of a high-risk pregnancy when the test result is normal.

Recently a new noninvasive technique has been developed in antepartum testing for the achievement of a CST. It is called the breast stimulation technique. This technique causes oxytocin to be released from the neurohypophysis and, if successful, the need for intravenous infusion of Pitocin is eliminated. With this new method, the nurse applies warm, moist towels over the woman's breast and instructs the patient to twist her nipples gently. This technique is similar to the nipple-rolling breast preparation that is recommended antepartally. If, after a reasonable time, sufficient contractions do not result, the nurse proceeds with the CST procedure.

Nonstress Testing

Observation of accelerated FHR associated with fetal movements led to the development of nonstress testing (NST). This form of testing does not require intravenous administration of drugs and thus can be safely and more quickly performed in an outpatient area. These features, coupled with the apparent reliability of the NST as a screening test, have resulted in a marked reduction in the number of CSTs performed.

Various criteria have been applied for interpreting the NST. The occurrence of five accelerations of >15 bpm for >15 seconds in 20 minutes was initially required as a normal or reactive test. More recent

The Contraction Stress Test*

A. Nursing Guidelines for Performing the CST:

1. Take patient to a labor room or antepartum testing unit.
2. Explain to the patient the testing procedure and the time involved. (The test itself requires an average of about 90 minutes but it is not uncommon for the procedure to take 3 hours.)
3. Have patient change into a gown.
4. Place patient in a semi-Fowler's position at a 30° to 45° angle with a slight left tilt.
5. Place patient on an external monitor. A phonotransducer or ultrasound transducer is used to record the FHR and a tokodynamometer to measure UC.
6. Record patient's blood pressure initially and at 5- to 10-minute intervals.
7. Obtain at least a 10-minute baseline recording of FHR and observe for spontaneous UC.
   If spontaneous uterine contractions without late decelerations are noted at a frequency of less than three (3) in 10 minutes or no spontaneous uterine activity is observed, proceed with oxytocin infusion.
8. Prepare and begin an oxytocin infusion according to the institutional protocol or as indicated by the physician.
   a. Start the oxytocin infusion (secondary line) by inserting the needle into the connector of the primary line at the connector most proximal to the primary line. Be sure to keep primary line running at a slow rate.
   b. Patient is evaluated by the physician when the dosage of oxytocin reaches 10 mU/minute. If the oxytocin infusion is to be continued, the physician must write an order to increase the dosage.

B. Guidelines for Interpretation of the CST:

1. Test is read as:
   a. Negative—no late deceleration of the FHR when an adequate frequency of three contractions in 10 minutes has been established, a "negative window"
   b. Positive—late decelerations occurring with three contractions in 10 minutes, a "positive window"
   c. Equivocal—no positive or negative window
   d. Hyperstimulation—excessive uterine activity is present in association with a deceleration of the FHR
   e. Unsatisfactory—inadequate UC or FHR record

*Courtesy of Patricia M. Graef, BSNEd.

studies have suggested that fewer accelerations of the same magnitude may be adequate. Because the fetus has cyclic periods of rest, external stimulation by manipulation has been used to elicit movement for the testing. Failure to demonstrate a reactive pattern owing either to lack of accelerations with movement or to lack of fetal movement is taken as an indication for further evaluation of the fetus by a CST (Fig. 41-14).

The NST and CST have been almost exclusively performed by nurses. Along with this function, nurses have assumed the role of educating the patients about the tests and screening the test results. A notable

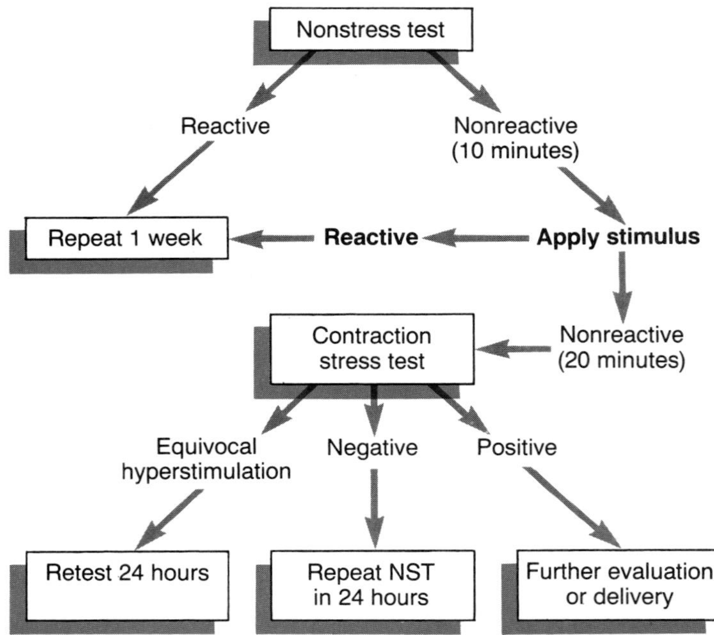

Figure 41-14.
An example of a protocol for antepartum fetal heart rate testing (NST and CST).

The Nonstress Test*

A. Nursing Guidelines for Performing the NST:

1. Take patient to the antepartum testing unit.
2. Explain the procedure to the patient, including the time involved. The test requires an average of 30 minutes.
3. Have patient change into a gown.
4. Place patient in a semi-Fowler's position at a 30° to 45° angle with a slight left tilt.
5. Place patient on an external monitor using ultrasound transducer or phonotransducer to record the FHR. A tokodynamometer is used to document fetal activity and spontaneous uterine activity.
6. Record patient's blood pressure initially and at 5- to 10-minute intervals.
7. The patient is asked to indicate each time fetal movement occurs by pressing the record button on the monitor. A 10- to 20-minute strip is obtained.

B. Interpretation of the NST:

1. Test is read as:
   a. Reactive—2 FHR accelerations greater than 15 bpm above the baseline and lasting 15 seconds or more with fetal movement in 10-minute period
   b. Nonreactive—no or one FHR acceleration greater than 15 bpm and lasting 15 seconds or more with fetal movement in a 10-minute period or accelerations less than 15 bpm or lasting less than 15 seconds

*Courtesy of Patricia M. Graef, BSNEd.

NC Nursing Care: Electronic Fetal Monitoring and Fetal Intensive Care*

Assessment	Intervention	Evaluation
Determination of need for electronic fetal monitoring (EFM)		
Assess current maternal physical status	Review maternal records and fetal data if available Check maternal vital signs and question regarding maternal subjective impressions and observations regarding physical status	If data within normal limits, EFM may not be needed If data show prenatal factors associated with possible fetal distress (*e.g.*, fetal growth retardation 3rd trimester bleeding, previous still births, hypertension, *etc.*), monitor is indicated
Assess labor progress	Review chart and question mother regarding onset and quality of contractions, condition of the membranes and other pertinent data Observe for behavioral manifestation of normal/abnormal labor progress Report and record as necessary (this to be done as indicated throughout)	If assessment indicates abnormal labor pattern, (hypertonic, hypotonic, *etc.*), monitor is indicated
Assess FHR	Auscultate FHR	FHR abnormalities, apply monitor
Assess amniotic fluid at time of rupture of membranes	Observe or review records as to quality and quantity	Scant, excessive, or meconium stained fluid may indicate fetal disease, abnormality or distress Monitor indicated
Assess couple's knowledge of EFM	Review records for evidence of prenatal preparation classes Question couple, allowing time for feedback	Couple exhibits satisfactory knowledge; if not, plan basic orientation to rationale and procedure of EFM
Assessment indicates application of EFM	Apply EFM—external or internal as indicated Explain (or reexplain) rationale for use Explain methods to be used	Parents understand rationale for use, procedure for monitoring, and interpretation of EFM data Allows participation in decision making Alerts parents for equipment failure
	Apply monitor so that mother is comfortable; explain about position changes Place monitor in mother's view; review initial tracings Review tracings with parents periodically; answer *all* questions	Mother able to be comfortable; understands need for position changes Allows use of data for breathing and relaxation techniques Parents better understand labor course Allows use of data to observe labor progress
Problem Assessment		
Determine baseline bradycardia by strip review and observations of mother's verbal and behavioral input	Confirm by auscultation	Confirmation and identification as arrhythmia permits verification of problem (this condition often associated with diminished

(Continued)

NC Nursing Care: Electronic Fetal Monitoring and Fetal Intensive Care (continued)

Assessment	Intervention	Evaluation
		baseline variability or late decelerations indicative of severe fetal distress)
	Evaluate FECG; identify arrhythmia Review tracing for periodic deceleration and baseline variability Review record for drugs	
	Institute remedial measures for fetal distress	Persistent and unexplained baseline bradycardia may indicate fetal hypoxia and acidosis; these measures should produce definitive relief if condition is not to progress
	Turn to left lateral recumbent position	Lateral position relieves venacaval occlusion, improves venous return to heart, and therefore improves cardiac output and uterine perfusion
	Discontinue oxytocin if applicable	Dairy oxytocin decreases contractions, which diminishes placental respiratory exchange and fetal oxygenation
	Administer O_2 by mask	O_2 by mask increases maternal oxygenation, which increases O_2 delivered to placental exchange
	Report and record verbally and in writing	
	Remain with patient; institute primary nursing (one-to-one); answer questions	Presence of nurse is supportive to patient and constant personal monitoring is necessary to watch for deterioration
	Comfort measures as necessary Be alert for possible deterioration, which may result in cesarean section Review strips frequently and regularly	
	Confirm by auscultation Evaluate FECG; identify arrhythmias	Confirmation and identification verifies problem
	Take maternal temperature	Maternal fever most frequent cause of fetal tachycardia
	Review drugs administered to mother	Certain drugs (ephedrine) may cause fetal tachycardia
	Review tracings for periodic decelerations and baseline variability	Fetal tachycardia may be sign of fetal distress; occasionally subtle late decelerations may be noted on review of tracing
	Institute remedial measures for fetal distress as outlined above	This condition, if persistent, may also indicate fetal hypoxia and acidosis; these measures should produce definitive relief if condition is not to progress

*Care plan revised by Mary Sullivan, R.N., M.N.

secondary benefit of these functions has been the opportunity for nurses working in both the antepartal and labor and delivery areas to establish a nurse–patient relationship with high-risk patients during the antepartum period. The benefits of this relationship in the delivery of nursing care during labor, delivery, and the puerperium should be obvious.

Conclusion

The development and application of continuous fetal monitoring has dramatically expanded the role of the nurse in caring for the family during labor and delivery. With this expanded role have come additional responsibilities in parent education, counseling, and patient care.

With consumerism becoming an increasingly important factor in the delivery of obstetrical care, the need for and the value of fetal monitoring are among the particular aspects of clinical practice that have been questioned. The principles of fetal monitoring and the scientific basis for interpreting the data have become well understood. It would seem logical to presume that the detection and alleviation of fetal stress (*e.g.,* due to excessive uterine activity or maternal hypotension) or the detection of fetal distress (hypoxia and acidosis) should be of benefit to the patient. Nevertheless, the long-term benefits of clinically applied fetal monitoring are not as yet well substantiated. In counseling patients, the nurse should not overstate the presumed benefits of monitoring, especially during normal pregnancy; nor should the potential risks, however infrequent, be ignored. Furthermore, continuing education in interpretation of data and the use of new equipment or tests is required. It is important, therefore, that the nurse be aware of the most current information regarding the risks, benefits, and applications of monitoring.

As fetal monitoring first became widely used, concerns were raised that there would develop a tendency to nurse the machine rather than the patients. This misgiving has not been substantiated in most instances. On the contrary, fetal monitoring has had the beneficial result of freeing the nurse from repetitious tasks and providing an opportunity for more and better quality care for the mother and the fetus. In applying monitoring, the nurse makes independent assessments of maternal and fetal pathophysiology and takes remedial action to correct abnormalities as they develop. These tasks have led to the concept of the nurse caring for a high-risk mother and fetus as an "intensivist." As a result, greater appreciation of the need for primary or one-on-one continuous nursing care during labor and delivery has developed. Thus, monitoring can be an important factor in enhancing the quality of nursing care during labor and delivery.

The care plan has been developed as an *overview* of EFM where there is a possibility of some fetal stress and distress. Hospitals may have more specific protocols and the nurse will become familiar with them.

Suggested Readings

General

Goodlin RC: History of fetal monitoring. Am J Obstet Gynecol 133:323, 1979

Haverkamp AD, Thompson HE, McFee JG, Cetrulo C: The evaluation of continuous fetal heart rate monitoring in high-risk pregnancy. Am J Obstet Gynecol 125:310, 1976

Haverkamp AD, Orleans M, Langendoerfer S, McFee J: A controlled trial of the differential effects of intrapartum fetal monitoring. Am J Obstet Gynecol 134:399, 1979

Hon EH: An Introduction to Fetal Heart Rate Monitoring, 2nd ed. Los Angeles, University of Southern California School of Medicine, 1975

Johnstone FD, Campbell DM, Hughes GJ: Has continuous intrapartum monitoring made any impact on fetal outcome? Lancet 1:1298, 1978

Neutra RR, Feinberg SE, Greenland S, Friedman EA: Effect of fetal monitoring on neonatal death rates. N Engl J Med 299:324, 1978

Paul RH, Hon EH: Clinical fetal monitoring: V. Effect on perinatal outcome. Am J Obstet Gynecol 118:529, 1974

Quilligan EJ, Paul RH: Fetal monitoring: Is it worth it? Obstet Gynecol 45:96, 1975

Renou P, Chang A, Anderson I, Wood C: Controlled trial of fetal intensive care. Am J Obstet Gynecol 126:470, 1976

Atlases of Fetal Monitoring

Klavan M, Laver AT, Boscola MA: Clinical concepts of fetal heart rate monitoring. Waltham, MA, Hewlett-Packard, 1977

Paul RH, Petrie RH, Rabello YA, Mueller EA: Fetal Intensive Care: I. An Introduction. North Haven, CT, William Mack, 1979

Paul RH, Petrie RH, Rabello YA, Mueller EA: Fetal Intensive Care: II. Case Management. North Haven, CT, William Mack, 1979

Paul RH, Petrie RH, Rabello YA, Mueller EA: Fetal Intensive Care: III. Case Management with Emphasis on Drug Effects. North Haven, CT, William Mack, 1979

Fetal Scalp Blood Sampling

Saling E: Fetal and Neonatal Hypoxia in Relation to Clinical Obstetric Practice. Baltimore, Williams & Wilkins, 1968

Seeds AE: Maternal-fetal acid-base relationships and fetal scalp blood analysis. In Makowski EL (ed): Clinical Obstetrics and Gynecology, High Risk Obstetrics, Vol. 21, No. 2, pp 579–591, New York, Harper & Row, 1978

Antepartum Testing

Evertson LR, Gauthier RJ, Schifrin BS, Paul RH: Antepartum fetal heart rate testing: I. Evolution of the nonstress test. Am J Obstet Gynecol 133:29, 1979

Gauthier RJ, Evertson LR, Paul RH: Antepartum fetal heart rate testing: II. Intrapartum fetal heart rate observation and newborn outcome following a positive contraction stress test. Am J Obstet Gynecol 133:34, 1979

Paul RH, Miller FC: Antepartum fetal heart rate monitoring. In Makowski EL (ed): Clinical Obstetrics and Gynecology, High Risk Obstetrics, Vol. 21, No. 2, pp 375–384, New York, Harper & Row, 1978

Ray M, Freeman R, Pine S, Hesselgesser R: Clinical experience with the oxytocin challenge test. Am J Obstet Gynecol 114:1, 1972

Rochard F, Schifrin BS, Goupil F, Legrand H: Nonstressed fetal heart rate monitoring in the antepartum period. Am J Obstet Gynecol 126:699, 1976

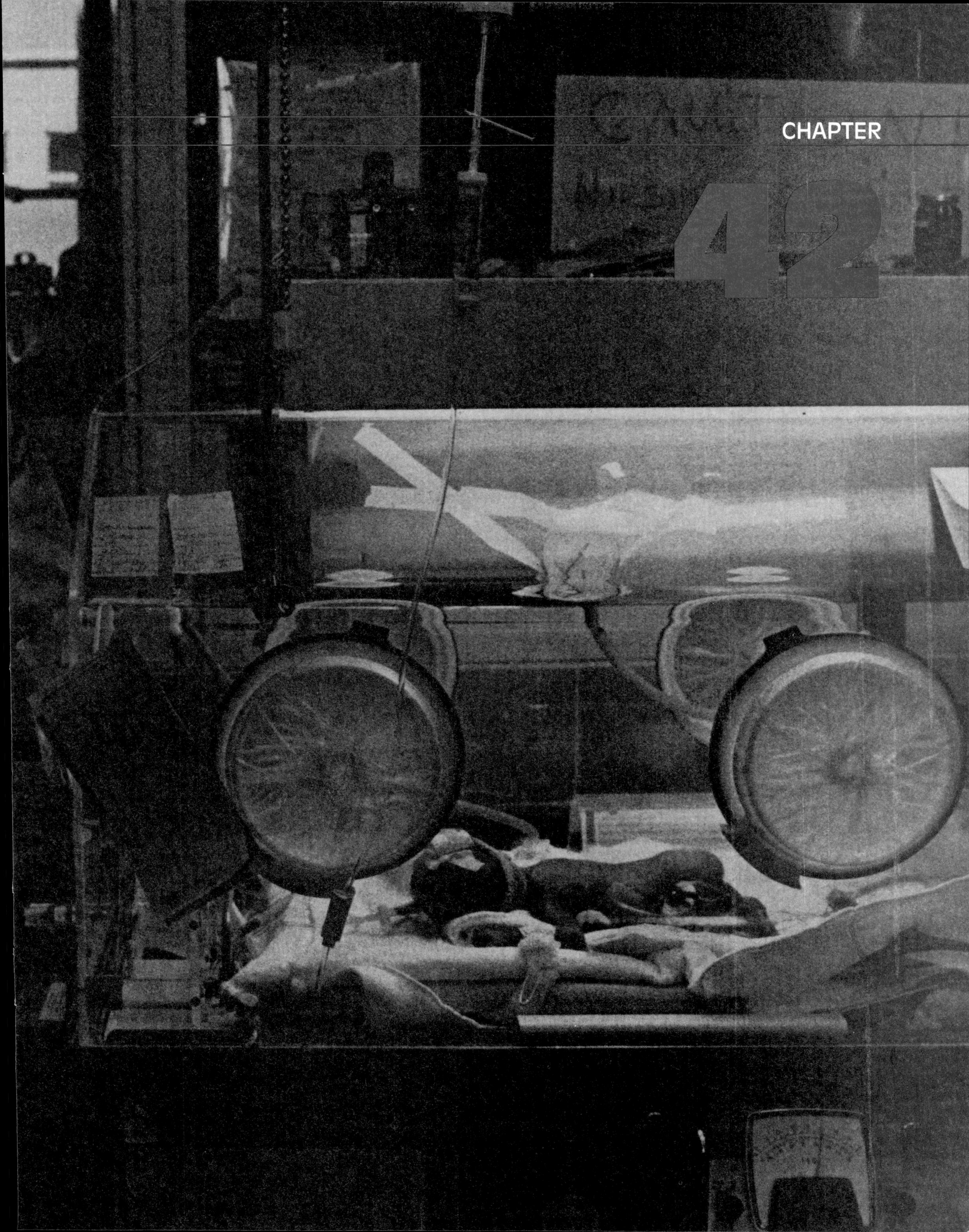

CHAPTER 42

CHAPTER 42

The High-Risk Infant: Disorders of Gestational Age and Birth Weight

The size of an infant at birth is influenced by many factors that affect the maternal and fetal environments. The relationship between low birth weight and perinatal morbidity and mortality has long been recognized. Only recently, however, have the different implications of birth weight relative to gestational age been established. Infants of low birth weight may be of appropriate size for their gestational age but immature because they are born before pregnancy has progressed to full term. These infants are classically "premature"—born before their organ systems have matured to the point of physiological functioning. Other low-birth-weight infants may be undersized for the length of their gestation, whether delivered before or at term. These infants are called "small for gestational age." Often they are physiologically mature but have not attained the size and weight appropriate for gestational age for numerous reasons.

Infants experiencing disorders of gestational age and birth weight also include those who are large for gestational age and who are postmature—born after pregnancy has progressed beyond full term. The associated problems and potential causes are different among these various types of altered fetal growth, requiring individualized assessment and approaches to management. The particular causes of alterations in fetal growth also determine the newborn's immediate and long-term prognosis. The challenge to effective assessment and management of fetal growth disorders begins with an understanding of the intricate and complex mechanisms that control normal fetal growth.

Classification of Infants by Birth Weight and Gestational Age

In the past, all newborns weighing 2500 g or less were termed premature, and those weighing more were designated full term. This approach assumed that intrauterine growth rates were essentially the same for all fetuses and that birth weight corresponded to gestational age. A considerable amount of data has now accumulated to demonstrate the inaccuracy of this assumption, and the two dimensions of *birth weight* and *gestational age* are now considered separately.

The World Health Organization (WHO) has designated a *term birth* as one occurring between 38 weeks' and 42 weeks' gestation, with age calculated from the date of the onset of the mother's last menstrual period. WHO advised that newborn infants not be classified as *premature* on the basis of weight alone. Gestational age must be used to assign categories of preterm, term, and postterm births. Also, it must be recognized that an infant weighing less than 2500 g is not necessarily premature.

Intrauterine growth standards are used to compare an infant's weight and gestational age with population averages. Although these have shortcomings in application to particular situations (*e.g.,* differences in weight due to race, parity, sex, altitude), they are useful as guides in the assessment of high-risk infants. The most widely used growth chart was developed in Colorado and gives percentiles of intrauterine growth for weight, length, and head circumference. However, the altitude effects made this estimate low for the rest of the country. A more recent fetal growth chart includes correction factors for parity, race, and sex and presents average fetal weights for the 10th, 25th, 50th, 75th, and 90th percentiles (Fig. 42-1). Infants may be classified in any one of nine groups (Fig. 42-2).

Weight serves in the assessment of growth, and gestational age in the assessment of maturity. An infant born at 40 weeks' gestation and weighing less than 2500 g (or below the 10th percentile for weight or length) would be mature but undergrown. This disorder is called *intrauterine growth retardation,* with the infant classified as *small for gestational age* (SGA). An infant born at 36 weeks' gestation and weighing 3500 g (above the 90th percentile for weight) would be immature but overgrown. Such *large for gestational age* (LGA) infants are typical for diabetic mothers. Although this infant has attained average term weight, it is actually premature, with incomplete maturation of organ systems.

The term *premature* seems appropriate for the *preterm,* immature infant, regardless of birth weight. Preterm infants may also be SGA, implying that at least two factors are involved: that causing the early delivery and that retarding the growth rate *in utero.*

The term *low-birth-weight infant* defines any liveborn infant weighing 2500 g or less. A *very-low-birth-weight infant* weighs 1500 g or less (Figs. 42-3 and 42-4).

(Text continues on page 934)

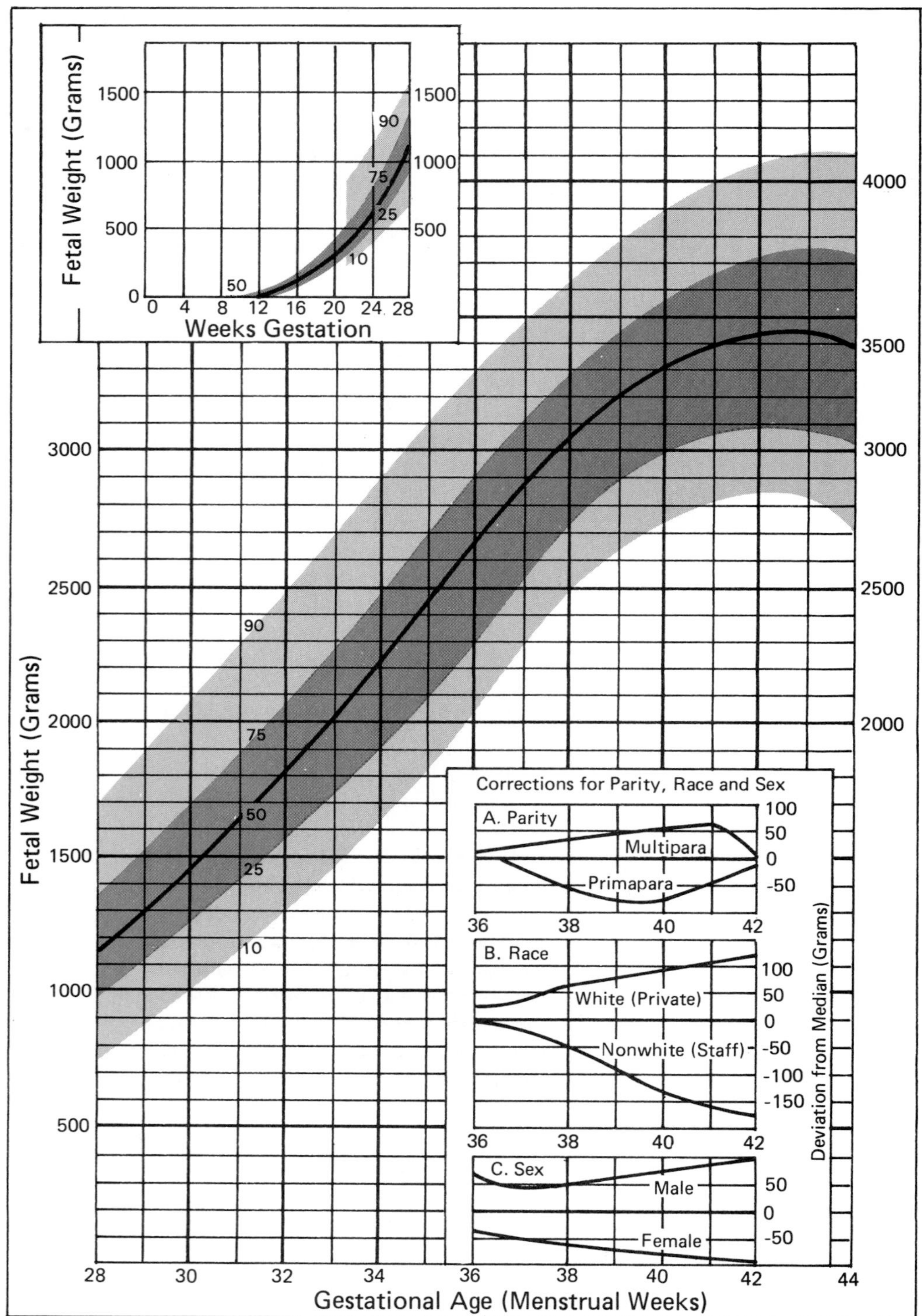

Figure 42-1.
Fetal weight. The 10th, 25th, 50th, 75th, and 90th percentiles of fetal weight in grams throughout pregnancy and correction factors for parity, race (socioeconomic status), and sex are graphed. Data obtained from 31,202 prostaglandin-induced abortions and spontaneous deliveries. (Courtesy of Brenner WE, Edelman DA, Hendricks CH: A standard of fetal growth for the United States of America. Am J Obstet Gynecol 126:555–564, 1976)

Weight (percentile)	Less than 38 wk	38–42 wk	Greater than 42 wk
Greater than 90	Preterm LGA	Term LGA	Postterm LGA
10–90	Preterm AGA	Term AGA	Postterm AGA
Less than 10	Preterm SGA	Term SGA	Postterm SGA

Figure 42-2.
Birth weight-gestational age groups as defined by Lubchenko et al. (Clewell WH: Prematurity. J Reprod Med 23, 5:237–244, 1979)

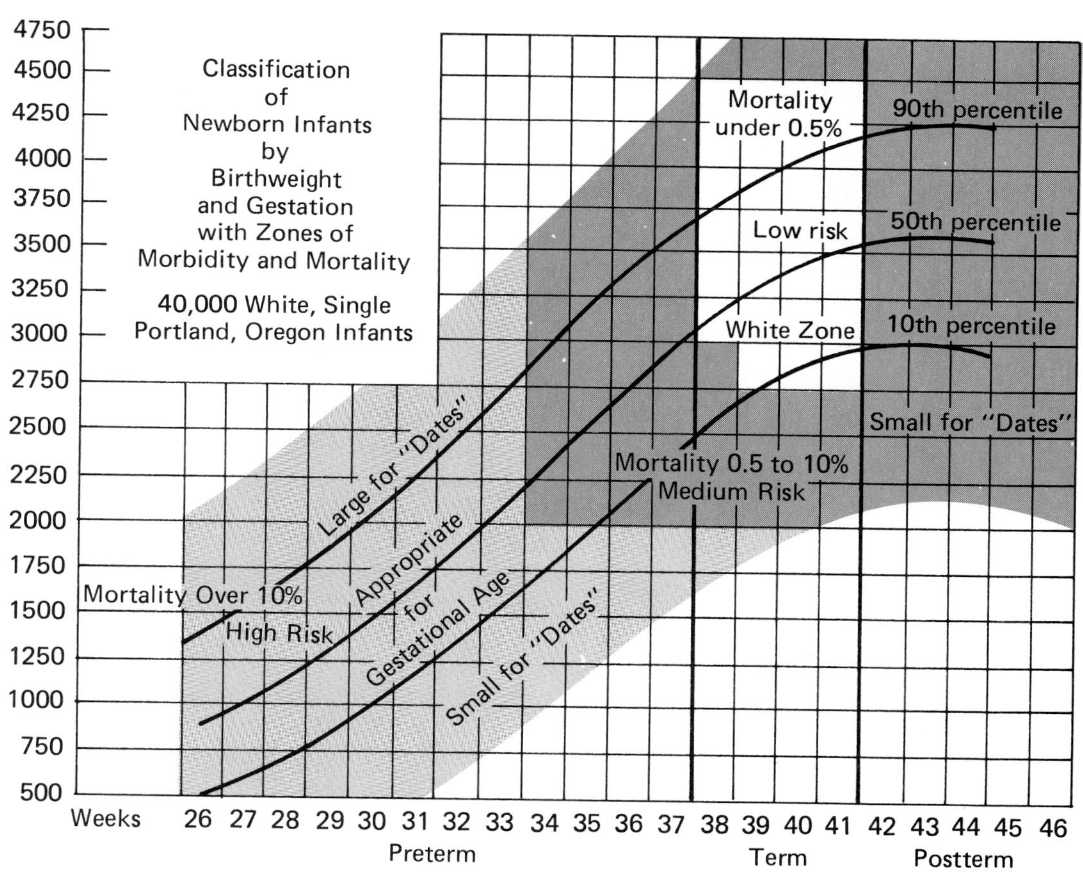

Figure 42-3.
Classification of newborn infants by birth weight and gestation with areas of morbidity and mortality. (Babson SG, Benson RC, Pernoll ML, Benda GI: Management of High-Risk Pregnancy and Intensive Care of the Neonate. St Louis, CV Mosby, 1975)

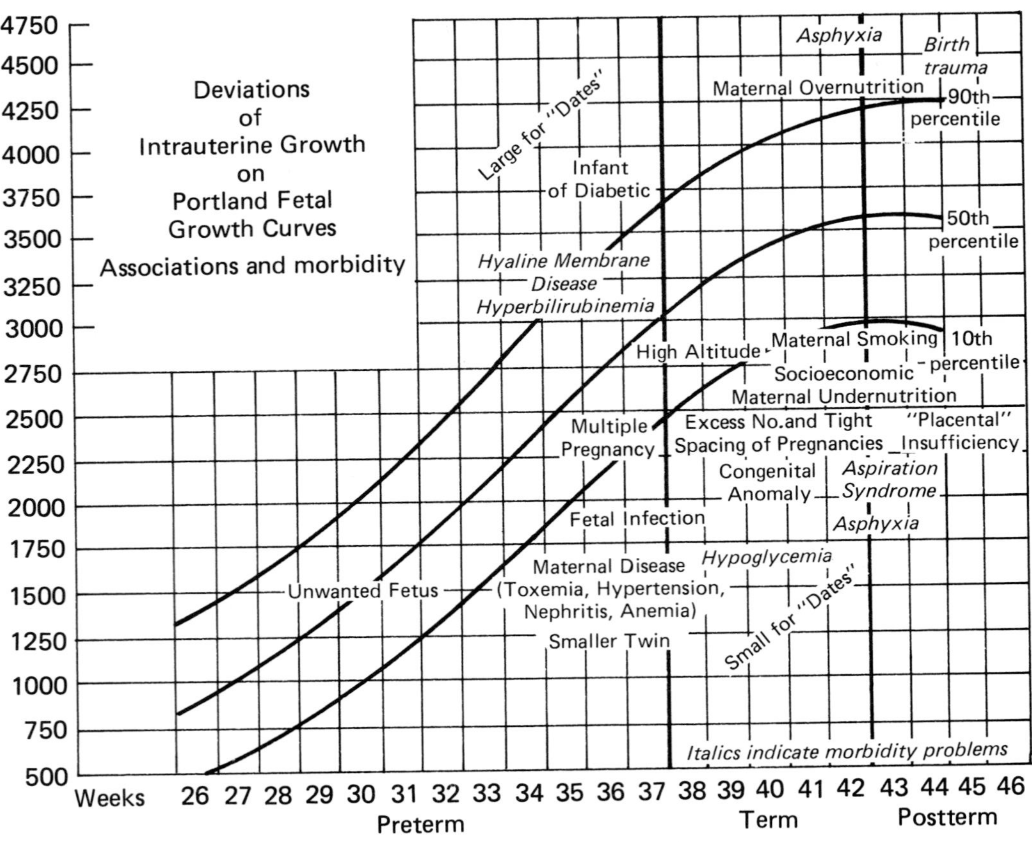

Figure 42-4.
Intrauterine growth curves and associations with perinatal mortality and morbidity. (Babson SG, Benson RC, Pernoll ML, Benda GI: Management of High-Risk Pregnancy and Intensive Care of the Neonate. St Louis, CV Mosby, 1975)

Etiology

Preterm or Premature

Premature or preterm infants are born before the 37th week of gestation, regardless of birth weight. Most babies who weigh less than 2500 g at birth are premature, as are almost all those weighing less than 1500 g. However, as previously stated, not all infants weighing less than 2500 g are necessarily premature. The main criterion is gestational age. The majority of these preterm infants are of appropriate weight for gestational age, but some are small-for-dates. The causes of early delivery in the cases of those infants who are appropriately sized remain obscure.

The majority of instances of premature labor have an unknown etiology. Conditions that have been clearly related to premature labor can be divided into categories of *maternal, fetal,* or *placental* etiology.

Maternal factors include preeclampsia, eclampsia, uterine anomalies or tumors, sepsis, cervical incompetence, cardiovascular or renal disorders, diabetes, and abdominal surgery.

Fetal factors include multiple pregnancy, hydramnios, rubella, toxoplasmosis, syphilis, and premature rupture of membranes.

Placental factors include placenta previa and abruptio placentae.

Mortality rates are inversely proportional to gestational age and birth weight.

Small-for-Gestational-Age Infants (Growth Retardation)

Infants whose weight falls below the 10th percentile for their gestational age have experienced impairment of the normal growth process during the prenatal period. Some physicians use the limiting criterion of birth weight of two standard deviations below the mean of gestational age. This condition may occur at any gestational age, but the majority of small-for-date infants are born at, or close to, term and weigh less than 2500 g. Under the old classification, these would have been called *premature,* although their period of intrauterine life was not significantly shortened. Though small, these infants are mature in comparison with infants of similar weight but lower gestational age.

Growth-retarded infants have an increased risk of perinatal morbidity and mortality and are estimated to account for about 25% of the entire perinatal mortality.[1] The infant's condition is a product of a process of intrauterine deprivation that begins many weeks before birth. It is often related to abnormalities of the pregnancy or of the fetus.

There are two types of growth retardation, which may occur separately or simultaneously. Fetal growth involves both an increase in the number of cells (hyperplasia) and an increase in the size of cells (hypertrophy). Embryonic growth involves a rapid increase in the number of cells as the organs and body structures are formed. These cells increase in size later in pregnancy. If an insult to the fetus occurs early in gestation, mitosis is impaired and fewer new cells are formed. This results in small organs of subnormal weight. The cells, however, are of normal size. If interference with growth occurs later, the cells are normal in number but smaller in size, again resulting in smaller organs but, in this instance, due to reduced amounts of cytoplasm. An intrauterine insult throughout both phases of growth results in cells that are fewer in number and smaller in size. The classic example of the latter condition is the infant with the rubella syndrome.

Maternal preeclampsia, which tends to be more prominent during later pregnancy, creates the second type of growth retardation in which cell numbers are normal, but cell size is reduced.

Factors That Affect Fetal Growth

Fetal growth is influenced by a variety of factors of maternal, placental, and fetal origins. Genetic predispositions, the mother's nutritional and health status, fetal nutrition, fetal and maternal endocrine functions, developmental insults, environmental stressors, and placental function are variably involved in this process. Maturation is affected by biochemical determinants, enzymes, genes, and hormones, particularly adrenal and thyroid. Development of the various organs follows a different time sequence, with hormonal action triggering a certain organ to grow and mature at a particular time during gestation. As different organs mature at different times, there are critical periods when stressors can significantly alter normal development. After these critical periods, the organ is less susceptible to damage and more capable of functioning in the extrauterine environment.

Maternal Factors

Genetic factors are important in determining fetal birth weight, but growth patterns are species-specific and follow a predictable course until the last several weeks of gestation. At this time, generally after 34 weeks' to 38 weeks' gestation, fetal weights differ significantly according to parity, race, and fetal sex.[2] In general, infants born to smaller parents tend to be smaller in length and weight than infants born to larger parents. However, the greatest influence on infant birth size appears to be related to the characteristics of the maternal environment as reflected in intrauterine development. These characteristics include prepregnancy weight, weight gain during pregnancy, parity, interval between pregnancies, and age at delivery. Other factors in the mother's environment affecting fetal growth include cigarette smoking, alcohol and drug use, infections, nutritional status, and socioeconomic conditions or changes. Finally, the occurrence of genetic defects exerts an influence on fetal growth that usually results in infants of low birth weight for their gestational age.[3]

Nutrition

The role of nutrition in pregnancy outcome is a continuing and perplexing concern for health-care providers. Although animal studies show direct causal relationships between inadequate maternal nutrition and reduced growth, altered organ function, and diminished rate of cell division in the brain and other organs in offspring, these data cannot be directly applied to humans. Malnutrition in humans is usually associated with other confounding factors such as poverty, low socioeconomic status, wars and famines, and other types of social and psychological stress. Although birth weight has been shown to be related to maternal prepregnancy weight and weight gain during pregnancy, the latter is not a good index of nutrition and may only indicate the relative adequacy of energy intake.

The question of which nutrients are of greatest importance is under examination. Recent primate studies do not support the view that protein and calories are the major factors in favorable versus unfavorable pregnancy outcome, as measured by impaired somatic or brain growth. Reduced protein intake prolongs primate pregnancy, resulting in a normal birth weight. This suggests a compensating mechanism between fetus and mother.[3] It has been suggested that energy (rather than protein, carbohydrates, or combinations thereof) is the most common nutritional factor affecting growth, and that primates conserve greater stores of nitrogen during pregnancy. These controlled studies could isolate the effects of protein or calorie restriction. Observations of human populations, on the other hand, must consider multiple factors.

The adequacy of diet is difficult to assess because of a lack of universally accepted standards of nutrition and health, imprecise determinations of needed nutrients, and limitations of study designs in research. In an examination of vitamin imbalance in low-birth-weight neonates with mothers showing no overt signs of malnutrition, no statistically significant differences in blood levels of vitamins were found between mothers with infants of normal birth weight and those with infants of low birth weight. However, when the blood level of vitamins in the infants was tested, three vitamins were significantly lower in low-birth-weight infants: folate, pantothenate, and vitamin B_{12}. Hematologic, neurologic, and immune system dysfunctions are related to deficiencies of these vitamins. The critical questions involve the cause–effect relationships; do the low vitamin levels result from the low birth weight, are they associated with it but not directly caused by low birth weight, or are they a factor causing the impaired fetal growth.[4]

Placental Function

Under normal conditions, the size of the placenta is a major determinant of fetal size. When there is severe maternal nutritional deprivation, it appears that the maintenance needs of the placenta are met first, leading to reduction of fetal growth. In a fetus with growth retardation, however, the placenta is relatively smaller than with a normally growing fetus of the same gestational age. This is associated with higher levels of asphyxia at birth and perinatal morbidity seen among SGA infants. Placental mechanisms for maintaining optimal transfer of nutrients and gases between maternal and fetal blood are necessary for an adequate supply of growth-promoting substances to the fetus. The diffusion capacity of the placenta increases proportionately with fetal weight during pregnancy. Any impairment of oxygen transfer has a deleterious effect on fetal growth. Transfer of minerals, electrolytes, and trace metals, which are necessary in an adequate supply for proper fetal growth, is also related to placental function.[3]

Decreased uteroplacental blood flow is believed to be a major mechanism in reduction of transfer of nutrients and oxygen to the fetus. This results in altered growth. Maternal vascular disease is associated with the highest frequency of growth-retarded fetuses in the United States (approximately 35% of these cases). Hypertensive mothers with significantly reduced blood volume have infants of smaller birth weight than nonhypertensive controls. Reduction of maternal blood volume apparently decreases uterine blood flow.[5]

There appears to be no single placental abnormality common to infants who are SGA, and placental and cord defects are present in only a small number of cases. When lesions are present, the most common are infarction, villous avascularity, fibrinosis, premature aging, and nonspecific chronic villous inflammation. Inadequate placental function is also associated with preeclampsia and diabetes.

Fetal Endocrine Influences

The hypothalamic-pituitary axis acts through the pancreas to modify fetal growth. This is an interactional situation between mother and fetus. In the normal-birth-weight fetus of a normal mother, the pancreas has 2% endocrine tissue with 40% beta cells. In infants of gestational diabetic mothers, endocrine tissue is 10% with 60% beta cells, leading to significantly higher fetal insulin levels. The percentages of endocrine tissue and insulin levels are directly proportional to the excess fetal weight observed in infants of diabetic mothers. There appears to be a competitive effect between adrenal cortical hormones and insulin. This relates to lung maturation and the formation of surfactant. Cortisol slows cell growth but enhances maturation of the fetal lung, whereas insulin acts as an antagonist to glucocorticoids. This effect seems related to the higher incidence of respiratory distress syndrome in infants of diabetic mothers. A similar relationship between insulin levels and glucocorticoids occurs with enzyme and glucose metabolism in the liver. Insulin, acting unopposed in the fetus, directly influences cytoplasmic growth and increases triglyceride concentrations in the brain, liver, and lung.[3]

Thyroid and adrenal hormones are important to fetal maturation. Inadequate levels of thyroid hormone are associated with decreased fetal size, delayed skeletal ossification, delayed maturation, and mental retardation. Infants of hyperthyroid mothers may have advanced neurologic development for gestational age, greater body weight, greater placental weight, and advanced skeletal development. They appear several weeks older than their gestational age. Corticosteroids are used to induce organ maturation, for instance, to promote lung maturation. They also affect maturation of the foregut (absorption of antibodies), pancreas, liver, and small bowel. Liver glycogen depends on the presence of corticosteroids. It is possible that growth hormone may play a role in brain growth. Somatomedins (growth hormone ancillary factors) may be important in cell multiplication in the fetus, as high levels are found in large infants at birth and low levels in infants small for gestational age. Through an endocrine chain, hormonal regulation of fetal growth may be finely regulated by the central nervous system.[3]

Infection

Certain intrauterine infections are known to cause decreased growth of the baby, for example, cytomegalic inclusion disease and rubella. For an in-depth discussion of the effects of viral diseases on infants see Chapter 44.

Genetic Factors

With the separation of true premature from small-for-date infants, it became apparent that most congenital malformations occur in undergrown infants. The smaller the infant was for its gestational age, the greater were the risks of congenital anomalies. Additionally, the highest incidence of severe malformations was found to occur in small-for-date infants with the longest gestation. Congenital malformations occur 10 to 20 times more frequently in SGA infants than in appropriate-for-gestational-age infants.[6] Congenital disorders such as dwarfism often occur in infants who are small-for-dates. In some families there are repeated births of infants who are small for gestational age without associated abnormalities except mental retardation.

Other Factors

Various other circumstances or conditions are associated with retarded intrauterine growth. Infants born of multiple pregnancies are usually small-for-dates if born after 35 weeks' gestation, presumably because the placenta can no longer supply the needs of the growing fetuses. Smoking is a significant statistical correlate to SGA babies, with moderate smokers having double the incidence, and heavy smokers a 3 times higher incidence of SGA babies than nonsmokers. Mothers who smoke more than 20 cigarettes per day give birth to growth-retarded infants 2 to 3 times more often than mothers who do not smoke. Living at higher altitudes tends to be related to lower birth weight for the duration of pregnancy. Certain noxious agents such as x-rays, aminopterin, and other antimetabolites result in growth impairment, malformations of the brain and cranial vault, and other anomalies, depending upon timing of exposure. Infants of drug addicts, notably heroin addicts, are often small-for-dates.

Identification of the High-Risk Neonate

Although the causes of prematurity and altered fetal growth are not completely understood, several associated factors have been identified that alert nurses and physicians to the possibility of these problems. Early recognition of mothers with high-risk pregnancies and careful prenatal care can often contribute to a better outcome for the infant and the mother.

Many of the factors contributing to the birth of a high-risk infant are not specific for a particular problem or condition, but are generally related to increased morbidity and mortality. Others have specific associations with neonatal disorders or fetal abnormalities. Those related to prematurity include diabetes, placental insufficiency, multiple pregnancy, preeclampsia and hypertensive disorders, and infection. Several overlap with increased incidence of SGA infants, including preeclampsia and hypertensive disorders, placental insufficiency, infections, discordant twin, and altitude. Congenital anomalies are more highly correlated to term SGA infants (Table 42-1).

Assessment of Gestational Age

Accurate assessment of an infant's gestational age is of immediate and critical importance in the proper management of problems and anticipation of needs for care. The clinical course, outcome, and problems are quite different for the preterm, SGA, and LGA infant. Preterm infants suffer more commonly from hyaline membrane disease, hyperbilirubinemia, apnea, and feeding problems. In SGA infants, frequent problems include hypoglycemia, hypocalcemia, congenital mal-

Table 42-1.
Identification of High-Risk Infant: Associated Factors

Antepartal Factors

Maternal Characteristics

Age less than 15 or over 35
Low socioeconomic status
Unmarried
Family or marital conflicts
Emotional illness or family history of mental illness
Persistent ambivalence or conflicts about the pregnancy
Stature under 5 feet
20% underweight or overweight
Malnutrition

Reproductive History

Parity greater than 8
Two or more previous abortions
Previous stillborn or neonatal death
Previous premature labor or low-birth-weight infant (<2500 g)
Previous excessively large infant (>4000 g)
Infant with isoimmunization or ABO incompatibility
Infant with congenital anomaly, genetic disorder, or birth damage
Preeclampsia or eclampsia
Uterine fibroids >5 cm or submucous
Abnormal Pap smear
Infertility
Prior cesarean section
Prior fetal malpresentations
Contracted pelvis
Ovarian masses
Genital tract abnormalities (incompetent cervix, subseptate or bicornate uterus)
Pregnancy occurring 3 months or less after last delivery
Previous prolonged labor or significant dystocia

Substances Abuse

Drugs
Alcohol
Heavy smoking (>2 packs day)

Medical Problems

Chronic hypertension
Renal disease (pyelonephritis, glomerulonephritis, polycystic kidney)
Diabetes mellitus (Classes B to F)
Heart disease (aortic insufficiency, pulmonary hypertension, diastolic murmur, cardiac enlargement, heart failure, arrhythmia)
Sickle cell trait or disease
Anemias with hemoglobin <9 g and hematocrit <32%
Pulmonary disease (tuberculosis, COPD)
Endocrine disorders (hypo- or hyperthyroidism, family history of cretinism, adrenal or pituitary problems)
Gastrointestinal or liver disease
Epilepsy
Malignancy (including leukemia and Hodgkin's disease)

Complications of Present Pregnancy

Low or excessive weight gain
Hypertension (mean arterial pressure >90, blood pressure 140/90, increase >30 mm Hg systolic or >20 mm Hg diastolic)
Recurrent glycosuria and abnormal fasting blood sugar or glucose tolerance test
Uterine size inappropriate for gestational age (either too large or too small)
Recurrent urinary tract infections
Severe varicosities or thrombophlebitis
Recurrent vaginal bleeding
Premature rupture of membranes
Multiple pregnancy
Hydramnios with a single fetus
Rh-negative with a rising titer
Late or no prenatal care
Exposure to teratogens (medications, x-ray, radioactive isotopes)
Viral infections (rubella, cytomegalovirus, herpes, mumps, rubeola, chickenpox, shingles, smallpox, vaccinia, influenza, poliomyelitis, hepatitis, Western equine encephalitis, Coxsackie B virus)
Syphilis, especially late pregnancy
Bacterial infections (gonorrhea, tuberculosis, listerosis, severe acute infection)
Protozoan infections (toxoplasmosis, malaria)
Postmaturity
Anemia with hemoglobin of 9 g or less
Severe preeclampsia, eclampsia
Abnormal CST
Falling urinary estriol levels

Intrapartal Factors

Complications of Labor and Delivery

Labor longer than 24 hours in primigravida
Labor longer than 12 hours in multigravida
Second stage longer than 1 hour
Ruptured membranes more than 24 hours
Abnormal presentation or position
Heavy sedation or injudicious anesthesia
Maternal fever or infection
Placenta previa or abruptio placentae
Cesarean section
Meconium-stained amniotic fluid
Fetal distress caused by monitoring or scalp blood sampling
Prolapsed cord
High or midforceps delivery, difficult or operative delivery
Premature labor
Severe preeclampsia, eclampsia
Precipitous labor less than 3 hours
Elective induction
Oxytocin (pitocin) augmentation

Immediate Problems of Infant

Malformation or other significant abnormality
Birth injury
Asphyxia (Apgar <6 at 5 minutes)

Neonatal Factors

Characteristics of Infant

Preterm or premature
SGA or LGA
Birth weight under 5½ pounds or over 9 pounds
Low-set ears
Enlargement of one or both kidneys
Single palmar crease
Single umbilical artery
Small head size

Clinical Problems

Feeding problems
Anemia
Hyperbilirubinemia
Temperature instability
Respiratory distress
Hypoglycemia
Polycythemia
Sepsis
Rh or ABO incompatibilities
Hypocalcemia
Hyperbilirubinemia
Persistent cyanosis
Shock
Seizures
Heart murmur

formations, aspiration, and polycythemia.[7] Among LGA infants, common problems are hypoglycemia, polycythemia, hyperviscosity syndrome, and birth trauma due to cephalopelvic disproportion.[8]

It may be important to determine gestational age during pregnancy (1) if fetal growth appears inappropriate for length of pregnancy, (2) if a high-risk condition exists in the mother, or (3) if premature labor threatens. After birth, determination of gestational age may be critical in anticipating problems and planning for care. This is especially true if the infant is of low birth weight, experiences neonatal complications, is premature, or has high-risk characteristics. A number of techniques and procedures have been developed to assess gestational age and fetal status during pregnancy and in the neonatal period.

Prenatal Assessment

This chapter focuses primarily on postnatal assessment of the gestational age of a newborn. For reference on prenatal techniques of estimating gestational age see Chapters 40 and 41.

Postnatal Assessment

After the infant's birth, a number of external physical characteristics and neurologic signs can be used to assess maturity. Standardized methods using these parameters have been developed and charts and scoring systems are available to make the procedures quicker and more accurate. Nurses involved in the care of high-risk infants should assess these physical characteristics and neurologic responses (Table 42-2).

Table 42-2.
Scoring System of External Physical Characteristics

External	Score*				
Sign	0	1	2	3	4
Edema	Obvious edema of hands and feet; pitting over tibia	No obvious edema of hand and feet; pitting over tibia	No edema		
Skin texture	Very thin, gelatinous	Thin and smooth	Smooth; medium thickness. Rash or superficial peeling	Slight thickening; superficial cracking and peeling, especially of hands and feet	Thick and parchment-like; superficial or deep cracking
Skin color	Dark red	Uniformly pink	Pale pink; variable over body	Pale; only pink over ears, lips, palms, or soles	
Skin opacity (trunk)	Numerous veins and venules clearly seen, especially over abdomen	Veins and tributaries seen	A few large vessels clearly seen over abdomen	A few large vessels seen indistinctly over abdomen	No blood vessels seen
Lanugo (over back)	No lanugo	Abundant; long and thick over whole back	Hair thinning especially over lower back	Small amount of lanugo and bald areas	At least ½ of back devoid of lanugo
Plantar creases	No skin creases	Faint red marks over anterior half of sole	Definite red marks over > anterior ½; indentations over < anterior ⅓	Indentations over > anterior ⅓	Definite deep indentations over > anterior ⅓
Nipple formation	Nipple barely visible; no areola	Nipple well defined; areola smooth and flat, diameter < 0.75 cm	Areola stippled, edge not raised, diameter < 0.75 cm	Areola stippled, edge raised, diameter > 0.75 cm	

(Continued)

Table 42-2.
Scoring System of External Physical Characteristics (continued)

External Sign	Score* 0	1	2	3	4
Breast size	No breast tissue palpable	Breast tissue on one or both sides, < 0.5 cm diameter	Breast tissue both sides; one or both 0.5 cm to 1 cm	Breast tissue both sides; one or both > 1 cm	
Ear form	Pinna flat and shapeless, little or no incurving of edge	Incurving of part of edge of pinna	Partial incurving whole of upper pinna	Well-defined incurving whole of upper pinna	
Ear firmness	Pinna soft, easily folded, no recoil	Pinna soft, easily folded, slow recoil	Cartilage to edge of pinna, but soft in places, ready recoil	Pinna firm, cartilage to edge, instant recoil	
Genitals: Male	Neither testis in scrotum	At least one testis high in scrotum	At least one testis right down		
Genitals: Female (with hips ½ abducted)	Labia majora widely separated, labia minora protruding	Labia majora almost cover labia minora	Labia majora completely cover labia minora		

Adapted by Dubowitz V, Dubowitz LMS, Goldberg C, Farr V et al: Clinical assessment of gestational age in the newborn infant. J Pediat 77:1, 1970. From Farr V, Mitchell RG, Neligan GA, Parkin JM et al: The definition of some external characteristics used in the assessment of gestational age of the newborn infant. Develop Med Child Neurol 8:507, 1966.

*If score differs on two sides, take the mean.

Physical Characteristics

During gestation, certain external physical characteristics develop and progress in an orderly fashion according to the age of the fetus. After birth, the gestational age can be determined by the presence or the absence of a number of these characteristics.

Breast Tissue and Areola. The nipples are present early in gestation, but the areola is barely visible until 34 weeks. After this time, the areola becomes raised and hair follicles become evident. Infants of less than 36 weeks' gestation have no breast tissue. At 36 weeks, a 1-mm to 2-mm nodule of breast tissue becomes palpable. This increases with gestational age under hormonal stimulation, until it reaches 7 mm to 10 mm at 40 weeks (Fig. 42-5).

Sole Creases. The soles of the feet become wrinkled first on the anterior portion, and then in the area extending toward the heel as gestation progresses. At 32 weeks, one or two creases can be seen; they become more numerous, crisscrossed, and deeper, covering the anterior two thirds of the sole by 37 weeks. The entire sole, including the heel, is covered at 40 weeks (Fig. 42-6). In the postterm infant, creases are deeper and there may be desquamation of the soles.

Ear Form and Cartilage. Infants of less than 33 to 34 weeks' gestation have relatively flat ears. After 34 weeks, the upper pinnae begin to curve inward. By 38 weeks, the upper two-thirds of the pinnae are incurved; this extends to the earlobe by 39 to 40 weeks. An extremely premature infant's ear remains folded over if pressed, due to the absence of cartilage. Cartilage is more reliable than ear form in estimating gestational age. It begins to appear at 32 weeks so that the ear slowly returns to its original position when folded over. By 36 weeks, the pinnae spring back when folded, and at term, they are firm, with the ear standing erect away from the head (Fig. 42-7).

Genitalia. The characteristics of both male and female genitalia change with gestational age. In the female, the clitoris is prominent at 30 to 32 weeks, while the labia majora are small and widely separated.

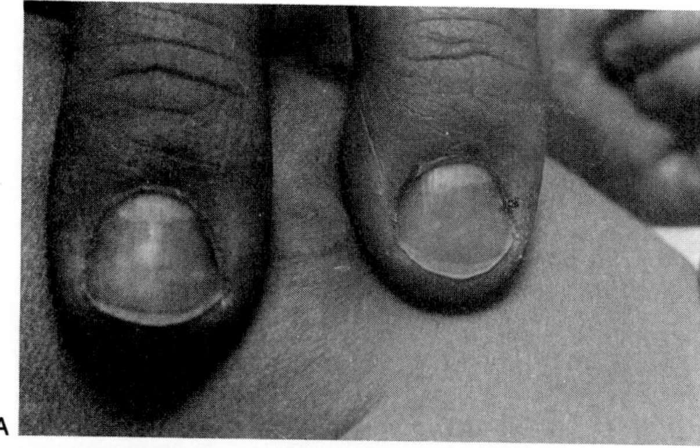

A

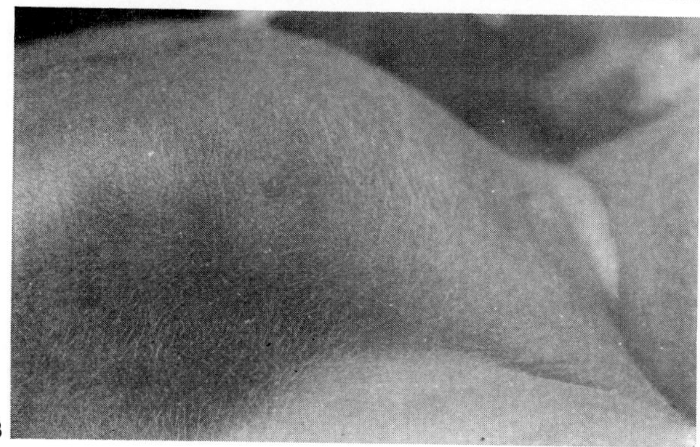

B

Figure 42-5.
Note the relatively distinct areola of the term infant *(A)* when compared to the preterm infant *(B)*. Also note the abundance of fine hair, lanugo, on the body of the preterm infant. (Whitley N: A Manual of Clinical Obstetrics. Philadelphia, JB Lippincott. In preparation.)

The labia majora increase in size and fullness with age, and at term they completely cover the labia minora and clitoris (Fig. 42-8).

In the male, the testes are high in the inguinal canal at about 30 weeks, gradually descend to be felt high in the scrotal sac at 37 weeks, and are well descended into the lower scrotal sac by 40 weeks. Rugae first appear on the scrotum anteriorly at 36 weeks and extend to cover the entire sac by 40 weeks. The postterm infant often has a pendulous scrotum covered with numerous rugae (Fig. 42-9).

Hair. Strands of hair are very fine in early gestation and tend to mat together like wool, with small bunches sticking out from the head. The full-term infant has silky hair that lies flat in single strands. In the postterm infant the hairline may recede. Important considerations to take into account when using hair as an assessment criterion are that hair varies in texture and characteristics with race and must be free of vernix before it is observed (see Fig. 42-7).

Skin and Vernix. The skin of premature infants is thin, pink, smooth, almost transparent with blood vessels visible, and thickly covered with vernix. The skin becomes thicker and more opaque with increasing age, until by 40 weeks it is pale with few vessels visible, with sparse vernix often occurring only in skin creases. In the postmature infant, there may be extensive desquamation of skin and absence of vernix (Fig. 42-10).

A

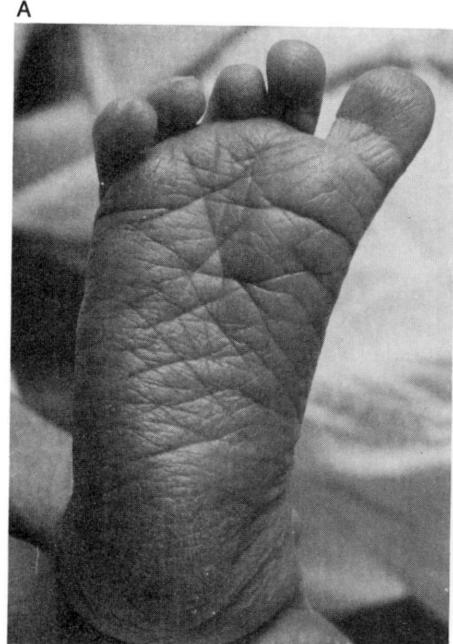

B

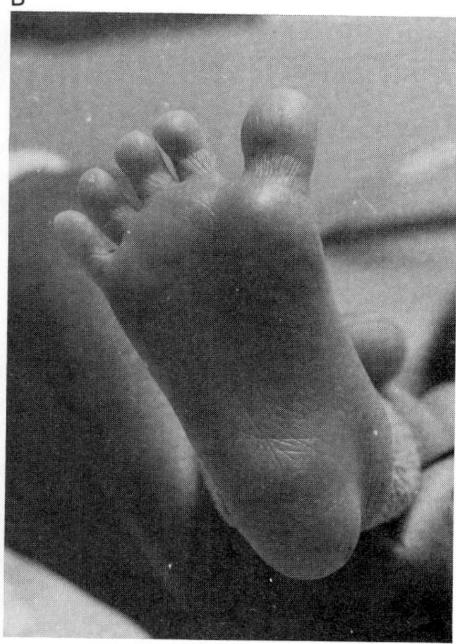

Figure 42-6.
A comparison of the sole creases on the foot of a term infant *(A)* with those of a preterm infant *(B)*. At 40 weeks' gestation, the entire foot, including the heel, is crisscrossed with creases. (Whitley N: A Manual of Clinical Obstetrics. Philadelphia, JB Lippincott. In preparation.)

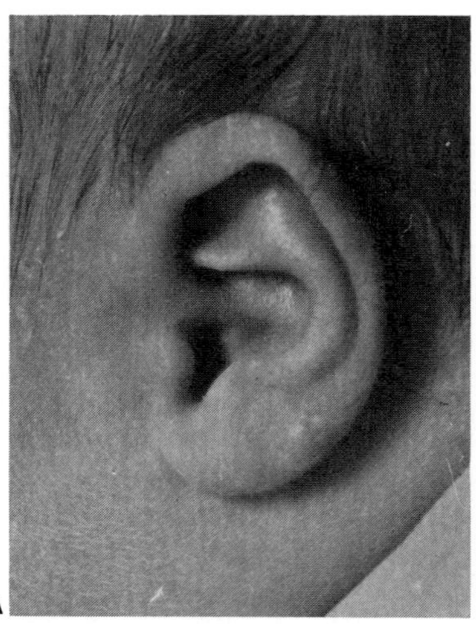

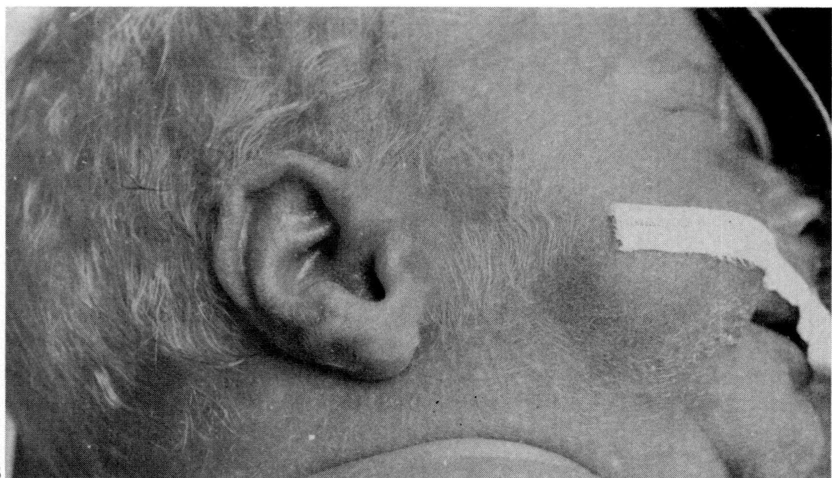

Figure 42-7.
Cartilage is well developed in the term infant *(A)* and the ear is erect, away from the head, while the ears of the preterm infant *(B)* lie flat against the head. Also note the matted hair and the presence of lanugo on the face of the preterm infant. (Whitley N: A Manual of Clinical Obstetrics. Philadelphia, JB Lippincott. In preparation.)

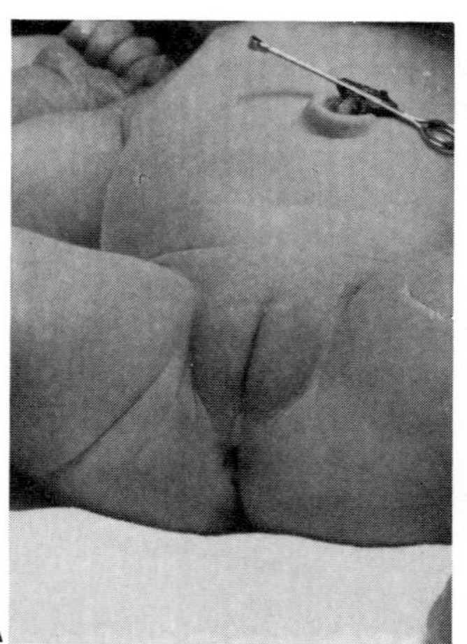

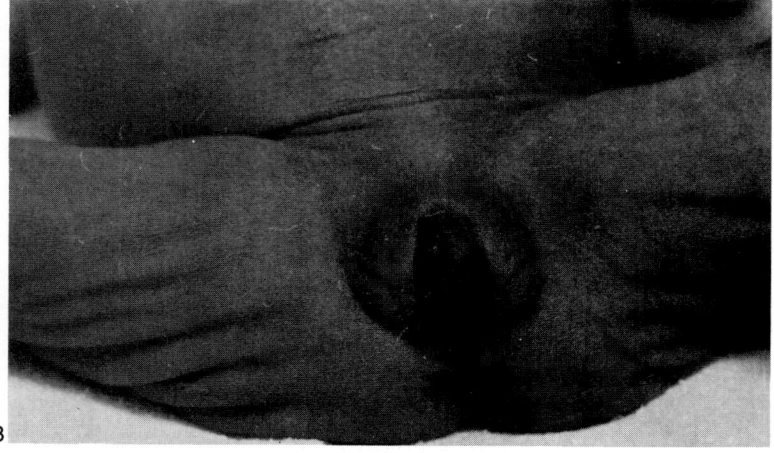

Figure 42-8.
The labia majora of the term infant *(A)* completely cover the labia minora and clitoris while they are small and widely separated in the preterm infant *(B)*. Also note the loose skin folds on the posterior thighs of the preterm infant. (Whitley N: A Manual of Clinical Obstetrics. Philadelphia, JB Lippincott. In preparation.)

Nails. At about 20 weeks the nails appear and gradually grow to cover the nailbed. At term, the nails extend beyond the fingertips slightly, but long nails well beyond the fingertips are characteristic of postmature infants.

Lanugo. This fine hair covers the infant's body at 20 weeks' gestation, and begins to disappear first from the face, then the trunk, and then the extremities (see Fig. 42-7). At term, hair, if present, tends to be located only over the shoulders.

Skull Firmness. The preterm infant has soft skull bones, particularly near the fontanels and sutures. The bones become firmer as gestation progresses, and at term the sutures are not easily displaced.

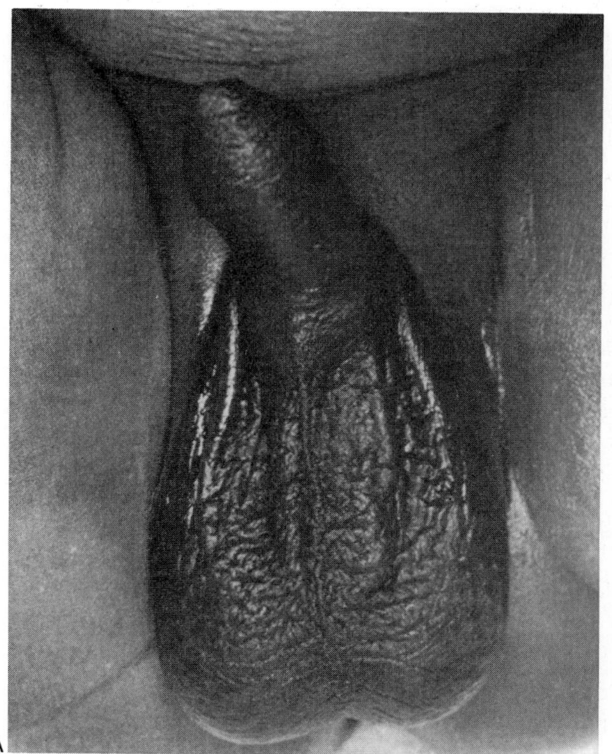

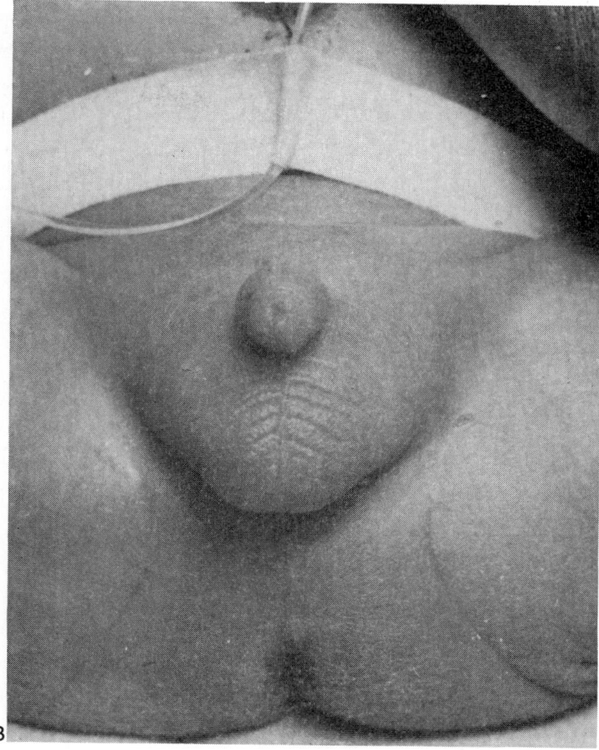

Figure 42-9.
The testes are well descended into the scrotal sac and the scrotum is covered with numerous rugae in the term infant *(A)* while the testes remain high in the inguinal canal and the rugae are largely undeveloped in the preterm infant *(B)*. (Whitley N: A Manual of Clinical Obstetrics. Philadelphia, JB Lippincott. In preparation.)

Neurologic Development

Gestational age may be assessed according to a number of neuromuscular responses of the newborn infant within the first few days of life. The infant's posture, the passive range of motion of certain parts, righting reactions, and various reflexes are evaluated.

The neurologic examination requires that the infant be in a quiet, rested state, although this may not be possible immediately after delivery. Most infants can be examined during the latter part of the first day of life, but others may not be ready until the second or third day. A shortened neurological examination including posture, tonicity, and recoil may be done during the first few hours after birth, with the more extensive examination delayed. Charts and scoring systems are also used for these parameters (Fig. 42-11). The development of muscle tone begins in the lower extremities and progresses in a cephalad direction.

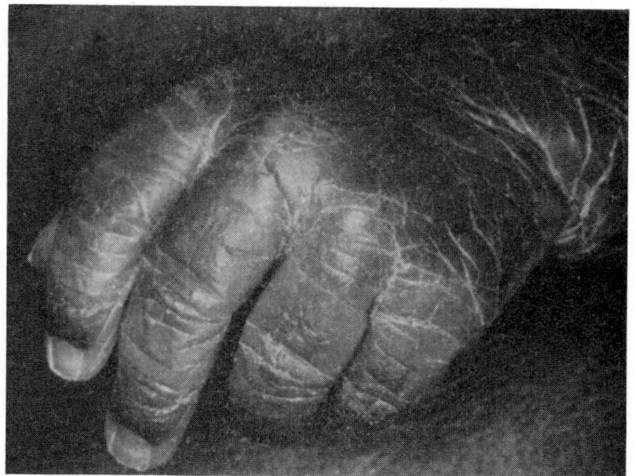

Figure 42-10.
Postterm infant's hand. Note dry, peeling, cracked skin. (Whitley N: A Manual of Clinical Obstetrics. Philadelphia, JB Lippincott. In preparation.)

Examination First Hours

PHYSICAL FINDINGS		20	21	22	23	24	25	26	27	28	29	30	31	32	33	34	35	36	37	38	39	40	41	42	43	44	45	46	47	48
Vernix		Appears				Covers body, thick layer														On back, scalp, in creases		Scant, in creases		No vernix						
Breast tissue and areola		Areola and nipple barely visible no palpable breast tissue														Areola raised		1–2 mm nodule		3–5 mm	5–6 mm	7–10 mm				?12 mm				
Ear	Form	Flat, shapeless														Beginning incurving superior		Incurving upper 2/3 pinnae			Well-defined incurving to lobe									
	Cartilage	Pinna soft, stays folded												Cartilage scant, returns slowly from folding				Thin cartilage, springs back from folding				Pinna firm, remains erect from head								
Sole creases		Smooth soles without creases												1–2 anterior creases			2–3 anterior creases	Creases anterior 2/3 sole		Creases involving heel				Deeper creases over entire sole						
Skin	Thickness & appearance	Thin, translucent skin, plethoric, venules over abdomen, edema												Smooth, thicker, no edema				Pink		Few vessels		Some desquamation pale pink		Thick, pale, desquamation over entire body						
	Nail plates	Appear												Nails to finger tips										Nails extend well beyond finger tips						
Hair		Appears on head			Eye brows and lashes					Fine, woolly, bunches out from head									Silky, single strands, lays flat					?Receding hairline or loss of baby hair, short, fine underneath						
Lanugo		Appears	Covers entire body												Vanishes from face					Present on shoulders				No lanugo						
Genitalia	Testes									Testes palpable in inguinal canal								In upper scrotum				In lower scrotum								
	Scrotum									Few rugae								Rugae, anterior portion				Rugae cover		Pendulous						
	Labia & clitoris											Prominent clitoris, labia majora small, widely separated						Labia majora larger, nearly cover clitoris				Labia minora and clitoris covered								
Skull firmness		Bones are soft								Soft to 1" from anterior fontanelle							Spongy at edges of fontanelle, center firm			Bones hard, sutures easily displaced				Bones hard, cannot be displaced						
Posture	Resting	Hypotonic, lateral decubitus						Hypotonic				Beginning flexion, thigh		Stronger hip flexion		Frog-like		Flexion, all limbs		Hypertonic				Very hypertonic						
	Recoil - leg	No recoil												Partial recoil						Prompt recoil										
	Arm	No recoil														Begin flexion, no recoil		Prompt recoil, may be inhibited				Prompt recoil after 30" inhibition								
		20	21	22	23	24	25	26	27	28	29	30	31	32	33	34	35	36	37	38	39	40	41	42	43	44	45	46	47	48

Figure 42-11.
Clinical estimation of gestational age. (Kempe HC, Silver HK, O'Brien D: Current Pediatric Diagnosis & Treatment, 5th ed. Palo Alto, CA, Lange Medical Publishers, 1978)

Resting Posture and Extremity Recoil. These two responses are sufficient to give a reasonable estimation of neurologic development in the first hour after birth. The remainder of the neurological examination is better carried out a day or two later to confirm the original findings. The resting posture of the premature infant is characterized by very little flexion of the upper extremities and only partial flexion of the lower. At about 30 weeks, there is slight flexion of the feet and knees. Flexion of the hips and thighs resulting in the characteristic frog position of the legs occurs at 34 weeks, but the arms are extended. At 36 to 38 weeks, the resting posture of the infant is one of complete flexion of all four extremities (Fig. 42-12).

Recoil of extremities lags behind flexion by about 2 weeks. At 36 to 37 weeks, the extremities remain extended but there is prompt recoil at 40 weeks.

To test recoil, flex the extremity and hold for 5 seconds, then extend for 30 seconds, and release. Brisk return to the flexed position indicates a full-term infant.

Heel to Ear. With the infant supine and hips flat, the foot is drawn as close to the ear as possible without forcing. In a premature infant, there is very little resistance and the foot may approximate the ear, with the leg well extended. There is marked resistance in the full-term infant, and it is impossible to draw the foot to the ear and extend the leg well (Fig. 42-13).

Popliteal Angle. Passive movement of the leg reveals an inverse relationship between muscle tone and popliteal angle, with a smaller angle with greater tone. Premature infants have larger popliteal angles than full-term infants.

Scarf Sign. In this test, the infant's arms are drawn across the neck as far across the opposite shoulder as

Confirmatory Neurologic Examination To Be Done After 24 Hours

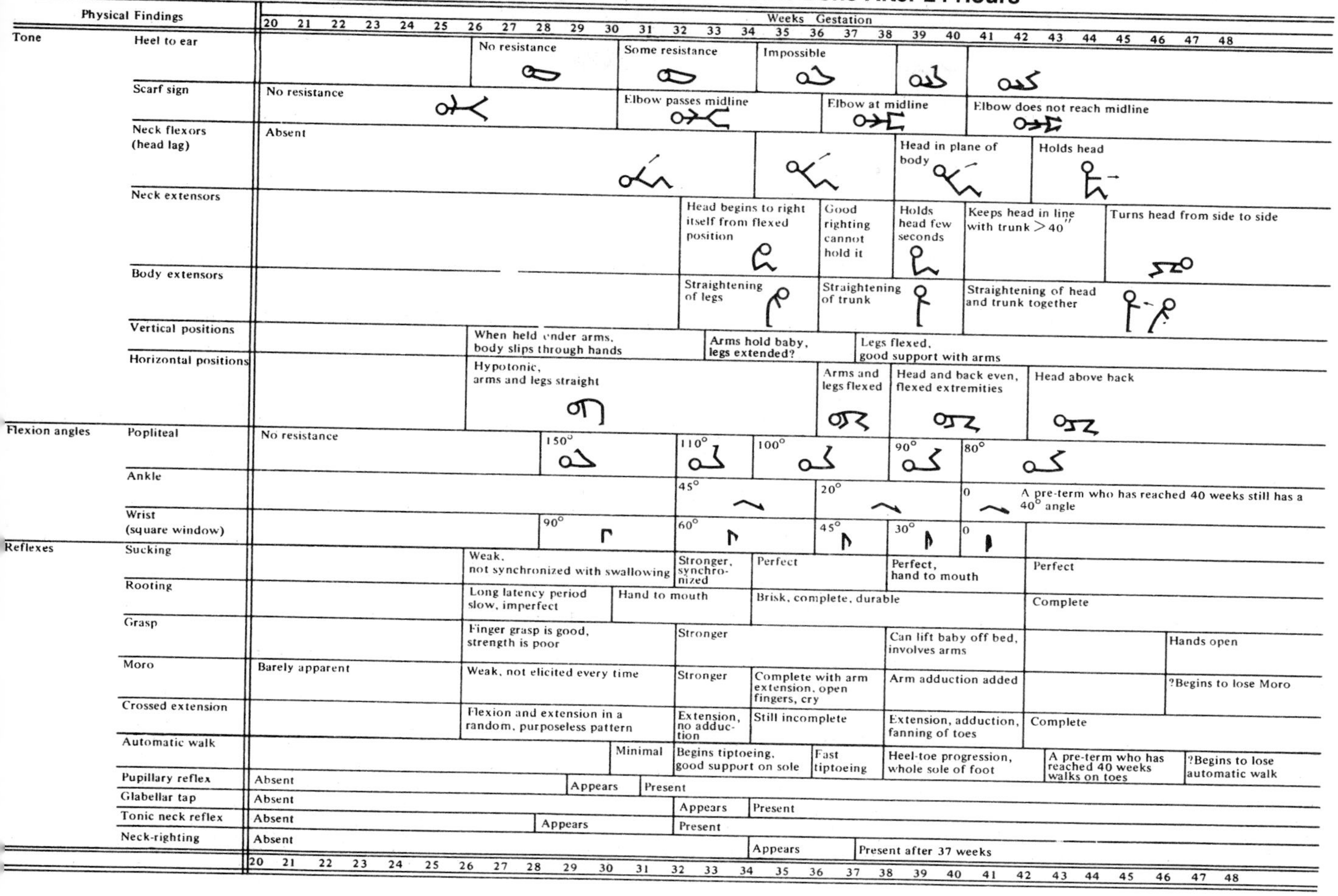

	Physical Findings	Weeks Gestation 20 21 22 23 24 25 26 27 28 29 30 31 32 33 34 35 36 37 38 39 40 41 42 43 44 45 46 47 48					
Tone	Heel to ear	No resistance	Some resistance	Impossible			
	Scarf sign	No resistance	Elbow passes midline	Elbow at midline	Elbow does not reach midline		
	Neck flexors (head lag)	Absent	Head in plane of body	Holds head			
	Neck extensors	Head begins to right itself from flexed position	Good righting cannot hold it	Holds head few seconds	Keeps head in line with trunk >40"	Turns head from side to side	
	Body extensors	Straightening of legs	Straightening of trunk	Straightening of head and trunk together			
	Vertical positions	When held under arms, body slips through hands	Arms hold baby, legs extended?	Legs flexed, good support with arms			
	Horizontal positions	Hypotonic, arms and legs straight	Arms and legs flexed	Head and back even, flexed extremities	Head above back		
Flexion angles	Popliteal	No resistance	150°	110°	100°	90°	80°
	Ankle	45°	20°	0	A pre-term who has reached 40 weeks still has a 40° angle		
	Wrist (square window)	90°	60°	45°	30°	0	
Reflexes	Sucking	Weak, not synchronized with swallowing	Stronger, synchronized	Perfect	Perfect, hand to mouth	Perfect	
	Rooting	Long latency period slow, imperfect	Hand to mouth	Brisk, complete, durable	Complete		
	Grasp	Finger grasp is good, strength is poor	Stronger	Can lift baby off bed, involves arms	Hands open		
	Moro	Barely apparent	Weak, not elicited every time	Stronger	Complete with arm extension, open fingers, cry	Arm adduction added	?Begins to lose Moro
	Crossed extension	Flexion and extension in a random, purposeless pattern	Extension, no adduction	Still incomplete	Extension, adduction, fanning of toes	Complete	
	Automatic walk	Minimal	Begins tiptoeing, good support on sole	Fast tiptoeing	Heel-toe progression, whole sole of foot	A pre-term who has reached 40 weeks walks on toes	?Begins to lose automatic walk
	Pupillary reflex	Absent	Appears	Present			
	Glabellar tap	Absent	Appears	Present			
	Tonic neck reflex	Absent	Appears	Present			
	Neck-righting	Absent	Appears	Present after 37 weeks			

possible (like a scarf). In the premature infant, there is less resistance and a greater draping (or scarf) effect. This maneuver is best carried out by lifting the elbow across the front of the body. Note how far across the chest the elbow will go. In the premature infant, the elbow reaches near or across the midline, whereas in the full-term infant it does not reach the midline (Fig. 42-14).

Ankle and Wrist Flexion. Pressure is applied to the foot to push it onto the anterior aspect of the leg, and the angle between the dorsum of the foot and the leg is measured. In premature infants this angle is 45° to 90°, whereas in the full-term infant the foot can be flexed until it touches the leg (Fig. 42-15). Similarly, the wrist is flexed with enough pressure to bring the hand as close to the forearm as possible. The angle between the hypothenar eminence of the wrist and the ventral aspect of the forearm is measured, with care taken not to rotate the wrist. In the premature infant this angle is 90°. In the full-term infant the wrist can be flexed onto the arm (Fig. 42-16).

Ventral Suspension. The infant is suspended in the prone position with the hand of the examiner supporting it under the chest (two hands may be used for a large infant). The degree of extension of the back and head, as well as the degree of flexion of the arms and legs, are noted. The premature infant hangs limply with arms and legs almost straight and back rounded. The full-term infant extends the head, straightens the back, and flexes the arms and legs (Fig. 42-17).

Head Lag. With the infant supine, grasp the hands or arms and pull him slowly to a sitting position. Observe the position of the head in relation to the trunk. The premature infant has no flexion of the neck. A gradual increase in flexion can be noted as gestation progresses. The full-term infant holds the head erect while being pulled to a sitting position (Fig. 42-18).

Reflexes. Although there are differences in reflexes according to the infant's age, these are often

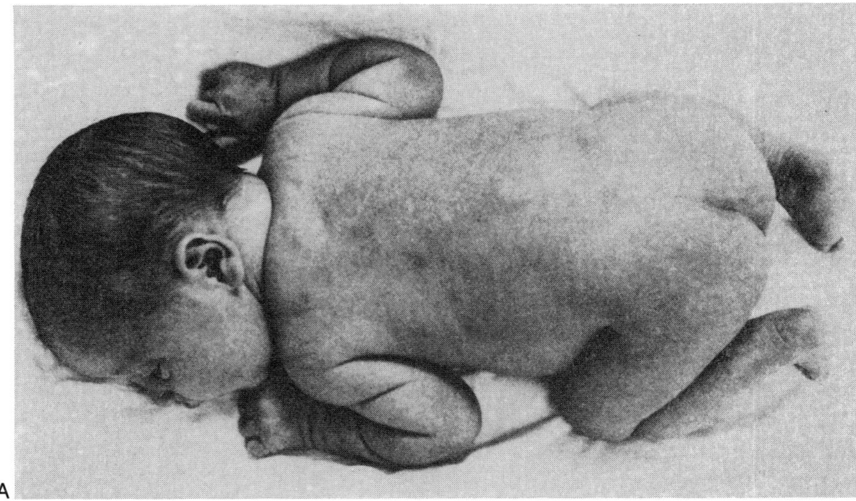

A

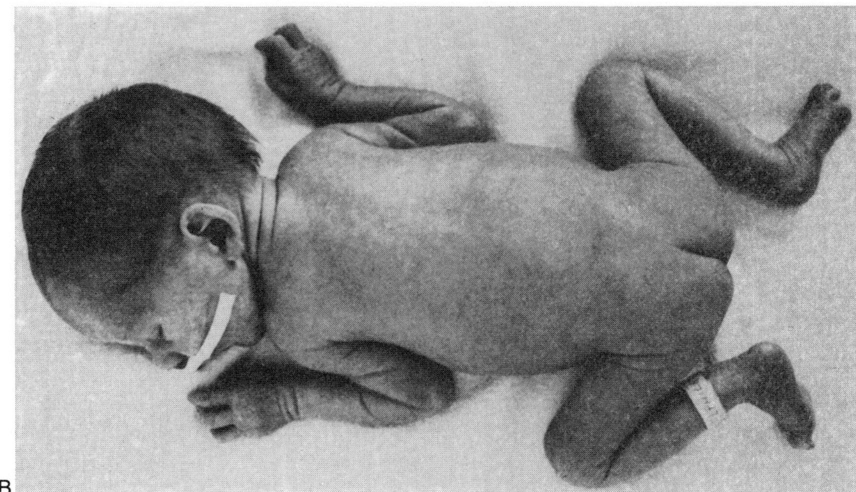

B

Figure 42-12.
Resting posture. Note the flexion of the extremities in the term infant *(A)* compared to the partial flexion in the preterm infant *(B)*, resulting in a froglike resting posture. (Whitley N: A Manual of Clinical Obstetrics. Philadelphia, JB Lippincott. In preparation.)

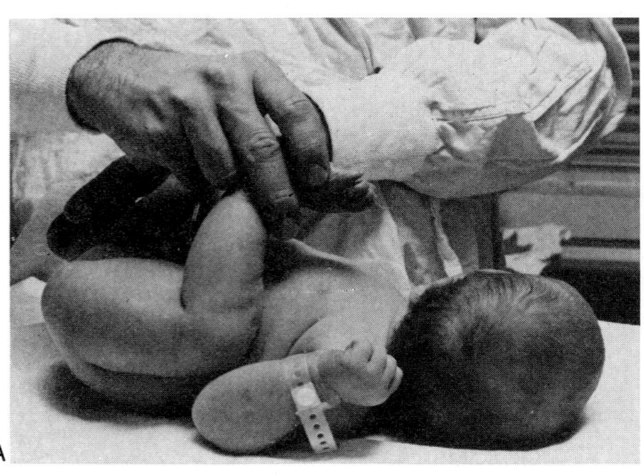

A

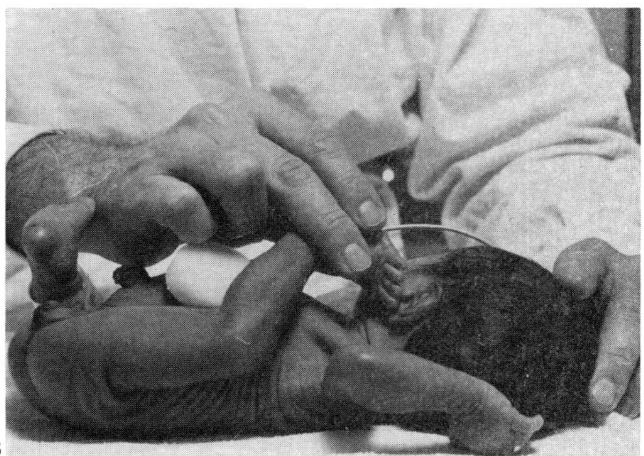

B

Figure 42-13.
Heel to ear. In the term infant *(A)* there is a marked resistance in the leg as the foot is gently drawn toward the ear, while in the preterm infant *(B)* very little resistance is noted. (Whitley N: A Manual of Clinical Obstetrics. Philadelphia, JB Lippincott. In preparation.)

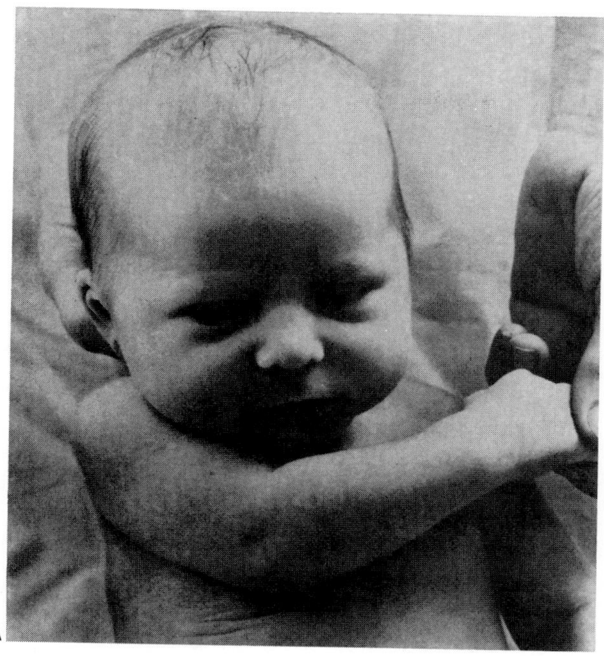

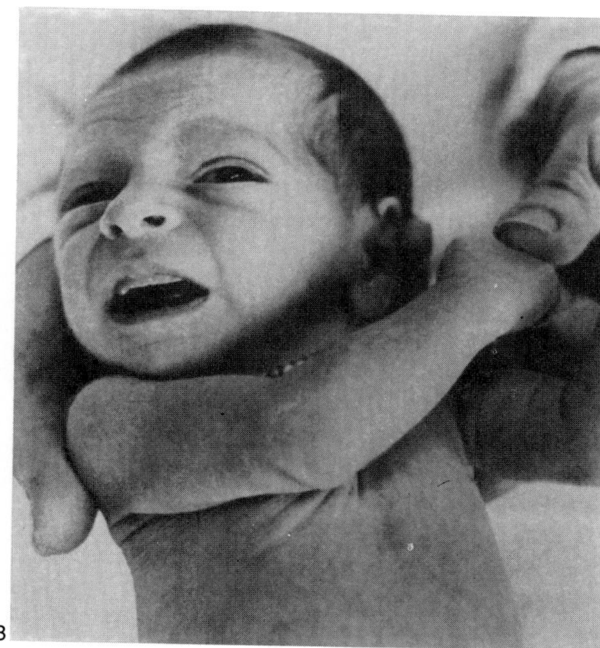

Figure 42-14.
Scarf sign. In the term infant *(A)* the elbow will not reach the midline, but in the preterm infant *(B)* the elbow will reach across the midline. (Whitley N: A Manual of Clinical Obstetrics. Philadelphia, JB Lippincott. In preparation.)

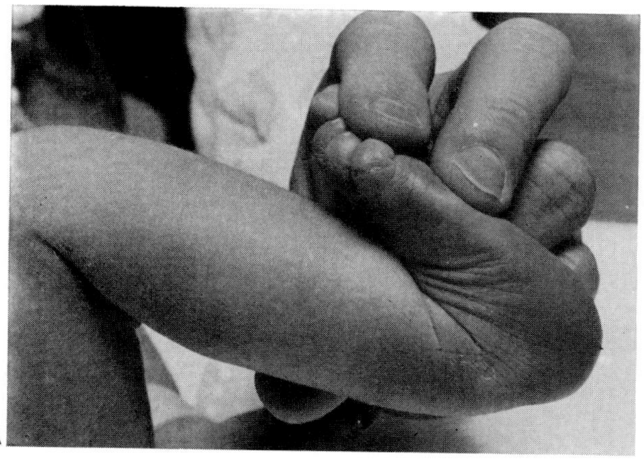

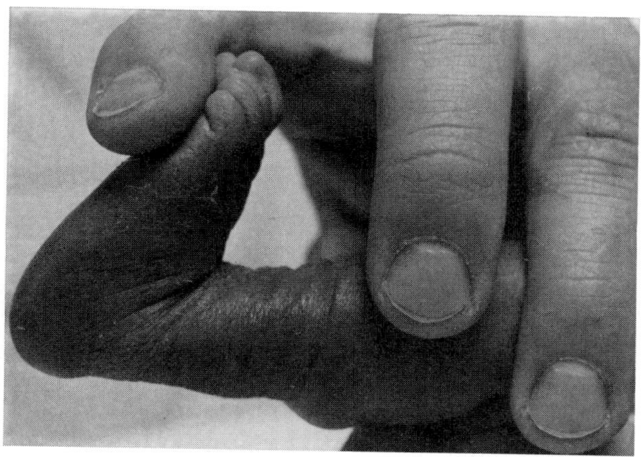

Figure 42-15.
Dorsiflexion of the ankle. In the term infant *(A)* the foot can be flexed until it touches the leg, but in the preterm infant *(B)* the foot can be flexed only to an angle of 45° to 90°. (Whitley N: A Manual of Clinical Obstetrics. Philadelphia, JB Lippincott. In preparation.)

not as pronounced as the other signs described above. The normal newborn's reflexes are discussed in Chapter 31, Assessment of the Newborn Infant. In the premature infant, the rooting reflex is less developed, as evidenced by the slower response in turning the head toward the stimulus. The sucking reflex is weak or absent, depending upon prematurity and condition. The grasp reflex is weak and the infant cannot be lifted off the bed while grasping the examiner's finger. The Moro reflex is also weak, and the walking reflex often absent. The sucking reflex, which is of particular importance because it is related to the ability to take adequate nourishment with nipple feedings, occurs at about 34 weeks.

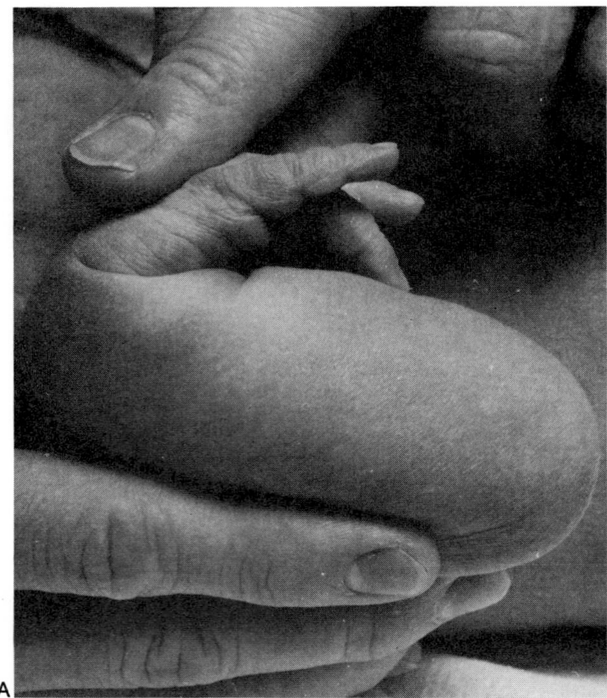

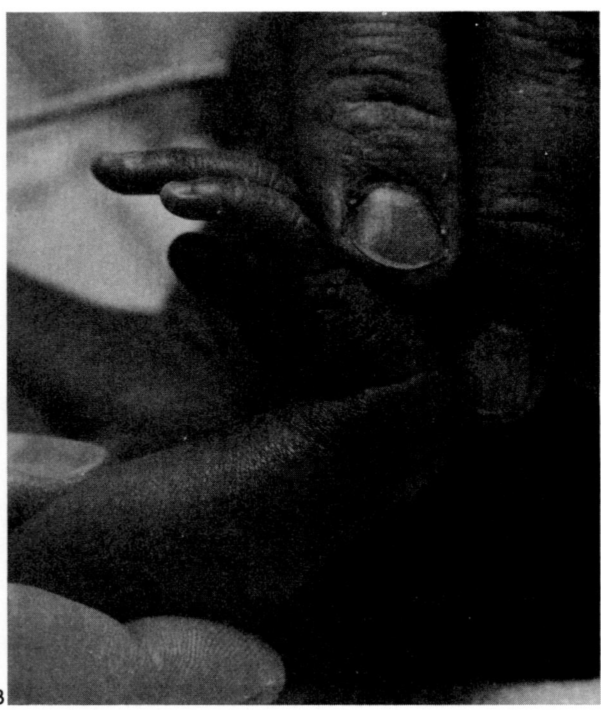

Figure 42-16.
Wrist flexion. In the term infant *(A)* the wrist can be flexed onto the arm, but the wrist can only be flexed to an angle of about 90° in the preterm infant *(B)*. (Whitley N: A Manual of Clinical Obstetrics. Philadelphia, JB Lippincott. In preparation.)

Nursing Assessment

The care of high-risk infants can be individualized by determining gestational age, as well as identifying particular neonatal complications or conditions. Many of the ante- and postnatal methods described for assessment of gestational age can be done by the nurse. The nonneurological portions should optimally be performed on all infants within a few hours of birth, so that the infant's needs can be anticipated early in the neonatal course. Nurses in the delivery room or nursery are the logical ones to carry out the assessment of physical characteristics and a brief initial neurological examination (posture and recoil tests) to establish gestational age.

Although the examinations appear long, a few of the criteria can be selected and used regularly, providing reliable assessment of the infant's age and related needs. For instance, observations of the breasts, ears, genitals, sole creases, posture, and recoil can be done rapidly and early. The correct age of the infant can usually be determined using these criteria. Recording these on a chart (see Fig. 42-11) speeds the process and simplifies the procedures. Once proficiency is developed in these selected criteria, it is easy to expand into more complete assessments. In this way, the nurse can anticipate problems and possibly prevent development of serious complications.[9]

Characteristics and Physiology of Small-for-Gestational-Age Infants

Appearance at Birth

Small-for-date infants appear thin and wasted, with skin that is loose, often dry, and, frequently, scaling. Meconium staining, involving the nails, skin, and umbilical cord, is common. Such infants have very little subcutaneous tissue, and the trunk and extremities do not appear to have as much musculature as would be expected. Their faces appear wizened and are not full and round, with sparse hair on the head. Although their weight is low, length is often

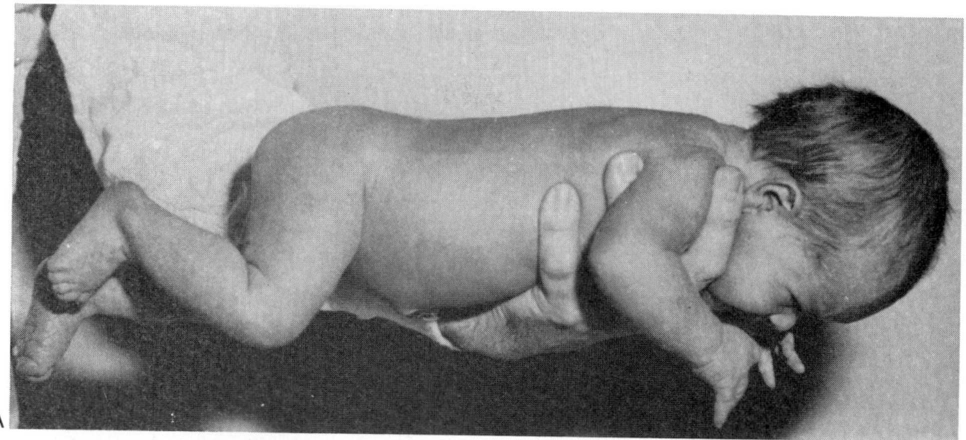

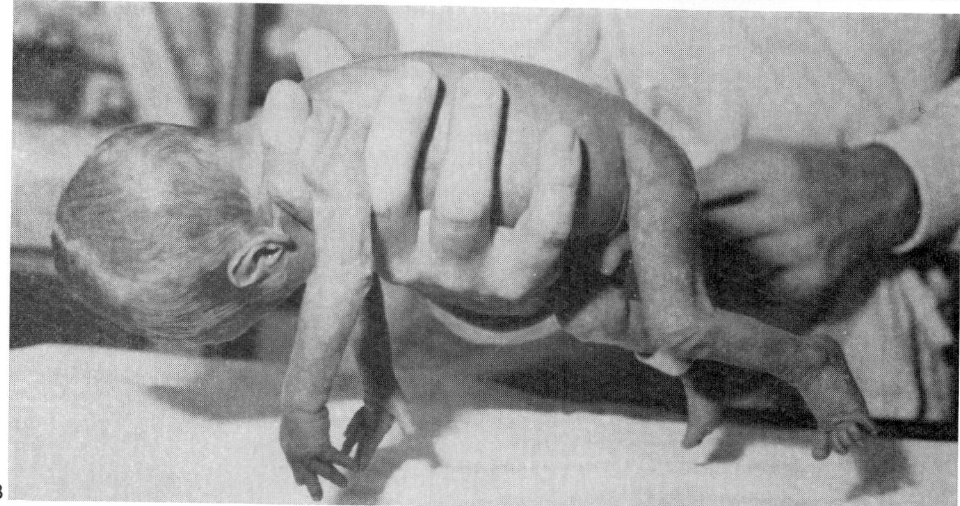

Figure 42-17.
Ventral suspension. When suspended in the prone position the term infant *(A)* will extend the head, straighten the back, and flex the arms and legs; however, the preterm infant *(B)* will hang limply with the arms and legs almost straight. (Whitley N: A Manual of Clinical Obstetrics. Philadelphia, JB Lippincott. In preparation.)

normal, as is head size. Shortly after birth, these infants are usually alert, active, and hungry. The umbilical cord may be thin and tends to dry more rapidly than that of normal infants. Some small-for-date infants appear proportionately small without wasting, meconium staining, or the other characteristics described. These babies appear old for their size and seem to have been undergrown for a long time; it is in this group that anomalies tend to occur.[6]

Physiological Problems

In adaptation to extrauterine life, the problems encountered by the SGA infant are different from those of the appropriate-for-gestational-age, preterm infant. If the problem of poor growth *in utero* has been detected during pregnancy, nurses and physicians skilled in resuscitation should be present at delivery.

Certain disorders tend to occur more frequently in the SGA infant and therefore should be anticipated by the care-giver.

Asphyxia

Perinatal asphyxia is the most serious complication faced by SGA infants, and generally occurs in those infants whose growth retardation is due to maternal or placental factors. Chronic hypoxia commonly has occurred *in utero* prior to labor, resulting from inadequate oxygen transfer from placenta to fetus.[7] Intra-

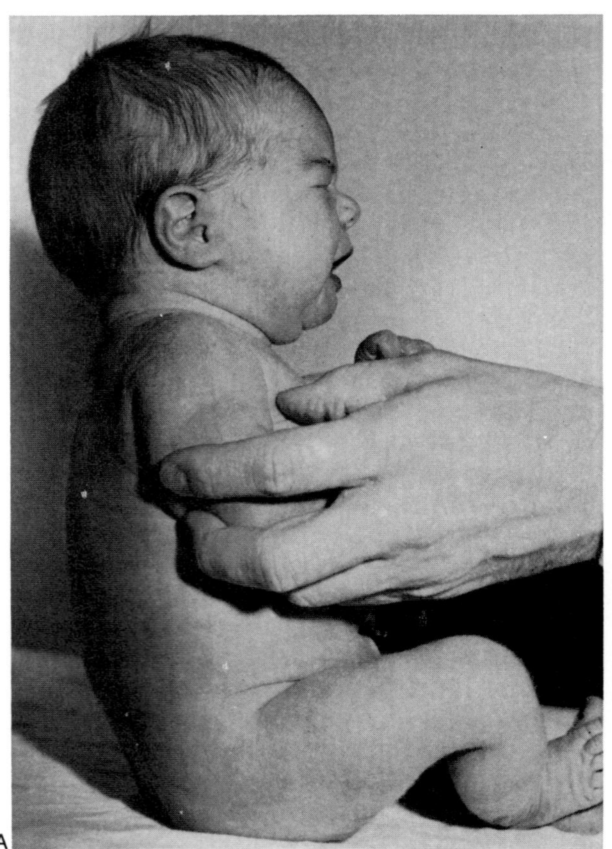

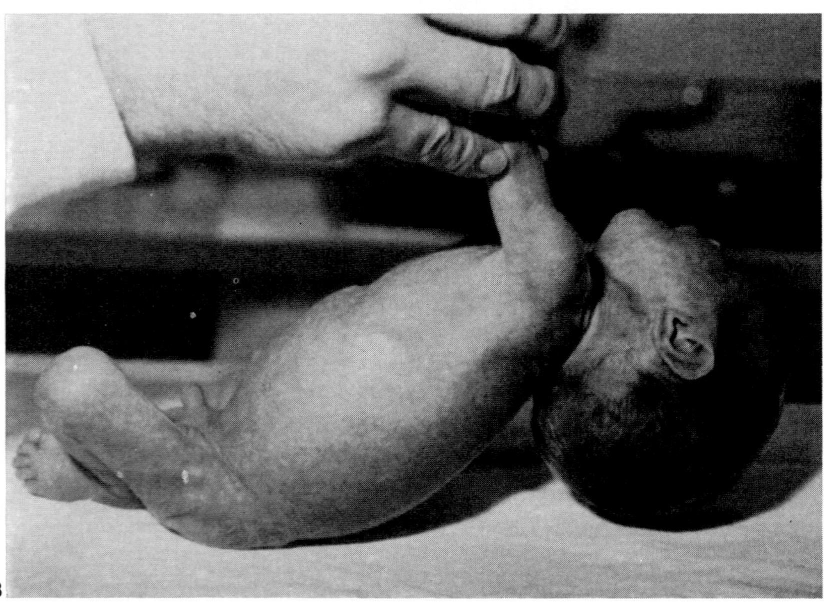

Figure 42-18.
Head lag. As the infant is slowly pulled from a supine to a sitting position, the term infant *(A)* will hold the head erect, but the preterm infant *(B)* will have no flexion in the neck. (Whitley N: A Manual of Clinical Obstetrics. Philadelphia, JB Lippincott. In preparation.)

Indicators of Intrauterine Hypoxia

- Meconium-stained amniotic fluid in a cephalic presentation
- Abnormal FHR patterns by monitoring
- Fetal acidosis as determined by scalp blood sampling

uterine hypoxia can often be diagnosed during labor. Three major indicators require preparation for resuscitation.

Immediate resuscitation is essential for an optimal outcome for the neonate. Perinatal asphyxia is a common denominator for most of the complications occurring in infants with growth retardation, and the occurrence, severity, and outcome of complications depend upon the severity of the asphyxia.

Meconium Aspiration Syndrome

Aspiration of meconium into the alveoli, occurring *in utero* or after birth, results from fetal hypoxia. The fetal response to hypoxia includes reflex relaxation of the anal sphincter and accelerated intestinal peristalsis, in addition to reflex gasping, which draws the meconium into the tracheobronchial system.[8]

Meconium in the respiratory tract acts like a foreign body and blocks the flow of air into the alveoli. Increasing inflation of the alveoli distal to the obstruction can lead to their rupture and the leakage of air into the interstitial tissue (Fig. 42-19). This initiates a series of complications such as pulmonary interstitial emphysema, pneumomediastinum, and pneumothorax. The asphyxia that results from these meconium effects on the lungs leads to the involvement of the central nervous system, kidney, erythropoietic system, and metabolism, which are associated with the meconium aspiration syndrome. The syndrome may be prevented or minimized through appropriate obstetric management of mothers in whom there is evidence of meconium-stained amniotic fluid and prompt removal of meconium from the infant's upper respiratory tract immediately after birth.

Hypoglycemia

Neonatal hypoglycemia is a frequent occurrence in SGA infants. Hypoglycemia is defined as a blood glucose level of 20 mg to 25 mg/dl in the low-birth-weight infant and 30 mg to 35 mg/dl in the term infant during the first 3 days of life. After 72 hours of life, glucose should be at 45 mg/dl. In actual practice, treatment is usually begun for any glucose level below 40 mg/dl.[6]

Although hypoglycemia usually occurs during the first 12 hours of life, it may appear as late as 48 hours. Blood sugars may be monitored by Dextrostix and verified by routine laboratory tests if abnormalities are suspected. Blood sugars must be carefully monitored and early feeding instituted as necessary. Intravenous glucose supplement may be necessary if the infant does not tolerate oral feedings.[6]

Infants are at increased risk of hypoglycemia if their growth retardation is due to maternal undernutrition or placental insufficiency. When the placental-fetal transfer of substrates is markedly reduced, the reserve for substrates (in this case, glycogen) is also reduced. At birth, increased amounts of glucose are used to supply the energy required for various physiologic adaptations. Increased glucose utilization, lack of substrate reserve, inefficient gluconeogenic mechanism, and insufficient intake of glucose then result in

Figure 42-19.
Severe meconium aspiration syndrome, showing shaggy heart border and irregular densities throughout both lungs, and having a wooly quality in this patient. (Avery GB: Neonatology: Pathophysiology and Management of the Newborn. Philadelphia, JB Lippincott, 1981)

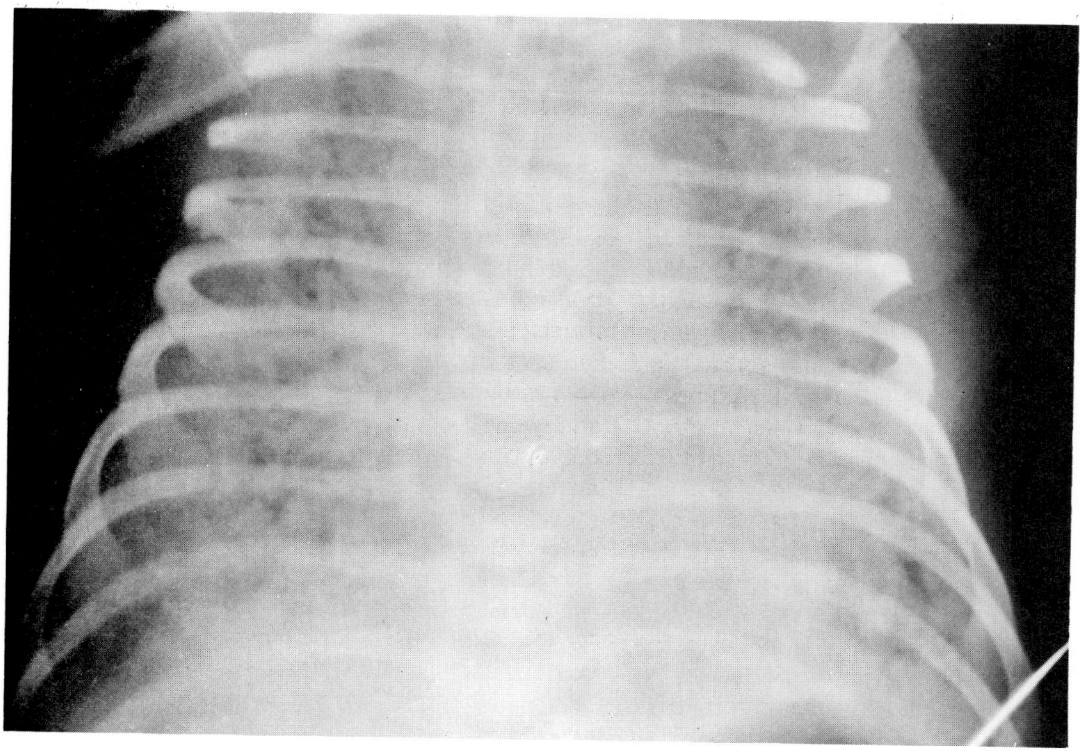

a fall in blood glucose with consequent hypoglycemia.

Symptoms such as tremors, cyanosis, convulsions, apnea, abnormal cry, cardiac arrest, hypotonia, hypothermia, and tachypnea are often nonspecific.[6] Continuous low blood sugar may result in increased risk of cerebral damage.

Hypocalcemia

The most common form of hypocalcemia is called *first-day hypocalcemia* and is often found in low-birth-weight infants (both premature and growth-retarded infants weighing less than 2000 g). The etiologic factor is probably not the low birth weight or status of nutrition, but the presence of asphyxia and related respiratory distress. This neonatal metabolic disorder is often found accompanying the meconium aspiration syndrome. Symptoms are nonspecific and similar to those found in hypoglycemia. There is no correlation between the symptoms and severity of hypocalcemia. Diagnosis is therefore based on clinical determinations of the serum calcium level. Serum calcium level should not be less than 7 mg/dl. Treatment consists of intravenous or oral supplements.

Polycythemia and Hyperviscosity

Infants with intrauterine growth retardation have been found to have increased red blood cell volume, elevated erythropoietin levels, a venous hematocrit greater than 65%, or hemoglobin in excess of 22 g/dl. Capillary measures may be higher than central measures. The cause is thought to be related to intrauterine hypoxia, because placental insufficiency leading to chronic fetal hypoxia may stimulate an increase in erythropoiesis. Hypoxia *in utero* can also cause redistribution of blood volume within the placental-fetal circuit with a transfer of blood from the placenta to the fetus. In view of the high probability of increased blood volume in infants with growth retardation, the cord should be clamped, or stripped, immediately after birth rather than later. This avoids the transfer of large amounts of placental blood to the infant.

Symptoms of polycythemia are related to

1. Increased destruction of red blood cells causing hyperbilirubinemia
2. Increased circulating blood volume causing congestive heart failure or pulmonary edema
3. The phenomenon of hyperviscosity

Hyperviscosity frequently accompanies a venous hematocrit in excess of 65%. Its clinical manifestations result from sludging of blood in the microcirculation of various organs. The most commonly observed signs involve the central nervous system and cardiopulmonary system. Cardiorespiratory signs include tachypnea, intercostal retraction, grunting, nasal flaring, tachycardia, and pleural effusion. Convulsions and other central nervous system manifestations may be present, as may scrotal edema and priapism. Treatment includes a partial exchange transfusion, replacing 10% to 15% of the infant's blood volume with plasma or other colloid solution.[10]

Congenital Anomalies

The incidence of congenital anomalies is 10 to 20 times higher in infants with intrauterine growth retardation, especially in instances involving the genitourinary and cardiovascular systems. A thorough physical assessment is necessary to rule out any anomalies.

Thermal Regulation

Lacking subcutaneous tissue and fat, SGA infants have difficulty maintaining body temperature. In addition to body composition, basal metabolic rates differ from normal newborns. The temperature setting in the isolette should be determined by closely monitoring the infant's temperature, with the goal of maintaining abdominal skin temperature between 36°C and 36.5°C. The effects of asphyxia are aggravated by the stress caused by cold.[6]

Postterm Infants

Characteristics

The postterm infant of over 42 weeks' gestation has the characteristic appearance of an infant of 1 to 3 weeks of age. Lanugo is absent and there is very little vernix. Scalp hair is abundant, fingernails are longer, and skin is whiter than in a term newborn. Often the skin is dry, cracked, and thin (see Fig. 42-10). There is little subcutaneous fat, which gives the infant a long, thin look. Vernix may be stained yellow or green. Postterm infants appear alert and wide-eyed.[11]

Clinical Problems

Common disorders of the postmature or postterm infant include hypoglycemia, polycythemia, and cold stress due to lack of subcutaneous fat. As with the SGA infant, congenital anomalies are more prevalent. Postmature infants may be hypoxic *in utero,* which may lead to meconium aspiration due to fetal distress or neonatal seizure activity.[8]

Large-for-Gestational-Age Infants

The best example of an LGA infant is the infant of a diabetic mother. For an extended discussion of this type of infant, see Chapter 44.

Characteristics and Physiology of the Premature Infant

Physical Characteristics

Since there are many degrees of prematurity, there are also various stages of anatomic and physiologic development. Many of the symptoms described below may vary in infants of approximately the same fetal age, depending on the factors associated with prematurity and the physical conditions of the mother and the infant.

At birth, the premature baby lacks the subcutaneous fat that is deposited during the last 2 months of intrauterine development. As a result, the skin appears transparent, with the blood vessels clearly visible. The skin is pink, smooth, and shiny. These premature babies are prone to develop icteric skin changes. Lanugo is usually abundant over the skin surface, but is sparse, fine, and fuzzy on the head.

The external ears and nose are very soft and pliable with underdeveloped cartilage. The ears lie very close to the head. The skull is round and relatively large, in contrast to the long anteroposterior skull diameter of the full-term infant. The bones of the skull and the ribs feel soft.[11]

The infant may be small or may approximate full-term weight; yet the internal organs may be imperfectly developed. These babies appear to be reluctant to assume the responsibility to live. The respiration is shallow and irregular owing to the lack of lung expansion and proper gaseous exchange. There are often periods of apnea.

Due to the irregular respiration and the poorly developed function of swallowing, there is danger of aspiration of milk or vomitus, causing cyanosis and predisposing the infant to pulmonary infections. The premature baby regurgitates food readily because the stomach is tubular and the sphincters are poorly developed.

The ability to excrete solute in urine is limited. The genitals are immature. The male testes are frequently undescended and scrotal rugae absent. In females, the labia minora and clitoris are prominent due to the underdeveloped labia majora.

The walls of the blood vessels are weak, and the tendency to hemorrhage is great. Because the central nervous system is not fully developed, the premature infant is sluggish and must be wakened to be fed. The muscular movements are feeble.

The extremities maintain an extended posture and tend to remain where they are placed (see Fig. 42-12). Reflexes are immature (*e.g.,* sucking is absent, weak, or inefficient).

The heat-regulating center is underdeveloped, resulting in a subnormal or fluctuating temperature. The cry is monotonous, whining, "kittenlike," and effortless, showing a lack of energy. All these characteristics are evidenced in varying degrees, according to the degree of immaturity.

Physiological Considerations

As discussed in Chapter 32, the newly born infant must make certain adaptations to extrauterine life. For the premature infant, adaptations will be even greater and more difficult owing to a variety of anatomic and physiologic deficiencies.

Respiratory System

The development of the lungs depends upon the degree of maturity of the newborn. For instance, the lungs of an infant weighing 2 lb (900 g) or less show small alveoli lined with cuboidal epithelium surrounded by a meager supply of capillaries (which prevent efficient gaseous exchange). The lungs of an infant weighing 6 lb (2730 g), on the other hand, show large alveoli, the walls of which are virtually formed by bare capillaries. There is a great increase in the capillary network between the 26th week and the 36th week of intrauterine life. For this reason, the ability of the lungs to sustain extrauterine life increases with each week of intrauterine existence. The more immature the infant, the less blood flow there is through the lungs, the remainder being shunted through the ductus arteriosus.

As noted with the mature newborn, the most critical event in the adjustment to extrauterine life is the establishment of ventilation by the previously unused lungs. The unexpanded lungs of any fetus are not just crumpled air sacs waiting to be filled. Rather, they are fluid-filled organs requiring a great deal of negative intrapleural pressure (up to 60 cm water has been used experimentally) for expansion. This great effort is necessary because of the viscosity of the fluid in the lungs, surface tension effects, and tissue resistance.

The premature baby is often not capable of this enormous task because of the previously mentioned inadequacy in the capillary anatomy that impedes appropriate gaseous exchange and because the respiratory centers of the brain that regulate depth and rate of respiration are not fully developed. In addition, these infants are hampered by weak respiratory muscles, a yielding thoracic cage, a decreased amount of pulmonary lipoprotein (surfactant), which reduces surface tension in the lungs, and a deficient amount of fibrinolysis. Hence, primary and secondary atelectasis are common to premature infants. The nasal passages are extremely narrow and the mucous membrane is easily injured. The cough reflex is poorly developed or absent, making the danger of inhalation of regurgitated fluids very real.[11]

In general, then, an unstable respiratory system is a result of these defects. Respiration tends to be irregular in rhythm and depth and there are periods of apnea during which cyanosis may develop. The infant uses the diaphragm more than the chest in breathing, and, if there is much atelectasis, the thoracic cage is dragged down with each inspiration. In severe cases, the sternum is sucked back toward the spine with inspiration, and expiration is accompanied by a short feeble grunt (Fig. 42-20). It is important to remember that with these infants, respirations must be counted for at least a minute if any accurate respiratory rate is to be determined.

Cardiovascular System

The *heart* is relatively large at birth and its action is often slow and feeble. Extrasystoles occur, and murmurs that may later disappear as the fetal openings gradually close, may be present at birth or soon after. As previously stated, there is a decrease in the density of capillaries available in vital organs to take up sufficient oxygen in babies under about 1000 g. The extreme capillary fragility, especially of the intracranial vessels, together with the low plasma prothrombin level, leads to a bleeding tendency in these infants. This tendency is evidenced by the frequency of ecchymosis of the skin, as well as by intraventricular hemorrhage and other internal bleeding.

The *systolic blood pressure* at birth is lower than that of the mature infant and decreases with the birth weight. Infants weighing between 2 lb and 4 lb (1000 g–2000 g) generally have a systolic pressure of 50 mm Hg as compared with 60 mm Hg to 70 mm Hg for term infants. The level rises with the age of the child, by about 20 mm by the end of the second week, and by an additional 5 mm by the age of 2 months.

The pulse rate ranges between 120 and 160, with the average around 140. Because of the tendency toward arrhythmia, the pulse rate is most accurately obtained with a stethoscope, counting the apical beat for a minute.

As with the mature baby, the premature infant has a relatively high hemoglobin concentration at birth,

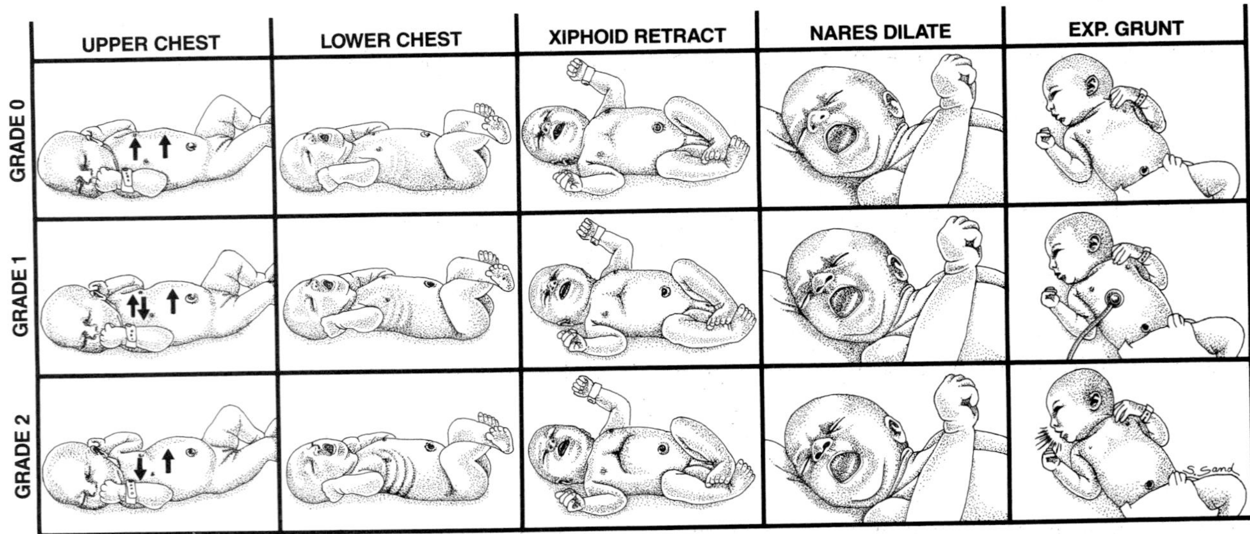

Figure 42-20.
Observation of retractions. An index of respiratory distress is determined by grading each of five arbitrary criteria. Grade 0 indicates no difficulty; grade 1 indicates moderate difficulty; and grade 2 indicates maximum respiratory difficulty. The retraction score is the sum of these values; a total score of 0 indicates no dyspnea, whereas a total score of ten denotes maximal respiratory distress.

which decreases to around 7 g/dl of blood at 4 to 8 weeks of age. This is due to the premature infant's inadequacy in manufacturing hemoglobin, together with the infant's relatively rapid rate of growth. After this time, the rate gradually increases until about 4 months, when there is a second fall, characterized by hypochromia of the red cells. If a severe enough anemia develops in the first phase of hemoglobin decline, it may be treated with iron therapy. Some investigators have found that *parenteral* (but not *oral*) administration of iron is useful in prevention of the first phase of anemia. However, the later phase responds well to oral iron therapy and it has become customary to institute the oral form of therapy from the third week onward.

White Blood Cells. The white blood cell count at birth is lower than that usually found in the term infant. There is a predominance of polymorphonuclear cells, as in the mature infant, and the same decrease in the total white cell count occurs during the first week of life. However, the change to lymphocytic predominance may occur slightly later for the mature infant.

Neurologic System

The stage of development of the nervous system at birth depends upon the degree of maturity. As with the normal newborn, all the premature infant's neurons are present, but they are not as fully developed and remain underdeveloped for months and sometimes years. The least mature infant tends to lie quietly unless disturbed, waking only at intervals for feeding. External stimulation results in weak, purposeless, jerky movements and perhaps a feeble cry. As the infant matures, movements tend to occur in bursts of activity, which can be quite vigorous, resulting in the infant wiggling from one end of the incubator to the other. At first, the less mature infant lies on his side in the fetal position; later he uncurls and after several days he lies on his back with his head rolled to one side, his hips flexed and abducted, and his knees and ankles flexed (frog position). The less mature the infant, the worse his muscle tone.

The vital centers controlling respiration and temperature are poorly developed, as are the centers controlling such important reflexes as coughing, swallowing, and sucking. The Moro and tonic neck reflexes are present in normal infants of both low birth weight and early gestational age, as are the Chvostek and Babinski signs. Tendon reflexes are variable in all immature infants.

Temperature Regulation. The premature infant's temperature-regulating mechanism is poorly developed at birth. Peripheral circulation is also poor, thus peripheral responses to heat and cold (*i.e.,* sweating and shivering) are inadequate. Furthermore, the premature infant does not flex his extremities like the term infant. The premature lacks this important conservation measure. Heat production is low and heat loss high because of the greater body surface relative to weight and the lack of subcutaneous fat.

Gastrointestinal System

Large premature infants may have fairly good sucking and swallowing ability. Less mature infants, however, generally have feeble reflexes which, in the very immature, may be lacking altogether. Because of the poorly developed mechanism for closing of the cardiac sphincter and the relatively strong pyloric sphincter, regurgitation is common.[6]

The powers of digestion depend on the degree of prematurity, being rudimentary in infants of 26 to 28 weeks' gestation, but becoming more efficient as the infant matures. The stomach of a 2-lb (900-g) infant at birth shows little folding of the mucosal surface (which reduces the surface area for absorption) and poor development of the secretory glands and muscle layers. A term baby shows a deeply folded mucosal layer and relatively well-developed glands and muscle tissue.

The premature infant appears to digest and absorb carbohydrates easily, proteins less well, and fats badly, even though fat-splitting enzymes are present at birth. This inability to manage fat causes the often seen greasy and foul-smelling steatorrheic stools. When the premature newborn uses glycogen stores, he depends, as usual, on body fat for energy; when food becomes available, more calories are used from the carbohydrates and less from the fats than in the term baby. The premature infant resembles the fetus more in this respect because the fetus also depends on carbohydrates as its main source of energy.

The musculature of the bowel is weak and easily distended, so that there may be a tendency to constipation. Because of the thin abdominal wall, gastric peristalsis is seen. If distention is present, intestinal peristalsis also becomes visible.

Urinary System

In comparison with the normal newborn, the premature infant's renal function is impaired because the kidney tubules continue to be formed until term; therefore kidneys in the premature infant are poorly developed. Thus, urine cannot be concentrated well (which becomes important when conditions involving an excessive loss such as diarrhea or vomiting occur) and sodium and chloride cannot be excreted well, resulting in early water retention and edema. It is believed by many that the tendency toward a more marked and prolonged acidosis in the newly born premature infant, and the inability to excrete many drugs, is probably due to the relatively poor development of the kidneys.

Low *p*H levels (normal is 7.42) are regularly found in apparently healthy immature infants and are not considered dangerous unless accompanied by conditions such as respiratory distress, vomiting, or diarrhea.

Urination may be scanty and infrequent for a few days after birth, until fluid intake is increased. Urates are commonly present in some excess, giving a false-positive for albumin by heat, acetic acid, or trichloracetic acid tests.

Hepatic System

The liver is relatively large in smaller infants, but its function is poorly developed. This immaturity of the liver predisposes the infant to jaundice because of the inability of the liver to conjugate and excrete bilirubin. It has also been suggested that the low blood sugar found in the premature infant is hepatogenic, due to small liver glycogen stores. Lower serum protein levels, deficiency of blood-clotting factors, and the deficient conjugation and detoxification of certain drugs are all attributed to liver immaturity.

Jaundice. Premature infants are more susceptible to tissue damage from high bilirubin levels than term infants. The immature liver is unable to process free bilirubin from the breakdown of red blood cells (RBCs). The nuclei of the cerebral cortex and thalamus, the last structures to be myelinated, are more susceptible to invasion by unconjugated bilirubin. The resultant neurologic damage (kernicterus) can bring about disorders such as mental retardation. Sick premature infants may not tolerate higher levels of bilirubin than 18 mg/dl. A safe level of bilirubin may be as low as 10 mg/dl.[12]

For further discussion of pathologic forms of jaundice, such as Rh incompatibility and ABO incompatibility, see Chapter 44.

Illnesses of the Premature Infant

The premature infant is particularly susceptible to certain pathophysiological conditions as a consequence of organ system immaturity, asphyxia during the perinatal period, and respiratory insult associated with the need for resuscitation and ventilation. The most common conditions seen in the premature infant include respiratory distress syndrome (hyaline membrane disease), bronchopulmonary dysplasia, pulmonary dysmaturity, and retrolental fibroplasia.

Respiratory Distress Syndrome

Also known as hyaline membrane disease (HMD), respiratory distress syndrome (RDS) is primarily a developmental disease of premature infants and rarely occurs in infants born at term. It is a leading cause of death (50%–70%) among premature infants, with incidence and severity increasing among infants of lower birth weight. Incidence depends on the stage of lung maturation rather than gestational age.

The greatest incidence of RDS occurs in preterm infants weighing between 1000 g and 1500 g, and it is observed in about 25% to 35% of all premature infants. It also occurs in infants of diabetic mothers and infants whose mothers experienced antepartal vaginal bleeding. The condition has also been noted in infants born by cesarean section. However, cesarean section in otherwise uncomplicated full-term deliveries is probably not associated with any increased incidence of the disease.

Pathophysiology

In RDS, the alveoli and the alveolar ducts are filled with a sticky exudate, a hyaline material, that prevents aeration. Although it is known that the hyaline material is a protein, the cause of hyaline membrane formation is not definitely known.

Three main theories have been postulated. The first proposes an alteration in the fibrinolytic enzyme system in the lung or blood that leads to the proliferation of the protein (fibrin) exudate. The second suggests alterations in or lack of the pulmonary surfactant that reduces alveolar ventilation and promotes atelectasis. The third indicates pulmonary hypofusion rather than surfactant deficiency. This hypofusion begins with intrauterine asphyxia and results in reduced alveolar ventilation and atelectasis. Whatever the exact causes and mechanisms, surfactant activity is indeed deficient, and, as a result, there is incomplete expansion of the lung and failure to establish normal, functional residual capacity (lack of alveolar stability). Thus, the lungs are atelectatic, and this is a hallmark of the disease.[13]

Several factors may result in a deficiency of surfactant, including

1. Immature cells lining alveoli
2. Decreased rate of production as a result of transient fetal or early neonatal stress

3. Inadequate release mechanism for surfactant from the lining of type II alveolar cells (usually functioning at 35 weeks)
4. Death of cells that produce surfactant[13]

Lecithin is thought to be the surface-active (surfactant) phospholipid responsible for maintaining alveolar stability. The production of lecithin normally begins around the 32nd week to 36th week of gestation, with the initial functioning of enzyme systems producing this phospholipid. The high glucocorticoid levels found in the fetus after the 34th week of gestation accelerate production and synthesis of surfactant and lead to lung maturation. It has been found that chronic stress conditions that increase cortisol levels, such as intrauterine infections, premature rupture of the membranes, maternal hypertensive disorders, and partial abruptio placentae, are associated with a lower incidence of RDS because these stressors lead to stimulation of earlier lung maturation. The use of the synthetic steroidal hormone betamethasone a few days prior to anticipated premature delivery stimulates maturation of the fetal lungs and holds promise of improving the outlook of RDS in the small premature infant.[13]

Clinical Manifestations

Pulmonary compliance, or the capacity of the lung to increase in volume in response to a given amount of applied pressure during inspiration, is diminished in RDS. The stiffness of the lungs and their limited distensibility contribute significantly to the work of breathing in these sick babies. Pulmonary vasoconstriction is another injurious factor of major importance. This vasoconstriction results in increased resistance within the pulmonary circuit and causes hypofusion of alveolar capillaries; hence, the lungs are ischemic as well as atelectatic. The fetal circulatory state persists in varying degrees and this becomes life-threatening to the neonate. After a few breaths, continued impairment of gas exchange enhances hypoxia, hypercapnia, and acidosis. This, in turn, increases the pulmonary vasoconstriction and ischemia; surfactant activity is further diminished and atelectasis becomes more extensive. Pulmonary compliance decreases and the energy required for the simple act of breathing increases intolerably. This leads to further impairment of gas exchange and a vicious cycle that soon becomes incompatible with life. Intensive treatment is necessary to remedy this situation.[13]

It was formerly believed that a free interval existed after birth before the onset of symptoms. However, when infants are observed closely and examined carefully, symptoms can be noted immediately after birth. A chest x-ray film usually confirms the diagnosis and rules out congenital cardiovascular disease (Fig. 42-21).

Expiratory grunting or whining (observable when the infant is not crying), sternal and subcostal retractions, nasal flaring, rapid respirations (more than 60 per minute), and low body temperatures are seen early and are diagnostic clues. Grunting, which is the most important and useful clinical sign, may be the only, or earliest, indication of the disease. Conversely, cessation of grunting is often the first sign of improvement

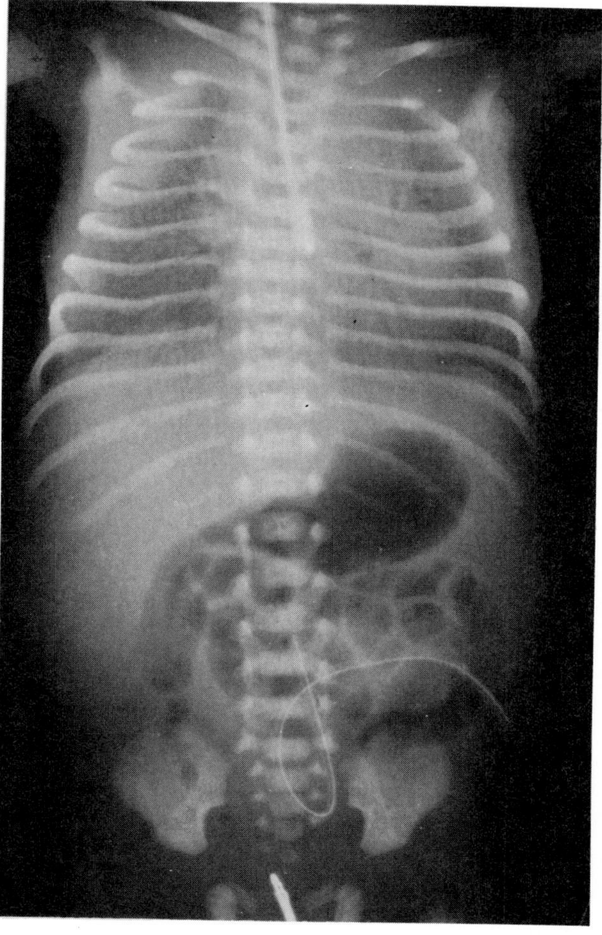

Figure 42-21.
Severe hyaline membrane disease (HMD). Note diffuse density of the lung fields compared with intestinal gas, with well-defined air bronchograms. Both lungs are uniformly involved. An umbilical artery catheter lies at the aortic bifurcation (third lumbar vertebra). (Avery GB: Neonatology: Pathophysiology and Management of the Newborn. Philadelphia, JB Lippincott, 1981)

The infant may be cyanotic in room air. Infants who are badly affected may be cyanotic even with oxygen therapy yet, paradoxically, exhibit a normal respiratory rate. Auscultation of the chest reveals poor air entry, decreased breath sounds, and, at times, fine rales. Arterial blood gases demonstrate decreased PO_2 and, often, metabolic and respiratory acidosis. There is reduced blood *p*H and increased nitrogen, phosphorus, and potassium. Bowel sounds are often diminished or absent in the early hours of the illness and the urine output is low during the first 2 or 3 days of life.

If the disease progresses, respiratory rate increases, chest retractions become more marked, and see-saw respirations ensue (see Fig. 42-20). Peripheral edema increases, and muscle tone decreases. With the increase in cyanosis, the body temperature tends to drop, and short periods of apnea are noted. The heart rate is often fixed except for periods of bradycardia accompanied by severe cyanosis and grunting.

Many symptoms are related to asphyxia, which depresses the respiratory center, causing apneic episodes and changes in the blood distribution throughout the body. This accounts for the pale gray skin color of the severely affected infant. In addition, the rate of heat production is also decreased.

If treatment is instituted promptly, modern care has resulted in about a 50% to 70% success rate in saving these infants. If treatment is not prompt or the infant is small and does not respond to treatment, death may occur within 48 hours.

It is important that the nurse make careful observations and recordings of the respiratory signs and symptoms of infants who are born prematurely. The outcome for the premature infant usually depends a great deal on his birth weight. The smaller the infant, the graver is the prognosis. For example, infants who weigh 1000 g or less generally succumb because their lungs are not developed enough to make the adjustment to extrauterine life.

Management

Since the cause and complete pathophysiology of RDS are not understood, the principles of management center on alleviation of the clinical manifestations. Thus, approaches to treatment are made directly, by treating the infant with oxygen and alkali, and indirectly, through influencing oxygen need and acid production by regulating the infant's body temperature, water balance, and caloric requirements. Treatment therefore involves

1. Regulation of body temperature
2. Intravenous feeding and base therapy
3. Oxygen therapy
4. Assisted ventilation, if necessary

The nurse is a key figure in all of these modalities. Accurate recording and reporting of all the data from the monitoring devices—skin, cardiac, apnea, and telethermometer—is necessary. The sites of attachment of the monitoring devices must be watched carefully for abrasions or skin breakdown. Adequate oxygenation of the infant is imperative.

With mild RDS, small amounts of oxygen administered by hood are often adequate, depending on the requirements demonstrated by arterial blood gas values. As RDS becomes more severe, ventilatory assistance is needed. This may be achieved by continuous positive airway pressure through an intratracheal tube, nasal prongs, mask, or hood; by continuous negative airway pressure by exerting pressure on the infant's body with the head exposed and oxygen administered by mask or prongs; or by continuous end-expiratory pressure with positive pressure exerted during expiration. Care must be taken in administration of oxygen and in ventilatory assistance because a number of complications can result from their injudicious use, as discussed below.

Prognosis

Infants with RDS generally show improvement within 72 hours after birth, or their condition deteriorates. If improvement occurs, slow recovery follows over a period of about 2 weeks. However, follow-up studies have shown an increased incidence of acute respiratory disease in infants less than 1 year old who were nonventilated victims of RDS.[14]

When the infant has remained stable for 12 to 24 hours, oral feedings are usually begun and advanced gradually. With the use of respiratory and metabolic interventions now available through new technology and equipment, premature infants with RDS can be sustained for longer time periods. The outcome may not be known for several weeks. Recovery or death may be postponed for varying lengths of time, creating both hope and longer periods of uncertainty for parents and health professionals.

Bronchopulmonary Dysplasia

Bronchopulmonary dysplasia (BPD) is a chronic lung disorder, an extension of RDS, with overall incidence of 10% to 15%. The incidence in very-low-birth-weight infants is 20% to 38%. Although reports vary as to etiology, in almost all cases four potential etiologic factors have been present: increased amounts of ambient oxygen, positive-pressure ventilation, endotracheal tube, and diseased or immature lungs. Furthermore, right to left shunting through a patent ductus arteriosus appears to increase the risk of occurrence of BPD.

These infants demonstrate tachypnea, subcostal retractions, rales, and cyanosis. It is often difficult to wean them from the respirator. Pathologic changes in the lung usually begin to occur at the transition stage in RDS, at about 10 to 20 days. Changes include alveolar necrosis, bronchiolar necrosis, and repair with bronchial metaplasia and interstitial fibrosis.[14] When improvement occurs, it develops gradually over several weeks with a diminishing need for oxygen. Some months may be needed for complete recovery. Prognosis is good for those surviving a year.

Retrolental Fibroplasia

Retrolental fibroplasia is an acquired disease, associated with prematurity, in which retinal pathology occurs in those infants receiving continuous oxygen therapy in high concentration. The incidence of the condition depends on the concentration of oxygen given, and the degree of immaturity of the eyes at the time when oxygen is given. Incidence is inversely proportional to birth weight.

The disease is characterized by spasm, then obliteration, of the developing retinal vessels, followed by neovascularization, hemorrhage, and retinal detachment. The disease has both an acute and a cicatricial phase. Both eyes are affected, although different stages may be present in the two eyes. Spontaneous arrest may occur at any stage.

The premature (but not the term) infant is susceptible to high oxygen concentrations because of the immaturity of retinal development. By 4 weeks' gestational age, the retinal vessels have grown about 6 mm from the optic nerve. Between 24 and 30 weeks no further growth occurs ("immature" fundus); after this time, however, growth again begins ("transitional" fundus). By about 34 weeks (weight 4 lb 6 oz or 2000 g) the fundus is usually mature. During the immature and transitional developmental stages of the fundus, infants are liable to become victims of the disease if injudicious concentrations of oxygen that initiate the above pathologic process are employed; hence the preponderance of this disease among the very-early-gestational-age and very-low-birth-weight infants.

The onset of the acute stage is usually between the ages of 10 days and 1 month, and the smaller the birth weight, the later the onset. Dilatation and tortuosity of the retinal blood vessels occur, with the fundus becoming pale. Hemorrhages appear adjacent to the vessels and spread into the vitreous; separation of the retina follows.

After several weeks, the acute stage passes into the cicatricial stage, characterized by formation of the retrolental membrane. The anterior chamber becomes shallow and impairment of vision may be accompanied by squint, photophobia, and nystagmus. In severe cases, microphthalmia and secondary glaucoma may be sequelae. Because most of the damage is mechanical, one cannot determine the extent of detachment that will occur.

Management

When the condition is detected early and proper measures are instituted promptly (*i.e.,* reduction in concentration of oxygen administered), the condition in the infant may regress at any stage of the disease; on the other hand, partial or complete blindness may result.

Extensive research, carried on during the years since retrolental fibroplasia was first described, has established the cause and the means of prevention of the disease. It is now known that almost all cases of retrolental fibroplasia in the premature infant are the result of intensive oxygen therapy. Today, oxygen is administered to an infant in the lowest concentration compatible with life and is discontinued as soon as feasible. Blood gases are monitored frequently in order to keep arterial oxygen pressure at acceptable levels (see Oxygen Therapy).

■■■

Care of the High-Risk Infant

Often, the first hours of the SGA or premature infant's life determine the outcome. These babies need warmth, meticulous physical care, gentle handling, precise and careful feeding, and protection from infection. Born either before the body systems have had enough time to develop and mature appropriately, or of a suboptimal uterine environment that has caused growth retardation, these infants must fight against almost insurmountable odds to make a viable adjustment to extrauterine life. The nurse is a key person in assisting these babies to maximize their resources in the struggle to live and grow, and in preventing the development of external complications that would further jeopardize their chances.

Resuscitation

All members of the delivery room team must be proficient at methods of ventilatory resuscitation. The necessary equipment should be readily available.

Preparation and checking of this equipment is

Equipment Needed for Resuscitation

- Overhead radiant warmer with servocontrol
- Bulb, syringe, vacuum suction with sterile catheters and tubing
- Pediatric laryngoscope, blades, and extra bulbs and batteries
- Oropharyngeal airways
- Endotracheal tubes—sizes 8, 10, and 14 with stylets
- Oxygen outlet
- Face mask and bags
- Connectors from bag and mask apparatus to endotracheal tubes
- Oxygen analyzer
- Umbilical catheterization tray
- Syringes, needles
- Light
- Stethoscope
- Doppler blood pressure apparatus
- ECG monitor and electrodes
- Clock with second hand
- Feeding tubes, sizes 5 and 8 French
- Drugs

essential for an organized, effective resuscitative effort.

The following principles of care must be kept in mind during the treatment of depressed infants with asphyxia.

Warmth

The infant's body should be dried and placed in a neutral thermal environment, such as an overhead radiant warmer. Temperature should be monitored by temperature probe or by frequent temperature-taking.

Posture

Some obstetricians hold the infant up by the feet momentarily after birth in order to expedite drainage of mucus from the trachea, the larynx, and the posterior pharynx. Others cradle the baby in the arm with the hand supporting the head, which is held down. After the first few breaths the baby is placed flat.

Clearing the Airway

Cleansing the air passages of mucus and fluid is essential because effective respiration cannot be accomplished through obstructed air passages. Suction of one type or another is frequently necessary. An ordinary catheter is used, size 8 to 10 French; in premature infants size 6 to 8 is advisable. Gentleness is essential because the mucous membrane of the infant's mouth is delicate. Mechanical suction devices are provided with most of the machines for infant resuscitation and are very convenient.

Indications for Resuscitation

A newborn with an Apgar score over 7 will usually not require any resuscitation unless there is a sudden drop in the score.

A newborn with an Apgar score of 3 to 6 probably has mild to moderate asphyxia. Usually suctioning followed by a bag and mask delivery of oxygen will be sufficient to effect improvement rapidly.

A newborn with an Apgar score of 0 to 2 is considered to be severely asphyxiated, and methods described below will be required.

In addition to low Apgar scores, other conditions that most likely will require the use of resuscitation include deficient lecithin/sphingomyelin (L/S) ratio, intrauterine growth retardation, fetal distress, maternal vaginal bleeding, birth weight less than 1500 g, and erythroblastosis fetalis.[15] Other high-risk factors may require the neonatal team to be in attendance and prepared to resuscitate at delivery.

Mask and Bag Resuscitation

With the infant in a supine position, a flattened rolled towel is placed under the shoulders to extend the neck slightly. Initially, a laryngoscope is inserted. With the larynx visualized, suction is applied through a catheter. The suction catheter is then removed and a curved plastic pharyngeal airway may be inserted between the tongue and palate to prevent the base of the tongue from falling backward over the glottic opening into the larynx. Use is optional in the neonate.

The mask is placed over the nose and mouth to create a seal. To avoid injury, care must be taken that it does not extend over the eyes. Initial insufflation pressure should be less than 30 mm H_2O. Humidified oxygen may be administered at 60% to 100% through the bag and mask. The bag should be squeezed at a rate of 40 to 60 times per minute. A nasogastric tube may be inserted to decompress the abdomen.

The chest of the baby will rise with each squeeze of the bag if the oxygen is delivered adequately. If this procedure is effective, spontaneous respirations should begin within 1 minute and cyanosis and hypotonicity should disappear. Oxygen should still be supplied by mask, however, until the infant is stable. If color and respirations have not improved after 1 minute or the heart rate falls below 100 beats per minute at any time, endotracheal intubation is urgently indicated.

Endotracheal Intubation

With the laryngoscope in place, an endotracheal tube is introduced through the glottis and advanced until the flange of the tube meets resistance, usually about 1 cm to 1.5 cm past the glottis (Fig. 42-22). The tube is held in place while the laryngoscope is carefully removed. Oxygen is delivered through a bag attached to the endotracheal tube. The bag is briskly squeezed

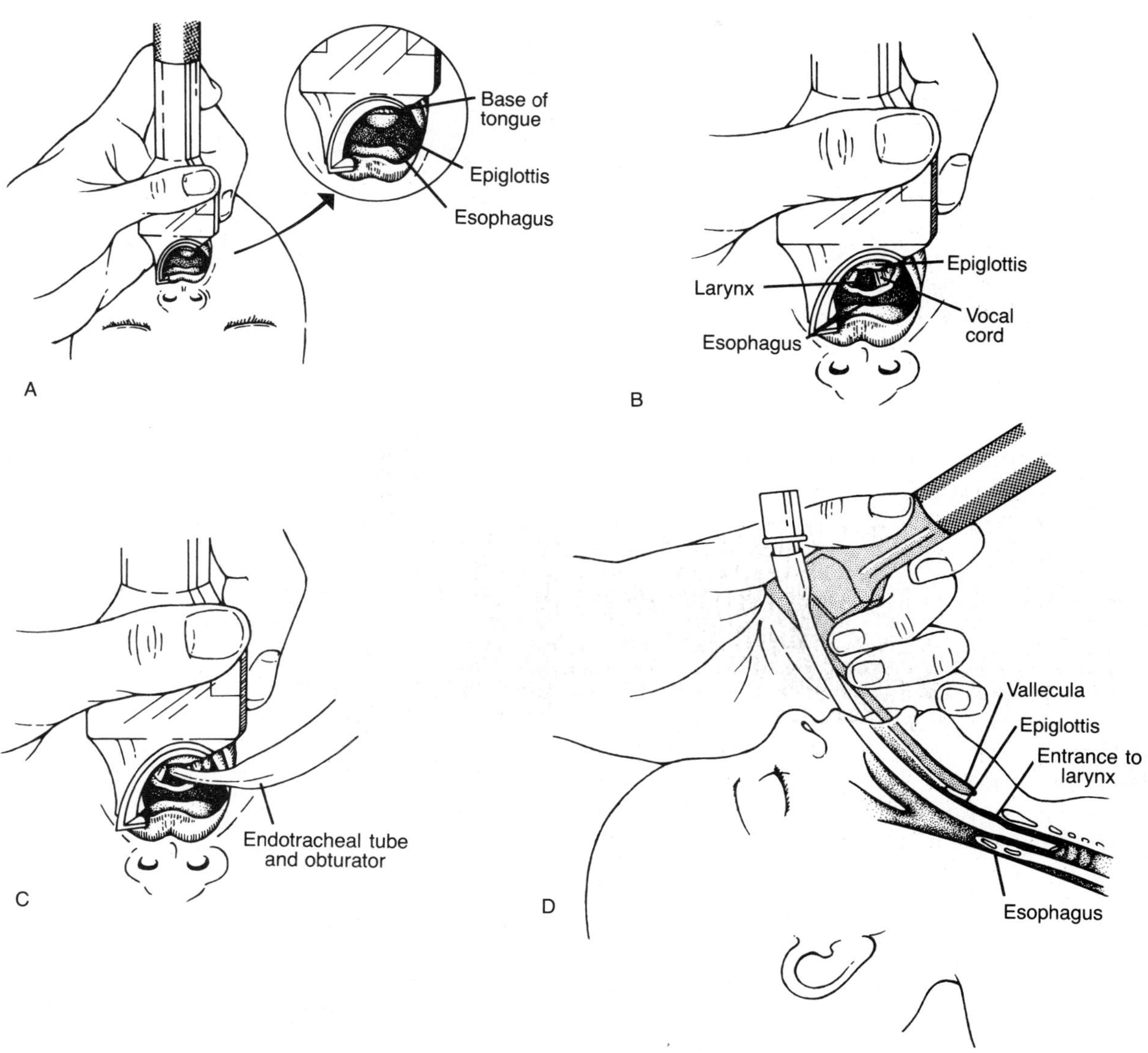

Figure 42-22.
Technique of endotracheal intubation. The Miller blade should be inserted near the midline and moved to the left side of the mouth, gently deflecting the tongue. As it is advanced, the base of the tongue and epiglottis are visualized. The blade should be advanced in the same plane of movement into the vallecula *(see D);* as the blade is gently raised, the epiglottis swings anteriorly, revealing the opening of the larynx. If secretions or meconium are noted, gentle suctioning should be done before insertion of the endotracheal tube. On certain occasions when the epiglottis is not adequately raised, the blade tip may be placed posterior to the epiglottis, which can then be gently raised to expose the vocal cords. The endotracheal tube is advanced from the right corner of the mouth and inserted while maintaining direct visualization. The laryngoscope blade is then carefully withdrawn while the position of the tube is maintained by the right hand on the infant's face. Note the tip of the blade in the vallecula.

and then released at a rate of about 50 times per minute. The chest should rise and fall with insufflation and rest. Breath sounds should be heard through the stethoscope on both sides of the chest.

Generally, once the lungs are oxygenated, the response is positive. Immediate improvement may be noted, although intubation for 10 minutes or longer is recommended. With the return of effective cardiac function, the baby becomes pink, and some muscle activity can be noted. If there is no pulse after 3 or 4 bag insufflations, external cardiac massage is mandatory. It is important to remember that only after cardiovascular function is restored is intravenous administration of sodium bicarbonate and dextrose essential. This is because the hypoxia causes metabolic acidosis and may produce hypoglycemia as a result of rapid depletion of glycogen stores.

External Cardiac Massage

If the heartbeat has not returned after 3 or 4 insufflations, external cardiac massage is instituted immediately. It should be performed by an assistant, leaving the primary operator free to manage ventilation. Downward pressure is applied at the midsternum, thereby compressing the heart (systole). When the pressure is released, the heart is dilated (diastole).

The index and middle fingers are placed on the midthorax at the level of the sternum and the area is pressed downward and released at a rate of 100 times per minute (Fig. 42-23). The total downward displacement of the chest wall should not exceed 1 inch. Excessive vigor may cause a laceration of the liver with severe blood loss.

It is imperative to maintain the cardiac massage and the ventilation. This can be accomplished by alternating the two maneuvers. A 5:1 ratio of cardiac massage to assisted ventilation of 100% oxygen should be used. The two procedures must not be performed simultaneously because the pressure applied during cardiac massage may rupture a lung that has just been inflated by the ventilation. If the procedure is effective, the femoral or temporal artery pulses are palpable in synchrony with depression of the sternum. The procedure is to be discontinued periodically to determine the presence of spontaneous cardiac activity. When this occurs, cardiac compression may be discontinued.

Drugs

Drugs that may be utilized in a resuscitative effort include the following:

narcan (narcotic antagonist)

albumin or plasmanate (volume expander)

10% dextrose in water (hydration, hypoglycemia)

sodium bicarbonate (severe metabolic acidosis)

calcium gluconate (severe bradycardia or arrhythmia, hypocalcemia)

epinephrine (cardiac arrest)[8]

General Measures

Critical observation of the infant before, during, and after any procedures is especially important. The completion of necessary recording is to be accomplished quickly because early transfer of the infant is usually requested.

The maintenance of body temperature is essential. The high-risk infant's temperature tends to fall even more precipitously than the normal infant's at birth because of poor heat-regulating ability. The baby should therefore be wrapped in a warmed blanket and placed in a warm environment (90° to 92° F or 32° to 33° C) or under radiant overhead heat.

After any immediate resuscitation efforts are concluded, the infant is generally transferred as quickly as possible to the high-risk unit to ensure a proper environment.

Continuing Management

Because of the magnitude of the high-risk problem, special nurseries and referral centers have been established for high-risk infants in many urban areas. Space in the hospital separate from the term-newborn nursery is usually allotted. In some cities, there is a large neonatal intensive care unit (NICU) located in a medical center. When these infants must be moved from a hospital to a medical center, or from a rural area to a hospital, effort is made to ensure safe transport to and from the hospital. A special transport incubator designed to maintain temperature and administer oxygen is generally used. It is strongly advised that the nurse who accompanies the infant be trained in resuscitative techniques.

As with initial management, continuing care revolves around maintaining temperature, preventing infection, and maintaining respiration and nutrition of the infant.

Neonatal Intensive Care Unit

NICUs, developed to provide highly skilled nursing and medical care to high-risk and sick neonates, require extensive and complicated equipment. Such life-support devices include reverse-isolation type incubators, radiant heaters, ECG–respiration–blood pressure monitors, head hoods, oxygen:air ratio controllers, oxygen analyzers, mechanical ventilators, heated nebulizers, infusion pumps, phototherapy

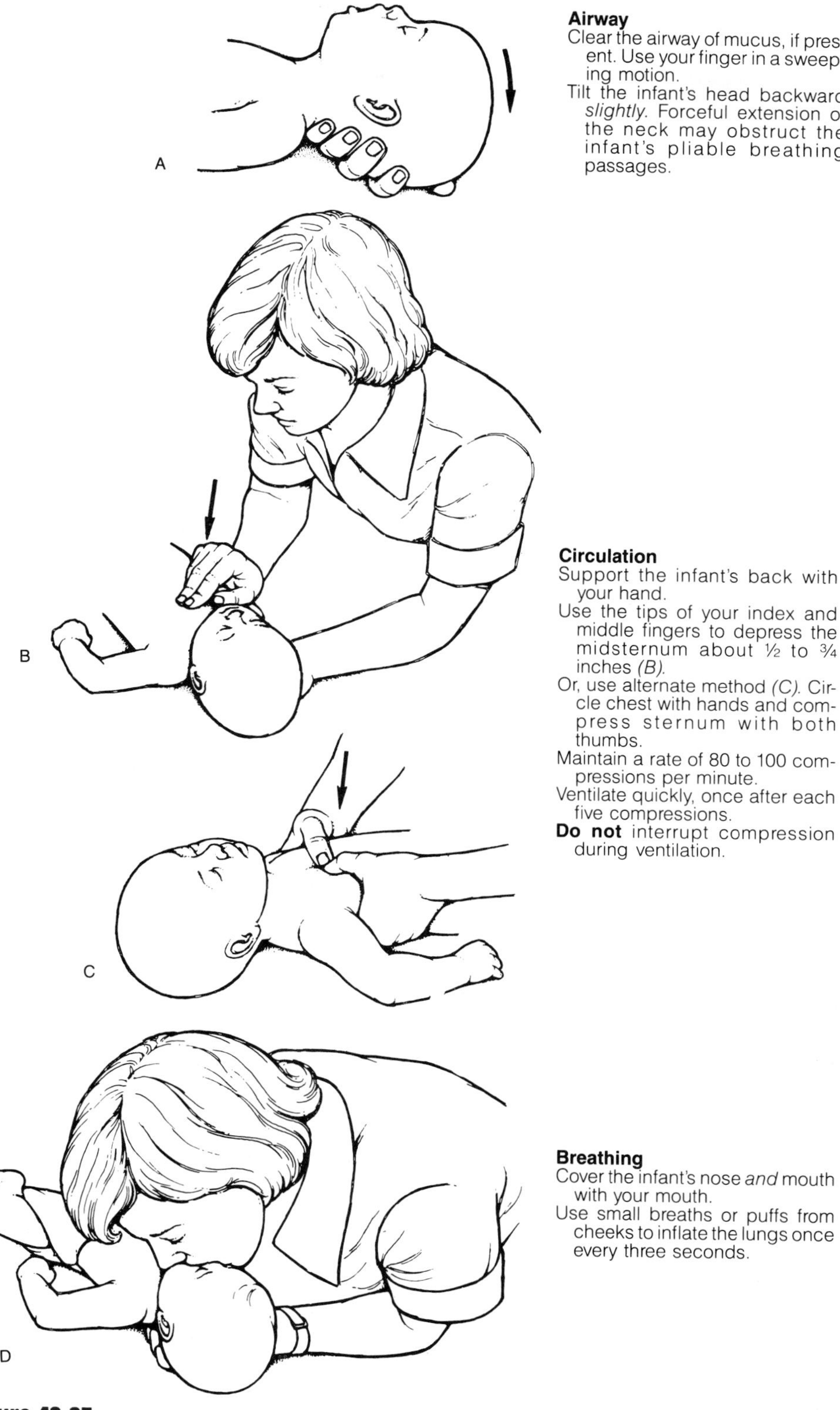

Figure 42-23.
Techniques of cardiopulmonary resuscitation in an infant. *(A)* Position. *(B)* Palpation of sternum. *(C)* Compression. *(D)* Ventilation. (Gildea JH: Techniques of cardiopulmonary resuscitation in an infant. Am J Nurs 78(2):265, 1978; original art by Neil Hardy. Copyright © 1978, American Journal of Nursing Company. Reproduced with permission from the American Journal of Nursing)

units, and amplifying stethoscopes. The maintenance and use of these machines are vitally important in the management of the patients. It is necessary to have technicians who can maintain this equipment in the NICU as well as in other special units throughout the hospital. Nurses should be free from the need to "nurse the equipment" because the critical condition of their tiny patients requires constant attention and full utilization of their special skills and knowledge.

Temperature Maintenance

Many babies have subnormal temperatures, sometimes as low as 90° F (32° C) when they arrive at the NICU. Bringing their temperature to normal and maintaining it is extremely important. High-risk infants whose temperatures are kept between 97° and 98° F (36° and 37° C) from birth have significantly higher survival rates.

It is important to remember that these infants increase their heat production in cooler environments; this requires more oxygen, which places an added and sometimes impossible burden on the immature and often diseased lungs.

The body temperature of the high-risk infant, as well as respiration, is maintained in the artificial environment of the incubator, or, as it is sometimes called, the *isolette.* The modern air-conditioned Isolette is a miniature room in which the infant can live and be cared for under ideal conditions (*i.e.,* desirable levels of heat, humidity, and oxygen). As the infant matures, the need for all three of these elements in such exactingly measured quantities will lessen. Eventually, the infant will be placed in a crib. There are several kinds of incubators currently in use, but the principle is the same. The differences are in the special construction details developed by various manufacturers.

Most incubators have controls on the outside of the unit to regulate the environment accurately and to adjust the bed from the horizontal to the tilted positions (Trendelenburg and reverse-Trendelenburg positions) to facilitate treatments and care. Some have the "Servo-Control" to adjust automatically to needed temperature and humidity settings by means of an automatic sensing device (thermistor) attached to the infant's skin. Special oxygen inlets provide adjustable oxygen concentrations (30%–40% is the usual recommended "maintenance" flow). Regardless of these built-in sensors, the nurse will want to check and record the oxygen concentration with a reliable

Figure 42-24.
Incubators for premature infants are constructed to provide easy access to the infant through the hand holes so that the carefully controlled environment will not be disrupted.

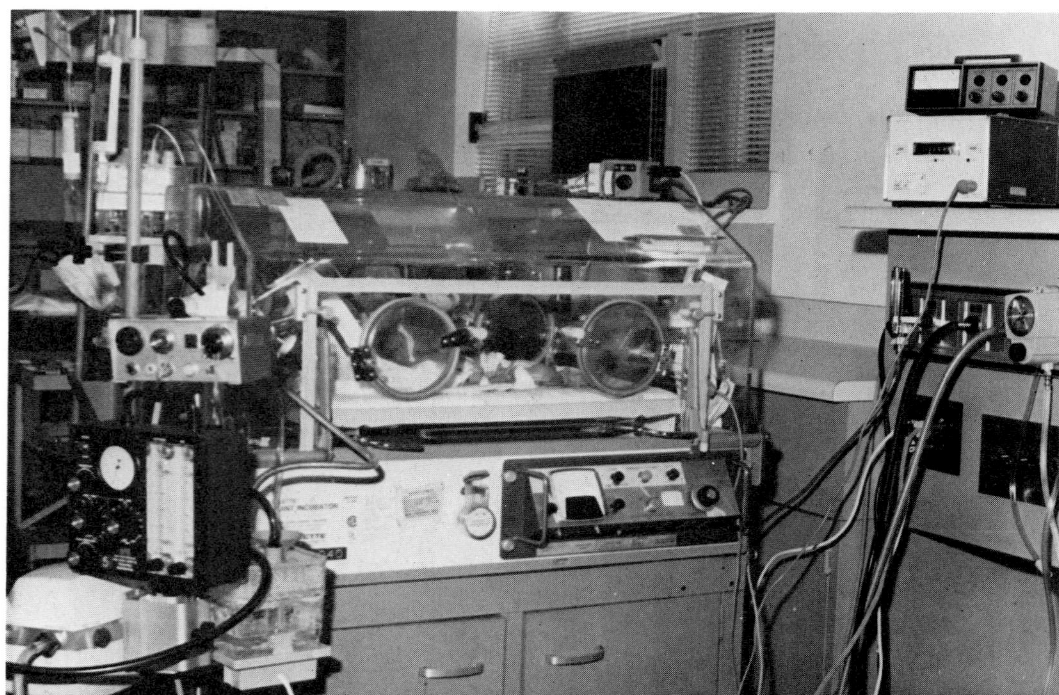

oximeter (oxygen analyzer) placed at the level of the infant's nose. A similar device can be used to ascertain the humidity level.

When oxygen therapy is no longer required, the incubator can be ventilated with fresh air from the room through a large, replaceable air filter, or through an outside air attachment. Humidity can be controlled, and, by means of a nebulizer, supersaturated atmosphere can be created. Constant temperatures within the incubator can be regulated and maintained with a double-thermoswitch-controlled, sealed heating unit.

These incubators are designed such that the infant can be observed from all sides through transparent windows. Moreover, hand holes with air-tight doors and self-adjusting sleeves permit the nurses and the physicians to care for the infant without disturbing the atmospheric conditions (Fig. 42-24). The incubators are made of stainless steel and plastic and are constructed for easy removal of all essential parts, without tools, to permit proper cleansing and sterilizing.

The overhead heating unit is another piece of equipment that is being used more now in the care of the high-risk neonate (Fig. 42-25). It adjusts the temperature automatically according to the infant's skin temperature, which is monitored by a probe. Advantages of the unit include easy access to the infant for nursing care and procedures and for parental contact. Disadvantages include insensible water loss, loss of heat by convection, and the inability to use the unit for isolation.

Prevention of Infection

Though the incubator provides a supportive environment, maintenance of asepsis in every detail is imperative for these fragile babies. Scrupulous handwashing and gowning technique is to be observed. Personnel are also cautioned to avoid contact with sources of infection that might be transferred to the babies. Usually, special nursery gowns are worn when one is assuming care of these infants. The gowning procedure varies from institution to institution, but the underlying principle is to keep anything that comes in contact with the high-risk infant as clean as possible. Masks are infrequently used, as they have been found to harbor a rich source of contamination; moisture and bacteria from the nasopharynx collect in the mask folds, and even ordinary conversation distributes the infectious contents throughout the environment.

Ancillary personnel assume the task of cleaning incubators, respirators, and suction equipment. All equipment is to be cultured after cleaning. Incubators that are in use are often cultured once a week and changed immediately if any bacterial growth is present. For long-term patients, it is well to change incubators once a week. For additional prophylaxis, a culture plate can be placed in each unit for 2 hours per day, and if any growth occurs the baby can be transferred to clean equipment.

Maintaining Respiration

As previously stated, the establishment and maintenance of respiration is of critical importance for infants with RDS. It is the nurse's responsibility to make careful, frequent observations and precise verbal and written recordings. It has been demonstrated that the first 5 minutes of life are crucial for the later successful outcome of the infant with respect to respiratory depression. Infants with unimproved respiratory function after these 5 minutes have a 4 times greater chance of dying in the first days than those infants whose condition improves or is good during this time.

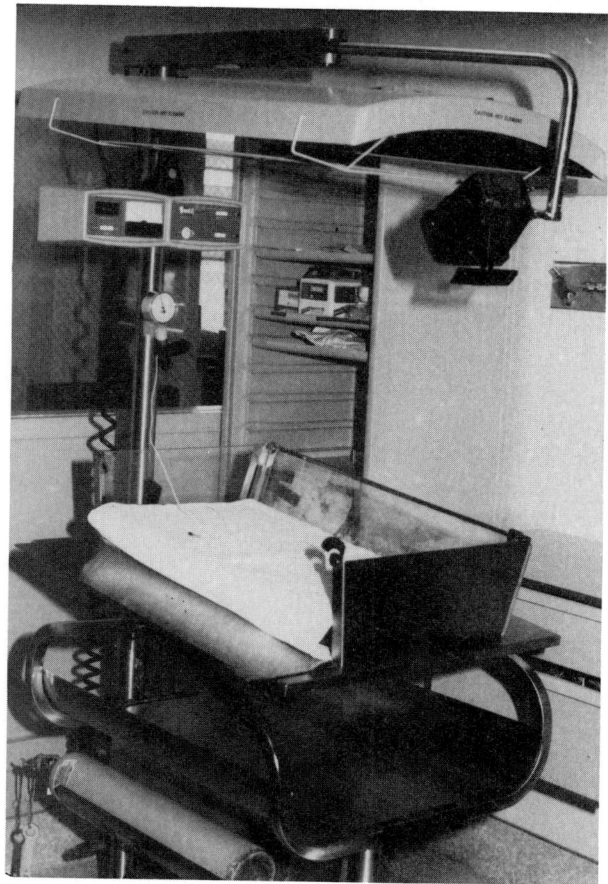

Figure 42-25.
Overhead heating unit.

Respiratory Patterns. In a quiet, large, healthy premature infant, the most common respiratory rhythm follows a steady pattern with no pause between inspiration and expiration. The next most common is the so-called adult rhythm, with its pattern of inspiration, expiration, and pause. Other patterns, such as inspiration–pause–expiration, also occur. Sighs that interrupt the regular pattern are common, and are often followed by apneic pauses. Periodic breathing, consisting of two or more periods of breathing per minute separated by an apneic pause of 3 seconds or more, is more common among small infants.

Normal respiratory rates are difficult to determine because it is difficult to define the "normal" premature and the "normal" conditions under which they prevail. Two patterns have been associated with a low mortality rate and have thus been described as normal. In the first pattern, about 40 respirations per minute occur from birth onward without any significant fluctuations. In the second pattern, rates over 60 respirations per minute occur in the first hour, with no significant increase, and subsequently decline. A significant increase is 15 or more respirations per minute above the average rate obtained in the first hour after birth.

The following patterns are always abnormal in the healthy term infant; they are also abnormal in the premature, but they are more expected because of the premature's developmental immaturity.

1. Simple retraction may be seen, in which the chest and abdomen rise together, with a slight indentation over the sternal area. When this occurs, observations must be increased and sharpened. This pattern is a warning sign and the physician may want to be alerted.
2. Paradoxical breathing is considered a critical condition; the abdomen rises while the chest sinks. There is a marked chin lag and an audible respiratory grunt, indicating respiratory distress. The physician should be alerted and informed of any progress in the condition. Therefore, exacting observation and frequent reporting are necessary.
3. Prolonged apnea (which is different from the periodic apnea discussed above) often occurs in cases of RDS, as well as in other pathologic conditions such as infection, pneumonia, and central nervous system injuries. Management usually consists of positive-pressure oxygen therapy and continuous observation because apneic spells are often repeated in these infants.

Nursing measures such as bathing and weighing are scheduled with the need to conserve the infant's strength and to prevent apnea due to exhaustion clearly in mind. Positioning the infant in a lateral Sims's position or supine position, with a rolled towel under the shoulder and neck extended, prevents mucus from reaching and remaining in the lungs. Changing position every 2 to 3 hours also aids in ventilating the lungs.

Oxygen Therapy

A majority of premature infants must receive oxygen initially because of respiratory depression, cyanosis, or concurrent pathologic conditions such as hemorrhage or erythroblastosis. Oxygen therapy is often a life-saving measure for the infant, but must be used judiciously. It is to be administered at the lowest concentration compatible with life, because the oxygen requirements for these infants will vary according to weight, maturity, and general condition.

The administration of oxygen must be closely monitored to avoid the serious and often irreversible problems that can result from oxygen toxicity, such as bronchopulmonary dysplasia and retrolental fibroplasia. The dosage of oxygen should be adequate to relieve cyanosis, and for apneic cyanotic episodes the oxygen can be administered by mask in dosages more concentrated than 40% for short periods of time. Dosage is determined by laboratory blood gas values.

An incubator provides a controlled source of oxygen and humidity, but it is difficult to maintain concentrations beyond 60% to 70%. A plastic hood is useful for oxygen levels at a constant 40% to 50% and can be used inside an incubator and outside during procedures (Fig. 42-26). Manual ventilatory assistance with the mask and bag is used for intermittent administration of concentrated oxygen therapy to maintain blood gas and acid–base balance within normal ranges. Continuous positive airway pressure is generally used to improve oxygenation when the infant's respiratory efforts are inadequate, to decrease pulmonary shunting, increase residual lung capacity, and prevent atelectasis on expiration by keeping alveoli open (Fig. 42-27).

Infants are weaned gradually from oxygen therapy by periodic decrements in dosage with monitoring of lab values and observations of heart rate, color, and respiratory effort.

Umbilical Catheterization

High-risk neonates often require insertion of an umbilical catheter to provide a route for parenteral fluid therapy or exchange transfusions, or to obtain

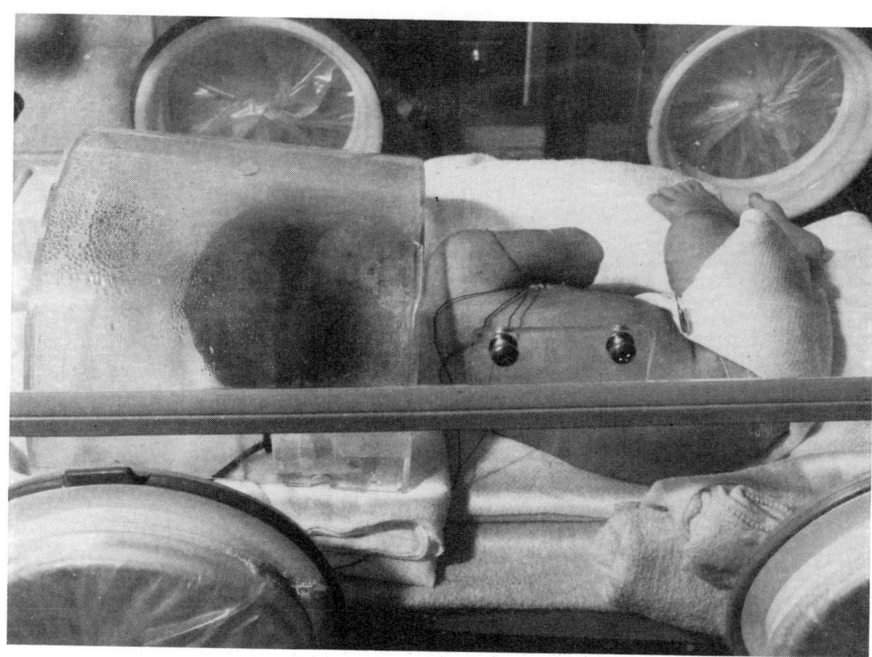

Figure 42-26.
Oxygen hood maintains level of oxygen delivered to the infant.

blood samples for gases and metabolic studies. This is a sterile procedure in which a catheter is inserted into the umbilical artery with radiographic confirmation of placement. The infant's response to the procedure is monitored and signs of complications assessed, including bleeding, emboli, infection, vasospasm, and blockage of the tubing.

Maintaining Nutrition

There is increasing evidence that delaying food and water in low-birth-weight infants lessens their chances for normal growth and development. Early feeding of these infants is associated with a reduced incidence of hyperbilirubinemia and symptomatic hypoglycemia.

Nutritional problems of low-birth-weight infants begin with an immature gastrointestinal system as well as immature reflexes. Sucking and swallowing reflexes, even though established before birth, are not coordinated until approximately 32 to 34 weeks of gestation. In addition, the gag reflex is poorly developed and the esophageal cardiac sphincter is incompetent. As a result, aspiration is a danger. Furthermore, the stomach of a premature infant has a limited capacity and is easily overdistended, yet caloric requirements are high.[16] The nutritional requirements of low-birth-weight infants are higher in calories per unit of body weight than normal infants (110–140 calories per kg per day) because their growth is more comparable to that of a fetus.

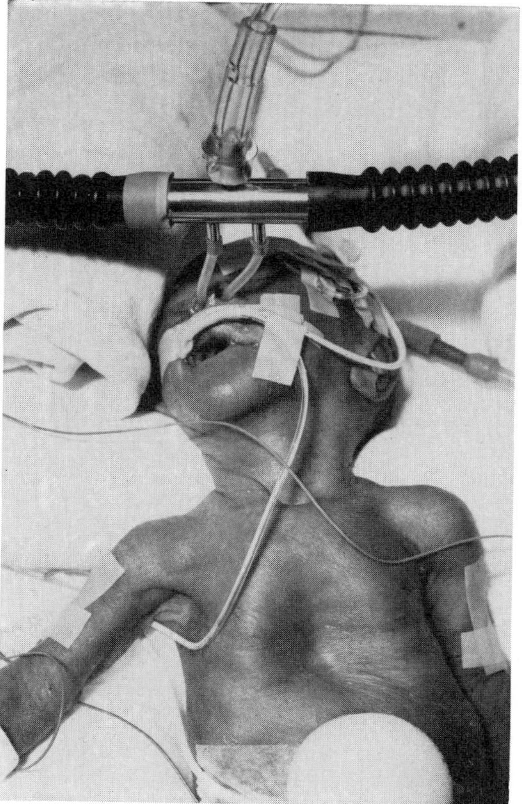

Figure 42-27.
Nasal continuous positive airway pressure (CPAP).

Similarly, the premature infant's nutritional requirements differ from term infant's requirements in several other areas. *Protein* requirements of 3 mg to 4 mg/kg/day are increased for the low-birth-weight infant. Water-soluble *vitamins B and C* and fat-soluble *vitamins A and D* are deficient, requiring supplementation by Poly-Vi-Sol, 1 ml daily. Low-birth-weight infants have low levels of *vitamin E* which is poorly absorbed in infants of less than 32 weeks' gestation. *Iron* intake also interferes with absorption of vitamin E. The recommendation is for a vitamin E supplement of 25 units per day orally. Iron stores are low, yet the timing of supplementation is a matter of some debate owing to its effect on vitamin E. Iron in the form of oral Fer-In-Sol may be begun at delivery or at 2 to 3 months of life at 2 mg to 3 mg/kg/day.[16] During the first few days, most of these babies will need intravenous infusion of a 10% glucose solution with appropriate electrolytes. Supplementation of calcium, magnesium, and phosphorus may be required because these elements are usually stored during the last trimester.

Extremely immature infants are usually given intravenous feedings. If the infant is somewhat more mature and healthy, oral feeding may start 3 to 6 hours after birth. A bottle with a soft nipple can be used if the infant is able to suck efficiently; if not, intermittent gavage is recommended. Breast-feeding may be tried for infants who have the ability to tolerate nipple feedings.

In planning the feeding schedule for the premature and low-birth-weight infant, it is important to establish a food tolerance, since the intestinal tract (as well as other organs) is underdeveloped. The caloric needs of the low-birth-weight baby are estimated according to the body weight. At first, the feeding should be in small amounts, increasing gradually to the amount that will produce a consistent gain. Vomiting and consequent aspiration, distention, and diarrhea may be due to overfeeding. Early and more nearly optimal feeding, in the case of the larger infant, will contribute to lessening mortality and morbidity by preventing nutritive depletion and maintaining biochemical homeostasis.

Those infants in good condition (these are usually but not always the larger infants) with active peristalsis may be started on oral 5% to 10% glucose or sterile water. Studies have shown that sterile water, if aspirated, is less damaging to the lung than dextrose water or milk.[17]

For the infant in poor condition, no matter what the cause, oral feedings are usually withheld for several days if necessary. Parenteral fluids are instituted instead. If the infant is fed orally, some physicians begin the infant on a trial of plain water; if it is retained, then glucose water or dilute modified cow's milk formula is instituted at 2-hour intervals. Thus, there is a gradual replacement of water feedings by milk feedings. A gradual increase in the amounts of milk and water at each feeding should continue until caloric and fluid requirements are met. If an infant is taking about 180 ml of full-strength modified cow's milk formula per kg of body weight per day, then he is getting about 120 calories per kg per day, which ensures an adequate weight gain (Table 42-3).

Table 42-3.
Daily Feeding Requirements of Low-Birth-Weight Infants and Premature Infants

Premature, appropriate for gestational age

Item	Calories/kg/24 hr	
Resting	40–50	(depending on age)
Activity	10–15	
Cold stress	5–10	(depending on environmental temperature)
Specific dynamic action	8–8	
Fecal loss	2†–12	
Growth	25–25	
Total	90–120	

Low birth weight

Nutrient requirements		First week of life	Active growth period
Water (ml)		80–200	130–200
Calories		50–100	110–150†
Protein	(gm)	1–2	3–4
Glucose	(gm)	7–12	12–15
Fat	(gm)	3–4	5–8
Sodium	(mEq)	1–2	2–3
Potassium	(mEq)	1–2	2–4
Chloride	(mEq)	1–2	2–3
Calcium	(mEq)	1–2	3–5
Phosphorus	(mEq)	1–2	2–4
Magnesium	(mEq)	—	0.5–1
Iron (mg)	(mEq)	—	1.5–2

†Above 120 calories/kg applies to infants with perinatal undergrowth.
(Source: Babson SG, Benson RC, Pernoll MI, and Benda GI: Management of High-Risk Pregnancy and Intensive Care of the Neonate. St. Louis, CV Mosby, 1975.)

Premature infants who weigh 1.4 kg (3 lb) or less may be fed every 2 or 3 hours. Infants who weigh over 1.6 kg (3½ lb) may be placed on a 3- to 4-hour feeding schedule. The stomach of the premature baby needs rest between feedings as much as that of the full-term baby; therefore, the interval should be regulated accordingly. The schedule should be as near that of a normal infant as is compatible with his progress.

Gavage Feeding

Feeding by gavage, whether intermittent or continuous, is a common means of feeding infants who cannot tolerate oral feedings for a period of time and whose gastrointestinal tract is intact. Infants who may require this feeding assistance include those of less than 32 weeks' gestation, or those with central nervous system depression and poor suck reflexes. Appropriate-for-gestational-age infants who become very tired may require gavage to avoid needless energy expenditure and loss of calories.

For intermittent gavage feeding, a 5 or 8 French feeding tube is chosen according to the infant's size and tolerance. Vagal stimulation with subsequent bradycardia may be a problem as the tube is introduced. The tube is measured from the tip of the nose or mouth to the tip of the earlobe, ending at the tip of the xiphoid process (Fig. 42-28). The tube may also be measured from the bridge of the nose to the umbilicus. The tube is then marked at the point of measurement, ensuring that it will be inserted only to that point.

The infant is positioned either on his back or on his side with his head elevated (Fig. 42-29). The infant may need to be restrained in a mummy restraint or held during the procedure.

After the tube is lubricated with sterile water, the infant's head is held still with one hand and the tube is inserted up to the mark with the other hand. Tubes may be inserted through the mouth or the nares. Nose insertion may obstruct the passage of a nose breather and irritate the nasal mucosa.

Correct placement of the feeding tube may be checked by aspiration of gastric residual and injection of 3 cc of air while listening with a stethoscope. Gastric residual should be measured and returned to the stomach unless otherwise ordered. If cyanosis, severe gagging, or coughing ensues, the tube may be misplaced and should be removed and reinserted properly.

Upon ascertaining correct placement, the syringe is separated from the tube. The plunger is then removed from the barrel and the barrel is reconnected to the tube. The desired amount of formula is poured into the syringe. The syringe is elevated 6 to 8 inches over the infant's head and the feeding is allowed to flow in by gravity.

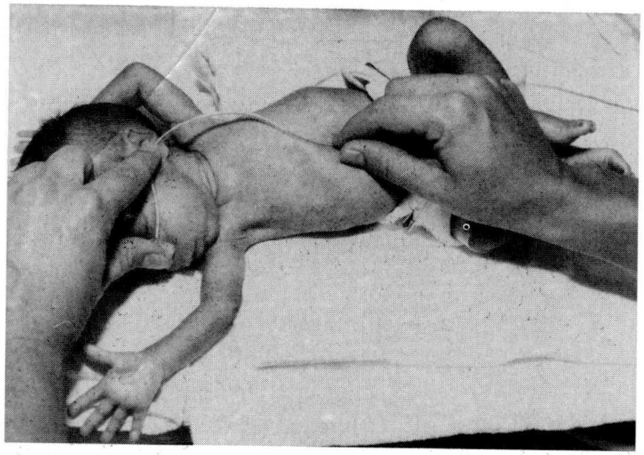

Figure 42-28.
Measurement for gavage feeding.

When the formula is absorbed, the tube is rinsed with 2 ml to 3 ml of sterile water. The tube is folded over onto itself and removed with one smooth motion.

If the infant could not be held during the feeding, this is an appropriate time to hold him. Some infants enjoy sucking on a pacifier during the feeding. Sucking helps the infant to practice the reflex and associate it with a full stomach.

The infant should be positioned on his right side or his abdomen with the head slightly elevated to facilitate digestion.

Continuous gavage feedings by nasogastric tube may minimize problems of distention and aspiration.[17] While a nasogastric tube is left securely taped in place, formula is pumped in by continuous drip. The tube may be clamped or removed when each feeding is complete. Residuals as well as abdominal circumferences are checked frequently.

Nasojejunal and Nasoduodenal Feedings

Continuous infusions by nasojejunal or nasoduodenal routes represent alternative methods of nutritional support. The tube is passed into the stomach, and placement is checked by x-ray film when gastric residual with a *p*H of 5 to 7 is obtained. Continuous infusion, advancing from glucose water to the infant's full fluid and caloric requirement, may be given. Hypertonic formulas should not be introduced directly into the small intestine. Perforations have been reported as polyvinyl or polyethylene catheters became stiff after a week or so of continuous usage. Oral feedings should be begun as soon as the infant's condition permits.[17]

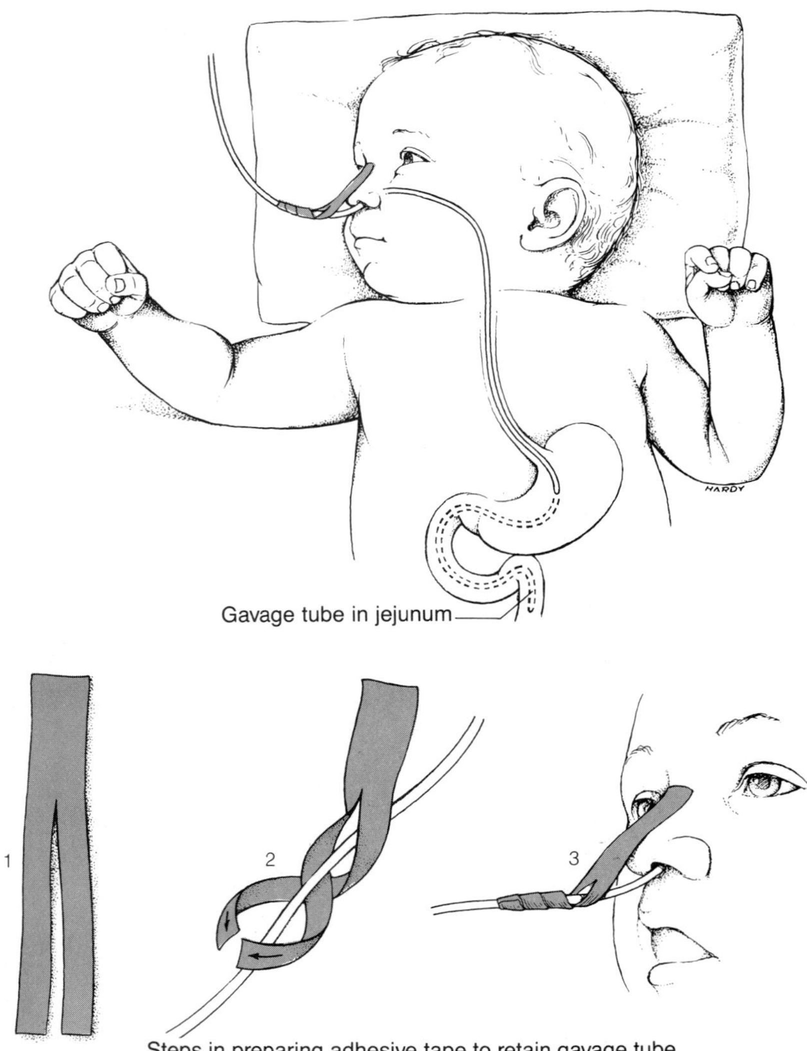

Figure 42-29.
Gavage feeding.

Gastrostomy

Gastrostomy tubes may be inserted, usually in surgical patients, in order to allow feedings to drip slowly into the stomach. Residuals are checked prior to feedings. The tubing is left open between feedings about 10 cm to 12 cm above the abdominal wall.[17]

Bottle-Feeding

Behaviors indicating that the infant may be ready to advance to bottle-feedings include a strong, vigorous suck, coordination of sucking and swallowing, sucking in response to the gavage tube, and wakefulness before feedings. The infant may be challenged with feedings slowly. Bottle-feedings could begin with once a day, then once a shift, then every other feeding, and so on, as tolerated. If the infant requires more than 30 minutes to finish the feeding, the next feeding should be a gavage feeding.[11]

A soft, average-sized nipple with an adequate opening is used. The infant may be helped to open his mouth to accept the nipple by applying gentle pressure on his chin and touching his lips with the nipple. Again, the infant is held in the semierect position to facilitate "burping" and nursing. After the feeding, the infant is positioned as described above.

There are several precautions to be aware of. The infant is not to be urged to accept more formula than is easily taken. Moreover, the bottle should be removed if the infant appears to be getting the milk too fast, in which case the infant usually gasps, chokes, or swallows so quickly as to interfere with respiration. Any infant who has been feeding well and shows reluctance to eat on two successive occasions needs critical reassessment.

Feedings are to be discontinued if the baby vomits, becomes cyanotic, overdistends, or develops frequent or diarrheal stools. Feedings should also be reevaluated if residuals are increasing.

Finally, the bottle of the premature infant is never to be propped. Any change of feeding habits in these infants is critical and may be the first sign of illness.

Total Parenteral Nutrition

Total parenteral nutrition (TPN, also known as *hyperalimentation*) is an aseptically prepared hypertonic solution composed of protein, carbohydrates, electrolytes, vitamins, and minerals (Table 42-4).

In cases where oral feedings must be delayed for a long period of time, TPN has been able to provide adequate nutrition to the neonate. Indications for the use of TPN include low-birth-weight infants, surgical infants in whom the gut needs to be rested, necrotizing enterocolitis, and prolonged diarrhea.[17]

Central catheters for TPN infusion may be inserted in various sites—external or internal jugular, or internal jugular into superior vena cava (Fig. 42-30). Peripheral lines may also be used. TPN is infused at a carefully calculated rate by way of an infusion pump. A filter is placed close to the insertion site to help prevent infection. A sterile dressing is placed securely over the insertion site. Neither medications nor blood should be given through the line.

Nursing care for the infant receiving TPN involves monitoring the equipment, the infusion, and the infant.

The solution bottle, tubing, and filter must be changed every 24 hours and labeled. The bottle label is carefully checked with the physician's order for proper ingredients and amounts. The insertion site dressing is changed at least 3 times a week using strict aseptic technique and following agency procedure. The infusion itself is maintained at the desired rate.

Various parameters are measured, such as Dextrostix, urine specific gravity, sugar and acetone, intake and output, and daily weights. Blood studies are done frequently to check electrolyte requirements. The infant's sucking needs may be satisfied by a pacifier.

Intralipid

Intralipid is a Swedish soybean oil–egg emulsion designed to deliver extra calories and lower glucose concentration in addition to TPN. Infants on TPN alone develop fatty-acid deficiencies quite rapidly. Intralipid should be infused slowly in a line separate from other intravenous solutions, but may be run in the same line through a Y connector close to the insertion site. Serum is checked for turbidity daily to ensure fat clearance.

Table 42-4.
Daily Requirements of Total Parenteral Nutrition

Protein	2–4 g/kg (2.5 g/kg for prematures)
Calories	100–120 cal/kg
H_2O	125 ml/kg or as needed
Na	3–4 mmol/kg
K	2–3 mmol/kg
Ca	2–2.5 mmol/kg
P	2.5 mmol/day*
Mg	1 mmol/day
Multivitamins (Multivit)	1 ml/day

*Blood levels may be watched at intervals and P as K_2PO_4 given as needed.
(From Avery GB, Fletcher AB: Nutrition. In Avery GB (ed): Neonatology, p 1034 Philadelphia, JB Lippincott, 1981)

Other Nursing Measures

Other necessary care of the infant, such as temperature taking, weighing, bathing, and dressing (if required), is usually done in conjunction with the feeding periods so that the infant may rest without interference at other times. The nurse should gather any materials needed and plan care carefully. Frequently entering the incubator is not in the interests of good aseptic technique and, of course, is very tiring to the infant.

The skin is extremely delicate and tender; if diapers are used, they should be changed as soon as they become wet or soiled. Sometimes only a small pad is placed under the baby. However, no clothing is really needed because of the controlled environment of the incubator.

Each institution has its particular procedures for routine care in the NICU, but the principles are the same as those involved in attending the normal newborn.

Growth and Development

Studies of high-risk infants born since the introduction of perinatal intensive care in the last two decades indicate that mortality and morbidity have significantly decreased. Contributing to this improvement have been early identification of high-risk pregnancies, maintenance of an appropriate thermal environment for the neonate, and early correction of neonatal acidosis, of hypoglycemia, and of hyperbilirubinemia. Refinement and widespread use of continuous dis-

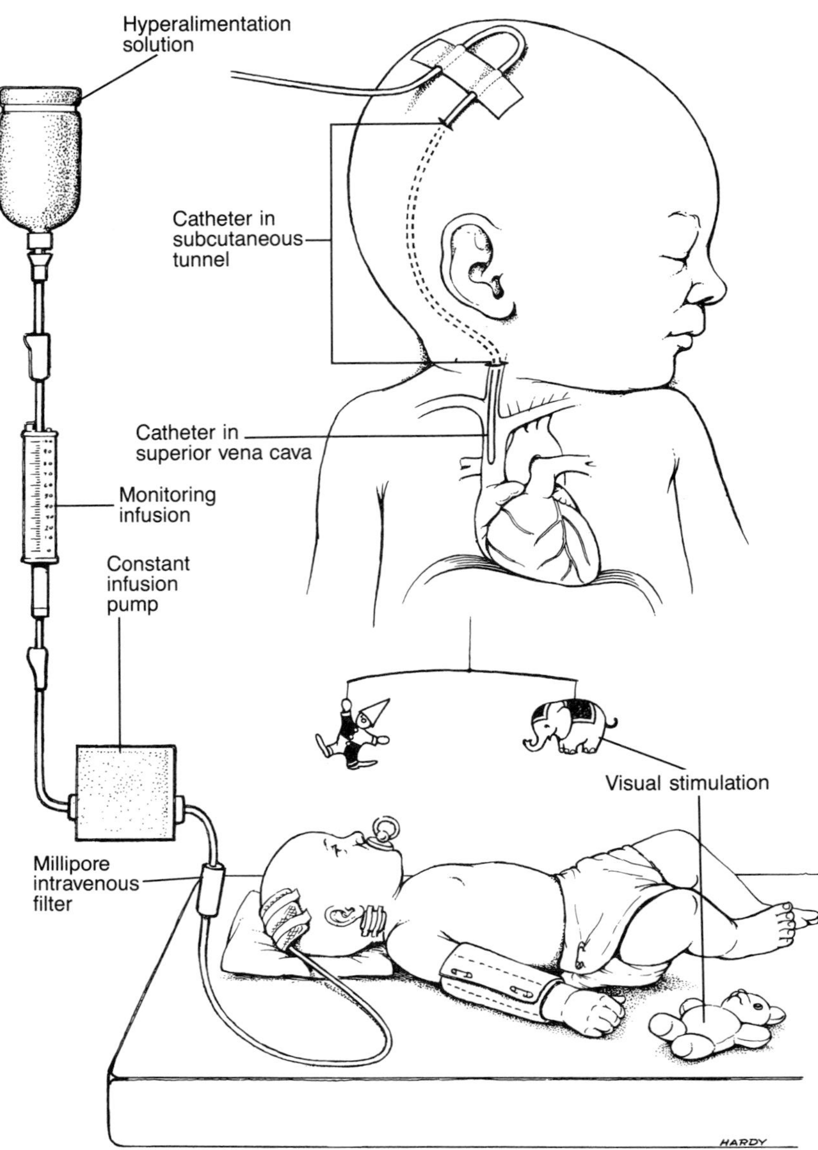

Figure 42-30.
Hyperalimentation.

tending pressure and ventilatory assistance methods have also been contributing factors.

In considering neurological and developmental deficiencies associated with low-birth-weight infants, data are confounded by the grouping together of premature (appropriate for gestational age) and SGA infants who also may have been born prematurely. In addition, varying criteria are used to define abnormalities, and the effects of socioeconomic status often are not included. With these limitations in mind, results of more recent studies indicate that low-birth-weight infants have IQ scores comparable to full-term infants at 2 to 5 years of age. Neurological studies indicate a decreased incidence of cerebral palsy, in the range of 3% to 4% compared to an average from previous studies of about 10%. Subtle neurologic deficiencies vary by study design, but it appears that visual impairments and speech abnormalities are not uncommon. Studies of growth generally demonstrate a lag in low-birth-weight infants compared to standard growth charts, with the SGA infants lagging in all parameters in comparison to appropriate-for-gestational-age infants of the same birth weight.[18]

Growth and development of the premature infant depend primarily on the degree of immaturity at birth. Much depends on the ability of the infant to meet the conditions attendant at birth and to adjust to the changes in the new environment. The majority (about 65%) of prematures weigh between 2000 g and 2500 g. Outcomes for these infants are good, barring complications. An additional 20% weigh 1500 g to 2000 g. If prompt good care is provided, they also have a chance of a good outcome. As birth weight decreases, chances of satisfactory growth and development also decrease, even though "survival" rates may be good. In general, infants who react well to prompt treatment and care usually make their adjustment by the end of the first year.

SGA infants with intrauterine growth retardation have different outcomes for growth and development depending upon the cause of retardation, the severity and duration of the intrauterine insult, the extent and management of perinatal asphyxia, and early diagnosis and management of various metabolic and physiological problems. Physical growth (weight, length, head circumference) does not catch up to normal infants during the first few years of life, even with adequate caloric intake. Studies have found that IQs of SGA infants are generally similar to those of normal children, and the incidence of overt neurological handicaps is low. However, there is a high incidence of abnormal electroencephalograms (EEGs), minimal brain damage, and school problems.[10]

The nurse is often asked by the parents if their premature or low-birth-weight baby will ever develop as well and become as strong and sturdy as a normal-sized newborn. Depending upon birth weight, the infant has a good chance of doing so.

The developmental level achieved by the small premature infant during his first year generally is lower than that expected for his chronologic age. For this reason, parents are encouraged to think of premature babies in terms of actual age since conception, which gives more realistic expectations for developmental level.

Parents of premature or low-birth-weight infants invariably need special guidance and support to help them develop confidence in their ability to care for their baby, particularly in anticipation of taking him home from the hospital. The nurse has a real responsibility to help them to be adequately prepared for the baby's homecoming.

■■■

Care of the Mother and Father

The parents of high-risk newborns often have adaptational needs or problems that necessitate sensitive and thoughtful nursing care. Not only are they making the transition to new parenthood with all its requirements, but they must cope with the unusual situation of a small, different, and often sick baby. The importance of the early postpartum period for the establishment of bonds between the parents and the newborn and the laying of the groundwork for healthy attitudes toward future relationships with the child must not be underestimated.

Interactional Deprivation

Prolonged mother–infant separation, such as is routine practice in most premature and high-risk nurseries, is currently under investigation for its effects on attachment. As soon as possible after the infant's birth, the mothers in the early contact group are admitted into the nursery and encouraged to touch their babies and to perform such caretaking duties as the infant's condition allows. Mothers in the late contact group are not permitted into the nursery until after their infants reach almost 1 month of age. Results to date reveal detectable differences in mothering performance between these two groups. In one study, high-contact mothers had higher scores on an attachment interview, maternal performance, *en face* feeding, and the amount of fondling of infants when tested 1 month after delivery.[19] In another study comparing late- and early-contact mothers 1 month after discharge of the infants, and after 200 feedings at home, the late-contact mothers held their babies differently, changed their positions and burped them less, and were not as skillful in feeding.[20] Some mothers who were barred from interaction with their babies in the nursery resumed prior interests when they returned home. The babies then had to compete with these interests when they were discharged.

Such studies suggest that prolonged separation may adversely affect commitment or attachment between mother and infant, reduce confidence in mothering abilities, and detract from the mother's ability to develop an efficient routine of care. When mothers were allowed into the high-risk nursery for early and frequent contact and caretaking of their infants, there was no increase in nursery infections or disruption of nursery routine.[21]

Modifying hospital routine to allow mothers early contact with their high-risk infants appears to have a positive effect on later maternal behavior (Figs. 42-31 and 42-32). This lends support to the concept of a sensitive time for bonding to occur between the mother and her infant. This time is probably within the first several hours of delivery. Greater maternal attentiveness and better caretaking seem related to later exploratory behavior in infants; thus, removing barriers to maternal attachment during the sensitive period may have a potent influence on the later development of these babies.

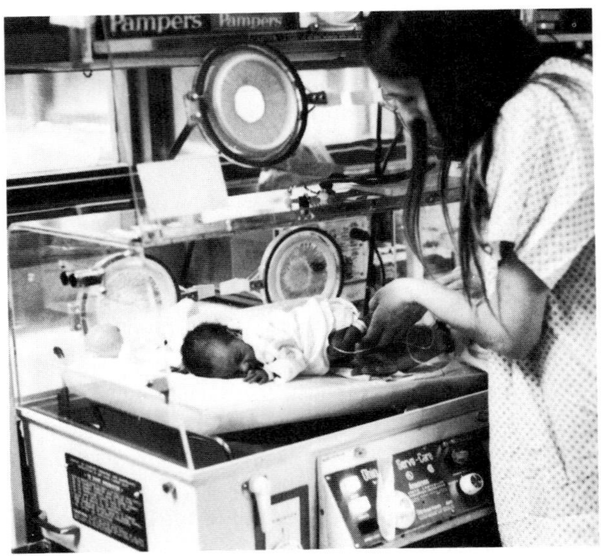

Figure 42-31.
Allowing the mother to attend to the infant in the incubator enhances mother-infant bonding.

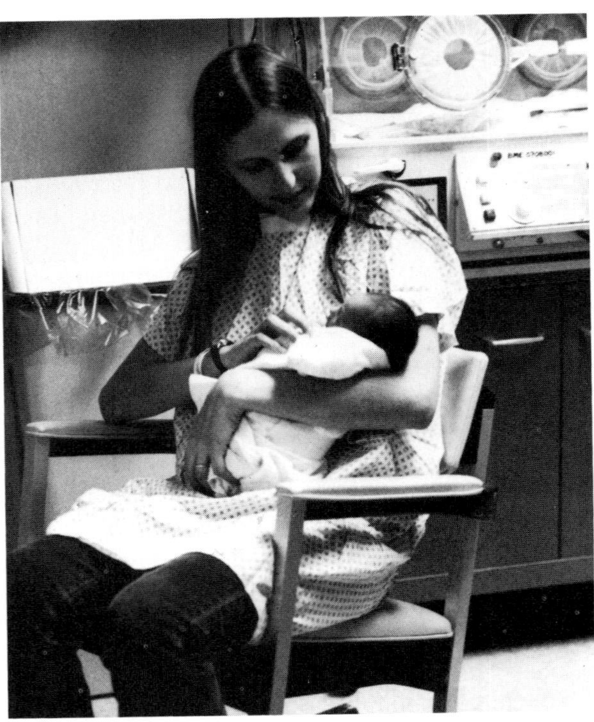

Figure 42-32.
En face contact between mother and infant should be encouraged when the infant is removed briefly from the incubator.

Parental Reactions and Psychological Tasks

The birth of a premature or high-risk infant is often experienced as an acute emotional crisis by the family. This causes a certain amount of disorganization in the parents before they are able to master their feelings and come to accept the event. Since the baby may be born before term, parents often are deprived of the last 6 to 8 weeks in which the final psychological (and sometimes material) preparation for the birth is made. Few of the physical and emotional signs of approaching labor (enumerated in Chap. 24) may happen. These are helpful to the mother in alerting her to the approach of another new phase in the childbearing process, and this awareness in turn assists her in achieving psychological preparation. The result may then be a rather abrupt arrival of the infant. The event may be surrounded by several anxiety-provoking features, such as an unattended delivery, a longer hospital stay for her baby and perhaps herself, separation from her infant, and most heart-rending of all, a delicate infant who may be in danger of death.

Guilt feelings and a certain amount of grieving in both parents are an invariable accompaniment. The parents ask themselves time and again such questions as, "What went wrong? What did we do? What made it happen? Can I really carry babies?" These guilt feelings and grief may be manifested in a variety of ways, including general anger with the whole situation, self-deprecation, numerous complaints, blaming the spouse or attendants, insistent bids for reassurance and attention, profuse crying, or extreme quiet and immobilization.

Loneliness is also a problem because the mother may have no opportunity to see, hold, feed, and examine her child as the other mothers have. We are all familiar with the wistful figure at the nursery window, gazing longingly through the glass, while the other mothers are occupied with feeding, changing, and cuddling their infants. The loneliness continues when the parents go home without their infant. Because of the continued separation, the task of integrating the new member into the household is delayed.

In addition, most mothers are concerned about whether they will be able to take adequate care of their babies when they do bring them home. The mother may still carry a picture of the frail infant surrounded by all the nursery paraphernalia and not realize that her baby will be reasonably mature when discharged from the hospital.

To cope with this concern, she may ask many questions while she is in the hospital and demand reassurance about the baby's condition; on the other hand, she may be quiet and uncommunicative, quite overwhelmed with the anticipated enormous responsibility.

The psychological processes the parents generally go through after the birth of a premature or high-risk infant include

Shock, disbelief and denial
Anger and searching self and others for causes
Grieving over loss of fantasized perfect infant
Grieving over own inability to produce perfect infant
Anticipatory worrying over loss of infant
Initiation of contact with infant
Belief and desire that infant will live
Readiness to establish caretaking relationship (Fig. 42-33)

Supportive Care

Although there is much that is specialized in the physical care activities for the premature infant, the mother's physical care remains generally the same as that for any normal postpartal course. Thus, the emphasis on care for these mothers is twofold: (1) they need help to facilitate their emotional adjustment (this holds true for the father as well) and (2) they need help in preparing for the care of the infant when they bring it home.

The nurse can do much to strengthen the mother's ego by helping her work through her guilt feelings and grief and thus reinforce her concept of herself as an adequate, worthy person. To do this, the nurse must provide opportunities for the mother to ventilate her feelings and to question the situation. It is often difficult for the nurse to answer all the questions the mother and father ask, especially if the prognosis for the baby is guarded. Yet, to avoid the questions or problems is to deprive the parents of a valuable avenue of coping with the problem. The fears and fantasies engendered by not knowing are often worse than the facts, even though the facts are unpleasant.

As the nurse listens to the mother and the father and reflects their concerns, they are helped to arrive

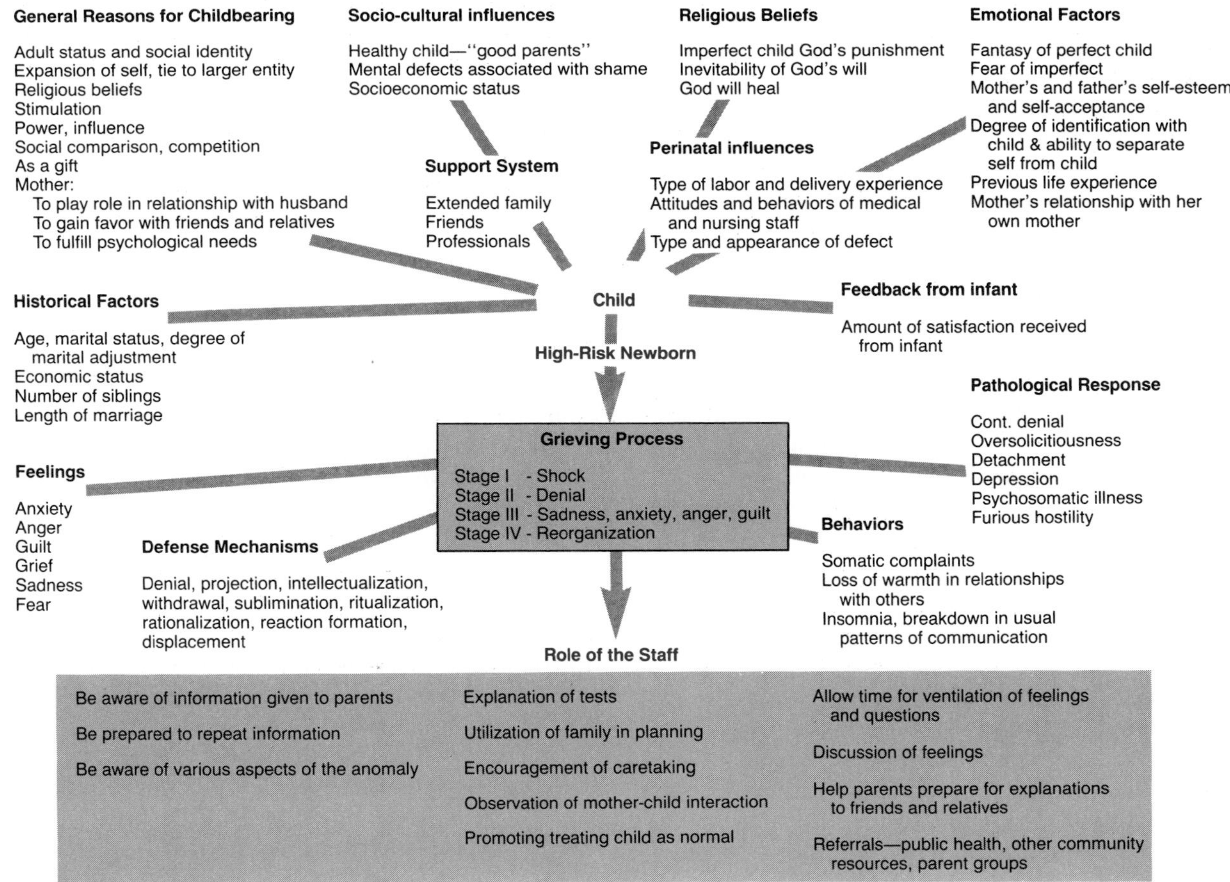

Figure 42-33.
Parental response to the high-risk newborn.

at a clearer notion of the reality of the situation. Thus they are able to separate fact from fancy and to work through to a more positive acceptance of their situation. The nurse can expect some negative feelings to be expressed, and the patient may go through a period of self-pity. An accepting, nonjudgmental attitude will help the patient move to a more positive frame of mind.

Keeping the lines of communication open between the nursery staff and the patient is another useful supportive measure. The nurse on the postpartal unit can be prepared with the latest reports regarding the baby's condition so that this information can be given to the parents. Especially when the mother cannot be taken to see her baby in the premature nursery, it is very helpful if the nurse in the premature unit can make regular visits to the mother on the ward to inform her of her infant's progress. If circumstances within the unit prevent this, contact with the mother by telephone may be substituted. This two-way communication between the floor and the nursery helps the patient to feel that everyone is "tuned in" to her situation and concerned about her. It also gives her the opportunity to know the personnel who are responsible for the care of her baby, and this is reassuring in itself.

Visiting the Nursery

When the mother is able, she can be allowed to visit the nursery, at least to observe her baby for a time. Some mothers find this difficult at first, especially if the infant is very small or ill. It is a wise nurse who allows the mother to indicate her readiness for such visits and gives appropriate encouragement as the mother becomes able to face the situation and take more responsibility.

Before the mother comes to the nursery, it is best to describe all the equipment surrounding the infant and what the baby will look like. The nurse's presence beside the mother when she first sees her baby permits any questions to be answered and provides support during this difficult period. If the infant is under the bilirubin light, it is important to remove the eye patches so the mother can see the baby's eyes.[20]

Other Sources of Support

All avenues of support are to be explored with the parents. If the mother seems to benefit from visitors or visiting with the other patients, then there need be no restriction on visiting privileges. There is no reason to isolate a mother in a room by herself (even if there has been a fetal demise) without ascertaining whether the mother needs to be alone for a time. If possible, the same nurse should be assigned to her care. If the mother is to work through her feelings, she must have time to build trust, and this takes at least several encounters.

Other personnel, such as the social worker, may be helpful if aid is needed financially or strict budgeting is necessary. Another source of help that can prove invaluable is the public health or visiting nurse. The need for a referral for these patients and their infants should never be overlooked. Most patients are delighted to have someone to rely on during the first difficult days when they bring the baby home. Furthermore, some patients cannot make much progress in expressing their feelings or in working the problem through during their short hospital stay. Thus, they need a competent person when they return home to help them in this, as well as in making necessary arrangements in preparation for the baby's homecoming.

Instructions for Home Care

Some hospitals encourage mothers to return to the nursery to feed and care for their babies until the time when the infant's condition permits discharge. Of particular help would be a counseling program on the feeding and psychological aspects of care that incorporates anticipatory guidance concerning the condition and the needs of the infant on arrival at home. Coping with sibling rivalry also may be included. This approach is very helpful, as it alleviates some of the separation and loneliness between mother and child and later fosters self-reliance and confidence in the mother at home.

Crisis Management

In implementing care, the nurse should remember that the advent of a high-risk birth is a crisis in itself; however, the parents may have to adjust to various related crises (*e.g.,* a sudden, downward turn in the baby's condition, financial embarrassment, unexpected developments regarding other children and relatives). Nurses must be prepared to help the parents to deal with these as they arise, and to seek appropriate resources for them if the matter lies beyond their competence. Knowledge of the principles of communication and supportive care will be utilized here as they would be in any other crisis. Willingness and ability to allow the parents to work through and vent their feelings about the situation is of prime importance. The nurse is one of the key persons in the care of high-risk infants and their parents.

NC **Nursing Care: The High-Risk Infant: Disorders of Gestational Age and Birth Weight**

Assessment	Intervention	Evaluation
Gestational age Thorough exam	Record indications of gestational age	
Respiratory distress	Monitoring vital signs Positioning Suctioning Provision of airway Administration of O_2 Chest physical therapy	Respiratory distress minimized
Nutritional needs	Daily weights Feedings as ordered—oral, gavage, nasojejunal Parental nutrition Administration of vitamins	Normal growth and development
Temperature instability	Use of appropriate "house"—isolette, open warmer	Stable temperature
Susceptibility to infection	Aseptic environment Hand-washing Appropriate isolation Aseptic care of equipment, intravenous lines, sites	No infection
Development needs Stimulation Nurturance Activity	According to development status of infant, provide balance of stimulation and rest. Hold and handle infant during feedings when condition permits.	Infant attains expected developmental landmarks for age, both neuromuscular and interactional.

(Continued)

Assessment	Intervention	Evaluation
Parent–infant bonding Contact Caretaking	Encourage bonding process through providing parents with information about status and characteristics of their infant, maximize parent–infant contact, support in caretaking activities, maintain telephone or written contact after mother is discharged, encourage visits to ICN for caretaking and holding.	Parents take active interest in progress and caretaking of their infant. Visit regularly after mother's discharge. Provide caretaking effectively.
Parental psychosocial needs Information and support Grief, reactions to anomalies Family adaptations	Provide information, discuss its meanings, encourage expression of feelings and reactions. Facilitate grieving process. Refer to other sources of support (parents groups, counseling, etc). Discuss family responses, needs of siblings, community resources.	Parents feel well informed and understand their infant's condition. Feelings of loss and grief are expressed as appropriate for the individual and family. Parents are able to interact and care for infant, or make decisions about alternate types of care. Family accepts and relates to infant, plans made for special care needs.

References

1. Hobbins JC, Berkowitz RL: Ultrasonography in the diagnosis of intrauterine growth retardation. Am J Obstet Gynecol 129, 5:957, November 1, 1977

2. Pilkin RM, Scott JR: The Yearbook of Obstetrics and Gynecology, p 1973, 1978. Chicago, Yearbook, 1978

3. Cheek DB, Graystone JE, Niall M: Factors controlling fetal growth. Clin Obstet Gynecol 20, 4:925–942, December 1977

4. Baker H, Thind IS, Frank O, DeAngelis B et al: Vitamin levels in low birth weight newborn infants and their mothers. Am J Obstet Gynecol 129, 5:521–524, November 1, 1977

5. Frigoletto FD, Rothchild SB: Altered fetal growth: An overview. Clin Obstet Gynecol 20, 4:918–919, December 1977

6. Klaus MH, Fanaroff AA: Care of the High Risk Neonate. Philadelphia, WB Saunders, 1973

7. Miner H: Problems and prognosis for the small-for-gestational-age and the premature infant. MCN 3, 4:221–226, July/August 1978

8. Olds SB, London ML, Ladewig PA, Davidson SV: Obstetric Nursing, pp 756–787, 805, Menlo Park, CA, Addison-Wesley, 1980

9. Sullivan R, Foster J, Schreiner RL: Determining a newborn's gestational age. MCN 4, 1:38–45, January/February 1979

10. Oh W: Considerations in neonates with intrauterine growth retardation. Clin Obstet Gynecol 20, 4:991–1003, December 1977

11. Whaley LF, Wong DL: Nursing Care of Infants and Children, pp 333–352. St Louis, CV Mosby, 1979

12. Usher RH: The special problems of the premature infant. In Avery GB (ed): Neonatology: Pathophysiology and Management of the Newborn, pp 230–261. Philadelphia, JB Lippincott, 1981

13. Stahlman MT: Acute respiratory disorders in the newborn. In Avery GB (ed): Neonatology: Pathophysiology and Management of the Newborn, pp 371–397. Philadelphia, JB Lippincott, 1981

14. Hodgman JE: Chronic lung disorders. In Avery GB (ed): Neonatology: Pathophysiology and Management of the Newborn, pp 398–411. Philadelphia, JB Lippincott, 1981

15. Phibbs RH: Delivery room management of the newborn. In Avery GB (ed): Neonatology: Pathophysiology and Management of the Newborn, p 189. Philadelphia, JB Lippincott, 1981

16. Avery GB, Fletcher AB: Nutrition. In Avery GB (ed): Neonatology: Pathophysiology and Management of the Newborn, pp 1002–1060. Philadelphia, JB Lippincott, 1981

17. Avery GB: The newborn. In Jelliffe DB, Jelliffe EF (eds): Nutrition and Growth, pp 129–152. New York, Plenum Press, 1979

18. Dangman BC, Driscoll JM: Impact of perinatal intensive care on outcome. In Aladjem S, Brown A (eds): Perinatal Intensive Care, pp 396–412. St Louis, CV Mosby, 1977

19. Klaus MH, Jerauld R, Kreger N, McAlpine W et al: Maternal attachment: Importance of the first postpartum days. N Engl J Med 286:460, 1972

20. Klaus, MH, Kennell JH: Mothers separated from their newborn infants. Pediatr Clin North Am 17:1015–1037, November 1970

21. Barnett C, Leidermann P, Grobstein R, Klaus M: Neonatal separation: The maternal side of interactional deprivation. Pediatrics 45:197, 1970

Suggested Reading

Bresadola C: One infant/one nurse/one objective: Quality care. American Journal of Maternal Child Nursing 2, 5:286–291, September/October 1977

Christensen AA: Coping with the crisis of a premature birth—one couple's story. American Journal of Maternal Child Nursing 2, 1:33–38, January/February 1977

Dubowitz LMS, Dubowitz V: Gestational Age of the Newborn. Menlo Park, CA, Addison-Wesley, 1977

Gabbe S: Recent advances in the assessment of fetal maturity. J Reprod Med 23, 5:227–234, November 1979

Hawkins–Walsh E: Diminishing anxiety in parents of sick newborns. American Journal of Maternal Child Nursing 5, 1:30–35, January/February 1980

Livingston R et al: Clinical assessment of gestational age. JOGN Nurs 6, 6:7–12, November/December 1977

Price E, Gyotoku S: Using the nasojejunal feeding technique in a neonatal intensive care unit. American Journal of Maternal Child Nursing 3, 6:361–366, November/December 1978

Rausch PB: Effects of tactile and kinesthetic stimulation on premature infants. JOGN Nurs 10, 1:34–42, January/February 1981

CHAPTER

43

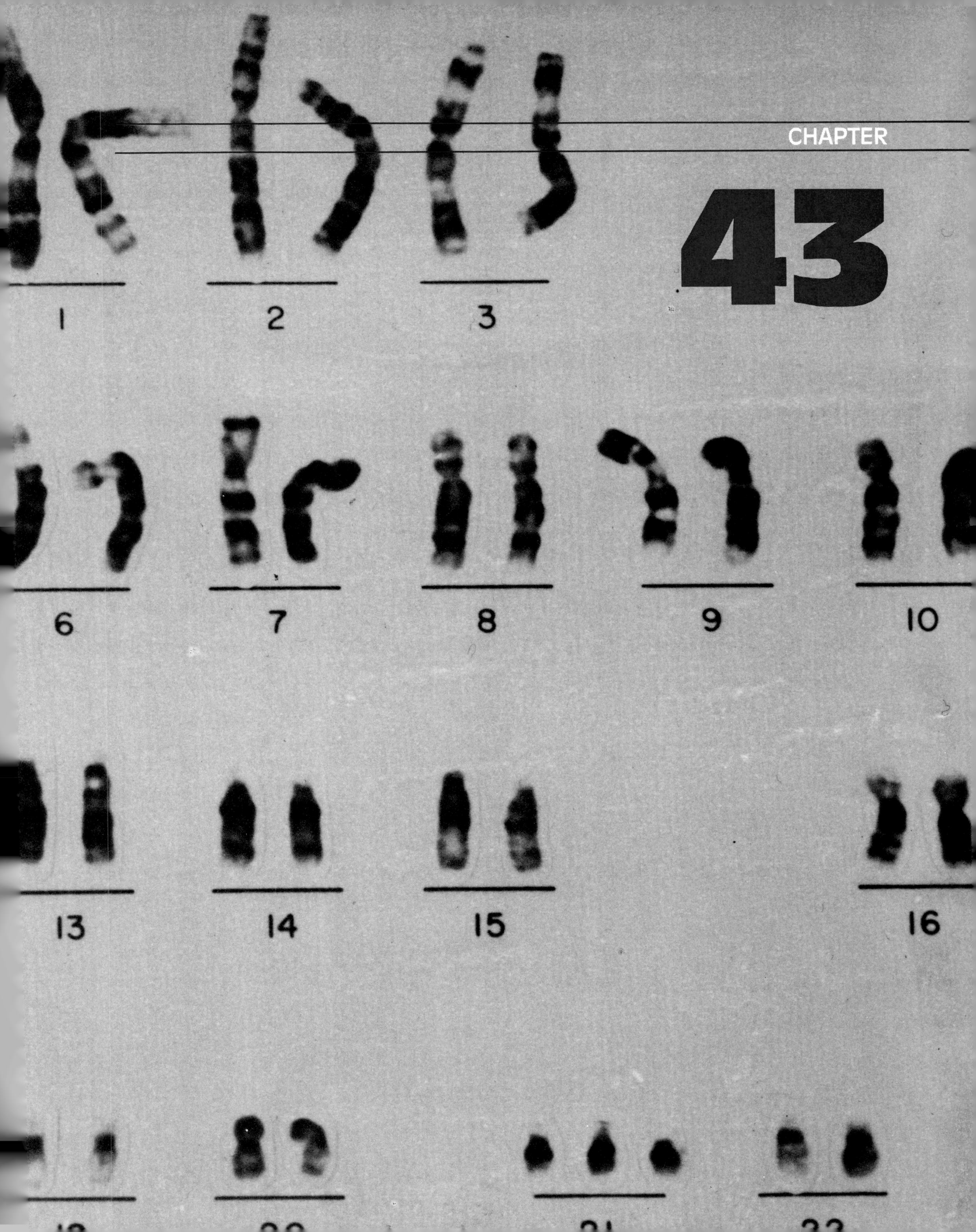

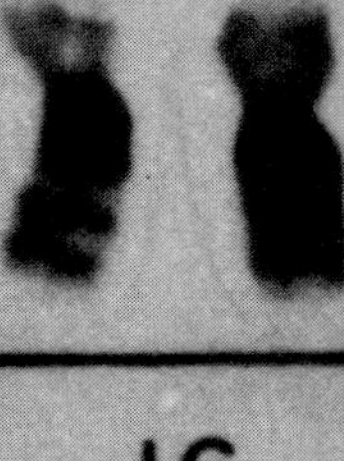

CHAPTER 43

The High-Risk Infant: Developmental Disorders

- **Parental and Staff Reactions to Defects and Disorders**
  - Working Through a Crisis
  - Avoiding Negative Communication
  - Telling the Parents
    - Realistic Appraisal and Reassurance
  - Acceptance of the Infant by the Staff
  - Grieving
    - Shock and Withdrawal
    - Denial and Disbelief
    - Anger and Sadness
    - Balance and Equilibrium
    - Reorganization and Restitution
  - Stillbirth or Neonatal Death
- **Congenital and Genetic Anomalies**
  - Congenital Heart Disease
    - Assessment of Manifestations
    - Murmurs
    - Oxygen Deficiency
    - Congestive Heart Failure
    - Types of Congenital Cardiac Anomalies
    - Nursing Care
    - Medical Management
  - Cleft Lip and Cleft Palate
    - Surgical Treatment
    - Nursing Management
  - Frenulum Linguae
  - Hypospadias and Epispadias
  - Ambiguous Genitalia
  - Spina Bifida
  - Hydrocephalus
  - Anencephaly
  - Microcephaly
  - Umbilical Hernia
  - Diaphragmatic Hernia
  - Obstructions of the Alimentary Tract
    - Atresia of the Esophagus
    - Pyloric Stenosis
    - Obstruction of the Duodenum and the Small Intestine
    - Omphalocele
    - Gastroschisis
    - Imperforate Anus
  - Chromosomal Abnormalities
    - Trisomy 13, or D
    - Trisomy 18, or E
    - Trisomy 21, or Down's Syndrome
    - Prevention and Management
  - Phocomelia
- **Inborn Errors of Metabolism**
  - Phenylketonuria
    - Diagnosis
    - Management
- **Musculoskeletal Disorders**
  - Talipes Equinovarus (Clubfoot)
  - Congenital Hip Dysplasia
  - Polydactyly
- **Conclusion**

NC Nursing Care: The High-Risk Infant

During labor, delivery, and the first several hours of neonatal life, many changes occur in the fetus and neonate that allow physiological adaptation to extrauterine life. Developmental characteristics of the infant may have significant influence on this process of moving from intrauterine to extrauterine life, such as genetic or congenital abnormalities and size and gestational age (see Chap. 42). Perinatal teams must be constantly alert to signs of complications in the neonate, with the objectives of identifying problems early, correcting disorders quickly (or minimizing subsequent effects), preventing permanent disabilities, and promoting the parental bonding process.

Parental and Staff Reactions to Defects and Disorders

The birth of an infant with congenital anomalies or developmental defects presents significant psychosocial stresses for the family and precipitates an adaptive crisis. A variety of emotional difficulties may interfere with the parents' relationship with the infant and disrupt functioning of the family. Parents often express feelings of anxiety, guilt, fear, inadequacy, helplessness, failure, and anger. The way in which parents cope with crisis and work through their feelings will influence how realistically they perceive their infant's medical condition and needs, how they are able to adapt to the infant's hospital environment, their ability to assume the primary caretaking role, their ability to assume responsibility for the infant's care after discharge, and, for some, how they will cope with the death of their infant (Fig. 43-1).[1]

Working Through a Crisis

Becoming a parent is a turning point in life, and it is particularly so for the parents of a child who has a disorder. They can emerge from this crisis less mentally and emotionally healthy than they were, or they can move on to increased maturity. If they utilize maladaptive coping mechanisms to deal with the crisis, the former no doubt will occur; if they can be helped to work through the problems positively, this experience will stand them in good stead for future stressful situations.

It is the responsibility of the members of the health team to help the parents cope with this situation adequately. However, staff members are only human, and at times they are hampered by their own anxieties, feelings, and fantasies. Thus, it is especially important for the staff to understand the psychodynamics occurring in both the parents and themselves so that they may choose a therapeutic course of action to help the parents.

During pregnancy, all women wish for and fantasize about a perfect child. They also fear that their babies might be abnormal. Their fantasies of the expected child are a composite of the images of the people who are important to or admired by them. When the infant deviates drastically from the anticipated child, the simultaneous occurrence of the sudden loss of the idealized child and the necessity of accepting a deviant child can be overwhelming. The greater the deviation from normal, the greater the impact of the experience can be.

It is important to remember that the parents have to grieve for the lost perfect child before they can form an attachment to the imperfect one. The process of grief involves anger, which can be directed toward anyone involved in the situation—including the infant. Mourning also impairs the capacity to recognize, evaluate, and adapt to reality appropriately. Thus, whenever possible, long-range planning for the infant should be delayed until the parents, particularly the mother, can participate in them; otherwise the mourning and depression may persist for an undue length of time.

Anxiety is another dominant reaction. It is thought that the sources of the most serious anxiety are the threats to the parents' sense of adequacy, self-esteem, and social status. One of the earliest questions expressed, "What caused this?" is charged with feelings of biological inadequacy. Indeed, what the parents are really asking is, "What's the matter with us as progenitors of children?" Particularly for the mother, her failure to produce what she has so long prepared herself to create may well be a threat not only to her femininity, but to her whole unique personhood as well. Moreover, these feelings hold true even for those who have not consciously planned the child or who have had several children. Procreating a defective child strikes at the very core of the woman's being. This is very understandable; the child just born is still, in effect, an extension of the mother, and a defect in him is tantamount to a defect in herself. The degree of the mother's anxiety is also related to a deep narcissistic wound, since the psychological work during pregnancy includes an increase in narcissism. Feelings of shame and embarrassment are the general accompaniment of personal feelings of inadequacy.[1]

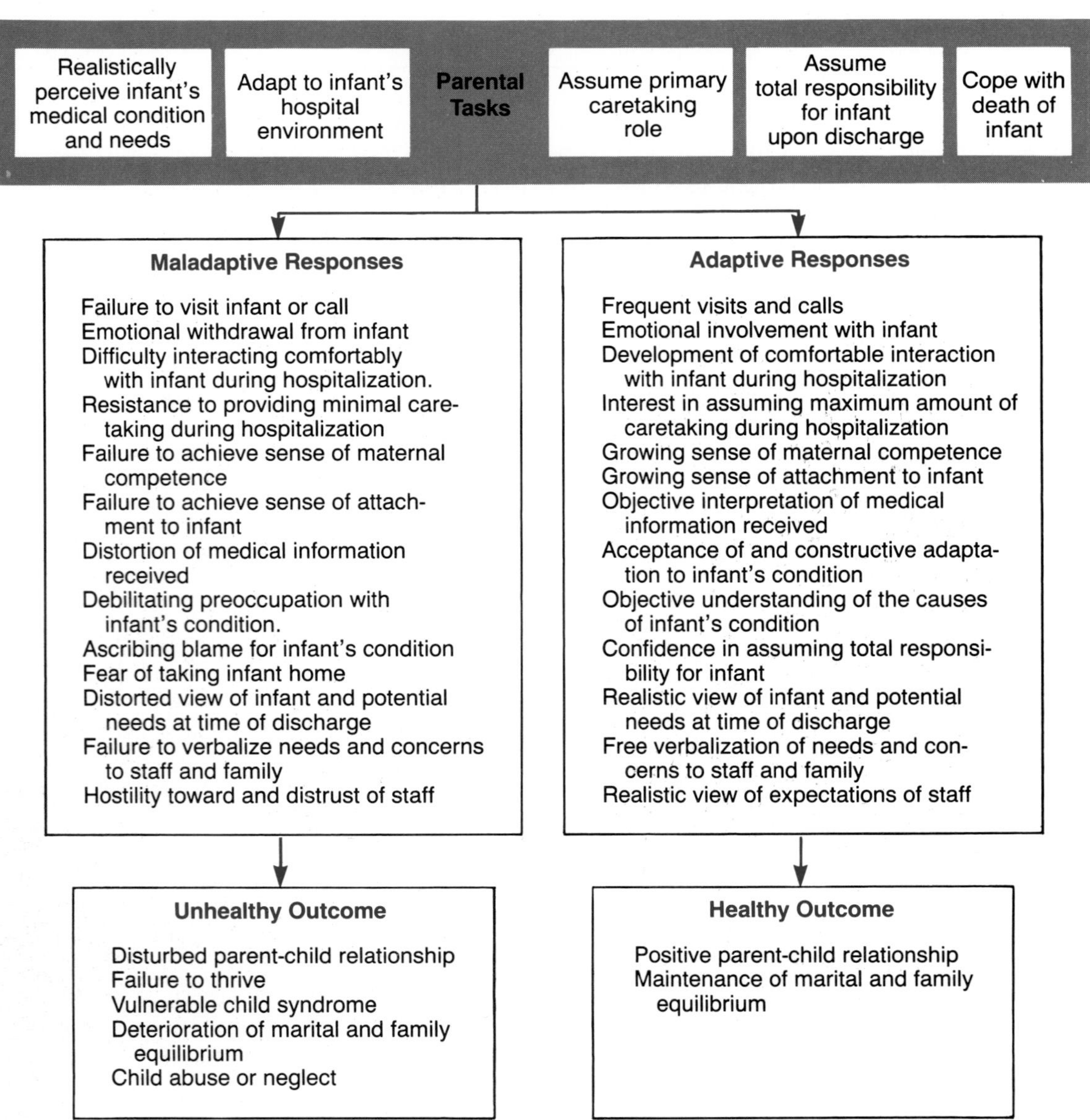

Figure 43-1.

Parental response during crisis period. (Grant P: Psychosocial needs of families of high-risk infants. Family and Community Health 1, 3:93, Nov 1978. An Aspen Publication. Article code 0160-6379/78/0013-0091.)

Some of the variables affecting the parents' coping behaviors include past experiences the parents have had in their own growing-up period. If their childhood experiences have fulfilled their needs for mastery, they will have gained trust, security in human relationships, feelings of optimism and the ability to cope, and freedom from crippling guilt and fear. They will also have learned tolerance for frustration. All of these will be of great help to them in their present crisis. Positive experiences with other handicapped or retarded adults and children can also affect the degree of concern and attitude the parents have. On the other hand, if they remember hostility directed toward a defective person, or if they (or others) responded to that person with guilt, pity, repugnance, or overprotectiveness, these feelings may become reactivated as they confront the abnormality of their child.

Another variable that may influence the response of the parents to their stress is the degree of energy they have at their disposal at the time of the crisis. The mother who has had a long, physically exhausting labor has less energy for coping with stress than the mother who has had a rapid, nonexhausting one. The father who has been at the mother's side coaching her during labor and delivery has less reserve than one who has not performed the physical and emotional effort that accompanies coaching. In addition, having to attend to other-related life situations, such as making emergency preparations for the care of other children or making arrangements for job-related problems and the like, also takes away valuable energy needed for coping.[2]

Many other variables such as differences in class, economic background, the physical and emotional maturity of the parents, the birth order of the child, its sex, appearance, and prognosis also influence the responses of the parents. All of these variables may have important bearing on the immediate significance the event will have for them.[2]

Avoiding Negative Communication

In the delivery room, the physician, patient, and nurse are intensely involved with one another. Interactions are characterized by intense alertness to behavioral cues.

Whenever a disorder is apparent at birth, especially if it is of any magnitude or of a long-term nature (an anomaly, acute respiratory distress), the tension may be prolonged and intensified instead of being released in the more customary ways. The physician and the nurse will know about the disorder immediately or shortly thereafter. Their verbal and nonverbal behaviors are apt to convey their shock and disappointment to the mother. Their posture may become rigid or they may use their bodies to shield the baby from the mother. Their conversation may dwindle or cease. If an emergency ensues, their actions quicken and conversation is exclusively directed to each other and is of a technical nature. The mother may sense this heightened tension and become increasingly aware that all is not well.

It is not always possible for the staff to stop their activities and to respond to the mother's questions; not only are their efforts often going into lifesaving measures for the infant, but they are having to cope with their own emotional reactions. For instance, it is not unnatural for the staff (and the parents later) to have, and perhaps to express, death wishes for a severely defective child. They feel frustrated and resentful toward a situation that they can neither control nor, in many cases, change. It may be an extremely difficult time for the physician, who may have a sense of failure because the patient cannot be "healed." The mother, in turn, may sense the attendants' frustration and misinterpret it as hostility or resentment toward her—that she also has "failed." This negative communication only intensifies the trauma that is experienced by all concerned. In addition, the new mother feels sadness, a completely different emotion from the joy she had anticipated; furthermore, it comes at a time when she may be physically and emotionally exhausted.

Telling the Parents

Most professionals agree that the mother and father should be informed as soon as possible (preferably immediately) of the disorder. However, some tend to seek or develop strategies for delaying the announcement of unpleasant news. If this occurs, it can mean significant and far-reaching consequences for the mother and father. The mother expects to see or at the very least be told about her infant. If this does not happen, she becomes suspicious and alarmed and eventually mistrustful. The important immediate establishment of a "trust" relationship will be impeded.

Sometimes, however, the abnormality makes the condition of the infant so critical that he must be transferred immediately to the intensive care nursery (ICN), and the mother may not see her baby. Therefore, *what* the parents are told about the condition and *how* they are told become critical issues. All too often, one hears parents complain bitterly about the bluntness, coldness, and unconcern that the staff demonstrated. Worse still is the "conspiracy of silence" that tortures the already overwrought pair, in which each professional avoids saying anything, pretending or assuming that the other will handle the matter, or that it is better left alone. It is important to recognize that the apparent coldness, avoidance, and so on, are not really manifestations of the staff members' true feelings, but rather are unsuccessful coping mechanisms to allay their feelings of helplessness, anxiety, and inadequacy. However, it is part of the nurse's professional responsibility to explore these feelings and to develop more effective ways of handling them.

Cues to the best type of intervention are obtained by observing the parents' behavior. The mother cannot invest feeling in the defective child until she can feel and talk about her disappointment, sense of failure, helplessness, or fears regarding the infant's health and future. The process of grieving is facilitated through repeated discussions before reality can be faced. Interpretations of the baby's condition must be synchronized with this mourning process so that the parents can assimilate facts and reality as they move through the process. When anger or guilt is not expressed, tremendous energy is utilized to contain it, and this energy can be better used later in forming a viable relationship with the child. Moreover, the lack of opportunity to discuss their feelings will hinder the parents' ability to test reality. Therefore, it is necessary that each fear be clarified as the parents are able to bring it into consciousness. In this way, distortions of thnking, feeling, and perception are reduced.

To accomplish this, nurses and other professional personnel want to encourage parents to react as fully as they desire by providing an emotional climate and physical environment where the parents are assured their behavior and feelings are accepted. An attitude of warmth and acceptance that is communicated by actions (physical care, comfort measures, simply sitting with the couple), as well as words, helps the couple regain self-esteem. It may be difficult for the professional personnel because our culture frowns on frank expression of deep feeling. Yet it is much easier for the parents to accept their own feelings if those feelings are accepted by the professionals around them. A mother feels understood if the nurse conveys to her that her feelings and behavior are natural.

The nurse wants to be particularly cognizant of maintaining communication regarding the parents' responses to their situation, the condition of the infant, and any other factors that have bearing on the situation. In this way, a coordinated effort can be made by all members of the health team for comprehensive care.

Realistic Appraisal and Reassurance

Many authorities think that, in order to be given a realistic appraisal of the situation, the parents should be informed immediately of the disorder and the prognosis, especially if repair or long-term care is involved. This information, of course, must be explained in terms that the couple can understand, and reinforcement over the days of hospitalization probably is necessary.

Whatever specifics are told, it is important that two aspects of realistic reassurance be given the mother and father: first, that they and their child are acceptable and, second, that the hospital and personnel are there to render any assistance possible. Particularly in the cases of some defects and deformities (*e.g.*, phocomelia or myelomeningocele) the parents must understand that, although their child may not be made whole, he usually can be helped to some degree. This kind of reassurance demonstrates an attitude of understanding and sharing of the parents' feelings of hurt and loss, and, at the same time, it does not minimize the gravity of the situation.

Acceptanc of the Infant by the Sta

The parents' ırst encounter with their infant is another crucial time. Particularly in cases in which there is an obvious anomaly, it is vitally important that the physician or the nurse who is showing the baby demonstrate an attitude of warmth and acceptance of the infant; if revulsion or rejection is manifested, the parents' own feelings of despair and ostracism will be intensified.

One way the staff can demonstrate to the parents that their child is valuable and important is to hold him close, cuddle him, and call him by name. At this time, if it seems to be indicated, the positive points in the prognosis can be reiterated or reinforced. This may be a difficult time for all concerned, as staff members are also trying to cope with their own possible feelings of rejection. Therefore, an attempt should be made to avoid a common kind of destructive behavior that tends to be demonstrated unconsciously, that of isolating the infant under the guise of protecting the mother.

Grieving

Grief can be considered a response to loss. It is most often known to us as a response to a loss through death or separation of a loved person, but it can occur following the loss of anything, tangible or intangible, that is highly valued. Grief is a universal, normal, developmentally evolved adaptive process. It progresses through predictable phases, and this progress enables the individual to deal adaptively with the disturbance of his psychological equilibrium that is inevitably caused by loss. The parents can be expected to show signs of grieving when a substantial defect in their infant (or death) occurs. The couple must come to terms with a difficult and perhaps unexpected situation, one in which the prognosis may be poor. Both parents demonstrate grief, and the father's needs, as well as the mother's, should be kept in mind.

Several phases are encountered in the grief reaction. How intensely the parents experience these varies according to the nature and the gravity of the disorder and their capacity for grieving.[3]

Shock and Withdrawal

The first phase of grief involves shock and difficulty in believing that their baby has a malformation or disorder. There is often a great urge to flee, and fathers may literally leave the situation. The parents may appear stunned or immobilized, or may try to carry on ordinary activities; intermittent flashes of anguish and despair occur as reality penetrates. Occasionally, there is an overtly intellectual response to the reality of the situation in which the mother or father may try to comfort the other, make any necessary arrangements, and so on. This type of response takes place only if the full emotional impact is not allowed to reach the consciousness. The loss is recognized, but its painful character is muted. This phase may last from minutes to days; the longings for a perfect child may be recalled, felt intensely, and discharged gradually. This process serves to free the parents' feelings so that they may proceed to the next phase.[3]

During the shock phase, the parents may initially withdraw. This is a strategy to escape the painful reality of the situation; hence, at times they want only silence and solitude. It is important not to label this behavior as "rejection of the child." If criticism of this kind is manifested or implied, the parents' anger may be directed toward the child so that they continue to not wish to see him. These parents are experiencing great psychic pain and their concerns naturally center on their own feelings. They are trying to sort out what this defect or illness means to them personally. Nurses can be of great assistance if they respond to withdrawal with understanding and a great deal of empathy, even in the face of seeming disinterest and apathy. This demonstration of generosity helps relieve the mother's feelings of guilt about her lack of motherliness if the nurse helps her to understand that such feelings always develop gradually as a mother cares for and handles her child.

On the other hand, the mother may indicate an *initial* overprotectiveness toward the infant. This behavior should also be respected because it is a defense against the mother's anxiety and disorganization. Self-pity may become displaced as pity for the child and, if the nurse is critical of this attitude, the defense will only be strengthened. Hence, the mother is not to be made to feel that others are trying to intrude between her and her infant. Those appropriate aspects of nurturance and care that she attempts to give can be reinforced and praised. Gradually she can be helped to realize the limits of her assistance.

Denial and Disbelief

The second phase is one of denial or disbelief that this could have happened to them. The parents wish to believe that their baby does not have a problem. This phase is affected by many factors, a significant one being the visibility of the malformation. The denial period may be longer with such conditions as Down's syndrome or other types of mental retardation that might not become clearly apparent for some time.[3] The more obvious defects demand more immediate recognition and admission that the problem does exist. The birth of a defective child may have grave implications for the marital bond. After the immediate shock of the birth, the parents, in this second stage of grieving, begin to reflect on the many problems facing them because of the defect. Often, one of them becomes very concerned about imparting information about the deviation to the other, and sometimes to close family or friends as well. This concern will be especially evident if the parent feels responsible in some way because of a family history of congenital defects, irresponsibility, or the like. This concern is manifested irrespective of whether the marriage is stable. Submergence of one's own feelings in deference to the partner's may occur in more stable unions, whereas blame may be attributed in less happy marriages. This latter response, particularly, only adds another source of stress. If either partner was afraid of what the birth of the baby might do to their relationship, the fears will only be intensified with the birth of a defective or ill child.

Anger and Sadness

The third phase involves anger and sadness, and often interweaves with the second period of denial. With developing awareness, there is often a feeling of loss and disappointment, accompanied at times by affective and physical symptoms (*i.e.,* emptiness in the epigastric or chest regions, sadness, and the like). Now the painful feelings are allowed to become conscious. The parents (particularly the mother) may cry, express anger toward a variety of persons and things, talk about the situation, or be unable to express any verbal emotions, although they may want to.[3]

A relationship between the nurse and the parents that is based on helping is most effective at this time; the nurse's approach should be dictated by the parents' reactions. By accepting and encouraging the expression of feelings (and providing privacy for their expression), the nurse helps to prepare the way for the next phase. Developing awareness may take a long time—days or months. The nurse in the hospital usually sees its beginning, but very infrequently sees its termination.

During the grieving process, the mother needs more physical rest than the usual postpartum patient because she needs increased energy to cope with the tragedy. Regression is natural at this time as dependency needs are increased in the presence of anxiety.

By responding to the mother's increased need for personal care, the nurse demonstrates acceptance of both the mother and the child. By caring for the baby and showing affection and interest in him, the nurse demonstrates a realistic investment in him. This reassures the mother that the child is worthwhile and others can love and accept him—this allays her feelings of inadequacy over time. The nurse wants to be alert to the times when the mother shows signs of wanting to learn to care for the infant. Fortunately, mothers are now given more opportunities to care for and feed their infants, even when the infants are in a special nursery.

Balance and Equilibrium

The fourth phase is a period of relative equilibrium during which some of the intense reactions have lessened. There may be little emotional resiliency at this time, however. Additional stresses can disrupt this tenuous balance, for example, the development of a new complication such as pneumonia in an infant with a congenital anomaly. With new stresses, the parents may lapse into the previous phase or begin the process over. Progression in the equilibrium phase is assisted by positive caretaking experiences.

The feeding experience is extremely significant for the mother. When she can feed her infant and sense some response in him, she will begin to have some tangible, positive reinforcement that she can perform a crucial nurturing activity for her baby. Thus, her self-esteem is increased. It must be remembered, however, that every time the mother does feed (or performs any other care-giving activity for) her infant, she must face the baby's defect or illness, and her initial feelings of anxiety, frustration, and guilt are apt to be reactivated. These initial feelings gradually diminish with successful trials of feeding or care giving. However, if the mother refuses to feed her infant or prefers to "skip" one or two feedings, it is wise to be unblaming. Nothing is to be gained by pushing the mother into prematurely caring for the infant. As the mother learns to feed her infant and do other specific activities for the infant, she channels some of her own dependency feelings into the activities and gradually gains confidence in her competence as a mother.

The arrival of a defective or ill child makes great demands on the father. This fact is often overlooked; attention is more frequently directed toward the mother because she is hospitalized. Often, the father's responsibilities are so overwhelming that he cannot perceive or provide the support his partner so earnestly needs. Unless he too receives assistance in coping with his feelings about the birth, he may have difficulty assuming his caretaking relationship. He needs to know that his feelings are important—that he is being considered as a person, not just as an expeditor. As he realizes that his grief is acceptable and that the professionals care about what he is experiencing, he is able to cope with his feelings better and able to offer more support to the mother.

Reorganization and Restitution

The fifth and final phase is that of reorganization, which over months and years may allow the parents to reach a better state of emotional organization than before they experienced this crisis. Self-esteem can often be improved, and such parents may be more able to tolerate other stresses and tragic events and be helpful to other parents and children.[3]

During restitution, mourning occurs, in which mutual grief and loss are expressed by the parents, sympathetic friends, and relatives. At this stage, religious beliefs and rituals are helpful in clarifying the ambiguity about suffering, eternity, and death. In this, the final phase of grief, resolution of the problem gradually occurs; this phase may take from 6 months to a year.

Stillbirth or Neonatal Death

Occasionally, parents and staff are faced with the unfortunate circumstance of a stillbirth or a neonatal death. All of the responses of both personnel and parents that have just been described may be apparent in these cases. Grief and mourning are noted particularly, and it becomes the nurse's responsibility to provide an environment in which the mother and father can express their feelings. Nursing care is essentially the same as that described above.

It appears that the length and intensity of mourning over the death of an infant is proportionate to the closeness of the relationship prior to death. Moreover, it has been found that caring for an infant who subsequently dies, or touching or fondling a dead infant is not unduly upsetting to an emotionally healthy mother (one who does not have a history of psychiatric problems). All too often, the reason given for not allowing the mother and father contact with their dying or dead infant is that it will be too upsetting. It is now known that affectional bonding is enhanced (as with all babies) with tactile stimulation and caretaking and that this type of contact does not result in pathologic grieving. It appears that affectional bonding is necessary in order that the parents may relinquish the dead child and work through the symbiotic relationship that existed before birth. Thus, a strong sense of grief appears to be a normal phenomenon of the grieving process and should not be considered pathologic or abnormal.

One of the most frequent complaints of parents, and especially mothers, is that the staff, including nurses, does not "know what to do with me." That is, the mothers are treated as if nothing has happened and no mention is made of the tragedy; this is part of the "conspiracy of silence" that was mentioned previously. It is difficult to outline specific nursing measures because the ability to interact and the depth of interaction depends to a great extent on the nurse's own feelings about death (or deformities) and personal experience in dealing with death and dying.

One approach is for the nurse to express sympathy or sorrow that the tragedy had to happen to the mother. This may start the mother crying, but this emotional demonstration need not be feared. The nurse may then put an arm around the mother and encourage her to continue, assuring her that this and other grieving behavior are acceptable. If the mother continues to cry, the nurse should gently reassure her. If the mother begins to talk about the tragedy, the nurse is able to pick up cues which may call for further reassurance that she was not "guilty" of anything. Factual information may also be called for. It may be that, initially, the nurse is able to express only sadness and ask if the mother would like to talk about it. The general goal is to meet the parents' spoken and unspoken cries for compassion, understanding, and factual information.[4]

The nurse must be careful not to offer the mother unhelpful platitudes, such as, "Please don't feel so bad. You have such lovely children at home," or "You can always have another baby." Statements of this kind not only are unhelpful but are detrimental to the situation. They convey to the patient the nurse's great lack of understanding and appreciation of the situation. The parents trust the nurse to the degree that they perceive an understanding and empathetic manner; to this same degree they trust and permit the nurse to help them arrive at a positive solution of their problem.

Congenital and Genetic Anomalies

The etiology of birth defects is not completely understood, but a multifactor etiology is generally accepted. It is recognized that most of these defects have an environmental component in their causes.

Malformations may arise from

1. Genetic factors such as change in the chromosome number, mutation, or structural abnormalities
2. Environmental factors, such as irradiation, infection, and drugs

It should be emphasized that the most frequent of the genetically influenced malformations are multifactorial. These defects result from interactions among multiple genetic and environmental factors.

There are approximately 250,000 babies born each year with abnormalities that cause a significant alteration in the structure or function of their bodies. The incidence of these disorders has not changed greatly over the decades; however, the techniques of prenatal diagnosis, repair, and correction have improved immensely, thus offering a great deal of hope and consolation to the parents and children who are afflicted with these conditions. Indeed, there is increasing specialization in *teratology*—the study of the relationship of genetic and environmental factors in the production of congenital abnormalities.

Congenital deformities may range from minor abnormalities, such as supernumerary digits, to grave malformations incompatible with life, which include *anencephalia* (absence of the brain), *hydrocephalus* (excessive amount of fluid in the cerebral ventricles with tremendous enlargement of the head), and various *heart abnormalities*. These grave defects are second only to accidents as a cause of death in childhood. Moreover, these youngsters represent a serious community health problem when one considers the numerous sequential surgical procedures and the attendant expense these families must undergo. In addition, the special rehabilitation and education that many require, plus the drain on the parents' time and emotional and physical reserves, can have a grave social impact.

Because these conditions are so numerous and varied, this section presents selected disorders—those more commonly seen that are apparent at birth or soon thereafter or those with which the maternity nurse will have to deal. The care of these infants and their parents presents a great challenge to the nurse, who must give competent and, at times, complex nursing care to the babies as well as help the parents to convert their feelings of disappointment and despair into constructive efforts at habilitation of the infant. In addition, the negative feelings that are aroused in the nurse must be controlled.

Congenital Heart Disease

At the time of birth and for weeks thereafter, there are great changes in the circulatory system of the newborn. When the cord is clamped and expansion of the lungs occurs, the pulmonary circulation increases in volume. The foramen ovale, the ductus arteriosus, and the ductus venosus are no longer needed and therefore close gradually over a period of several months.

Usually, the foramen ovale is closed by the third month of life and the ductus by the second; during the period of closure, signs or symptoms of patency rarely occur. When they do, they may be an indication of defects in these structures or other parts of the heart.

Congenital heart disease has an incidence of about 7.5 per 1000 at birth. Cardiovascular malformations account for approximately 1.2 deaths in 1000 births during infancy.

The role of heredity as an etiologic agent is not yet well understood. Congenital lesions may be recorded in as many as three generations, and siblings seem to manifest the disease more often than in the preceding or succeeding generations. *Maternal disease* during pregnancy, such as rubella or diabetes, influences the bodily structures of the developing fetus. Yet the etiology and dynamics of cardiovascular lesion are not known definitively. However, there is a higher incidence of other congenital defects such as Down's syndrome among infants with congenital heart disease. Thus, the infant may suffer from multiple disorders.

Assessment of Manifestations

Distress from congenital heart disease is often hard to distinguish from the distress that is secondary to pulmonary disease, such as respiratory distress syndrome (RDS). Yet accurate diagnosis is essential so that effective cardiac surgery can be instituted when indicated.

The physical signs of the normal and the abnormal newborn infant, such as right ventricular overactivity, behavior of the second heart sound, and color, are governed largely by the pulmonary artery pressure level, the rate of constriction of the ductus arteriosus, and the amount of placental transfusion. These are important and can mask the signs of congenital heart disease.

Murmurs

Murmurs are abnormal heart sounds usually caused by turbulent blood flow being shunted between two heart chambers or vessels. The auscultation of a murmur is a common sign of congenital heart disease. Murmurs must be followed by a workup—chest x-ray film, electrocardiogram (ECG), and echocardiogram in order to rule out more serious cardiac disease. Various types of murmurs represent significant findings in certain cardiac defects, such as ventricular septal defect (VSD), atrial septal defect (ASD), and patent ductus arteriosus (PDA).

Oxygen Deficiency

It must be remembered that peripheral cyanosis occurs a great deal in the newborn period; arterial blood oxygen tensions are significantly lower shortly after birth than they are several days later. Thus, cardiac malformations associated with severe arterial oxygen desaturation later in the neonatal period may be present in a relatively acyanotic form. This is due to the good mix of oxygenated and unoxygenated blood that results temporarily from continued patency of the ductus arteriosus or foramen ovale.

Cyanosis, however, is a much more threatening sign than a murmur. One third of infants with potentially lethal congenital heart disease have cyanosis as a major sign.

Congestive Heart Failure

In addition to murmurs and cyanosis, the newborn with congenital heart disease frequently presents with signs of congestive heart failure.

Clinical Manifestations of Congestive Heart Failure. Some signs noted by the nurse may be failure to feed well as a result of easy fatigability, diaphoresis, failure to gain weight, tachypnea, respiratory distress, hepatomegaly, tachycardia, decreased systemic arterial pulses, and edema.[5,6]

Diagnosis is established from the history, physical findings, and roentgenographic and electrocardiographic examinations. If doubt still exists, cardiac catheterization, angiocardiography, and aortography usually supply the needed confirmatory data.

Types of Congenital Cardiac Anomalies

Transposition of the Great Vessels. The aorta originates in the right ventricle rather than the left, and the pulmonary artery originates in the left ventricle rather than the right. There must be an abnormal communication between these vessels to maintain life.[5]

Atrial Septal Defect. An abnormal opening between the right and left atria persists after birth, with left to right shunting of blood. This may result from failure of the foramen ovale to close properly, or there may be other defects high in the ostium secundum or basally in the ostium primum.[5]

Patent Ductus Arteriosus. The vascular connection between the pulmonary artery and aorta, which is functional during fetal life, persists after birth, rather than closing as it normally does. When the duct remains patent after birth, the direction of blood flow through it is reversed because of the higher pressure in the aorta, thus shunting oxygenated aortic blood into the pulmonary vasculature. During fetal life, the shunt is from the pulmonary artery to the aorta.[5]

Ventricular Septal Defect. There is an abnormal opening between the right and left ventricles. This varies in size and may occur in the muscular or membranous portion of the septum. Shunting of blood from the left to right ventricles occurs during systole because of higher left ventricular pressure. If, however, pulmonary vascular resistance produces pulmonary hypertension, the shunt is reversed, and occurs right to left with resultant cyanosis.[5]

Coarctation of the Aorta. There is a constriction of the aorta, causing narrowing of the lumen; this partially obstructs blood flow, creating increased left ventricular pressure and work load. The coarctation may occur before or after the ductus arteriosus, and there are great variations in anatomic features of coarctations.[5]

Tetralogy of Fallot. Four defects are combined in this anomaly, which is the most common defect causing cyanosis in children who survive beyond 2 years of age. There is pulmonary stenosis, ventricular septal defect, overriding aorta, and hypertrophy of the right ventricle. The severity of symptoms depends on the size of the ventricular septal defect, degree of pulmonary stenosis, and degree to which the aorta overrides the septal defect.[5] Figure 43-2 illustrates these types of congenital cardiac anomalies.

Other Cardiac Defects. There are other types of cardiac anomalies, including tricuspid atresia, pulmonary and aortic stenosis, overriding aorta and truncus arteriosus, and anomalous venous return. Surgery can repair some of these defects, and, in some instances, restore the infant to normal cardiac functioning. Others cannot be repaired and often are incompatible with life.

Nursing Care

Nursing care of infants afflicted with congenital heart disease is directed at offsetting those factors that aggravate symptoms.

The following nursing goals must be kept in mind:

1. Reduction of the work of the heart
2. Maintenance of nutrition
3. Reduction of respiratory distress
4. Prevention of respiratory and other infection
5. Reduction of the parents' anxiety, and their support and teaching

Every precaution is taken to protect the infant from exposure to infection. The principles discussed in the chapter on care of the immature infant apply here. In addition, unnecessary disturbance is to be kept at a minimum because startling or physical effort often distresses these babies.

When the infant shows signs of severe respiratory distress, relief is sometimes achieved by elevating the head of the bed or placing the baby in an infant seat.

Profuse diaphoresis is often seen and sponge baths with tepid water can supplement the daily bath.

Feedings are usually given more frequently and in smaller amounts than to the healthy term infant. The aim, of course, is to avoid undesirable pressure of a distended stomach on the diaphragm and heart. If the infant can suck without distress, a bottle is the best feeding method. If bottle feeding results in cyanosis or impaired respiration, gavage feeding may be necessary. Strict intake and output are vital nursing measurements to be taken, as well as daily weights. Supportive care is necessary for the parents of these babies; keeping lines of communication open between the parents and the staff (*i.e.,* obstetrician, pediatrician, heart surgeon, nursery nurses, and pediatric nurses) does much to help alleviate anxiety and help in the adjustment to the idea of having a child with cardiac disease.

Medical Management

Drugs that may be utilized in congestive heart failure include morphine, digoxin, oxygen, and lasix. Low-sodium formula may be given, such as Similac Pm 60/40.[5]

Cleft Lip and Cleft Palate

The cleft lip and the cleft palate, which may occur separately or in combination, result from the failure of the soft or bony tissues of the palate and the upper jaw to unite during the fifth to tenth weeks of gestation. The defect may be unilateral or bilateral (Fig. 43-3). Only the lip may be involved, or the disunion may extend into the upper jaw or the nasal cavity.

Each year about 1 in 1000 white infants and 1 in 2000 black infants are born with a cleft lip or cleft palate; thus, this condition is one of the most common of birth defects. More males than females appear to be affected by the combination cleft lip and cleft palate disorder. Cleft palate alone has an increased incidence in females.

A clear-cut etiologic pattern for these deformities remains obscure. Variables found to be associated with them include genetic factors, drugs (particularly corticosteriods), radiation, hypoxia *in utero,* maternal illness during pregnancy, and dietary influences. The hypothesis has been put forward that palatolabial defects may be due to sex-modified multifactorial inheritance.[7]

Transposition of the great arteries

This anomaly is an embryologic defect caused by a straight division of the bulbar trunk without normal spiraling. As a result, the aorta originates from the right ventricle, and the pulmonary artery from the left ventricle. An abnormal communication between the two circulations must be present to sustain life.

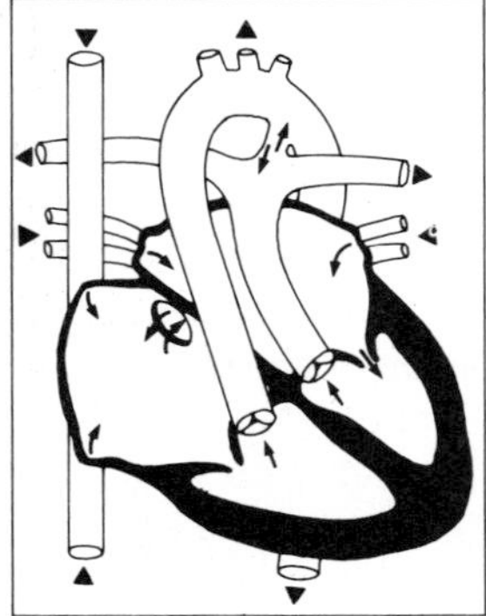

Atrial septal defect

An atrial septal defect is an abnormal opening between the right and left atria. Basically, three types of abnormalities result from incorrect development of the atrial septum. An incompetent foramen ovale is the most common defect. The high ostium secundum defect results from abnormal development of the septum secundum. Improper development of the septum primum produces a basal opening known as an ostium primum defect, frequently involving the atrioventricular valves. In general, left to right shunting of blood occurs in all atrial septal defects.

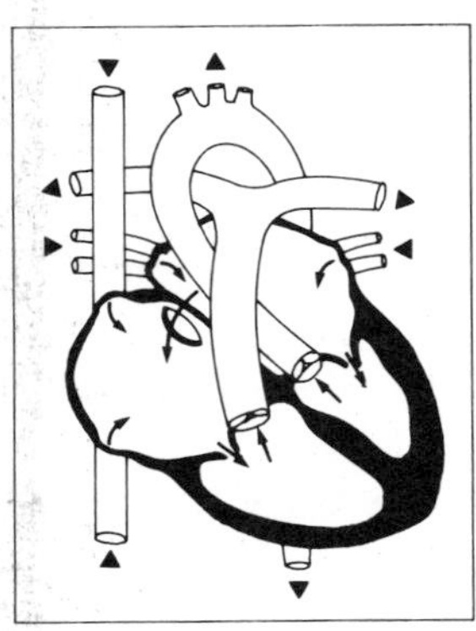

Patent ductus arteriosus

The patent ductus arteriosus is a vascular connection that, during fetal life, short circuits the pulmonary vascular bed and directs blood from the pulmonary artery to the aorta. Functional closure of the ductus normally occurs soon after birth. If the ductus remains patent after birth, the direction of blood flow in the ductus is reversed by the higher pressure in the aorta.

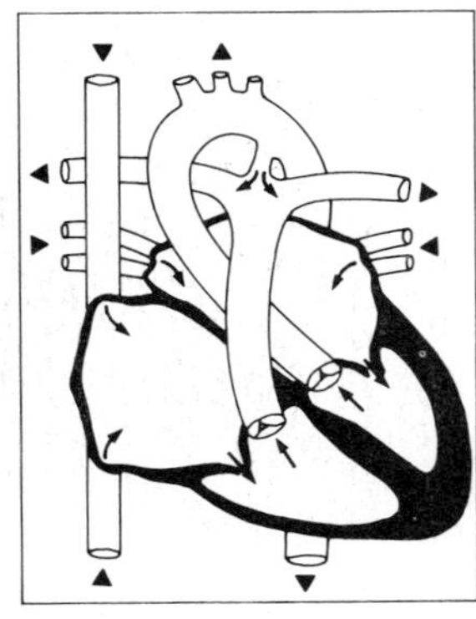

Ventricular septal defect

A ventricular septal defect is an abnormal opening between the right and left ventricle. Ventricular septal defects vary in size and may occur in either the membranous or muscular portion of the ventricular septum. Due to higher pressure in the left ventricle, a shunting of blood from the left to right ventricle occurs during systole. If pulmonary vascular resistance produces pulmonary hypertension, the shunt of blood is then reversed from the right to the left ventricle resulting in cyanosis.

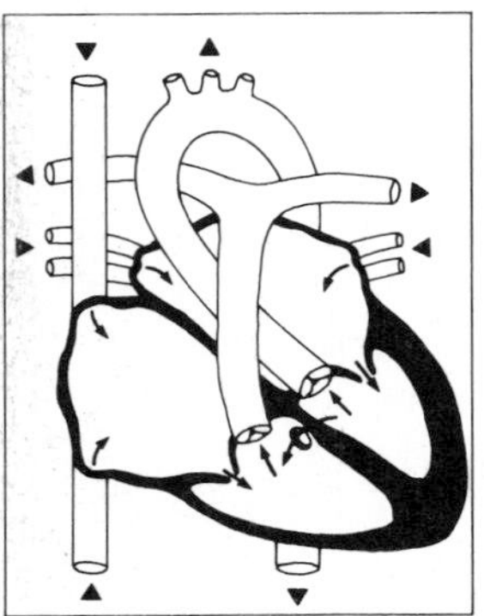

Coarctation of the aorta

Coarctation of the aorta is characterized by a narrowed aortic lumen. It exists as a preductal or postductal obstruction, depending on the position of the obstruction in relation to the ductus arteriosus. Coarctations exist with great variation in anatomical features. The lesion produces an obstruction to the flow of blood through the aorta causing an increased left ventricular pressure and work load.

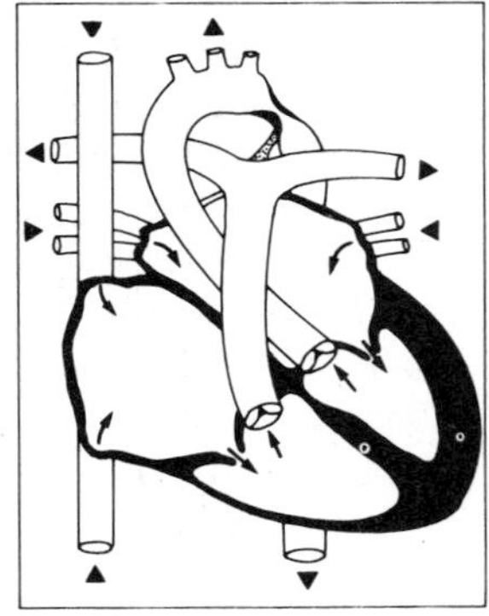

Tetralogy of Fallot

Tetralogy of Fallot is characterized by the combination of four defects—(1) pulmonary stenosis, (2) ventricular septal defect, (3) overriding aorta, and (4) hypertrophy of right ventricle. It is the most common defect causing cyanosis in patients surviving beyond two years of age. The severity of symptoms depends on the degree of pulmonary stenosis, the size of the ventricular septal defect, and the degree to which the aorta overrides the septal defect.

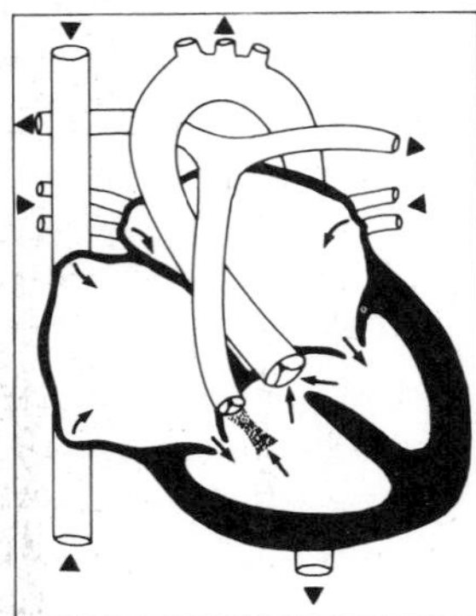

Figure 43-2.
Six types of congenital anomalies. (Courtesy of Ross Laboratories)

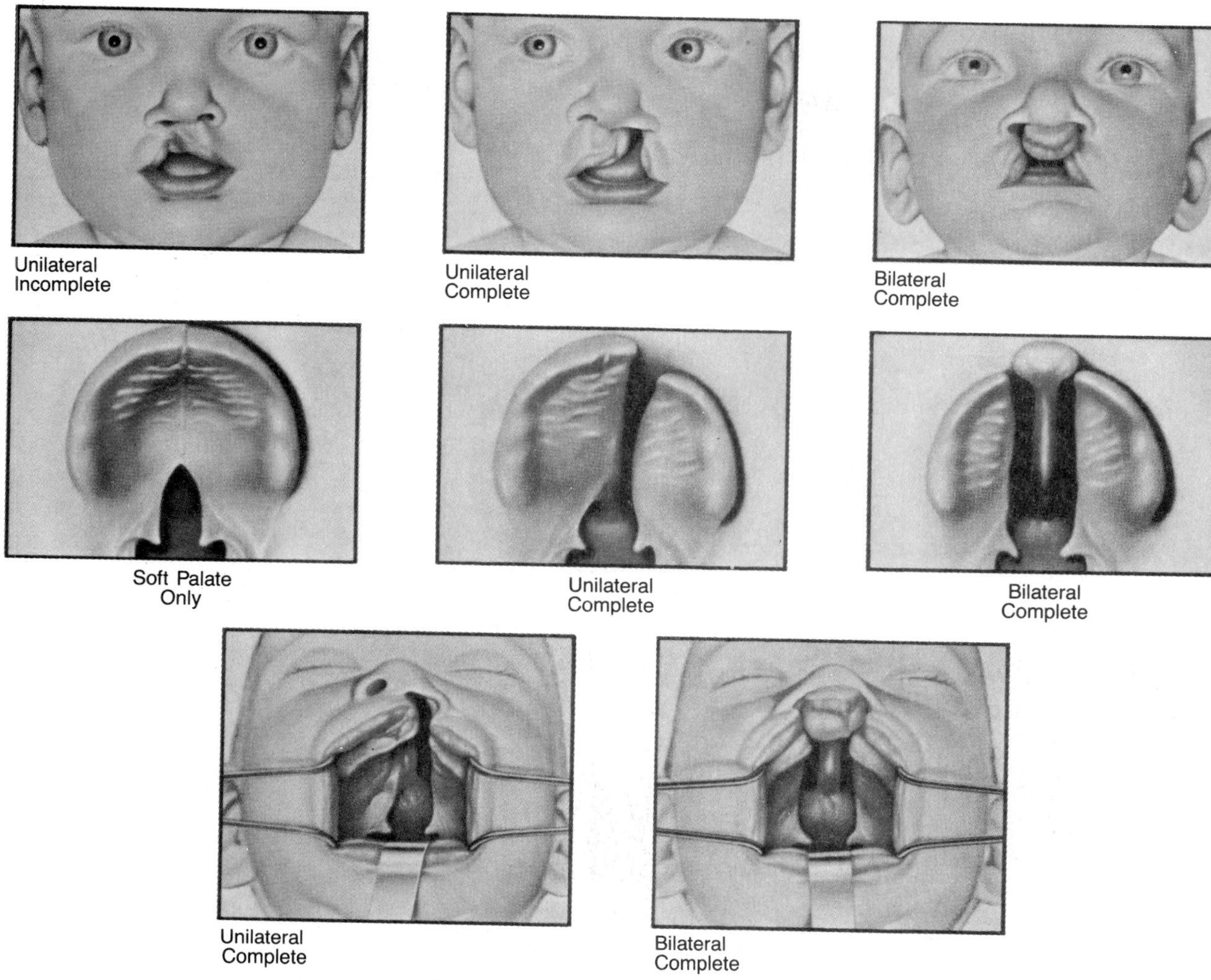

Figure 43-3.
Illustrations of cleft lip and cleft palate. (Redrawn from drawing provided by Ross Laboratories)

Surgical Treatment

The plan of treatment and outcome depends on the severity of the condition. If only the lip is involved, surgery may take place within the first few days, although some physicians prefer to wait until the child is 8 to 12 weeks of age because they feel that there is more tissue available at that time to facilitate operative precision. When the palate is involved, the repair is usually postponed until the child has aged from 6 months to 5 years. Time is not the only salient variable; it is even more important that the child be free of infection and nutritionally sound.

When surgery is performed later, a prosthetic speech device usually is fitted so that speech development may not be hindered. Cleft palates usually involve other difficulties, such as frequent respiratory infections and orthodontia and speech problems. Therefore, the care of these children involves the coordinated activities of the pediatrician, plastic surgeon, orthodontist, hospital and community health nurses, speech therapists and, very often, the social worker. Fortunately, modern treatment is so effective that these defects become a relatively minor handicap.

The parents require a great deal of supportive help initially, especially since this disorder is so disfiguring. In our culture, a high value is put on physical attractiveness. When this condition occurs, particularly if the baby is a girl, it may come as a tremendous shock and burden to the parents. However, repair is generally successful, and it is very helpful if the parents know and understand this. Members of the team involved in the reconstruction process can visit the parents after a comprehensive assessment of the infant has been made. To assure them that the defect is correctable, color transparencies are shown of an infant with a similar defect and the results of the surgery. Such visual reassurance has been found to be more effective than any verbal explanation.

The pattern of treatment is explained so parents can understand and begin to participate in the feeding and care of their child.

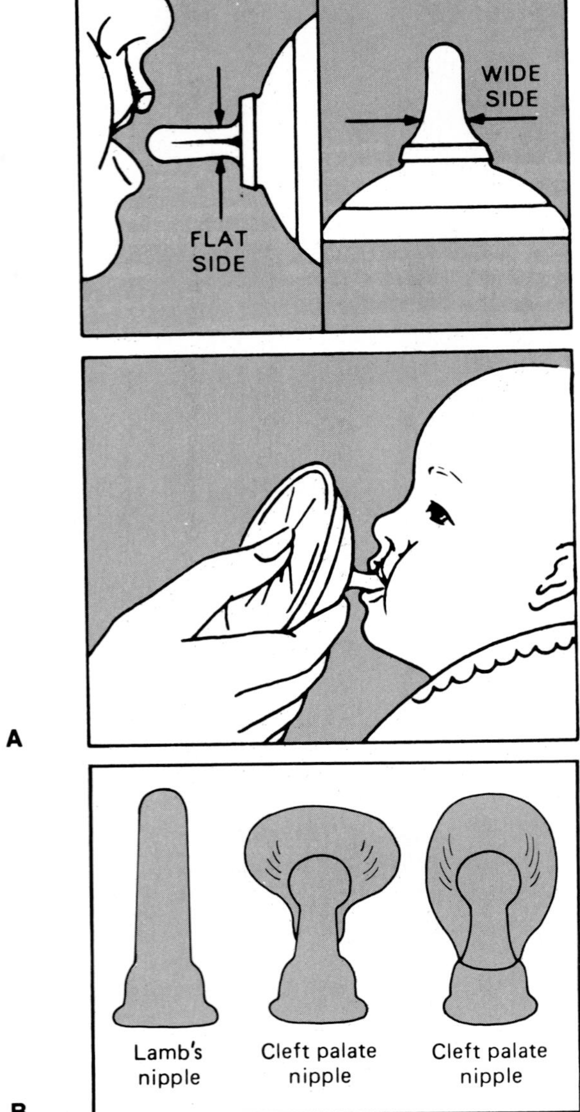

Figure 43-4.
Nipples used for feeding babies with cleft lip and palate. *(A)* Beniflex Nurser. *(B)* Other types of nipples. (Beniflex Nurser courtesy of Mead–Johnson)

Nursing Management

Feeding is usually one of the most immediate and difficult problems in the daily care of the infant with a cleft lip or cleft palate. It can best be accomplished by placing the infant in an upright position and directing the flow of milk against the side of the mouth. This will decrease the possibility of aspiration as well as the amount of air swallowed during feeding.

Since sucking strengthens and develops the muscles needed for speech, a nipple is used for feeding whenever possible. A variety of nipples may be tried, including a regular nipple with enlarged holes, a soft rubber nipple, a presoftened "preemie" nipple, a Beniflex nurser, a cleft-palate nipple, or a duck-bill nipple (Fig. 43-4). The last two are more expensive. Specific instructions are necessary with their use. If the infant cannot use any of the nipples, then a spoon or a rubber-tipped asepto syringe may be tried. The flow of milk must be adjusted to the infant's swallowing and should not be stopped until the infant attempts to suck.

The feedings are given at a pace that neither causes the infant to become unduly tired nor results in aspiration of the liquid. Thickened formulas are often used. Since these infants tend to swallow large amounts of air, they should be bubbled at frequent intervals. The mother needs to be instructed in this technique.[8]

The nurse should help the mother to attain ease in feeding her baby and should arrange to stay with her during several of the sessions. This is one way of assessing how well the mother is progressing.

Gavage feeding usually is unnecessary and should be used only when the other methods fail, since it does not stimulate the sucking and swallowing reflexes, and promotes aspiration.

The mother may want to breast-feed her infant, and there is no contraindication as long as the milk can be given in a way that the baby can take it. This may mean that the mother may have to express her milk and offer it in a bottle.

Frenulum Linguae

The frenulum of the tongue is a sharp, thin ridge of tissue that arises in the midline from the base of the tongue and is attached to its undersurface for varying distances toward the top. When the attachment extends far forward, a concavity or groove is apparent at the tip of the tongue on its upper surface. This has been called tongue-tie. It rarely interferes with feeding nor produces a speech impediment, as formerly thought. Therefore, incising the frenulum is not indicated because it provides a portal of entry for infection and there is danger of severing the large vein in the area of the frenulum.

Hypospadias and Epispadias

In *male hypospadias,* the urethra opens on the under surface of the penis proximal to the usual site. Minor degrees of this condition are quite common, and no surgical intervention is necessary. If the opening is at the base of the penis or far back on the shaft, plastic surgical repair is necessary.

In *male epispadias,* the urethral opening is on the dorsal surface of the penis. If the defect is pronounced, it also will require repair. Surgical correction is usually made by 2 years of age.[8] Definitive urethroplasty should be performed before the boy enters school so that it will be possible for him to urinate in the standing position. Since the foreskin is used in the repair, boys with hypospadias are not to be circumcised (Fig. 43-5).

In *female hypospadias,* the urethral meatus opens into the vagina, whereas in *female epispadias,* the upper urethral wall is absent, with possible exstrophy of the bladder. Serious types of genitourinary abnormalities often occur with numerous other anomalies.

Ambiguous Genitalia

Infants may be born with ambiguous or uncertain genitalia, or with characteristics of both male and female genitals (Fig. 43-6). Abnormal sexual differentiation in fetal development can be due to genetic defects (adrenogenital syndrome, Klinefelter's syndrome, Turner's syndrome) or to the intrauterine hormonal environment (steroid sex hormone therapy given to the mother to prevent abortion). It is important for the nurse to report any instances of questionable genitalia because establishment of genetic sex and sexual rearing are critical to later compatible psychosexual development. Chromosomal sex, as well as the morphologic characteristics of internal and external sex organs, are taken into consideration in sex assignment.

Often surgery to convert genitalia to one or the other sex is necessary, as well as later hormonal therapy to promote the development of secondary sex characteristics. Intersex problems represent an area of specialty, and appropriate referrals to experts in this field are indicated.

Spina Bifida

Spina bifida is a rather common malformation (1:500 live births) and is due to the congenital lack of one or more vertebral arches, usually at the lower part of the spine (Fig. 43-7*A*). When the membranes covering the spinal cord bulge through the opening, the condition is known as *meningocele* (Fig. 43-7*A*). It forms a soft, fluctuating tumor filled with cerebrospinal fluid. The tumor can be diminished by pressure. It enlarges

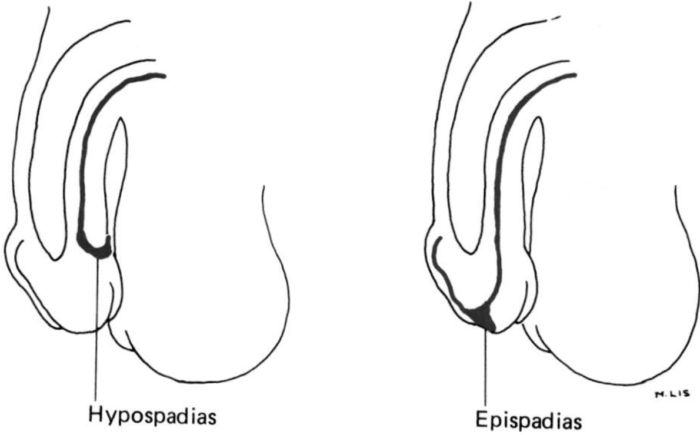

Figure 43-5.
Illustration of hypospadias and epispadias.

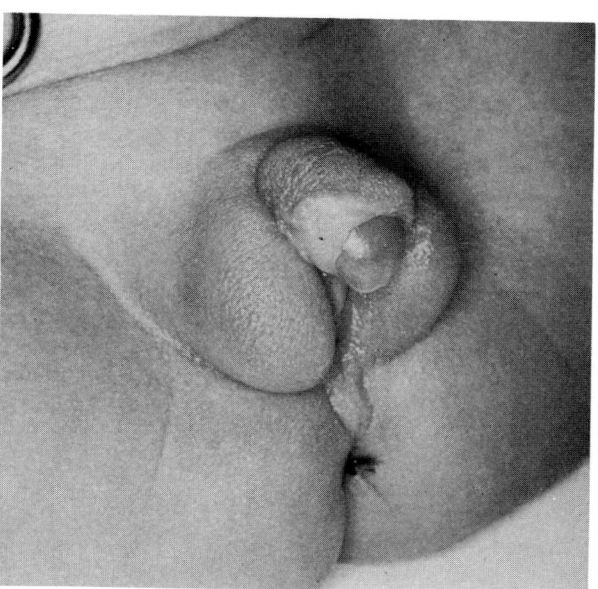

Figure 43-6.
Infant born with ambiguous genitalia. From this photograph it is difficult to tell whether this patient has an atypical penis with penoscrotal hypospadias or whether there is extreme masculinization of the clitoris and scrotal changes of the labia majora (Avery GB: Neonatology: Pathophysiology and Management of the Newborn, 2nd ed. Philadelphia, JB Lippincott, 1981)

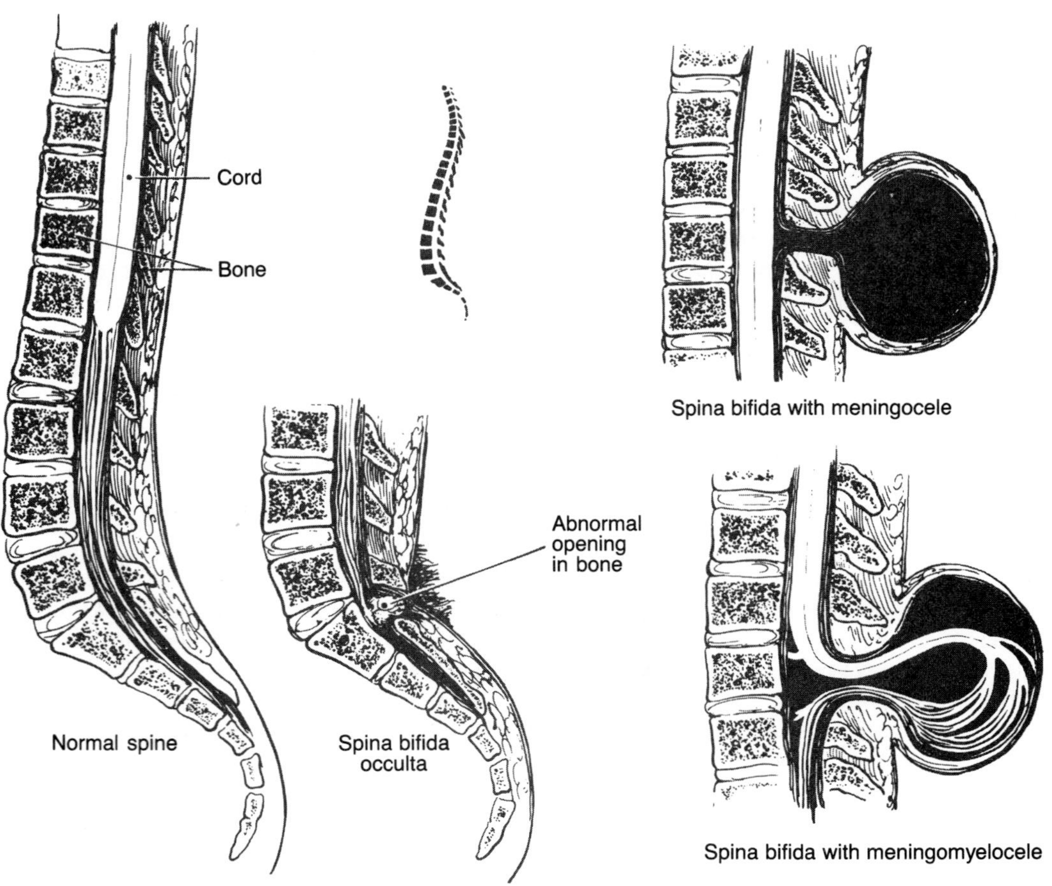

Figure 43-7A:
Spina bifida. (Spina Bifida: Hope through Research. PHS Pub. No. 1023, Health Information Series No. 103, 1970)

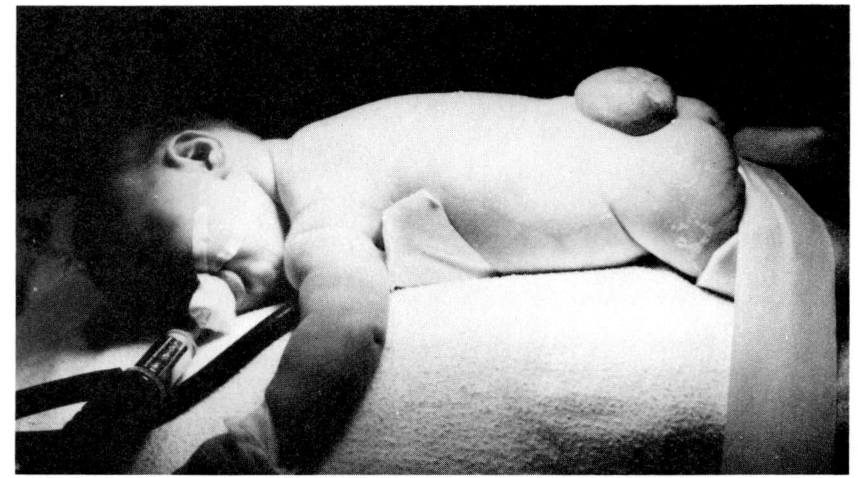

Figure 43-7B.
Meningomyelocele in the lumbosacral area. The patient is in a prone position with supporting blanket rolls beneath a heating blanket. (The heating blanket is not shown. Mayer BW: Pediatric Anesthesia: A Guide to Its Administration. Philadelphia, JB Lippincott, 1981)

when the baby cries. The extrusion of the cord along with the coverings is known as *meningomyelocele* (Fig. 43-7*A* and *B*). Most surgeons advocate early surgical closure, in the first 12 to 18 hours after birth.

When the repair is massive, the outlook can be discouraging. Hydrocephalus may occur if not already present. The situation and prognosis for the infant may be guarded, and the parents need a good deal of support and instruction about the continuing care of their infant.

Many infants with neural tube defects die or suffer from neuromuscular impairments if they survive. Permanent impairment depends upon the level of the defect and the extent of central nervous system tissue involvement. Prenatal diagnosis can identify neural tube defects through use of ultrasound, amniography, or increased levels of α-fetoprotein in the amniotic fluid or maternal serum. Anencephaly can also be diagnosed prenatally by these techniques.

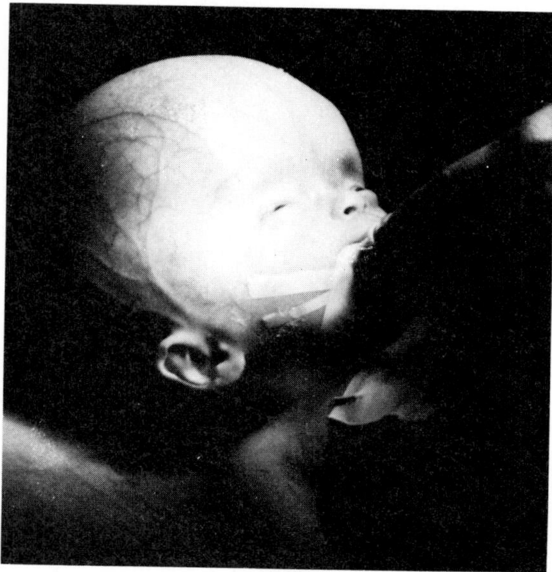

Figure 43-8.
Hydrocephalus. Note the enlargement of the head, the prominent veins in the skin, and the "setting sun" appearance of the eyes (Mayer BW: Pediatric Anesthesia: A Guide to Its Administration. Philadelphia, JB Lippincott, 1981)

Hydrocephalus

An abnormal accumulation of fluid in the cranial vault causes enlargement of the head, atrophy of the brain, prominence of the forehead, and the typical "setting sun" appearance of the eyes due to downward pressure (Fig. 43-8). Hydrocephalic infants frequently have other anomalies, are subject to perinatal complications, and have a high incidence of mental retardation, neuromuscular defects, and convulsions. The incidence is about 1 per 2000 deliveries. The abnormal accumulation of fluid may occur between the brain and dura mater or within the ventricles of the brain. Because of the enlarged head, these infants are often breech and require delivery by cesarean section.[8]

Surgical shunting of cerebrospinal fluid is the treatment indicated to reduce pressure within the cranial vault; otherwise there will be irreversible neurologic damage and death. Not all cases are operable, however, and observations over time are necessary to determine therapy.

Anencephaly

In anencephaly, there is complete or partial absence of the infant's brain and of the skull overlying the brain. The cause is not known. Although there is a familial tendency in occurrences, multiple environmental factors seem to be involved. About 70% of anencephalic infants are female. Often the pregnancy involves polyhydramnios. Many infants die during labor and delivery, but if they survive these, their life expectancy is quite short. Supportive care is provided the infant; it seldom lives more than a few days. The parents also need much support in grieving and integrating this traumatic situation.

Microcephaly

The microcephalic infant has a head that is considerably smaller than normal, and a smaller brain with accompanying mental retardation. Several causes of microcephaly have been identified, including exposure of the pregnant woman to x-rays or radiation, rubella infections during pregnancy, and cytomegalic inclusion virus infection or other prenatal infections. Many of these infants survive and need varying amounts of custodial care depending upon the extent of retardation. As with Down's syndrome, parents need assistance with decisions involving caring for the infant or child at home or seeking placement for institutional care.

Umbilical Hernia

Umbilical hernia, or rupture at the umbilicus, may occur during the first few weeks of life. The associated protrusion of intestinal contents may disappear entirely if pressure is applied, but it reappears when

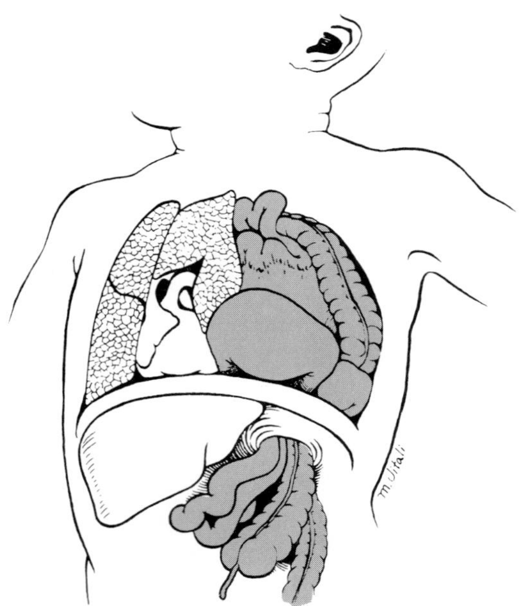

Figure 43-9.
Diaphragmatic hernia showing abdominal contents within the thoracic cavity. This is considered a true pediatric emergency (Mayer BW: Pediatric Anesthesia: A Guide to Its Administration. Philadelphia, JB Lippincott, 1981)

the pressure is removed, or when the baby cries. This is due to a weakness or an imperfect closure of the umbilical ring and is often associated with nonunion of the recti muscles. The condition usually disappears spontaneously by the age of 2 to 3 years. If the hernia persists beyond 3 years, surgical repair is necessary.

Adhesive dressings with coins and metal or plastic objects are ineffective and merely cover the defect and irritate the skin.

Diaphragmatic Hernia

Diaphragmatic hernia is caused by a defect in the development of the diaphragm that allows abdominal organs to herniate into the thoracic cavity (Fig. 43-9). Neonates present with cyanosis and severe respiratory distress.

If the defect is small, it can be easily repaired. This must be done soon after birth because the herniated abdominal organs interfere with adequate respiration. Large defects in the diaphragm allow extensive herniation, which can prevent normal intrauterine development of pulmonary tissue, and can be incompatible with life. The outcome depends upon the size of the defect, the amount of normal pulmonary development, and the success of surgery to close the hernia.

Obstructions of the Alimentary Tract

Atresia of the Esophagus

Atresia of the esophagus, although less common than some that have been mentioned, is quite serious, and immediate steps must be taken to prevent aspiration. The defect occurs during embryonic development and results in the esophagus ending in a blind pouch rather than in the stomach. A fistula usually occurs into the trachea near the bifurcation of the esophagus and the trachea. When the baby attempts to swallow liquids or even normal secretions, there is an overflow into the trachea from the blind pouch (Fig. 43-10).

This malformation should be suspected whenever the infant demonstrates excessive drooling, coughing, gagging, or respiratory distress during feeding. Abdominal distention may occur as air travels through the fistula to the esophagus and into the stomach. The nurse must report these symptoms immediately.

Figure 43-10.
Esophageal atresia. *(A)* The most common form of esophageal atresia. *(B)* Both segments of the esophagus are blind pouches. *(C)* Esophagus is continuous, but with narrowed segment. *(D)* Upper segment of esophagus opens into trachea.

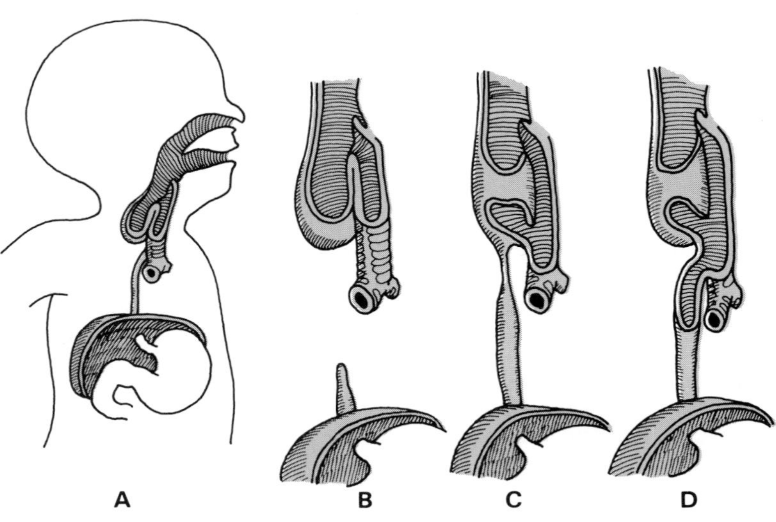

Unless necessary surgery to correct the defect is prompt, the baby will contract bronchitis or pneumonia from repeated aspiration of milk and secretions.

The infant is placed in the supine position, with his head elevated 30° or more to prevent any gastric secretions from rising into the trachea through the fistula. The baby usually is placed in a heated, humidified incubator after surgery. This atmosphere is needed to liquefy the tenacious mucus that collects. A sump suction catheter (Replogle tube) is placed in the upper pouch to eliminate mucus. The nurse should watch carefully for any cyanosis or labored respiration that indicates the need for this measure. Blood, plasma, parenteral fluids, and antibiotics are also given. The extent of the repair and the condition of the baby determine when oral feeding should begin.[8]

Pyloric Stenosis

Pyloric stenosis is a congenital anomaly with an incidence of 1 in 300 to 1 in 1000. It usually manifests its symptoms from the first week to the second or third week by the onset of vomiting that becomes projectile and occurs within 30 minutes after every feeding. The infant loses weight, the bowel elimination lessens, highly colored urine becomes scanty, and the symptoms of dehydration appear. Upon examination, gastric peristalsis is found to be present, and the pyloric "acornlike" tumor may be palpated. Surgery is the treatment of choice.

The operation is not usually an emergency, leaving sufficient time for supportive treatment, in order to correct any dehydration or electrolyte imbalance beforehand. Fluids, electrolytes, and blood replacement may be necessary, depending on the condition of the infant. Gastric lavage, from 1 to 2 hours before operation may be done until returns are clear. Maintaining body heat before and after the operation is essential.

Postoperative feedings are resumed gradually, beginning with glucose water, in limited amounts, at about 6 hours. Feedings are advanced slowly to full-strength formula with close observation and recording of the infant's tolerance.

As soon as the infant is tolerating feedings, breastfeeding may be resumed. With an uncomplicated course, an infant should be discharged within 4 to 6 days postoperatively.[9]

Obstruction of the Duodenum and the Small Intestine

These congenital conditions are relatively easy to diagnose. Vomiting occurs with the first feeding, and no meconium is eliminated. The vomitus may be bile-stained, depending on whether the obstruction is high or low in the intestinal tract. If the obstruction is low, usually there is marked distention. A roentgenogram is used to confirm the diagnosis, and immediate surgery is indicated.

The operation is usually accompanied by continuous parenteral fluids, and blood should be available if needed. Postoperative care includes maintaining body temperature and providing intravenous fluids until peristalsis is established (about a week). This is followed by feedings as given in pyloric stenosis. If distention occurs, nasoduodenal suction may be necessary.

Omphalocele

Omphalocele is a congenital abdominal wall defect, occurring in 1 in 6000 births, in which an amount of abdominal contents protrudes through a wide umbilical ring (Fig. 43-11). The mass is covered with a layer of peritoneum and amnion and may rupture at delivery.

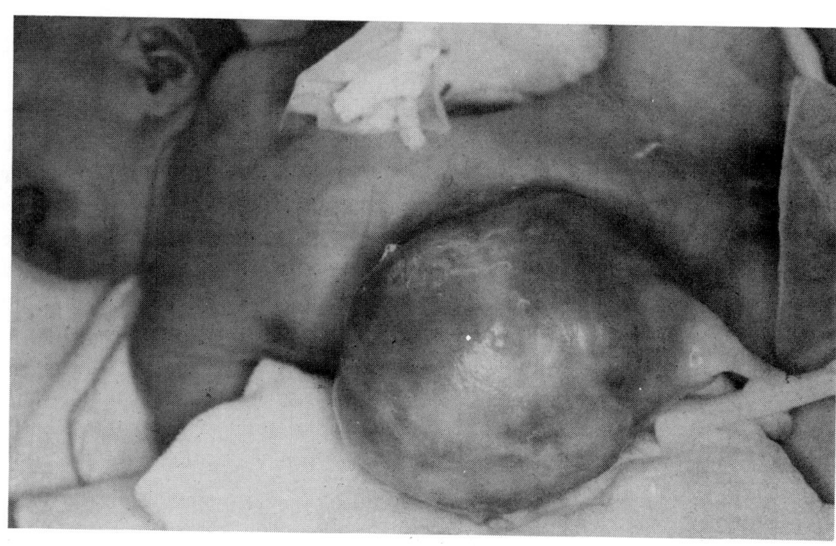

Figure 43-11.
Large omphalocele. Note covering of the sac and its relationship to the umbilicus which protrudes from the lower portion (Avery GB: Neonatology: Pathophysiology and Management of the Newborn, 2nd ed. Philadelphia, JB Lippincott, 1981)

Treatment requires covering of the mass with sterile gauze soaked in saline, nasogastric tube placement, and immediate surgical repair. Sepsis is a serious and potential complication.[8,10]

Gastroschisis

Gastroschisis is a similar defect that occurs less frequently than omphalocele, with incidence of about 1 in 50,000 or less. The lesion is not covered with membrane and the umbilical cord protrudes lateral to the defect in the abdominal wall (Fig. 43-12).[10,11]

Imperforate Anus

Imperforate anus consists of atresia of the anus, with the rectum ending in a blind pouch. Careful examination of the infant in the delivery room usually reveals the condition. Surgical treatment is, of course, imperative. Later continence depends upon the nature of the anorectal abnormalities and effectiveness of surgery. Incidence is 1 in 5000 births.

More males are affected by imperforate anus than females. Most females who are affected have a small fistula. This is uncommon in males (Fig. 43-13). The fistulous connection may be into the vagina, bladder, or urethra, or through the perineum. Male fistulas may lead into the bladder or urethra or through the perineum (Fig. 43-14). If there appears to be an anal opening, the nurse can check for patency by inserting a well-lubricated probe (thermometer, tubing, small finger), and observe physiologic functioning by stroking the anus and watching for the normal "wink" response of the sphincter. X-ray examination confirms definitive diagnosis.

Chromosomal Abnormalities

When a particular chromosome is in triplicate rather than the usual duplicate (pair), it is called *trisomy*. Three such trisomies—trisomy 13 (D trisomy), trisomy 18 (E_1 trisomy), and trisomy 21,22 (Down's syndrome)—have typical clinical pictures and can be recognized in the delivery room or in the nursery.

As discussed in Chapter 10, in the normal person, there are 46 chromosomes in 23 pairs: one pair of sex-determining chromosomes and 22 pairs of autosomes. The extra chromosome found in trisomy results from nondisjunction (see Chap. 16) which can occur at any time in a cell's lifetime, during either meiosis or mitosis. Two different cytologic pictures emerge in trisomic cells. In the first, there is a free extra chromosome, giving 47 chromosomes, or a chromosome is lacking, giving only 45. This is called nondisjunction. In the second, the extra chromosome is translocated, that is, attached to another chromosome. The total number is 46, but one of the chromosomes is the size of 2 chromosomes combined.

There is an increased incidence of all three types of trisomy with advanced maternal age. This phenomenon is thought to be related to the long storage of oocytes in the mother. These germ cells are laid down during the mother's own fetal life; they wait, however, until the time of their individual ovulation to complete their meiotic divisions. Thus, it appears that nondisjunction tends to occur in older oocytes.

Trisomy 13, or D

Trisomy 13 is characterized by an extra chromosome in the D group, which includes pairs 13 through 15 (see Chap. 16). Infants with this abnormality frequently have difficulty establishing and maintaining respiration. One of the most striking features is the abnormal cranial development. The cranium is usually small with a sloping forehead. The ears may be malformed and low-set and the eyes usually have some defect (cataracts, iris defects, unusual smallness), often bilaterally. Cleft palate and lip are commonly present. In addition, the hands and feet are often grossly deformed. Extra digits are common on both hands and feet. The thumbs may be retroflexible (double-jointed). The foot frequently has a posterior prominence of the heel sometimes accompanied by a convex sole known as "rocker bottom" foot. Other defects may include a bulbous nose, umbilical and diaphragmatic hernias, abnormal genitalia, scalp defects, and extensive capillary hemangiomata far in excess of what is usually found in the normal newborn.[5]

Neurologic examination reveals these infants to have a weak or absent Moro reflex and little or no response to loud noises; hence they appear to be deaf. They are prone to develop myoclonic seizures. All suffer from apneic spells of unknown origin. Autopsy often reveals the complete lack of olfactory nerves and tracts. All of these infants are mentally retarded and the majority have severe cardiac defects (dextroposition of the heart, VSD), which are the major contributors to death in these infants. The average life span for these youngsters is less than a year, although several have lived to the age of 5 years.

Trisomy 18, or E

Trisomy 18 is characterized by an extra chromosome in the E group, which includes pairs 17 and 18 (see Chap. 16). These babies are usually born at term but are small, averaging about 2 kg (5 lb). Their placentas are often very small. The head is small with a prominent occiput, but is in proportion to the body size. The eyes are usually normal but the ears are generally

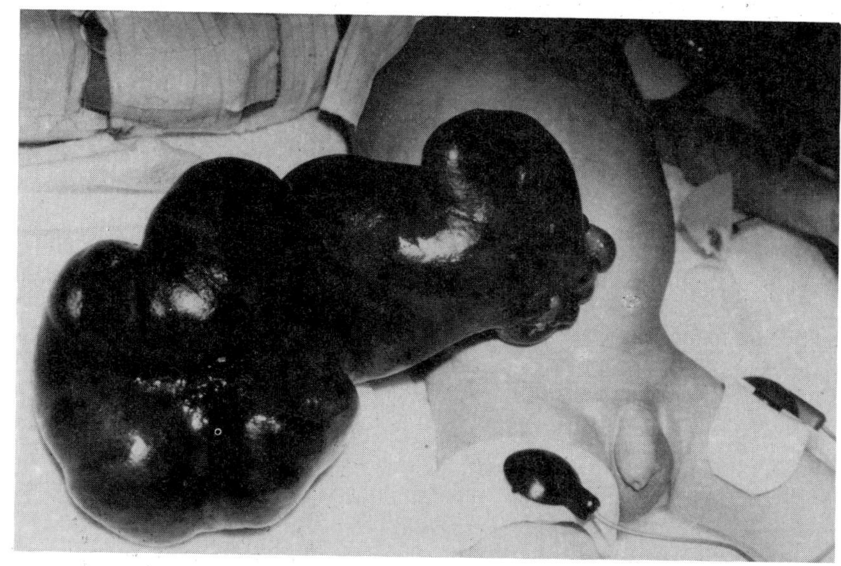

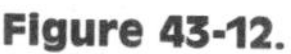

Figure 43-12.
Patient with gastroschisis. Note edematous, matted bowel, the result of the intestines floating freely in the amniotic fluid. Remarkably, these distorted viscera will ultimately fit back into the abdominal cavity and will finally assume a normal appearance and function (Avery GB: Neonatology: Pathophysiology and Management of the Newborn, 2nd ed. Philadelphia, JB Lippincott, 1981)

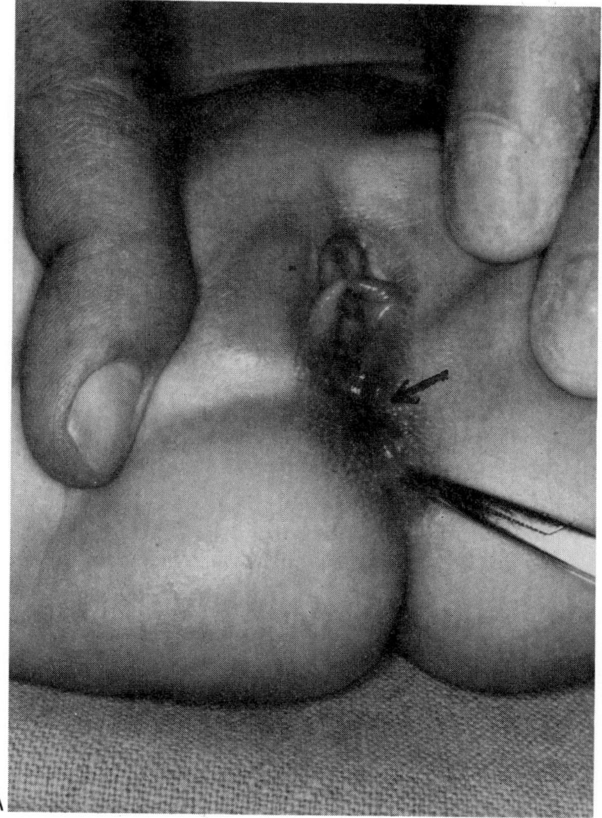

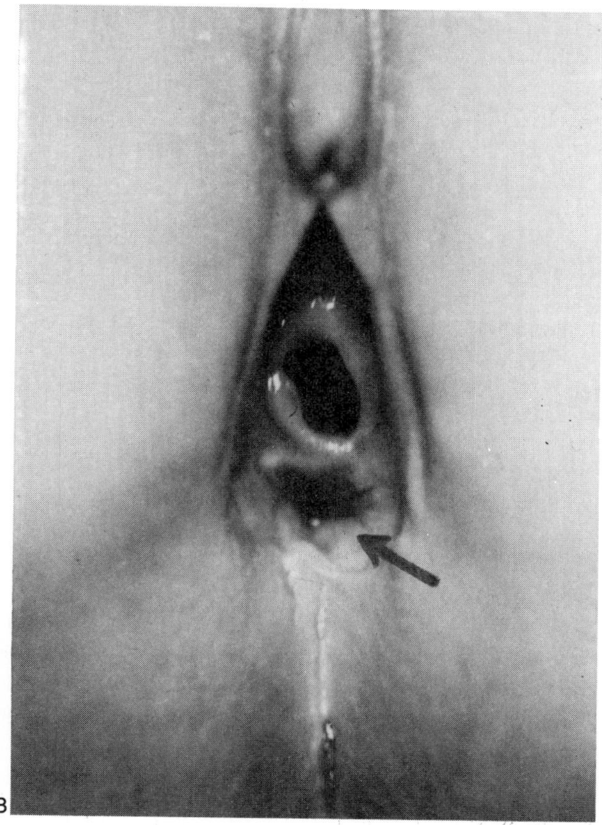

Figure 43-13.
(A) Female with imperforate anus. The arrow demonstrates perineal fistula opening. The clamp is at the point where a normal anus would open. *(B)* Close-up of female with imperforate anus and an introital fistula just inside the labia minora and immediately beneath the hymenal ring. This is the most common form of fistulous opening in female imperforate anus (Avery GB: Neonatology: Pathophysiology and Management of the Newborn, 2nd ed. Philadelphia, JB Lippincott, 1981)

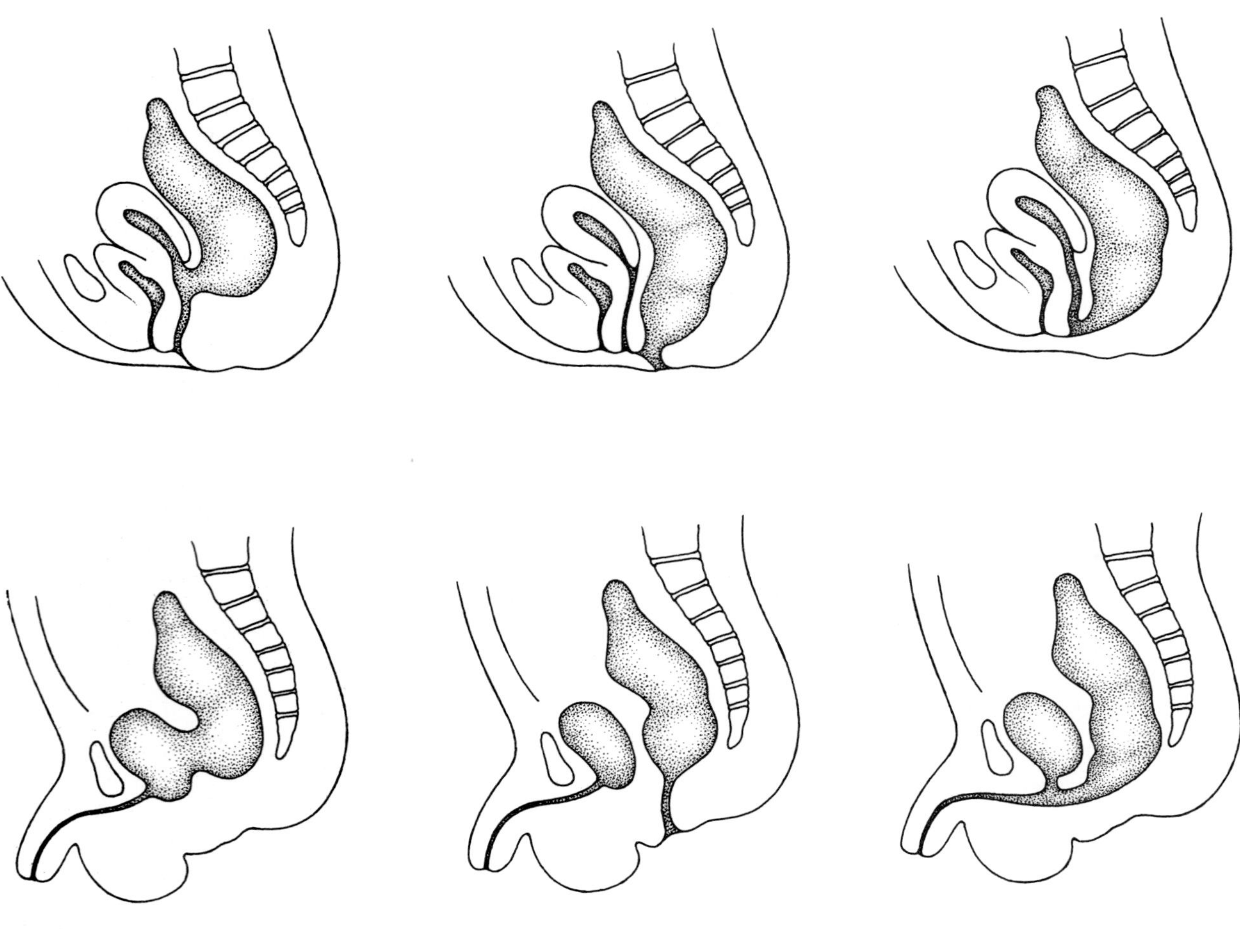

Figure 43-14.
Types of imperforate anus.

malformed and low-set. The mouth appears small because of the short upper lip and the mandible is small, giving a receding chin.

The hands of these babies are always malformed but in a different way from the trisomy 13. They give the best diagnostic clue to the condition. These babies keep their fists clenched most of the time, with the index finger overlying the third finger.

Profuse lanugo covers the forehead, back, and extremities, and the skin usually has a mottled appearance. The sternum is very short, thus the abdomen appears long. The pelvis is small with limited abduction of the hips. There also may be abnormal genitalia. Inguinal and umbilical hernias are frequent; diaphragmatic eventration (elevation of a thinned portion of the diaphragm) occurs more often in these patients rather than frank hernia.

Neurologic examination reveals abnormal muscle tone. These babies progress from a hypertonic state to frank opisthotonus. Since the sucking reflex is poor, gavage feeding is often instituted. Unlike trisomy 13, trisomy 18 demonstrates no gross brain abnormalities. Cardiac abnormalities are common and either these or aspiration accounts for the demise of these babies.

The life span of these infants is less than 6 months on the average. During this time they become progressively undernourished and present a failure-to-thrive syndrome. As with trisomy 13, some infants have survived to childhood, so that death in infancy cannot be predicted.

Trisomy 21, or Down's Syndrome

In Down's syndrome, an extra chromosome belonging to pair 21 or pair 22 or a translocation of 15/21 is found (see Chap. 16). Although these babies are apt to have congenital defects and are more susceptible to infection, they can be expected to live much longer and have less severe mental retardation (although it can be very severe) than the other trisomies. The term *mongolism* was formerly used to refer to this syndrome, but *Down's syndrome* is the preferred nomenclature because the word *mongolism* bears a negative connotation and is descriptively inaccurate for these infants.

The eyes of these infants are set close together and are slanting, and the palpebral fissures are narrow. The nose is flat. The tongue is large and fissured, and usually is very obvious because it protrudes from the open mouth. The head is small, and posteriorly the occiput appears flat above the broad, pudgy neck (Fig. 43-15). The hands are short and thick, especially the fingers (the little finger is curved), with simian creases apparent on the palmar surfaces. In addition to having defective mentality and the deformities mentioned above, these infants have underdeveloped muscles, loose joints, and heart and alimentary tract abnormalities. Although these infants sometimes live past the age of puberty, the majority succumb earlier to some infection.

Incidence and Etiology. The incidence of Down's syndrome has been estimated at 1 in 500 births. However, this ratio has dropped with the lowering of maternal age. In mothers under 35 years, the incidence is about 1 in 1500 births; in those 35 to 40 years of age it is 1 in 300 births; and in those over 40 years of age, it rises to 1 in 30 to 50 births.[8]

Types. The most common chromosomal defect of the ovum in Down's syndrome is trisomy of the chromosome 21 or chromosome 22. This results in a total chromosomal count of 47 instead of the normal number of 46. This type, commonly referred to as *standard trisomy,* usually occurs in infants born to older women and is rarely familial. The incidence of standard trisomy is 1 in 600 births.

The second type of abnormality results from a 15/21 translocation; in this type the actual chromosomal count is 46. The translocation type of Down's syndrome usually occurs in infants born to younger parents, is of the familial type, and is rare.

The third type of the disorder, mosaicism, is very rare. A unique factor in mosaicism is that one person may have cells with different chromosomal counts. Laboratory tests may demonstrate that the affected person's blood cells, for example, have 47 chromosomes, whereas his skin cells may show 46 chromosomes. This is not a familial type of Down's syndrome, and, moreover, the abnormalities may be less.

Prognosis. The usual causes of death in these babies are heart defects and infectious illnesses. The survival rate is variable. Children with Down's syndrome are essentially retarded but have been found to be far more educable than was previously thought.

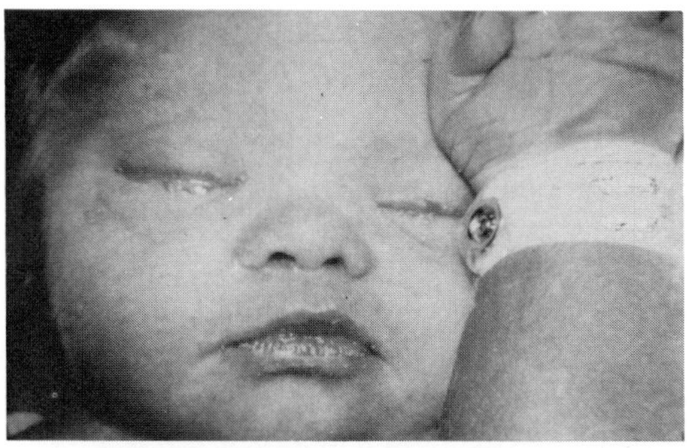

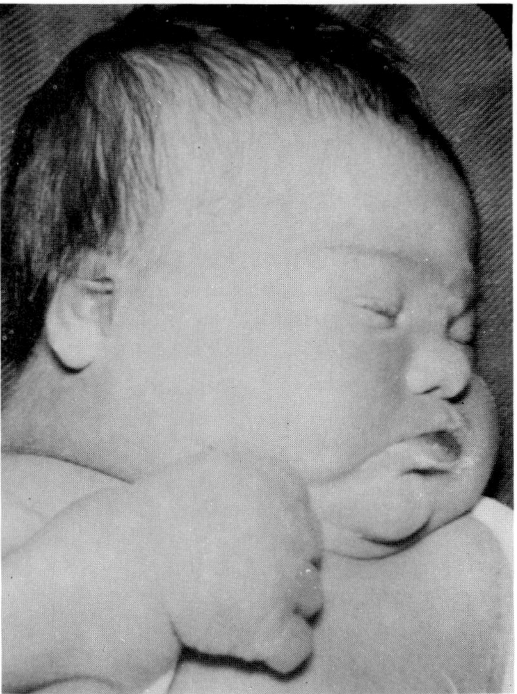

Figure 43-15.
Patient with Down's syndrome (Avery GB: Neonatology: Pathophysiology and Management of the Newborn, 2nd ed. Philadelphia, JB Lippincott, 1981)

Thus, the decision to institutionalize the child is an exceedingly difficult one and should not be forced on the parents by well-meaning professionals.

Prevention and Management

The key approach to trisomy conditions lies in prevention because treatment does not alter the long-range prognosis. Education of the public regarding the effect of maternal age is the key issue in prevention. The incidence of all three trisomies goes up with increased maternal age. The later 30s and 40s are less safe for childbearing (from many points of view). Childbearing is less risky when the mother is younger.

Genetic counseling is another aspect of public education (see Chap. 16). Parents who have had a trisomic child (or if trisomy has appeared among their siblings) would benefit from counseling concerning the risk of having another affected child. In some families, trisomies are not the result of nondisjunction and therefore have an appreciable chance of recurring. This depends on the interaction of the variables of family history, maternal age, and chromosomal arrangement.

Immediate care is supportive for the infant. Warmth, prevention of infection, fluid and electrolyte balance, and, often, oxygen therapy are provided. Nursing therapy is aimed primarily at supporting the parents in helping them to work through their grief. This latter aspect is particularly important because of the grave prognosis for these babies. It is often helpful to institute community health or visiting nurse referrals because the parents may need technical help upon arriving home with the infant. If a fetal demise occurs, supportive help from a public health nurse is also helpful.

Phocomelia

Phocomelia (seal limbs) is a defect in one or several limbs. Thalidomide has caused the lack of an intermediate part or a deformity of a distal part. Since the early 1960s, the United States Food and Drug Administration has tightened the regulation of drugs. Often, the etiology of stunting or amputation of limbs is unknown. Nurses need to be supportive of parents while they attempt to cope with this crisis. Multiprofessional referrals are needed in order to begin the complicated rehabilitative process.[5]

Inborn Errors of Metabolism

Numerous metabolic disorders, so-called inborn errors of metabolism, are now known to originate from mutations in the genes that alter the genetic constitution of a person to the extent that normal function is disrupted. These biochemical disorders arise because of the disturbance (mutation) in a molecule of the gene itself. They *do not* stem from some mishap or alteration during the embryonic development of tissue or organs. The mode of transmission of these inborn errors usually is recessive; that is, a child, to be affected, must receive a pair of defective genes (one from the mother and one from the father). The mother and the father in these cases would be carriers of the defective genes but would not be affected by the resulting disorder *per se*. Fortunately, defective genes are found rather infrequently in the general population, and the chance of their joining is rare; hence, the diseases they produce are commensurately rare.

Some of the more familiar hereditary metabolic disorders and resulting conditions include

1. Defects in metabolism and transport of amino acids
   a. Phenylketonuria
   b. Maple sugar urine disease
2. Defects in protein metabolism
   Agammaglobulinemia
3. Defects in metabolism and transport of carbohydrates
   a. Diabetes mellitus
   b. Gargoylism (Hurler's disease)
   c. Galactosemia
   d. Arachnodactyly (Marfan's syndrome)
4. Defects in metabolism and transport of lipids
   a. Cerebroside lipidosis (Gaucher's disease)
   b. Ganglioside lipidosis (Tay-Sachs disease)
   c. Sphingomyelin lipidosis (Niemann-Pick disease)

It is important to remember that these inborn errors of metabolism do not produce symptoms that are apparent at birth. Therefore, the maternity nurse rarely will see evidence of these disorders although she is involved in the testing for phenylketonuria.

Phenylketonuria

Phenylketonuria, commonly known as PKU, is an inborn error of metabolism of the essential amino acid phenylalanine. It is characterized by a deficiency in the liver enzyme phenylalanine hydroxylase, which is essential in phenylalanine metabolism. High blood levels of phenylalanine occur, and phenylketone bodies are excreted in the urine. Phenylalanine makes up 5% of the protein factor of all foods.

Normally, phenylalanine is converted to tyrosine in the liver and then is further metabolized. The child with PKU is able to digest protein and to absorb the resulting amino acids. However, there is a block in the normal metabolic pathway at this point, and the excess dietary phenylalanine, unable to be converted to tyrosine, builds up in the tissues (blood levels of this amino acid reach as high as 60 mg/dl as compared with the normal 1 mg to 3 mg/dl) and spills into the urine in the form of phenylpyruvic acid, excess phenylalanine, phenylacetic acid, and orthohydroxyphenylacetic acid. These components, excreted in the urine and the perspiration, give the child a characteristic musty odor.[8]

Without treatment, the condition usually results in mental retardation, although the rest of the clinical picture varies. Typically, the child with PKU is hyperactive and demonstrates unpredictable, erratic behavior. Usually he does not relate well in interpersonal contacts, either within the family or with strangers, and he appears very immature and overly dependent.

The main foci of management are early detection of the condition and dietary management restricting the phenylalanine intake.

Diagnosis

PKU may be diagnosed from both blood and urine tests. The former are more advantageous because they can be done before the infant leaves the hospital, and they give a low rate of false-positive reactions. One of the easiest and most efficient tests to perform is the microbiological assay (MIA), more commonly known as the Guthrie method. In this test, 1 or 2 drops of blood are secured from the infant's heel from the second day to the day of discharge and are immediately placed on filter paper. The laboratory then uses a bacterial inhibition assay method on the serum phenylalanine to determine the phenylalanine level. A result of 8 mg/dl or above is considered to be diagnostic of PKU. This method is also used to monitor children on the PKU diet.

Other blood tests have been developed (LaDuMichael, McCaman, and Robins methods) that require more blood. They are as reliable as the Guthrie method and, with proper laboratory facilities, are often used.

The urine tests use ferric chloride as the testing agent; this solution is dropped on a freshly saturated diaper, or a prepared test stick is pressed against a wet diaper or dipped in urine. A green reaction indicates probably PKU. The urine tests are effective only after the infant is 6 weeks old; they are useful in screening large populations of infants and are most often done in well-baby clinics.

Since early diagnosis is imperative, the blood tests are the tests of choice. However, since about 10% of newborns affected by PKU do not have high phenylalanine blood levels during the first 3 to 4 days of life, screening should be repeated in about 2 weeks. Diagnosis should be established and dietary treatment begun before the infant is 3 months old.

Management

Restriction of phenylalanine intake is the basis of treatment, yet enough protein must be available for growth and development; hence the child's diet becomes all-important. Commercial products (*e.g.*, Lofenalac, a special food that is mixed with water) that provide adequate protein for growth with minimal phenylalanine content are available. The plan of dietary treatment should be reviewed carefully with both parents, so that they have an understanding of how to prepare the formula, and how to use the meal guides and food exchange lists and prepare menus from them.

Requesting that the parents review their understanding of the problem, diet, and so on often elicits the areas that need clarification. The parents must be supported until they feel comfortable discussing the problem; until this happens, they cannot be receptive to further teaching. Because this is a long-term condition and requires consistent counseling and follow-up, the need for a referral to the public health nurse is evident.

Care should be taken so that the parents of an affected child are not led to believe that all babies treated will have the usual pattern of growth and development (intellectual development may be slow, for instance). This cannot be guaranteed. *Early detection* and *prompt treatment* prevent mental retardation. The control of this condition demands consistent and disciplined supervision and follow-through on the part of the parents.

■■■

Musculoskeletal Disorders

Talipes Equinovarus (Clubfoot)

Clubfoot occurs twice as often in males as in females, with an overall incidence of 1 in 1000 births. The three elements of this deformity are equinus or plantar flexion of the foot at the ankle, varus or inversion deformity of the heel, and forefoot adduction (Fig. 43-16). All three are present in classic talipes equinovarus. Infants with this deformity should be examined for associated anomalies, especially those of the spine. There is a hereditary pattern in some families. Clubfoot may also be part of a generalized neuromuscular syndrome.

Therapy begins early, often while the infant is still in the nursery, and consists of applying plaster casts after the affected foot structures have been stretched and manipulated. Casts are applied sequentially, correcting first the forefoot adduction, then inversion of the heel, and lastly the equinus flexion at the ankle. Serial casting is needed as the infant grows. After correction is obtained, braces are usually needed for months to years to prevent recurrences of the deformities. About half of these children require an operation to lengthen tightened foot structures.

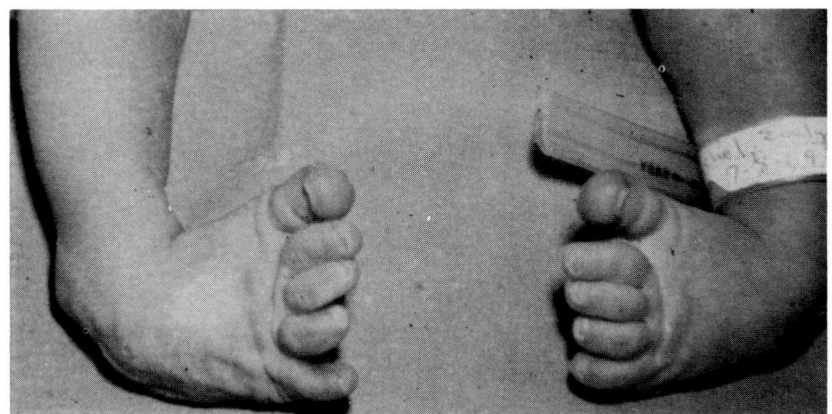

Figure 43-16.
Talipes equinovarus foot (clubfoot) (Avery GB; Neonatology: Pathophysiology and Management of the Newborn, 2nd ed. Philadelphia, JB Lippincott, 1981)

Congenital Hip Dysplasia

Congenital hip dysplasia refers to malformations of the hip involving various degrees of deformity that are present at birth. Congenital hip dysplasia occurs in 1 in 500 to 1000 births. It occurs more frequently in females than in males. One fourth of the cases are bilateral; if unilateral, it more often involves the left hip than the right.

There is an association between congenital hip disorders and breech deliveries and cesarean sections due to the abnormal position *in utero*.

Three categories of congenital hip can be noted. The first is *acetabular dysplasia* (or preluxation). In this instance, there is bony hypoplasia of the acetabular roof. The femoral head remains in the acetabulum. The second is *subluxation,* involving a majority of dysplasias. There is incomplete dislocation, in which the femoral head remains in contact with the acetabulum but is slightly displaced. In *dislocation,* the femoral head loses contact with the acetabulum and is displaced posteriorly and superiorly over the fibrocartilaginous rim.[10]

Prognosis is best if diagnosis is established while the newborn is still in the nursery. Ortolani's sign demonstrates that the femoral head can be lifted into the acetabulum as the thigh is abducted in flexion, and that it dislocates as the hip is adducted (Fig. 43-17).[12]

Treatment should begin promptly for best outcome. The longer treatment is delayed, the poorer is the prognosis.

In infants less than 1 year of age, treatment may be any method designed to keep the hip in full abduction. Methods range from triple diapering to a device made of plastic, metal, leather, or a soft pillow (Frejka pillow splint, Fig. 43-18). If these methods are ineffective, a hip spica cast may be applied followed by a brace. Successful treatment is usually accomplished within a year.[10]

Parents need education and support in applying corrective measures or appliances, using adaptive feeding and holding techniques, and understanding the course of treatment and expected results. If identified and treated early, the long-term prognosis for correction is good.

Polydactyly

This hereditary condition consists of extra digits on the hands or feet. If the digits do not include bones, ligation with a silk suture during the neonatal period is often adequate to cause sloughing of the tissue, leaving only a small scar after a few days. Surgery is required if bones are present in the extra digits. Surgery should wait until the function of each of the duplicated digits is certain.

■ ■ ■

Conclusion

Developmental disorders present a devastating problem for the family of a high-risk neonate. Supportive nursing care and referral at this time are essential to the resolution of these problems.

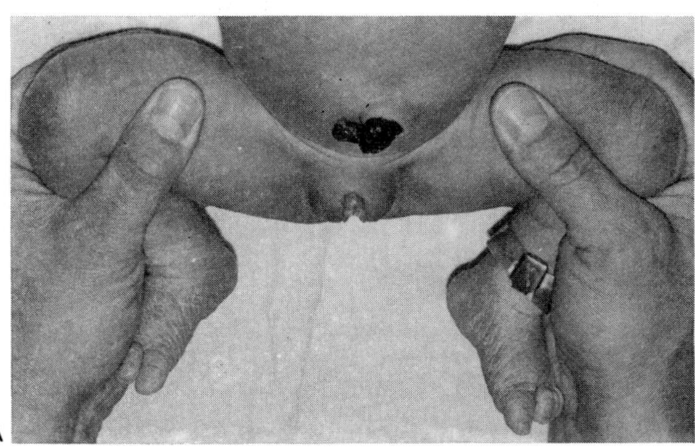

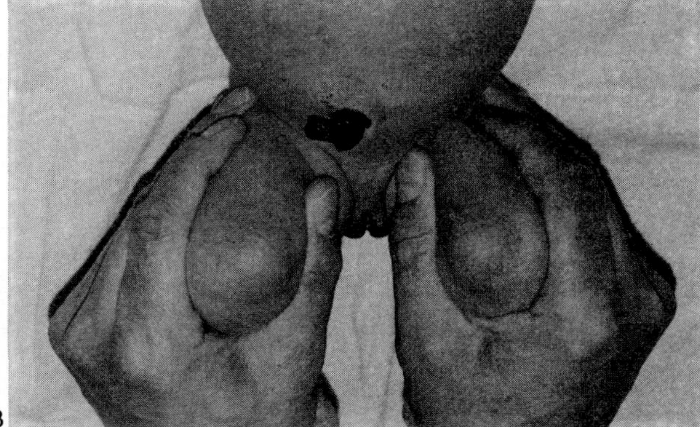

Figure 43-17.
(A) Ortolani's sign. The fingers are on the trochanter and thumb grips the femur as shown. The femur is lifted forward as the thighs are abducted. If the head was dislocated it can be felt to reduce. *(B)* The thighs are adducted and if the head dislocates it will be both felt and seen as it suddenly jerks over the acetabulum (Avery GB: Neonatology: Pathophysiology and Management of the Newborn, 2nd ed. Philadelphia, JB Lippincott, 1981)

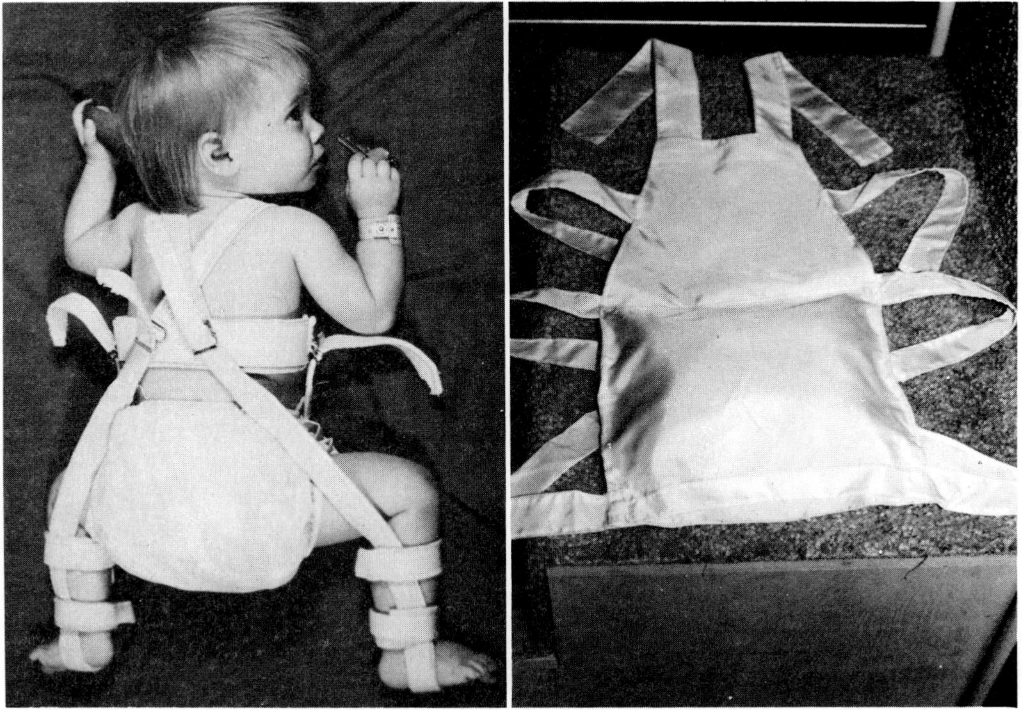

Figure 43-18.
Nonrigid Frejka apron, an abduction device used to correct a dislocated hip (Coleman S: Congenital Dysplasia and Dislocation of the Hip. St Louis, CV Mosby, 1978)

NC **Nursing Care: The High-Risk Infant**

Assessment	Intervention	Evaluation
Physiological Status of Newborn		
Immediate care Respiration and oxygenation Respiratory characteristics Skin color, heart rate, cry, muscle tone Birth injury and trauma Signs of depression from central nervous system injury Symmetry of reflexes, facies Neuromuscular tone Symmetry of limbs Condition of skin (edema, hematoma, ecchymosis) Hemorrhage or shock Overt bleeding, source Depression, tachycardia, respiratory distress Congenital anomalies Type and characteristics Disease or illness Signs present at birth Gestational age Initial exam (posture, tonicity, recoil)	Assist ventilation (intubation, resuscitation, oxygen). Assist suctioning. Assist drawing specimens for blood gases and electrolytes. Assist maintenance of circulation (intravenous lines, transfusions, umbilical catheter). Assist or administer emergency medications (cardiac, bicarbonate). Assist cardiac massage. Record signs of birth injury. Record congenital anomalies. Record signs of disease or illness, hemorrhage or shock. When anomaly is present, examine infant carefully for other less obvious defects. Report anomalies, signs of injury or disease to members of neonatal team. Record indications of gestational age. Monitor vital signs. Conserve warmth during procedures.	Respiration maintained, spontaneous or assisted Skin color, heart rate, muscle tone, cry improve Condition stabilizes (control of hemorrhage, tremors, seizures, depression, etc.)
Continuing care Respiratory exchange (apnea) Later manifestations of trauma (irritability, convulsions) Signs and symptoms of disease Hypoglycemia, hypocalcemia, polycythemia, jaundice	Maintain assisted ventilation. Monitor oxygen levels. Monitor vital signs. Report and record signs and symptoms of disease, behavior indicating central nervous system trauma, or neurologic damage.	Adequate ventilation maintained, assisted or spontaneous Vital signs stable Behavior and functions within normal limits for gestational age Treatments restore to greater physiological equilibrium
Gestational age (thorough exam) Sleep patterns, restlessness, irritability Feeding needs and response Temperature regulation Hematologic problems Hemorrhage, polycythemia, anemia	Administer treatments (medications, positioning, exchange transfusion, phototherapy, intravenous feeding or hydration, gavage feeding, etc.). Record and report variations in sleep patterns.	Sleep patterns normal for gestational age Takes adequate nourishment and retains feedings Temperature remains within normal limits Infant gains weight Elimination normal

Assessment	Intervention	Evaluation
Renal and bowel function Signs of infection Central nervous system problems Musculoskeletal and soft tissue trauma	Provide and record type, route, and amounts of feedings, responses. Record and report elimination. Report signs of infection, central nervous system, musculoskeletal, and soft tissue problems. Maintain warmth in isolette, prevent heat loss during procedures.	
Development Needs		
Stimulation Nurturance Activity	According to developmental status of infant, provide balance of stimulation and rest. Hold and handle during feedings when condition permits.	Infant attains expected developmental landmarks for age, both neuromuscular and interactional
Parent–Infant Bonding		
Contact Caretaking	Encourage bonding process through providing parents with information about status and characteristics of their infant, maximize parent–infant contact, support caretaking activities, maintain telephone or written contact after mother is discharged, encourage visits to ICN for caretaking and holding.	Parents take active interest in progress and caretaking of their infant Visit regularly after mother's discharge Provide caretaking effectively
Parental Psychosocial Needs		
Information and support Grief, reactions to anomalies Family adaptations	Provide information, discuss its meanings, encourage expression of feelings and reactions. Facilitate grieving process. Refer to other sources of support (parents' groups, counseling, etc.). Discuss family responses, needs of siblings, community resources.	Parents feel well informed and understand their infant's condition. Feelings of loss and grief are expressed as appropriate for the individual and family. Parents able to interact and care for infant, or make decisions about alternate types of care. Family accepts and relates to infant, plans made for special care needs.

References

1. Grant P: Psychosocial needs of families of high-risk infants. Fam Community Health 1, 3:91–102, November 1978
2. Waechter EH: Bonding problems of infants with congenital anomalies. Nurs Forum 16, 3, and 4:298–318, 1977
3. Kennell JH: Birth of a malformed baby: Helping the family. Birth Fam J 5, No. 4:219–222, Winter 1978
4. Schuman H: Thoughts and comment. JOGN Nurs 3, 3:48–49, May/June 1974
5. Olds SB, London ML, Ladewig PA, Davidson SV et al: Obstetric Nursing, pp 189–190, 878–892. Menlo Park, CA, Addison-Wesley, 1980
6. Smith K: Recognizing cardiac failure in neonates. American Journal of Maternal Child Nursing 4, 2:98–104, March/April 1979
7. Walton RL: A study of etiological variables in palatolabial malformations. J Kans Med Soc 73:370–377, August 1972
8. Whaley LF, Wong DL: Nursing Care of the Infant and Children, pp 187, 316, 369–399, 401–412. St Louis, CV Mosby, 1979
9. Randolph JG, Altman RP, Anderson KD: Surgery of the neonate. In Avery GB (ed): Neonatology: Pathophysiology and Management of the Newborn, pp 790–831, Philadelphia, JB Lippincott, 1981
10. Babson SG, Pernoll ML, Benda GI: Diagnosis and Management of the Fetus and Neonate at Risk, pp 284–285. St Louis, CV Mosby, 1980
11. Hazle N: An infant who survived gastroschisis. American Journal of Maternal Child Nursing 6, 1:35–40, January/February 1981
12. Griffin PP: Orthopedics in the newborn. In Avery GB (ed): Neonatology-Pathophysiology and Management of the Newborn, pp 890–909. Philadelphia, JB Lippincott, 1981

Suggested Reading

Arney WR, Nagy JN, Little GA et al: Caring for parents of sick newborns. Obstet Gynecol Surv 33, 9:603–605, September 1978

Bresadola C: One infant/one nurse/one objective: Quality care. MCN—Am J Maternal Child Nurs 2, 5:287–290, September/October 1977

Eager M: Long-distance nurturing of the family bond. MCN—Am J Maternal Child Nurs 2, 5:293–294, September/October 1977

Erdman D: Parent-to-parent support: The best for those with sick newborns. MCN—Am J Maternal Child Nurs 2, 5:291–292, September/October 1977

Kennell JH: Parenting in the intensive care unit. Birth Fam J 5, No. 4:223–226, Winter 1978

Korones SB: High-Risk Newborn Infants, The Basis for Intensive Nursing Care. St Louis, CV Mosby, 1978

Wyatt DS: Phenylketonuria: The problems vary during different developmental stages. MCN—Am J Maternal Child Nurs 3, 5:296–302, September/October 1978

CHAPTER 44

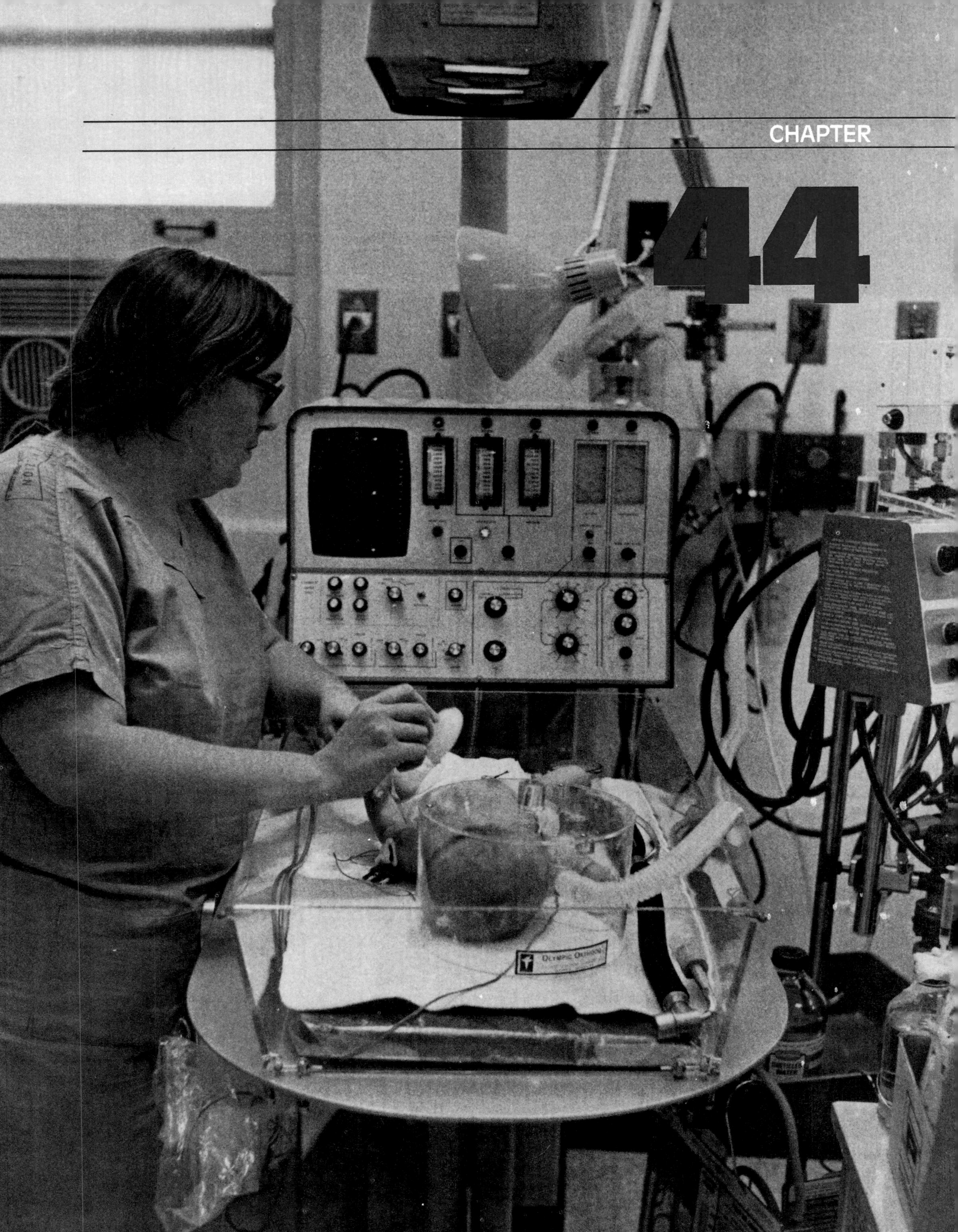

CHAPTER 44

The High-Risk Infant: Acquired Disorders

Certain factors have an impact upon the neonate's transition to extrauterine life. These include maternal disorders, birth trauma and anoxia, and postnatal infections and physiological processes as affected by the newborn's environmental systems. Most neonates make the transition to extrauterine life smoothly. For those neonates that do not, the professionals' skills in the delivery room and the nursery are important to their future development.

Birth Trauma and Anoxia

Immediate observation of the newborn in the delivery room usually permits the nurse to identify injuries or anoxia resulting from the birth process. Some kinds of birth trauma require emergency intervention to save the infant's life; others can be treated later or resolve spontaneously in several days. A thorough neonatal assessment, alertness to subtle changes in the newborn's behavior and condition, efficient communication, careful recording of observations, and facility with emergency techniques enable the nurse to promote the well-being of high-risk infants. Communicating with parents by providing information and support is also a major nursing responsibility (see Chap. 43).

Neonatal Asphyxia

The neonate may be a victim of asphyxia during labor or delivery or immediately after birth. The etiology of asphyxia during this stressful time may fit into one of four categories:

1. Fetal asphyxia from lack of umbilical circulation
2. Fetal asphyxia from lack of placental exchange, as in abruptio placentae
3. Fetal asphyxia from inadequate perfusion of the maternal side of the placenta
4. Neonatal asphyxia from failure to inflate the lungs

Neonatal asphyxia may be a result of excess fluid in the lungs, airway obstruction, or ineffective respiratory effort. It may also be a result of one of the three fetal asphyxia mechanisms.[1]

The failure to initiate or maintain normal respiratory patterns at birth is a severe life-threatening emergency requiring immediate intervention to prevent anoxic cellular damage and to save the infant's life. Usually, normal respiratory patterns are established almost immediately, and by 1 minute the infant is pink, crying, and active, with a heart rate of 120 to 160 beats per minute, normal reflexes and muscle tone, and an Apgar score of 8 to 10. If asphyxia has occurred, the infant is apneic.

Primary apnea occurs when asphyxia has been prolonged over 1 minute to 2 minutes, with mild bradycardia and hypotension. The newborn is cyanotic with diminished reflexes, bradycardia of 60 to 100 per minute, and an Apgar score of 3 to 5. Following gentle suctioning and the administration of oxygen, gasping respirations usually begin after about 2 minutes. Rapid improvement often follows, with the 5-minute Apgar score reaching 8 to 10. Without other complicating conditions, these infants have an excellent immediate and long-term prognosis.

Secondary apnea occurs when there is severe bradycardia and hypotension, and death follows shortly if there is not immediate resuscitation. The newborn is ashen, heart sounds are distant with weak pulses and bradycardia between 20 and 60 beats per minute, reflexes are absent, and the Apgar score is 1 to 3. No gasping movements are initiated with stimulation, and the infant must be resuscitated (see Chap. 42). Spontaneous respiration may not begin for 5 to 15 minutes after resuscitation is started. There is danger of irreversible effects of anoxia with long-term disabilities.[2]

The three causes of intrauterine injury of the central nervous system—narcosis, hypoxia, and brain hemorrhage—all produce a similar clinical syndrome of asphyxia, characterized by apnea. The course and prognosis of this syndrome vary with the degree of hypoxia, the location and extent of the hemorrhage, and the degree of hypercapnia and acidosis. This acidotic asphyxial state is more injurious and difficult to correct than hypoxia alone.

The normal oxygen saturation of the arterial blood of the fetus at birth is approximately 60% but in severe cases may drop as low as 12%. In addition, the blood of these infants has a high concentration of lactic acid and a very low *p*H.

Management is aimed at correcting metabolic acidosis as well as maintaining tissue oxygenation. Any underlying disorder (hypoglycemia, anemia) must also be identified and corrected.

Prevention of asphyxia begins with the first antepartal visit when the pelvis is measured to make sure that it is large enough to allow passage of the infant's head without compression. Good diet and hygiene contribute greatly to the health of the infant at birth.

During labor, asphyxia of the infant can be prevented through careful use of analgesic and anesthetic drugs and by avoiding as much as possible the more difficult types of operative delivery. Moreover, by monitoring the fetal heart tones, the nurse may detect early signs of impending fetal distress (slow or irregular rate). With this warning, it may be possible for the infant to be delivered before serious trouble develops. The passage of meconium-stained amniotic fluid in a cephalic presentation is another sign of fetal distress.

Caput Succedaneum

Prolonged pressure on the head during a protracted first stage of labor, when the membranes rupture before the cervix is fully dilated, causes an edematous swelling of the soft tissues of the scalp over the area where it is encircled by the cervix (Fig. 44-1). This condition is called *caput succedaneum,* and in its milder forms is very common—so common that it may be regarded as normal.

It is due to an extravasation of serum into the tissues of the scalp at the portion surrounded by the cervix. The term is not confined to vertex cases; the corresponding swelling that forms on any presenting part is also, for the sake of uniformity, known as caput succedaneum.

The condition always disappears within a few days without treatment. A prompt and simple explanation should be given to the parents, because this condition, although benign, can be somewhat disfiguring. Once the parents know that the caput succedaneum will disappear of its own accord, they usually are reassured and will not press for treatment.

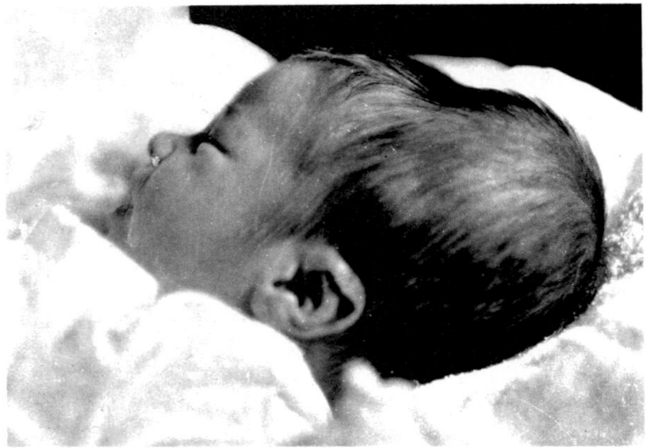

Figure 44-1.
Caput succedaneum. (MacDonald House, University Hospitals of Cleveland)

Cephalhematoma

Cephalhematoma is another swelling of the scalp. It resembles caput succedaneum in certain respects (Fig. 44-2). It is caused by an effusion of blood between the bone and the periosteum (Fig. 44-3). This explains why the swelling appears directly over the bone. Cephalhematoma is most common over the parietal bones. It is usually unilateral, but occasionally bilateral. It does not cross suture lines. It is seldom visible when the infant is born and may not be noticed for several hours or more after delivery because subperiosteal bleeding occurs slowly.

The cephalhematoma increases gradually in size until about the seventh day after birth, when it remains stationary for a time and then begins to disappear. The infant usually recovers without treatment in 2 weeks to 3 weeks.

Cephalhematoma may be due to pressure exerted in normal labor or by forceps. It is also seen occasionally in breech cases in which no instruments were used nor prolonged pressure exerted on the aftercoming head. Such cases, however, are not common.

Occasionally hyperbilirubinemia may result from the breakdown of the accumulated blood. Again, the parents should receive assurance regarding the temporary nature of this condition and its spontaneous disappearance.

Intracranial Hemorrhage (Cerebral Hemorrhage, Subdural Hematoma)

In contrast to the two conditions just described, ***intracranial hemorrhage*** is one of the gravest complications encountered in the newborn. It may occur any place in the cranial vault, but is particularly likely to take place as the result of tears in the tentorium cerebelli with bleeding into the cerebellum, the pons, and the medulla oblongata. Because these structures contain many important centers such as the respiratory center, hemorrhage in these areas is very often fatal.

Intracranial hemorrhage occurs most often after prolonged labor, especially in primiparae, and is particularly likely to take place in a traumatic forceps delivery. It is also seen more commonly in precipitate deliveries as the result of the rapid and abrupt propulsion of the infant's head through the birth canal. It is due primarily to excessive or unduly prolonged pressure on the fetal skull. This causes excessive molding of the head and such overriding of the cranial bones that the delicate supporting structures of the brain (tentorium cerebelli, falx cerebri) are torn, with consequent rupture of blood vessels.

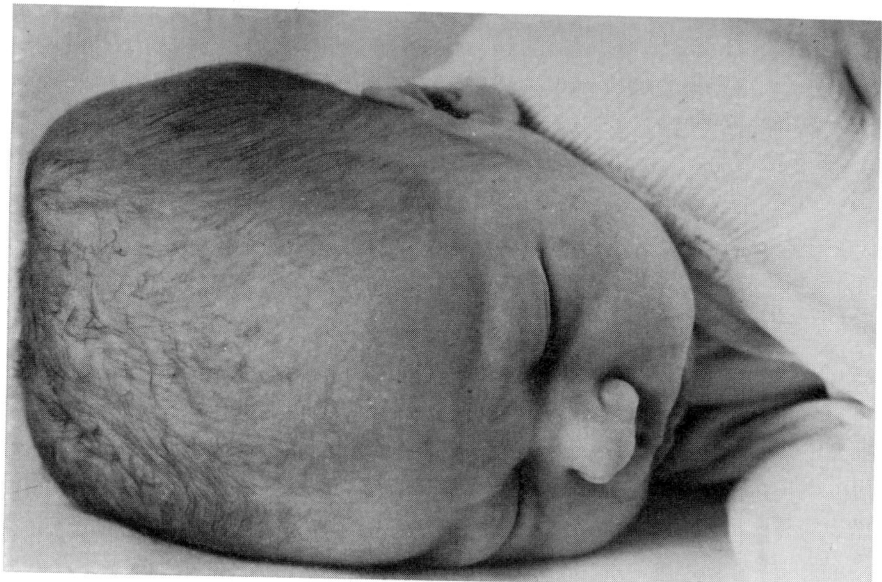

Figure 44-2.
Cephalhematoma. (Courtesy of Mead–Johnson Laboratories)

Manifestations

The development of symptoms in cerebral hemorrhage may be sudden or gradual. If the hemorrhage is severe, the infant is usually stillborn. If it is less marked, apnea of the newborn may result, often with fatal outcome. Many infants who are resuscitated with difficulty at birth succumb later from brain hemorrhage. On the other hand, the infant may appear normal after delivery and develop the first signs of intracranial hemorrhage several hours or several days later.

If any of the following common signs of cerebral hemorrhage occur, they should be reported immediately.

1. *Convulsions.* Convulsions may vary from mild, localized twitchings to severe pain spasms of the whole body. Twitching of the lower jaw is characteristic, particularly when associated with salivation.
2. *Cyanosis.* Cyanosis may be persistent but is more likely to occur in repeated attacks.
3. *Abnormal respiration.* Grunting respiration is characteristic; or it may be irregular, of Cheyne-Stokes type, very rapid and shallow, or very slow. Very slow breathing, usually associated with cyanosis, suggests respiratory paralysis due to pressure on the medulla oblongata and is a grave sign.
4. *A sharp, shrill, weak cry.* This cry is similar to that seen in meningitis.
5. *Flaccidity or spasticity.* If this condition is present, it usually portends a fatal outcome. Somnolence

Figure 44-3.
Comparative diagram of the underlying pathophysiology in caput succedaneum *(Left),* and cephalohematoma *(Right).*

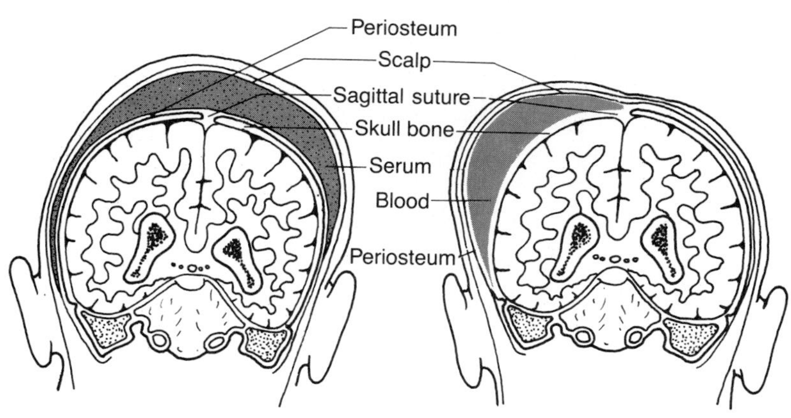

also may be present. In other cases there may be generalized spasticity with backward arching of the head and neck and extension of the legs *(opisthotonos)*.

Management

Prevention is most important and is largely the responsibility of the health-care provider conducting the delivery. It consists of protecting the infant from trauma, particularly in difficult or precipitate deliveries. A small dose of water-soluble vitamin K_1 (1 mg) may be given the infant after birth.

Curative treatment can be effective if damage is not too extensive.

Complete rest with the very minimum amount of handling is imperative. Infants suspected of having a cerebral hemorrhage are placed in intensive care. Supportive measures such as maintaining heat and oxygenation and monitoring vital signs are employed along with intravenous feeding or gavage. If a subdural hematoma is suspected, a spinal tap is done for diagnostic purposes. Excess subdural bloody fluid may be removed as a therapeutic measure. Usually, the physician will order some form of sedative for convulsions. Vitamin C and water-soluble vitamin K may be used to control the hemorrhage, and antibiotics may be given prophylactically. The infant may be placed in a modified reverse Trendelenberg because this position is believed to lower intracranial pressure and facilitate respirations.

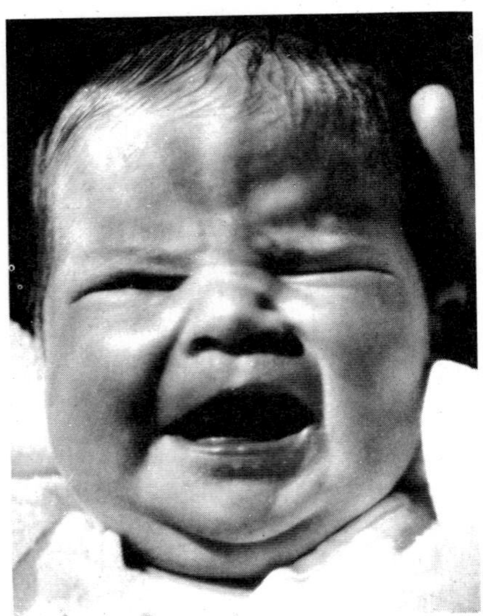

Figure 44-4.
Facial nerve paralysis. Note the asymmetry of the mouth during crying.

The outcome for the infant depends upon the location and extensiveness of the hemorrhage, the amount of central nervous system (CNS) damage, and other complicating conditions such as respiratory and metabolic problems. The prognosis is guarded, and among those infants who live, there is the risk of mental retardation and cerebral palsy.

Perinatal Hemorrhage and Shock

The neonate with a hemorrhagic condition may have suffered intrauterine hemorrhage or hemolysis. Because the average blood volume of a term infant is about 80 ml per kg, rapid blood loss of as little as 50 ml can cause shock. Intrauterine bleeding can occur from fetal to maternal circulation, from one twin to another, or from placental problems such as rupture of abnormal vessels, abruptio placentae, and placenta previa.

The newborn with severe *hypovolemic shock* appears collapsed and presents a clinical picture similar to that of asphyxia, except that tachycardia is usually seen with hemorrhage and bradycardia with asphyxia. Symptoms include pallor and cyanosis, hypotonia, hypotension, decreased or absent pulses, gasping and retractions, tachypnea, tachycardia, and weak or absent cry.

Treatment is instituted immediately with placement of an umbilical catheter and withdrawal of blood for hemoglobin and hematocrit values, platelet count, Coombs' test, cross-matching, and coagulation screen. Blood volume is then rapidly expanded by transfusion, usually with group O Rh-negative blood, plasma (fresh or substitute) or volume expanders such as albumin. Subsequent management depends upon identification of the source of hemorrhage.

Facial Paralysis

Facial paralysis may occur as a result of a difficult vaginal delivery or by pressure by forceps on the facial nerve, which may cause temporary paralysis of the muscles of one side of the face so that the mouth is drawn to the other side. This will be particularly noticeable when the infant cries. The condition is usually transitory and disappears in a few days, often in a few hours. Because the infant can look grotesque, the parents will need an explanation concerning the temporary nature of this affliction (Fig. 44-4).

If the mother is allowed to feed the baby, the nurse should be with her consistently during the first feedings to help her as necessary. Sucking may be difficult for the infant, and the mother needs to develop patience and skill in the feeding of her baby.

If one eye remains open because of the affected muscles, the physician prescribes such treatment as is appropriate.

Artificial tears may need to be instilled daily to prevent drying. Any necessary instruction regarding continuing care after discharge should be given the mother before she leaves the hospital.

Very often parents are afraid to handle their infants when disorders occur for fear of hurting the child. This may happen even if the condition is short-term and fairly innocuous. Thus, parents should be encouraged to hold and cuddle their infants whenever the condition permits.

Arm Paralysis (Erb-Duchenne's Paralysis, Brachial Palsy)

This condition results from excessive stretching of the nerve fibers that run from the neck through the shoulder and down toward the arm (brachial plexus). It is a result of the shoulders having been forcibly pulled away from the head during delivery, which can occur in a vertex or breech delivery.

Generally, only the muscles of the upper arm are involved, and the infant holds his arm at the side with the elbow extended and the hand rotated inward (Fig. 44-5). The hand and fingers may not be involved. If the nerves are merely stretched, recovery occurs in several weeks; if they are broken within their sheaths, healing is not complete for several months. If healing fails to occur within that time, surgery is indicated; the outcome for recovery in these cases is guarded.

To reduce tension on the brachial plexus, the physician usually places the arm in a splint or cast in an elevated, neutral position. While the arm is healing, the physician orders gentle manipulation and massage of the muscles to prevent contractures. The mother is to be instructed in these procedures so that she may continue the care.

Fractures and Dislocations

Fractures of long bones may occur as a result of a difficult shoulder delivery or difficult upper extremity delivery in the vertex position. Incidence increases with increase in birth weight. Fractures of the clavicle or of the jaw, or dislocation of either of these bones, may follow forcible efforts to extract the aftercoming head in cases of breech presentation.

Fracture or dislocation of the cervical spine, usually accompanied by damage to the spinal cord, may also be the consequence of a difficult breech extraction. The vertebrae most often affected are C5 and C6. If the cord is not completely severed, surgical repair is often effected. These babies have a flaccid paralysis of the trunk and extremities and breathe abdominally because the diaphragm is innervated by the nerves that have been injured in the dislocation or fracture.

Management

Fractures in the newborn baby, particularly in the long bones, usually heal rapidly, but it is often difficult to keep the parts in good alignment during repair. Immobilization of the part often can be achieved by swaddling and positioning the infant on his side. Splints, slings, and other apparatus are useful. However, these devices often make handling of the infant difficult and cumbersome; hence, parents tend to avoid touching the infant for fear of hurting him. Care should be taken by the staff to encourage the parents to give their infant adequate love and attention if these apparatuses are used. This means that the parents have to be shown how to manipulate the apparatus effectively to avoid traumatizing the injury.

Dislocation should be reduced at once, or there is great danger of permanent deformity in the joint. Follow-up supervision is necessary to prevent permanent deformity. Physiotherapy under orthopedic direction is important.

Diaphragmatic Paralysis

Injury to the phrenic nerve can occur as a result of lateral hyperextension of the neck, often during a difficult breech delivery. Spinal nerve roots at C3 to C5

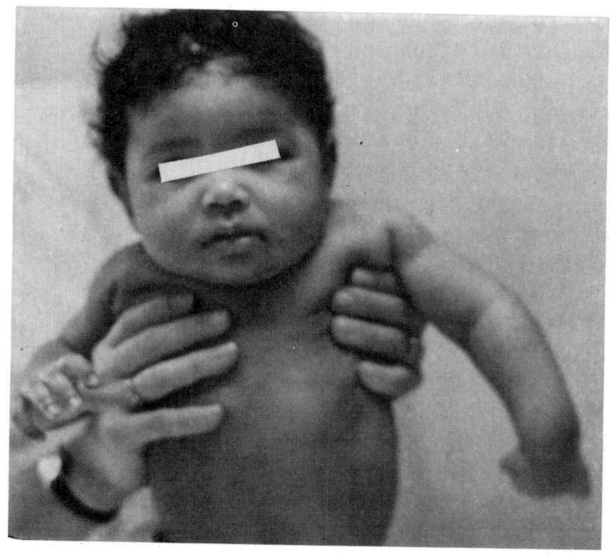

Figure 44-5.
A 2-month-old baby girl with a left Erb's palsy (Avery GB: Neonatology: Pathophysiology and Management of the Newborn, 2nd ed. Philadelphia, JB Lippincott, 1981)

are involved. Paralysis of the diaphragm is usually one-sided, with irregular thoracic respirations, no abdominal movement on inspiration on the affected side, and cyanosis. The elevated diaphragm, which is displaced upward and which also displaces thoracic organs, can be demonstrated by roentgenogram.

Unless there is respiratory distress, in which case surgery to lower the diaphragm is necessary, the treatment consists of positioning the infant on the affected side, administering oxygen if needed, and providing nutrition by the route most appropriate to the infant's condition. In order to prevent pneumonia, atelectasis of the involved lung should not be allowed to develop. Spontaneous recovery within 6 weeks to a year is usual.

Infections

The neonate is particularly vulnerable to infection, with incidence of 0.6 to 2 in 1000 live births. Preterm infants tend to be in the higher range. Infection is responsible for 10% of all neonatal deaths, thus making it a significant problem to be aware of for health professionals.

Maternal IgG antibody is the only immunoglobin that crosses the placenta. Maternal IgM antibody does not cross the placenta. The small neonate is particularly vulnerable to infection due to its relative immaturity.

Infections may be acquired transplacentally, as in viruses, and from ascending organisms that pass through the cervix and infect the fetus, particularly after prolonged rupture of the membranes. Infections may also be acquired during delivery itself when the fetus meets maternal, perineal, fecal, and vaginal flora on its passage through the birth canal. Finally, infections may be acquired in the nursery from exposure to personnel and equipment.[3]

Nursing Responsibilities

A primary nursing responsibility is to report any suspected change in behavior that may be indicative of sepsis. A wide range of symptoms in all body systems may be demonstrated. Significant examples are seizures, respiratory distress, vomiting, jaundice, and hypothermia.[4] An additional vital responsibility is the maintenance of an aseptic environment (see Chap. 32). Finally, nurses need to be able to reinforce physicians' explanations of diagnosis and treatment. Because most septic infants need to be isolated, the mother needs support during the period of separation.

Bacterial Infections

Diarrhea of the Newborn

A change in feeding practices in young infants is most directly linked to newborn diarrhea, not to pathogenic organisms. However, a few bacterial agents can cause diarrhea. The most common is the enteropathic *Escherichia coli.* Other bacteria such as *Salmonella, Shigella,* and *Staphylococcus* are not so commonly implicated.

Stools may be green, watery, and approximately 7 to 10 in number per day. Blood and mucus in the stool are rare except in shigellosis. Dehydration and electrolyte imbalances are the major sequelae. Complications are rare, provided diagnosis and therapy are appropriate.[5]

Management and Prevention

Any infant suspected of harboring an infection should be isolated, following agency procedure. In the case of diarrhea, rectal swabs for culture should be taken from the suspect infant, as well as from others in the nursery. Prior to receiving culture reports, therapy for the primary infant and prophylactic therapy for other infants may be instituted. Medications of choice are *neomycin* or *colistine sulfate.*[6] Other therapy includes fluid and electrolyte maintenance through parenteral or oral routes.

An outbreak of diarrhea in the nursery may necessitate closure of the nursery to any new admissions and a thorough cleaning of the physical environment. All personnel who come in contact with newborns should review infection-control techniques as a preventive measure against future outbreaks.

Cutaneous Infections

As opposed to the benign *erythema toxicum* (see Chap. 32), most infections of the skin in neonates follow invasion by the organism *Staphylococcus aureus.* The most common signs are *pustules* and *furuncles,* which may appear isolated or in groups. Location of lesions is more often around the umbilicus and diaper area. However, lesions may spread to other areas of the body following the primary outbreak.

Management and Prevention

Once cultures are taken, treatment may vary, depending on the number of lesions and condition of the infant.

Small numbers of pustules may be treated topically with hexachlorophene. More skin involvement or systemic infection may require treatment with parenteral antibiotics, such as penicillin. Prevention of further infection involves identification and isolation of suspect infants.[5]

Syphilis

Transmission of syphilis to the fetus occurs by transplacental passage, or contact with active genital lesions at birth.[6] Untreated early syphilis occurring during pregnancy may cause midtrimester abortion, fetal death *in utero,* or premature labor and delivery. The extent of the disease in the newborn depends on when the mother became infected. If this infection occurred less than 1 to 2 years before conception, there are serious consequences for the fetus. When the disease onset is at conception or early pregnancy, the infant may be seriously deformed. When the onset is during the second half of pregnancy, the fetus may be spared.[3]

Ophthalmia of the Newborn

This is a serious condition that may result in partial or complete loss of vision as a result of corneal ulceration. If suitable treatment is adopted at the very outset of the disease and intelligently carried out, the sight can usually be saved.

State laws making the use of an antibacterial prophylaxis compulsory for all infants at birth have reduced the incidence of this infection immeasurably. Before eye prophylaxis became mandatory, however, 25% to 30% of all children in schools for the blind suffered impaired sight as a result of the infection. This condition is of gonorrheal origin and is characterized by a profuse, purulent discharge in the eyes due to infection, generally from the genital canal at the time of birth.

The most common reason for delay in the diagnosis is the assumption by inexperienced persons that all conjunctivitis in the first few days of life is a consequence of the prophylactic silver nitrate (or the antibiotic ointment). A degree of conjunctival inflammation with catarrhal discharge may occur with silver nitrate and, to a lesser degree, with the various antibiotic preparations. However, the nurse should give primary consideration to infection in the presence of purulent exudate during the first days of life or to catarrhal conjunctivitis persisting longer than three days. Chemical conjunctivitis disappears in 24 hours, but ophthalmia neonatorum becomes more severe on the third or fourth day. It is well to remember also that the widely used procedure of phototherapy for neonatal hyperbilirubinemia necessitates shielding the infant's eyes during the procedure and may result in obscuring this disease—thus, the pads should be removed regularly and the eyes examined.

If the infection occurs at the time of birth, the disease appears within 2 or 3 days; but as the septic discharge may be introduced into the eye at a later period because of improper care of the infant, the onset may be later. Both eyes are usually affected. At first they are suffused with a watery discharge and considerable inflammation of the eyelids. Within 24 hours, the lids become very much swollen, and a thick, creamy, greenish pus is discharged. Later, unless treatment has been instituted early, the swelling becomes so marked that the eyes cannot be opened, opacities of the cornea occur, the conjunctiva is ulcerated and then perforated, and the eye collapses and finally atrophies.

Preventive treatment consists of using an antibacterial agent, usually 1% silver nitrate, or erythromycin or tetracycline ophthalmic ointment, which is instilled immediately after birth. However, if infection does occur, penicillin intramuscular injections may be given. The swelling and the purulent discharge usually disappear within 12 to 24 hours after treatment is begun. As gonorrheal conjunctivitis is infectious, isolation technique is essential to prevent spread to other patients and staff.

Thrush

Thrush is an infection of the mouth caused by the organism *Candida albicans,* the organism that causes monilial vaginitis in the mother. The infant may acquire the infection as it passes through the birth canal of a mother so infected. However, the infection may be transferred from infant to infant on the hands of attendants and is favored by lack of cleanliness in feeding, in the care of the mother's nipples, or in the care of the bottles and the nipples. It is most likely to occur in weak, undernourished babies and in those receiving antibiotic therapy because the use of certain antibiotics alters the oral flora, making it more susceptible to this opportunistic organism.

The condition appears as small white patches (due to the fungus growth) on the tongue and in the mouth. These white plaques may be mistaken at first for small curds of milk. The infant's mouth must be kept clean, but great gentleness is required to avoid further injury to the delicate epithelium. Any attempt to wipe away the plaques usually causes bleeding.

Management

Nystatin (Mycostatin) is the drug of choice in treating oral monilia infections. It is applied directly to the mucosa with cotton-tipped applicator or given as an oral instillation (100,000 units per ml), 1 ml four times a day at intervals of 6 hours. The solution is slowly and gently instilled so that there is an opportunity for it to be widely distributed throughout the oral cavity before it is swallowed. It is important to keep equipment used for this baby such as linen, clothing, diapers, and feeding equipment especially clean. Breast-feeding mothers may be instructed to treat their nipples with topical nystatin.

Pneumonia

Pneumonia is a significant factor in 10% of neonatal deaths. Three types of pneumonia exist, depending on the time of presentation and route of acquisition.

Transplacental pneumonitis is a congenital infection acquired *in utero*. Symptoms manifest themselves early and may be connected with infections such as cytomegalovirus, herpes, rubella, toxoplasmosis, and *Listeria monocytogenes*.

Aspiration pneumonia, acquired as part of the birth process, manifests itself in the first few days of life. Organisms most often involved are: group B beta-hemolytic streptococci, group D streptococci, pneumococci, and coliform organisms.

Acquired pneumonia at delivery or in the postpartum period is the third type. *Staphylococcus aureus* and coliform organisms are commonly implicated in postnatally acquired pneumonia. Symptoms characteristic of neonatal pneumonia are poor color, hypotonia, and irritability. Symptoms of respiratory distress may vary, but include nasal flaring, tachypnea, retractions, diminished breath sounds, and rales.

Diagnosis is based on white blood cell (WBC) count, blood and tracheal cultures, and chest roentgenogram.

Treatment consists of appropriate antibiotic therapy, oxygen, and supportive measures. Many newborns with aspiration pneumonia do not require antibiotic therapy.[5]

Group B Streptococci

Infections of this nature are now the leading cause of early neonatal sepsis. Previously, coliform organisms retained this distinction. Five types of group B streptococci have been isolated. Sites of culture of the organisms are the throat, stools, and genital tract.[4,7] The maternal carrier rate is about 30%, remaining relatively the same regardless of trimester. Incidence is about 2 in 1000 live births with mortality of 40% to 75%.

Two separate clinical syndromes have been identified. Early onset has a higher mortality rate than late onset. Early-onset disease usually manifests itself within 3 to 5 days of life and most often within 12 to 24 hours. Early-onset symptoms closely resemble those of respiratory distress syndrome (RDS).[3,4]

The late-onset syndrome, occurring between 10 and 50 days of age, presents with nonspecific signs of irritability, lethargy, apnea, failure to nurse, and fever.[3] Meningitis often is the consequence of late-onset disease.

Diagnosis is presumed based on isolation of the organism from the neonate's gastric contents and confirmed by positive blood or cerebrospinal cultures.

Treatment is supportive in addition to appropriate therapy following laboratory studies.[3]

Necrotizing Enterocolitis

Necrotizing enterocolitis (NEC) has become the most common surgical emergency in neonates. Incidence is 2% of all neonates admitted to neonatal intensive care units, with mortality rates of 30% to 50%.[8]

The stressed, low-birth-weight infant seems to be most at risk for NEC. Other associated factors are premature rupture of membranes, placenta previa, maternal sepsis, and preeclampsia.[9] Infants already stricken with RDS, congenital heart disease, and sepsis are also at risk. The disease has been diagnosed in term infants.

Etiology

The basic cause of NEC is unknown, although many factors have been implicated as contributors.

Three factors appear to be essential in the progression of the disease: intestinal ischemia, invasion of the intestine by gas-forming bacteria, and formula feeding which irritates the intestine.

A popular theory for the cause of intestinal ischemia is the shunting of blood to the brain and heart in response to hypoxia. Vasospasm may also be induced by umbilical catheterization. However, NEC has also been diagnosed in infants who have never been catheterized.

Bacteria that have been cultured from infants with NEC include *Salmonella, E. coli, Klebsiella, Clostridium, Staphylococcus,* and coxsackie virus.[9]

Although NEC has developed in breast-fed infants and in infants who have never been fed, it is still thought that breast milk provides immunity in most cases.

Diagnosis

Diagnosis is based upon observation of clinical signs and radiographic findings. Onset is between the first and tenth day of life in a majority of infants.

Clinical Signs

Clinical signs, in order of frequency, are abdominal distention, lethargy, gastric retention, temperature instability, vomiting and regurgitation, apnea, and gastrointestinal bleeding.[9,10]

Radiographic Findings

Diagnosis is confirmed by the presence of intramural bowel gas—"pneumatosis intestinalis" is a classic sign.[10]

Medical Management

Medical management is geared toward resting the bowel and counteracting sepsis. All feedings are held and nasogastric suction is begun. Following blood, urine, and stool cultures, antibiotic therapy is begun, either parenteral or by gavage. Fluid therapy is initiated, often utilizing total parenteral nutrition. Serial abdominal roentgenograms are obtained.

Surgical Intervention

The timing of surgical intervention is variable, but the critical indicators are evidence of free perforation of the intestine and intestinal gangrene. The procedures performed are resection of the necrotic bowel and double-barrelled enterostomy.

Nursing Care

Preventive nursing care of infants receiving early feedings include abdominal evaluation for distention by measurement of abdominal girth and measurement of gastric residuals prior to feedings.[10]

Following diagnosis of NEC, the infant is observed closely for changes in abdominal status. This can be accomplished most efficiently by exposing the infant's entire abdomen. The abdomen is observed for distention by measurement of abdominal girth and visual inspection for tight, shiny skin. Any changes in vital signs may be indicative of shock secondary to intestinal perforation. Careful intake and output measurements are essential, especially measurement and description of gastric contents. All stools must be hematested. Postoperative care is similar to that of other abdominal surgeries, with special attention to stoma care. Infants with NEC usually are placed on long-term total parenteral nutrition therapy until the bowel is re-anastomosed.

Parents of infants with NEC require simple explanations of the baby's condition, opportunity for frequent contact, and increasing care-taking of the infant over the long course of therapy.

Nonbacterial Infections—The TORCH Complex

Toxoplasmosis

Toxoplasmosis may result from transplacental transfer of the parasite *Toxoplasma gondii* to the fetus. From 2 to 7 women in 1000 acquire the active disease in pregnancy, resulting in 30% to 40% having infected infants.

Early symptoms in the neonate are hepatosplenomegaly with jaundice, chorioretinitis, lethargy or seizure or both. Later manifestations are hydrocephalus or microcephaly, mental retardation, or cerebral calcification.[3,11]

Diagnosis may be based on IgM fluorescent antibody test.[3] Drug therapy is questionable as to effectiveness. Sulfadiazine and pyrimethamine are drugs of choice. Folinic acid may be given to counteract effects of pyrimethamine such as thrombocytopenia or leukopenia. Once the diagnosis is confirmed, strict isolation is not necessary.[11]

Rubella

Although rubella is usually considered to be a relatively mild illness, for the fetus whose mother has been exposed, the consequences may be disastrous. Damage to the fetus may occur without obvious illness in the mother. Consequences in the fetus depend on the virulence of the virus and the gestational age of the fetus. The fetus is at a crucial period in the first 4 weeks of pregnancy, when there is a 50% chance of a resulting anomaly. From the fifth to eighth week chances decrease to 25%. Finally, there is an 8% to 17% chance during the ninth week to twelfth week.[12]

Major defects identified with infection occurring up to 4 weeks prior to pregnancy or during the first trimester are cardiac defects, cataracts, and deafness. There is a higher rate of spontaneous abortions and stillbirths.[12] Some additional problems of infants infected in the first trimester are intrauterine growth retardation, glaucoma, hepatosplenomegaly, hepatitis, lesions in long bones, meningitis, and pneumonia.[3,12] Psychomotor retardation, microcephaly, and deafness result from second trimester infection. Infection during the last trimester of pregnancy may also result in problems.[12]

Diagnosis of rubella is made by the rapid rubella virus hemagglutinin-inhibition (HI) test.

Treatment of the neonate consists of supportive management, surgical correction of defects as feasible, and multidisciplinary referral.

Strict isolation and care by immunized personnel are essential. Pregnant women must not handle these infants because the virus may be shed through tears, saliva, and other body secretions for years.[11]

The potential risk to the fetus of susceptible pregnant women is great, particularly in the first 3 to 4 months of pregnancy. Inclusion of rubella testing as part of the routine prenatal laboratory panel can identify nonimmune women and precautions to avoid exposure to possible cases of rubella can be advised. Immunizing nonpregnant susceptible women is the most important preventive measure, but they should not become pregnant for 3 months following vaccination. Immune globulin injections will not prevent rubella. They may suppress the external evidence but a subclinical rubella may result.[3]

Cytomegalovirus

Cytomegalovirus appears to be the most common among the known pathogens. Positive cervical cultures occur in 3% to 28% of pregnant women. Infections are usually transmitted transplacentally and intrapartally, and, less frequently, through breast milk and other contact. Intrapartal or postpartal infections are usually asymptomatic. Classic signs occurring at birth or within 24 hours are jaundice, thrombocytopenia with petechiae, hepatosplenomegaly, chorioretinitis, and microcephaly with intracranial calcifications.[3,11]

Diagnostic tools include immunofluorescence IgM, rising antibody titers, and virus isolation from throat, urine, or cerebrospinal fluid.[3]

Treatment is supportive. Long-term followup is essential to follow growth and development that may be impaired. Isolation while in the nursery is essential.

Herpes Simplex Virus

Herpes simplex (type II) in the neonate may be transmitted through contact with the mother's infected birth canal at delivery, from infection ascending from the cervix during pregnancy, or from possible transplacental passage. The first mode mentioned is by far the most frequent and likely. Risk of acquisition of infection in a neonate of a genitally infected mother could be as high as 50%.[13]

The neonate is in greater jeopardy for acquired HSV type II when a primary infection exists in the mother at time of delivery, delivery is vaginal, membranes were ruptured 4 to 6 hours before delivery, or infant is preterm.[13]

Several forms of disease are possible. The first is the very serious *disseminated herpes* with high mortality of 60% to 90%. Disseminated herpes mainly affects the liver, adrenals, and possibly CNS. The second form is the *localized herpes,* in which lesions are found in the eyes, skin, mouth, and brain. A third form is the *asymptomatic herpes* infection, with symptoms developing up to 21 days of life. Symptoms are basically the same for all forms, except for the timing of appearance.

Diagnosis is difficult because initial symptoms are very nonspecific—poor eating, listlessness, restlessness, and diarrhea. As severity of symptoms increases, characteristic skin lesions occur. Other symptoms that may be seen include fever or hypothermia, productive or nonproductive coughing, vomiting, dyspnea, tachypnea, tachycardia, cyanosis, jaundice, seizures, bleeding tendencies, and shock.[3,11,13]

Diagnosis is made by smears from skin vesicles and viral isolation from vesicle fluid, throat, urine, blood, or cerebrospinal fluid. Specimens for passive hemagglutination assay and detection of IgM antibodies are also diagnostic tests.[3]

Treatment of the infant with drugs has not been encouraging because antiviral drugs are so toxic. Adenine arabinoside (ara-A) is not as toxic and may be utilized. Strict isolation of the neonate is essential.

Preventive measures include recognition of active herpes in the mother and recommendation of cesarean delivery for all pregnant women at the time of labor or 3 weeks prior.

Neonatal Problems Secondary to Maternal Disorders

Infant of a Diabetic Mother

The successful control of diabetes with insulin has led to survival and fertility of an increasing number of pregnant women. Incidence of infants of diabetic mothers (IDM) is 4 in 1000 pregnancies, and the incidence of infants born to mothers with gestational diabetes is 6 in 1000. The neonatal mortality rate for all classes of diabetes has decreased from 40% to approximately 5% to 10%.[14]

Perinatal mortality and morbidity are generally attributed to the increased number of pregnancy complications, stillbirths, cesarean sections, and preterm births.

Appearance

IDMs are large for gestational age, having a cushinoid-type of appearance—round face, soft skin, and abundance of subcutaneous fatty tissue (Fig. 44-6).[3]

Pathophysiology

The basic cause of the IDM's clinical appearance and problems can be narrowed down to a combination of hyperinsulinism and epinephrine depletion. Hyperglycemia in the pregnant woman stimulates fetal beta cells in the islets of Langerhans to increase secretion of insulin. Consequently, utilization of glucose and protein anabolism are increased. Insulin may be inhibited by secretion of epinephrine. When the IDM is born, glucose supply is shut off, resulting in a neonatal hypoglycemic state.[15]

Clinical Problems and Related Management

Macrosomia is increased body weight due to deposition of fat, not increased total body weight.

Hypoglycemia is the most common metabolic problem. Glucose levels are the lowest at 1 hour to 2 hours of life, consequently blood sugars should be monitored at an early age. Symptoms that may be observed include jitteriness, tremors, seizures, high-pitched or weak cry, refusal to feed, and hypotonia. Frequent monitoring of glucose levels is essential while treatment is carried out. Treatment most likely will be a constant infusion of 10% to 15% glucose in a volume appropriate for weight and gestational age. In addition, some centers may administer a bolus of 25% or 50% glucose. Intravenous infusions may be tapered according to the success of oral feedings.[15]

Congenital anomalies may be serious, and anencephaly, meningocele, transposition of the great vessels, ventricular septal defect, and coarctation of the aorta predominate.[15]

Respiratory distress syndrome incidence is high, possibly due to the fetal hyperinsulinism state. This state may antagonize cortisol's action on lung maturation. Management is the same as for preterm infants who have RDS (Chap. 42).

Hyperbilirubinemia incidence is relatively high, possibly due to decreased extracellular fluid volume, hyperviscosity of blood, premature state, and traumatic delivery.

Hypocalcemia symptoms are jitteriness, convulsions, and twitching. One theory regarding etiology is that maternal hypercalcemia produces a neonatal hypoparathyroidism. Management consists of intravenous or oral supplemental calcium.[15]

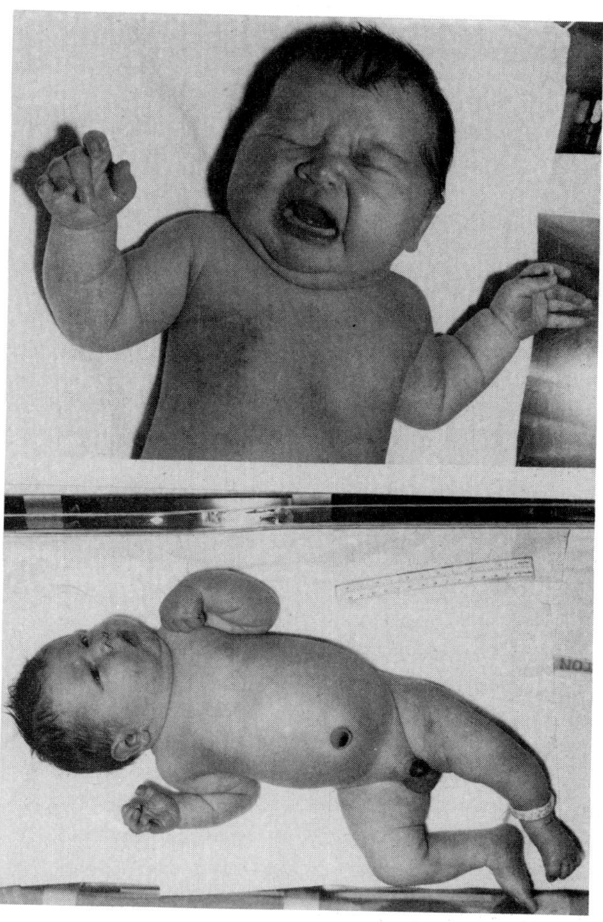

Figure 44-6.
The infant of a diabetic mother showing typical features (Avery GB: Neonatology: Pathophysiology and Management of the Newborn, 2nd ed. Philadelphia, JB Lippincott, 1981)

Pathologic Jaundice in the Neonate

Hyperbilirubinemia in the neonate may occur due to numerous causes. Physiological jaundice, evident after 24 hours of age, is a common phenomenon (see Chap. 31).

Pathological forms of jaundice may be the result of a variety of factors. Hemolytic disease of the newborn (*e.g.*, Rh or ABO incompatibility) is significant but decreasing in severity due to preventive measures. The administration of anti-D globulin (Rhogam) to eligible women has been an important intervention combating Rh incompatibility and erythroblastosis fetalis. ABO incompatibility has always been less of a threat to the newborn than the Rh problem. For extensive discussion of the pathophysiology of these entities see Chapter 40.

Other factors which may produce hyperbilirubinemia by the overproduction of unconjugated bilirubin are:

Enclosed hemorrhage, for example, cephalhematoma

Ecchymosis from bruising, as in a breech delivery

Congenital enzyme deficiency, as in glucose-6-phosphate-dehydrogenase deficiency (G6PD)

Drug-induced hemolytic anemia, such as that produced by excessive amounts of vitamin K

The following factors delay or alter bilirubin conjugation into water-soluble form:

Immaturity of glucuronyl transferase enzyme system

Asphyxia, hypoglycemia, hypothermia

Liver cell damage due to sepsis or medications[3]

Finally, hepatitis, biliary duct obstruction, and galactosemia can lead to impaired excretion of bilirubin.

Pathological forms of jaundice pose a serious threat to the neonate due to the possibility of the complication of kernicterus. Kernicterus results from the accumulation of unconjugated and unbound bilirubin in brain cells. Neurologic signs occur and ultimately intellectual function is impaired. The exact bilirubin level at which kernicterus occurs varies with each individual infant, occurring sooner in the preterm infant.

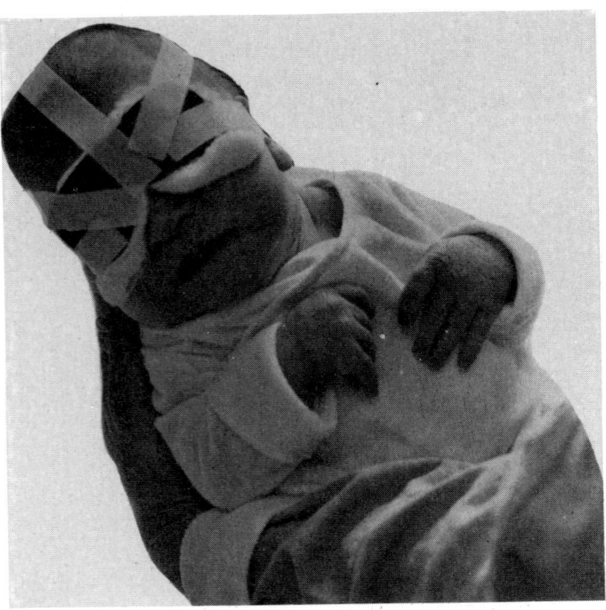

Figure 44-7.
Infant prepared with eye shield in place for phototherapy treatment.

Clinical Signs

Pathological disease may be suspected if jaundice is evident within the first 24 hours of life, lasts more than 7 days in the term infant or 10 days in the preterm, or serum bilirubin increases by greater than 5 mg/dl every 24 hours. Further investigation is also needed if bilirubin levels are greater than 12 mg/dl in the term infant and 15 mg/dl in preterm infants during the first 48 hours.[16] Finally, infants with erythroblastosis fetalis (severe isoimmunization) present with generalized edema, pallor, hepatosplenomegaly, hydrothorax, and severe anemia.

Diagnostic tests that may be utilized are direct and total serum bilirubin, blood typing of mother and baby, complete blood count, total serum protein, and direct Coombs' test. The Coombs' test is performed on neonatal cord blood, measuring whether neonatal red blood cells (RBCs) are coated with maternal antibodies. A positive Coombs' test may prompt immediate phototherapy, without waiting for a rise in bilirubin. Treatment may involve immediate exchange transfusion with serious cases, such as erythroblastosis fetalis, although more often conservative treatment of phototherapy is utilized.

An exchange transfusion alternately removes a small amount of blood from the infant and replaces it with the same amount of donor blood. An infusion is started either in the umbilical stump or by cutdown into the jugular or femoral arteries. The procedure is sterile and done with minimization of cold stress to the infant. The donor blood is warmed, and amounts of 5 ml to 20 ml at a time are slowly exchanged. Following every 100 ml, calcium gluconate is usually given, then the exchange transfusion procedure proceeds.

A 50% glucose solution and sodium bicarbonate should also be available for management of hypoglycemia and acidosis. Cardiac arrhythmias are also a danger. Use of warmed blood in small amounts with calcium gluconate minimizes this risk. Careful monitoring of vital signs, time, type, and amount of medication, increments of blood exchange, and infant response is essential.

Phototherapy. The use of intense fluorescent light to reduce serum bilirubin has gained acceptance in the treatment of hyperbilirubinemia (Fig. 44-7). Blue light decomposes bilirubin by photo-oxidation, which appears to take place in the skin. The chemical nature of the products formed in the breakdown of bilirubin has not been precisely determined, nor have long-term outcomes been evaluated as well as the theoretic effects of intense light upon a wide spectrum of biological processes. For these reasons, there are some reservations about the unqualified use of this treatment for all jaundiced babies.

Phototherapy is applied by exposing the nude infant to fluorescent daylight bulbs that supply 200 to 400 foot-candles on the skin surface. Phototherapy success is measured by serial bilirubin levels. The infant's eyes are shielded from the light by means of patches. The nurse should make sure that the lids are closed when the blindfold is applied. The bandages are to be removed at least once each shift to inspect the eyes for conjunctivitis, and to allow eye contact with parents and visual stimulation.

Some centers cover the genital areas with a face mask as a "bikini diaper," while others do not. Effects of exposure to light, particularly with male genitalia, are unknown. Monitoring of temperature is important because additional heat from the light necessitates adjustments in environmental temperature. Infants in open cribs may exhibit heat loss. Fluids need to be increased to compensate for insensible water loss. Expected changes in elimination patterns are loose green stools and green urine. Evaluation of skin color with the light turned off is necessary. The newborn needs frequent repositioning in order to expose all skin surfaces to light. Finally, the neonate needs to have tactile stimulation as often as possible, whether with parents or the nursing staff. Parental contact will provide reassurance to the family of the infant's progress.

Breast Milk Jaundice

Rarely (about 1 in 200 breast-fed babies) jaundice is caused by breast milk. Breast milk jaundice does not produce a rise in bilirubin levels until the second week, and peaks in the third week, but may persist as long as 6 weeks.

The exact etiology has not been determined but several theories are in existence. The most popular theory points to pregnanediol, a steroid present during the last 3 months of pregnancy and possibly high in breast milk for 6 weeks postpartum. Pregnanediol antagonizes the enzyme glucuronyl transferase, which converts bilirubin to excretable form.[17]

Controversy exists over the length of time necessary to discontinue breast-feeding. The range is between 12 to 24 hours and 2 to 4 days. Bilirubin levels rarely climb higher than 15 mg/dl to 20 mg/dl. The mother needs instructions on how to pump her breasts during the time the infant receives formula feedings.

Addiction Syndromes

Drug Addiction in the Newborn

Drug addiction in the newborn is being seen more frequently with the rise of drug addiction in the general population. Furthermore, it is the nurse who may be the first to discover this condition. The symptoms of the infant are due to withdrawal rather than narcosis. They may appear almost immediately after birth or be delayed for several hours, depending on the time of the mother's last injection of narcotic, the dose, and the interval between the administration of the narcotic and the delivery.

The infant may manifest restlessness, tremors, shrill crying, convulsions, or twitchings of the extremities or face. The Moro reflex may be incomplete, and the deep tendon reflexes may be increased. Diarrhea, vomiting, anorexia, yawning, sneezing, and excessive mucus also may be present. These symptoms parallel somewhat those found in the adult undergoing withdrawal symptoms from narcotics. If the signs of withdrawal are unrecognized, the baby may die; if the infant is treated (hydration, supportive measures, and diminishing doses of sedatives), recovery and permanent cure are ensured because the infant does not have a psychic dependence on narcotics.

Heroin or methadone are the narcotic drugs most commonly involved in neonatal drug addiction. Withdrawal symptoms occur in 70% to 90% of infants born to addict mothers. Many of these babies are also small for gestational age. In addition to CNS hyperirritability, these infants have sleep disturbances including absence of quiet sleep and inability to sleep. These problems may persist past 1 year of age. Abnormalities of crying (high-pitched, shrill, and continuous crying) strain the mother's endurance, as do sleep disturbances. Addicted infants have a high sucking need, although sucking may be disorganized or depressed. Overfeeding because of this need to suck can compound gastrointestinal problems such as vomiting, regurgitation, and diarrhea. It is advisable to provide a pacifier to meet the infant's nonnutritive sucking needs and reduce tension levels.[18] Infants of barbiturate-addicted mothers manifest the same types of symptoms, but with later onset.

Addicted babies are harder to hold, less cuddly, and more difficult to console, and show depressed visual response and exaggerated auditory response. They appear to be less alert, are more irritable, have increased muscle tone, and are more labile in alternating between hyperactivity and lethargy. These characteristics make addicted infants harder to mother in a situation where every support is needed to enhance mother–infant bonding. Minimizing separation of infant and mother and assisting the mother in experiencing satisfying caretaking episodes are critical in promoting the relationship. An honest and open approach in discussing the effects of addiction on the baby and his needs may help the mother feel more confident in her mothering ability. She may experience guilt and anxiety, and the question of care for the infant after discharge must be discussed. A multidisciplinary approach involving drug counselors, social workers, and community health nurses is useful in providing follow-up care for both mother and baby.

Fetal Alcohol Syndrome

Maternal alcohol intake above 3 oz of absolute alcohol or 6 drinks per day can result in congenital anomalies of the infant with typical craniofacial and limb defects, cardiovascular defects, intrauterine growth retardation, and developmental delay. It is not certain whether alcohol or its breakdown, acetaldehyde, is responsible for the fetal damage. Alcohol interferes with protein synthesis and the absorption of numerous nutrients, and heavy consumption is most likely to affect fetal development during the first trimester when organogenesis is occurring. Spontaneous abortion is common among alcoholics, but improved nutrition and vitamin fortification now allow many of these pregnancies to continue. If excessive alcohol consumption occurs during the second trimester, infant weight is most affected, which leads to growth retardation.

One study found that daily consumption of 1 oz of absolute alcohol before pregnancy is associated with a decrease in birthweight of 91 g. The same amount in late pregnancy is associated with a decrease in birthweight of 160 g.[19]

Characteristic anomalies seen in the fetal alcohol syndrome include microcephaly, short palpebral fissures, epicanthal folds, cleft palate, maxillary hypoplasia, altered palmar creases, joint defects, cardiac defects, anomalous genitalia, fine-motor dysfunction, and capillary hemangiomas. Postnatally, there often is developmental delay and growth deficiency. There may be severe mental retardation with depressed sucking and swallowing reflexes, or slight retardation which is not detected until later when developmental problems occur. The extent of immediate fetal depression at birth depends upon the time and amount of the mother's last intake of alcohol, as well as such problems as anoxia or aspiration perinatally. Difficulties in feeding and disturbances of sleep are common in the newborn with this syndrome. Prenatal detection of excessive alcohol consumption and counseling to stop or reduce drinking are the most important preventive measures.[20]

Conclusion

Infants with acquired disorders may be only mildly affected, or they may be confined to intensive care for months. Parents of these infants need teaching from nurses in order to be able to cope with any unexpected illness of the infant. Parents also need assistance in dealing with guilt associated with this traumatic experience.

References

1. Phibbs RH: Delivery room management of the newborn. In Avery GB (ed): Neonatology: Pathophysiology and Management of the Newborn, pp 182–201. Philadelphia, JB Lippincott, 1981

2. MacDonald MG, Risenberg HM: Neonatal emergencies: Fetal neonatal transition, acute intensive care. In Bolognese RJ, Schwartz RH (eds): Perinatal Medicine: Management of the High Risk Fetus and Neonate, pp 279–299. Baltimore, Williams & Wilkins, 1977

3. Babson SG, Pernoll ML, Benda GI: Diagnosis and Management of the Fetus and Neonate at Risk, pp 211–274. St Louis, CV Mosby, 1980

4. Daum RS, Smith AL: Bacterial sepsis in the newborn. Clin Obstet Gynecol 22, 2:391–395, June, 1979

5. McCracken GH: Bacterial and viral infections in the newborn. In Avery GB (ed): Neonatology: Pathophysiology and Management of the Newborn, pp 723–747. Philadelphia, JB Lippincott, 1981

6. Reynolds DW, Stagno S, Alford CA: Chronic congenital and perinatal infections. In Avery GB (ed): Neonatology: Pathophysiology and Management of the Newborn, pp 748–789. Philadelphia, JB Lippincott, 1981

7. Mizer HE: Group B streptococci in neonatal infection. American Journal of Maternal Child Nursing 3, 1:21–24, January/February 1978

8. Avery GB, Fletcher AB: Nutrition. In Avery GB (ed): Neonatology: Pathophysiology and Management of the Newborn, pp 1002–1060. Philadelphia, JB Lippincott, 1981

9. Kosloske AM: Necrotizing enterocolitis in the neonate. Surg Gynecol Obstet 148:261–263, February 1979

10. Flores RN: Necrotizing enterocolitis. Nurs Clin North Am 13, 1:41, March 1978

11. Visintine AM, Nahmias AJ: The TORCH syndrome of perinatal infection. In McNall LK (ed): Contemporary Obstetric and Gynecologic Nursing, pp 94–95. St Louis, CV Mosby, 1980

12. Brown SG: The devastating effects of congenital rubella. American Journal of Maternal Child Nursing 4, No. 3:171–173, May, June 1979

13. Bahr JE: Herpes virus hominis type 2 in women and newborns. American Journal of Maternal Child Nursing 3, No. 1:16–21, January/February 1978

14. Fletcher AB: Infant of a diabetic mother. In Avery GB (ed): Neonatology: Pathophysiology and Management of the Newborn, pp 287–302. Philadelphia, JB Lippincott 1981

15. McAteer J: Diabetic pregnancy and neonatal outcome. Crit Care Q 4:69, December 1979

16. Maisels MJ: Neonatal jaundice. In Avery GB (ed): Neonatology: Pathophysiology and Management of the Newborn, pp 473–544. Philadelphia, JB Lippincott, 1981

17. Ward JM: Breast milk jaundice. Cent Afr J Med 24:73–74, 1978

18. Kantor GK: Addicted mother, addicted baby—a challenge to health care providers. American Journal of Maternal Child Nursing 2, No. 5:281–289, September/October 1977

19. Lindor E, McCarthy AM, McRae MG: Fetal alcohol syndrome. JOGN Nurs 9, No. 4:222–228, July/August 1980

20. Luke B: Maternal alcoholism and fetal alcohol syndrome. Am J Nurs 77, No. 12:1924–1926, December 1977

Suggested Reading

Bliss VJ: Nursing care for infants with neonatal necrotizing enterocolitis. American Journal of Maternal Child Nursing 1, 1:37–40, January/February 1976

Gennaro S: Listeria infection: Nursing care of mother and infant. American Journal of Maternal Child Nursing 5, 6:390–392, November/December 1980

Gennaro S: Necrotizing enterocolitis: Detecting it and treating it. Nursing 80 10, 1:52–55, January 1980

Picaud FJ, Francois R, Ruitton-Ugliengo A, David A: The newborn of diabetic mothers. Biol Neonate 24, 1 and 2:1–30, 1974

Stephens CJ: The fetal alcohol syndrome: Cause for concern. American Journal of Maternal Child Nursing 6, 4:251–256, July/August 1981

Vogel M: When the pregnant woman is diabetic: Care of the newborn. Am J Nurs 79, 3:458–460, March 1979

Study Aids for Unit VIII: Assessment and Management of Perinatal Disorders

Conference Material

1. In your own hospital setting, evaluate the facilities for and the care of the newborn infants in relation to the prevention of infection.

2. A mother's firstborn infant has a cleft lip and cleft palate. The infant is apparently normal otherwise. The distraught mother can see only "my poor deformed baby girl" and blames herself for this "tragedy," because she did not follow her physician's instructions during pregnancy, particularly in relation to good nutrition. How might the nurse handle the nursing problems in this situation?

3. How do you account for the high infant mortality during the neonatal period?

4. What community agencies in your city render services for handicapped children? What is the procedure for making the referral to such agencies? How can the public health nurse function most effectively in such cases?

5. What legislation in your city or state has contributed to reducing the incidence of congenital syphilis?

6. What methods are used by your hospital, well-baby clinics, or other community agencies for the detection of phenylketonuria?

Multiple Choice

Read through the entire question and place your answer on the line to the right.

1. Which of the following factors may predispose to the production of an erythroblastotic infant?
   - A. Rh-negative mother
   - B. Rh-positive father
   - C. Rh-positive fetus
   - D. Rh-positive substance from the fetus finds its way into the mother's bloodstream to build up antibodies.
   - E. Mother has had a previous Rh-positive pregnancy or transfusion.

   Select the number corresponding to the correct letters.
   1. A and D
   2. A, C, and D
   3. B, C, and E
   4. All of the above ______

2. Which of the following statements concerning diabetes complicated by pregnancy are correct?
   - A. The size of the placenta tends to be in direct relationship to the size of the infant.

B. Toxemia occurs more frequently than in nondiabetic pregnancies.
C. Deliveries are always performed by cesarean section, usually 2 weeks prior to term.
D. The fetus tends to be large.
E. Hypoglycemia occurs in the infant following delivery.

Select the number corresponding to the correct letters.
1. A and B
2. B, D, and E
3. B, C, D, and E
4. All of the above ____

3. The most effective treatment of erythroblastosis is accomplished by blood transfusion. Which of the following is the best method to use?
A. Exchange transfusion with Rh-negative blood
B. Exchange transfusion with Rh-positive blood
C. Exchange transfusion with blood plasma
D. Repeated small transfusions with Rh-negative blood
E. Repeated small transfusions with Rh-positive blood
F. Repeated small transfusions with blood plasma ____

4. Hemolytic disease of the newborn may be produced by the union of parents with which of the following blood types?
A. Rh-positive mother with Rh-negative father
B. Rh-negative mother with Rh-negative father
C. Rh-negative mother with Rh-positive father
D. Type O mother with Type A father
E. Type A mother with Type B father

Select the number corresponding to the correct letters.
1. A and C
2. B and D
3. C and D
4. All of the above ____

5. Which one of the following infectious diseases, when contracted by the mother during the first trimester of pregnancy, will most often produce congenital anomalies in the infant?
A. Scarlet fever
B. Rubella
C. Diphtheria
D. Rubeola
E. Typhoid fever ____

Multiple Choice (continued)

6. Some disorders that affect the infant in the neonatal period are manifestations of inborn errors of metabolism. Which of the following conditions would this include?

A. Phenylketonuria
B. Icterus neonatorum
C. Galactosemia
D. Down's syndrome
E. Erythroblastosis fetalis

Select the number corresponding to the correct letter or letters.

1. A only
2. A and C
3. B, C, and D
4. B, D, and E ____

7. What has recently become the best method to prevent erythroblastosis fetalis?

A. Injection of the mother soon after delivery with Rh-immune globulin to prevent maternal sensitization
B. Transfusing the mother during pregnancy
C. Transfusing all Rh-negative fathers
D. Transfusing all Rh-negative babies
E. Repeated small transfusions of Rh-positive blood to the mother

Select the number corresponding to the correct letter or letters.

1. A only
2. A and B
3. B, C, and D
4. C, D, and E ____

8. Sampling of amniotic fluid can be useful in determining fetal lung maturity. The determination that is carried out for this purpose is

A. Bilirubin
B. Cytology
C. Creatinine
D. Lecithin-sphingomyelin (L/S) ratio ____

9. Certain behaviors indicate that a preterm infant may be ready to advance from gavage feedings to nipple feedings. Which of the following are those behaviors?

A. Strong, vigorous suck
B. Sucking and swallowing coordinated
C. Competent gag reflex
D. Sucking on gavage tube
E. Wakefulness before feeding time

Select the number corresponding to the correct letters.

1. B, C, and E
2. C and D
3. A and C
4. All of the above ____

10. Nursing care for an infant receiving TPN includes which of the following interventions?

- **A.** Changing tubing every 48 hours
- **B.** Changing the insertion site dressing once a week
- **C.** Frequent checking of Dextrostix
- **D.** Measuring head circumference
- **E.** Offering pacifier to infant

Select the number corresponding to the correct letters.

1. A, B, and E
2. B and C
3. A and D
4. All of the above ____

11. Small-for-gestational-age infants exhibit which of the following clinical problems?

- **A.** Hyperglycemia
- **B.** Anemia
- **C.** Congenital disorders
- **D.** Hypercalcemia
- **E.** Temperature instability

Select the number corresponding to the correct letter or letters.

1. A and B
2. B, C, and E
3. C and E
4. All of the above ____

12. When the mother learned that her preterm infant was receiving gavage feedings she asked the nurse why this was being done. Which of the following reasons may be correct for the nurse to reply?

- **A.** "This method of feeding your baby was indicated because he became exhausted when he tried to swallow."
- **B.** "Feeding your baby this way prevents him from vomiting and thus eliminates the danger of his aspirating formula into his lungs."
- **C.** "Feeding your baby this way conserves his strength and permits him to receive food into his stomach when sucking or swallowing may be difficult."
- **D.** "Your baby can be given his formula quickly this way and thus he does not have to be handled as much."
- **E.** "A tiny baby's resistance to infection is poor, so gavage feeding is really a protective measure against such infections as thrush, which he might acquire if he were bottle-fed."

Select the number corresponding to the correct letter or letters.

1. A only
2. C only
3. B, C, and D
4. B, D, and E ____

Multiple Choice
(continued)

13. Signs of neonatal congestive heart failure include
A. Tachypnea
B. Bradycardia
C. Hepatomegaly
D. Edema
E. Sternal retractions

Select the number corresponding to the correct letters.
1. A, C, D, and E
2. B, C, and E
3. A and D
4. B and E ____

14. Which of the following conditions are congenital disorders?
A. Patent ductus arteriosus
B. Brachial palsy
C. Hydrocephalus
D. Retrolental fibroplasia
E. Caput succedaneum

Select the number corresponding to the correct letter or letters.
1. A and C
2. B, C, and D
3. B, D, and E
4. All of the above ____

15. Factors that may produce hyperbilirubinemia by the overproduction of unconjugated bilirubin are
A. Rh incompatibility
B. Asphyxia
C. Ecchymosis from bruising
D. Liver cell damage due to sepsis
E. Hepatitis

Select the number corresponding to the correct letters.
1. B, C, and D
2. A, D, and E
3. A and C
4. All of the above ____

16. The following are examples of viral infections in the neonate:
A. Herpes simplex type II
B. Rubella
C. Syphilis
D. Toxoplasmosis
E. Cytomegalovirus

Select the number corresponding to the correct letters.
1. A, B, D, and E
2. B, C, D, and E
3. A and C
4. All of the above ____

17. Which of the following clinical problems are possible in the infant of a diabetic mother?
   A. Small-for-gestational-age
   B. Respiratory distress syndrome
   C. Hyperglycemia
   D. Hyperbilirubinemia
   E. Hypercalcemia

   Select the number corresponding to the correct letters.
   1. A, C, and E
   2. B and D
   3. B, C, and E
   4. All of the above _____

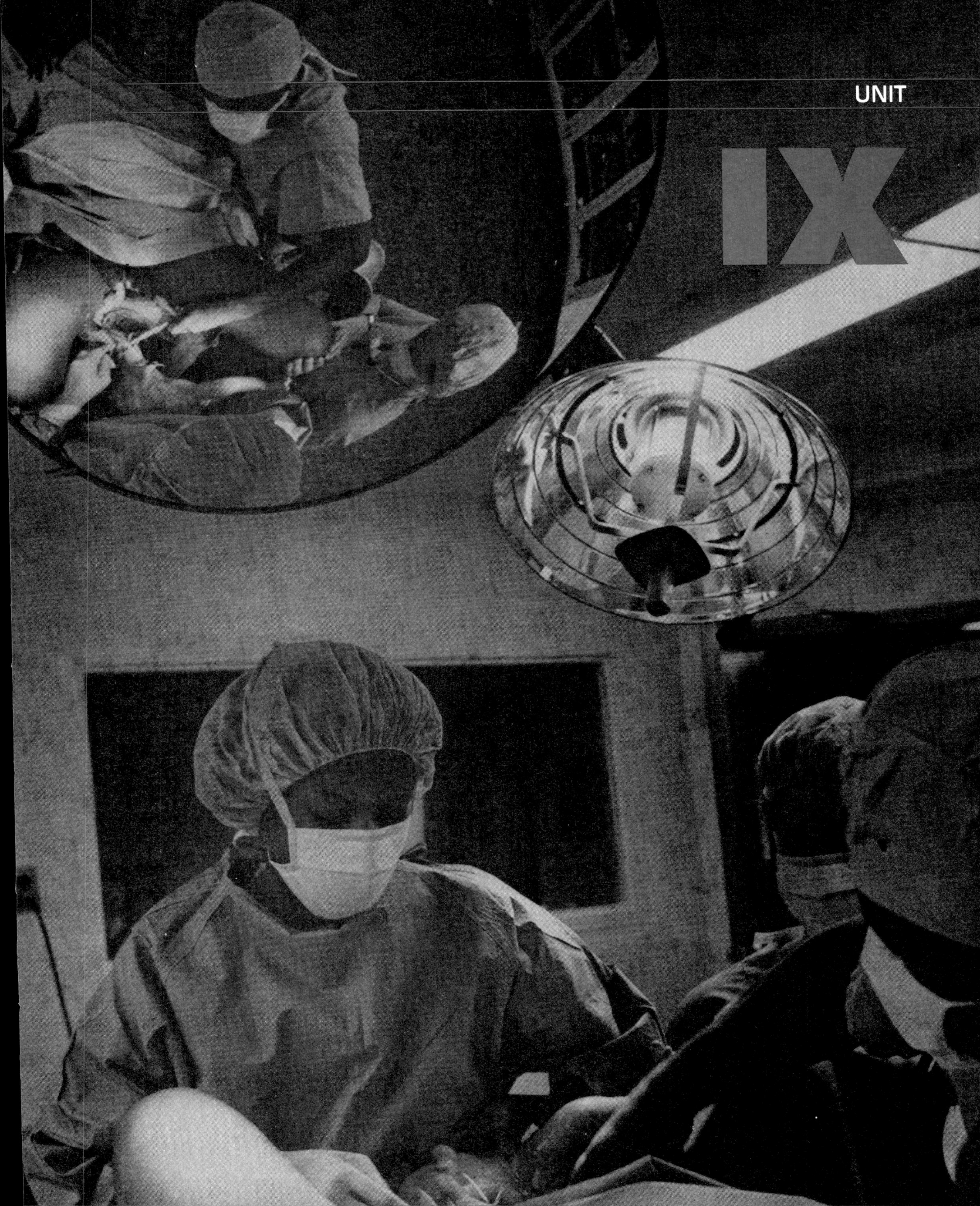

UNIT

IX

UNIT IX

Special Considerations in Maternity Nursing

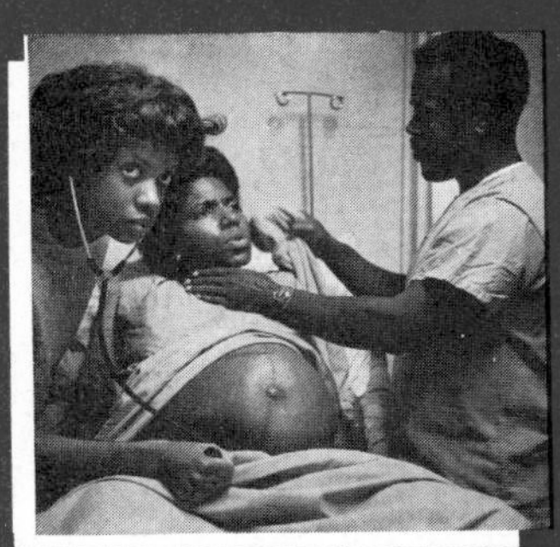

45 Alternatives in Maternity Care

History of Family-Centered Maternity Care

Resurgence of Home Births

Alternative Birth Centers

Nurse-Midwifery

Options Available for Cesarean Births

Options in Maternity Nursing

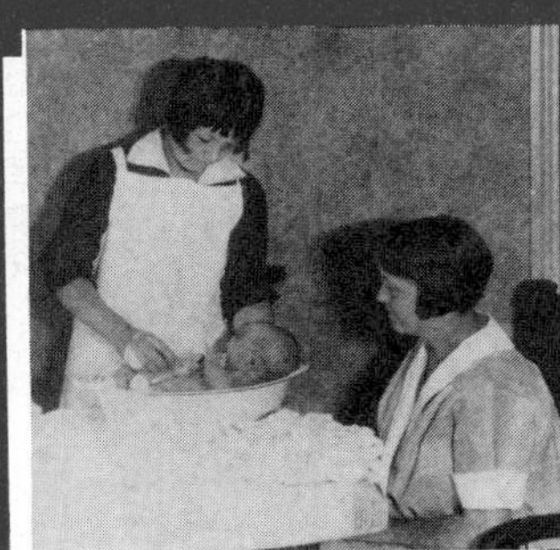

46 Evolution of Maternity Nursing

Obstetrics Over the Centuries

Development of Maternal and Infant Care in the United States

The Emergence and Development of Maternity Nursing

Future Possibilities

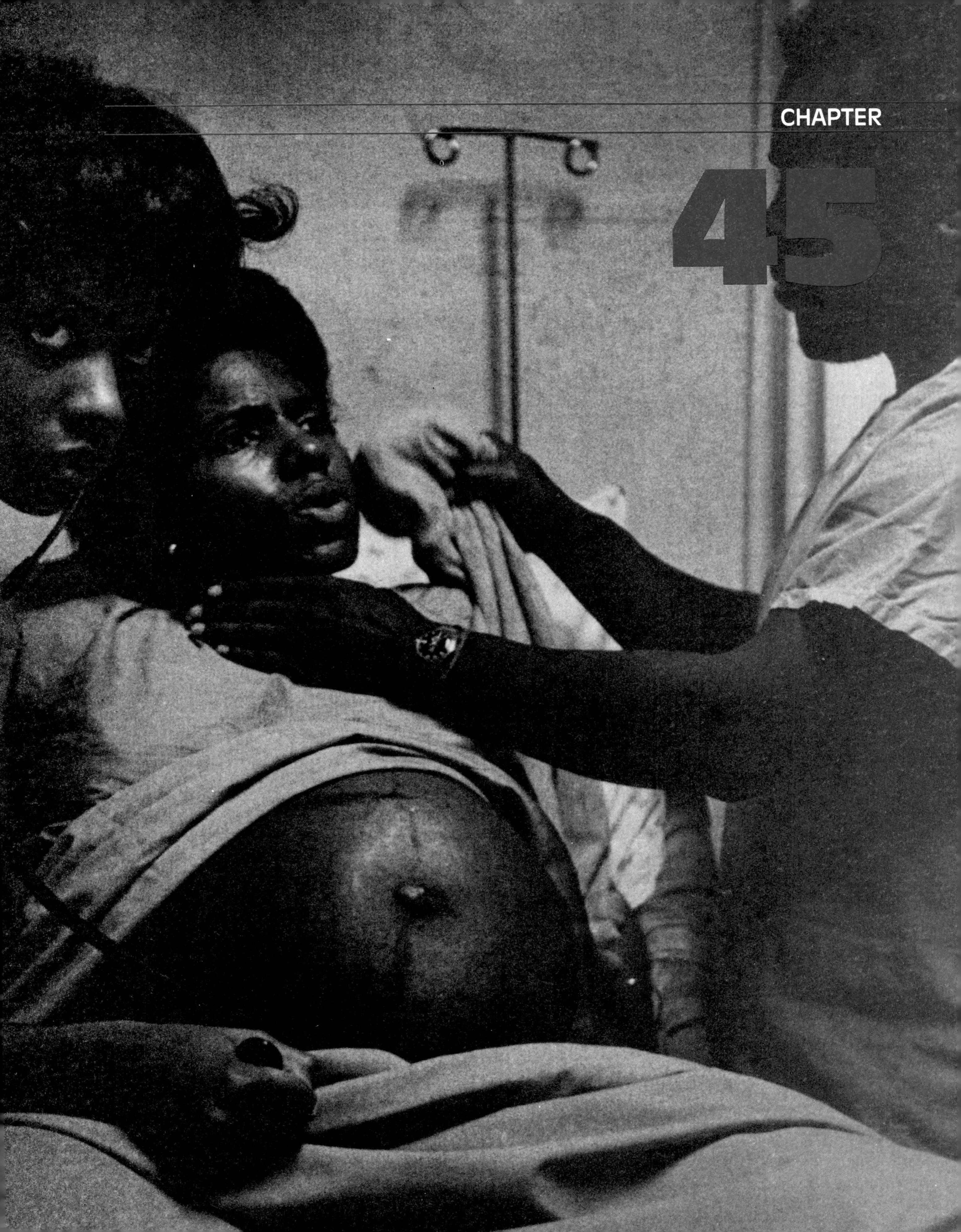

CHAPTER

45

CHAPTER 45

Alternatives in Maternity Care

The birth of a baby was once a family and community event. Labor and delivery usually took place in the home, with the mother attended by a midwife, and with the support of family members and close friends. Children were familiar with birth and death, as were all family members, because these events occurred within their living environment. The acceptance of the childbearing process, with its inherent risks and joys, was a common part of the fabric of life. The institution of prenatal care and hospital deliveries, and the entrance of the medical profession into the maternity field, undoubtedly contributed to the marked decrease in maternal and neonatal mortality that has characterized the 20th century. However, improved maternal nutrition, improved sanitation, and the declining birth rate may be even more significant factors in reducing the mortality of mothers and neonates.

Cultural traditions surrounding and supporting childbearing have been replaced by professional norms and standards, particularly in Western countries. Folk wisdom has largely been lost, as has familiarity with the childbearing and childrearing processes, and the efforts of health professionals to replace these traditional supports have not yielded outstanding successes in numerous instances. Often, professional interventions have created additional problems that are still affecting the physical and emotional well-being of childbearing families. The history of the United States reveals a gradual transition from maternity care by trained midwives to care by medical doctors (allopathic medicine). In the 17th and 18th centuries, midwives were held in equal esteem as "physicians and chirurgeons."[1] In the early 19th century, the use of physicians as childbirth attendants became a new vogue, leading to the use of forceps and a trend toward selection of the hospital as the location for delivery and for physician training in obstetrics. At the beginning of the 20th century, urban areas experienced a decline in social and health conditions, with increased maternal and infant mortality. These effects, combined with the low status of women, led to gradual discouragement of midwife practice in urban areas. The proportion of babies delivered by midwives in New York City decreased from 40% in 1905 to less than 10% in 1936.[2]

As physicians increasingly dominated the maternity field, and as hospitals replaced the home as the place for care of the sick and the parturient woman, the public's knowledge of these areas decreased. The chemical revolution brought about by growing use of powerful drugs, and the explosion of technology in medicine further removed the public from understanding the processes and management of illness and potentially hazardous biological events such as childbearing. The uninitiated public viewed the complex and mysterious medical field with awe, and through the values of professionals and the beliefs of the lay public, people came to abdicate their responsibility for health and the management of illness to the medical and health professionals.

As a result, until the early 1960s a woman felt generally in the dark regarding her pregnancy, labor, and delivery. There was usually little or no exchange of educational information between the physician and the pregnant woman, and most of the decisions made about the pregnancy were made by the physician. Much of the information that a woman might obtain about childbearing and childbirth was provided by family members and friends who would share their experiences with the woman. Often these stories would emphasize the pain and suffering women had to endure to give birth—information that only increased the pregnant woman's feelings of anxiety and apprehension about her forthcoming labor and delivery.

When a woman's labor started, she was usually taken to the hospital. Home births became less commonplace during this time because of sociological and medical pressure against this practice.[3] Once the woman was admitted to the hospital, she was usually separated from the father. Except for short visiting periods during labor, the labor and delivery rooms were off-limits to the father, relatives, and friends of the woman for the duration of the intrapartum period. With little knowledge about the usual course of labor and birth, and having been isolated from the father (and other support persons), the laboring woman relied heavily on the advice of the obstetrical staff to help her cope with the discomfort and apprehension she was experiencing. Analgesics and anesthetics that were administered by the well-meaning obstetrical staff to relieve the woman's pain, also relieved her of her sense of control and self-esteem. More often than not, a woman would awaken after childbirth unaware that she had, in fact, given birth. It was not uncommon for the father, not the mother, to be the first to become acquainted with the newborn infant, though usually only through the nursery room window.

During the postpartum period, the mother would bathe and feed her infant according to the hospital schedule. When these tasks were completed, the infant was usually returned to the nursery where the father, mother, and the other children could gather to view the newborn infant. In some hospitals, fathers were not allowed to touch their infants until the infant was discharged. The importance of efficiency and competency at specific medical tasks was often emphasized in the nurse's role during this period, and patient advocacy and education had little or nothing to do with maternity nursing. It is not difficult to understand why consumers became dissatisfied with this kind of maternity care. They began to question health-care professionals about the rationales for some of these practices; gradually their demands for more involvement in pregnancy and childbirth began to have a significant impact on maternity care in this country.

History of Family-Centered Maternity Care

Family-Centered Care

The concept of *family-centered maternity care* began to gain support among nursing circles during the 1960s. This approach advocated consideration of other members of the family, particularly the father, during pre- and postdelivery care. The pregnant woman, who had been viewed largely in isolation as a medical problem, was recognized as having social and emotional needs that deserved the nurse's attention as did her physical needs. It seems strange now that nurses had to be reminded that pregnant women had families with psychological needs for some involvement in this most momentous event, as well as very real practical problems and social concerns that often could be helped by nursing attention. But this had been the outcome of years of emphasis on efficiency and routinization on the one hand, and influence of the medical model on the other.

Prepared Childbirth

Contributing to family-centered maternity care was the *participant childbirth movement,* which brought about significant changes in the practice of obstetrics through consumer pressure. Its purposes closely paralled the family-centered approach, but even greater involvement of the father was advocated. As the ideas and techniques of Dick-Read, Lamaze, and Bradley caught on in the United States, childbearing women and their partners began to seek knowledge and demand a right to make choices in the conduct of their own pregnancies, labors, and deliveries. Women wanted to be aware and awake, to feel a central part of the process, to become equipped to cope with the stress of labor without heavy medication, and to have their partners by their side to share the experience. Prepared childbirth usually involved education about the processes of parturition and instruction in techniques to reduce pain perception and enhance the sense of control over the process (see Chaps. 18 and 26).

Fathers frequently served as labor coaches, and through this type of involvement pressure was brought to bear on hospitals to allow their presence in the labor room. It seemed ludicrous to allow fathers to assist their partners during labor, only to dismiss them at the climax of the entire process. This gain was not achieved easily, and took a period of some years before reluctant physicians and nurses accepted the fact that prepared fathers were not going to faint or become irate over necessary procedures or during unexpected complications.

Mother–Baby Couple Care

Following increased concern about family involvement in the childbearing process, *mother–baby couple care* was instituted in many postpartum units to facilitate development of the early mother–infant relationship. The forerunner of this practice was *rooming-in,* when mothers who elected to do so (and could afford a private room or could be placed with a roommate who also wanted rooming-in) would have their babies placed in the room with them during the hospitalization period. Rooming-in had a varying course over the years, with persistent professional resistance that mothers had to overcome, often only to be left largely on their own with their new babies.

Mother–baby couple care represents a commitment on the part of the postpartum and nursery staff to restructure the hospital units so mothers and babies may be together the greater part of the day and night. Usually satellite nurseries are developed to serve each wing of the maternity unit, and postpartum and nursery nurses move back and forth within the wing or area. Babies are with their mothers except for specified times when they are in the nursery for physical examinations, tests, or procedures, or if the mother or baby is temporarily sick.

Although the logistics of mother–baby couple care require some working out, and although nurses need some retraining in the area of their lesser experience, the benefits of each mother–baby couple having the same nurse responsible for their care are enormous. In this way, the same nurse knows the condition and needs of both mother and baby, enhancing the development of the mother–infant relationship through intimacy and close contact, immediate response to needs or problems, and elimination of the communication gap.

Breast-Feeding

The back-to-nature movement that was an expected reaction to the increasing use of artificial substances and chemical additives in a wide variety of materials and products served as an impetus to the rediscovery of *breast-feeding*. Organizations such as the LaLeche League were formed to assist mothers relearn the art of breast-feeding and encourage success through information and support. In response to maternal need, postpartum nurses began to learn how to help mothers initiate satisfactory breast-feeding patterns during their first days of nursing their babies in the hospital.

Resurgence of Home Births

Family-centered maternity care has evolved over several years; and to some consumers the changes that have occurred seem conservative. Today, routine maternity care in some areas of the country includes expensive, sophisticated tests and procedures which many women, and their partners, regard as invasive and interfering manuevers on the part of health-care professionals. The increasing reliance of obstetricians on such procedures as routine fetal monitoring, amniotomy, administration of intravenous fluids, and oxytocic drugs during the course of uncomplicated labors and births illustrates the still prevalent belief that pregnancy and childbirth are pathological, not normal, processes.[4,5] Furthermore, the increasing cost of maternity and obstetrical services, especially when unnecessary tests and procedures are used routinely, is a very real concern of expectant families. As a result, there has been a gradual increase in the number of home births occurring in this country during the past decade.[6]

This current trend concerns both the consumers and providers of maternity care. The primary concern of both these groups is the potential complications that can occur during any normal birth but that can be even more life-threatening to either the mother or the fetus when the birth occurs at home without adequate medical back-up or quick access to emergency equipment. Although some physicians and nurses are proponents of home births that utilize good medical and emergency back-up systems, most health-care professionals regard this practice as exposing the mother and the fetus to unnecessary danger.[7,8]

For a small but increasing number of women, however, home birth remains the birth alternative of choice. Although there are many different types of women choosing to deliver at home, the general profile has been found to be a white, married, 25-year-old woman who has attended college. The five most important reasons given by women for electing a home birth are:

1. Desire to have the baby close to the mother after birth
2. Desire to have the father present during birth
3. Viewing pregnancy as a normal process and hence out of place in a hospital
4. Having more control over the childbirth experience at home
5. Wanting to give birth in familiar surroundings[9]

Mistrust of the hospital and negative feelings about the hospital environment are important factors in the decision to give birth at home. The main issues involved are fear of medical intervention, loss of control over the labor process, the delivery, and postdelivery environment, and dislike of hospital routines and professional attitudes. Many women view their labor as a vulnerable time and want their energies free to focus on this demanding process. They do not want a confrontation over such practices as using drugs for pain relief, stimulation of labor with oxytocins, use of monitoring devices, use of amniotomies, or such medical interventions as forceps or episiotomies at delivery. Many women also feel that they cannot maintain as much control over their environment at the hospital, even in birthing centers. There is an inherent tension in the hospital atmosphere that is perceived as increasing a woman's pain and complications. Hospital routines are seen as more in the interest of the institution and its staff than in the interest of the childbearing family. Women are concerned about early and continued physical contact with the infant, early cutting of the umbilical cord, use of silver nitrate in the infant's eyes, and giving babies sugar water to supplement breast-feedings. They also want to be able to use the delivery position of their choice and to avoid being moved just before delivery.

Birth to such women is a natural, normal phenomenon, and home is the natural setting when there are no medical problems. The hospital is seen as a place for the ill, not the healthy undergoing a normal physiological process. The hospital poses additional dangers in some women's views. Medical intervention during labor and delivery is associated with increased risks for the mother and infant, and women fear unnecessary intervention when in an atmosphere supportive of it. The risk of infection is seen as greater in the hospital because of virulent germ strains (as has been often seen in nosocomial infections) and staff errors and oversights leading to breaks in technique or exposure to contamination. Alternative birth centers are unattractive to some women for many of these same reasons. The hospital atmosphere still prevails, and if there are any complications (even minor ones) the woman is transferred to the regular labor unit. One woman expressed her concerns as follows:

> They charge a lot of money to pretend you're having the birth at home. People there are still trained in complications. I was afraid they'd think, since the machinery's here, why not use it?[9]

Women who give birth at home generally find that the experience surpasses their expectations. It is a powerful reinforcement of their ability to undergo childbirth and to maintain control without much pain. The bonding between mother, father, and infant has been described as "unbelieveable." Siblings observing the birth also undergo remarkable bonding. It is described as a very strengthening experience for the family.

Because the home offers many qualities not available in hospitals, women continue to choose to deliver at home. Health practitioners who oppose home births deny this alternative to their clients and eliminate a practice option for themselves; their expertise cannot be brought to bear in assisting women to have optimal birth experiences. Greater responsibility for providing emergency obstetrical equipment and transportation in the event of complications has been suggested as an appropriate response by health professionals.

Alternative Birth Centers

In 1978, a joint statement entitled "The Development of Family-Centered Maternity/Newborn Care in Hospitals" was issued by the Interprofessional Task Force on Health Care of Women and Children.[10] This task force was composed of representatives from the American College of Nurse-Midwives, the American Nurses' Association, the Nurses' Association of the American College of Obstetricians and Gynecologists, the American College of Obstetricians, and the American Academy of Pediatrics. The representatives from these groups collaborated and agreed upon the following definition of family-centered maternity/newborn care:

> Family-centered maternity/newborn care can be defined as the delivery of safe, quality health care while recognizing, focusing on, and adapting to both the physical and psychological needs of the client-patient, the family, and the newly born. The emphasis is on the provision of maternity/newborn health care which fosters family unity while maintaining physical safety.[10]

The joint statement prepared and issued by this group of professionals also provided guidelines for implementing family-centered maternity/newborn care in hospitals interested in incorporating such programs into their obstetrical units. The statement advocated the establishment of such services as:

1. Childbirth classes for the entire family
2. Continuing education for maternity staff including information on current childbirth trends and techniques
3. A more liberal definition of family to include other supportive persons important to the mother
4. Development of birthing rooms as options in addition to standard labor and delivery rooms
5. Development of the option of early discharge of mother and infant with appropriate follow-up visits to assess early postpartum progress

This professional statement in 1978 reflects increased awareness of consumer demands and changing client values related to maternity care. As a result of a number of forces, childbearing couples are more knowledgeable and concerned consumers. The prepared childbirth movement, the women's health movement, and the rise of consumer consciousness are among these forces.[11] Two common themes are the emphasis on client control and decision-making power, and the desire for highly personalized health care. The unmet needs of a large group of uncomplicated, low-risk pregnant patients within the traditional hospital obstetrical service led to demands for alternatives; the concept of a *birth center* was one alternative that emerged recently. For many expectant families, the alternative birth center (ABC) provides an acceptable option to the traditional medical delivery of an infant in the hospital, as well as a safe alternative to giving birth at home.

Physical Set-Up and Procedures

An ABC usually consists of one or more private birthing rooms where a woman labors and gives birth to her infant. The woman can be accompanied by the father and, in some ABCs, by her children and other family members or friends. The physical set-up of the birthing room is quite different from the standard labor and delivery rooms used in traditional obstetrical units. Usually there is a bed that is large enough for the mother, father, and their newborn to recline comfortably. Chairs and a dresser are included in the furnishings, as are plants and pictures. In some ABCs parents are encouraged to bring their own pictures and wall hangings to decorate the room so that the room is similar to their own home environment. Often a stereo is provided in the room for the laboring woman to listen to her favorite music as a means of relaxing and maintaining inner calm during the labor and birth. Private bathroom facilities are incorporated into each birthing room for the convenience and comfort of the mother. The standard equipment used during childbirth is usually stored in cabinets in the room until it is needed. Emergency equipment that might be needed during the intrapartum period is readily available to the staff and is similarly stored.

ABCs are subject to the organizational demands of their hospital; therefore considerable variation occurs in appearance as well as policies and procedures. The room decor ranges from unmodified labor rooms to very homelike bedrooms. Policies and procedures vary less and usually include options for the presence of family and friends, minimal medical intervention, no separation of parents and infant, and early discharge (usually 6–24 hours after birth). The choice of attendant for the birth varies with hospital policy and professional availability, but may include nurse-midwives, family-practice physicians, obstetricians, and specially trained nurse practitioners or physician's assistants.

Patient Selection

Most ABCs are located within hospitals, and are designed for use by women who have had normal pregnancies and who are experiencing uncomplicated intrapartal periods. Strict criteria are used by physicians, nurse-midwives, and nurse practitioners during the prenatal and intrapartal periods to evaluate women who desire to give birth in an ABC. If a woman is considered to be in a high-risk category during her pregnancy, she is usually not eligible for an ABC. When a woman with a normal prenatal course is initially admitted to an ABC but develops a complication during labor, she is usually transferred to the regular obstetrical unit of the hospital.

There is considerable variation in policies for determining risk factors that exclude a patient from the ABC or complications that require a transfer out of the ABC. In some hospitals, a woman will be transferred if she requires any or more than a small amount of analgesia (*e.g.,* 25 mg of nisentil or Demerol), whereas in others any procedures short of forceps delivery can be done in the ABC.[12] Examples of factors excluding patients from an ABC, and criteria requiring transfer out of the ABC after labor admission are given below.

Supportive Atmosphere

In an ABC, a woman is free to move about during her labor. She is allowed to drink fluids, and is often encouraged to bring beverages to the ABC from her home so she will have the type of fluids she desires. Analgesics are available in some ABCs; however, most couples are required to attend childbirth classes during the pregnancy so that the women will learn some

High-Risk Factors Excluding Admission to ABC Programs

- Preeclampsia or chronic hypertension
- Premature labor (occurring prior to 37 weeks' gestation)
- Abnormal presentations (other than vertex) or multiple births
- Third trimester bleeding
- Prolonged rupture of membranes (greater than 24 hours before onset of labor)
- Previous cesarean section
- History of postpartum hemorrhage
- Genital herpes (at the time of labor)
- Postdatism (41 to 43 weeks' gestation)
- Maternal history of heart disease, kidney disease, psychiatric disorder or severe emotional problems, previous stillbirths, Rh-sensitization, diabetes, tuberculosis, chronic or acute pulmonary problems
- Estimated fetal weight less than 5 lb or greater than 9 lb
- Anemia (Hb less than 9.5 g–10 g)
- Primiparas over 35 years old or multiparas over 45 years old
- Polyhydramnios or olighydramnios
- Treatment during pregnancy with any drugs that could adversely affect the infant

(Patterson KA, Peterson VL: The alternative birth center movement in the San Francisco and Bay area. J Nurse-Midwifery 25 (2):26, March/April 1980)

Criteria Requiring Transfer Out of ABC After Labor Admission

Anemia (Hb less than 9.5 g–10 g)

Temperature elevation (greater than 38°C)

Significant variation in maternal blood pressure from prenatal values

Signs of preeclampsia (hypertension, proteinuria, edema, visual disturbances)

Meconium-stained amniotic fluid

Abnormal fetal heart rate or pattern—development of need for continuous fetal heart rate monitoring

Prolonged labor (greater than 24 hours)

Second state arrest (greater than 2 hours for primigravidas or greater than 1 hour for multiparas)

Significant vaginal bleeding

Mother's desire for repeated medication or regional anesthesia

Any condition of mother or infant that birth attendant feels requires greater management than ABC provides

(Patterson KA and Peterson VL: The alternative birth center movement in the San Francisco and Bay area. J Nurse-Midwifery 25 (2):26, March/April 1980)

breathing techniques to decrease or eliminate her need for analgesics during labor. Although one-to-one nursing care is provided for the woman, active participation of the father (or coach) is encouraged and supported by the nurse. In some ABCs, children are allowed to be present during the birth, but a responsible adult (other than the parents or nursing staff) must accompany the child or children to observe them and attend to their needs throughout this event.

The atmosphere in an ABC is usually relaxing and congenial as a woman labors and gives birth. Because nursing care is provided on a one-to-one basis, the opportunity for establishing rapport between the expectant family and the nurse is excellent. Often a nurse meets the family during the prenatal period and contracts with that family to be their obstetrical nurse throughout the labor and birth of their child. The nurse becomes familiar with the members of the family prior to the birth and is better able to assess their special needs and intervene appropriately to meet these needs during the intrapartum period.

Labor and Delivery Practices

In an ABC, the goal of the staff is to meet the individual desires and needs of the woman during a safe, normal childbirth while they carefully monitor the progress of her labor and the birth of her child. Enemas, pubic shaving, and stirrups are not routine in the majority of ABCs. Similarly, episiotomies are not routinely done; rather, attempts are made to stretch the woman's perineum naturally through gentle massaging of the vaginal introitus during the second stage of labor. The actual birth of the infant can occur in any position that is safe and comfortable for the mother. Since much of the amniotic fluid contained in the infant's lungs, trachea, and nasal passages is squeezed out as the infant passes through the birth canal, suctioning of the newborn's mouth and nose is not standard after the birth, but is performed only when necessary.

With the safe emergence of the infant's head and shoulders, many birth attendants encourage the mother (or the father) to actually complete the birth by lifting the newborn onto the mother's abdomen (Fig. 45-1). While the mother, father, and children become acquainted with the newborn infant through sight and touch, the nurse observes and assesses the newborn's transition to extrauterine life without interfering in the parent–infant bonding process (Fig. 45-2). In some ABCs, the instillation of silver nitrate in the newborn's eyes is delayed for 30 minutes to 1 hour so that the infant can have eye-to-eye contact with the mother and father—an important factor in the bonding process. Breast-feeding soon after the birth is encouraged because it enhances maternal attachment and increases uterine contractions, which facilitates placental separation. After the umbilical cord pulsations cease, the birth attendant clamps and cuts the umbilical cord (or allows the father to do this), and then delivers the placenta.

During the postpartum period, the mother and her newborn infant are carefully observed for several hours. If there are no complications, the mother and her infant may be discharged after the infant has been examined by a pediatrician or the family physician. Many ABC programs employ nurses who make follow-up home visits during the first week postpartum to assess the health of the mother and the infant. Samples for such tests as the PKU and T4 can be obtained during one of these homes visits.

Growth of ABCs

The positive responses of families that have used alternative birthing centers, combined with the economic advantages of the lower cost for obstetrical care in this type of facility, have contributed to the feasibility of

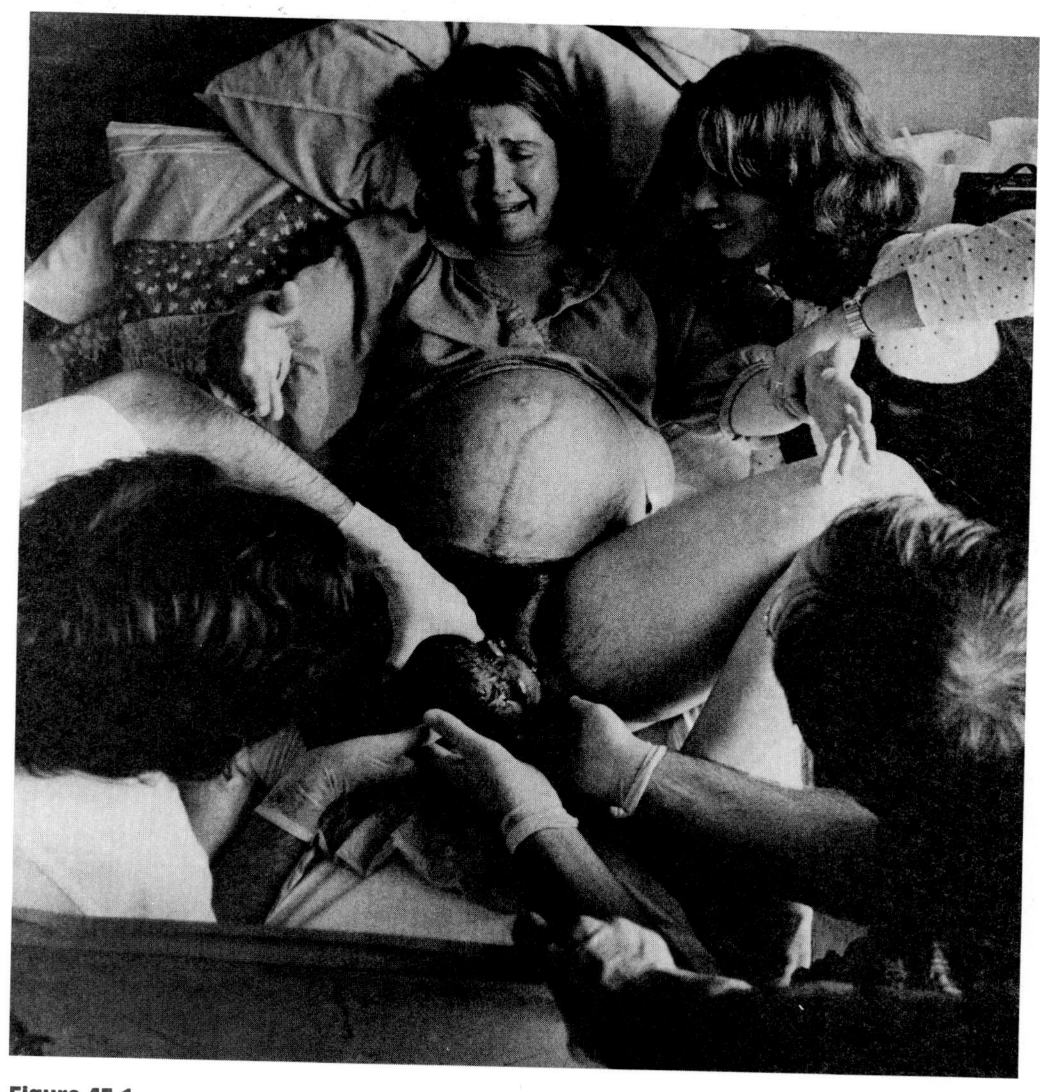

Figure 45-1.
Delivery in the alternative birth center is usually conducted in the labor bed. The father and the obstetrician both participate in the delivery while the mother watches the birth of her baby in the mirror being held in the foreground. Note that the nurse in this particular alternative birth center does not wear a traditional uniform. (Photo by Michael Alexander, 1979)

establishing such programs within the traditional setting of the hospital and in out-of-hospital settings (Fig. 45-3).[13–17]

Women are very interested in options in childbearing, as demonstrated by a study in which there was an increase from 33% to 66% of women preferring nontraditional facilities after reading a brief description of the characteristics of a birth center or birthing suite. There was no significant difference in age, education, religion, annual income, and parity among women preferring traditional services and women preferring various nontraditional options. There is a variety of interested, potential ABC clients. A market was demonstrated for the alternative birth center. Emphasis was placed on the need to educate women regarding its availability and characteristics.[18]

Nurse-Midwifery

Another alternative in maternity care that is returning in many parts of the country is the nurse-midwife as childbearing attendant. Throughout most of the

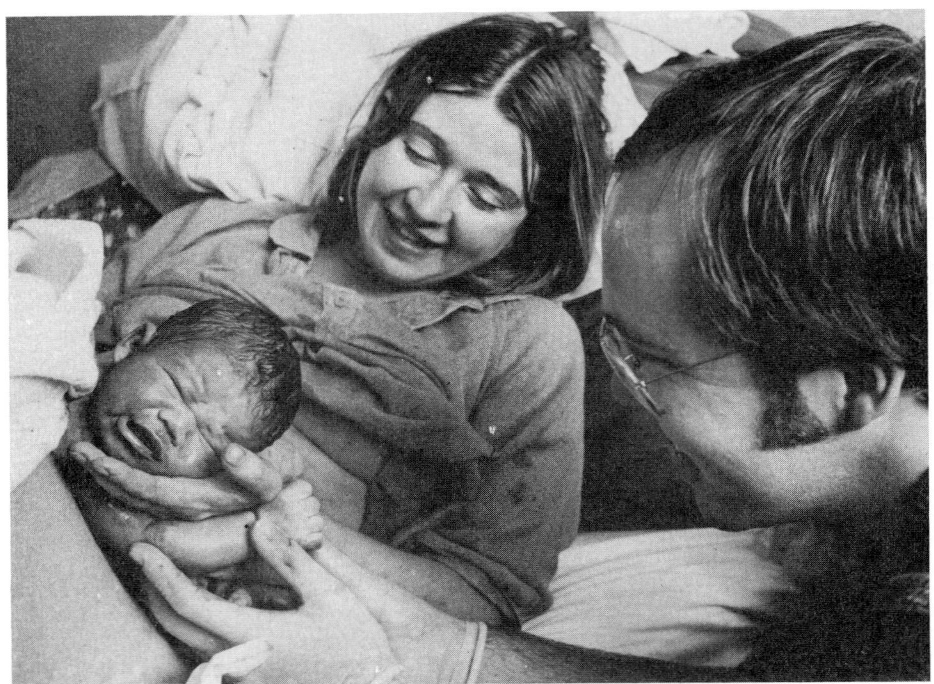

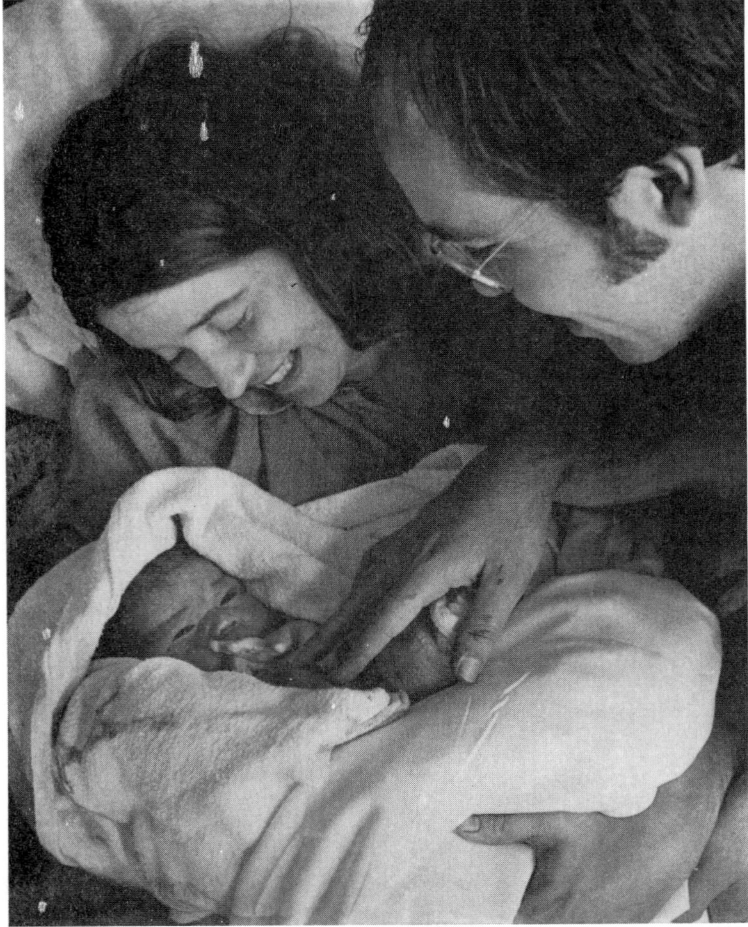

Figure 45-2.

The parents have the opportunity to become acquainted with their new baby immediately after delivery. (Photos by Michael Alexander, 1979)

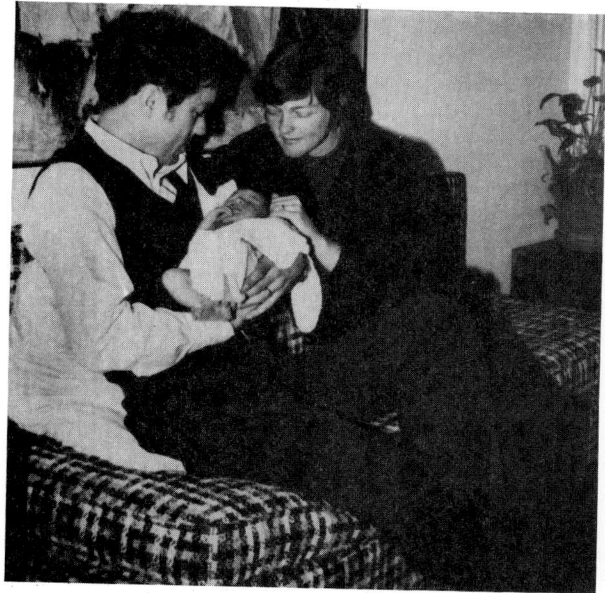

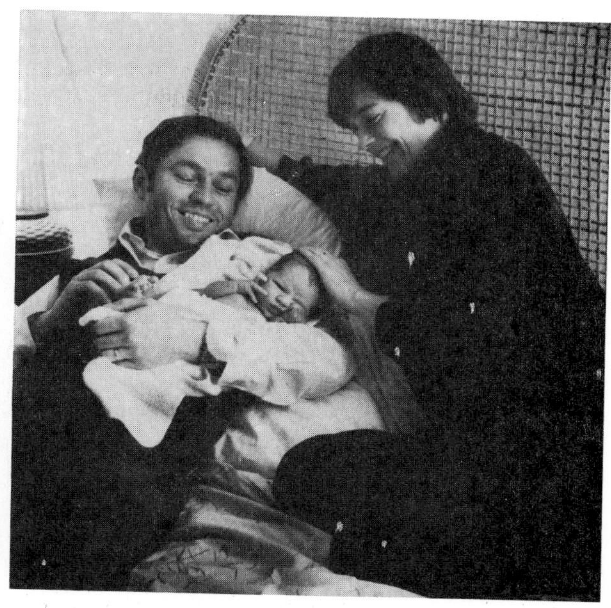

Figure 45-3.
Parents enjoy their new baby in the homelike setting of the Alternative Birth Center, Alta Bates Hospital, Berkeley, California. (Photos by Jeff Weissman. By permission of Alta Bates Hospital, Berkeley, California)

world, nurse-midwives or lay midwives provide the preponderance of maternity care. In the United States, nurse-midwives are registered nurses who have completed a recognized program of study and clinical experience leading to a certificate in nurse-midwifery. They are prepared to give comprehensive care to childbearing couples, including physical management and educational-counseling aspects. Nurse-midwives are prepared to assume primary responsibility for prenatal, intrapartal, and postpartal care of women having normal pregnancies.

History of Nurse-Midwifery in the United States

In early colonial times, midwives were important to the continued growth of the newly settled territories. Midwife services were guaranteed by several charter companies to induce women to travel to the colonies. Midwives were given first transportation on ferry boats (along with physicians) as an indication of their status and the importance of their services. Between the 17th and 20th centuries, the midwife's status and functions in maternity care were gradually eroded by the emergence of scientific medicine and the predominance of hospitals as the site of treatment of illness and of childbirth.

The first nurse-midwifery service in the U.S. was founded by Mary Breckenridge as the Frontier Nursing Service. Its purpose was to provide primary health care and maternity services in the mountain counties of Kentucky. Begun in 1925, this rural health service has a medical center and outpost clinics that are staffed by nurse-midwives and nurse practitioners. Traveling rough country roads, usually by jeep, nurse-midwives at times need to travel by horseback to reach families in the more remote areas. This organization has demonstrated that nurse-midwives can help lower mortality rates in a large population in rural and isolated areas. The Frontier Nursing Service also operates a graduate school of midwifery and a family nurse practitioner program.

The Maternity Center Association was founded in New York in 1918, and in 1932 established a school of nurse-midwifery for graduate nurses in association with the Lobenstine Midwifery Clinic. Consolidated as the Maternity Center Association 3 years later, this organization graduated and certified over 400 nurse-midwives over the next 30 years. The school was transferred to the Kings County Hospital in affiliation with Downstate University of New York in Brooklyn in 1958. This move initiated hospital-based formal midwifery education. Other midwifery schools were developed at Yale, Johns Hopkins, Columbia, Catholic

Nurse-Midwifery

What is a Certified Nurse-Midwife?

A certified nurse-midwife (CNM) is an individual educated in the 2 disciplines of nursing and midwifery, who possesses evidence of certification according to the requirements of the American College of Nurse-Midwives.

What is Nurse-Midwifery Practice?

Nurse-midwifery is the independent management of care of essentially normal newborns and women, antepartally, intrapartally, postpartally, and/or gynecologically, occurring within a health care system which provides for medical consultation, collaborative management, or referral and is in accord with the *Functions, Standards, and Qualifications for Nurse-Midwifery Practice* as defined by the American College of Nurse-Midwives.

The nurse-midwife provides care for the normal mother during pregnancy and stays with her during labor, providing continuous physical and emotional support. She evaluates progress and manages the labor and delivery. She evaluates and provides immediate care for the normal newborn. She helps the mother to care for herself and for her infant; to adjust the home situation to the new child, and to lay a healthful foundation for future pregnancies through family planning and gynecologic services. The nurse-midwife is prepared to teach, interpret, and provide support as an integral part of her services.

(J Nurse-Midwifery 26 (2):42, March/April 1981)

University, several state universities, Loma Linda, Emory, Meharry Medical College, New Jersey College of Medicine, and by the U.S. Air Force.

The American College of Nurse-Midwifery was established in 1955 as an organization of nurse-midwives to study and evaluate midwifery activities, plan and develop educational programs, and respond to professional needs. The college is a member of the International Confederation of Midwives. In 1969, the name was changed to the American College of Nurse-Midwives, with objectives including improving services to mothers and newborn babies in cooperation with other groups, establishing qualifications for midwifery activities, developing educational programs, establishing communications channels with other groups, and sponsoring research and literature.

Although physicians had long opposed widespread use of nurse-midwives, and many barriers to practice through restrictive legislation and denial of hospital privileges had been created, the American College of Obstetricians and Gynecologists took a positive stance in 1970. Together with the Nurses Association of the American College of Obstetricians and Gynecologists (NAACOG) and the American College of Nurse-Midwives, the physician's organization issued a "Joint Statement of Maternity Care," published in 1971, which allowed midwifery to reenter the mainstream of American health care. The statement provided that, as part of a medically directed health team, "qualified nurse-midwives may assume responsibility for the complete care and management of uncomplicated maternity patients."[19] Also in 1971, the American College of Nurse-Midwives initiated a National Certification Examination to standardize the level of basic competency among nurse-midwives.

Nurse-Midwifery Practice

Nurse-midwifery practice encompasses the care of essentially normal women and emphasizes the promotion and maintenance of health. Most midwives offer a comprehensive approach to maternity care, functioning as a member of a health-care team. In addition to managing the complete care for mothers with normal pregnancies, the certified nurse-midwife (CNM) is prepared to function in all areas of women's health maintenance including family planning and childbirth, and also provides perinatal care and newborn management. The CNM in the United States usually delivers in the hospital setting, where most American births take place. The CNM is an employee of a hospital or medical center, or works for a community-based maternal and child health service, or is in private practice with an obstetrician or family physician.

A recent examination of the content and process (methods) used by nurse-midwives in providing prenatal care found that the clinical practice of CNMs reflected their philosophy of comprehensive, personalized maternity care. The nurse-midwives had longer visits with clients than most physicians, and varied the content according to the patient's needs. They discussed topics including health status and pregnancy, preventive health care, preparation for labor and parenthood, and treatments prescribed for the patient. Table 45-1 shows the content of topics discussed in prenatal visits as well as the proportion of visits in which the topics were covered. Some type of physical examination was included in every visit and used as participative care. The nurse-midwife would have the woman or partner palpate fetal parts or listen to the fetal heart beat, and often use this as a departure point for parent education. A significant other (usually husband or partner) was present in about one third of the

Table 45-1.
Content of Topics Discussed by Nurse-Midwives and Proportion in 40 Prenatal Visits

Topic		Visits where present	
		Number	Percent
Health Status	Pregnancy progress interim history	40	100
	Danger signs	13	32.5
	Exercise/rest	19	47.5
	Explain illness	14	35
	Signs/symptoms of labor	11	27.5
	Discomforts of pregnancy	32	80
	Laboratory tests/results	28	70
	Nutrition/diet history	17	42.5
	Breast care	7	17.5
	Weight gain/weight loss	27	67.5
	BP/vital signs	6	15
	Emotions of pregnancy	5	12.5
	Other	13	32.5
Preventive Health Care	Accident prevention	1	2.5
	Dental care	1	2.5
	Family planning	4	10
	Community health resources	3	7.5
	Smoking	3	7.5
	Ultrasound	5	12.5
	Other	5	12.5
Treatments	Vitamins or iron	19	47.5
	Other medications	17	42.5
	Other	2	5
Preparation for Labor	Conduct of labor and delivery	10	25
	Alternate birth options/orientation	7	17.5
	Prenatal education classes	30	75
	Reading by client	5	12.5
	Cesarean section	3	7.5
	Job/employment	11	27.5
	Explain CNM role	5	12.5
	Other	9	22.5
Preparation for Parenthood	Breast feeding	10	25
	Infant care	1	2.5
	Rooming-in	4	10
	Pediatrician	7	17.5
	Circumcision	5	12.5
	Attitudes toward pregnancy/parenting	4	10
	Other	6	15
Miscellaneous	Charting/Paperwork	5	12.5
	Hospital admission procedures	3	7.5
	Other	0	0

(After Lehrman EJ: Lehrman Nurse-Midwifery Practice: Descriptive Study of Prenatal Care. Journal of Nurse Midwifery 26/3:33, 1981) visits. Patient and family education was a dominant focus in most visits, with the midwives showing openness to working with the woman and family in meeting their wishes for alternatives for hospital birth.[20]

Many nurse-midwives have assumed nonclinical positions because of the restriction on or prohibition of their practice that was common until recently. In a 1977 survey of graduates of the Yale nurse-midwifery program, it was found that 32% of the graduates were clinicians, 32% were teachers, 14% were administrators, 10% had both clinical and teaching positions, 2.3% were other, and 13% were not working. Those who were clinicians provided primary care for groups of patients, which included health checks and screening, health supervision and maintenance, maternity care, family planning, and diagnosis and management of acute illness.[21] Another study of midwives in the 11 Western states who were in practices that included provision of prenatal care revealed the following areas of employment:[22]

Hospital	39.1%
Nurse-midwifery maternity service	30.4%
Private nurse-midwifery practice	30.4%
Private practice with a physician	21.7%
Nurse-midwifery educational program	17.4%
Public health agency	8.6%
Prepaid health plan	4.3%
Military	4.3%*

Nurse-Midwives and Pregnancy Outcome

The aggressive management of human parturition that is characteristic of obstetrics in the 1970s and 1980s is not generally in the best interests of the great majority of mothers and infants. In developed countries that have a significantly lower incidence of infant mortality than that of the United States, highly trained nurse-midwives provide most of the family planning and obstetrical services. Nurse-midwives who are well trained practice nonintervention obstetrics that integrates updated scientific research, while respecting and supporting the delicately balanced natural mechanisms of the labor process. The medical expertise of the physician is used only when the pregnant woman develops a significant illness, or when labor and birth is anticipated to be, or found to be, abnormal.

Many obstetrical practices are known to be or are suspected of being potentially injurious to the mother, infant, or their developing relationship. Electronic or ultrasonic devices used to ascertain and monitor fetal status may pose dangers to the fetus. Animal studies have revealed delayed neuromuscular development, EEG changes, altered emotional behavior, and anomalies when such devices are used. Amniotomy has been associated with increased risk of umbilical cord compression and prolapse, and increased pressure on the fetal brain. Confining a woman to bed during labor tends to prolong labor by 2.5 hours, and increases the woman's need for analgesics, uterine stimulants, and forceps deliveries, and increases the incidence of abnormal fetal heart rates and poor infant Apgar scores. Drugs that are potentially teratogenic or carcinogenic may depress the infant's cardiovascular, respiratory, and thermoregulatory mechanisms, and may have subtle permanent effects on the infant's brain circuitry.[22]

Data from the North Central Bronx Hospital in New York indicate that the outcome of pregnancy may be significantly improved, even among higher-risk patients, with the use of nurse-midwives. The maternity service is essentially run by nurse-midwives, with appropriate physician consultation. About 30% of the patients are clearly medically high risk, and their care is much the same as for low-risk patients. If there is a medical indication for intervention, care is provided by a board-certified obstetrician or chief pediatric resident. Only severely Rh-sensitized expectant mothers were transferred to another hospital. A review of 2,608 birth records during 1979 showed an outstanding maternal and infant outcome, including the high-risk patients. Of the total population of mothers, 83% were successfully delivered by midwives; these were spontaneous vaginal deliveries without fundal pressure. Fewer than 30% of all labors required analgesia or anesthesia. Of infants above 1000 g, 93% had Apgar scores of 7 or above at 1 minute, and 98.3% had such scores at 5 minutes. The neonatal mortality rate among infants 1000 g or heavier was 4.2 in 1000. The incidence of instrumental deliveries (forceps, vacuum extraction) was 2.34%, and the cesarean section rate was 9% (7% primary and 2% repeat). All mothers who had delivered previously by cesarean section were allowed to labor spontaneously; of these, 37% gave birth vaginally. Fewer than 50% of patients were monitored electronically, including the 30% who were high risk. Episiotomy was done in only 26% of births; 45% of patients gave birth over an intact perineum, and 26% had first- or second-degree tears. Uterine stimulants (oxytocin) were used in only 3% of labors, and only when there was a medical indication.[22]

The skilled and supportive care provided by nurse-midwives made possible these low-interven-

*Total is more than 100% because of part-time work in more than one type of position. Figures indicate a significant amount of dual positions or holding of more than one job in this nurse-midwife population.

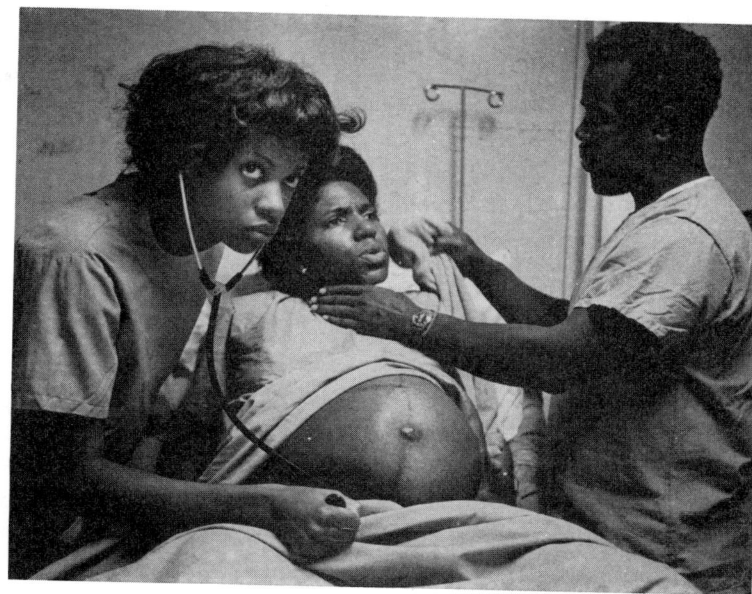

Figure 45-4.
A labor conducted by a nurse-midwife. The nurse-midwife monitors the fetal heart, while the father coaches the mother to keep her Lamaze breathing light and high in the chest. (Photo by Alison Wachstein)

tion and positive-outcome rates (Fig. 45-4). Childbirth education was a key component of the program, and presence of loved ones for support during labor was important. Other practices during labor and delivery included allowing low-risk mothers to eat and drink during labor, avoiding enemas, not prepping or shaving the perineum, minimizing vaginal examinations (3–5 times per labor), taking great care not to rupture membranes, having most mothers give birth in their labor beds in the labor room, allowing mothers to give birth in the semisitting position without stirrups, and delivering low-birth-weight infants over an intact perineum unless there was insufficient stretch (Fig. 45-5). On this service, there were no elective inductions of labor.

Although the highly trained obstetrician's skills are critical in medically complicated childbirth, and although the neonatologist contributes significantly to saving very premature, ill, and defective infants, care during pregnancy and childbirth that is noninterventionist and supportive of health and well-being remains the most important factor in most normal pregnancies. Nurse-midwives are particularly suited by training and philosophy to provide such care (Fig. 45-6).

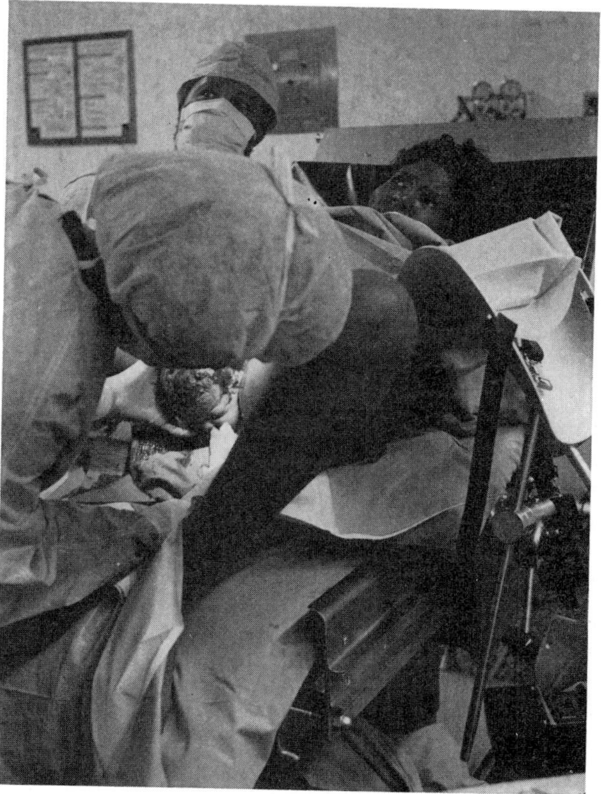

Figure 45-5.
The nurse-midwife delivers the baby with the mother out of stirrups in the semi-upright position. The parents watch the birth in the overhead mirror. (Photo by Alison Wachstein)

Options Available for Cesarean Births

The woman undergoing a cesarean birth is in need of the same sensitive and supportive care recommended for vaginal births by the Interprofessional Task Force

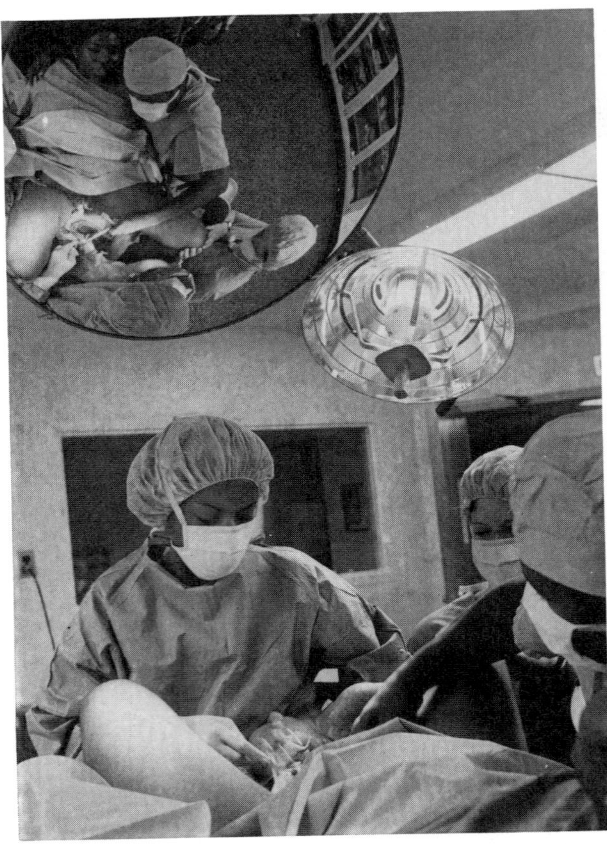

Figure 45-6.
The nurse-midwife supervises the father as he cuts the umbilical cord. (Photo by Alison Wachstein)

on Health Care of Women and Children. There is considerable professional and public concern over the dramatically rising cesarean section rate which has occurred in this country over the past 2 decades. Before 1965, cesarean birth rates remained relatively stable at about 4.5%. The rate has more than tripled within 15 years, and now stands at 17% to 18% nationally, even reaching 25% in some institutions.[23] This rise has occurred all over the country, in all types of hospitals (although larger hospitals have higher and more rapidly increasing rates), in all racial and ethnic groups, practice settings, and methods of payment. Cesarean rates in Europe have also been rising, but at a lower rate and from a lower baseline.[24]

Numerous factors are involved in this rising rate, and understanding their interrelations and relative importance is a complex task. Standards of obstetrical practice in managing certain labor complications contribute significantly to the increased cesarean birth rate. Four diagnostic categories account for about 80% of all cesareans and for 80% to 90% of the rise in the rate: repeat cesareans, dystocia, breech presentation, and fetal distress. There is also a changing attitude on the part of physicians to operative delivery, partly based upon scientific evidence, partly on changes in medical training programs, and partly due to legal and economic concerns.

Factors Contributing to Increased Cesarean Births

Childbirth Complications

The purpose of operative intervention in cases of maternal disease or labor complications is to improve the fetal outcome. A virtual explosion of obstetrical technology has occurred to assist physicians in monitoring the condition of the fetus and diagnosing the presence of a dangerous situation. Included are such procedures and equipment as amniotomy, prenatal stress testing, chemical induction and stimulation of labor, amniocentesis, electronic fetal monitoring, internal pressure transducers for measuring the strength of uterine contractions, assessment of fetal scalp blood *p*H, and various other blood and chemical studies. In nearly all cases, the technology itself has inherent risks, both direct and indirect, to the well-being of mother and infant. The following are the most common indications for cesarean section.

Previous Cesarean Birth. About 98% of women in the United States with a previous cesarean birth have operative deliveries with subsequent births. Almost one third of all cesarean sections are done for this indication, and it accounts for 25% to 30% of the rise in the cesarean rate. This practice has been standard in American obstetrics since 1916, although in Europe vaginal delivery after cesarean section is not uncommon. Because of the increasing rate of primary cesareans, this category multiplies the overall rate increase. Several studies have documented the safety of allowing selected patients to deliver vaginally after a cesarean birth. These studies also found that between 50% to 60% deliver successfully involving the same or fewer risks than repeat cesareans.[25,26] The NIH Consensus Development Task Force on Cesarean Childbirth recommended in its 1980 report that labor and vaginal delivery is a safe, relatively low-risk choice following a previous low segment transverse uterine incision. It also recommended that trials of labor take place in facilities with capability of an immediate emergency cesarean section if necessary.[27] See Report of the NIH Concensus Development Task Force on Cesarean Childbirth for further information.

Report of the NIH Consensus Development Task Force on Cesarean Childbirth

In 1979 the National Institutes of Health convened a Consensus Development Task Force to examine cesarean childbirth. A group of experts from medicine, research, law, social sciences, and the public examined all available evidence about cesareans, and arrived at consensus recommendations for practice. In 1980, their report was published with these recommendations for lowering the cesarean birth rate:

1. Labor and vaginal delivery is a safe, relatively low-risk choice following a previous low-segment transverse uterine incision.
2. Trials of labor after previous cesareans should take place in facilities with the capability of a prompt emergency cesarean if necessary. Hospitals that lack such facilities should inform patients in advance, and refer them to the nearest fully equipped hospital.
3. Prolonged labor (dystocia) should be treated with such measures as rest, hydration, sedation, ambulation, and oxytocin stimulation before resorting to cesarean.
4. Research should continue into means for evaluating the progress of labor, the effects of conservative treatment of dystocia, and the effects of emotional support and regional anesthesia.
5. Vaginal breech delivery should continue to be an accepted practice with a full-term baby not expected to be over 8 lb, normal pelvis, frank breech presentation without hyperextended head, and an experienced obstetrician.
6. All patients should have the choice of regional anesthesia.
7. Fathers should be allowed to be present at cesarean births.
8. Parents and infants should not be routinely separated after birth, unless indicated by the mother's or infant's condition.
9. Parent education and information about cesareans should be provided during pregnancy by childbirth educators and health professionals.

Dystocia. Dystocia includes such diagnoses as cephalopelvic disproportion (CPD), prolonged labor, uterine dysfunction, and failure to progress in labor. It accounts for 30% of the rise in the cesarean rate, the largest single category for primary operations. Several factors are involved in the increased rate for dystocia. Absolute CPD is rare. Much of the increase stems from a change in obstetrical management from less anatomical emphasis to a functional definition of the progress of labor. Labor graphs are used that set parameters for normal progress in terms of time, centimeters dilatation, and effectiveness of contractions. When women in labor deviate from graphic definitions of normal progress, indications arise for cesarean delivery. Suggestions have been made to reduce the incidence of cesareans in this category. Approaches include managing prolonged labor with rest, hydration, sedation, ambulation, and, if effective labor does not ensue, use of oxytocin stimulation with discretion. The amount of time allowed for response to treatment of dysfunctional labor needs to be evaluated; the implication is that intervention comes too soon. Childbirth preparation, a supportive labor environment, more freedom of maternal movement and choices, and avoidance of technological intervention are associated with decreases in cesarean births for dystocia.[28]

Breech Presentation. Changes in the medical philosophy of breech management have led to an increase of cesareans for breech presentation. About 10% to 15% of the rise in cesarean rate is due to breech presentation. Many studies have indicated increased morbidity and mortality among breech-born infants, but there is other evidence that overall perinatal mortality is not significantly lessened with cesarean sections. When mothers of equal parity with infants in equal weight groups are compared, there is no significant decrease in perinatal mortality in infants delivered by cesarean in the great majority of groups.[26] The NIH Task Force recommended that vaginal breech delivery continue to be an accepted practice with a full-term baby not over 8 lb, a normal pelvis, frank breech presentation without hyperextended head, and an experienced obstetrician. This last requirement is becoming more and more difficult to fulfill, however, because of the diminishing experience of resident physicians in delivering breech infants vaginally. Because of policies tending toward cesarean delivery as standard for all breech presentations, residents have less and less experience with vaginal breech deliveries. They become reluctant to do this when in practice later, and are also concerned with possible lawsuits for not doing cesareans if the infant is injured by vaginal birth.

Fetal Distress. Over the past 10 years the most rapidly increasingly indication for cesarean section has been fetal distress. This category has had an eightfold increase, and now accounts for 10% to 15% of all cesareans. The association of fetal distress, cesarean birth, and electronic fetal monitoring (EFM) is complex and controversial. Although the increased cesarean rate and introduction of widespread EFM occurred about the same time, there is no proof of causality, and this may only reflect a greater reliance on technology and intervention in obstetrics generally. The key question is whether EFM permits more accurate identification of fetal distress than auscultation, or whether fetal distress is being overdiagnosed. It is recognized that the monitors malfunction, that physicians and nurses misread the tracings, and that abnormal tracings do not always correlate with low Apgar scores or low scalp *p*H. In addition, EFM appears involved indirectly in increasing cesarean rates for other indications than fetal distress. Some studies have found a higher incidence of dystocia in women who are monitored during labor. The stress produced by procedures used to insert monitors, by tension in the environment, and by fear of the implications of EFM could contribute to reduced uteroplacental perfusion and general muscular tension in the woman. Having to lie stationary on her back to accommodate the equipment's needs is detrimental to effective labor and the woman's ability to cope with contractions. Monitors might also lead to premature diagnosis of failure to progress, with physicians allowing less time to determine effective labor.

Changing Attitudes Toward Operative Delivery

Obstetricians are more willing to perform operative deliveries now than in the past, for a number of reasons. Cesarean birth is relatively safe for the mother, with maternal mortality reported between 20 and 70 per 1000 operations. Maternal mortality rates have continued to decline despite sharply rising cesarean birth rates. Perinatal mortality has also decreased, and is less than one third that of 30 years ago. It has continued to decline even with the increase in cesarean deliveries. Improved diagnosis of fetal maturity has helped to prevent premature delivery by the physician. The development of EFM and functional (graphic) definitions of labor have provided more scientific rationales for operative deliveries. Although overall perinatal mortality rates are higher for abdominal than vaginal delivery, the selective use of cesarean sections can improve the fetal prognosis in a number of conditions. Some of the drawbacks of cesarean section are listed in the Maternal Risks in Cesarean Birth chart. The patient should also be made aware of the ways of avoiding unnecessary cesarean birth (see chart on Avoiding Unnecessary Cesarean Birth).

Changes in medical training are also important. Obstetrical residents receive less preparation and experience in the use of forceps, especially mid-forceps. They deliver fewer breech presentations vaginally and are taught to rely more on cesarean sections. Obstetrical residents learn values which support more active physician intervention in the childbirth process and are less inclined to wait and encourage natural processes to take place. Extreme adherents of such values hold that normal birth is dangerous for infants owing to forces and pressures on the fetal head that lead to risk of brain damage, and suggest that the majority of women will eventually be delivered by surgery.[29]

Certain changes in characteristics of the obstetrical population may also lead to greater inclination by physicians to perform cesareans. The proportion of nulliparous mothers has increased, and the average age of the obstetrical population has risen recently. Both of these groups have higher incidences of cesarean births. Changes in the health-care delivery system have occurred, allowing more low-income patients to undergo operative deliveries owing to better health benefits. A greater proportion of maternity care is being provided by obstetricians (rather than family or general practice physicians), who perform cesarean sections more frequently than non-obstetricians. The trend toward more deliveries occurring in larger hospitals also contributes to the increased number of cesarean sections, as these larger hospitals have higher cesarean birth rates. Economic factors may be involved; cesareans are about three times more costly than vaginal deliveries, but the evidence concerning cesarean births in prepaid, military, and governmental facilities (where there should be no fee incentive) is mixed. The threat of malpractice suits appears to be an enormous concern for many physicians, who fear loss of community trust and goodwill even in unsuccessful suits. However, suits involving cesareans are related more to events occurring during the operation, rather than failure to perform the cesarean.

Alternatives for Women Undergoing Cesarean Birth

Many women feel overwhelmed by an unexpected cesarean birth and are completely unprepared for their physical and emotional responses. They express feelings of anxiety for themselves or the baby. They experience anger or depression because they expected a normal birth. They tend to feel a sense of

Maternal Risks in Cesarean Birth

Maternal mortality, although rare, is 4 times higher with cesarean delivery than with vaginal delivery. Half of this increase is due to complications leading to the cesarean or to maternal disease. The other half is due to the surgery itself.

Maternal mortality in repeat cesarean is about twice that in vaginal deliveries.

Maternal morbidity is much greater after cesarean, the major risks are from:
- Infection of uterus and other genital tract structures
- Infection of respiratory or urinary tract
- Hemorrhage

Postoperative discomforts occur frequently, including incisional pain, gas, weakness, and difficulty in movement.

Maternal–infant bonding is interfered with through common hospital practices such as:
- General anesthesia during surgery
- Separation of mother and infant during recovery and first day
- Analgesics given the mother for pain relief
- Isolation necessary for infections

Development of mothering skills is interfered with because of:
- Disorientation following anesthesia and surgery
- Pain limiting activities and requiring sedation
- Weakness which limits the energy the mother can give to infant caretaking
- Postoperative complications further reducing mother–infant contact
- Emotional turmoil and the need to process feelings (anger, loss, confusion, fear, inadequacy, etc.) associated with undergoing cesarean birth and operative procedures
- Delay and increased difficulty gaining a sense of mastery over the mother's body

Breast-feeding is more difficult or impossible because of:
- Pain, weakness, limited activities
- Infections or other serious complications
- Medications that may be excreted in breast milk
- Sense of inadequacy related to childbearing capabilities

loss over not experiencing vaginal delivery, not witnessing the birth, and not having their partner's or family's participation. There are often altered body perceptions as well as many concerns surrounding mothering the infant during their recovery from surgery.[30] The nurse has a large responsibility in providing explanations of events and decisions, and in giving support through physical contact, calmness, comfort measures, verbal reassurances, and assisting the mother to gain mastery of her body and infant-care tasks.

Nurses who have prenatal contact with pregnant couples can effect change in these experiences by preparing them for the possibility of cesarean delivery. Nearly one fourth of all deliveries are by cesarean in some medical centers, and it is not unreasonable to include education in childbirth and parenting classes about this type of birth. There are also organizations, books, and audiovisual media which can assist parents to better understand and cope with cesarean births. (See Resources for Consumers and Professionals.)

Women and their partners need to become aware of the alternatives that may be available to them if they undergo a cesarean birth. These alternatives are supportive of parent participation in the birth, parent–infant bonding, and minimizing the stress and trauma of operative delivery. Some alternatives available to women undergoing cesarean birth include the following:

1. Regional (epidural) anesthesia so the mother can be awake during the birth
2. Presence of the father (partner, other support person) during the surgery and birth
3. Having hands freed from restraints for touch contact with father and baby
4. Dropping the screen (which prevents the mother and father from seeing the mother's abdomen during surgery) at the time of delivery
5. Having an advocate (usually a nurse) who describes to parents what is going on during the operation and delivery

Resources for Consumers and Professionals

Organizations

C/SEC (Cesareans Support Education and Concern, Inc.)
66 Christopher Rd., Waltham, Mass. 02154
(617) 547-7188

Cesarean Birth Association
125 North 12th Street, New Hyde Park, N.Y. 11040
(212) 523-8991

Local childbirth education groups through health department

Books

Donovan B: The Cesarean Birth Experience: A Practical, Comprehensive, and Reassuring Guide for Parents and Professionals. Boston, Beacon Press, 1977 ($8.95 hardback, $4.95 paperback)

Hausknecht R, Hausknecht H: Having a Cesarean Baby. New York, Dutton Publishing, 1978 ($4.95 paperback)

Bestal L (ed): The Cesarean Celebration. Madison, Cesarean Families of Madison, 1977 (available through Debbie Loughrin, 6009 Meadowood Drive, Madison, Wis. 53711; $2.95 paperback)

Young D: Unnecessary Cesareans: Ways to Avoid Them. ICEA, P.O. Box 20048, Minneapolis, Minn. 55420 ($1.50 paperback)

International Childbirth Education Association (ICEA) Book Center, P.O. Box 70258, Seattle, Wash. 98107 (has selection of childbirth literature)

Audiovisuals

"Having a Cesarean Is Having a Baby." Polymorph Films, 118 South Street, Boston, Mass. 02111 (28 minute slide–tape, $120 purchase, $35 rental)

6. Touching or holding the baby immediately after birth
7. Delaying instillation of silver nitrate drops into the baby's eyes for the first hour after birth
8. Continual contact between mother, father, and baby during first hour of life if the baby is stable
9. Breast-feeding the infant immediately after birth in delivery or recovery room
10. Initiation of rooming-in as soon as the mother desires this (often this begins in the recovery room after the birth)
11. Extended or unlimited visiting privileges for the father (or support person) during the postpartum period so that the mother can have help with the care of the infant
12. The utilization of medications (when necessary) that are not secreted in significant amounts in the mother's breastmilk[31,32]

The psychological sequelae of cesarean section births are just being investigated. It is now known that the woman who undergoes a cesarean section, especially when it is not a planned event, often has feelings of failure and guilt about not having a normal or natural childbirthing experience.[33] Furthermore, the physical discomfort of the mother after the surgery, combined with her feelings of disappointment or guilt, can interfere with her ability to bond to her infant. The long-term consequences of inadequate or delayed maternal–infant bonding can range from poor growth and development of the infant to blatant child abuse.

Mothers who were allowed early and continuous contact with their infants following cesarean birth (with spinal anesthesia and delivery of a healthy, normal infant) were found to have significantly more positive perceptions of their infants in the early postpartal period. They also displayed more maternal behavior in caretaking at this time and when the infant was 1 month old than cesarean mothers who only had brief contact in the first 12 hours after birth.[34]

Nursing Intervention

Labor and delivery nurses can play a very important role in helping the mother and father integrate the events that precede and follow a cesarean section birth. Explaining the need for such procedures as surgical preps and catheterizations before attempting to perform them helps to decrease the anxiety and apprehension the couple may feel about these invasive procedures. When the father is not allowed to accompany the mother to surgery, the nurse can accompany the woman and stay with her so the mother has the support of at least one familiar person during this very stressful event. If the father is allowed to be with the mother during the surgery, the nurse's presence can still provide the couple with a sense of reassurance and familiarity in the foreign, sterile environment of an operating room. After the birth, the nurse can encourage and foster the parent–infant bonding process by providing the mother (when she is awake) and the father the opportunity to touch and hold the newborn. When it is difficult for the mother to actually hold the infant herself, the nurse can hold the infant in an *en face* (face-to-face) position in order to facilitate the maternal–infant bonding process.

Avoiding Unnecessary Cesarean Birth

Cesarean births are necessary for a small proportion of women with serious conditions threatening fetal or maternal life, or both (such as placenta previa and abruptio, and other emergencies). For many other women, a series of events takes place which, in their combined effects, leads to an inevitable decision for cesarean birth which is usually necessary at that time, but which might have been prevented had different choices been made. Some approaches to minimizing the risk of cesarean birth include:

1. Carefully considered choice of birth attendant who will be most supportive of parents' needs and desires for the birth experience. A nurse-midwife, if available, might be more compatible with parents' chosen style of birth.
2. Selection of a birth environment that provides the type of setting compatible with the parents' objectives for the birth experience. For some couples, this may be the home, an alternate birth center, or a hospital with policies permitting many choices for the parents
3. Taking responsibility to be well informed about childbearing, its potential risks, choices available at various decision points, and legal rights and responsibilities
4. Participation in childbirth-preparation classes, which increase knowledge and reduce fear, provide tools for positive management of labor and delivery, and help the mother attain optimal physical and emotional condition for undergoing labor and birth
5. Maintaining general health through appropriate nutrition, exercise, weight, and activities; avoiding habits or practices that increase risk (such as smoking, alcohol or drug use)
6. When the birth attendant is an obstetrician, discussing his or her beliefs and practices related to cesareans, such as indications for surgery, induction or labor stimulation, and the percentage of deliveries done by cesarean section (above 10% increases risk)
7. When birth occurs in a hospital, finding out the hospital's policies relating t cesarean operations and fetal monitoring, and what percentage of deliveries are by cesarean section (above 30% increases risk)

One or two days after the birth, a visit from the labor and delivery nurse who assisted the couple during the childbirth is often beneficial and necessary for the integration of the event into their lives. The filling in of missing pieces is important for all women who experience gaps in their memories of the labor and births of their infants.[35] This may be more important when the woman is attempting to understand the reasons for surgical intervention in what is often expected to be a natural process. Visits such as this also provide the couple with the opportunity to discuss any feelings of failure, guilt, or anger they may be experiencing. A sensitive and responsive nurse can effectively help the couple work through such feelings by remaining open to their comments and honestly addressing their concerns. If the family unit is to be strengthened through the childbearing process, and if childbirth is to be a family-centered event, then every attempt should be made by the obstetrical staff to help families incorporate this experience into their lives—regardless of whether the childbearing event is categorized as normal or abnormal according to medical criteria.

Options in Maternity Nursing

Nurses today are in a unique position to foster family-centered maternity/newborn care both in the hospital setting and in out-patient facilities. The recognition of the need for expanded nursing roles to meet consumer demands for adequate, personalized health care has provided several choices for nurses pursuing careers in maternal–child health care. One such option that has been available to nurses for a number of years is nurse-midwifery.

Maternity Clinical Specialists

A new specialty emerging within the last decade is the *maternity clinical specialist.* These clinicians undergo advanced study of maternity nursing at the graduate level and are able to provide in-depth intervention for many of the adaptational and physiological problems encountered in maternity care. Frequently, clinical specialists have an area of expertise within the specialty field, such as a maternity clinical specialist with special expertise in the care of pregnant diabetics, breast-feeding mothers, parents experiencing neonatal death or abnormalities, Rh-sensitized mothers, and so on. These nurses with master's degrees also serve as consultants to other maternity nursing staff, assisting them to plan care for difficult problems or special situations encountered in the unit. Although clinical specialists may also be involved in staff education, their primary function is direct patient services using a high degree of knowledge, skill, and competence in their area of specialty.[36]

Nurse Practitioner

The latest new role to emerge on the nursing scene is that of the *nurse practitioner.* Beginning around 1965, physicians and nurses started working together in several settings to broaden the role of the nurse in the provision of care to patients in ambulatory and outpatient settings. Impetus for such changes was provided by the health manpower crisis and disillusionment of the American public with its health-care system during the mid-1960s.

With an undersupply of physicians that was predicted to get worse, and underutilization of the knowledge and skills of hundreds of thousands of registered nurses, many voices cried out for an extension of the scope of nursing practice to help meet the health needs of the nation.

Some nurses had previously been identifying health problems and providing limited treatment, notably in community health and private office settings, but their effectiveness was reduced by lack of a systematic approach and a body of knowledge to enable them to carry out treatment.

As the nurse practitioner role evolved, it encompassed additional skills in the techniques of physical diagnosis that were formerly in the realm of medicine, as well as the knowledge base to diagnosis and treat common problems and minor illness. Health prevention and maintenance, including examination, testing, and education, as well as management of stabilized chronic illness are also included in nurse practitioner functions. The nurse practitioner combines the nurse's sensitivity to emotional needs and focus on adaptation and social aspects of patient care with the techniques and knowledge of medicine to diagnose and treat pathophysiological problems. These nurses usually practice in a primary-care setting, defined as the first contact in any given episode of illness with the health-care system, and are responsible for continuance of care including maintenance of health, evaluation and management of symptoms, and appropriate referrals.[37,38]

The Maternity Nurse Practitioner

The maternity nurse practitioner, or OB-GYN nurse practitioner, provides prenatal care for uncomplicated pregnancies in conjunction with a physician consultant. The nurse takes a health and pregnancy history, performs the physical and obstetrical examination, orders and interprets laboratory and other diagnostic studies, plans for necessary treatments and medications in conjunction with the physician, and assesses family relationships and psychosocial needs.

Throughout the pregnancy, the maternity nurse practitioner sees the woman on antepartal visits, sometimes alternating with the physician, evaluates the progress of the pregnancy, and manages minor physical problems. Information and counseling related to pregnancy and childbirth and assessment of the couple's adjustments and family problems are also part of the nurse practitioner's role. Referrals to community agencies, prepared childbirth classes, and other medical specialties may also be made. Most maternity nurse practitioners are skilled in provision of contraception and can select appropriate methods for the patient, including oral contraceptives, insertion of intrauterine devices, fitting for diaphragms, and teaching about other methods.

Family nurse practitioners also provide care during pregnancy. They are generalists who care for all family members similarly to family-practice physicians. In addition to the functions described above for maternity nurse practitioners, family nurse practitioners provide postdelivery care for the baby as it grows, thus providing continuity throughout the reproductive process except during the intrapartal phase.

References

1. Fox CG: Toward a sound historical basis for nurse-midwifery. Bull Am College Nurse-Midwifery 14, 3, pp 76+, August 1969

2. Harris D: The development of nurse-midwifery in New York City. Bull Am College Nurse-Midwifery 14, 1, pp 4+, Feb. 1969

3. Devitt N: The transition from home to hospital birth in the United States, 1930–1960. Birth Fam J 4, 2:47–58, Summer 1974

4. Anderson SF: Childbirth as a pathological process: An American perspective. MCN—Am J Maternal Child Nurs 2, 4:240–244, July/August, 1977

5. Arms S: Immaculate Deception. Boston, Houghton-Mifflin, 1975

6. Hazell LD: A study of 300 elective home births. Birth Fam J 2,1:11–15, Winter 1974/1975

7. Estes MN: A home obstetric service with expert consultation and back-up. Birth Fam J 5, 3:151–157, Fall 1978

8. Epstein JL, McCartney M: A home birth service that works. Birth Fam J 4, 2:71–75, Summer 1977

9. Searles C: The impetus toward home birth. J Nurse-Midwifery 26, 3:51–56, May/June 1981

10. The development of family-centered maternity/-newborn care in hospitals. A joint position statement prepared by the Interprofessional Task Force on Health Care of Women and Children. New York, The National Foundation/March of Dimes, June 1978

11. Patterson KA, Peterson VL: The Alternative Birth Center Movement in the San Francisco and Bay Area. J Nurse-Midwifery 25, 2:23–27, March/April 1980

12. DeVries R: The development and future of the hospital-based alternative birth center. J Nurse-Midwifery 24, 6:37–38, November/December 1979

13. Ernst EKM, Forde MP: Maternity care: An attempt at an alternative. Nurs Clin North Am 10, 2:241–249, June 1975

14. Goldschmidt J, Mann R: Choices in childbirth—The nurse-midwifery service at San Francisco General Hospital. Birth Fam J 4, 3:120–122, Fall 1977

15. Kerner J, Ferris CB: An alternative birth center in a community teaching hospital. Obstet Gynecol 51, 3:371–373, March 1978

16. Lubic RW: The childbearing center. J Nurse-Midwifery 21, 3:24–25, Fall 1976

17. Rising SS: A consumer-oriented nurse-midwifery service. Nurs Clin North Am 10, 2:251–262, June 1975

18. Mather S: Women's interests in alternative maternity facilities. J Nurse-Midwifery 25, 3:3–8, May/June 1980

19. American College of Obstetricians and Gynecologists; the Nurses Association of the American College of Obstetricians and Gynecologists; and the American College of Nurse-Midwives: Joint statement on maternity care. ACOG Newsletter February 1971

20. Lehrman EJ: Nurse-Midwifery practice: Descriptive study of prenatal care. J Nurse-Midwifery 26, 3:27–40, May/June 1981

21. Burgess HA: Nurse-midwives from Yale—what are they doing now? J Nurse-Midwifery 25, 5:43–45, September/October 1980

22. Haire D: Improving the outcome of pregnancy through increased utilization of midwives. J Nurse-Midwifery 26, 1:5–8, January/February 1981

23. Young D: Unnecessary cesareans: Ways to avoid them. Birth Fam J 8, 1:47+, Spring 1981

24. Shearer E: NIH Consensus Development Task Force on cesarean childbirth: The process and the result. Birth Fam J 8, 1:25–30, Spring 1981

25. Bottoms SF, Rosen MG, Sokol RJ: The increase in the cesarean birth rate. N Engl J Med 302, 10:559–563, March 6, 1980

26. Minkoff HL, Schwarz RH: The rising cesarean section rate: Can it safely be reversed? Obstet Gynecol 56, 2:135–143, August 1980

27. Final Report of the NIH Consensus Task Force on Cesarean Childbirth. Office of Research Reporting, Bldg. 31, NICHD, 9000 Rockville Pike, Bethesda, MD 20205, 1980

28. Beck NC, Hall D: Natural childbirth: A review and analysis. Obstet Gynecol 52:371–379, 1978

29. Corea G: The cesarean epidemic. Mother Jones V, VI:28–35, July 1980

30. Affonse DA, Stichler JF: Cesarean birth: Women's reactions. American Journal of Nursing 80, 3:468–470, March 1980

31. Enkin MW: Having a section is having a baby. Birth Fam J 4, 3:99–102, Fall 1977

32. Hedahi KJ: Cesarean birth: A real family affair. American Journal of Nursing 80, 3:471–472, March 1980

33. Marut JS: The special needs of the cesarean mother. MCN—3, 4:202–206, July/August 1978

34. McClellan MS, Cabianca WA: Effects of early mother–infant contact following cesarean birth. Obstet Gynecol 56, 1:52–55, July 1980

35. Affonso D: 'Missing pieces'—a study of postpartum feelings. Birth Fam J 4, 4:159–164, Winter 1977

36. Riehl JP, McVay JW: The Clinical Nurse Specialist: Interpretations. New York, Appleton–Century–Crofts, 1973

37. National Commission for the Study of Nursing and Nursing Education, Jerome Lysaught, Director: An Abstract for Action. New York, McGraw–Hill, 1970

38. Extending the Scope of Nursing Practice. A Report of the Secretary's Committee to Study Extended Roles for Nurses. Washington, DC, Department of Health, Education and Welfare, November 1971

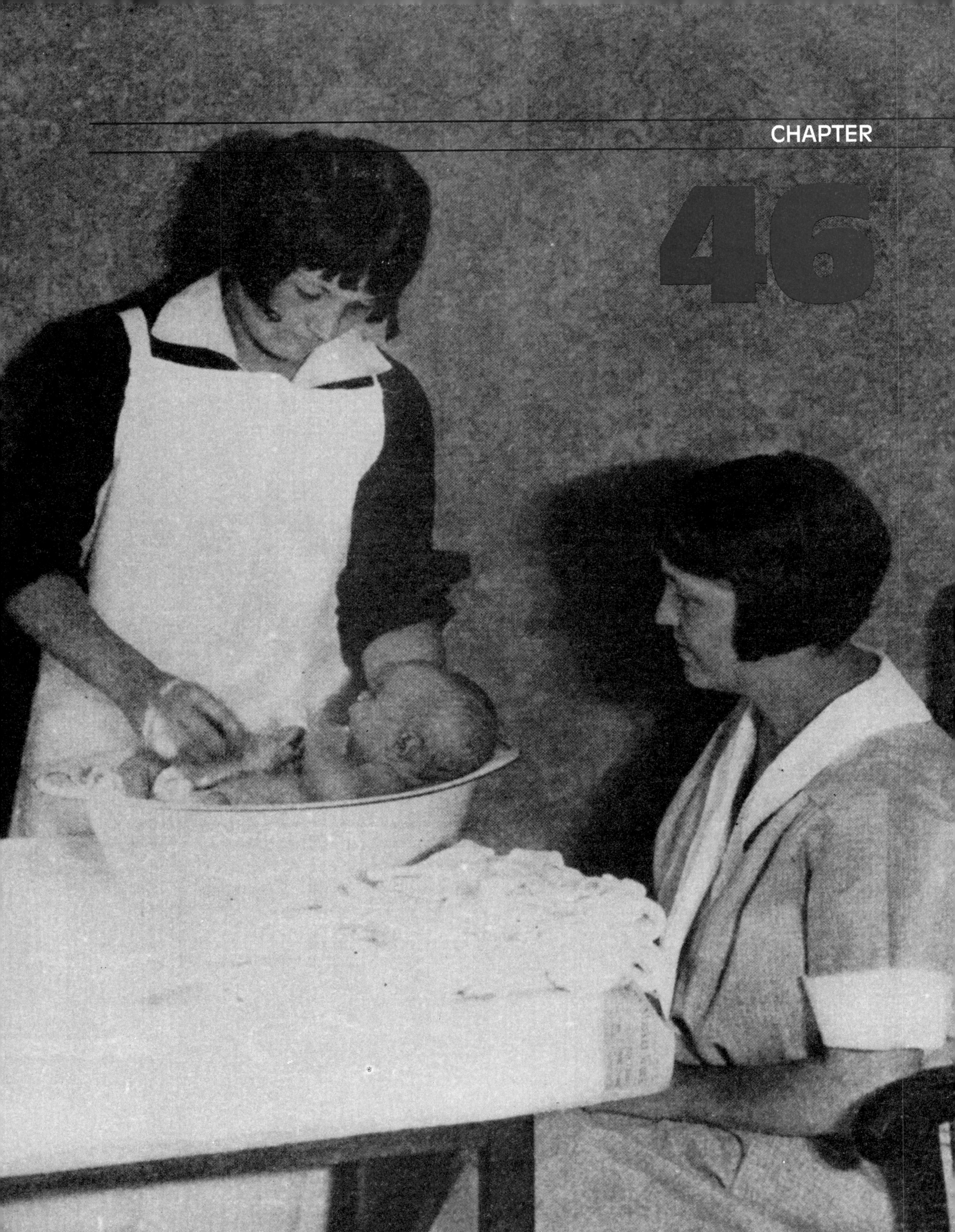

CHAPTER 46

CHAPTER 46

Evolution of Maternity Nursing

Obstetrics Over the Centuries

The bearing of children is an event of enormous social significance and has certain symbolic meanings for all peoples. Traditions, rites, and practices have been developed around this event to encourage positive outcomes for the individual and society. Roles for attendants during the reproductive process are formalized in one way or another, and differ greatly among cultures. Involvement of the sciences in childbearing grew gradually through the ages, but continued to be interwoven with folk beliefs and customs. In the less-developed countries, ancient folk practices continue to prevail in the care provided during pregnancy, delivery, and the postpartum period.

In Western societies, there has been a reawakening of interest in childbearing practices that are more natural and minimize technical intervention. Family and friends once again are assuming a central role in attending laboring women, with new support roles emerging for health professionals (see Chap. 45, Alternatives in Maternity Care). As knowledge continues to advance, there is a growing appreciation of the fine balance of natural ecosystems and the wisdom of restraint in applying technology to the reproductive process. Although much of the modern history of obstetrical care has seen an increasing scientific treatment of difficulties in the natural process, a point of diminishing returns has been reached in which continued interventions frequently lead to iatrogenic problems and associated morbidity. A balance is required, in which technology is applied more discriminately in instances of complications, so that the normal reproductive process can proceed with the least amount of interference.

A brief account of the history of obstetrics follows, including an outline of the major stages in the development of medical involvement in care during the reproductive process.

Obstetrics Among Primitive Peoples

We know little about obstetrics among primitive peoples, but careful study of the customs of the aboriginal American Indians and the African peoples has shed some light on some aspects of obstetrical practice of simple societies. Childbirth in primitive times was a relatively simple process. The mother retired to a place apart from the tribe and there gave birth to her child without great difficulty.

It is known that intertribal marriages were relatively rare; therefore, there was not the miscegenation that occurs today. A realization of this fact alone makes possible an understanding of the relative simplicity of childbirth under these circumstances. The fetal head and body were accommodated satisfactorily within the anatomic range of the maternal pelvis. The lack of mixed marriages prevented the resultant disproportion between passenger and pelvic passages.

It became customary for some women to attend other women in labor, and they became the primitive counterpart of our present-day midwife. The only real danger a primitive mother faced was that of abnormal presentation, which usually terminated fatally for both mother and child. Toxemias and other complications are largely the products of more advanced civilization and were rarely if ever encountered by primitive peoples.

Egyptian Obstetrics

In ancient Egypt, a highly organized state of society existed, and with it there arose a more complicated, if not more advanced, type of obstetrics. The priesthood in Egypt was interested in all the activities of society, including obstetrics. It had a supervisory interest in it and took an active part in the care of abnormal or operative cases. Ancient Egyptians are known to have had obstetric forceps, to have performed cesarean sections on dead mothers, and to have carried out podalic version.

There were special rooms in temples for giving birth to a pharaoh or divinity, and reliefs on temple walls give a visual idea of the Egyptian method of delivery. Parturient women are shown kneeling, sitting on their heels, or sitting on two bricks with a space between them. One midwife supported the woman from behind, and another received the infant. Ancient papyrus documents contained remedies for assisting labor, including vaginal suppositories, manual massage, and oral potions. There seems to have been a large body of gynecological and obstetrical knowledge in Egyptian society, with many approaches to assisting women in conception, pregnancy, and childbirth, as well as with gynecological problems.

Oriental Obstetrics

Hindu medicine was probably the first authentic system of medicine to be introduced in the world. Among the earliest Hindus of whom there is written record was Surata, one of the most prolific of Hindu writers. The exact date of his existence is still a matter of dispute, but he is variously stated to have worked and written between 600 B.C. and 500 A.D., more probably about the latter date. His knowledge of menstruation and gestation was quite modern. He knew and described intelligently the management of normal and abnormal labor. He described the use of forceps and cesarean section upon dead mothers to remove living children, and gave excellent antepartal and postpartal advice. He advised cleanliness on the part of the obstetrician: cutting the beard, the hair, and the nails closely, wearing clean gowns, and disinfecting the operating rooms prior to operation or delivery. His surgical antiseptic technique seems remarkable to modern students.

Chinese obstetrics was largely based on folk lore until the publication of a Chinese household manual of obstetrics, *Ta Sheng P'Ien,* which, according to the author's own statement, "is correct and needs no change or addition of prescription." There were monographs on obstetrics prior to this, but none so complete. Many of the statements are unfounded; in fact the knowledge is scanty or incorrect in many places, but the author had the saving grace of objecting to unnecessary interference and counseled patience in the treatment of labor.

Grecian Obstetrics

Prior to Hippocrates. The Asclepiads, or followers of Aesculapius, the father of medicine, had a largely supervisory interest in obstetrics. Abortions were not illegal. There is little definite knowledge concerning this period, but it seems probable that obstetrical treatment was primitive.

The Hippocratic Period. During this age, normal obstetrical cases were handled by midwives under the supervision of physicians. Abnormal labor was entirely in the hands of the medical profession. To Hippocrates is accredited the Hippocratic oath, which is still a part of the exercises for all students graduating from medical school. Treatises on obstetrics attributed to Hippocrates are the oldest records available of the Western world's obstetrical methods.

Greco-Roman Obstetrics. The Greco-Roman period was one of progress, which was due largely to the work of Celsus, Aëtius, and Soranus (second century) (Fig. 46-1). Soranus reintroduced podalic version and is responsible for the first authentic records of its use in the delivery of living children. He gave an excellent technical description of the procedure and the indications for its use.

Figure 46-1.
Bas-relief (second or third century A.D. near Rome) depicting birth scene. Note that the physician (center) holds a pair of obstetric forceps aloft in his right hand. (Danforth DN (ed): Obstetrics and Gynecology. Philadelphia, Harper & Row, 1982)

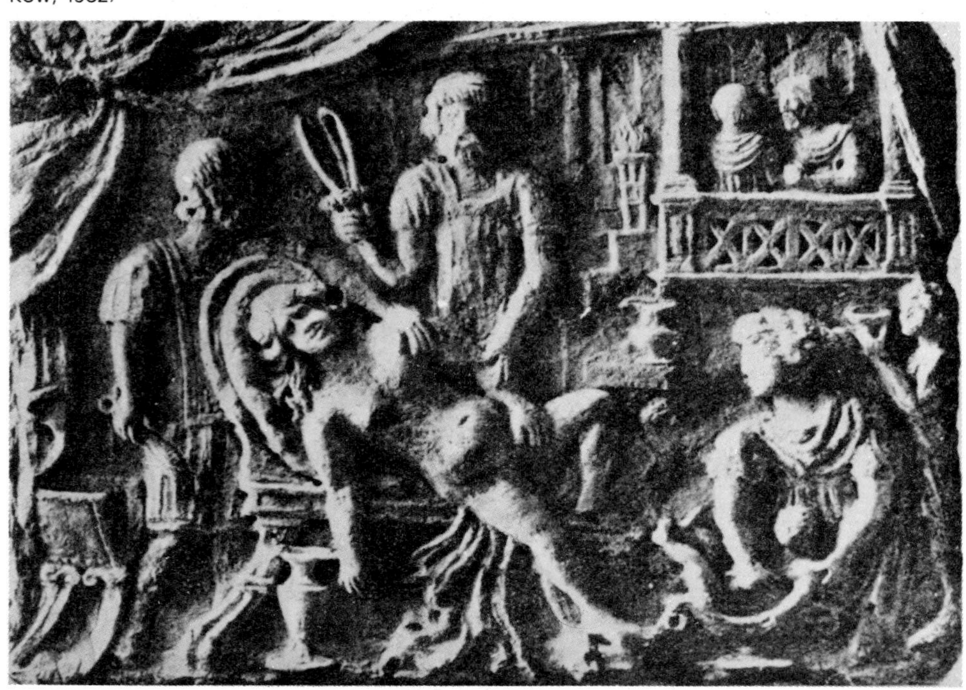

Byzantine, Mohammedan, Jewish, and Medieval Periods

These periods are characterized by a retrogression and loss of previously known practice. This was due in large part to the general inadequacy of science in the medieval period and the inhibiting effects of religious institutions. The paucity of operative treatment in difficult labor may be judged from the recommendations contained in the only textbook of the day on obstetrics and gynecology, which reads as follows: "Place the patient in a sheet held at the corners by four strong men, with her head somewhat elevated. Have them shake the sheet vigorously by pulling on the opposite corners, and with God's aid she will give birth." Despite this almost superstitious attitude toward childbirth, hospitals and nursing services were organized in this age.

Although the ancient Jews specified little assistance to the woman during labor and delivery, they were interested in the hygiene of pregnancy and cleanliness at the time of childbirth. Hygiene and sanitation were practices integrated into religious law. In instances of difficult deliveries, the women "were comforted until they died." The stool or obstetrical chair was used at this time and continued to be used until about the 19th century A.D. Reference is made to this chair in the Bible, in the first chapter of Exodus, "when you do the office of the midwife to the Hebrew women, and see them upon the stools. . . ."

The Renaissance Period

The Renaissance was characterized by advances in medicine and obstetrics commensurate with those in other fields. During this time the first English text on obstetrics, the *Byrthe of Mankynde,* was published by Raynalde. Both it and its German counterpart by Roesslin are copies of Soranus, and with their publication podalic version was reintroduced to obstetrical practice (Fig. 46-2). Many famous men were responsible for the progress in obstetrics—among them Leonardo da Vinci (who made the first accurate

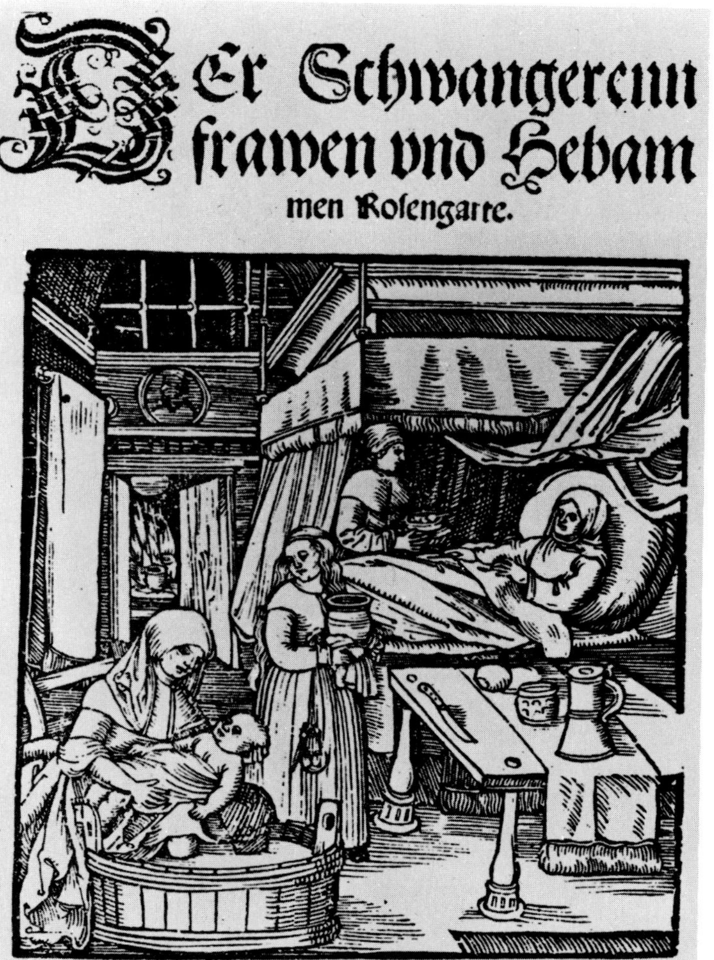

Figure 46-2.
Title page of an early text for midwives. (Henrich Steiner's 1537 edition of Rösslins Rosengarte)

sketches of the fetus *in utero*) and Vesalius (who accurately described the pelvis for the first time).

To Ambrose Paré, the dean of French surgeons and obstetricians, must go the chief credit for making podalic version a useful and practicable procedure to be used in preference to cesarean section in difficult labor. Through his studies, a significant part of obstetrical practice was removed from the hands of the midwives, where it had rested since the fall of the Roman Empire. Obstetrics was thereby established as an independent branch of medicine. Schools were established during this period to train midwives, and laws passed to regulate their practice. Paré's work on podalic version and his discouragement of cesarean section were opportune.

Cesarean sections had been practiced upon dead mothers since antiquity, but the first authentic cesarean section performed upon a living mother is credited to Trautman, of Wittenberg, in 1610. According to the records, the woman had a large ventral hernia which contained the uterus. Prior to this, Nufer, a sow gelder, is reputed to have performed the operation on his wife after obstetricians and midwives had failed to deliver her. It has been stated that Jane Seymour was delivered by a cesarean section done by Frère, a noted surgeon of the time, at the request of Henry VIII. That she died a few days after the birth of Edward VI adds credence to the story, but no absolute confirmation is available. Due to the frightful mortality from hemorrhage, sepsis, and so on, cesarean sections did not become popular in spite of the advocacy of the Church. Through the following centuries it was done occasionally, but not until the advent of uterine sutures and aseptic technique did it become a practical procedure.

The origin of the name has been ascribed to Julius Caesar, who is said to have been delivered by cesarean section. However, as his mother lived many years after his birth, this seems improbable—considering the high mortality of all abdominal operations before the time of Lister. A more accurate explanation is that Numa Pompilius, one of the earlier Roman kings, passed a law making it compulsory to perform the operation upon all mothers who died while pregnant so that the mother and the child might be buried separately. This was known as the *Lex Regis* and with the advent of the Caesars as the *Lex Caesaris* and subsequently the term *cesarean section* was coined. The name has also been attributed to *cedere,* the Latin verb meaning to cut, but the former explanation seems to be more reasonable.

The 17th century was notable for many famous obstetricians. Mauriceau, of Paris, was the first to correct the view that the pelvic bones separated in normal labor. He was also the first man to refer to epidemic puerperal fever. His description of an obstetrician, or rather of the qualities an obstetrician should possess, is both interesting and amusing. He stated

> He must be healthful, strong and robust; because this is the most laborious of all the Operations of Chirurgery; for it will make one sometimes sweat, so he shall not have a dry Thread, tho' it were the coldest day in Winter. . . . He ought to be well shaped, at least to outward appearance, but above all, to have small hands for the easier Introduction of them into the Womb when necessary; yet strong, with the Fingers long, especially the Fore-finger, the better to reach and touch the inner orifice. He must have no Rings on his Fingers, and his Nails well pared, when he goeth about the Work, for fear of hurting the Womb. He ought to have a pleasant Countenance, and to be as neat in his Clothes as in his person, that the poor women who have need for him be not affrighted at him. Some are of the opinion, that a Practitioner of this Art ought on the contrary to be slovenly, at least very carless, wearing a great Beard, to prevent the Occasion of the Husband's Jealousy that sends for him. Truly some believe this Policy augments their Practice but 'tis fit they should be disabused; for such a Posture and Dress resembles more a Butcher than a Chirurgeon, whom the woman apprehends already too much, that he needs not such as Disguise. Above all he must be sober, no Tipler, that he may at all times have his Wits about him. . . .

Van Deventer, of Holland, has been called the father of modern obstetrics and is credited with the first accurate description of the pelvis, its deformities and their effect on parturition. He also shares with Ould, of Dublin, the first description of the mechanism of labor.

As time passed, customs changed, and the term *accoucheur* replaced the objectionable *midman* and *man-midwife*. Obstetrical forceps were invented, probably about 1580, by Peter Chamberlen, but were kept as a family secret until 1813 in an effort of the Chamberlens to monopolize the field. By the time the Chamberlen forceps were finally revealed to the profession, other types of forceps had been developed.

The 16th century witnessed severe population losses due to plagues, wars, and natural disasters. In England, William Pelty realized that controlling communicable diseases and saving infant lives would prevent continued diminution of the population. To this end he recommended isolation of plague patients and maternity hospitals for unmarried pregnant women. Such ideas were too far in advance of the time, however, and had no immediate consequences.

The Eighteenth Century

Population continued to be a great general concern to the governments of the world. Those who were concerned with general matters of health felt that governments ought to take a more active role in overseeing health matters. Between 1779 and 1817, Johan Peter Frank in Germany wrote several volumes entitled *System einer vollstandigen medicinischen Polezey.* This work is even today considered a landmark in the history of thought on the social relations of health and disease. His recommendations concerning childbirth were many and, as with Pelty, farsighted for his time. He insisted that all childbirth be attended by trained persons, and further urged that a midwife be consulted prior to the expected date of confinement. In addition, he proposed legislation to enforce a reasonable period of bed rest during the puerperium and to free the mother for several weeks from any work in or outside the house that might prevent her from giving the necessary attention to her infant. When necessary, he felt that the state should support parturients for the first 6 weeks after delivery. He then expanded upon the above and outlined a detailed child welfare program. Acceptance of his work and ideas spread to all countries in close cultural contact with Germany.

The 18th century was also marked by a succession of famous men connected with obstetrics such as Palfyne, the Hunters, Smellie, White, and others. Palfyne is credited with the invention of a type of obstetrical forceps because in 1770 he presented a copy to the Academy of Medicine of Paris.

Smellie taught obstetrics with a manikin and made improvements on the obstetrical forceps in use at the time, adding a steel lock and curved blades. He also laid down the first principles for their use and differentiated by measurement between contracted and normal pelves.

William Hunter, though a pupil of Smellie, was opposed to the use of forceps, and frequently exhibited his rusted blades as evidence of their uselessness. In conjunction with his brother he laid the foundation of modern knowledge of placental anatomy.

Charles White published a thesis on obstetrics advocating the scrubbing of the hands and general cleanliness on the part of the accoucheur; he was the pioneer in aseptic midwifery. John Harvie, 90 years before Credé, advocated external manual expression of the placenta. It is known that a similar procedure was in use in Dublin at that time. One of the most active and famous English obstetricians of the time, John Clarke, had his fame commemorated in this epitaph:

> Beneath this stone, shut up in the dark
> Lies a learned man-midwife y'clep'd Dr. Clarke.
> On earth while he lived by attending men's
> wives,
> He increased population some thousands of
> lives;
> Thus a gain to the nation was gain to himself,
> An enlarged population, enlargement of pelf.
> So he toiled late and early, from morning to
> night,
> The squalling of children his greatest delight;
> Then worn with labours, he died skin and bone
> And his ladies he left all to Mansfield and Stone.

There were many famous obstetricians on the Continent during this period. Chief among them was Baudelocque, who invented the pelvimeter and named and described various positions and presentations. In America, prejudices against men in midwifery were carried over from Europe; as late as 1857 a demonstration before the graduating class at Buffalo roused such a storm of criticism that the American Medical Association had to intervene. Their judgment was that any physician who could not conduct labor by touch alone should not undertake midwifery.

The 18th century produced such men as Moultrie, Lloyd, and Shippen. Shippen was a pupil of Smellie and Hunter. In 1762, he opened a school for midwifery in Philadelphia, and, because he provided convenient lodgings for the accommodation of poor women during confinement, he may be said to have established the first lying-in hospital in America. With Morgan, he founded the School of Medicine of the University of Pennsylvania, becoming its first Professor of Anatomy, Surgery, and Midwifery.

The Nineteenth and the Twentieth Centuries

The increased knowledge, interest, and ability that physicians brought to obstetrics were largely offset by the increased mortality due to puerperal fever. During the 17th, 18th, and 19th centuries it became a pestilence, at times wiping out whole communities of puerperal women. The mortality rates varied in the best European clinics at Paris and Vienna from 10% to 20%. The origin and the spread of the disease were little understood or studied. Obstetricians spent futile hours on a study of minor alterations in instruments or technique and ignored the vast loss of life from puerperal fever. Oliver Wendell Holmes, of Harvard, first presented his views on the contagiousness of puerperal fever in 1843. In 1855 he reiterated them in a monograph on *Puerperal Fever as a Private Pestilence.* This was, and still remains, a medical classic on the subject. His statements aroused great controversy in America, and he received a great deal of abuse and criticism from Meigs and Hodge, two of the foremost American obstetricians of the day. One of them stated that it was ridiculous to conceive of any gentleman carrying contamination on his hands from patient to patient.

Whereas Holmes first conceived the correct idea of the nature of the disease, it is to Ignaz Philipp Semmelweiss that the glory for finally proving without question the nature of its source and transmission must go. He was an assistant in the Viennese clinic for women. While his associates were fussing with details of technique, he was studying and mourning the tremendous death rate among puerperal women in the clinic. He observed that the death rate in Clinic I, where women were delivered by medical students or physicians, was always higher than in Clinic II, where midwives officiated and received instruction. After fruitless study and manifold changes in technique in order to follow more closely that of Clinic II, the cause of the disease was brought home to him in a desperate and startling fashion. His friend, Kalletschka, an assistant in pathology, died after performing an autopsy upon a victim of puerperal fever, during which Kalletschka had sustained a slight cut on his finger.

At postmortem the findings were identical with those of puerperal sepsis, and Semmelweiss concluded that the disease was transmitted from the dead by contact from the physicians and the students, who often went directly from the postmortem room to deliveries. Accordingly, he immediately instituted and enforced a ruling that made it obligatory that all physicians and students wash their hands in a solution of chloride of lime after attending autopsies and before examining patients or delivering babies. In 7 months he had reduced the mortality in Clinic I from 12% to 2%. In the subsequent year Clinic I had a mortality lower than Clinic II, a hitherto unheard-of feat. Subsequently, he observed that puerperal sepsis could be transmitted from patient to patient, or from attendants to patient, by contact of contaminated material, as well as from the postmortem room. In 1861 he published his immortal work on *The Cause, Concept, and Prophylaxis of Puerperal Fever.*

The history of medicine provides pitiful figures in profusion, but none, it seems, met such a cruel reception and ultimate fate as Semmelweiss. His colleagues (for the most part, but with a few notable and loyal exceptions) distorted and criticized his teachings. Had they stopped there, it might have been bad enough, but they carried their distaste for his views to the stage of persecution. He was forced to leave Vienna and go to Budapest, where a similar attitude—if possible a more malignant one—awaited him. A disappointed man, he died in 1865 from a brain abscess which may have originated in an infection similar to that of his friend Kalletschka. His work, however, has lived on; Pasteur and Lister added to it; and with the advent of a more modern and tolerant age his worth has been recognized.

The 19th and the 20th centuries were largely notable for their use of drugs to alleviate the pains of childbirth. The use of ether as an anesthetic was first discovered in America, but it was first used for childbirth by Simpson in Great Britain. He brought back the lost art of podalic version by making it a safer procedure. Eventually he substituted chloroform for ether. As with almost every advance in medicine, it was opposed bitterly. The opposition was loudest and most vehement from the clergy, but, in 1853, Queen Victoria accepted it for delivery and by her action silenced most of the criticism. Nitrous oxide had been used in 1880 and has continued to be popular since that time.

Obstetrical analgesia and anesthesia have made great strides during the 20th century (see Chap. 27, Analgesia and Anesthesia for Childbirth).

The present century may be remembered largely for the development of antepartal clinics and the more concentrated care of the expectant mothers that came with them. The application of advances in general medicine, metabolism, and public health to obstetrics has led to a marked decrease in mortality and morbidity from cardiac, pulmonic, metabolic, venereal, and associated medical conditions complicating pregnancy. The consideration of adequate vitamin, mineral, and caloric contents in connection with the diet of pregnant and puerperal women not only has decreased the morbidity but also has enhanced the health of all mothers and children who receive adequate obstetrical care.

Many other contributions have been made and are being added constantly to the science of obstetrics, not the least of which is more intensive training and study in this specialty demanded by the public as well as by the medical profession. The advent of routine external expression of the placenta, antibacterial prophylaxis in the eyes of the newborn, purified ergot, and pituitary preparations in hemorrhage control and prevention are but a few of the methods and medications that marked the early 20th century.

The morphological and anthropological studies of Naegele, Roberts, Williams, Goodwin, Caldwell, Moloy, and others have done much to improve our understanding of the various types of pelves and some of their importance in labor. Roentgenological pelvimetry, cephalometry, and tokodynamometry have greatly advanced our knowledge of the probable course of labor and delivery. Thoms, Caldwell and Moloy, Hanson, Jarcho, and countless others have contributed to our advances in this field.

Development of Maternal and Infant Care in the United States

As we know it today, maternal and child care developed into its present status through various avenues of investigation and many by-paths of interrelated activity and work. Individuals, both from the profession and the laity, as well as private and municipal organizations, contributed time, money, and interest until, at last, government action was obtained.

1866. When a story was written concerning cruelty to a child, some thoughtful person referred the case to The Society for the Prevention of Cruelty to Animals. Henry Bergh, a former diplomat to Russia, was the founder and director of this association and was influential in having the judgment pronounced on the ground that a child was a human animal. This incident stimulated interest in the general treatment of children.

1873. *The New York Diet Kitchen Association,* the oldest public health organization in America, was opened at the request of doctors from "de Milt Dispensary" on the lower East Side of New York City. It was first organized as a soup kitchen, and milk, gruel, beef tea, and cooked rice were taken to the sick in their homes, with the idea of restoring health. In 1892, they began to make formulas for sick babies and still later dispensed free milk, or sold it at 3 cents a quart. Maria L. Daniels, the first nurse director, contributed a great deal to public health progress. In 1926, this group was organized as The Children's Health Service of New York. The organization grew with the times, changing its program from curing the sick to preventive work—keeping well babies well. Although the organization devoted its major effort to work with babies and preschool children, it also included antepartal care in its program.

1876. The beginning of child-welfare legislation in the United States was the act passed by the New York State Legislature, granting to *The Society for the Prevention of Cruelty to Children* a charter that gave it wide power in the protection of child life. The inception of this legislation was based on the incident of the "child as a human animal" (1866).

1893. The first *Infant Milk Station* in the United States was established in New York City by Nathan Strauss. Through his persistence, milk was finally made safe through pasteurization, and many such stations were set up.

1900. *The United States Census Bureau* was made a permanent organization. Up to this time, vital statistics were considered to be of so little importance in the United States that, as soon as the population was tabulated and classified, the bureau was disbanded, to be reestablished and reorganized every ten years.

1906. *The United States Census Bureau* published mortality statistics that drew attention to the appalling loss of life among babies and children. Up to this time, very little thought had been given to maternal and infant protection.

1907. Due to growing interest, Mr George H. F. Schrader gave money to *The Association for Improving Conditions of the Poor* (now the *Community Service Society*) for the salaries of two nurses to do antepartal work. This was the first consistent effort to prevent deaths of babies by caring for the mothers *before* the babies were born. Two reasons were given as to why antepartal care would be of value: (1) nurses in convalescent homes for postpartal mothers thought that if patients had better care during pregnancy, the health of mothers would be improved; (2) social workers going into the homes felt that they were not adequately prepared to advise pregnant mothers.

1907. *The New York Milk Committee* was organized. Its object was the reduction of infant mortality through the improvement of the city's milk supply. It established milk depots that proved beyond question their great value in the reduction of infant mortality by dispensing clean, pasteurized milk and by educating mothers.

1908. In this year the *Division of Child Hygiene* was established in New York City, the first in the United States, and it was important enough to be recognized nationally. Josephine Baker, M.D., was appointed chief. This was a pioneer achievement, and the methods that evolved had no precedent.

1909 to 1914. At approximately this time, Mrs William Lowell Putnam, of Boston, promoted a demonstration of organized antepartal care. It was called *The Prenatal Care Committee* of the Women's Municipal League. The members of this committee worked in cooperation with the Boston Lying-In Hospital through Robert L. DeNormandie, M.D., of Harvard Medical School, Dr. Ruggles, of the then Homeopathic Hospital, and the Instructive District Nurses Association. The committee functioned long enough to establish the fact that good obstetrical care was not possible without antepartal care.

1909. In this year *The American Association for the Study and Prevention of Infant Mortality* was organized and held its first meeting in New Haven, Connecticut. This committee was composed of both professional and lay members and devoted itself entirely to problems connected with child life, particularly to studying and trying to correct the high mortality rate. At this time there were no records of births or deaths, and the causes of deaths were unknown. The education of physicians and nurses was shamefully unsatisfactory; there was no public health in the schools, and practically no activity on the part of municipal, state, or federal government to prevent infant mortality. The first president of this association was J. H. Mason Knox, M.D. Gertrude B. Kipp was the first secretary. The committee consisted of the Honorable Herbert Hoover, Livingston Ferrand, M.D., L. Emmet Holt, M.D., Richard Bolt, M.D., and Philip Van Ingen, M.D. The work of this organization was of profound significance. In 1918, its expanding activities caused it to change its name to *The American Child Hygiene Association,* and in 1923 the name was changed to *The American Child Health Association.* In 1935, after having contributed to every angle of this pioneer work, the association was disbanded.

1909. *The First White House Conference,* on "The Dependent Child," was called by President Theodore Roosevelt. These investigations resulted in the establishment of the U.S. Children's Bureau in 1912. According to some authorities, this conference was called through the influence of a public health nurse.

1910. *The Census Bureau* published another report, this time on the mortality of infants under 1 year of age and at "special ages." As a result of this report maternity hospitals made an effort to improve the care given to infants.

1911. In New York City *the first strictly municipal baby-health stations* were organized under the jurisdiction of the Department of Health. The full cost of the work was borne by the municipality. Soon the dispensing of milk came to be of minor importance, and emphasis was placed on prevention. They are now called *Child-Health Stations.*

1911. *The New York Milk Committee* (1907) made an investigation at the baby-health stations and found that 40% of all infant deaths (112 in 1000) occurred within the first month of life before the mothers registered their babies at the health stations. This indicated the necessity for care *before* birth. The committee then decided to carry out an experiment in antepartal work. (See 1917.) They were convinced that much could be hoped for as a result of organized antepartal care.

1912. *The Babies' Welfare Association* (formerly *The Association of Infant Milk Stations* [1893]) represents the first comprehensive and successful attempt to coordinate the various child-welfare agencies in any community. All of the organizations of this type agreed to coordinate their activities by preventing duplication and overlapping without interfering with the organizations. In 1922, the name was changed to the *Children's Welfare Federation* of New York City. It continued to act as a clearinghouse and, among its other activities, managed the *Mother's Milk Bureau.*

1912. The *United States Children's Bureau* was established. It began in the Department of Commerce and Labor; in 1913 it was made a part of the Department of Labor and, in 1946, was transferred to the Federal Security Agency. This was created by Congress through a federal act (government sanction). This bureau was to set up special machinery to study and protect the child and to study all matters pertaining to the welfare of children and child life among all classes of our people, to assemble and accumulate factual information and to disseminate this information throughout the country. Miss Julia Lathrop was chosen as chief. Much of the success of this bureau is credited to Miss Lathrop's vision. Fortunately, her successor, Miss Grace Abbott, continued the work with equal zeal.

1915. *The Birth Registration Area* was established by a federal act. The information is compiled in a uniform manner, giving the birth and the death statistics on which our information on mortality rates are based.

1915. Dr. Haven Emerson, Health Commissioner of New York City, appointed a special committee (Ralph W. Lobenstine, M.D., Clifton Edgar, M.D., and Philip Van Ingen, M.D.), in cooperation with the New York Milk Committee, to make an analysis of the facilities for maternity care in the city. The result of the survey showed that there was little antepartal work and no uniformity, and that only a very small number of pregnant mothers were receiving care. It showed also that hospitals took care of 30% of the deliveries, midwives delivered 30%, general practitioners delivered 30%, and private physicians, who might be classified as obstetricians, delivered 10%. Previous to this time, little or nothing had been done to regulate or control the midwives.

1916. *The National Society for the Prevention of Blindness* was created after much pioneer work and investigation, locally and throughout the states, by Carolyn Van Blarcom, R.N. She was chosen to be the executive secretary. Through these investigations it was learned that by far the greatest cause of blindness was ophthalmia of the newborn. This finding led to the passing of a law compelling all physicians and midwives to use prophylaxis in newborn babies' eyes. Also, as a direct result of Miss Van Blarcom's surveys, a school for lay midwives, Belleview School for Midwives (no longer in existence), was started. Miss Van Blarcom took out a midwife's license and was the first nurse in the United States so to register. The first obstetrical nursing textbook to be written by a nurse is credited to Miss Van Blarcom. Her later contribution to the better care of mothers and babies was to secure for Johns Hopkins Hospital the E. Bayard Halsted Fund for medical research.

1917. The Women's City Club of New York City and the New York Milk Committee opened three antepartal centers. The one sponsored by the Women's City Club was organized as the *Maternity Service Association* and, with Francis Perkins as the first executive secretary and Miss Mabel Choate as president, provided stimulating leadership. Dr. Ralph W. Lobenstine, a famous obstetrician, gave much time, labor, authority, and direction as chairman of the medical board. In 1918, this organization was incorporated as the *Maternity Center Association* and carried out the first extensive piece of organized antepartal work in the United States. Miss Anne Stevens was director. Miss Annie W. Goodrich's wise counsel, as a member of the nursing committee, gave impetus to the organization's accomplishments. Louis I. Dublin, Ph.D., associated with this movement from the beginning, made an analysis of the first 4000 records collected by the association. This revealed the startling fact that, through antepartal care, 50% of the lives of mothers might be saved and 60% of the lives of babies. Antepartal training and experience were extended to nurses throughout the world. This piece of intensive antepartal work fired increased interest in the care of mothers and babies. In 1929, the Maternity Center Association opened a school for the training of nurse midwives.

1919. *The Second White House Conference* was called by President Woodrow Wilson as a result of the activities of the U.S. Children's Bureau. It was organized in five sections. Each section was interested in a different phase of maternity and child care.

1919. *The American Committee on Maternal Welfare* was founded. The object of the committee was to stimulate interest of the medical profession in cooperating with public and private agencies to protect the lives and health of mothers and infants. The committee also sought to teach principles and practice of personal hygiene and health to parents, physicians, nurses, and others dealing with the problems of maternity. The Committee was incorporated as a non-profit organization in 1934 for the purpose of studying the maternal mortality rate in the United States and the management of obstetrical problems generally. For more recent progress, see 1957 and 1964.

This organization publishes the magazine *The Bulletin of Maternal and Child Health.* It also promoted the American Congress of Obstetrics and Gynecology, which was held every 3 years.

1921. *The Sheppard–Towner Bill* was passed by Congress, an act for the promotion of the welfare and hygiene of maternity and infancy, to be administered by the United States Children's Bureau. This bill was introduced in the 65th Congress by Congresswoman Jeanette Rankin of New Jersey. It was reported out of committee favorably but failed to pass. A second bill was introduced in the 66th Congress. It passed in the Senate but, through delays, was not considered by the House. In the first session of the 67th Congress the bill was again introduced by Senator Sheppard and Congressman Towner and, after much agitation, finally passed—an epoch in child-welfare legislation. An appropriation of $1,240,000 per year was granted for 5 years. The Cooper Bill, passed in 1927, extended it for 2 more years. This law was accepted by all of the states except three. This legislation gave a tremendous impetus to the education not only of laity but also of physicians. Because of this legislation there was created at once, in the states that did not already have them, departments that now are quite uniformly labeled Divisions or Bureaus of Maternal and Child Health. In 1935, the Social Security Act was passed, following the plan of the Sheppard-Towner Bill. This Act appropriated $3,800,000. In 1939, the Social Security Act was amended, increasing the appropriation to $5,820,000. The amount has been increased gradually, and by 1952 (the 82nd Congress), $30,000,000 was appropriated for Maternal and Child Health, Crippled Children and other Child Health Services.

1923. *The National Committee for Maternal Health* was formed with Robert L. Dickinson, M.D. as secretary and later as president. This was a clearinghouse and a center of information on certain medical aspects of human fertility. The object was to gather and analyze material, to stimulate research, to issue reports to the medical profession, and to persuade it to take a leading part in the scientific investigations of these problems in preventive medicine. No other group existed for this purpose. It was dissolved in 1950.

1923. *The Margaret Sanger Research Bureau* came into being, an affiliation of the Planned Parenthood Federation of America, Inc., for research in the field of infertility, contraception, and marriage counseling.

1923. Mary Breckinridge began her investigations in Kentucky, which led to the organization of the *Frontier Nursing Service.* With this concentrated effort of all phases of maternity and infant care, the striking results proved the value of prenatal care. Through her vision, determination, and unfaltering energy, Mary Breckinridge has made this organization one of worldwide renown. In 1936, the Frontier Nursing Service opened a school for the training of nurse midwives.

1925. *The Joint Committee on Maternal Welfare* was formed. This consisted of the American Gynecological Society, the American Association of Obstetrics and Gynecology and Abdominal Surgeons, and the American Child Health Association (1909). Later, the section of Obstetrics, Gynecology and Abdominal Surgeons of the American Medical Association was represented. The Committee issued a pamphlet entitled *An Outline of Delivery Care.* This stimulated the Children's Bureau to publish a concise pamphlet, *Standards of Prenatal Care* (1925), an outline for the use of physicians that did much to standardize routine procedures.

1930. *The Third White House Conference* was called by President Herbert Hoover. Mr. Hoover's interest in child welfare was very evident. The conference was very comprehensive and far-reaching and was devoted to all aspects of maternity and child care. The Children's Charter was adopted and became a federal act. To show the paramount importance of care during pregnancy and the early years, 45,000,000 children were analyzed in chart form.

1938. *The Conference on Better Care for Mothers and Babies* was called by the Children's Bureau. This was the first time that representatives from the states, private and public organizations, both lay and professional people, met to pool ideas.

1939. *The Maternity Consultation Service* in New York City was organized to further antepartal education and care.

1940. *The Fourth White House Conference* on Children in a Democracy was called by President Franklin D. Roosevelt. It considered the aims of American civilization for the children in whose hands its future lies—how children can best be helped to grow into the kind of citizens who will know best how to preserve and protect our democracy. By 1940, the 48 states, the District of Columbia, Puerto Rico, Alaska, and Hawaii (then territories) were cooperating with the Children's Bureau in its administration of child-welfare services.

1940. *The Cleveland Health Museum* was opened to the public—the first health museum in the Western hemisphere. It is significant in the maternity field because, in its workshops, it is reproducing the *Dickinson-Belskie models,* acquired in 1945. Dr. Bruno Gebhard, Director, says that, in his belief, the use of this sculptural series in professional and lay education will advance knowledge on this all-important subject more quickly and more accurately than any other visual means thus far available.

1943. *The Emergency Maternity and Infancy Care Program* was launched to care for the wives and the babies of men enlisted in the armed forces. From $17,000,000 to $45,000,000 per year was appropriated. This act also furthered interest in prenatal and child care.

1944. *The Public Health Service Act* was signed on July 3, 1944, and brought together all existing laws affecting the public health service. In addition, the act revised existing laws, provided authority for grants, and authorized expansion of the federal–state cooperative public health programs that had bearing on maternal and child health programs. This act was to have a great indirect influence on the care of mothers and infants because of its provisions funding research and education of personnel needed in these areas.

1946. The *World Health Organization*—an agency of the United Nations—became a reality. At the first meeting in Paris, 64 nations signed the constitution. The membership as of 1965 totaled 117 countries. The object of the organization is "the attainment of the highest possible level of health of all the peoples." So far, much has been accomplished toward that end.

1950. *The Fifth White House Conference,* with emphasis on children and youth, was called by President Harry S. Truman.

1950. *The Fred Lyman Adair Foundation* of the American Committee on Maternal Welfare was established. Its purpose is to collect funds from charitable sources to underwrite research and educational projects in this field.

1955. *The American College of Nurse-Midwifery* was established as an organization of nurse-midwives to study and evaluate the activities of nurse-midwives, to plan and develop educational programs meeting the requirements of the profession, and to perform other related functions. In 1957, the College became a member of the International Confederation of Midwives, a midwifery organization with members from some 30 countries throughout the world.

1957. *The American Association for Maternal and Infant Health* (formerly the American Committee on Maternal Welfare) was activated at the Seventh American Congress held in July. Prompted by the spectacular improvements and advances in maternity care that have taken place since its founding, the board of directors of the committee voted unanimously to change the name, the role, and the character of the organization. The new American Association for Maternal and Infant Health provides close integration of the various disciplines that participate in providing modern maternity care, and serves as a forum for their mutual problems related to maternal and infant health.

1960. *The Sixth White House Conference,* concerned with the nation's children and youth, was called by President Dwight D. Eisenhower. The theme of this Golden Anniversary Conference was "Opportunities for Children and Youth to Realize Their Full Potential for Creative Life in Freedom and Dignity."

1962. *The Conference on Maternal and Child Health Teaching in Graduate Schools of Public Health* was convened in response to the reports of the lack of qualified personnel with any public health background in the area of maternal and child health. The conference recommended that a maternal and child health career development program be established to offset the existing and predicted shortages of personnel. Such a program was established at the University of California at Berkeley with financial aid from the federal government (U.S. Children's Bureau) in 1965. The objectives of early recruitment of qualified physicians and the provision for specialized training in obstetrics or pediatrics with general community, maternal, and child health content has been realized.

In 1962 *The National Institute of Child Health and Human Development* was authorized. The goal of this Institute was support of research and training in special health problems and needs of mothers and children. This Institute also conducts and supports research in the basic sciences relating to the processes of human growth and development, including prenatal development. Five conferences were held in 1967 which sought to find the problems involved in maternal and infant mortality and morbidity and to establish guidelines for change toward optimal care.

1963. *The Maternal and Child Health and Mental Retardation Planning Amendments of 1963* was enacted. This law makes it possible for the Children's Bureau to carry out some of the major recommendations of the President's panel.

1964. *The American Association for Maternal and Child Health* (formerly the American Association for Maternal and Infant Health), as a multidisciplinary organization, is one of the most potentially valuable groups interested in matters concerning infant, child, and maternal health. The board of directors of the Association altered the official title of the organization, not to imply any change in its proposed program, but to present a more accurate definition of the organization's aims and objectives.

1964. *The Nurse Training Act,* one of the amendments of the Public Health Act, was an indirect aid to maternal and infant care. This act authorized grants for the expansion and improvement of nurse training, assistance to nursing students, scholarship grants to schools of nursing, and the establishment of a National Advisory Council on Nurse Training.

1965. *Amendments to the Social Security Act* provided for a new 5-year program of special project grants for comprehensive health care and services for school and preschool children, particularly in low-income family areas. These amendments also increased the authorization for money to support maternal and child health service programs. There are now 54 such projects in existence due to this legislation.

1965. *PKU testing* became mandatory for all infants in the states of Illinois and Michigan, thus setting a precedent for other states.

1966. *The Department of Health, Education and Welfare* issued a policy statement on birth control that stated that the Department would support, on request, health programs making family planning information and services available. Due to this unique statement, federally supported family planning programs have since slowly begun to evolve.

The Federal Food, Drug and Cosmetic Act was instituted on June 14, 1966. This legislation required labeling of ingredients of food represented for special dietary use. Infant foods, particularly, were specified.

The Child Protection Act of 1966 banned the sale of toys and children's articles containing hazardous substances, regardless of labeling.

1967. *The Public Health Law 89–749* is considered by health authorities to be one of the most significant health measures passed by Congress because it provides for increasing flexibility at state and regional levels to attack special health problems which have regional or local impact.

1967. *Medicaid* programs were increasing among the states (30 in 1967) to provide health care for low-income families. Care during pregnancy and child care were included.

1968. Head Start programs provided educational opportunities for underprivileged children of preschool age. These programs are often associated with nutritional and health screening programs.

1968. The second part of the *President's Committee on Mental Retardation* noted that three fourths of the country's mental retardation was found in isolated and impoverished urban and rural areas. It cited evidence of a close relationship between diet and mental and nervous disorders. It recommended federal action to improve manpower shortages and develop facilities for care of the mentally retarded.

1968. *The Citizens' Board of Inquiry into Hunger and Malnutrition in the United States* issued its report "Hunger—U.S.A." which verified the presence of widespread hunger among millions of United States citizens.

1969. A live-virus vaccine for *rubella* (German measles) was released and the United States Public Health Service began immunization programs.

1969. *The National Center for Family Planning* was established under the Health Services and Mental Health Administration, Department of Health, Education and Welfare (DHEW), to serve as a clearinghouse for information about contraception.

1969. *Neighborhood Health Centers* pilot projects began in many Southern states and Northern urban slums to provide medical care to the poor.

1969. Nurses and physician's assistants were being trained as *Pediatric Assistants* in several university pediatrics departments.

1969. *Amniocentesis* was used to diagnose hereditary disease in the fetus.

1969. *The White House Conference on Food, Nutrition and Health* was charged with formulating a national nutritional program, based on reports of malnutrition among the lower-income population and the consequences of nutritional deficiency for the growth and development of infants.

1970. A nationwide drive was spearheaded by the *Center for Disease Control* in Atlanta, Georgia, to vaccinate children against rubella.

1970. *The Seventh White House Conference on Children and Youth* met, and recommended the establishment of a child advocacy agency by the federal government with full ethnic, cultural, racial, and sexual representation.

1969–1970. The *Office of Child Development* was established within DHEW to administer child development programs (Head Start, day care) and coordinate activities of governmental and private agencies involved in programs for children and youth.

1970. New York state liberalized its *abortion law* to leave the decision up to the woman during the first 24 weeks of pregnancy, permitting abortion after that time only to save the woman's life.

1971. *National Commission for the Study of Nursing and Nursing Education,* Jerome Lysaught, director, reported a study of nursing roles and recommended that nursing roles be expanded, educational systems repatterned, and nursing input into health care increased.

1971. The American Nurses Association (ANA) and American Academy of Pediatrics jointly developed guidelines for *training pediatric nurse associates,* and held a national conference to implement these. The ANA and American College of Obstetricians and Gynecologists also met to draw up guidelines for training clinical nurse specialists in obstetrics–gynecology.

1971. Funds were awarded to six innovative *child advocacy demonstration projects* by two agencies of DHEW.

1972. *Home Start* programs were inaugurated to help disadvantaged parents to provide child development services in their own homes and to be the primary educators of their own children.

1972. The *Office of Child Development* sponsored programs to help teenagers learn how to become good parents, and in coordinated efforts with Head Start and Community Mental Health Centers strove to improve the quality of mental health care, including prevention, diagnosis, and treatment of mental health problems for Head Start children and their families.

1972. *The Committee to Study Extended Roles for Nurses* reported to the secretary of DHEW that functions of nurses "need to be broadened [so they can] assume broader responsibility in primary care, acute care, and long-term care." The new nurse practitioner was functioning in expanded nursing roles in many areas including obstetrics, pediatrics, psychiatry, and medical–surgical nursing.

1972. *Professional Standards Review Organizations* (PSRO) were required by an amendment to the Social Security Act to be set up to oversee care given by physicians to Medicare and Medicaid patients in hospitals.

1973. The *United States Supreme Court* struck down almost all state statutes prohibiting or restricting abortion, leaving the abortion decision to the woman and her physician during the first 3 months of pregnancy; after this time the state could only regulate abortion procedures in the interest of maternal health. Essentially, the decision to abort became the right of the individual woman, with the state unable to interfere in her choice except to ensure that the abortion be performed under safe conditions.

1973. The *Child and Family Resource Program* began as an experimental project designed to strengthen the role of the family in the birthing process by providing or making available prenatal health and nutritional education, after-school tutoring for primary grade children, and mental health services to parents about child development.

1973. Data showed that immunization of women with *anti-Rh antibodies* shortly after delivery was highly effective in preventing Rh-sensitization in the Rh-negative mother (Rhogam).

1973. *The National Commission for the Study of*

Nursing and Nursing Education, directed by Jerome Lysaught, reported on the implementation phase of its study. To encourage the expansion of nursing practice, it conducted educational and informational activities aimed at nursing professionals and the public, developed a national joint practice commission between medicine and nursing with state counterparts, and developed statewide planning committees to generate changes in patterns of education and practice.

1973. *National Center on Child Abuse and Neglect* was established in DHEW's Office of Child Development to act as clearinghouse on information about child abuse. A *National Commission* was formed to study the role of the federal government in this area and the adequacy of state laws. Funds were made available to regional child-abuse prevention and treatment demonstration programs.

1974. *Guidelines on Short-Term Education Modules for the Obstetric-Gynecologic Nurse Practitioner* were drawn up by the Interorganizational Committee of Obstetric–Gynecologic Health Personnel.

1974. Federal *Child Health Screening Programs* were strengthened (Public Law 92–603), requiring states to inform Medicaid families about availability of child-health screening services and provide these when requested.

1974. Funds made available to study *Sudden Infant Death Syndrome* by the National Institute of Child Health and Human Development.

1975. The Division on Maternal and Child Health Nursing Practice of the ANA issued a *guide for short-term continuing education programs* for nurse clinicians in neonatal and maternal–fetal care, an outgrowth of a joint effort among several organizations.

1975. The ANA Commission on Nursing Education offered *accreditation for nondegree-granting nurse practitioner programs,* including the OB–GYN nurse practitioners.

1975. *The National Advisory Council on Maternal, Infant and Fetal Nutrition* was established. Annual reports submitted to the President and Congress make continuing recommendations for administrative and legislative changes in programs aimed at low-income individuals at nutritional risk (PL 94–105).

1975. The *WIC* program (Special Supplemental Food Program for Women, Infants and Children) was intended to provide low-income families with supplemental foods and nutrition education through local agencies, as an adjunct to good health during critical times of growth and development.

1975. *Title XX,* a comprehensive amendment to the Social Security Act, provided funds for family-planning services, child care services, child protective services, and foster care for children (as well as other benefits and services for adults).

1976. *The Early and Periodic Screening, Diagnostic and Treatment* program (EPSDT) provided Medicaid-eligible children with regular health screening and treatment through federal funding.

1975. Landmark legislation was passed, the *National Health Planning and Resources Act* (PL 93–641), which set the framework for establishing a system of national health policy, planning, and development. Health Service Areas were to be established throughout the United States to coordinate health-care resources and services. To avoid duplication and overlapping services and to combat the rising costs of health care, regulations indicate that to justify a hospital having an obstetrical section there should be 75% occupancy in the unit where there are more than 1500 births per year. Exceptions to these regulations are provided for rural or geographically isolated communities, and for other special situations.

1976. The *Food and Drug Administration* (FDA) required pharmaceutical companies to withdraw the sequential oral contraceptives from the market because studies indicated there was an increased risk of endometrial cancer.

1976. The *FDA* ordered warning labels for physicians and pharmacists on the risks of oral contraceptives, including birth defects, tumors, blood clots, and heart attack in women over 40 years of age.

1976. The *FDA* recommended *gonad shielding* for men and women of reproductive age as a routine practice for protection from x-rays, and issued proposed guidelines.

1977. A *national symposium on immunization* sponsored by the March of Dimes urged renewed attention to immunization. An estimated 20 million children of the 52 million under age 15 were not immunized against one or more childhood diseases; a nationwide campaign was undertaken by the ANA, March of Dimes, and the federal government to improve the level of immunization among children.

1977. The *Child Health Assessment Act* (CHAP) extended the early and periodic screening program (EPSDT) to broaden eligibility and to require that treatment be given for conditions discovered during assessment, with exceptions of mental retardation, mental health, developmental problems, and dental care. This legislation also expanded and improved community health centers.

1977. *ANA and NAACOG* offered a national

examination for maternal–gynecological–neonatal nurses.

1977. The *FDA* required patient labeling for estrogenic drug products, except those used for contraception, related to cancer risks.

1977. The *FDA* required manufacturers' labeling of IUDs for patients, describing potential risks and side-effects and requiring physicians to have patients read the brochure before insertion of the IUD.

1977. *The National Institute on Alcohol Abuse and Alcoholism* issued a warning that pregnant women who have more than 2 drinks per day risk deformed or retarded children (the fetal alcohol syndrome).

1977. Legislation was passed (the Hyde Amendment) and upheld that *federal funds could not be used for abortions* except in cases where low-income women's lives would be endangered by continuing the pregnancy, or where birth would cause severe and long-lasting damage to the woman's physical health. Victims of rape and incest could also receive funds.

1978. The *Civil Rights Act* of 1974 was amended to protect working women from occupational discrimination because of pregnancy, requiring employers with medical disability plans to provide pregnancy disability payments on an equal basis with other medical conditions.

1978. The *Rural Health Clinic Services Act* (PL 95–210) provided for the reimbursement of nurse practitioners under Medicare and Medicaid without a physician being present on site, under jointly developed protocols, in clinics that qualified as rural.

1978. The *Committee on Maternal Health Care and Family Planning* of the American Public Health Association published guidelines to address the problems of quality, quantity, and cost of prenatal, postpartum, and interconceptional care, family planning, adolescent pregnancy, health education, nutritional and social services, human resources, facilities and equipment, and evaluation.[1]

1979. The United Nations designated 1979 as the *International Year of the Child,* encouraging all nations to upgrade the care and well-being of children. Their Declaration of the Rights of the Child includes the following:

- The right to affection, love, and understanding
- The right to adequate nutrition and medical care
- The right to free education
- The right to full opportunity for play and recreation
- The right to a name and nationality
- The right to special care, if handicapped
- The right to be among the first to receive relief in times of disaster
- The right to learn to be a useful member of society and to develop individual abilities
- The right to be brought up in a spirit of peace and universal brotherhood
- The right to enjoy these rights, regardless of race, color, sex, religion, or national or social origin[2]

1979. The *World Health Organization* targeted the year 2000 for bringing all citizens of the world to a state of positive health. Key to this goal is making primary care universally accessible. There is also need to work toward solution of problems related to nutrition, water, immunization, maternal and child health, and mental health.

1979. By this year *all 50 states had enacted laws* requiring every child to be immunized as a condition of entry into school. Approximately 85% to 90% of children ages 5 to 14 were immunized against measles, rubella, polio, and DPT.

1980. Congress passed the *Child Health Assurance Program (CHAP)* designed to improve health screening of poor children. This program was intended to expand the EPSDT programs previously enacted.

1980. The Maternity Care Association and John A. Hartford Foundation began a *collaborative study* of a sample of 4000 births at 11 *alternate birth centers,* comparing results with a national sample of hospital births.

1980. The *Children's Bureau* was disbanded after 68 years of significant contributions to the welfare of United States children. This is viewed by many as evidence of weakening of child advocacy in America.

1981. Congress authorized *Medicaid payments for services of nurse-midwives,* making this alternate care available to many women who previously lacked access.

1981. The *White House Conferences on Children* were discontinued by the Reagan Administration. These decennial national conferences are to be replaced by smaller state meetings that will reflect the Administration's commitment to federalism.

1981. *Abortion statistics* released by the Center for Disease Control reported the smallest increase in 5 years, reflecting decreased public funding for abortions, increased sterilization or other contraception, or decreased reporting. Publicly funded abortions decreased by more than one third.

1981. *Federal budget cuts* in health-care spending led to states' reducing Medicaid services, eligibility, and reimbursement, resulting in less health-care coverage for the poor.

1981. The *federal health-care program* included a maternal and child health-care block and categorical programs in family planning and childhood immunization, as well as an adolescent family life program providing services to pregnant teenagers and storefront counseling centers. The reductions in the budget totaled $8.5 billion in health care over the next 3 years.

1981. The World Health Organization adopted a *code to discourage use of infant formulas in developing countries* where the conditions of life are poor and clean water or other facilities for safe formula use are lacking. The United States was the only nation to vote against these voluntary international guidelines, reflecting industry pressure to protect marketing opportunities.

1981. The Maternity Center Association initiated a program to develop *low-cost maternity care birth centers* outside the hospital setting. A manual of birth-center standards, creation of a cooperative resources and information network, and promotion of wider public understanding are included in the program.

1981. The *Select Panel for Promotion of Child Health* made a report to Congress recommending reorganization of health services to stress prevention and primary care. They announced that the government must ensure universal access to prenatal care, comprehensive care for children from birth to the age of 5 years, and family-planning services.

1981. The *Cesarean Birth Task Force* report, issued by the National Institute of Child Health and Human Development (NIH), documented that cesarean births had tripled since 1970. The report questioned improvement in neonatal mortality related to cesareans, as well as the need for repeat cesareans.

1982. The *Centers for Disease Control* reported record low incidence of measles, with most states having less than one case per 100,000 population.

1982. The *March of Dimes Birth Defects Foundation* sponsored an experimental screening and preventive care program which reduced premature births by 63%, through patient education to detect early signs of labor and prompt medical treatment to delay delivery.

1982. The FDA issued *warnings on the use of aspirin* by children who have chicken pox or viral influenza, due to the increased danger of Reye's syndrome, which may be fatal.

1982. The *Centers for Disease Control* reported a 36.7% reduction in the mean level of lead in the population's blood, creating a greater margin of safety for high-risk young children living in environments with high-dose sources of lead.

■■■

The Emergence and Development of Maternity Nursing

From time immemorial women have taken care of other women during pregnancy and childbirth; most cultures, both primitive and modern, have a well-developed "motherlore" that keeps alive instructions and practices to be used during the childbearing period.

Midwifery

In every primitive society, there seems to have been someone present to care for the mother and the infant. Usually this task fell to women who, in essence, were the ancient forerunners of maternity nurses. Midwives no doubt have existed for centuries untold; Homer made reference to a nurse-midwife in the *Iliad.* They continued to attend the majority of deliveries in Roman and medieval times, although the role of physicians was enlarging. During the 18th century maternity cases began to receive more attention as many lying-in charities were formed and midwives were included in training programs in London and Paris.

As midwifery assumed a more scientific status, special lying-in hospitals increased, and the last 50 years of the 18th century saw a remarkable decrease in maternal and infant deaths in these hospitals owing to better techniques of nursing management. The male physicians remained mostly uninvolved in parturient care unless needed for special procedures in difficult labors.[3] It was not until the 19th century that physicians participated extensively in obstetrics, and much opposition had to be overcome from both physician and the public before the man-midwives were widely accepted. In the United States, a school for midwifery was started in 1762 by a physician from Philadelphia. Both nurse-midwives and physician-midwives practiced during the 18th and 19th centuries, though the nurse-midwives predominated (see Chap. 45).

Emergence of Professional Maternity Nursing

A variety of factors, cultural, social, and technological, have had important roles in shaping the growth and development of maternity nursing. One of the most important and most direct of these factors was the shift from home to hospital delivery. At the turn of the century, almost all women were delivered at home by a midwife or a physician. At the present time, more than 90% of mothers deliver in the hospital. Two other factors, in turn, brought about this change to hospital delivery and helped shape the kind of care received there. An increase in the understanding of asepsis made physicians much more attentive to this aspect of care, particularly for maternity patients. A growing conviction developed that delivery in a hospital was mandatory. As more women began delivering in hospitals, provision had to be made for quick, efficient, aseptic care. Certain time-saving devices and work-simplification procedures were borrowed from industry. "Assembly-line care" soon flourished. Compliance with time-saving techniques, performance of the somewhat ritualistic procedures called for to maintain asepsis, and the increasingly bureaucratic structure generated by the complex, modernizing hospital all went into defining and shaping the very essence of maternity care. Hence, there arose the ritualistic, rigid adherence to rules and procedures (with rather little thought to the patient) that characterizes so much of maternity care even today. It was during these early times that antepartal care was conceived and developed as an aspect of preventive medicine. Thus, women increasingly had longer contact with their physicians during the childbearing time and this, together with the still prevalent Victorian notion of dependency, served to cement the obstetrical relationship. In order to justify this relationship, physicians began to insist even more strongly on hospital deliveries.

Maternity nursing developed as obstetrics developed and, not surprisingly, was based on the medical model of obstetrics in which pathology was the main focus. Thus, the nursing student's experiences were oriented to the physical care of her patients, with emphasis on technical competence. Moreover, a good deal of the student's patient experiences was in reality service to the hospital. The early hospitals were, in fact, staffed largely by students. This type of service-to-the-institution, technical competence orientation produced a nurse who was efficient in organizing care for many patients. However, because of the great numbers of patients, no in-depth nursing therapy was either attempted or possible. Little or no public health experience was offered, and the nurse gradually became more institution (*i.e.,* hospital) oriented. The nurse became the physician's veritable right arm (Table 46-1).

Nursing Roles and Women's Status

Undoubtedly, part of the reason why nursing was so subjugated by medicine was the powerless status of women and the distaste with which working women were viewed. It is unfortunate that maternity nursing split so completely with nurse-midwifery that two different fields were eventually formed. Midwives were also suppressed by medicine. Their practice became illegal in some states, and was generally discredited and maligned. Maternity nurses have conducted, with more or less vigor, the long struggle toward more responsibility and autonomy that parallels the women's movement for full and equal status.

Compartmentalization and Routinization

In the third and fourth decades of this century, hospitals became larger and more complex and the nurse gradually had to assume more and more administrative and organizational duties. Similarly, medical science enlarged and with the new knowledge and progress, more functions, formerly in the province of the physician, were delegated to the nurse. These factors, together with the acute hospital personnel shortage precipitated by World War II, combined to develop and promote impersonal routinized care for the mother and her infant.

As more became known about the transmission and control of pathogenic organisms, various subunits were designated for the use of the mother, the well newborn, the sick newborn, and the premature infant. Thus, restrictions and compartmentalization of nursing function (nursery nurse, postpartum nurse, and so on) proliferated in the name of better technique but at the expense of unity in the mother–infant relationship. Perhaps even worse was the compartmentalization of thinking and communication that also evolved. The postpartum nurse knew and cared about the progress of the particular mothers in her charge while they were on the ward. She rarely knew how they responded to their pregnancy in general. She might know something about how they had withstood their labors, but only in the physical sense, and then only in relation to their immediate postpartum course. The nursery nurse knew about the babies in her nursery, but very little about the parents who would take them home or the environment into which they would go.

The experience of childbearing, once common to all members of the social group and centered in the home, with involvement of most family members, had now become a disjointed, technical, and alien process about which parents were generally ignorant. Complex and mystical, childbirth had become the province of physicians and specialized nurses, to be enacted in a strange, threatening institution in which the parents were the most powerless members. It is not hard to understand why there was widespread dissatisfaction with this state of affairs, leading to the many far-reaching and sometimes radical changes that have occurred over the last 20 years.

Table 46-1.
Characteristics of Maternity Care and Emergence of Maternity Nursing

Maternity Care	Maternity Nursing
Birth a family and community event, integrated into every day life	Midwives usual birth attendants, precursors to maternity nurse
↓	↓
Development of scientific medicine and physician participation in childbirth	Gradual replacement of midwives by physicians as birth attendants
↓	↓
Increasing understanding of asepsis and increased technology in obstetrics	Nursing emerged as women's occupation, paralleling growth of scientific medicine
↓	↓
Growing emphasis on hospital deliveries rather than home births	Nurses in obstetrics taught by medical (pathological) model
↓	↓
Increasing numbers of women delivering in the hospital	Nursing students focused upon technical competence and physical care of patients in hospitals
↓	↓
Necessity for efficient, organized aseptic care in hospitals, due to organizational structure	Nursing students provided service to hospitals where trained
↓	↓
Borrowing of time-saving approaches and work-efficient procedures from industry	Nursing orientation was toward efficient care of a number of patients, without in-depth nursing therapy (as there was no theoretical foundation)
↓	↓
"Assembly-line care" in hospitals	Institution-oriented nurses became the physician's "right arm"
↓	↓
Ritualistic practices, rigid adherence to rules and procedures	Development of the humanistic-supportive nursing model as distinct from the pathological–intervention medical model
↓	↓
Impersonal, routine care	Expansion of the maternity nurse's role to include personalized care, parent education, counseling and psychosocial support, advocacy, alternative care services to childbearing families
↓	↓
Resurgence of family and participant focus in childbearing, through natural childbirth and consumer movements	Emergence of new roles (nurse practitioner, clinical specialist) and resurgence of nurse-midwifery
↓	
Pressure for change in hospital routines and procedures, alternative birth approaches	
↓	
Development of family-centered maternity care, participant childbirth, rooming-in, alternate birth centers	

Recent Developments. Many factors, social, economic, political, and technical, have contributed to the significant changes in maternity care that have occurred since the midcentury. Such concepts as family-centered maternity care, participant childbirth, natural childbirth, rooming-in, birth without violence, alternate birthing, and a resurgence of home births have refocused attention on childbirth as a social and family process. Less technical interference, greater humanism, a wider range of choices and options, and reaffirmation of the natural birth process have become more typical of current maternity care. More sophisticated technology has led to the development of specialty centers for management of complicated pregnancy, neonatal intensive care units, and the new field of neonatology. However, recognition of the importance of maternal–infant bonding in the first hours and days of the newborn's life has led to practices encouraging maximal mother–child contact. Many of the newer alternative approaches to maternity care are covered in Chapter 45, Alternatives in Maternity Care.

Future Possibilities

In speculating about the future of maternity nursing, several significant recent developments in health care and social patterns must be taken into consideration.

Perhaps the most far-reaching is the declining birthrate in the United States, with its associated slowing of the rate of population increase.

The most overt manifestation of the decrease in birthrate was the closing of maternity units in many small to moderate-sized hospitals in this country. It became economically impossible to maintain these units because of a falling census, so consolidation of obstetrical services in a few designated hospitals became common. In some of the larger cities with higher concentrations of physicians, some obstetricians and pediatricians were hard-pressed to find enough business. However, the maldistribution of health-care services continued as before, with lower income and inner city or outlying rural populations still left with inadequate services.

Trends in population location show significant increases in nonmetropolitan counties, indicating the need for increased attention to health services in rural areas, and emphasis on the regional impact of health resources. Population profiles suggest that the mix of medical and health care will need to be modified during the 1980s to take into account the existence of fewer infants and more older people.[4]

Regionalized Perinatal Health Care

As a result of changing population profiles and the widespread concern over cost, quality, and availability of health-care services, and with the additional impetus of PL 93–641 (National Health Planning and Resources Act), there is a strong trend toward providing a regionalized system of perinatal care for mothers and infants. The goals of this system are to make complex care available to entire populations within the constraints of geography, costs, population distribution, and availability of specialists and subspecialists.

The regionalized structure consists basically of four types (or levels) of facilities: physicians' offices and clinics, local facilities for uncomplicated deliveries, larger urban facilities providing a fairly full range of obstetrical and neonatal services, and perinatal centers and specialized units offering the full range of services for maternal and neonatal complications. Primary care units for mothers during pregnancy, and mothers and infants following delivery, are generally physicians' offices and maternal–child health clinics. These provide primary perinatal care, including promotion and support for maintenance of health status, screening for complications of pregnancy, and treatment of intercurrent diseases and problems.

Level 1 facilities are generally community hospitals that are designed to provide care for mothers and neonates without major complications. These are local facilities that relate closely to the community. Because all complications cannot be identified in advance, level 1 units must be able to provide emergency services of a more complex nature until the mother or infant can be transferred to a facility with greater capacity. Level 2 facilities are hospitals in larger, usually urban, communities that offer a wider range of maternal and neonatal services. These serve as referral sources to local hospitals and physicians for high-risk pregnancies or neonatal care. They provide an intermediate level of complex services and can manage the more common complications of childbearing and the newborn.

Level 3 facilities are the regional perinatal centers that provide the full range of services for perinatal complications of both mother and infant. These units can generally meet most maternal or neonatal needs related to high-risk conditions and may contain specialized units such as children's cardiac centers, units for management of pregnant diabetics, or units for intrauterine exchange transfusions in the cases of severe Rh-sensitization. To make such a regionalized structure workable, it is necessary for health providers to develop and maintain a network through communication, consultation, transportation, and outreach education (Table 46-2).[5]

Directions for Maternity Nursing

To remain congruent with such changes in the health-care delivery system, maternity nursing must also adapt and grow in new and diverse directions. The desires of the consumers of maternity care also signify a growing need for changes. This is because the routinized and standardized care organized in settings more convenient for the providers than for the consumers of care are less and less acceptable. Parents are asking for full participation in all phases of childbearing, the right to be involved in decisions affecting their bodies and health, and the right to institute practices that they believe are important for the happiness and well-being of parents and baby. (See The Pregnant Patient's Bill of Rights.)

A growing body of literature and research is reaffirming the importance of early and continued close contact between mother and baby, a situation many of our modern hospital practices have made impossible to attain. The importance of natural practices, such as breast-feeding and avoidance of highly processed and chemically preserved foods, suggests that health professionals support rather than discourage parents who wish to follow these practices.

The appropriateness of routine delivery of normal,

Table 46-2.
Regionalized Perinatal Health Care

Primary Care	Level 1 Facilities	Level 2 Facilities	Level 3 Facilities
Physician's offices **Prenatal clinics** **Well-child clinics**	**Community hospitals (local facilities)**	**Larger, urban hospitals**	**Regional Perinatal centers**
Provide primary perinatal care, including health promotion, identification of complications, treatment of intercurrent diseases and problems	Provide maternal and neonatal care of uncomplicated patients, with emergency services of more complex nature until transfer to another facility with greater capacity can occur	Provide wider range of maternal and neonatal services, serve as referral source for local hospitals and physicians for high-risk pregnancies and neonatal care; intermediate level of complexity, manage the more common complications of childbearing and the newborn	Provide full range of services for perinatal complications of mother and infant, can care for most high-risk conditions, may contain specialized units for neonatal problems or pregnancy complications

Relate through a network involving communication, consultation, transportation, and outreach education

uncomplicated maternity patients in the hospital with its focus on disease and illness is being questioned. However, new data about the importance of immediate, active intervention in delivery of high-risk pregnancies and the postdelivery care of depressed, sick, or anoxic infants reinforce the need for highly trained personnel and well-equipped delivery rooms and intensive care nurseries. The situation appears paradoxical, and answers will not be easy. It is safe to say that what have come to be accepted as routine practices in the care of maternity and newborn patients are being seriously questioned by both the experts and the public.

Maternity nursing must enlarge its scope if it is to remain viable. Narrow concentration on the processes of childbearing and newborn care limit the services the maternity nurse can offer the patient and family. Because reproduction is basically a sexual event, both physiologically and in terms of role and identity, the most obvious areas for extension of maternity are into sexuality and contraception. To some extent, this is now occurring. Abortion care is another natural extension, as it is a variation within the process of reproduction.

Increasing expertise in early childhood development and familiarity with the normal growth and development of children equips the nurse to provide much-needed assistance to families beyond the immediate childbearing period. Skill in counseling families and knowledge of family dynamics permit the nurse to be of service when problems or needs arise not only in integrating the new baby, but also with relationships between parents and other children and relatives.

Another area with potential for involvement of maternity nurses is that of women's search for a satisfying identity and sense of productivity and self-realization, generally thought of as the "women's movement." With an inquisitive mind and open attitudes, and a willingness to question personal and social tenets, both nurse and patient could attain more satisfying levels of existence.

It is hard to predict what the role of the nurse-practitioner will be, but it will certainly entail an enlargement of the scope of maternity and other nursing practice. One possibility is an eventual merging of maternity nurse practitioner with the nurse-midwife, resulting in provision of the full range of childbearing services by such nurses to uncomplicated cases. Should this occur, relationships with the medical profession would have to be altered because physicians would primarily provide care to high-risk and complicated cases, perform gynecological surgery, and serve as consultants to the nurses providing care during normal childbearing.

Perhaps maternity nursing will split off into two separate specialties, one the nurse practitioner type involved in prenatal and postpartal follow-up, and the other the acute hospital nurse involved in intrapartal and immediate postdelivery care. Nurse-midwifery

The Pregnant Patient's Bill of Rights*

American parents are becoming increasingly aware that health professionals do not always have scientific data to support common American obstetrical practices and that many of these practices are carried out primarily because they are part of medical and hospital tradition. In the last forty years many artificial practices have been introduced which have changed childbirth from a physiological event to a very complicated medical procedure in which all kinds of drugs are used and procedures carried out, sometimes unnecessarily, and many of them potentially damaging for the baby and even for the mother. A growing body of research makes it alarmingly clear that every aspect of traditional American hospital care during labor and delivery must now be questioned as to its possible effect on the future well-being of both the obstetric patient and her unborn child.

One in every 35 children born in the United States today will eventually be diagnosed as retarded; one in every 10 to 17 children has been found to have some form of brain dysfunction or learning disability requiring special treatment. Such statistics are not confined to the lower socioeconomic group but cut across all segments of American society.

New concerns are being raised by childbearing women because no one knows what degree of oxygen depletion, head compression, or traction by forceps the unborn or newborn infant can tolerate before that child sustains permanent brain damage or dysfunction. The recent findings regarding the cancer-related drug diethylstilbestrol have alerted the public to the fact that neither the approval of a drug by the U.S. Food and Drug Administration nor the fact that a drug is prescribed by a physician serves as a guarantee that a drug or medication is safe for the mother or her unborn child. In fact, the American Academy of Pediatrics Committee on Drugs has recently stated that there is no drug, whether prescription or over-the-counter remedy, which has been proven safe for the unborn child.

The Pregnant Patient has the right to participate in decisions involving her well-being and that of her unborn child, unless there is a clear-cut medical emergency that prevents her participation. In addition to the rights set forth in the American Hospital Association's "Patient's Bill of Rights" (which has also been adopted by the New York City Department of Health) the Pregnant Patient, because she represents TWO patients rather than one, should be recognized as having the additional rights listed below.

1. *The Pregnant Patient has the right,* prior to the administration of any drug or procedure, to be informed by the health professional caring for her of any potential direct or indirect effects, risks or hazards to herself or her unborn or newborn infant which may result from the use of a drug or procedure prescribed for or administered to her during pregnancy, labor, birth, or lactation.
2. *The Pregnant Patient has the right,* prior to the proposed therapy, to be informed, not only of the benefits, risks, and hazards of the proposed therapy but also of known alternative therapy, such as available childbirth education classes which could help to prepare the Pregnant Patient physically and mentally to cope with the discomfort or stress of pregnancy and the experience of childbirth, thereby reducing or eliminating her need for drugs and obstetric intervention. She should be offered such information early in her pregnancy in order that she may make a reasoned decision.
3. *The Pregnant Patient has the right,* prior to the administration of any drug, to be informed by the health professional who is prescribing or administering the drug to her that any drug which she receives during pregnancy, labor and birth, no matter how or when the drug is taken or administered, may adversely affect her unborn baby, directly or indirectly, and that there is no drug or chemical which has been proven safe for the unborn child.
4. *The Pregnant Patient has the right,* if cesarean section is anticipated, to be informed prior to the administration of any drug, and preferably prior to the hospitalization, that minimizing her and, in turn, her baby's intake of nonessential preoperative medicine will benefit her baby.

undoubtedly will increase as restrictive laws change and programs develop to more equitably distribute care to all the American population.

Whatever the future portends, its hallmark will be change. Health care, medical care, and nursing care are all undergoing major upheavals. The issues of national health insurance, the role of third-party payers, problems with malpractice insurance, federal controls, and peer review organizations, changing practice laws of nursing and medicine, the exorbitant costs of health care and the increasingly vociferous consumer advocacy movement, and the development of health maintenance organizations and community health networks, all signify that health care in this country is experiencing radical changes. Maternity nursing must ride the winds of change, and nursing leaders must take the initiative in shaping the new form this specialty will take in the years to come to serve the best interests and needs of families during all phases of childbearing.

5. *The Pregnant Patient has the right,* prior to the administration of a drug or procedure, to be informed if there is NO properly controlled follow-up research which has established the safety of the drug or procedure with regard to its direct and/or indirect effects on the physiological, mental and neurological development of the child exposed, via the mother, to the drug or procedure during pregnancy, labor, birth, or lactation (this would apply to virtually all drugs and the vast majority of obstetric procedures).
6. *The Pregnant Patient has the right,* prior to the administration of any drug, to be informed of the brand name and generic name of the drug in order that she may advise the health professional of any past adverse reaction to the drug.
7. *The Pregnant Patient has the right* to determine for herself, without pressure from her attendant, whether she will accept the risks inherent in the proposed therapy or refuse a drug or procedure.
8. *The Pregnant Patient has the right* to know the name and qualifications of the individual administering a medication or procedure to her during labor or birth.
9. *The Pregnant Patient has the right* to be informed, prior to the administration of any procedure, whether that procedure is being administered to her for her or her baby's benefit (medically indicated) or as an elective procedure (for convenience or teaching purposes).
10. *The Pregnant Patient has the right* to be accompanied during the stress of labor and birth by someone she cares for, and to whom she looks for emotional comfort and encouragement.
11. *The Pregnant Patient has the right* after appropriate medical consultation to choose a position for labor and for birth which is least stressful to her baby and to herself.
12. *The Obstetric Patient has the right* to have her baby cared for at her bedside if her baby is normal, and to feed her baby according to her baby's needs rather than according to the hospital regimen.
13. *The Obstetric Patient has the right* to be informed in writing of the name of the person who actually delivered her baby and the professional qualifications of that person. This information should also be on the birth certificate.
14. *The Obstetric Patient has the right* to be informed if there is any known or indicated aspect of her or her baby's care or condition which may cause her or her baby later difficulty or problems.
15. *The Obstetric Patient has the right* to have her and her baby's hospital medical records complete, accurate, and legible and to have their records, including Nurses' Notes, retained by the hospital until the child reaches at least the age of majority, or, alternatively, to have the records offered to her before they are destroyed.
16. *The Obstetric Patient,* both during and after her hospital stay, *has the right* to have access to her complete hospital medical records, including Nurses' Notes, and to receive a copy upon payment of a reasonable fee and without incurring the expense of retaining an attorney.

It is the obstetric patient and her baby, not the health professional, who must sustain any trauma or injury resulting from the use of a drug or obstetric procedure. The observation of the rights listed above will not only permit the obstetric patient to participate in the decisions involving her and her baby's health care, but will help to protect the health professional and the hospital against litigation arising from resentment or misunderstanding on the part of the mother.

*Reprinted by permission of the Committee on Patient's Rights, Box 1900, New York, N.Y. 10001.

References

1. Barnes FEF (ed): Ambulatory Maternal Health Care and Family Planning Services: Policies, Principles, Practices. Committee on Maternal Health Care and Family Planning, Maternal and Child Health Section, American Public Health Association, New York 1978

2. Bishop B: Editorial. "International Year of the Child" MCN—Am J Maternal Child Nurs 9, 4, January/February 1979

3. Bullough VL, Bullough B: The Emergence of Modern Nursing, pp 4, 17, 28–29, 76–78. Toronto, Macmillan, 1969

4. Green BL: Rural health delivery systems of the 1980s. Fam Community Health 1, 2:95–108, July 1978

5. Graven SN: Perinatal health promotion: An overview. Fam Community Health 1, 3:1–11, November 1978

Suggested Reading

American College of Obstetrics and Gynecologists: Proceedings: Health Care for Mothers and Infants in Rural and Isolated Areas. Chicago, 1978

Anderson EM, Leonard BJ, Yates JA: Epigenesis of the nurse practitioner role. Am J Nurs 74:1812–1816, October 1974

Barrett J: The nurse specialist practitioner: A study. Nurs Outlook 20:524–527, August 1972

Changing patterns of obstetric care. Am J Nurs 73:1723–1727, October 1973

Committee on Fetus and Newborn: Standards and Recommendations for Hospital Care of Newborn Infants, 6th ed. Evanston, IL, American Academy of Pediatrics, 1977

Committee on Perinatal Health: Toward Improving the Outcome of Pregnancy: Recommendations for the Regional Development of Maternal and Perinatal Health Services. New York, The National Foundation/March of Dimes, 1975

Contemporary Nursing Series: Maternal and newborn care: Nursing interventions. Compiled by Browning MH, Lewis EP. Am J Nurs New York, 1973

Fowler MM: The maternity nurse clinician in practice. In Anderson EH (ed): Current Concepts in Clinical Nursing, pp 210–215. St Louis, CV Mosby, 1973

Lubic RW: Myths about nurse-midwifery. Am J Nurs 74:268–269, February 1974

Lynaugh JE, Bates B: Physical diagnosis: A skill for all nurses? Am J Nurs 74:58–59, January 1974

Martin LM: I like being an FNP. Am J Nurs 75:826–828, May 1975

McCormack GB: The visiting nurse becomes a nurse practitioner. Nurs Outlook 22:119–123, February 1974

National Health Planning and Resources Development Act of 1974, PL 93–641, 88 Stat. 2225, 1975

Study Aids for Unit IX: Special Considerations in Maternity Nursing

Conference Material

1. One of the responsibilities of the nurse in an antepartal clinic is to provide childbirth education classes to parents. In preparing material for these classes, you have decided to include a class on cesarean birth, even though the women are having normal pregnancies and are generally low-risk patients. Part of your reason for doing this is the knowledge of the rising cesarean rate, which in some medical centers is one of every four deliveries. Discuss in detail (a) how you decide which areas of content related to cesarean births you include in this 1-hour class, and (b) write a brief content outline of these topics and the specific points you plan to make in each area.

2. Alisa K. is a 22-year-old primigravida in the first trimester, who is in excellent health with no apparent risk factors. She and her husband Ron have sought your advice as a community health nurse regarding childbirth options. They believe strongly in natural birth with full family participation in a supportive and comfortable setting. The couple has been considering a home birth and is seeking information about this as well as other options and about having a nurse-midwife as a birth attendant. How do you counsel Alisa and Ron about (a) advantages and risks of various childbirth options, and (b) advantages and disadvantages of various childbirth attendants?

3. Discuss the changing emphasis of practice that occurred in nursing from the late 1800s to the present, taking into consideration social and cultural conditions, the status of women, the growth of scientific medicine, the development of the hospital as an institution, and the evolution of nursing as a profession. Give specific examples relevant to maternity nursing and the care of childbearing families.

4. Discuss future directions for maternity nursing practice based upon recent developments in the maternal–infant care field and the nursing profession. Take into consideration population and demographic changes, consumer preferences, economic considerations, trends in health-care system organization, and other relevant factors you may identify. Create a scenario of what the nurse's practice might be like (*e.g.,* setting, types of clients, services provided, compensation, interprofessional relaions, etc.) if a particular future direction is realized.

5. What do you see as the coming trends in maternity nursing in the next 10 years? What past social trends and technologies are shaping the evolution of maternity nursing?

Discussion

1. What are the main concepts in family-centered maternity care?

2. Name four reasons why a woman might choose to have a home birth.

Discussion
(continued)

3. What is an alternative birth center (ABC)?

4. Name four factors that would exclude a woman from labor and delivery in an ABC.

5. Name four criteria requiring transfer out of an ABC after labor admission.

6. What does the scope of practice of the nurse-midwife include?

7. Describe three advantages to the patient in having a nurse-midwife attend at labor and delivery.

8. What four diagnostic categories account for the vast majority of cesarean births?

9. Discuss three factors contributing to the marked increase in cesarean births that have occurred over the past 15 years.

10. Discuss three recommendations of the NIH Consensus Task Force on Cesarean Birth to reduce the cesarean birth rate.

11. Name three physical and three psychological risks to the mother who has a cesarean birth.

12. Compare the role of the maternity clinical specialist with that of the maternity nurse practitioner.

13. Name two ancient cultures that appeared to have some knowledge of forceps and cesarean sections.

14. How did Semmelweiss deduce the causality of puerperal fever?

15. Briefly describe the work of two organizations that were formed to promote maternal or infant health in the early 20th century in America.

16. Briefly describe three organizations, laws, or programs that promoted maternal or infant health initiated within the last 30 years.

17. What were some factors leading to the transition from primarily home to primarily hospital deliveries?

18. How did the structure of the hospital affect the type of care provided to patients by nurses?

19. What are some factors that have occurred in recent years leading to relaxation of many hospital policies and routines related to maternity care?

20. Briefly explain the concept of regionalized perinatal health care.

21. List four rights that are included in the Pregnant Patient's Bill of Rights.

22. What are two new roles that have emerged for maternity nurses?

Appendix

Glossary

Note: The pronunciations indicated follow Webster's Second International Dictionary.

āle, cha᷵otic, câre, ădd, *ă*ccount, ärm, ȧsk, sof*ȧ*; ēve, hẹre, e᷵vent, ĕnd, sil*ĕ*nt, makẽr; īce, ĭll, char*ĭ*ty; ōld, o᷵bey, ôrb, ŏdd, soft, c*ŏ*nnect; food, foot; out; oil, cūbe, u᷵nite, ûrn, ŭp, circ*ŭ*s, menü; chair; go; sing; then, thin; natu᷵re; verdu᷵re; k = ch in German ich or ach; bon; yet zh = z in azure

ABC. Abbreviation for *alternate birth center.*

abdominal (ăb-dŏm'ĭn*ă*l). Belonging to or relating to the abdomen.

- **a. delivery.** Delivery of the child by abdominal section. See *cesarean section.*
- **a. gestation.** Ectopic pregnancy occurring in the cavity of the abdomen.
- **a. lifting.** The lifting of the abdominal wall with the hands to reduce abdominal pressure on the uterus during a contraction in labor.
- **a. pregnancy.** See *a. gestation.*

abduction (ăb-dŭk'sh*ŭ*n). The drawing or pulling away (of a part of the body) from the median axis.

ablatio placentae. See *abruptio placentae.*

abortion. The termination of pregnancy at any time before the fetus has attained a stage of viability (*i.e.,* before it is capable of extrauterine existence).

- **a. rate.** The number of abortions per 1000 women between the ages of 15 and 44.
- **a. ratio.** 1. The number of abortions per 1000 live births during a given period. 2. The number of abortions during a given period per 1000 live births 6 months later.
- **complete a.** An abortion in which all the products of conception are passed and identified.
- **criminal a.** An abortion performed illegally, often under less than desirable aseptic conditions by an unskilled person.
- **incomplete a.** An abortion in which some but not all the products of conception are passed.
- **induced a.** An abortion that is produced deliberately and intentionally.
- **inevitable a.** The condition that precedes an abortion that will proceed naturally. Vaginal bleeding is profuse, the membranes may have ruptured, and the cervix may have become dilated.
- **missed a.** The condition in which the embryo has died and subsequently the products of conception are retained in the uterus.
- **spontaneous a.** An abortion that starts of its own accord; commonly called a miscarriage.
- **threatened a.** The condition in which vaginal bleeding or spotting occurs in early pregnancy and the cervix is not dilated. The symptoms may subside and the pregnancy may proceed to full term.

abruptio placentae (ăb-rŭp'shĭ-ŏ pl*ȧ*-sen'tē). Premature separation of normally implanted placenta.

acetonuria (ăs"*ĕ*-to᷵-nū'rĭ-*ȧ*). The presence of excessive acetone bodies in the urine.

acidosis (ăs″ĭ-dō′sĭs). A condition resulting in the accumulation of acids or depletion of alkaline reserve in the blood and body tissues. This condition may be exhibited by a newborn infant who is cold stressed.

acinus cell (ăs′ĭ-nŭs). Pl. *acini cells* (ăs′ĭ-nī). Milk-secreting cell contained in a lobule of the breast.

acromion (ȧ-krō′mĭ-ŏn). An outward extension of the spine of the scapula, used to explain presentation of the fetus.

acrosome (ăk′rō-sōm). The caplike structure at the head of a sperm cell that contains enzymes which are believed to play an important role in the entrance of the sperm cell into the ovum.

adduction (ă-dŭk′shŭn). The drawing or pulling (of a part of the body) toward the median axis.

adenoma (ăd″ĕ-nō′mȧ). An epithelial tumor, usually benign, with a glandlike structure.

adhesion (ăd-hē′zhŭn). 1. The property of remaining in close proximity. 2. The joining of normally separate tissues.

adnexa (ăd-nĕk′sȧ). Appendages.

a., uterine (ū′tĕr-ĭn). The fallopian tubes and ovaries.

adolescence (ăd″ō-lĕs′ĕns). The period of life beginning at puberty, when the secondary sex characteristics begin to develop and the capacity for reproduction is reached, and ending with adulthood.

adrenogenital syndrome (ăd-rĕn″ō-jĕn′ĭ-tăl sĭn′drōm). See *syndrome, adrenogenital.*

aerobic exercise (ā″ĕr-ō′bĭk). A physical activity that increases oxygen consumption and action of the cardiovascular system.

afferent (ăf′ĕr-ĕnt). Centripetal; bringing toward a central part, as afferent nerves convey stimuli to the central nervous system.

afibrinogenemia (ă-fī″brĭn-ō-jĕn-ē′mē-ă). Lack of fibrinogen in the blood.

afterbirth (ăf′tĕr-bûrth″). The structures cast off after the expulsion of the fetus, including the membranes and the placenta with the attached umbilical cord; the secundines.

afterpains (ăf′tĕr-pāns″). Those pains, more or less severe, after expulsion of the afterbirth, which result from the contractile efforts of the uterus to return to its normal condition.

agalactia (ăg′ȧ-lăk′shĭ-ȧ). Absence or failure of the secretion of milk.

albuminuria (ăl-bū″mĭ-nū′rĭ-ȧ). The presence of albumin in the urine.

alkalosis (ăl″kȧ-lō′sĭs). A condition resulting from the loss of base, or depletion of acid without comparable loss of base, from body fluids.

allantois (ă-lăn′tō-ĭs). A tubular diverticulum of the posterior part of the yolk sac of the embryo; it passes into the body stalk through which it is accompanied by the allantoic (umbilical) blood vessel, thus taking part in the formation of the umbilical cord; and later, fusing with the chorion, it helps to form the placenta.

allele (ă-lēl′). One of two or more alternate genes that occur at a particular locus of a chromosome which decide alternate inherited characteristics.

alternate birth center (ABC). An organization of a hospital or a free-standing labor and delivery area that provides a homelike atmosphere. It has liberal policies regarding the presence of family and friends, labor practices, no separation of parents and infant, and early discharge.

amenorrhea (ā-mĕn″ŏ-rē′ȧ). Absence or suppression of the menstrual discharge.

amnesia (ăm-nē′zhĭ-ȧ). Loss of memory.

amniocentesis (ăm″nĭ-ō-sĕn-tē′sĭs). The perforation by surgery of the amniotic sac to obtain amniotic fluid for purposes of fetal genetic diagnosis.

amnion (ăm′nĭ-ŏn). The most internal of the fetal membranes, containing the waters that surround the fetus in utero.

amnioscope (ăm′nĭ-ō-skōp). An instrument for examination of the fetus and amniotic fluid by passage through the maternal abdominal wall into the amniotic cavity, thus permitting direct visualization.

amniotic (ăm″nĭ-ŏt′ĭk). Pertaining to the amnion.

a. cavity. The area between the amnion and the fetus containing the amniotic fluid.

a. fluid. The clear fluid that is 98% water contained in the amnion. This fluid provides protection to the fetus, keeps the temperature constant, and provides some nourishment to the fetus. Also called *liquor amnii.*

a.f. embolism (ĕm′bō-lĭzm). The blocking of a maternal artery with amniotic fluid forced into it by strong uterine contractions.

a. sac. The "bag of membrane" containing the fetus before delivery.

amniotomy (ăm″nĭ-ŏt′ō-mĭ). The artificial rupture of the amniotic sac to induce labor.

analgesic (ăn″-ăl-jē′zĭ-ĭk). Drug that relieves pain, used during labor.

analog (ăn′ȧ-lŏg). A chemical compound with a structure similar to that of another but differing from it with respect to a certain component. It may have similar or opposite action metabolically.

androgen (ăn′drō-jĕn). Any hormonal substance that possesses masculinizing activities, such as the testis hormone.

android (ăn′droid). The term adopted for the male type of pelvis.

andrology (ăn-drŏl′ō-jĭ). The scientific study of the male constitution and diseases, especially male reproductive problems.

anemia (ă-nē′mĭ-ȧ). A condition of the blood in which there is a deficiency in the red blood cells per unit volume, in the quantity of hemoglobin, or in the total volume.

anencephalia (ăn-ĕn″sē-fā′lĭ-ȧ). Form of monstrosity with absence of a brain.

anesthesia (ăn″ĕs-thē′zĭ-ȧ). The loss of sensation or feeling, especially the feeling of pain.

anomaly (ă-nŏm′ȧ-lĭ). A deviation from the expected standard, especially as a result of a congenital defect.

anorexia (ăn″ō-rĕk′sĭ-ȧ). The loss of appetite.

anovular (ăn-ŏv′ū-lĕr). Not accompanied with the discharge of an ovum; said of cyclic uterine bleeding.

anoxia (ăn-ŏks'ĭ-*ȧ*). Oxygen deficiency; any condition of absence of tissue oxidation.

anteflexion (ăn"tē-flĕk'sh*ŭ*n). The tipping or bending forward of the uterus on its axis.

antenatal (ăn"tē-nā'*tă*l). Occurring or formed before birth.

antepartal (ăn"tē-pär'*tă*l). Before labor and delivery or childbirth; prenatal.

anterior (ăn-tẹr'ĭ-ŏr). Situated in the front or forward part of a body or organ.

anthropoid pelvis (ăn'thrō-poid pĕl'vĭs). See *pelvis, anthropoid.*

antibody (ăn"tĭ-bŏd"ĭ). Any of the body immunoglobulins that interact with antigens, neutralize toxins, and agglutinate bacteria or cells.

Apgar scoring system (ăp'gär). A system for appraising the condition of a newborn infant on the basis of heart rate, respiratory effort, muscle tone, reflex irritability, and color. The maximum score is 10. The evaluation may be made at 60 seconds after birth, then again at 3, 5, and 10 minutes.

apnea (ăp-nē'*ȧ*). The cessation of breathing.

arachnodactyly (ă-răk"nō-dăk'tĭ-lĭ). A hereditary metabolic disorder characterized by abnormally long and slender fingers and toes. Also called Marfan's syndrome.

areola (*ȧ*-rē'ō-l*ȧ*). The ring of pigment surrounding the nipple.

  secondary a. A circle of faint color sometimes seen just outside the original areola about the fifth month of pregnancy.

articulation (är-tĭk"ū-lā'sh*ŭ*n). The fastening together of the various bones of the skeleton in their natural situation; a joint. The articulations of the bones of the body are divided into two principal groups—*synarthroses,* immovable articulations, and *diarthroses,* movable articulations.

artificial feeding (är"tĭ-fĭsh'*ă*l). Feeding an infant by bottle rather than at the mother's breast.

artificial insemination (ĭn-sĕm"ĭ-nā'sh*ŭ*n). The introduction of semen into the cervix or vagina by artificial means.

artificial menopause (mĕn'ō-päs). The cessation of menstruation by artificial means such as surgery or irradiation.

Aschheim–Zondek test (ăsh"hīm–tsŏn'dek). See *test, Aschheim–Zondek.*

Asclepiad (ăs-klē'pĭ-ăd). A member of a guild of physicians in ancient Greece who were followers of Aesculapius, the mythical god of healing and father of medicine. These physician–priests had a slight and largely supervisory interest in obstetrics.

asexual (ā-sĕk'shoo-*ă*l). Having no sex or functional sexual organs.

Asherman's syndrome (ă'shēr-mănz sĭn'drōm). See *syndrome, Asherman's.*

asphyxia (ăs-fĭk'sĭ-*ȧ*). Suspended animation; anoxia and carbon dioxide retention resulting from failure of respiration.

  a. neonatorum (nē"ō-n*ȧ*-tō'r*ŭ*m). "Asphyxia of the newborn," deficient respiration in newborn babies. Also called *neonatal asphyxia.*

asthma (ăz'm*ȧ*). A condition marked by recurring attacks of spasmodic dyspnea with wheezing. May be caused by allergies, vigorous exercise, psychological stress, and so on.

atelectasis (ăt"ĕ-lĕk't*ȧ*-sĭs). The incomplete expansion of a lung or the collapse of a lung.

atonic (ă-tŏn'ĭk). Lacking the tone or strength that is normally present.

atrial septal defect (ā'trĭ-*ă*l sĕp'*tă*l dē'fĕkt). A congenital cardiac anomaly in which there is an abnormal opening between the right and left atria of the heart.

attitude (ăt'ĭ-tūd). A posture or position of the body. In obstetrics, the relation of the fetus members to each other in the uterus; the position of the fetus in the uterus.

auscultation (äs"kŭl-tā'sh*ŭ*n). The act of listening for sounds within the body. Used to ascertain the fetal position and condition of the fetal heart.

autosome (ä'tō-sōm). Any of the 22 ordinary paired chromosomes as distinguished from the 2 sex chromosomes.

axis (ăk'sĭs). A line about which any revolving body turns.

  pelvic a. The curved line that passes through the centers of all the anteroposterior diameters of the pelvis.

azoospermia (ă-zō"ō-spûr'mĭ-*ȧ*). The absence of spermatozoa in the semen.

back labor. A condition that occurs in one fourth of all labors when the position of the fetus is such that the back of the head is directed to the mother's back or turned toward her sacrum. Extreme discomfort is felt by the mother as labor progresses.

bag of waters. The membranes that enclose the liquor amnii of the fetus. See *amniotic sac.*

ballottement (b*ă*-lŏt'm*ĕ*nt). Literally means tossing. A term used in examination when the fetus can be pushed about in the pregnant uterus.

Bandl's ring (Băn'dls). A groove on the uterus at the upper level of the fully developed lower uterine segment; visible on the abdomen after hard labor as a transverse or slightly slanting depression between the umbilicus and the pubis. Shows overstretching of lower uterine segment. Resembles a full bladder.

Barr body (bär). The persistent mass of the material of the inactivated X chromosome in cells of normal females. Also called *sex chromatin.*

Bartholin's glands (Bär'tō-lĭn). Glands situated one on each side of the vaginal canal opening into the groove between the hymen and the labia minora.

basal body tempeature (BBT) (bā's*ă*l). The resting temperature taken in the morning before arising or performing any activity. Characteristic changes in BBT that usually occur in fertile women are used to identify the time ovulation has occurred.

BBT. Abbreviation for *basal body temperature.*

bicornate uterus (bī-kôr'nāt). Having two horns that, in the embryo, failed to attain complete fusion.

bilirubin (bĭl"ĭ-roo'bĭn). The principal pigment of the bile, reddish yellow in color.

bilirubinemia (bĭl″ĭ-roo-bĭ-nē′mĭ-*ȧ*). The presence of bilirubin in the blood.

bimanual (bī-măn′ū-*ă*l). Performed with or relating to both hands.

b. palpation. Examination of the pelvic organs of a woman by placing one hand on the abdomen and the fingers of the other in the vagina.

birth rate. The number of births per 1000 population.

bisexuality (bī-sĕk′shoo-ăl′ĭ-tĭ). The experiencing of sexual eroticism and genital intimacy with partners of both sexes.

blastocyst (blăs′tō-sĭst). The product of conception after the morula stage and before the embryonic stage.

blastoderm (blăs′tō-dûrm). The outer layer of cells of a fertilized ovum in the blastula stage.

b. vesicle. Hollow space within the morula formed by the rearrangement of cells, and by proliferation.

blastula (blăs′tū-l*ȧ*). The fertilized ovum in the stage in which the cells are arranged in a hollow ball.

body image (bŏd′ĭ ĭm′ĭj). The way one pictures one's body.

boggy (bŏg′ĭ). Inadequately contracted and having a spongy rather than firm feeling, descriptive of the postdelivery uterus.

bonding. The process by which the human infant becomes attached to his parents.

brachial palsy (brā′kĭ-*ă*l). See *palsy, brachial.*

Bracht maneuver (bräkt m*ȧ*-noo′vēr). See *maneuver, Bracht.*

bradycardia (brăd″ĭ-kär′dĭ-*ȧ*). Slowness of the heartbeat below normal.

Braxton–Hicks contractions. Uterine contractions occurring periodically during pregnancy, thereby enlarging the uterus to accommodate the growing fetus. During the third trimester, they are felt as a painless hardening or tightening of the uterus. They can become painful and are often difficult to differentiate from labor. Also called *B.–H. sign.*

B.H. version. One of the types of operation designed to turn the baby from an undesirable position to a desired one.

breakthrough bleeding. Vaginal spotting or bleeding that occurs between menstrual periods, due to failure of oral contraceptive to support the endometrium adequately.

breast milk jaundice (jän′dĭs). A condition that occasionally occurs due to a substance in breast milk that inhibits the conjugation of bilirubin. May be treated by temporary or permanent cessation of breast feeding.

breech (brēch). Nates or buttocks.

b. delivery. Labor and delivery marked by breech presentations.

bregma (brĕg′m*ȧ*). The point on the surface of the skull at the junction of the coronal and sagittal sutures.

brim (brĭm). The edge of the superior straight or inlet of the pelvis.

bronchopulmonary dysplasia (brŏng″kō-pûl′mō-nĕr-ĭ dĭs-plā′sĭ-*ȧ*). A chronic lung disease in infants believed to be associated with oxygen toxicity. It is often preceded by severe RDS and treatment in a high-oxygen environment.

cachexia (k*ȧ*-kĕk′sĭ-*ȧ*). Weight loss and wasting associated with systemic illness.

caked breast. See *engorgement.*

Candida albicans (kăn′dĭ-d*ȧ* ăl′bĭ-kăns). A yeastlike fungus that causes infections in the human being, commonly involving the mucous membranes of the mouth and vagina. During pregnancy, women are more susceptible to candidal infections due to the changed *p*H of the vagina and increased glycogen in vaginal cells.

candidiasis (kăn″dĭ-dī′*ȧ*-sĭs). A vaginal infection caused by *Candida albicans* with characteristic increased discharge and pruritus.

capacitation (k*ȧ*-păs″ĭ-tā′sh*ŭ*n). The process by which a spermatozoon is conditioned to fertilize an ovum after it is exposed to the female reproductive tract.

caput (kā′p*ŭ*t). 1. The head, consisting of the cranium, or skull, and the face. 2. Any prominent object, such as the head.

c. succedaneum (sŭk″sē-dā′nē-ŭm). An edematous swelling that sometimes appears on the presenting head of the fetus during labor.

carcinogen (kär-sĭn′ō-jĕn). A chemical or other substance that can induce or promote cancer.

cardiac anomalies (kär′dĭ-ăk *ă*-nŏm′*ă*-lĭs). Anomalies that result from congenital heart defects. These include transposition of the great vessels, atrial septal defect, patent ductus arteriosus, ventrical septal defect, coarctation of the aorta, the tetralogy of Fallot, and others.

catamenia (kăt-*ȧ*-mē′nĭ-*ȧ*). See *menses.*

catheterization (kăth″ĕ-tĕr-*ĭ*-zā′shŭn). The use of a tubular instrument for withdrawing fluids from (or introducing into) a body cavity, especially the bladder through the urethra for the withdrawal of urine.

caudal (kô′d*ă*l). The term applied to analgesia or anesthesia resulting from the introduction of the suitable analgesic or anesthetic solution into the caudal canal (nonclosure of the laminae of the last sacral vertebra).

caul (kôl). A portion of the amniotic sac that occasionally envelops the child's head at birth.

cellulitis (sĕl″ū-lī′tĭs). Inflammation of cellular tissue.

cephalhematoma (sĕf″*ȧ*l-hē″m*ȧ*-tō′m*ȧ*). A tumor or swelling between the cranium and the periosteum caused by an effusion of blood.

cephalic (sē-făl′ĭk). Belonging to the head.

c. presentation. Presentation of any part of the fetal head in labor.

cephalopelvic disproportion (CPD) (sĕf″*ȧ*-lō-pĕl′vĭc). A condition in which the fetal head is disproportionately large for passage through the maternal pelvis.

cerebral palsy (sĕr′*ĕ*-br*ă*l, sĕ-rē′br*ă*l). See *palsy, cerebral.*

cerebroside lipidosis (sĕr′ĕ-brō-sīd″ lĭp″ĭ-dō′sĭs). See *disease, Gaucher's.*

cervical mucus (sûr′vĭ-k*ă*l mū′kŭs). The secretion of the mucous membrane of the cervix.

cervical dilation. See *dilation, cervical.*

cervix (sûr′viks). Neckline part; the lower and narrow end of the uterus, between the os and the body of the organ.

cesarean delivery (sē-zâ′rē-*ă*n). Delivery of the fetus by an incision through the abdominal wall and the wall of the uterus.

classical c.d. A cesarean delivery that involves a vertical incision in the abdomen over the fundus and baby and then a vertical incision into the upper uterine segment.

extraperitoneal c.d. (ĕks″trȧ-pĕr″ĭ-tō-nē′ăl). A cesarean section performed when intrauterine infection is present. The incision is low, and the bladder must be dissected off the uterus.

low-segment c.d. A cesarean delivery in which the incision is made into the lower uterine segment, either transversely or vertically.

Chadwick's sign (tshăd′wĭks). The violet color on the mucous membrane of the vagina just below the urethral orifice, seen after the fourth week of pregnancy.

change of life. See *climacteric.*

chloasma (klō-ăz′mȧ). Pl. *chloasmata* (klō-ăz-ma′tȧ). A cutaneous affection exhibiting spots and patches of a yellowish brown color. The term chloasma is a vague one and is applied to various kinds of pigmentary discoloration of the skin.

c. gravidarum, c. uterinum. Chloasma occurring during pregnancy.

cholelithiasis (kō″lē-lĭ-thī′ȧ-sĭs). The formation of gallstones.

choriocarcinoma (kō″rĭ-ō-kăr″sĭ-nō′mȧ). See *chorioepithelioma.*

chorioepithelioma (kō′rĭ-ō-ĕp-ĭ-thē-lĭ-ō′mȧ). Chorionic carcinoma; a tumor formed by malignant proliferation of the epithelium of the chorionic villi.

chorion (kō-rĭ-ŏn). The outermost membrane of the growing zygote, or fertilized ovum, which serves as a protective and nutritive covering.

chorionic villus (kō″rĭ-ŏn′ĭk vĭl′ŭs). Pl. *villi* (vĭl′ī) One of the villi growing in tufts on the external surface of the chorion.

chromosomal sex (kro″mō-sō′măl sĕks). The determination of the sex of an individual by the configuration of chromosomes in his cells (*i.e.,* XY is the male configuration, and XX is the female configuration).

chromosome (kro′mo-sōm). One of several small, dark-staining and more or less rod-shaped bodies that appear in the nucleus of the cell at the time of cell divisions and particularly in mitosis.

cilium (sĭl′ē-ŭm). Pl. *cilia* (sĭl′ē-ȧ). One of the hairlike projections of a structure such as the fallopian tube. The cilia of the fallopian tube beat in such a manner as to direct any overlying fluid in the direction of the uterine cavity. Thus, the cilia are partially responsible for the transportation of an ovum along the tube.

circumcision (sûr″kŭm-sĭzh′ŏn). The removal of all or part of the prepuce, or foreskin, of the penis.

claiming behavior. The conduct of a new mother in developing by early contact the feeling that her infant is emotionally hers.

cleavage (klēv′ĭj). The series of cell divisions that occur during the development of a fertilized ovum into an embryo when the structure remains the same size while the cleavage cells become smaller and smaller.

cleft palate (klĕft păl′ĭt). Congenital fissure of the palate and the roof of the mouth.

climacteric (klī″măk-tĕr′ĭk). A particular epoch of the ordinary term of life at which the body undergoes a considerable change, especially the menopause or "change of life."

climax (klī′măks). See *orgasm.*

clitoris (klī′tō-rĭs). A small, elongated, erectile body situated at the anterior part of the vulva. An organ of the female homologous with the penis of the male.

clubfoot (klŭb′foot). A congenitally deformed foot. See *talipes equinovarus.*

coarctation of the aorta (kō″ărk-tā′shŭn) (ā-ôr′tȧ). A congenital cardiac anomaly in which there is a constriction of the aorta, causing narrowing of the lumen. This partially obstructs blood flow, creating increased left ventrical pressure and work load.

coccyx (cŏk′sĭks). The bone at the caudal end of the spine. In a child the coccyx consists of four or five separate vertebrae; in an adult these bones are fused into one.

coitus (kō′ĭt-ŭs). Sexual intercourse; copulation.

c. interruptus (ĭn″tĕr-rŭp′tŭs). The practice of withdrawal as a means of contraception. The penis is withdrawn from the vagina before ejaculation.

colostrum (kō-lŏs′trŭm). The thin, yellow fluid, high in protein and inorganic salts, which is secreted from the breasts during the last weeks of pregnancy and the 3 days after delivery before milk is produced.

c. corpuscles. Large granular cells found in colostrum.

colporrhaphy (kŏl-pōr′ȧ-fī). 1. The operation of suturing the vagina. 2. The operation of denuding and suturing the vaginal wall for the purpose of narrowing the vagina.

colposcope (kŏl′pō-skōp). A viewing instrument designed for close examination of the tissues of the cervix, similar to a low-magnification microscope with binocular vision.

colpotomy (kŏl-pŏt′o-mĭ). Any surgical cutting operation upon the vagina.

commissure (kŏm′ĭ-shūr). A site of union of corresponding parts.

complete abortion. See *abortion, complete.*

conception (kŏn-sĕp′shŭn). The impregnation of the female ovum by the spermatozoon of the male, whence results a new being.

condyloma (kŏn″dĭ-lō′mȧ). Pl. *condylomata* (kŏn″dĭ-lō-ma′tȧ). A wartlike excrescence near the anus or the vulva; the flat, moist papule of secondary syphilis.

confinement (kŏn-fīn′mĕnt). Term applied to childbirth and the lying-in period.

congenital (kŏn-jĕn′ĭ-tăl). Born with a person; existing from or from before birth, as, for example, congenital disease, a disease originating in the fetus before birth.

conjugate (kŏn′joo-gāt). The anteroposterior diameter of the pelvic inlet.

conjunctivitis (kŏn-jŭngk″tĭ-vī′tĭs). Inflammation of the conjunctiva, the membrane lining the eyelids, generally associated with a discharge.

constipation (kŏn″stĭ-pā′shŭn). The infrequent or difficult passage of feces.

contraception (kŏn″trȧ-sĕp′shŭn). The prevention of conception or impregnation.

contracted pelvis (kŏn-trăk′tĕd). See *pelvis, contracted.*

contraction (kŏn-trăk′shŭn). The intermittent shortening of a muscle, especially the uterus during labor in order to expel the contents.

convulsion (kŏn-vŭl′shŭn). An involuntary and violent contraction of voluntary muscles.

coronal (kō-rŏ′năl). Belonging to, or relating to, the crown of the head.

c. suture. The suture formed by the union of the frontal bone with the two parietal bones.

corona radiata (kō-rō′nȧ rā″dī-ā′tȧ). The layer of follicular cells arranged in a radial pattern that envelop the zona pellucida of the ovum.

cor pulmonale (kôr pŭl-mō-nā′lē). Heart disease secondary to disease of the lungs or lung blood vessels; a type of heart failure.

corpus albicans (kôr′pŭs ăl′bĭ-kănz). The white fibrous tissue that replaces the corpus luteum in the ovary as it shrinks in the last stages of pregnancy.

corpus luteum (kôr′pŭs lū′tē-ŭm). The yellow mass found in the graafian follicle after the ovum has been expelled.

cotyledon (kŏt″ĭ-lē′dŭn). Any one of the subdivisions of the uterine surface of the placenta.

couvelaire uterus (koo″vĕl-ār′). A severe uterine condition seen in some cases of placenta separation, when coagulation is impaired and there is extensive bleeding into the uterine muscle.

Cowper's gland (kow′pĕrz). One of two glands located at the base of the prostrate gland and on either side of the membranous urethra that produce a mucinous substance that lubricates the urethra and coats its surface.

CPD. Abbreviation for cephalopelvic disproportion.

cramp (krămp). A painful contraction of a muscle.

creatinine (krē-ăt′ĭ-nine). The end product of metabolism, found in muscle and blood, and excreted in the urine.

criminal abortion. See *abortion, criminal.*

crowning (krown′ĭng). The phase in the second stage of labor when a large part of the top of the fetal head is visible in the vaginal opening. The anus is open, and the perineum is distended.

cul-de-sac (kool′dē-săk′). [Fr.] A pouch or sac having only one end open.

Douglas' c. A sac or recess formed by a fold of the peritoneum dipping down between the rectum and the uterus. Also called *pouch of Douglas* and *rectouterine pouch.*

culdoscopy (kŭl-dŏs′kō-pĭ). A visual examination of the organs of a female pelvis with an endoscope.

cumulus oophorus (kū′mū-lŭs ō-ŏf′ō-rŭs). A loosely arranged solid mass of cells surrounding the ovum in the ovarian follicle.

curanderas (kū″rän-dĕr′ăs) f.; **curanderos** (kū″rän-dĕr′ōs) m. Mexican-American folk healer.

curettage (kū″rĕ-täzh′). [Fr.] The removal of substances from the wall of a cavity, especially the uterine cavity, with a spoon-shaped instrument called a curet.

cyanosis (sī″ȧ-nō′sĭs). A bluish discoloration of the skin or mucous membranes as a result of an excessive concentration of hemoglobin that is not combined with oxygen in the blood.

cyesis (sī-ē′sĭs). Pregnancy.

cystitis (sĭs-tī′tĭs). An infection or inflammation of the urinary bladder.

cystocele (sĭs′tō-sĕl). The pouching downward of the bladder through the vaginal wall.

cytomegalic inclusion disease. See *disease, cytomegalic inclusion.*

cytomegalovirus (sī″tō-mĕg″ȧ-lō-vī′rŭs). A herpesvirus that produces unique large cells bearing intranuclear inclusions.

D & C. Abbreviation for dilatation and curettage.

D & E. Abbreviation for dilatation and evacuation.

decidua (dē-sĭ′dū-ȧ). The endometrium of a pregnant uterus, which, except for the deepest layer, is shed during childbirth.

d. basalis. The part of the decidua directly underneath the chorionic vesicle and attached to the myometrium, the main muscular mass of the uterus.

decrement (dĕk′rē-mĕnt). Decrease; also the stage of decline.

delivery (dē-lĭv′ĕr-ĭ). [Fr., *délivrer,* to free, to deliver.] 1. The expulsion of a child by the mother, or its extraction by the obstetric practitioner. 2. The removal of a part from the body, for example, *delivery* of the placenta.

dermatitis (dûr″mȧ-tī′-tĭs). An inflammation of the skin.

detumescence (dĕ″tū-mĕs′ĕns). The subsidence of swelling, congestion, or turgor; the period in which the organ or passage decreases in size and returns to its original state.

diabetes (dī″ȧ-bē′tēz) or **diabetes mellitus** (mĕ-lĭ′tŭs). An endocrine disorder that involves disruption of normal carbohydrate metabolism caused by a deficiency of insulin. Because there is a significant change in the course of diabetes when pregnancy intervenes, close supervision of the prenatal care of a diabetic gravida is required.

diagonal conjugate measurement. The chief internal pelvic measurement made to determine the actual diameter of the pelvic passage. It is the distance between the sacral promontory and the lower margin of the symphysis pubis.

diamniotic dichorionic twins. See *twins, diamniotic dichorionic.*

diamniotic monochorionic twins. See *twins, diamniotic monochorionic.*

diaphragm (dī′ȧ-frăm). 1. The partition separating the abdominal and thoracic cavities made of muscle and membrane. 2. A contraceptive device made of rubber that is inserted in the vagina to act like a cap over the cervix. To be effective, the device is used with spermicidal cream or jelly.

diaphragmatic (dī″ȧ-frăg-mă′tĭc). Pertaining to the diaphragm.

d. hernia (hûr′nĭ-ȧ). A defect in the development of the diaphragm, which allows the abdominal organs to herniate into the thoracic cavity.

d. paralysis (pȧ-răl′ĭ-sĭs). A condition resulting from injury to the phrenic nerve during a difficult breech delivery. The paralysis is usually one sided, with irregular thoracic respirations, no abdominal movement on inspiration on the affected side, and cyanosis.

diarrhea (dī″*ă*-rē′*ă*). Abnormally frequent and liquid fecal discharges.

diastasis (dī-ăs′t*ă*-sĭs). A separation, as of the rectus muscle of the abdomen, away from the median line.

Dick–Read approach to childbirth. The approach that is based on the understanding that fear of pain produces muscular tension, which produces pain and greater fear. This approach includes an educational program to teach physiological processes of labor, exercise to improve muscle tone, and techniques to assist in relaxation and prevent the fear–tension–pain mechanism. Also called *Read method of childbirth preparation.*

dilatation and curettage. [D & C] A method of emptying the contents of the uterus by utilizing cervical dilatation and curettage. The technique is widely used for first trimester abortions.

dilatation and evacuation. [D & E] See *suction curettage.*

dilation (dī-lā′sh*ŭ*n). The act of dilating or stretching.

cervical d. The opening of the cervix to accommodate the birth of the fetus.

dimorphism (dī-môr′fĭsm). The manifestation in the same species of two forms, such as male and female; refers to both bodily form and appearance and to sex differences in behavior and language.

disease (dĭ-zēz′). Any departure from health of a structure, organ, or system.

Gaucher's d. (gō-shāz′). A lipidosis in which the fatty accumulation in the body is largely kerasin. In the infant form, it is characterized by yellow pigmentation of the skin and marked impairment of the central nervous system. It is also known as *cerebroside lipidosis* and is a hereditary defect of the metabolism.

hemolytic d. (hē″mō-lĭt′ĭk). Anemia in a fetus or newborn caused by antibodies that are transmitted from the mother due to the incompatibility between the blood group of the mother and her child.

Hurler's d. (hûr-lērz) (gargoylism). A hereditary disorder caused by an enzyme deficiency. It is characterized by gargoylelike features of the head (depressed bridge of the nose, large prominent tongue, and widely spaced teeth), dwarf structure, short neck, broad short hands, severe mental retardation, blindness, deafness, and cardiovascular defects.

hyaline membrane d. (HMD) (hī′*ă*-lĭn). A disease of premature infants characterized by the formation of a translucent membrane in the respiratory passages and the incapacity of the lungs to expand adequately. Also known as respiratory distress syndrome (RDS).

Niemann–Pick d. (nē′m*ă*n). A lipidosis characterized by brownish yellow discoloration of the skin and nervous system involvement. It is a hereditary disease and is also known as *sphingomyelin lipidosis.*

Tay–Sachs d. A hereditary metabolic disorder also known as *ganglioside lipidosis.* It is characterized by a degeneration of brain cells, a red spot on each retina, and eventually by dementia, blindness, paralysis, and death.

venereal d. (vē-nē′rē-*ă*l). One of a number of infectious diseases that are transmitted through sexual contact and may be localized or systemic. Common types are gonorrhea, syphilis, condylomata (venereal warts), and herpes simplex type II.

Wilson–Mikity d. See *pulmonary dysmaturity.*

disseminated intravascular coagulation (dĭs-sĕm′ĭ-nāt″ĕd ĭn″tr*ă*-văs′kū-l*ă*r kō-ăg″ū-lā′sh*ŭ*n). A disorder in the clotting mechanism of the blood in which there is widespread clotting through the blood vessels. The condition may occur in a newborn baby secondary to sepsis, hypoxia, acidosis, and maternal eclampsia.

diuresis (dī″ū-rē′sĭs). An increased excretion of urine.

diuretic (dī″ū-rĕt-ĭk). An agent that promotes urine excretion.

dizygotic (dī″zī-gŏt′ĭk). Pertaining to or proceeding from two zygotes (ova).

d. twins. See *twins, dizygotic.*

Döderlein's bacillus (dĕd′ĕr-līnz). The large gram-positive bacterium occurring in the normal vaginal secretion.

dominant inheritance (dŏm′ĭ-n*ă*nt ĭn-hĕr-ĭ-t*ă*ns). The acquiring of a characteristic by transmission in a gene from parents to their offspring regardless of the state of the corresponding allele.

Douglas' cul-de-sac. See *cul-de-sac, Douglas.*

Down's syndrome. See *syndrome, Down's.*

ductus (dŭk′t*ŭ*s). A duct.

d. arteriosus (är-tēr″rĭ-ō′s*ŭ*s). "Arterial duct," a blood vessel peculiar to the fetus, communicating directly between the pulmonary artery and the aorta.

d. venosus (vē-nō′s*ŭ*s). "Venous duct," a blood vessel peculiar to the fetus, establishing a direct communication between the umbilical vein and the inferior vena cava.

Duncan mechanism (dŭng′k*ă*n). The position of the placenta, with the maternal surface outermost; to be born edgewise.

dyscrasia (dĭs-krā′zē-*ă*). A diseased condition.

dysmenorrhea (dĭs″mĕn-ō-rē′*ă*). Painful menstruation.

dyspareunia (dĭs″p*ă*-roo′nĭ-*ă*). Painful intercourse, which can result from penetration, frictional movement, and deep thrusting.

dysplasia (dĭs-plā′sĭ-*ă*). Abnormality of the development of cells or a part.

dyspnea (dĭsp′nē-*ă*). Labored breathing.

dystocia (dĭs-tō′shĭ-*ă*). Difficult, slow, or painful birth or delivery. It is distinguished as maternal or fetal (*i.e.,* the difficulty is due to some deformity on the part of the mother or on the part of the child).

d., placental. Difficulty in delivering the placenta.

eclampsia (ĕk-lămp′sĭ-*ă*). Acute toxemia of pregnancy characterized by convulsions and coma, which may occur during pregnancy, labor, or the puerperium.

ectocervix (ĕk″tō-sûr′vĭks). The outer portion of the cervix visible on examination.

ectoderm (ĕk′tō-dŭrm). The outer layer of cells of the primitive embryo.

ectopic (ĕk-tŏp′ĭk). Out of place.

e. gestation. Gestation in which the fetus is out of its normal place in the cavity of the uterus. It includes gestations in the interstitial portion of the tube, in a rudimentary horn of the uterus (cornual pregnancy), and cervical pregnancy as well as tubal, abdominal, and ovarian pregnancies. Also known as *ectopic pregnancy* and *extrauterine pregnancy.*

e. pregnancy. Same as *ectopic gestation.*

ectropion (ĕk-trō′pĭ-ŏn). Eversion of an edge or margin, as of the columnar epithelium of the endocervical canal onto the ectocervix. The tissue appears darker pink-red and bumpy compared to the smooth pink squamous epithelium of the ectocervix.

EDC. Abbreviation for *expected date of confinement.*

edema (ĕ-dē′mȧ). Abnormal swelling owing to large amounts of fluid in the tissues.

effacement (ĕ-fās′mĕnt). Obliteration. In obstetrics, refers to thinning and shortening of the cervix.

efferent (ĕf′ēr-ĕnt). Centrifugal; conveying away from a center, as efferent nerves convey stimuli to the peripheral nervous system.

effleurage (ĕf-loo-razh′). [Fr.] A rubbing movement, as in massage.

ejaculation (ē-jăk″ū-lā′shŭn). A sudden act of expulsion, as of semen.

electronic fetal monitor. A system for monitoring fetal heart rate and uterine activity by electrically operated instruments.

embolism (ĕm′bō-lĭzm). The sudden blocking of an artery or vein by a blood clot or other obstruction that was brought there by the blood current.

embolus (ĕm′bō-lŭs). A clot or other obstruction brought to a vein or artery by the blood from a larger vessel.

embryo (ĕm′brĭ-ō). The product of conception in utero from the third through the fifth week of gestation; after that length of time it is called the fetus.

embryonic disc (ĕm″brĭ-ŏn′ĭk dĭsk). The flattish portion of a fertilized ovum in which the first traces of an embryo are seen.

empathy (ĕm′pȧ-thĭ). The projection of one's own consciousness into that of another. Empathy may be distinguished from sympathy in that the former state includes relative freedom from emotional involvement.

encephalopathy (ĕn-sĕf″ȧ-lŏp′ȧ-thĭ). Any degenerative brain disease.

endocervical (ĕn″dō-sûr′vĭ-kăl). Pertaining to the interior of the cervix of the uterus.

endocervix (ĕn″dō-sûr′vĭks). 1. The mucous membrane lining of the cervical canal. 2. The region of the opening of the cervix into the uterine cavity.

endometritis (ĕn″dō-mĕ-trī′tĭs). Inflammation of the endometrium.

endometrium (ĕn″dō-mē′trĭ-ŭm). The mucous membrane that lines the uterus.

endorphin (ĕn′dor-f ĭn). An opiatelike substance produced by the body.

endoscope (ĕn′dō-skōp). An instrument used for viewing the interior of a hollow organ; as the bladder.

endotracheal intubation (ĕn″dō-trā′kē-ăl ĭn″tū-bā′shŭn). The insertion of a tube into the trachea to be used to administer anesthesia, maintain an airway, or ventilate the lungs.

enema (ĕn′ĕ-mȧ). A liquid injected into the rectum.

enface (ĕn fäs). [Fr.] The position in which the mother's face is rotated so that her eyes and those of her infant meet fully.

engagement (ĕn-gāj′mĕnt). In obstetrics, applies to the entrance of the presenting part into the superior pelvic strait and the beginning of the descent through the pelvic canal.

engorgement (ĕn-gôrj′mĕnt). Hyperemia; local congestion; excessive fullness of any organ or passage. In obstetrics, refers to an exaggeration of normal venous and lymph stasis of the breasts, which occurs in relation to lactation.

entoderm (ĕn′tō-dûrm). The innermost layer of cells of the primitive embryo.

enzygotic (ĕn-zī-gŏt′ĭk). Developed from the same fertilized ovum.

epididymis (ĕp″ĭ-dĭd′ĭ-mĭs). Pl. *epididymides* (ĕp″ĭ-dĭd′ĭ-mĭ-dēz) A part of the canal system of the testes, made up of numerous seminiferous tubules. Its long coiled duct provides for storage, transit, and maturation of spermatozoa.

epidural anesthesia (ĕp″ĭ-dū′răl). Anesthesia produced by injecting between the vertebral spines and beneath the ligamentum flavum into the extradural space. It is used in obstetric anesthesia to alleviate maternal pain with minimal danger to the infant. It requires the expertise that is afforded a surgical patient.

epinephrine (ĕp″ĭ-nĕf′rĭn). A chemical hormone that is secreted by the adrenal medulla. It is released in response to hypoglycemia. This chemical is injected in infants of diabetic mothers to treat hypoglycemia.

episiotomy (ĕ-pĭz″-ĭ-ŏt′ō-mĭ). Surgical incision of the vulvar orifice for obstetric purposes.

epispadias (ĕp″ĭ-spā′dĭ-ăs). The congenital absence of the upper wall of the urethra.

Epstein's pearls. Small white cysts on the hard palate or gums of the newborn. They are not abnormal.

Erb's paralysis. Partial paralysis of the brachial plexus, affecting various muscles of the arm and the chest wall.

ergonovine (ûr″gō-nō′vĭn). An alkaloid of ergot and a powerful oxytocic. May be administered intravenously, orally, or intramuscularly. This drug will cause an elevation of blood pressure.

ergot (ûr′gŏt). A drug having the remarkable property of exciting powerfully the contractile force of the uterus, and chiefly used for this purpose, but its long-continued use is highly dangerous. Usually given in the fluid extract.

erotic (ĕ-rŏt′ĭk). Pertaining to sensuousness or sensual arousal.

erythema toxicum (ûr″i-thē′mȧ tŏks′ĭ-cŭm). A blotchy rash that may appear in the first few days of life. It develops more frequently on the back, shoulders, and buttocks. No treatment is necessary, and it will disappear in a day or so. It is also called *"newborn rash."*

erythroblastosis fetalis (ē-rĭth″rō-blăs-tō′sĭs). A severe hemolytic disease of the newborn usually due to Rh incompatibility.

esophageal atresia (ĕ-sŏf″ă-jē′ăl ă-trē′zĭ-ă). A congenital defect in which the esophagus ends in a blind pouch rather than a continuous tube to the stomach. It is characterized by excessive drooling, gagging, coughing, vomiting when fed, cyanosis, and dyspnea. The condition is corrected by surgery.

estradiol (ĕs″tră-dī′ŏl). An estrogen produced in ovarian follicles. It inhibits the release of follicle-stimulating hormones prior to ovulation.

estrogen (ĕs′trō-jĕn). The generic term for the female sex hormones. It is a steroid hormone produced primarily by the ovaries but also by the adrenal cortex. It is responsible for the development of secondary sex characteristics and the cyclic nature of female reproductive physiology.

expected date of confinement (EDC). The calculated date for the birth of the fetus.

external rotation. In childbirth, a change in the position of the fetus following the birth of the head during which the shoulders are born.

extraction, vacuum. In assisted childbirth, the use of a metal cup applied to the fetal head by creating a vacuum between it and the head to assist in the delivery of a fetus. Traction is exerted by means of a short chain attached to the cup, with a handle at its far end.

extraperitoneal (ĕks″tră-pĕr-ĭ-tō-nē′ăl). Situated or occurring outside the peritoneal cavity.

extrauterine (ĕks″tră-ū′tĕr-ĭn). Outside of the uterus.

- **e. pregnancy.** See *ectopic gestation.*

face presentation. A less common head presentation in which the fetal face is presented in labor.

facies (fā′shĭ-ēz). Pl. *facies.* [L.] A term used in anatomy to refer to the front of the head from forehead to chin.

fallopian (fă-lō′pĭ-ăn). [Relating to G. *Fallopius,* a celebrated Italian anatomist of the 16th century.]

- **f. tubes.** The oviducts—two canals extending from the sides of the fundus uteri.

false labor. A condition in the latter weeks of some pregnancies in which irregular uterine contractions are felt but the cervix is not affected.

false pelvis. See *pelvis, false.*

family-centered care. Maternity care that takes into account other members of the family, particularly fathers and children, in prenatal, intrapartal, and postpartal care of pregnant women.

fecundation (fē″kŭn-dā′shŭn). The act of impregnating or the state of being impregnated; the fertilization of the ovum by means of the male seminal element.

fecundity (fē-kŭn′dĭ-tĭ). The ability to produce offspring in large numbers in a short period of time.

fertility (fĕr-tĭl′ĭ-tĭ). The ability to produce offspring; power of reproduction.

- **f. awareness.** The development of familiarity with the bodily signs of impending ovulation and bodily signs after ovulation, which enables a woman to anticipate her fertile period and its ending.
- **f. rate.** The number of births per 1000 women aged 15 through 44 years.

fertilization (fûr-tĭ-lĭ-zā′shŭn). The fusion of the spermatozoon with the ovum; it marks the beginning of pregnancy.

fetal (fē′tăl). Pertaining to a fetus.

- **f. acidosis.** A condition of a fetus resulting in the accumulation of acids or depletion of alkaline reserve in the blood and body tissues.
- **f. alcohol syndrome.** See *syndrome, f. alcohol.*
- **f. bradycardia.** Slowness of the fetal heartbeat.
- **f. distress.** A condition of fetal difficulty during labor. Signs are persistent rapid heartbeat, slowing of the heartbeat, which bears no relationship to contractions, or change in heartbeat, and meconium in the amniotic fluid in a vertex presentation.
- **f. habitus** (hăb′ĭ-tŭs). The attitude of the fetus, or the relation of the fetal parts to each other.
- **f. heartrate (FHR).** The heartrate of the fetus. Normally, it can be heard about the middle of pregnancy and may vary between 120 to 160 beats per minute.
- **f. heart tones (FHT).** The sounds of a fetal heart as heard by auscultation.

fetoscope (fē′tō-skōp). 1. A head stethoscope designed especially for listening to fetal heart tones. 2. An endoscope for viewing a fetus.

fetus (fē′tŭs). The baby in utero from the end of the fifth week of gestation until birth.

FHR. See *fetal heart rate.*

FHT. See *fetal heart tones.*

fibroid (fī′broid). See *myoma.*

fimbria (fĭm′brĭ-ă). A fringe; especially the fringelike end of the fallopian tube.

fissure (fĭsh′ĕr). A cleft or groove, which may be normal or abnormal. Anal fissures are painful linear ulcers at the margin of the anus.

fistula (fĭs′tū-lă). An abnormal passage between two internal organs or between an organ and the surface of the body.

flatulence (flăt′ū-lĕns). An excess amount of gas in the stomach or intestines.

flexion (flĕk′shŭn). The act of bending. In obstetrics, the process in the mechanism of labor referring to the bending of the fetal head so that the chin is in contact with the chest, thus presenting the smallest anteroposterior diameter to the pelvis.

foam, contraceptive. A spermicidal preparation that is inserted vaginally prior to intercourse to prevent conception. Its effectiveness is enhanced when it is used with a diaphragm.

follicle (fŏl′lĭ-k′l). A sac or pouchlike cavity.

follicle stimulating hormone (FSH). A gonadotropic hormone secreted by the anterior pituitary, which stimulates the development of graafian follicles.

fontanel (fŏn″tă-nĕl′). The diamond-shaped space between the frontal and two parietal bones in very young infants. This is called the *anterior f.* and is the familiar "soft spot" just above a baby's forehead. A small, triangular one (*posterior f.*) is between the occipital and parietal bones.

footling breech. A breech presentation in which one or both feet or the knees extend below the buttocks. It is also known as incomplete breech presentation.

foramen (fō-rā′mĕn). A hole, opening, aperture or orifice—especially one through a bone.

f. ovale (ō-vā′lē). An opening situated in the partition that separates the right and left auricles of the heart in the fetus.

forceps (fōr′sĕps). A two-bladed instrument with a handle used for grasping tissues or sterile dressings in surgery. In obstetrics, one of several kinds of instruments used for assisting in the delivery of an infant after the cervix is dilated and the vertex of the fetal head is engaged.

foreskin (fōr′skĭn). The prepuce—the fold of skin covering the glans penis.

fornix (fôr′nĭks). Pl. *fornices* (fôr′nĭ-zēz). An arch; any vaulted surface.

f. of the vagina. The angle of reflection of the vaginal mucous membrane onto the cervix uteri.

fourchette (foor-shĕt). [Fr., "fork"] The posterior angle or commissure of the labia majora.

frenulum linguae (frĕn′ū-lŭm lĭng′gwē). A sharp, thin ridge of tissue that arises in the midline from the base of the tongue and is attached to its undersurface for varying distances. Depending upon this distance of attachment, it restrains the movement of the tongue. Also called *lingual frenum.*

frenum (frē′nŭm). A fold of mucous membrane that checks, curbs, or restrains the movements of a part.

lingual f. (lĭng′gwăl). See *frenulum linguae.*

Friedman's curve (frēd′măn). A graph designed to describe and record progress during labor.

Friedman's test. See *test, Friedman's.*

FSH. Abbreviation for *follicle-stimulating hormone.*

fundus (fŭn′dŭs). The upper rounded portion of the uterus between the points of insertion of the fallopian tubes.

funic souffle (fū′nĭc soo′f'l). A soft, blowing sound, synchronous with the fetal heart sounds and supposed to be produced in the umbilical cord.

funis (fū′nĭs). A cord—especially the umbilical cord.

galactagogue (gȧ-lăk′tȧ-gŏg). 1. Causing the flow of milk. 2. Any drug that causes the flow of milk to increase.

galactorrhea (gă-lăk-tō-rē′ă). Prolonged and abnormal lactation, often profuse.

gamete (găm′ēt). A sexual cell; a mature germ cell, as an unfertilized egg or a mature sperm cell.

Gamper method of childbirth preparation. One of a number of methods employed by parents for handling the discomforts of labor.

ganglioside lipidosis (găng′glĭ-ō-sīd lĭp″ĭ-dō′sĭs). See *disease, Tay–Sachs.*

gargoylism (gär′goil-ĭzm). See *disease, Hurler's.*

gastroenteritis (găs″trō-ĕn-ter-ī′tĭs). Inflammation of the stomach and intestines.

gastrula (găs′troo-lȧ). The early embryonic stage that follows the blastula; the cuplike stage with two layers of cells.

gate control theory. A theory proposed in 1965 by Melzack and Wall to explain the neurophysical mechanism underlying the sensation of pain.

Gaucher's disease (gō-shāz′). See *disease, Gaucher's.*

gavage feeding (gȧ-väzh′). Forced feeding, as through a tube into the stomach.

gender identity. The sameness, unity, and persistence of one's individuality as male or female, or ambivalent, especially as experienced in self-awareness and behavior. Gender identity is the private experience of gender role.

gender role. Everything one says and does to indicate to others or the self the degree to which one is male or female, or ambivalent. It includes but is not restricted to sexual arousal and response. Gender role is the public expression of gender identity.

gene (jēn). A hereditary germinal factor in the chromosome that carries on a hereditary transmissible character.

genetic anomaly (jĕ-nĕt′ĭk ă-nŏm′ă-lĭ). A marked deviation from the expected standard as a result of an inherited defect.

genetic counseling. A process in which individuals or families are given information that is needed to understand a hereditary disorder.

genetics. The study of heredity.

genitalia (jĕn″ĭ-tăl′ĭ-ȧ). The reproductive organs.

genital herpes (jĕn-ĭ-tȧl hûr′pēz). A viral skin disease of the genitals marked by groups of vesicles 3 to 6 mm in diameter.

genotype (jĕn′ō-tīp). An individual's entire hereditary constitution.

gestation (jĕs-tā′shŭn). The condition of pregnancy; pregnancy; gravidity.

gestational age. The age of the product of conception between fertilization and birth.

glucose tolerance test (GTT) (gloo′kōs tŏl′ûr-ăns). See *test, glucose tolerance.*

glycosuria (glī″kō-sū′rĭ-ȧ). The presence of glucose (sugar) in the urine.

gonad (gŏn′ăd). A gamete-producing gland; an ovary or testis.

gonadal sex (gō-năd′ăl sĕks). The sex of an individual determined by the presence of either testes or ovaries as gonads, or in the case of a true hermaphrodite, the presence of gonads of both sexes.

gonadotropin (gŏn″ȧ-dō-trō′pĭn). A substance produced by the anterior pituitary and placenta that has an affinity for or a stimulating effect on the gonads.

gonorrhea (gŏn″ō-rē′ȧ). A disease spread by sexual contact that affects the mucosa of the genital tract. The disease may be asymptomatic in women, except for a vaginal discharge. It can produce puerperal infection if present in the cervix at the time of delivery. The infection can infect the infant's eyes at birth.

gonorrheal conjunctivitis (gŏn″ō-rē′ăl kŏn-jŭngk″tĭ-vī′tĭs). A severe form of conjunctivitis caused by the bacteria of gonorrhea.

gonorrheal salpingitis (săl-pĭn-jī′tĭs). An infection of the fallopian tube caused by the gonorrhea bacteria. It may cause a narrowing of the fallopian tube, which may subsequently prevent the passage of a fertilized ovum down the tube, resulting in a tubal pregnancy.

Goodell's sign (good'ĕlz). Softening of the cervix, a probable sign of pregnancy.

gossypol (gŏs'ĭ-pŏl). A derivative of cottonseed oil that has male contraceptive actions by suppressing sperm production and affecting sperm structure and mobility.

graafian follicles or **vesicles** (grăf'ĭ-ăn). Small spherical bodies in the ovaries, each containing an ovum.

grasp reflex. See *reflex, grasp.*

gravid (grăv'ĭd). Pregnant.

gravida (grăv'ĭ-dȧ). A pregnant woman.

GTT. Abbreviation for *glucose tolerance test.*

Guthrie method in PKU (gŭth'rē). A method of diagnosing PKU. It is a blood test in which one or two drops of blood may be taken from an infant's heel; then the blood is tested to determine the phenylalanine level.

gynecoid pelvis (gī'nē-koid). See *pelvis, gynecoid.*

gynecology (gī"nē-kŏl'ō-jĭ). The branch of medicine that studies and treats women's diseases, especially of the genital tract.

Haase's rule (häz'ez). A method for calculating the length of an embryo or fetus. During the first 5 months, the number of months should be squared to approximate the length in centimeters (*e.g.,* second month of pregnancy, the fetus is about 4 cm in length). After the fifth month, the number of months should be multiplied by 5.

habitus (hăb'ĭt-ŭs). Attitude, disposition, or tendency; to act in a certain way; position acquired by frequent repetition.

Harvard pump (här'värd). A constant infusion pump used to administer oxytocin in labor.

HCG. Abbreviation for *human chorionic gonadotropin.*

Health Systems Agency (HSA). A regional agency within a state that has primary responsibility for health planning and development of health services, manpower, and facilities to meet the needs of its service areas.

Hegar's sign (hā'gärz). Softening of the lower uterine segment; a sign of pregnancy.

hematocrit (hē-măt'ō-krĭt). The volume percentage of red blood corpuscles in whole blood. Formerly, it meant the procedure used to determine this number; now it is the result of that determination.

hematoma (hĕm"ȧ-tō'mȧ). A tumor caused by effused blood. Continued bleeding from lacerations or an episiotomy can cause vaginal or vulvar hematomas in postpartum patients.

hemoglobinopathy (hē"mō-glō"bĭ-nŏp'ȧ-thĭ). A disorder of the blood resulting from a genetically caused altered molecular structure of hemoglobin.

hemolytic disease (hē"mō-lĭt'ĭk). See *disease, hemolytic.*

hemophilia (hē"mō-fĭl'ĭ-ȧ). An inherited condition that is due to a deficiency in a coagulation factor in the blood. It is characterized by subcutaneous and intramuscular hemorrhages, bleeding from the mouth, gum, lips, and tongue, and blood in the urine. It affects males but is transmitted by females.

hemorrhage (hĕm'ŏr-ĭj). Bleeding.

hemorrhagic diathesis (hĕm"ō-răj'ĭk dī-ăth'ĕ-sĭs). A predisposition to abnormal bleeding.

hemorrhoid (hĕm'ō-roid). A varicose dilatation of a vein in the rectal area. It may occur around the anus or internally higher in the rectum.

hepatitis (hĕp"ȧ-tī'tĭs). Inflammation of the liver.

hermaphroditism (hûr-mŏf'rō-dī-tĭz'm"). A congenital condition of ambiguity of reproductive structures so that the sex of the individual is not clearly defined as exclusively male or female. The condition is named for Hermes and Aphrodite, the Greek god and goddess of love.

hernia (hûr'nĭ-ȧ). The protrusion of an organ through an abnormal opening in the wall of the cavity that contains it.

diaphragmatic h. See *diaphragmatic hernia.*

umbilical h. (ŭm-bĭl'ĭ-kăl). The protrusion of the intestines through a rupture at the navel. In an infant, the condition usually disappears spontaneously by 1 year of age.

herpesvirus (hûr"pēz-vī'rŭs). One of a large group of DNA viruses that cause a variety of conditions, as genital herpes, varicella (chickenpox), and herpes zoster (shingles).

heterosexuality (hĕt"ĕr-ō-sĕk"shoo-ăl'ĭ-tĭ). The selection of partners of the opposite sex for sexual eroticism and genital intimacy; the predominant mode of sexual partner preference.

high risk. Pertaining to an individual, especially an infant, whose medical and physical history, or that of his parents, indicates that the likelihood is great for his having physiological problems.

hip dysplasia (dĭs-plā'sĭ-ȧ). A hereditary condition involving dislocation with partial or complete loss of contact between the femoral head and the cup-shaped cavity on the lateral surface of the hip bone.

histology (hĭs-tŏl'ō-gĭ). The branch of anatomy that deals with the study of the minute structure, composition, and function of the tissues.

HMD. Abbreviation for *hyaline membrane disease.*

HMG. Abbreviation for *human menopausal gonadotropin.*

Homan's sign (hō'mănz). An indication of thrombophlebitis if with leg extended and foot flexed, pain and tenderness are produced in the calf.

homologous (hō-mŏl'ō-gŭs). Corresponding in structure or origin; derived from the same source.

homologue (hōm'ō-lŏg). An organ similar in structure, position, and origin to another organ.

homosexuality (hō"mō-sĕk"shoo-ăl'ĭt-tĭ). The selection of partners of the same sex for sexual eroticism and genital intimacy. There are many degrees of its expression.

hormonal sex (hôr'mō-năl sĕks). The sex of an individual determined by the preponderance of either estrogen (female) or testosterone (male) sex hormones.

hormone (hôr'mōn). A chemical substance produced in an organ, which, being carried to an associated organ by the bloodstream, excites in the latter organ a functional activity.

HPL. Abbreviation for *human placental lactogen.*

HSA. Abbreviation for *health systems agency.*

human chorionic gonodotropin (HCG) (kôr"ĭ-ŏn'ĭk gŏn"ȧ-dō-trō'pĭn). A hormone secreted by the placenta that prolongs the life of the corpus luteum. It is excreted in the mother's urine and makes possible the standard tests for pregnancy.

human menopausal gonodotropin (HMG) (mĕn"ō-pä'zȧl). A hormone excreted in the urine of postmenopausal women that has the property of stimulating growth and maturity of ovarian follicles.

human placental lactogen (HPL) (plȧ-sen'tal lăk'tō-jĕn). A hormone secreted by the placenta that influences somatic growth and facilitates preparation of the breasts for lactation.

Hurler's disease (hûr-lērz). (gargoylism). See *disease, Hurler's.*

hyaline membrane disease (HMD) (hī'ȧ-lĭn mĕm'brān). See *disease, hyaline membrane.*

hydatidiform mole (hī"dȧ-tĭd'ĭ-fôrm). Cystic proliferation of chorionic villi, resembling a bunch of grapes.

hydramnios (hī-drăm'nĭ-ŏs). An excessive amount of amniotic fluid.

hydrocephalus (hī-drō-sĕf'ȧ-lŭs). An excessive accumulation of cerebrospinal fluid in the ventricles of the brain with consequent enlargement of the cranium.

hymen (hī'mĕn). A membranous fold that partially or wholly occludes the external orifice of the vagina, especially in the virgin.

hyperalimentation (hī"pĕr-ăl"ĭ-mĕn-tā'shŭn). The ingestion of more than adequate amounts of nutrients.

hyperbilirubinemia (hī"pĕr-bĭl"ĭ-roo"bĭ-nē'mĭ-ȧ). The presence of excessive amounts of bilirubin in the blood, which may lead to jaundice.

hyperemesis gravidarum (hī"pĕr-ĕm'ĕ-sĭs gră-vĭ-dā'rŭm). Pernicious vomiting of pregnancy. This condition is present when vomiting is excessive, continues beyond the fourth month, and causes a marked loss of weight and acetonuria.

hyperemia (hī"pĕr-ē'mĭ-ȧ). An excess of blood in a part.

hyperestrogenic (hī"pĕr-ĕs-trō-gĕn'ĭk). Pertaining to a state of exaggerated estrogen response created by high levels of estrogen secretion.

hypernatremia (hī"pĕr-nȧ-trē'mĭ-ȧ). Excessive amounts of sodium in the blood.

hyperplasia (hī"pĕr-plā'zĭ-ȧ). Abnormal multiplication or increase in the number of cells in the normal arrangement in tissue.

hypertension (hī"pĕr-tĕn'shŭn). Persistent high blood pressure, especially arterial blood pressure.

hypertonic (hī"pĕr-tŏn'ĭk). 1. Having high osmotic pressure. 2. Having abnormally high muscle tone.

h. saline (sā'lēn). A concentrated salt solution, as is instilled into the amniotic fluid for a midtrimester abortion.

h. uterine dysfunction (ū'tĕr-ĭn dĭs-fŭngk'shŭn). An abnormality in the functioning of the uterus to propel the fetus through the birth canal. Uterine action is incoordinate; although there is constant tension in the muscle, the contractions are of poor quality.

hyperventilation (hī"pĕr-vĕn"tĭ-lā'shŭn). The condition that results from rapid and deep breathing and is marked by confusion, dizziness, numbness, and muscular cramps.

hypnosis (hĭp-nō'sĭs). An artificially induced state of extreme suggestibility in which the patient is insensible to outside impressions.

hypocalcemia (hī"pō-kăl-sē'mĭ-ȧ). Reduction of blood calcium below normal.

hypofibrinogenemia (hī"pō-fī-brĭn"ō-jen-ē'mĭ-ȧ). Deficiency of fibrinogen in the blood.

hypogalactia (hī"pō-gă-lăk"shĭ-ȧ). Deficiency in the secretion of milk.

hypoglycemia (hī"pō-glī-sē'mĭ-ȧ). An abnormally diminished content of glucose in the blood.

hypoprothrombinemia prophylaxis (hī"pō-prō-thrŏm"bĭ-nē'mĭ-ȧ prō"fĭ-lăk"sĭs). The administration of vitamin K, intramuscularly, to a newborn infant as a preventive measure against neonatal hemorrhagic disease.

hypospadias (hī"pō-spā'dĭ-ȧs). A developmental anomaly in which the urethra opens on the underside of the penis.

hypotension (hī"pō-tĕn'shŭn). Abnormally low blood pressure.

hypothalamus (hī"pō-thăl'ȧ-mŭs). A specialized structure within the brain located just above the pituitary that regulates and controls a number of autonomic activities, including the release of gonadotropic hormones by the pituitary gland.

hypothermic reaction (hī"pō-thûr'mĭk). A reaction of low body temperature of the mother after delivery.

hypotonic uterine dysfunction (hī"pō-tŏn'ĭk ū'tĕr-ēn dĭs-fŭngk'shŭn). An abnormality in the functioning of the uterus to propel the fetus through the birth canal in which contractions decrease in strength and the tone of the uterine muscles is less than usual.

hypovolemia (hī"pō-vō-lē'mĭ-ȧ). An abnormally decreased volume of liquid (plasma) circulating in the body.

hypoxia (hī-pŏks'ĭ-ȧ). Insufficient oxygen to support normal metabolic requirements.

intrauterine h. (ĭn"trȧ-ū'tĕr-ĭn). A condition of hypoxia in the fetus that can be determined in labor by indicators such as meconium-stained amniotic fluid, abnormal fetal heart rate, and fetal acidosis.

hysterectomy (hĭs"tĕ-rĕk'tō-mĭ). The surgical removal of the uterus by cutting either through the abdominal wall or through the vagina.

hysterosalpingography (hĭs"tĕr-ō-săl"pĭng-gŏg"rȧ-fĭ). The making of a record by x-ray of the uterus and uterine tubes after injecting them with opaque material.

hysterotomy (hĭs"tĕr-ŏt'ō-mĭ). A method of midtrimester abortion involving an incision into the uterus by a surgical procedure. Also called *minicesarean section.*

icterus neonatorum (ĭk'tĕr-*ŭ*s nē"ō-nā-tō'r*ŭ*m). The jaundice of a newborn infant.

identification (ī-dĕn"t*ĭ*-fĭ-kā'sh*ŭ*n). The process whereby an individual likens himself to another person.

iliopectineal line (ĭl"ĭ-ō-pĕk-tĭn'ē-*ă*l). The linea terminalis.

ilium (ĭl'ĭ-*ŭ*m). Pl. *ilia* (ĭl'ĭ-*ȧ*). The upper and largest portion of the hip bone.

imperforate anus (ĭm-pĕr'fō-rāt ā'n*ŭ*s). An abnormal closing of the anus.

impotence (ĭm'pō-tĕns). A male sexual dysfunction involving impairment of erection; an inability to attain or sustain an erection and have intercourse in 25% of the attempts.

impregnation (ĭm"prĕg-nā'sh*ŭ*n). The act of becoming pregnant. See *fertilization.*

incompetent cervical os (ĭn-kŏm'pē-tĕnt sûr'vĭ-kăl ŏs). A mechanical defect in the cervix, which causes late habitual abortion or preterm labor.

incomplete abortion. See *abortion, incomplete.*

incontinence (ĭn-kŏn'tĭ-nĕns). Inability to control the excretion of urine or feces.

increment (ĭn'krē-mĕnt). That by which anything is increased.

induced abortion. See *abortion, induced.*

induration (ĭn"dū-rā'sh*ŭ*n). The process or quality of hardening.

inertia (ĭn-ûr'sh*ĭȧ*). Inactivity; inability to move spontaneously. Sluggishness of uterine contractions during labor.

inevitable abortion. See *abortion, inevitable.*

infant (ĭn'f*ă*nt). A baby; a child under 2 years of age.

i. mortality rate. The number of infant deaths per 1000 live births.

infertility (ĭn-fûr-tĭl'ĭ-tĭ). The condition of being unfruitful or barren; sterility.

inlet (ĭn'lĕt). The upper limit of the pelvic cavity (brim).

intercourse (ĭn'tĕr-cōrs). A mutual exchange, especially sexually; coitus.

internal rotation (ĭn-tûr'n*ă*l rōtā'sh*ŭ*n). The process in the delivery of a baby in which the fetal head is rotated so that it enters the pelvis in the transverse position and exits in the anteroposterior position.

interstitial pregnancy (ĭn"tĕr-stĭsh'*ă*l). An ectopic pregnancy that develops in that portion of the tube that passes through the uterine wall.

interval minilaparotomy (ĭn'tĕr-v*ă*l mĭn"ĭ-lăp"*ȧ*-rŏt'ō-mĭ). A sterilization technique in which a small incision is made below the pubic hair line for tubal ligation.

interval of fertility. Those days during the menstrual cycle during which a woman can conceive, determined by considering the life span of both ova and sperm and the cyclic variability. It ranges from about 8 to 15 days in duration.

intracranial hemorrhage (ĭn"tr*ȧ*-krā'nĭ-*ă*l hĕm'ŏr-ĭj). Bleeding within the cranium. When it occurs in a newborn as a result of a long labor or difficult delivery, it is extremely grave. Also called *subdural hematoma.*

intrauterine (ĭn"tr*ȧ*-ū'tĕr-ĭn). Inside the uterus.

i. device (IUD) (dē-vīs'). A small, flexible appliance that is inserted into the uterine cavity to prevent conception. It may be in various shapes (spirals, loops, rings) and of various materials, (plastic tubing, nylon thread, stainless steel).

i. growth retardation (IUGR). The condition of an infant born at 40-weeks gestation and weighing less than 2500 g (or below the tenth percentile for weight or length).

i. hypoxia. See *hypoxia, intrauterine.*

i. parabiosis (păr"*ȧ*-bī-ō'sĭs). The joining of fetal twins anatomically and physiologically.

introitus (ĭn-trō'ĭ-t*ŭ*s). A term applied to the opening of the vagina.

in utero. Inside the uterus.

inversion (ĭn-vûr'sh*ŭ*n). A turning upside down, inside out, or end for end.

i. of the uterus. The state of the womb being turned inside out, caused by violently drawing away the placenta before it is detached by the natural process of labor.

involution (ĭn"vō-lū'sh*ŭ*n). 1. A rolling or pushing inward. 2. A retrograde process of change that is the reverse of evolution: particularly applied to the return of the uterus to its normal size and condition after parturition.

ischial tuberosity (ĭs'k*ĭ*-*a*l too"bĕ-rŏs'ĭ-tĭ). A protuberance on either side of the ischium.

ischium (ĭs'kĭ-*ŭ*m). The posterior and inferior bone of the pelvis, distinct and separate in the fetus or the infant, or the corresponding part of the hip bone in the adult.

isotonic (īs"ō-tŏn'ĭk). Having the same osmotic pressure, especially a salt solution having the same osmotic pressure as blood.

IUD. Abbreviation for *intrauterine device.*

IUGR. Abbreviation for *intrauterine growth retardation.*

jaundice (jôn'dĭs). A condition characterized by hyperbilirubinemia and yellowness in the skin, eyes, and mucous membranes.

jelly (jĕl'ĭ). A soft substance that is coherent, tremulous, and more or less transparent.

contraceptive j. A spermicidal preparation that is inserted vaginally prior to intercourse to prevent conception. Its effectiveness is enhanced when it is used with a diaphragm.

j. of Wharton (hwôr't*ŭ*n). See *Wharton's jelly.*

kalemia (k*ȧ*-lē'mĭ-*ȧ*). The presence of potassium in the blood.

karyotype (kăr'ē-ō-tīp). The chromosome makeup of the nucleus of a human cell; also, the photomicrograph of chromosomes arranged in an organized way.

Kegel's exercise (kā'g'l). The tightening and relaxing of the pubococcygeal muscle. It aids in toning the vagina, strengthening the perineum, preventing hemorrhoids, and controlling stress incontinence of urine.

ketamine (kĕt'*ȧ*-mēn). A dissociative intravenous analgesic that, used in proper doses during labor, is associated with a minimal newborn depression, no appreciable effects on uterine activity, and few bad dreams or hallucinations.

Klinefelter's syndrome (klĭn′fĕl-tẽrz). See *syndrome, Klinefelter's.*

labia (lā′bĭ-ȧ). The nominative plural of *labium.* Lips or liplike structures.

l. majora (mȧ-jō′rȧ). The folds of skin containing fat and covered with hair that form each side of the vulva.

l. minora (mĭ-nō′rȧ). The nymphae, or folds of delicate skin inside the labia majora.

labor (lā′bẽr). Parturition; the series of processes by which the products of conception are expelled from the mother's body.

lack of arousal. A female sexual dysfunction formerly called frigidity. It involves failure to respond adequately with congestion and lubrication even with appropriate sexual stimulation.

lactation (lăk-tā′shŭn). The act or period of giving milk; the secretion of milk; the time or period of secreting milk.

lactosuria (lăk″tō-sū′rĭ-ȧ). The presence of lactose in the urine, a condition common during lactation.

LaLeche League (lä lĕ-shā′ lēg). An organization that holds classes about breast feeding for women either before or after the baby is born.

Lamaze method of delivery (lȧ-mäz′). The most widely used prepared childbirth method in the United States. It uses an individualized approach with classes for both parents in the anatomy and neuromuscular activity of the reproductive system, breathing techniques in labor, and exercises. Sometimes other subjects such as nutrition, hygiene, and child care are taught. Also called *psychoprophylactic method of prepared childbirth.*

lambdoid (lăm′doid). Having the shape of the Greek letter λ (lambda).

l. suture. The suture between the occipital and two parietal bones.

laminaria (lăm″ĭ-nâ′rĭ-ȧ). A genus of seaweeds. Also, a small stick of hygroscopic material that absorbs moisture rapidly and expands. It is used to begin initial dilation of the cervix prior to abortion.

lanugo (lȧ-nū′gō). The fine hair on the body of the fetus. The fine, downy hair found on nearly all parts of the body except the palms of the hands and the soles of the feet.

laparoscopy (lăp″ȧ-rŏs′kō-pĭ). The introduction of a slender, long surgical instrument (the laparoscope) into the abdominal cavity through very small incisions, not involving actual opening of the abdominal cavity. This procedure is often used for female sterilization.

laparotomy (lăp-ȧ-rŏt′ō-mĭ). Surgical entry into the abdominal cavity.

large for gestational age (LGA). Pertaining to an infant born at 36 weeks gestation and weighing 3500 g (about the 90th percentile for weight). LGA infants are immature but overgrown and are typical of diabetic mothers.

layette (lā-ĕt′). The complete outfit of clothing for a newborn infant.

Leboyer method of delivery (lĕ-boi-yā′). A method of delivery based on theories of a French obstetrician, Frederick Leboyer. The method avoids harsh, sudden sensory stimulation of the newborn by having a quiet, dimly lit delivery room and warm bath for the infant to make birth less of a traumatic event for the newborn.

Leopold's maneuver (lā′ō-pŏldz mȧ-noo′vẽr). See *maneuver, Leopold's.*

Let-down reflex. See *reflex, let-down.*

leukorrhea (lū″kŏ-rē′ȧ). A whitish discharge from the female genital organs.

LGA. Abbreviation for *large for gestational age.*

LH. Abbreviation for *luteinizing hormone.*

LHRF. Abbreviation for *luteinizing hormone releasing factor.*

lie. Lie of the fetus. It is the relation of the long axis of the fetus to that of the mother. It is either longitudinal or transverse.

ligation (lī-gā′shŭn). The binding or tying of a vessel with a substance such as string or catgut.

tubal l. (tū′bȧl). The sterilization of a woman by surgically interrupting her fallopian tubes to prevent ova from being transported to the uterus and to prevent sperm from fertilizing the ovum. The method may involve ligation, crushing, burning, coagulating, or embedding the ends of the tubes.

lightening (līt′ĕn-ĭng). The sensation of decreased abdominal distention produced by the descent of the uterus into the pelvic cavity, which occurs from 2 to 3 weeks before the onset of labor.

linea (lĭn′ē-ȧ). Pl. *lineae* (lĭn′ē-ē). A line or thread.

l. alba (ăl′bȧ). The central tendinous line extending from the pubic bone to the ensiform cartilage.

l. nigra (nī′grä). A dark line appearing on the abdomen and extending from the pubis toward the umbilicus—considered one of the signs of pregnancy.

l. terminalis (tẽr″mĭ-năl′ĭs). The oblique ridge on the inner surface of the ilium, continued on the pubis, which separates the tube from the false pelvis. Formerly called the iliopectineal line.

lingua (lĭng′gwȧ). Tongue.

l. frenata (frĕ-nä′tȧ). Tongue-tie.

lipid (lĭp′ĭd). One of a group of fats in the body that is easily stored and serves as a source of fuel, is an important part of cells, and serves other useful functions. It may be a fatty acid, neutral fat, wax, or steroid.

lipidosis (lĭp″ĭ-dō′sĭs). A disorder of cellular lipid metabolism that involves abnormal accumulation of lipid. The lipidoses include Tay–Sachs disease, Niemann–Pick disease, and Gaucher's disease.

liquor (lī′kwôr). A liquid.

l. amnii (lī′kwôr ăm′nĭ-ī). The fluid contained within the amnion in which the fetus floats. See *amniotic fluid.*

lithotomy (lĭ-thŏt′ō-mĭ). The surgical incision of an organ or duct, especially the bladder.

l. position. The bodily posture of a patient lying down

with hips and knees flexed and thighs abducted and rotated.

lochia (lō'kī-*ă*). The discharge from the genital canal during the first or second week following delivery.

low birth weight. The weight of an infant at birth of 2500 g or less.

L/S ratio. The ratio of lecithin to sphingomyelin in the amniotic fluid. It increases suddenly at 35 to 36 weeks gestation and indicates pulmonary maturity.

lumbar sympathetic block (lŭm'bēr sĭm"p*ă*-thĕt'ĭk blŏk). The blocking of neuropathways of pain by injecting a local anesthetic at L2. It abolishes pain in the uterus only.

lunar month (loo'năr). A period of four weeks. Because a lunar month usually corresponds to the length of the menstrual cycle, it is often used for calculating fetal development.

luteinizing hormone (LH) (loo"tē-ĭn-īz'ĭng hôr'mōn). A hormone released by the pituitary gland to bring about the final ripening of the graafian follicle and ovulation.

l. h. releasing factor (LHRF). A substance secreted by the hypothalamus that causes the pituitary gland to release luteinizing hormone.

luteolysis (loo"tē-ŏl'ĭ-sĭs). The destruction of the corpus luteum through the dissolution of cellular structure. Thus, luteolysis interferes with the function of the corpus luteum in progesterone secretion.

lysozyme (lī'sō-zīm). A crystalline, basic protein present in many body fluids that functions as an antibacterial enzyme.

maneuver (m*ă*-noo'vēr). A planned process involving dexterity; in obstetrics, a procedure used by an obstetrician in assisting manually in delivery.

Bracht m. (bräkt). A method of assisting with the delivery of the aftercoming head in a breech delivery. The back is gently arched to the mother's abdomen when the scapulas are seen. The arms then tend to deliver spontaneously. Suprapubic pressure is applied to assist descent of the head into the pelvis, and the suspended body continues to be brought slowly to the mother's abdomen. The face and occiput should then deliver spontaneously.

Leopold's m. (lā'ō-pŏldz). Four maneuvers for diagnosing the fetal position by external palpation of the mother's abdomen.

Mauriceau–Smellie–Veit m. (mō'rē-sō smĕl'ē vīt). A method of assisting with the delivery of the aftercoming head in a breech delivery. Two fingers of the left hand are placed firmly over the mandibles to flex the head. The right hand is placed over the back, with the fingers over the shoulders to guide the shoulders and head. The torso is elevated slowly with flexion of the head maintained by the maxillary pressure. Suprapubic pressure is applied by an assistant during these maneuvers to aid the descent of the head into the pelvis, and eventually with the suprapubic and maxillary pressure, the occiput is delivered.

Ortolani's m. (Or'tō lânēz). A diagnostic procedure performed on the newborn to determine congenital hip dysplasia.

Ritgen m. (rĭt'gĕn). Delivery of the infant's head by lifting the head upward and forward through the vulva, between contractions, by pressing with the tips of the fingers upon the perineum behind the anus.

Sellick's m. (sĕl'ĭks). A technique in which pressure is applied to the ring of cartilage at the lower part of the larynx to prevent aspiration of gastric contents during anesthesia induction.

Marfan's syndrome (mär'fänz sĭn'drōm). See *arachnodactyly.*

marginal sinus rupture (mär'jĭ-n*ă*l sī'nŭs rŭp'tūr). A disorder of placental attachment, a mild type of abruptio placentae in which slight separation occurs at the edge of the placenta in the region of the marginal sinus of the mother.

mask of pregnancy (măsk). See *chloasma.*

mastitis (măs-tī'tĭs). Inflammation of the breast.

masturbation (măs"tûr-bā'sh*ŭ*n). Self-stimulation of the genitals in men or women, usually to attain orgasm.

maternal infant bonding. See *bonding.*

maternity clinical specialist. A graduate registered nurse with special expertise in adaptational and physiological problems in maternity care.

maternity nurse practitioner. A specialty nurse practitioner who provides prenatal care for uncomplicated pregnancies, postpartal care, contraception counseling, and management of minor problems. Also called *OB–GYN nurse practitioner.*

maturation (măt"ū-rā'sh*ŭ*n). In biology, a process of cell division during which the number of chromosomes in the germ cells is reduced to one half the number characteristic of the species.

Mauriceau–Smellie–Veit maneuver (mō'rē-sō smĕl'ē vīt m*ă*-noo'vēr). See *maneuver, Mauriceau–Smellie–Veit.*

McDonald's measurement (măk-dŏn'*ă*ldz). Measurement of the height of the uterine fundus with a tape measure; the distance from symphysis pubis to fundus.

meatus (mē-ā't*ŭ*s). A passage; an opening leading to a canal, duct, or cavity.

m. urinarius (ū"rĭ-nā'rĭ-*ŭ*s). The external orifice of the urethra.

mechanism (mĕk'*ă*-nĭz'm). The manner of combinations that subserve a common function. In obstetrics refers to labor and delivery.

meconium (mē-kō'nĭ-*ŭ*m). The dark green or black substance found in the large intestine of the fetus or newly born infant.

meiosis (mī-ō'sĭs). The special method for cell division that a sex cell undergoes through which it is matured and its genetic material, or chromosomes, is prepared for fertilization.

menarche (mē-när'kē). The establishment or the beginning of the menstrual function.

Mendelian disorder (měn-dē′lē-*ă*n). A genetic disorder that follows the inheritance patterns described by Mendel (*i.e.,* dominant, recessive).

meningomyelocele (mě-nĭng″gō-mī′ĕ-lō-sēl″). A malformation that accompanies spina bifida when the membranes covering the spinal cord as well as the cord bulge through the opening in the spine.

menopause (měn′ō-pôz). The period at which menstruation ceases; the "change of life."

menorrhagia (měn″ō-rā′jĭ-*ȧ*). Excessive uterine bleeding occurring at the regular time of menstrual flow.

menses (měn′sēz). [Pl. of Latin *mensis,* month.] The periodic monthly discharge of blood from the uterus; the catamenia.

menstrual extraction (měn′stroo-*ă*l ěks-trăk′sh*ŭ*n). The aspiration of the endometrium performed in very early pregnancy without cervical dilatation using a small cannula and syringe or other low-pressure suction.

menstruation (měn″stroo-ā′sh*ŭ*n). The cyclic, physiologic uterine bleeding that normally recurs at approximately 4-week intervals, in the absence of pregnancy, during the reproductive period.

mentum (měn′t*ŭ*m). The chin.

mesoderm (měs′ō-dûrm). The middle layer of cells derived from the primitive embryo.

metrorrhagia (mē-trŏ-rā′jĭ-*ȧ*). Uterine bleeding that occurs at irregular intervals; the amount of flow is usually average.

microcephaly (mī″crō-sĕf′ă-lĭ). Abnormal smallness of the head, usually accompanied by mental retardation.

micropill (mī′krō-pĭl). An oral contraceptive that contains a lower dosage (50 mcg or less) of estrogen than the standard pill.

micturition (mĭk″tū-rĭsh′*ŭ*n). Urination.

midwifery (mĭd′wī-fĕr-ĭ). The practice of assisting at childbirth. See *nurse–midwife.*

migration (mī-grā″sh*ŭ*n). In obstetrics refers to the passage of the ovum from the ovary to the uterus.

milia (mĭl′ĭ-*ȧ*). Plural of milium.

milium (mĭl′ĭ-*ŭ*m). A small white nodule of the skin, usually caused by clogged sebaceous glands or hair follicles.

milk ejection reflex. See *reflex, milk ejection.*

milk-leg. See *phlegmasia alba dolens.*

milk let-down. See *reflex, milk ejection.*

minicesarean section. See *hysterotomy.*

minipill (mĭn′ĭ-pĭl). An oral contraceptive that contains only progestin and no estrogen.

miscarriage (mĭs-kăr′ĭj). Abortion.

missed abortion. See *abortion, missed.*

mittelschmerz (mĭt′ĕl-shmārts). Painful discomfort sometimes experienced during ovulation or in the middle of the menstrual cycle.

molding (mōld′ĭng). The shaping of the baby's head so as to adjust itself to the size and shape of the birth canal.

mongolian spots (mŏn-gō′lĭ-*ă*n). Gray-blue pigmented areas seen on some infants, especially those with dark skins. These have no relationship to mongolism and disappear spontaneously later.

mongolism (mŏn′gō-lĭz′m). See *syndrome, Down's.*

monilial infection (mō-nĭl′ĭ-*ă*l). An infection caused by a genus of fungi formerly called *Monilia,* now called *Candida.* Examples are thrush and monilial vaginitis.

monoamniotic monochorionic twins (mŏn″ō-ăm″nĭ-ŏt′ĭk mŏn″ō-kō″rĭ-ŏn′ĭk). See *twins, monoamniotic monochorionic.*

monotropy (mŏn″ôt′trō pĭ). The principle, stated by Bowlby in 1958, that the structure of the attachment process is such that parents become attached to only one infant at a time.

monozygotic (mŏn″ō-zī-gŏt′ĭk). Pertaining to or derived from one zygote.

m. twins. See *twins, monozygotic.*

mons veneris (mŏnz vĕn′*ĕ*-rĭs). The eminence in the upper and anterior part of the pubes of women.

Montgomery's tubercles (m*ŭ*nt-gŭm′ēr-ĭz). Small, nodular follicles or glands on the areolae around the nipples.

morning-after pill. A method of contraception not in general use. The postcoital pill, diethylstilbestrol (DES) is a synthetic estrogen with severe side-effects including nausea, vomiting, and headache. It is used only in emergency situations, such as rape, because it has been shown to cause vaginal cancer in some offspring of mothers who took it.

morning sickness. A symptom of pregnancy in some women, characterized by waves of nausea and sometimes vomiting. It usually occurs in the early part of the day and subsides in a few hours. It may appear 2 weeks after the first missed menstrual period and subside 6 or 8 weeks later.

Moro reflex (mō′rō). See *reflex, Moro.*

morphological sex (môr″fō-lŏj′ĭ-k*ă*l sěks). The sex of an individual as determined by the body shape and characteristic with appropriate secondary sex characteristics. In the case of a true hermaphrodite, the individual has a mixture of the body and secondary sex characteristics of both sexes.

morula (mŏr′ū-l*ȧ*). The fertilized ovum at the 16-cell stage 3 days after conception. It is traveling from the fallopian tube into the uterine cavity prior to implantation.

mother–baby couple care. An organization of postpartum units that includes rooming-in or satellite nurseries, with the same nurse caring for mother and baby.

mucous membrane (mū′k*ŭ*s měm′brān). The lining of a body cavity or passageway that is connected to the exterior and is protected by a slimy substance it secretes called mucus.

mucous plug. A plug that closes the cervical canal during pregnancy. It is made of mucous secretions of the cervix.

multigravida (mŭl″tĭ-grăv′ĭ-d*ȧ*). A woman who has been pregnant several times, or many times.

multipara (mŭl-tĭp′*ȧ*-r*ȧ*). A woman who has borne several, or many, children.

multiple pregnancy. The condition in which two or more embryos develop in the uterus at the same time.

mutagen (mū′t*ȧ*-jěn). A chemical or substance that causes a change in gene structure or alteration of genetic information.

myoma (mī-ō′m*ȧ*). Pl. *myomata* (mī-ō′m*ȧ*-t*ȧ*). A uterine tumor made up of muscular elements; a benign tumor of the uterine muscle. Also called a *fibroid.*

myomotomy (mī″ō-mŏt′ō-mĭ). An incision into a myoma.

myotonia (mī″ō-tō′nĭ-*ȧ*). Increased muscle tension and tone; increased contractility of muscles.

myxedema (mĭk″sĕ-dē′m*ȧ*). A condition characterized by a dry, waxy type of swelling, with abnormal deposits of the glycoprotein mucin, in the skin. The facial changes are often associated with hypothyroidism.

Naegele's rule (nā′gĕ-lēz). A method of calculating the expected date of confinement. The date is calculated by subtracting 3 calendar months from the first day of the last menstrual period and adding 7 days.

natural childbirth See *prepared childbirth.*

natural method of birth control. An approach to contraception that relies upon identification of the fertile period and avoidance of intercourse during this time. Such a method may involve predicting ovulation by use of a menstrual calendar, identifying changes in cervical mucus, or identifying when ovulation has occurred using a basal body temperature chart, or a combination of these. Some couples use other contraceptive methods during the fertile period rather than avoid intercourse.

nausea (nä′sē-*ȧ*). An unpleasant feeling vaguely in the area of the upper abdomen that often culminates in vomiting.

navel (nāv′ĕl). The umbilicus.

neonatal (nē″ō-nā′t*ă*l). Pertaining to the newborn, usually considered the first 4 weeks of life.

- **n. asphyxia** (ăs-fĭk′sĭ-*ȧ*). Respiratory failure in a newborn infant; also called *asphyxia neonatorum.*
- **n. period.** The period from birth through the 28th day of life

neonatology (nē″ō-nā-tŏl′ō-jĭ). The study of the diagnosis and treatment of disorders of the newborn infant.

neurohormonal (nū″rō-hŏr′mō-n*ă*l). Pertaining to both a nerve or nerves and a hormone.

nevus (nē′v*ŭ*s). A natural mark or blemish; a mole, a circumscribed deposit of pigmentary matter in the skin present at birth (birthmark).

nidation (nĭ-dā′sh*ŭ*n). The implantation of the fertilized ovum in the endometrium of the pregnant uterus.

Niemann–Pick disease (nē′măn–pĭk). See *disease, Niemann–Pick.*

nocturnal ejaculation (nŏk-tûr′n*ă*l ē-jăk″ū-lā′sh*ŭ*n). An orgasm with ejaculation of seminal fluid that occurs during sleep particularly in adolescent boys. Also called *"wet dreams."*

nonorgasm (nŏn-ŏr′găzm). A female sexual dysfunction in which sexual arousal with congestion and lubrication occurs but orgasm is inhibited.

norm (nŏrm). Rule, generally for behavior.

nuclear family (nū′klē-*ă*r). A family group that consists of the father, mother, and children.

nulligravida (n*ŭ*″lĭ-grăv′ĭ-d*ȧ*). A woman who has never been pregnant.

nullipara (nŭ-lĭp′*ȧ*-r*ȧ*). A woman who has not borne children.

nurse–midwife. A registered nurse who has completed a recognized program of study and clinical experience leading to a certificate in nurse–midwifery.

nurse practitioner. A registered nurse with additional preparation in physical and psychosocial assessment, who provides primary care management for patients with common acute and chronic illnesses and developmental needs.

OB–GYN nurse practitioner. See *maternity nurse practitioner.*

obstetrics (ŏb-stĕt′rĭks). The branch of medicine that is concerned with the management of women during pregnancy, childbirth, and the puerperium.

occipitobregmatic (ŏk-sĭp″ĭt-ō-brĕg-măt′-ĭk). Pertaining to the occiput (the back part of the head) and the bregma (junction of the coronal and sagittal sutures).

OCT. Abbreviation for *oxytocin challenge test.*

oligohydramnios (ŏl″ĭ-gō-hī-drăm′nĭ-ŏs). Deficiency of amniotic fluid.

oligospermia (ŏl″ĭ-gō-spûr′mĭ-*ȧ*). Deficiency in the number of sperm cells in the semen.

oliguria (ŏl″ĭ-gū′rĭ-*ȧ*). Suppression of urinary excretion.

omphalic (ŏm-făl′ĭk). Pertaining to the umbilicus.

oocyesis (ō′ō-sī-ē′sĭs). Ovarian pregnancy.

oocyte (ō′ō-sīt). A developing egg cell in one of two stages. A primary oocyte develops from an oogonium, which subsequently divides into a secondary oocyte and a polar body. Ovulation follows, and the mature ovum and a second polar body develops.

oophorectomy (ō″ŏf-ō-rĕk′tō-mĭ). The surgical removal of an ovary or ovaries.

ophthalmia neonatorum (ŏf-thăl′mĭ-*ȧ*). Acute purulent conjunctivitis of the newborn usually due to gonorrheal infection.

oral contraceptive (ō′r*ă*l). A conception preventive taken by mouth.

organogenesis (ôr″g*ȧ*-nō-jen′ĕ-sĭs). The beginning and development of organs.

orgasm (ôr′găzm). The culmination of sexual excitement. Also called *climax.*

orgasmic platform (ŏr-găz′mĭk plăt′fôrm). The thickened area of congested tissue that builds up in and surrounds the lower third of the vagina during high levels of sexual arousal and just preceding orgasm.

Ortolani's maneuver (Or′tō lânēz). See *maneuver, Ortolani's.*

os (ŏs). Pl. *ora* (ō′r*ȧ*). Mouth.

- **o. externum** (*external os*). The external opening of the canal of the cervix.
- **o. internum** (*internal os*). Internal opening of canal of cervix.
- **o. uteri.** "Mouth of the uterus."

osmolality (ŏz″mō-lăl′ĭ-tĭ). A property of a solution that depends on the concentration of the substance dissolved per unit of solvent.

ova. Plural of ovum.

ovary (ō′v*ȧ*-rĭ). The sexual gland of the female in which the ova are developed. There are two ovaries, one at each side of the pelvis.

ovulation (ō-vū-lā'shŭn). The growth and discharge of an unimpregnated ovum, usually coincident with the menstrual peiod.

ovum (ō'vŭm). The female reproductive cell. The human ovum is a round cell about 1/120 of an inch in diameter, developed in the ovary.

oxytocic (ŏk"sĭ-tō'sĭk). 1. Accelerating parturition. 2. A medicine that accelerates parturition.

oxytocin (ŏk"sĭ-tō'sĭn). A hormone produced by the hypothalamus that stimulates contraction of the uterus, used to induce or intensify labor.

  o. challenge test. See *test, oxytocin challenge.*

pain (pān). A localized sensation of hurt. In clinical practice, it can be defined as whatever the experiencing person says it is, existing whenever he says it does.

  p. intensity. The severity of the pain sensation.

  p. tolerance. The intensity or duration of pain that the patient is willing to endure without making further efforts to relieve it.

palpation (păl-pā'shŭn). The act of feeling with the hands and fingers portions of the body for purposes of diagnosis.

palsy (pôl'zĭ). A synonym for paralysis, used in connection with certain special forms.

  Bell's p. Peripheral facial paralysis due to lesion of the facial nerve, resulting in characteristic distortion of the face.

  brachial p. (brā'kĭ-ăl). Paralysis of an arm.

  cerebral p. (sûr'ĕ-brăl, sē-rē'brăl). A motor and speech disorder resulting from an injury to the brain at birth or earlier.

  Erb's p. (ûrbz). The upper-arm type of brachial birth palsy.

Papanicolaou smear (păp"ă-nĭk"ō-lā'oo). Cytology test of cervical cells used as a screening for cervical cancer.

para (pär'ä). The term used to refer to past pregnancies that have produced an infant that has been viable, whether the infant is alive at birth or not.

paracervical block (păr"ă-sûr'vĭ-kăl blŏk). The blocking of neuropathways of pain by injecting a local anesthetic into the parametrium at sites in the cervix. It abolishes pain in the uterus only.

parametritis (păr"ă-mē-trī'tĭs). Inflammation of the parametrium. Also called *pelvic cellulitis.*

parametrium (păr-ă-mē'trĭ-ŭm). The fibrous subserous coat of the supravaginal portion of the uterus, extending laterally between the layers of the broad ligaments.

parenteral feeding (pă-rĕn'tĕr-ăl). Feeding by routes other than through the alimentary canal, such as intravenously.

parity (păr'ĭ-ti). The condition of a woman with respect to her having borne children.

parovarian (pär-ō-vâr'ĭ-ăn). Pertaining to the residual structure in the broad ligament between the ovary and the fallopian tube.

parturient (pär-tū'rĭ-ĕnt). Bringing forth; pertaining to childbearing. A woman in childbirth.

parturition (pär'tū-rĭsh'ŭn). The act or process of giving birth to a child.

patent ductus arteriosus (pă'tĕnt dŭk'tŭs ăr-tēr"ĭ-ō'sŭs). A congenital cardiac anomaly in which the vascular connection between the pulmonary artery and aorta, which is open during fetal life, does not close after birth as it should, causing the recirculation of arterial blood through the lungs.

patulous (păt'ū-lŭs). Spreading somewhat widely apart; open.

pedigree (pĕd'ĭ-grē). A record of an individual's ancestors. In genetics, it is used for analyzing Mendelian traits.

pelvic (pĕl'vĭk). Pertaining to the pelvis.

  p. axis. See *axis, pelvic.*

  p. cellulitis (sĕl"ū-lī'tĭs). See *parametritis.*

  p. congestion (kŏn-jĕst'yŭn). Excessive accumulation of blood in the pelvic region.

pelvimeter (pĕl-vĭm'ĕ-tĕr). An instrument for measuring the diameters and capacity of the pelvis.

pelvimetry (pĕl-vĭm'ĕ-trĭ). The measurement of the dimensions and capacity of the pelvis.

pelvis (pĕl'vĭs). The lower part of the body bounded by the two hip bones, the sacrum, and the coccyx.

  android p. (ăn'droid). One of the four main types of female pelvis, generally characterized as resembling the pelvis of a male and having a wedge-shaped inlet and narrow anterior segment.

  anthropoid p. (ăn'thrō-poid). One of the four main types of female pelvis, generally characterized by a long anteroposterior diameter of the inlet.

  contracted p. (kŏn-trăk'tĕd). A pelvis that measures 1 to 3 cm shorter than normal in any important diameter.

  false p. (fäls). The part of the pelvis superior to a plane passing through the linea terminalis.

  gynecoid p. (gī'nĕ-koid). The most prevalent of the four main types of female pelvis having a rounded oval shape.

  platypelloid p. (plăt"ĕ-pĕl'oid). One of the four main types of female pelvis having a flattened pelvic inlet.

  true p. (troo). The part of the pelvis inferior to a plane passing through the linea terminalis.

penis (pē'nĭs). The male organ of copulation.

perinatal (pĕr"ĭ-nā'tăl). Pertaining to the time before and after birth; variously defined as beginning at conception through the 28th day of life or conception through the first year of life.

perineorrhaphy (pĕr"ĭ-nē-ŏr'ăfĭ). Suture of the perineum; the operation for the repair of lacerations of the perineum.

perineotomy (pĕr"ĭ-nē-ot'ō-mĭ). A surgical incision through the perineum.

perineum (pĕr"ĭ-nē'ŭm). The area between the vagina and the rectum.

peritoneoscopy (pĕr"ĭ-tō"nē-ŏs'kō-pĭ). Direct visualization of the tubes and ovaries with an endoscope.

peritoneum (pĕr"ĭ-tō-nē'ŭm). A strong serous membrane investing the inner surface of the abdominal walls and the viscera of the abdomen.

peritonitis (pĕr"ĭ-tō-nī'tĭs). Inflammation of the peritoneum.

phenylketonuria (PKU) (fĕn"il-kē"tō-nū'rĭ-ă). An inborn

error of metabolism resulting in a deficiency in liver enzyme. It may be detected by blood or urine tests. Early treatment will prevent mental retardation.

phimosis (fī-mō'sĭs). Tightness of the foreskin.

phlebitis (flĕ-bī'tĭs). Inflammation of a vein.

phlegmasia alba dolens (flĕg-mā'zhĭ'*ȧ* ăl'b*ȧ* dō'lĕnz). "Milk leg." Phlebitis of the femoral vein, occasionally following delivery.

phocomelia (fō"kō-mē'lĭ-*ȧ*). A developmental anomaly characterized by total absence or stunting of the arms or legs.

phospholipid (fŏs"fō-lĭp'ĭd). Any lipid that contains phosphorus; the major form of lipid in all cell membranes.

phototherapy (fō"tō-thĕr'*ȧ*-pĭ). The use of light to treat a disease, especially the use of intense fluorescent light to reduce serum bilirubin in the treatment of hyperbilirubinemia.

physiologic jaundice (fĭz"ē-ō-lŏj'ĭk jôn'dĭs). Mild icterus neonatorum lasting a few days.

pica (pī'k*ȧ*). The abnormal intake of specific substances such as clay dirt, cornstarch, or plaster. It may characterize the behavior of malnourished children or pregnant women.

pit drip. The administration of Pitocin (usually during the third stage of labor) by intravenous drip.

Pitocin (pī-tŏ'sĭn). A proprietary solution of oxytocin.

PKU. Abbreviation for *phenylketonuria.*

placenta (pl*ȧ*-sĕn't*ȧ*). The circular, flat, vascular structure in the impregnated uterus forming the principal medium of communication between the mother and the fetus.

- **ablatio p.** See *abruptio placentae.*
- **abruptio p.** Premature separation of the normally implanted placenta.
- **previa p.** A placenta that is implanted in the lower uterine segment so that it adjoins or covers the internal os of the cervix.

platypelloid pelvis (plăt"ĭ-pĕl'oid pĕl'vĭs). See *pelvis, platypelloid.*

plexus (plĕks'*ŭ*s). A network or tangle, such as a network of veins, lymphatic vessels, or nerves.

polycythemia (pŏl"ē-sī-thē'mĭ-*ȧ*). An increased red blood cell volume.

polydactyly (pŏl"ē-dăk't*ĭ*-lĭ). A developmental anomaly characterized by extra digits on the hands or feet.

polygalactia (pŏl"ē-g*ă*-lăk'shē-*ȧ*). Excessive secretion of milk.

polyhydramnios (pŏl"ĭ-hī-drăm'nĭ-ŏs). Hydramnios.

polyp (pŏl'ĭp). A protrusion growing from a mucous membrane.

position (pō-zĭsh'*ŭ*n). The situation of the fetus in the pelvis; determined by the relation of some arbitrarily chosen portion of the fetus to the right or the left side of the mother's pelvis. Thus, each presentation has either a right or left position.

postasphyxia encephalopathy (pōst"ăs-fĭks'ĭ-*ȧ* ĕn-sĕf"*ȧ*-lŏp'*ȧ*-thĭ). One of various central nervous system symptoms caused by injury resulting from episodes of perinatal asphyxia.

postcoital test (pōst-kō'*ĭ*-t*ă*l). See *test, postcoital.*

postmaturity (pōst"-mă-tū'rĭ-tĭ). Overdevelopment, as of a postmature infant who was born after pregnancy has progressed beyond full term.

postnatal (pōst-nā't*ă*l). Occurring after birth, referring to the infant.

postpartal (pōst-pär't*ă*l). After delivery or childbirth, referring to the mother.

postpartum period. The period occurring after childbirth, referring to the mother.

PPM. Abbreviation for *psychoprophylactic method of prepared childbirth.*

precipitate delivery (prē-sĭp'*ĭ*-tāt dē-lĭv'ĕr-ĭ). A delivery that occurs with undue rapidity (less than 3 hours) and usually without the benefit of asepsis.

preeclampsia (prē-ĕk-lămp'sĭ-*ȧ*). A disorder encountered during pregnancy or early in the puerperium, characterized by hypertension, edema, and albuminuria.

pregnancy (prĕg'n*ă*n-sĭ). [Latin, *praeg'nans,* literally "previous to bringing forth."] The state of being with young or with child. The normal duration of pregnancy in the human female is 280 days, or 10 lunar months, or 9 calendar months. See also *abdominal.*

- **p., ectopic p., interstitial p., multiple p., tubal p.**

premature infant. An infant that weighs 2500 g or less at birth.

premature ejaculation. A male sexual dysfunction in which difficulty is met in controlling orgasm for a sufficient period of time to enable his partner to attain sexual satisfaction.

prematurity. Underdevelopment, as of a premature infant.

premenstrual tension (prē-mĕn'stroo-*ă*l tĕn'sh*ŭ*n). A syndrome sometimes experienced during the 10 days preceding menstruation. It is characterized by irritability, insomnia, headache, pain in the breasts, abdominal distention, nausea, anorexia, constipation, emotional instability, and urinary frequency.

prepared childbirth. The methods by which parents actively participate in childbirth. Some approaches include the concepts and techniques of Dick–Read, Lamaze, and Bradley. Also called *natural childbirth.*

prepuce (prē'pūs). The fold of skin that covers the glans penis in the male.

- **p. of the clitoris.** The fold of mucous membrane that covers the glans clitoris.

presentation (prĕ"zĕn-tā'sh*ŭ*n). Term used to designate that part of the fetus nearest the internal os; or that part that is felt by the physician's examining finger when introduced into the cervix.

presumptive signs of pregnancy (prē-sŭmp'tĭv). Signs that strongly suggest that a healthy woman is pregnant. These include menstrual suppression, nausea, vomiting, frequency of micturition, tenderness and other changes of breasts, "quickening", Chadwick's sign, pigmentation of the skin, and abdominal striae.

primigravida (prī"mĭ-grăv'ĭ-d*ȧ*). Pl. *primigravidae* (prī"mĭ-grăv'ĭ-dē). A woman who is pregnant for the first time.

primipara (prī-mĭp'*ȧ*-r*ȧ*). Pl. *primiparae* (prī"mĭ-grăv'ĭ-dē). A woman who has given birth to her first child.

primordial (prī-môr'dĭ-*ă*l). Original or primitive; or the simplest and most undeveloped character.

probable signs of pregnancy. Signs that the likelihood of pregnancy is great. These include enlargement of the abdomen, changes in the size, shape, and consistency of the uterus, fetal outline felt by palpation, changes in the cervix, Braxton–Hicks contractions, and a positive pregnancy test.

prodromal (prŏ-drō'măl). Premonitory; indicating the approach of a disease.

p. labor. The latent or early phase in which there is some effacement and slow dilatation of the cervix. It lasts perhaps an averge of 8½ hours in a nullipara.

progesterone (prō-jĕs'tĕr-ōn). The pure hormone contained in the corpora lutea whose function is to prepare the endometrium for the reception and development of the fertilized ovum.

progestin (prō-jĕs'tĭn). Any of the synthetic progesterone preparations that are used in oral contraceptives. The common types include norethynodrel, norethindrone, ethynodiol diacetate, and norgestrel.

prolactin (prō-lăk'tĭn). A proteohormone from the anterior pituitary that stimulates lactation in the mammary glands.

prolan (prō'lăn). Zondek's term for the gonadotropic principle of human-pregnancy urine, responsible for the biologic pregnancy tests.

prolapse of umbilical cord (prō-lăps' ŏv ŭm-bĭl'*i*-*kăl* kōrd). Delivery of the umbilical cord in labor prior to the delivery of the fetus.

promontory (prŏm'*ŭ*n-tō"rĭ). A small projection; a prominence.

p. of the sacrum. The superior or projecting portion of the sacrum when in situ in the pelvis, at the junction of the sacrum and the last lumbar vertebra.

prostaglandin (prŏs"t*a*-glăn'dĭn). Any of a group of fatty acids found in semen, which are effective abortifacients at any stage of pregnancy. These are the most common agents for inducing midtrimester abortion through instillation into the amniotic fluid.

prostate gland (prŏs'tāte). A gland in the male that surrounds the neck of the bladder and urethra.

proteinuria (prō"tē-ĭn-ū'rĭ-*a*). The presence of protein in the urine.

pseudocyesis (sū"dō-sī-ē'sĭs). An apparent condition of pregnancy; the woman really believes she is pregnant when, as a matter of fact, she is not.

psychogenic sexual stimuli (sī"kō-gĕn'ĭk sĕk'shoo-*ă*l stĭm'ū-lī). Stimuli processed through the higher brain centers that cause sexual arousal. These include sensory stimuli such as sight, sound, taste, smell, and touch, and cognitive events such as thoughts, fantasies, memories, and images.

psychophysiology (sī"kō-fĭz"ĭ-ŏl'ō-gĭ). The interaction between psychological and physiological processes, that is, between higher mental processes and the responses of muscles, glands, and organs.

psychoprophylactic method of prepared childbirth (PPM) (sī"kō-prō"fĭl-ăk'tĭc). See *Lamaze method of delivery*.

psychosexual method of childbirth (sī"kō-sĕks'ū-*ă*l). A method of childbirth prepartion developed by Sheila Kitzinger based on a method using sensory memory and the Stanislavsky method of acting. Sexuality is seen as part of the larger whole encompassing family relationships, birth, cuddling, and feeding.

puberty (pū'bĕr-tĭ). The age at which the generative organs become functionally active.

pubic (pū'bĭk). Belonging to the pubis.

pubiotomy (pū'bĭ-ŏt'ō-mĭ). The operation of cutting through the pubic bone lateral to the median line.

pubis (pū'bĭs). The os pubis or pubic bone forming the front of the pelvis.

pudenda (pū-dĕn'd*a*). [L.] The plural of pudendum.

pudendal (pū-dĕn'd*ă*l). Relating to the pudenda.

p. block. The blocking of neuropathways of pain by injecting a local anesthetic into the pudendal nerve. It abolishes pain in the vagina and perineum.

pudendum (pū-dĕn'd*ŭ*m). [Latin, *pudere,* to have shame or modesty.] The external genital parts of either sex, but especially of the female.

puerperal fever (pū-ĕr'pĕr-*ă*l). Infection, accompanied by fever, which develops in a wound to the birth canal during delivery.

puerperium (pū"ĕr-pē'rĭ-*ŭ*m). The period elapsing between the termination of labor and the return of the uterus to its normal condition, about 6 weeks.

pulmonary dysmaturity (pŭl'mō-nĕr"ĭ dĭs-m*a*-tūr'ĭ-tĭ). An insidious disease of premature infants beginning with mild respiratory symptoms after the first week of life. The cause is thought to be collapse of the bronchial tree, with partial airway obstruction following aspiration of small amounts of milk as a result of a poorly developed gag reflex. Also known as *Wilson–Mikity disease*.

pyelonephritis (pī"ĕ-lō-nĕ-frī'tĭs). Inflammation of the kidney due to bacterial infection. In pregnancy, hormonal and anatomical changes cause narrowing of the lower ureter and dilation of the upper ureter and renal pelvis, thus increasing the risk of infection.

pyloric stenosis (pī-lôr'ĭk stĕn-ō'sĭs). A congenital anomaly manifested in an infant from the first to the second or third week by projectile vomiting 30 minutes after feeding. Surgery removes a stricture of the pylorus that is the cause.

quickening (kwĭk'ĕn-ĭng). The mother's first perception of the movements of the fetus.

rabbit test. See *test, Friedman's*.

radioimmunoassay test. See *test, radioimmunoassay*.

RDS. Abbreviation for *respiratory distress syndrome*. See *disease, hyaline membrane*.

Read method of childbirth preparation. See *Dick–Read approach to childbirth*.

reanastomosis (rē"*a*-năs"tō-mō'sĭs). The reestablishing of a connection between vessels, such as surgically reconnecting the severed vas deferens or fallopian tubes following sterilization. The purpose of this surgery is to reestablish fertility, but success rates are variable.

recessive inheritance (rē-sĕs′ĭv ĭn-hĕr′ĭ-tăns). The acquisition of a characteristic from both parents that is the result of an allele that must be carried by both members of a pair of homologous chromosomes.

rectocele (rĕk′tō-sēl). The protrusion by hernia of a part of the rectum into the vagina.

reflex (rē′flĕks). An involuntary activity.

grasp r. The reflex present at birth in an infant's hands and feet causing the fingers and toes to curl around an object placed touching them.

let-down r. See *milk ejection r.*

milk ejection r. The activation of a process by which contractions of the myoepithelial cells in a mother's breast propel milk along the duct into the lactiferous sinuses. Also called *let-down reflex* and *milk let-down.*

Moro r. (mō′rō). See *startle r.*

rooting r. The tendency of an infant to open his mouth and turn toward an object that is gently stroking his cheek or the corner of his mouth.

startle r. The reflex that is present from birth to age 3 months that indicates an awareness of equilibrium by a symmetrical drawing up of legs and grasping of arms in response to a sudden jarring of his crib or clothes. Also known as *Moro reflex.*

stepping r. The reflex that is present at birth but disappears soon after that causes an infant to make little stepping or prancing movements when he is held upright with his feet touching a surface.

sucking r. The reflex in infants to suck anything that comes in contact with their lips. It seems to be a great need for the first 2 months of life, is present while sleeping, and need not be nutritive.

swallowing r. The reflex present at birth to swallow food that an infant sucks into his mouth.

tonic neck r. (tŏn′ĭk). The tendency of an infant while lying on his back to turn his head to one side and extend the arm and leg on that side, flexing the arm and leg on the other side.

reflexogenic sexual stimulus (rē-flĕk″sō-jĕn′ĭk). A direct stimulation of an erogenous area that causes sexual arousal in a reflexive, or automatic, manner.

respiratory distress syndrome (RDS) (rē-spī′ră-tō″rī). See *disease, hyaline membrane.*

resuscitation (rē-sŭs″ĭ-tā′shŭn). The restoring to life of a patient who is apparently dead or dying.

retinal vein thrombosis (rĕt′ĭ-năl vān thrŏm-bō′sĭs). The presence of an obstruction caused by an aggregation of blood factors in the retinal vein. This clotting disorder may be partially the result of the use of oral contraceptives.

retroflexion (rĕt″rō-flĕk′shŭn). The bending backward of an organ on its axis, specifically the tipping backward of a uterus upon itself.

retrolental fibroplasia (rĕ″trō-lĕn′tăl fī″brō-plā′sĭ-ă). An acquired disease of a premature infant resulting in eye injury as a result of continuous oxygen therapy in high concentration.

retroversion (rĕt″rō-vûr′zhŭn). The tipping backward of an entire organ; in the case of retroversion of the uterus, the turning back of the entire uterus in relation to the pelvic axis.

Rh. Abbreviation for *Rhesus,* a type of monkey. This term is used for a property of human blood cells, because of its relationship to a similar property in the blood cells of Rhesus monkeys.

Rh factor. A term applied to an inherited antigen in the human blood.

RhoGAM (rō′găm). A preparation of anti-Rh antibodies administered by injection to unsensitized Rh negative women following childbirth or abortion, to prevent the development of endogenous antibodies which could later lead to erythroblastosis fetalis (Rh disease of the fetus) in a subsequent pregnancy.

rhythm method (rĭth′m). A birth control method relying upon abstinence from sexual intercourse before, during, and after the period of time the ovum is capable of being fertilized.

Ritgen maneuver (rĭt-gĕn mă-noo′vĕr). See *maneuver, Ritgen.*

roentgenogram (rĕnt-gĕn′ō-grăm). A record of the internal structure of a body by the use of x-ray photography.

role complementarity (rōl kŏm″plĕ-mĕn-tăr′ĭ-tī). The learning of roles in pairs.

role differentiation (rōl dĭf″ĕr-ĕn″shē-ā′shŭn). The process by which roles are structured and delineated.

roll over test. See *test, roll over.*

rooming-in. The hospital practice in which postpartum mothers have their infants in their rooms all the time, except for necessary examinations or procedures.

rooting reflex. See *reflex, rooting.*

rotation (rō-tā′shŭn). The turning on an axis; specifically, in labor, the turning of the fetal head through a right angle so that the longest diameter of the head corresponds to the longest diameter of the pelvic outlet.

rubella (roo-bĕl′ă). German measles.

r. syndrome. See *syndrome, rubella.*

Rubin's test (roo′bĭnz). See *test, Rubin's.*

rupture of the membranes (rŭp′tūr). The breaking of the amniotic sac, which may occur spontaneously and be the first indication of approaching labor. If the membranes have not ruptured previously, they must be broken before the fetal head is delivered to prevent aspiration of fluid when the infant takes its first breath.

sacral promontory (sā′krăl prŏm′ŭn-tō″rī). The marked projection in the pelvis formed by the junction of the last lumbar vertebra with the sacrum.

sacrococcygeal articulation (sā″krō-kŏk-sĭj′ē-ăl är-tĭk″ū-lā′shŭn). The joint or juncture of the sacrum and coccyx.

sacroiliac articulation (sā″krō-il′ĭ-ăk är-tĭk″ū-lā′shŭn). The two joints or junctures of the sacrum and the ilium on either side of the pelvis.

sacrum (sā′krŭm). A triangular wedge-shaped bone, consisting of five vertebrae fused together, which serves as the back part of the pelvis.

saddle block (săd′'l blŏk). The blocking of neuropathways of pain by injecting a local anesthetic into the subarachnoid space in the spine. A *true saddle block* blocks pain in the perineum. A *modified saddle block* abolishes both uterine and perineal discomfort.

Saf-T-coil. One of the commonly used intrauterine devices.

salpingitis (săl″pĭn-jī′tĭs). Inflammation of the fallopian tubes.

scarf sign (skärf sīn). A test to assess infant maturity. The infant's arms are drawn across the neck and as far across the opposite shoulder as possible. In the premature infant there is less resistance and greater draping (or scarf) effect; the elbow will reach near or across the midline. In the full term infant, the elbow will not reach the midline.

Schultze's mechanism (shoolt′sĕz). The expulsion of the placenta with the fetal surfaces presenting.

sebum (sē′bŭm). The secretions of the sebaceous glands of the skin; a thick, semifluid substance composed of fat and epithelial cell debris.

secondary areola. See *areola, secondary.*

secundines (sĕk′ŭn-dīn). The afterbirth; the placenta and membranes expelled after the birth of a child.

segmentation (sĕg″mĕn-tā′shŭn). The process of division by which the fertilized ovum multiplies before differentiation into layers occurs.

Sellick's maneuver (sĕl′ĭks mȧ-noo′vĕr). See *maneuver, Sellick's.*

semen (sē′mĕn). 1. A seed. 2. The fluid secreted by the male reproductive organs.

sex chromatin (sĕks krō′mȧ-tĭn). See *Barr body.*

sex chromosome (sĕks krō′mō-sōm). One of two chromosomes in human cells that are associated with the determination of the sex of the individual. A male cell normally contains one X and one Y chromosome, a female cell contains two X chromosomes.

sex-linked inheritance trait. An inheritance trait in which the gene is carried on the X chromosome and is expressed in the male offspring. (Males do not possess another X chromosome to offset the effects of the X chromosome that carries the gene.)

sexologist (sĕks-ŏl′ō-jĭst). A specialist in the area of human sexuality; one engaged in sex research or particularly learned in the physiological, behavior, or psychoemotional aspects of sexuality.

sex role. The public expression of gender identity; all actions used to convey one's maleness or femaleness.

sex therapy. A short-term therapy aimed at relief of the sexual symptom, which uses systematically structured sexual experiencing with conjoint therapeutic sessions. It is designed to modify immediate obstacles to sexual functioning, although intrapsychic and transactional conflicts are also dealt with to some extent.

sexual dysfunction (sĕk′shoo-ăl dĭs-fŭnk′shŭn). A psychosomatic disorder that makes it impossible for an individual to have or enjoy intercourse. There is inadequate sexual response involving both vasocongestive and orgasmic components either together or separately. See also *impotence, premature ejaculation, vaginismus, lack of arousal, nonorgasm,* and *dyspareunia.*

sexuality (sĕk′shoo-ăl′ĭ-tĭ). The complex of emotions, attitudes, preferences, and behaviors related to the individual's expression of the sexual self and eroticism. Components of sexuality include the individual's genetic, hormonal, gonadal, and morphological sex gender identity, sex role, and sexual partner preference.

SGA. Abbreviation for *small for gestational age.*

Shake test. See *test, shake.*

Shirodkar technique (shĭ-rŏd′kär tĕk-nēk). A treatment in the early part of the second trimester for incompetent cervical os to prevent relaxation and dilation of the cervix. The vaginal mucous membrane is elevated, and the internal os of the cervix is encircled by a thin strip. Then the vaginal membrane is restored to its original position and sutured. The suture is removed for a vaginal delivery or, if it is in good position, it is maintained and cesarean section may be elected.

shoulder dystocia (shŏl′dĕr dĭs-tō′sĭ-ȧ). A serious complication in the birth of an oversized infant whose unusually large shoulders arrest at either the pelvic brim or the outlet.

shoulder presentation (shŏl′dĕr prē″zĕn-tā′shŭn). A serious complication of birth in which the infant lies crosswise in the uterus instead of longitudinally. The risk of perinatal mortality is reduced by a cesarean delivery.

show (shō). Popularly, the blood-tinged mucus discharged from the vagina before or during labor.

sickle cell anemia (sĭk′'l sĕl ă-nē′mĭ-ȧ). A hereditary, genetically determined hemolytic anemia. It is generally manifest before childbearing, and crises may occur in the nonpregnant as well as pregnant state. One must consider not only the impact of pregnancy in precipitating crises in a patient with sickle cell anemia but also the genetic outlook and limited life expectancy of the patient.

sitz bath (sĭtz). A treatment for perineal or perianal discomfort in which the patient sits for 20 minutes three to four times per day in very warm water that may have astringents or solutions added.

Skene's gland. One of two glands just within the meatus of the female urethra; regarded as the homologue of the prostate gland in the male.

smegma. A thick cheesy secretion found under the prepuce and in the region of the clitoris and the labia minora.

small for gestational age (SGA). Pertaining to infants whose weight falls below the tenth percentile for their gestational age. These infants have experienced growth retardation during the prenatal period and may be born close to term but weigh less than 2500 g.

socialization (sō″shăl-ĭ-zā′shŭn). The process by which an individual learns society's expectations for behavior.

souffle (soof′f'l). A soft, blowing auscultatory sound.

funic s. A hissing souffle; synchronous with the fetal heart sounds and supposed to be produced in the umbilical cord.

placental s. A souffle supposed to be produced by the blood current in the placenta.

spermatid (spûr′mȧ-tĭd). A developing sperm cell that results from fission of a secondary spermatocyte. With development of a tail, it becomes a mature spermatozoon.

spermatocyte (spûr′mȧ-tō-sīt). A developing sperm cell in one of two stages. A primary spermatocyte develops from a spermatogonium and subsequently divides into two secondary spermatocytes. Each spermatocyte divides into two spermatids.

spermatogenesis (spûr′mȧ-tō-jĕn′ĕ-sĭs). The process of forming spermatozoa.

spermatogonium (spûr′mȧ-tō-gō′nĭ-ŭm). Pl. *spermatogonia* (spûr′mȧ-tō-gō′nĭ-ȧ). The undivided male germ cell that develops into the seminiferous tubes. Each will eventually develop into four spermatozoa.

spermatozoon (spûr′mȧ-tō-zō′ŏn). Pl. *spermatozoa* (spûr′mȧ-tō-zō′ȧ). A mature male germ cell; the mobile microscopic sexual element that resembles in shape an elongated tadpole.

spermicide (spûr′mĭ-sīd). An agent that destroys spermatozoa; used as a contraceptive.

sphingomyelin lipidosis (sfĭng″gō-mī′ĕ-lĭn lĭp″ĭ-dō′sĭs). See *disease, Niemann–Pick.*

spina bifida (spī′nȧ bĭf′ĭd-ȧ). A rather common malformation due to the congenital absence of one or more vertebral arches, usually at the lower part of the spine.

s. b. occulta (ŏk-ŭl′tȧ). Spina bifida in which the defect to the spinal canal does not include protrusion of the cord and meninges.

spinal anesthesia (spī′năl an″ĕs-thē′zĭ-ȧ). Relief of pain by injecting a local anesthetic into the subarachnoid space in the spine.

spontaneous abortion (spŏn-tā′nē-ŭs ă-bŏr′shŭn). See *abortion, spontaneous.*

Stanislavsky method (stăn″ĭ-släf′skĭ). A technique used in acting in which the actor tries to empathize with the character he is portraying. It is used in teaching relaxation in the psychosexual (Kitsinger) method of childbirth preparation.

startle reflex (stăr′t′l rē′flĕks). See *reflex, startle.*

stenosis (stĕ-nō′sĭs). The narrowing of a duct or canal. See *pyloric stenosis.*

stepping reflex. See reflex, stepping.

sterilization (stĕr″ĭ-lĭ-zā′shŭn). 1. A process of eliminating microbial viability. 2. A permanent method of contraception; process by which an individual is made incapable of reproduction.

stillborn (stĭl′bôrn″). Born without life; born dead.

stork bite. A cluster of small capillaries that may be apparent on the nape of the neck, the eyelids, or over the bridge of the nose of a newborn infant. These usually disappear spontaneously during infancy.

stria (strī′ȧ). Pl. *striae* (strī′ē). A Latin word signifying a "groove," "furrow," or "crease."

striae gravidarum (grăv-ĭ-där′ŭm). Shining, reddish lines upon the abdomen, thighs, and breasts during pregnancy.

subdural hematoma (sŭb-dū′răl hĕm″ȧ-tō′mȧ). A hemorrhage under the tough outer covering (periosteum) of the skull or cranium.

subinvolution (sŭb′ĭn-vō-lū′shŭn). Failure of a part to return to its normal size and condition after enlargement from functional activity, as subinvolution of the uterus which exists when normal involution of the puerperal uterus is retarded.

succedaneum (sŭk′sē-dā′nē-ŭm). See *caput.*

sucking reflex. See *reflex, sucking.*

suction curettage (sŭk′shŭn kū″rĕ-täzh′). A method of first trimester abortion utilizing cervical dilation and suction evacuation of uterine contents. Also known as *dilatation and evacuation (D&E).*

superfecundation (sū′pĕr-fē-kŭn-dā′shŭn). The fertilization at about the same time of two different ova by sperm from different males.

superfetation (sū′pĕr-fē-tā′shŭn). The fecundation of a woman already pregnant.

suppository, contraceptive (sŭ-pŏz′ĭ-tō-rĭ). A suppository containing a spermicide that is inserted in the vagina prior to intercourse for purposes of contraception.

suprapubic (soo″prȧ-pū′bĭk). Located above the pubic area; slightly above the symphysis pubis in the midlower abdomen.

surfactant (sûr-făk′tȧnt). A mixture of the secretions of the lungs and air passages that reduces the surface tension of pulmonary fluids and thus contributes to the elastic properties of lung tissue.

swallowing reflex. See *reflex, swallowing.*

symphysis (sĭm′fĭ-sĭs). The union of bones by means of an intervening substance; a variety of synathrosis.

s. pubis (pū′bĭs). "Symphysis of the pubis," the pubic articulation or union of the pubic bones, which are connected with each other by interarticular cartilage.

symptothermal method (sĭmp″tō-thêr′măl). Combination of the ovulation, or Billings, method (based on symptoms that provide clues as to when ovulation is occurring) and the BBT method. This approach tends to improve effectiveness of the fertility awareness approach to birth control. It also decreases the number of days on which a couple is permitted to have sexual intercourse.

synchondrosis (sĭng″kŏn-drō′sĭs). A union of bones by means of a fibrous or elastic cartilage.

syncope (sĭng′kō-pē). A temporary loss of consciousness; a faint.

syndrome (sĭn′drōm). A set of symptoms characterizing a particular state of abnormality or illness.

adrenogenital s. (ăd-rĕn″ō-jĕn′ĭ-tăl). A hyperfunction of the adrenal cortex. It is manifested by virilism in the female at birth and precocious sexual development in the male 3 or 4 years after birth.

Asherman's s. (ă′shēr-mănz). Amenorrhea due to adhesions within the uterine cavity, usually as a result of postpartal or postabortal infection or pelvic tuberculosis.

Down's s. (downz). A chromosomal abnormality characterized by slanting eyes set close together; narrow palpebral fissures; flat nose; protruding large fissured tongue; small head and flat occiput; broad pudgy neck; short, thick hands with simian creases on the palms; defective mentality; underdeveloped muscles, loose joints; and heart and alimentary tract abnormalities. The syndrome may be inherited although its incidence increases with maternal age. Also called *trisomy 21* and, formerly, *mongolism.*

fetal alcohol s. A congenital anomaly resulting from maternal alcohol intake above 3 oz of absolute alcohol per day. It is characterized by typical craniofacial and limb defects, cardiovascular defects, intrauterine growth retardation, and developmental delay. No *safe* alcohol limit has been determined.

Klinefelter's s. (klīn'fĕl-tĕrz). A genetic defect characterized by variable degrees of masculinization, small testes, or uncertain genitalia.

Marfan's s. (mär'fănz). See *arachnodactyly.*

respiratory distress s. See *disease, hyaline membrane.*

rubella s. A congenital syndrome caused by a rubella infection suffered by the mother during the first 16 weeks of pregnancy. It is characterized by varying combinations of cardiac anomalies, eye defects, developmental ear defects, encephalitis, immunologic defects, jaundice, osteomyelitis, pneumonitis, and other problems.

Turner's s. (tûr'nērz). A genetic defect characterized by undifferentiated gonads, short stature, and other abnormalities which may include webbing of the neck, low posterior hairline, and cardiac defects.

synergistic (sĭn"ĕr-jĭs'tĭk). Acting together in a way that one agent enhances the effect of the other, and their combined effect is greater than the sum of their individual effects.

syphilis (sĭf'ĭ-lĭs). A serious contagious venereal disease that is transmitted by direct intimate contact or congenitally. It is divided into three stages (primary, secondary and tertiary) that have different characteristics, lesions being apparent in the primary and secondary stages. It is treatable by penicillin.

talipes equinovarus (tăl'ĭ-pēz ē-kwī"nō-vā'rŭs). The typical clubfoot. Its elements are equinus or plantar flexion of the foot at the ankle, varus or inversion deformity of the heel, and forefoot adduction.

Tay–Sachs disease (tā-săks'). See *disease, Tay–Sachs.*

TENS. Abbreviation for *transcutaneous electric nerve stimulation.*

teratogen (tĕr'ă-tō-jĕn). A chemical or substance that interferes with fetal development after conception.

teratogenic (tĕr"ă-tō-jĕn'ĭk). Tending to produce anomalies of formation or physical defects in an embryo or fetus.

test (tĕst). An examination, trial, or method of assessment.

Aschheim–Zondek t. (ăsh"hīm–tsŏn'dĕk). A test for the diagnosis of pregnancy. Repeated injections of small quantities of urine voided during the first weeks of pregnancy produce in infantile mice, within 100 hours, (1) minute intrafollicular ovarian hemorrhage and (2) the development of lutein cells.

Friedman's t. (frēd'măn). A modification of the Aschheim–Zondek test for pregnancy; the urine of early pregnancy is injected in 4-ml doses intravenously twice daily for 2 days into an unmated mature rabbit. If, at the end of this time, the ovaries of the rabbit contain fresh corpora lutea or hemorrhagic corpora, the test is positive.

glucose tolerance t. (GTT) (gloo'kōs tŏl'ĕr-ăns). A test of carbohydrate metabolism in which 100 g of glucose is given orally while fasting; blood sugar should return to normal in 2 to 2½ hours. It is a test for diabetes.

oxytocin challenge t. (ŏk"sĭ-tō'sĭn). A test providing information about uteroplacental function, fetal response, and indications of fetal distress.

postcoital t. (pōst-kō'ĭ-tăl). A test of the cervical mucus within 12 hours following intercourse. It permits evaluation of placement of spermatozoa, the quality of cervical secretions, and their ability to support the life of spermatozoa.

rabbit t. (răb'ĭt). See *Friedman's test.*

radioimmunoassay t. (rā"dĭ-ō-ĭm"ū-nō-ăs'ā). A test for pregnancy of blood serum. It is very accurate from the eighth day after fertilization.

rollover t. A simple test for preeclampsia in which the diastolic blood pressure is recorded with the patient in a lateral recumbent position, then on her back. A positive result is indicated if diastolic blood pressure increases by 20 mm Hg or more.

Rubin's t. (roo'bĭnz). A test for evaluating tubal function using uterotubal insufflation with carbon dioxide. If the manometer registers no higher than 100 mm Hg, the tubes are patent. If it rises to 200 mm Hg, the tubes are completely occluded.

Shake t. (shāk). The foam stability test to measure precisely the L/S ratio in the fetus. It is relatively simple and quick. The test depends on the ability of the surfactant in the amniotic fluid when mixed with ethanol to generate stable foam at the air–liquid interface.

testicle (tĕs"tĭ-k'l). One of the two glands contained in the male scrotum.

testosterone (tĕs-tŏs'tĕ-rōn). The principal male sex hormone produced in the testes in response to the luteinizing hormone. It is believed to be responsible for regulating spermatogenesis, male characteristics, and maintaining muscle mass and bone tissue in the adult.

tetralogy of Fallot (tĕ-trăl'ō-jĭ ŏv făl-ō'). A combination of four congenital cardiac anomalies including ventrical septal defect, pulmonary stenosis, overriding aorta, and hypertrophy of the right ventricle.

theoretical effectiveness of a contraceptive method. The maximum effectiveness of a contraceptive method in preventing pregnancy under ideal conditions and when it is completely understood.

thermacogenesis (thûr"mă-kō-jĕn'ĕ-sĭs). The elevating of body temperature by the action of a drug.

thermal regulation (thûr'măl reg"ū-lā'shŭn). Regulation of body heat. Pertains particularly to the newborn's ability to regulate his temperature.

threatened abortion. See *abortion, threatened.*

thromboembolic disorder (thrŏm″bō-ĕm-bō′lĭc). A disorder involving the obstruction of a blood vessel with thrombotic material brought by the blood to the site from its origin.

thromboembolism (thrŏm″bō-ĕm′bō-lĭzm). The blocking of a blood vessel with a thrombus that has broken loose from its site of formation.

thrombophlebitis (thrŏm″bō-flē-bī′tĭs). A condition in which inflammation of the wall of a vein has preceded the formation of a thrombus.

thrombus (thrŏm′bŭs). A coagulation of blood elements, often causing an obstruction at the point of formation.

thrush. An infection caused by the fungus *Candida albicans,* characterized by whitish plaques in the mouth.

tocodynamometer (tō″kō-dī″nă-mŏm′ĕ-tĕr). An instrument that measures the expulsive force of uterine contractions in childbirth.

tomography (tō-mŏg′ră-fī). The recording of internal body images in a particular plane by using an x-ray source.

tongue-tie (tŭng′tī). A condition in which the attachment of the thin ridge of tissue in the middle of the base of the tongue (the frenulum linguae) extends far forward causing a concavity at the tip of the tongue on its upper surface. Also called *lingua frenata.*

tonic neck reflex. See *reflex, tonic neck.*

TORCH infections. An acronym for toxoplasmosis, rubella, cytomegaly, and herpes infections.

toxemia (tŏks-ē′mī-ă). The toxemias of pregnancy are disorders encountered during gestation, or early in the puerperium, which are characterized by one or more of the following signs; hypertension, edema, albuminuria, and, in severe cases, convulsions and coma.

toxoplasmosis (tŏk″sō-plăz-mō′sĭs). A congenital disease characterized by lesions of the central nervous system, which may lead to blindness, brain defects, and death.

transcutaneous electric nerve stimulation (trăns″kū-tān′ē-ŭs). The use of a mild electric current through the skin to relieve pain.

transposition of the great vessels (trăns″pō-sĭ′shŭn). A congenital cardiac anomaly in which the aorta originates from the right ventricle rather than the left, and the pulmonary artery originates from the left ventricle rather than the right.

transsexualism (trăns-sĕk′shoo-ă-lĭz′m). Behaviorally, the act of living and passing in the role of a member of the opposite sex, before or after having attained hormonal, surgical, and legal sex reassignment. Psychically, the condition of people who have the conviction that they belong to the opposite sex and are driven by a compulsion to have the body, appearance, and social status of a member of the opposite sex.

transverse arrest (trăns-vûrs′ ă-rĕst′). An abnormal fetal position in which rotation of the head is incomplete and the head is stopped in the transverse position.

Trendelenburg's position (trĕn-dĕl′ĕn-bĕrg). A position in which a patient lies on his back with his head tilted downward 15° to 40° with the bed at an angle at his knees.

trichomonas (trĭk-ŏm′ō-năs). A genus of parasitic flagellate protozoa.

t. vaginalis (văj″ĭ-nă′lĭs). A species sometimes found in the vagina.

t. vaginitis (văj″ĭ-nī′tĭs). A vaginal infection caused by trichomonas vaginalis with characteristic increased discharge and pruritus, or itching.

trisomy (trī′sō-mĭ). A chromosomal abnormality in which a particular chromosome is in triplicate rather than the usual pair.

t. 21. See *syndrome, Down's.*

trophectoderm (trŏf-ĕk′tō-dûrm). The outer layer of cells of the early blastodermic vesicle; it develops the trophoderm—the feeding layer.

true pelvis. See *pelvis, true.*

tubal ligation (tū′băl lī-gā′shŭn). See *ligation, tubal.*

tubal pregnancy. An ectopic pregnancy in which the fertilized ovum is embedded in one of the fallopian tubes rather than the wall of the uterus.

tuberischii (tū″bĕr-ĭs′kĭ-ī). Pertaining to the ischial tuberosities, the protuberances at the sides of the pelvic outlet.

Turner's syndrome. See *syndrome, Turner's.*

twins. Two offspring produced in the same pregnancy.

diamniotic dichorionic t. (dī″ăm-nĭ-ŏt′ĭk dī″kôr-ĭ-ŏn′ĭk). Twins that develop within separate amniotic sacs and have separate chorions.

diamniotic monochorionic t. (mŏn″ō-kō″rĭ-ŏn′ĭk). Twins that develop within separate amniotic sacs and have one chorion.

dizygotic t. (dī″zī-gŏt′ĭk). Twins that develop from separate zygotes, or fertilized ova; dichorionic twins; fraternal twins.

monoamniotic monochorionic t. (mŏn″ō-ăm″nĭ-ŏt′ĭk). Twins that develop within the same amniotic sacs and have one chorion.

monozygotic t. (mŏn″ō-zī-gŏt′ĭk). Twins that develop from the same zygote; monochorionic twins; identical twins.

ultrasonography (ŭl″tră-sŏn″ŏg′ră-fī). The visualization of structures within the body by recording echoes of ultrasonic waves directed into the tissues. Used for fetal assessment because it poses a minimal risk.

umbilical (ŭm-bĭl′ĭ-kăl). Pertaining to the umbilicus.

u. arteries. The two arteries that accompany and form part of the umbilical cord.

u. catheterization (kăth″ĕ-tĕr-ĭ-zā′shŭn). A method of inserting a catheter into the umbilicus of a high-risk neonate to provide a route for parenteral feeding, exchange transfusion, or obtaining blood samples.

u. cord [Latin, *funis umbilicalis*]. The cord connecting the placenta with the umbilicus of the fetus, and at the close of gestation principally made up of the two umbilical arteries and the umbilical vein, encased in a mass of gelatinous tissue called "Wharton's jelly."

u. hernia. Hernia at or near the umbilicus.

u. vein. Forms a part of the umbilical cord.
umbilicus (ŭm-bĭl'ĭ-kŭs, ŭm"bĭ-lī'kŭs). [L.] The navel; the cicatrix or scar that marks the attachment of the umbilical cord to the placenta.
ureter (ū-rē'tĕr). The tube through which urine passes from the kidney to the bladder.
use effectiveness of a contraceptive method. The effectiveness of a contraceptive method under actual conditions of use, in which some people use it correctly and others use it carelessly or incorrectly.
uterine souffle. See *souffle, uterine.*
uterotubal insufflation (ū"tĕr-ō-tū'băl ĭn"sŭf-flā'shŭn). A procedure used in Rubin's test involving the introduction of carbon dioxide into the uterus by way of a cannula. If one or both tubes are patent, the carbon dioxide flows through the uterus and tubes into the peritoneal cavity. When the patient sits up, the carbon dioxide rises to the diaphragm, causing pain in the shoulder referred there by way of the phrenic nerve.
uterus (ū'tĕr-ŭs). The hollow muscular organ in the female designed for the lodgement and nourishment of the fetus during its development until birth.

vacuum aspiration (văk'ū-ŭm ăs"pĭr-ā'shŭn). A method used for first trimester abortions in which the contents of the uterus are removed by applying a vacuum through a hollow curet or cannula inserted into the uterus.
vacuum extraction. See *extraction, vacuum.*
vagina (vȧ-jī'nȧ). [Latin, a sheath.] The canal in the female, extending from the vulva to the cervix of the uterus.
vaginismus (văj"ĭ-nĭz'mŭs). A female sexual dysfunction that involves a painful spasm of the vagina preventing penetration.
vaginitis (văj"ĭ-nī'tĭs). An infection involving the mucous membrane of the vagina, commonly associated with increased malodorous discharge, itching, and burning.
trichomonas v. See *trichomonas vaginitis.*
varicosity (văr"ĭ-kăs'ĭ-tĭ). The condition of a vein that is unnaturally and permanently distended.
vasectomy (vă-sĕk'tō-mĭ). The surgical interruption and ligation of the vas deferens, the spermatic duct, in order to prevent sperm from being in the ejaculate. It is the method of male sterilization.
vasocongestion (văs"ō-kŏn-jĕst'yŭn). Excessive accumulation of blood in the blood vessels.
venereal disease. See *disease, venereal.*
venous thrombosis (vē'nŭs thrŏm-bō'sĭs). The presence of a thrombus in a vein.
ventricular septal defect (vĕn-trĭk'ū-lĕr sĕp'tăl dēfĕct). A congenital cardiac anomaly in which there is an abnormal opening between the right and left ventricles.
vernix caseosa (vûr'nĭks kā"sē-ō'sȧ). "Cheesy varnish." The layer of fatty matter that covers the skin of the fetus.
version (vûr'shŭn). The act of turning; specifically, a turning of the fetus in the uterus so as to change the presenting part and bring it into more favorable position for delivery.
vertex (vûr'tĕks). The summit or top of anything. In anatomy, the top or crown of the head.
v. presentation. Presentation of the vertex of the fetus in labor.
vestibule (vĕs'tĭ-būl). A triangular space between the labia minora; the urinary meatus and the vagina open into it.
viable (vī'ȧ-b'l). A term in medical jurisprudence signifying "able or likely to live"; applied to the condition of the child at birth.
villus (vĭl'ŭs). Pl. *villi* (vĭl'ī). A small vascular process or protrusion growing on a mucous surface, such as the chorionic villi seen in tufts on the chorion of the early embryo.
vulva (vŭl'vȧ). The external genitals of the female.

weaning (wēn'ĭng). The discontinuance of breast feeding of an infant and the substitution of other forms of nourishment.
Wharton's jelly (hwôr'tŭnz). [Thomas *Wharton,* English anatomist, died 1673.] The jellylike mucous tissue composing the bulk of the umbilical cord.
Wilson–Mikity disease. See *pulmonary dysmaturity.*
witches' milk (wĭch'ĕz). A milky fluid secreted from the breast of the newly born.
withdrawal. The practice of retracting the penis from the vagina in intercourse prior to ejaculation, used as a method of contraception.
womb (woom). The uterus.
Wright method. A method of childbirth preparation based on psychoprophylaxis but using less active breathing than the Lamaze method.

X-ray pelvimetry (pĕl-vĭm'ĕ-trĭ). The measurement of pelvic size by x-rays. Although it is the most accurate method of measuring the pelvis, the exposure to x-rays precludes its regular use.

Zatuchni–Andros prognostic index. (ză-tŭch'nē–ăn'drōs prŏg-nŏs'tĭk ĭn'dĕks). A system to evaluate the feasibility of vaginal delivery in breech presentations.
zona pellucida (zō'nȧ pĕll-ū'sĭd-ä). A transparent belt; translucent or shining through.
zygote (zī'gōt). A cell resulting from the fusion of two gametes.

Conversion Table for Weights of Newborn

(Gram equivalents for pounds and ounces)

For example, to find weight in pounds and ounces of baby weighing 3315 grams, glance down columns to figure nearest 3315 = 3317. Refer to number at top of column for pounds and number to far left for ounces = 7 pounds, 5 ounces.

Pounds→ Ounces↓	**3**	**4**	**5**	**6**	**7**	**8**	**9**	**10**
0	1361	1814	2268	2722	3175	3629	4082	4536
1	1389	1843	2296	2750	3203	3657	4111	4564
2	1417	1871	2325	2778	3232	3685	4139	4593
3	1446	1899	2353	2807	3260	3714	4167	4621
4	1474	1928	2381	2835	3289	3742	4196	4649
5	1503	1956	2410	2863	3317	3770	4224	4678
6	1531	1984	2438	2892	3345	3799	4252	4706
7	1559	2013	2466	2920	3374	3827	4281	4734
8	1588	2041	2495	2948	3402	3856	4309	4763
9	1616	2070	2523	2977	3430	3884	4338	4791
10	1644	2098	2551	3005	3459	3912	4366	4819
11	1673	2126	2580	3033	3487	3941	4394	4848
12	1701	2155	2608	3062	3515	3969	4423	4876
13	1729	2183	2637	3090	3544	3997	4451	4904
14	1758	2211	2665	3118	3572	4026	4479	4933
15	1786	2240	2693	3147	3600	4054	4508	4961

Or, to convert grams into pounds and *decimals* of a pound, multiply weight in grams by .0022. Thus, 3317 × .0022 = 7.2974 (*i.e.*, 7.3 pounds, or 7 pounds, 5 ounces).

To convert pounds and ounces into grams, multiply the pounds by 453.6 and the ounces by 28.4 and add the two products. Thus, to convert 7 pounds, 5 ounces, 7 × 453.6 = 3175; 5 × 28.4 = 142; 3175 + 142 = 3317 grams.

Aid for Visualization of Cervical Dilatation

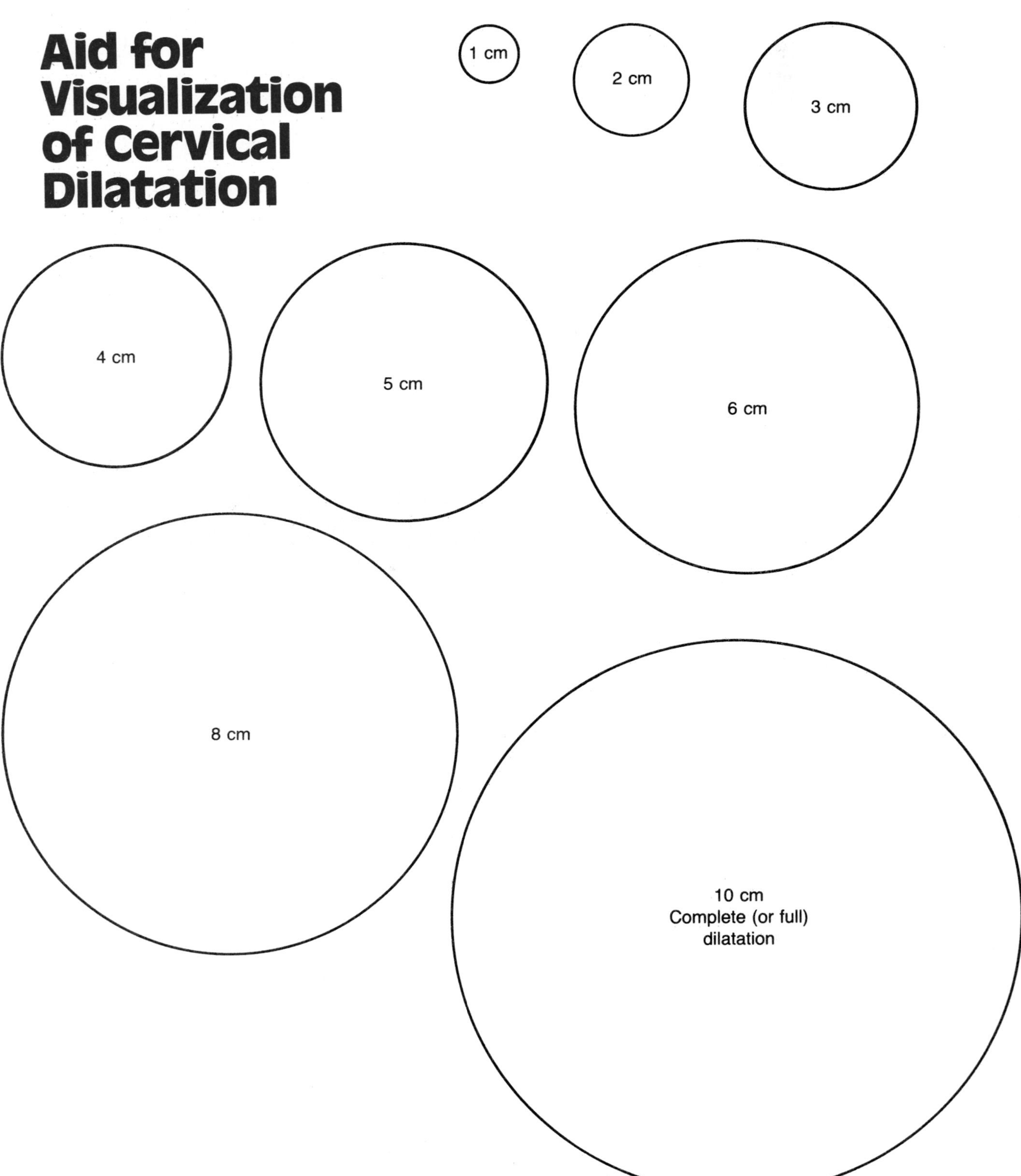

Index

Numbers followed by an *f* indicate a figure;
t following a page number indicates tabular material.
Glossary definitions are indicated by **bold face**.

Photo credits

The following sources are gratefully acknowledged for the use of the photographs found on the unit and chapter opening pages specified:

Michael Alexander—pages 456 (middle and right), 469, and 483

D. Atkinson—pages 742 (right) and 853

Augusta General Hospital, Augusta, Maine—pages 2 (left) and 5

Tracy Baldwin—pages 3 (left), 45, 186 (middle), 189, 290 (right), 291 (middle), 309, and 359

Michael Boyette—pages 290 (middle) and 293

Richard Weymouth Brooks—pages xxvi and 741

Carnegie Institution of Washington, Department of Embryology, Davis Division—pages xv, 85, 87 (middle and right), 151, and 161

Cooper Medical Devices Corporation—pages 187 (left) and 233

Hewlett-Packard Company—pages 882 (right) and 905

Ted Hill—pages 186 (right) and 207

David Holtz—pages 2 (center), 3 (center and right), 19, 61, 73, 86 (middle), 89, 742 (middle), and 771

Marcia Lieberman—pages xxix, 881, 883 (left and right), 929, and 1011

Osteopathic Hospital of Maine—pages 742 (left) and 817

H. Armstrong Roberts—pages xiii and 1

St. Petersburg Times—pages 457 (middle) and 535

Edward Siemens—87 (left) and 129

Mike Strueber—pages 457 (left) and 523

University of Michigan—pages 1037 (right) and 1063

Alison Wachstein—pages xxxii, 1035, 1037 (middle), and 1039

Jeff Weissman—pages xxiv and 597

Peter T. Whitney—page ii